**2002**



**Leonard L. Lance, RPh, BSPharm**
*Senior Editor*
Pharmacist
Lexi-Comp Inc.
Hudson, Ohio

**Charles F. Lacy, PharmD, FCSHP**
*Editor*
Facilitative Officer, Clinical Programs and Business Affairs
Nevada College of Pharmacy
Coordinator of Clinical Services
Department of Pharmacy
Cedars-Sinai Health System
Los Angeles, California

**Morton P. Goldman, PharmD, BCPS**
*Associate Editor*
Assistant Director, Pharmacotherapy Services
Department of Pharmacy
Cleveland Clinic Foundation
Cleveland, Ohio

**Lora L. Armstrong, PharmD, BCPS**
*Associate Editor*
Manager, Clinical Services
Caremark Rx, Inc.
Northbrook, Illinois

# NOTICE

This handbook is intended to serve the user as a handy quick reference and not as a complete drug information resource. It does not include information on every therapeutic agent available. The publication covers 1572 commonly used drugs and is specifically designed to present certain important aspects of drug data in a more concise format than is generally found in medical literature or product material supplied by manufacturers.

Although great care was taken to ensure the accuracy of the handbook's content when it went to press, the editors, contributors, and publisher cannot be responsible for the continued accuracy of the supplied information due to ongoing research and new developments in the field. Further, the *Quick Look Drug Book* is not offered as a guide to dosing. The reader, herewith, is advised that information shown under the heading **Usual Dosage** is provided only as an indication of the amount of the drug typically given or taken during therapy. Actual dosing amount for any specific drug should be based on an in-depth evaluation of the individual patient's therapy requirement and strong consideration given to such issues as contraindications, warnings, precautions, adverse reactions, along with the interaction of other drugs. The manufacturers most current product information or other standard recognized references should always be consulted for such detailed information prior to drug use.

The editors and contributors have written this book in their private capacities. No official support or endorsement by any federal agency or pharmaceutical company is intended or inferred.



This manual was produced using the FormuLex™ Program —
a complete publishing service of Lexi-Comp Inc.

lexi-comp

**Lexi-Comp, Inc**
**1100 Terex Road**
**Hudson, Ohio 44236**
**(330) 650-6506**

# TABLE OF CONTENTS

# ABOUT THE AUTHORS

**Leonard L. Lance, RPh, BSPharm**

Leonard L. (Bud) Lance has been directly involved in the pharmaceutical industry since receiving his bachelor's degree in pharmacy from Ohio Northern University in 1970. Upon graduation from ONU, Mr Lance spent four years as a navy pharmacist in various military assignments and was instrumental in the development and operation of the first whole hospital I.V. admixture program in a military (Portsmouth Naval Hospital) facility.

After completing his military service, he entered the retail pharmacy field and has managed both an independent and a home I.V. franchise pharmacy operation. Since the late 1970s, Mr Lance has focused much of his interest on using computers to improve pharmacy service and to advance the dissemination of drug information to practitioners and other health care professionals.

As a result of his strong publishing interest, he serves in the capacity of pharmacy editor and technical advisor as well as pharmacy (information) database coordinator for Lexi-Comp. Along with the *Quick Look Drug Book*, he provides technical support to Lexi-Comp's *Drug Information Handbook for the Allied Health Professional*, and many other titles published by Lexi-Comp, Inc. Mr Lance has also assisted approximately 120 major hospitals in producing their own formulary (pharmacy) publications through Lexi-Comp's custom publishing service.

Mr Lance is a member and past president (1984) of the Summit Pharmaceutical Association (SPA). He is also a member of the Ohio Pharmacists Association (OPA), the American Pharmaceutical Association (APhA), and the American Society of Health-System Pharmacists (ASHP).

**Charles F. Lacy, PharmD, FCSHP**

Dr Lacy received his doctorate from the University of Southern California School of Pharmacy. With over 19 years of clinical experience at one of the nation's largest teaching hospitals, Cedars Sinai Medical Center, he has developed a reputation as an acknowledged expert in drug information and critical care drug therapy.

Dr Lacy is the current Facilitative Officer for Clinical Programs and professor at the Nevada College of Pharmacy. In his current capacity, Dr Lacy oversees the clinical curriculum, clinical faculty activities, the computer information systems, student experiential programs, residency programs, continuing education programs, entrepreneurial activities, and all of the drug information needs for the college. Additionally, as Coordinator of Clinical Services for the Department of Pharmacy at Cedar-Sinai Health System in Los Angeles, Dr Lacy plays an active role in the education and training of the medical, pharmacy, and nursing staff. He administrates over the Drug Information Network, he coordinates the development of medical center clinical pathways, the pharmacists' clinical certification and staff development program, the department's continuing education program, and the pharmacy residency clinical assessment, training, and longitudinal experience program. He also supervises the activities of clinical specialists in medication use evaluation, antibiotic use review, infection control, investigational drug protocols, transplant pharmacy services, the Adverse Drug Reaction Monitoring Program, the Medical Center's Medication Error Detection and Remedy Program, and directs the maintenance of the Medical Center Formulary Program. He is co-editor of the Medical Center's *Drug Formulary Handbook*, and associate editor of the drug information newsletter *Prescription*.

Presently, Dr Lacy holds teaching affiliations with the Nevada School of Pharmacy, the University of Southern California School of Pharmacy, the University of California at San Francisco School of Pharmacy, the University of the Pacific School of Pharmacy, Western University of Health Sciences School of Pharmacy, and the University of Alberta at Edmonton, School of Pharmacy and Health Sciences.

Dr Lacy is an active member of numerous professional associations including the American Society of Health-System Pharmacists (ASHP), the American College of Clinical Pharmacy (ACCP), the American Society of Consultant Pharmacists (ASCP), the American Association of Colleges of Pharmacy (AACP), American Pharmaceutical Association (APhA), and the California Society of Hospital Pharmacists (CSHP), through which he has chaired many committees and subcommittees.

**Morton P. Goldman, PharmD, BCPS**

Dr Goldman received his bachelor's degree in pharmacy from the University of Pittsburgh, College of Pharmacy and his Doctor of Pharmacy degree from the University of Cincinnati, Division of Graduate Studies and Research. He completed his concurrent 2-year hospital pharmacy residency at the V.A. Medical Center in Cincinnati. Dr Goldman is presently the Assistant Director of Pharmacotherapy Services for the Department of Pharmacy at the Cleveland Clinic Foundation (CCF) after having spent over 4 years at CCF as an Infectious Disease pharmacist and 4 years as Clinical Manager. He holds faculty appointments from Case Western Reserve University, College of Medicine; The University of Toledo, College of Pharmacy; and The University of Cincinnati, College of Pharmacy. Dr Goldman is a Board-Certified Pharmacotherapy Specialist.

In his capacity as Assistant Director of Pharmacotherapy Services at CCF, Dr Goldman remains actively involved in patient care and clinical research with the Department of Infectious Disease, as well as the continuing education of the medical and pharmacy staff. He is an editor of CCF's *Guidelines for Antibiotic Use* and participates in their annual Antimicrobial Review retreat. He is a member of the Pharmacy and Therapeutics Committee and many of its subcommittees. Dr Goldman has authored numerous journal articles and lectures locally and nationally on infectious diseases topics and current drug therapies. He is currently a reviewer for the *Annals of Pharmacotherapy* and the *Journal of the American Medical Association*, an editorial board member of the *Journal of Infectious Disease Pharmacotherapy*, and coauthor of the *Infectious Diseases Handbook*, the *Drug Information Handbook*, and the *Drug Information Handbook for the Allied Health Professional* produced by Lexi-Comp, Inc. He also provides technical support to Lexi-Comp's Clinical Reference Library™ publications.

Dr Goldman is an active member of the Ohio College of Clinical Pharmacy, the Society of Infectious Disease Pharmacists, the American College of Clinical Pharmacy, and the American Society of Health-Systems Pharmacists.

**Lora L. Armstrong, PharmD, BCPS**

Dr Armstrong received her bachelor's degree in pharmacy from Ferris State University and her Doctor of Pharmacy degree from Midwestern University. Dr Armstrong is a Board-Certified Pharmacotherapy Specialist (BCPS).

In her current position, Dr Armstrong serves as manager of the Pharmacy and Therapeutics Committee process at Caremark Rx, Inc, Prescription Services Division. Caremark is a prescription benefit management company (PBM). Dr Armstrong is responsible for coordination of the Caremark National Pharmacy & Therapeutics Committee and she chairs the Caremark Pharmacy & Therapeutics Subcommittee. Dr Armstrong is also responsible for coordinating the Caremark Clinical Practice Committee, monitoring the pharmaceutical product pipeline, monitoring drug surveillance, and communicating Pharmacy & Therapeutics Committee Formulary information to internal and external customers.

Prior to joining Caremark Rx, Inc, Dr Armstrong served as the Director of Drug Information Services at the University of Chicago Hospitals. She obtained 17 years of experience in a variety of clinical settings including critical care, hematology, oncology, infectious diseases, and clinical pharmacokinetics. Dr Armstrong played an active role in the education and training of medical, pharmacy, and nursing staff. She coordinated the Drug Information Center, the medical center's Adverse Drug Reaction Monitoring Program, and the continuing Education Program for pharmacists. She also maintained the hospital's strict formulary program and was the editor of the University of Chicago Hospitals' *Formulary of Accepted Drugs* and the drug information center's monthly newsletter *Topics in Drug Therapy*.

Dr Armstrong is an active member of the Academy of Managed Care Pharmacy (AMCP), the American Society of Health-Systems Pharmacists (ASHP), the American Pharmaceutical Association (APhA), and the American College of Clinical Pharmacy (ACCP). Dr Armstrong wrote the chapter entitled "Drugs and Hormones Used in Endocrinology" in the 4th edition of the textbook *Endocrinology*. She also serves on the Editorial Advisory Board of the *Drug INFO Line* Newsletter.

# EDITORIAL ADVISORY PANEL

## EDITORIAL ADVISORY PANEL

## EDITORIAL ADVISORY PANEL

# PREFACE

Working with clinical pharmacists, hospital pharmacy and therapeutics committees, and hospital drug information centers, the editors of this handbook have directly assisted in the development and production of hospital-specific formulary documentation for several hundred major medical institutions in the United States and Canada. The resultant documentation provides pertinent detail concerning use of medications within the hospital and other clinical settings. The most current information on medications has been extracted, reviewed, coalesced, and cross-referenced by the editors to create this *Quick Look Drug Book*.

Thus, this handbook gives the user quick access to data on 1572 medications with cross referencing to 4896 U.S. and Canadian brand or trade names. Selection of the included medications was based on the analysis of those medications offered in a wide range of hospital formularies. The concise standardized format for data used in this handbook was developed to ensure a consistent presentation of information for all medications.

All generic drug names and synonyms appear in lower case, whereas brand or trade names appear in upper/lower case with the proper trademark information. These three items appear as individual entries in the alphabetical listing of drugs and, thus, there is no requirement for an alphabetical index of drugs.

Mailing and WEB site addresses for Pharmaceutical Manufacturers and Drug Distributors are provided in the appendix section of this book.

The Indication/Therapeutic Category Index is an expedient mechanism for locating the medication of choice along with its classification. This index will help the user, with knowledge of the disease state, to identify medications which are most commonly used in treatment. All disease states are cross-referenced to a varying number of medications with the most frequently used medication(s) noted.

— L.L. Lance

# ACKNOWLEDGMENTS

The *Quick Look Drug Book* exists in its present form as the result of the concerted efforts of the following individuals: Robert D. Kerscher, publisher and president of Lexi-Comp, Inc; Lynn D. Coppinger, managing editor; Barbara F. Kerscher, production manager; Daniel L. Krinsky, director, pharmacotherapy sales and marketing; Ginger S. Stein, project manager; and David C. Marcus, director of information systems.

Special acknowledgment goes to all Lexi-Comp staff for their contributions to this handbook.

# USE OF THE HANDBOOK

The *Quick Look Drug Book* is organized into a drug information section, an appendix, and an indication/therapeutic category index.

The drug information section of the handbook, wherein all drugs are listed alphabetically, details information pertinent to each drug. Extensive cross referencing is provided by brand name and synonyms.

Drug information is presented in a consistent format and for quick reference will provide the following:

| | |
|---|---|
| Generic Name | U.S. Adopted Name (USAN) or International Nonproprietary Name (INN)<br><br>If a drug product is only available in Canada, a ***(Canada only)*** will be attached to that product and will appear with every occurrence of that drug throughout the book |
| Pronunciation Guide | Subjective aid for pronouncing drug names |
| Synonyms | Official names and some slang |
| U.S./Canadian Brand Names | Common trade names used in the United States and Canada (Can) |
| Therapeutic Category | Lexi-Comp's own system of logical medication classification |
| Controlled Substance | Drug Enforcement Agency (DEA) classification for federally scheduled controlled substances |
| Use | Information pertaining to appropriate use of the drug |
| Usual Dosage | The amount of the drug to be typically given or taken during therapy |
| Dosage Forms | Information with regard to form, strength and availability of the drug |

### Appendix

The appendix offers a compilation of tables, guidelines, and conversion information that can often be helpful when considering patient care.

### Indication/Therapeutic Category Index

This index provides a listing of accepted drugs for various disease states thus focusing attention on selection of medications most frequently prescribed in relation to a clinical diagnosis. Diseases may have other nonofficial drugs for their treatment and this indication/therapeutic category index should not be used by itself to determine the appropriateness of a particular therapy. The listed indications may encompass varying degrees of severity and, since certain medications may not be appropriate for a given degree of severity, it should not be assumed that the agents listed for specific indications are interchangeable. Also included as a valuable reference is each medication's therapeutic category.

# SAFE WRITING

Health professionals and their support personnel frequently produce handwritten copies of information they see in print; therefore, such information is subjected to even greater possibilities for error or misinterpretation on the part of others. Thus, particular care must be given to how drug names and strengths are expressed when creating written health care documents.

The following are a few examples of safe writing rules suggested by the Institute for Safe Medication Practices, Inc.*

1. There should be a space between a number and its units as it is easier to read. There should be no periods after the abbreviations mg or mL.

| **Correct** | **Incorrect** |
|---|---|
| 10 mg | 10mg |
| 100 mg | 100mg |

2. Never place a decimal and a zero after a whole number (2 mg is correct and 2.0 mg is incorrect). If the decimal point is not seen because it falls on a line or because individuals are working from copies where the decimal point is not seen, this causes a tenfold overdose.
3. Just the opposite is true for numbers less than one. Always place a zero before a naked decimal (0.5 mL is correct, .5 mL is **in**correct).
4. Never abbreviate the word "unit." The handwritten U or u, looks like a 0 (zero), and may cause a tenfold overdose error to be made.
5. IU is not a safe abbreviation for international units. The handwritten IU looks like IV. Write out international units or use int. units.
6. Q.D. is not a safe abbreviation for once daily, as when the Q is followed by a sloppy dot, it looks like QID which means four times daily.
7. O.D. is not a safe abbreviation for once daily, as it is properly interpreted as meaning "right eye" and has caused liquid medications such as saturated solution of potassium iodide and lugol's solution to be administered incorrectly. There is no safe abbreviation for once daily. It must be written out in full.
8. Do not use chemical names such as 6-mercaptopurine or 6-thioguanine, as 6-fold overdoses have been given when these were not recognized as chemical names. The proper names of these drugs are mercaptopurine or thioguanine.
9. Do not abbreviate drug names (5FC, 6MP, 5-ASA, MTX, HCTZ CPZ, PBZ, etc) as they are misinterpreted and cause error.
10. Do not use the apothecary system or symbols.
11. Do not abbreviate microgram as µg; instead use mcg as there is less likelihood of misinterpretation.

---

*From "Safe Writing" by Davis NM, PharmD and Cohen MR, MS, Lecturers and Consultants for Safe Medication Practices, 1143 Wright Drive, Huntingdon Valley, PA 19006. Phone: (215) 947-7566.

12. When writing an outpatient prescription, write a complete prescription. A complete prescription can prevent the prescriber, the pharmacist, and/or the patient from making a mistake and can eliminate the need for further clarification. The legible prescriptions should contain:
    a. patient's full name
    b. for pediatric or geriatric patients: their age (or weight where applicable)
    c. drug name, dosage form and strength; if a drug is new or rarely prescribed, print this information
    d. number or amount to be dispensed
    e. complete instructions for the patient, including the purpose of the medication
    f. when there are recognized contraindications for a prescribed drug, indicate to the pharmacist that you are aware of this fact (ie, when prescribing a potassium salt for a patient receiving an ACE inhibitor, write "K serum leveling being monitored")

# ALPHABETICAL LISTING OF DRUGS

**A-200™ Lice [OTC]** *see* permethrin *on page 462*

**A-200™ Shampoo [OTC]** *see* pyrethrins *on page 510*

**A and D™ Ointment [OTC]** *see* vitamin A and vitamin D *on page 630*

## abacavir (a BAK a veer)

**U.S./Canadian Brand Names** Ziagen®

**Therapeutic Category** Antiretroviral Agent, Nucleoside Reverse Transcriptase Inhibitor (NRTI)

**Use** Treatment of HIV infections in combination with other antiretroviral agents

**Usual Dosage** Oral:

Children: 3 months to 16 years: 8 mg/kg body weight twice daily (maximum: 300 mg twice daily) in combination with other antiretroviral agents

Adults: 300 mg twice daily in combination with other antiretroviral agents

**Dosage Forms**

Solution, oral: 20 mg/mL (240 mL)

Tablet: 300 mg

## abacavir, lamivudine, and zidovudine

(a BAK a veer, la MI vyoo deen, & zye DOE vyoo deen)

**U.S./Canadian Brand Names** Trizivir™

**Therapeutic Category** Antiretroviral Agent, Nucleoside Reverse Transcriptase Inhibitor (NRTI)

**Use** Treatment of HIV infection (either alone or in combination with other antiretroviral agents) in patients whose regimen would otherwise contain the components of Trizivir™ (based on analyses of surrogate markers in controlled studies with abacavir of up to 24 weeks; there have been no clinical trials conducted with Trizivir™)

**Usual Dosage** Adolescents and Adults: Oral: 1 tablet twice daily; **Note:** Not recommended for patients <40 kg

**Dosage Forms** Tablet: Abacavir 300 mg, lamivudine 150 mg, and zidovudine 300 mg

**Abbokinase®** *see* urokinase *on page 618*

**ABCD** *see* amphotericin B cholesteryl sulfate complex *on page 37*

## abciximab (ab SIK si mab)

**Synonyms** c7E3

**U.S./Canadian Brand Names** ReoPro®

**Therapeutic Category** Platelet Aggregation Inhibitor

**Use** Adjunct to percutaneous transluminal coronary angioplasty or atherectomy (PTCA) for the prevention of acute cardiac ischemic complications; prevent cardiac ischemic complications in a wider range of percutaneous coronary interventions (PCIs), including balloon angioplasty and stent placement, and without qualification of high risk for abrupt vessel closure; unstable angina that does not respond to conventional therapy when PCI is planned with 24 hours

**Usual Dosage** I.V.: 0.25 mg/kg bolus followed by an infusion of 10 mcg/minute for 12 hours

**Dosage Forms** Injection: 2 mg/mL (5 mL)

**Abelcet®** *see* amphotericin B lipid complex *on page 38*

**Abenol® (Can)** *see* acetaminophen *on next page*

**ABLC** *see* amphotericin B lipid complex *on page 38*

**Abreva™ [OTC]** *see* docosanol *on page 197*

**absorbable cotton** *see* cellulose, oxidized *on page 119*

**absorbable gelatin sponge** *see* gelatin (absorbable) *on page 270*

**Absorbine® Antifungal *(Discontinued)*** *see page 750*

**Absorbine® Antifungal Foot Powder [OTC]** *see* miconazole *on page 390*

**Absorbine® Jock Itch *(Discontinued)*** *see page 750*

**Absorbine Jr® Antifungal *(Discontinued)*** *see page 750*

## acarbose (AY car bose)

**U.S./Canadian Brand Names** Prandase® (Can); Precose®

**Therapeutic Category** Antidiabetic Agent, Oral

**Use** Treatment of noninsulin-dependent diabetes mellitus (NIDDM); as monotherapy or in combination with a sulfonylurea when diet plus acarbose or a sulfonylurea does not result in adequate glycemic control; also used with insulin or metformin in patients with noninsulin-dependent diabetes mellitus (NIDDM)

**Usual Dosage** Adults: Oral: Dosage must be individualized on the basis of effectiveness and tolerance while not exceeding the maximum recommended dose of 100 mg 3 times/day

Initial dose: 25 mg 3 times/day with the first bite of each main meal

Maintenance dose: Should be adjusted at 4- to 8-week intervals based on 1-hour postprandial glucose levels and tolerance. Dosage may be increased from 25 mg 3 times/day to 50 mg 3 times/day; some patients may benefit from increasing the dose to 100 mg 3 times/day; maintenance dose ranges: 50-100 mg 3 times/day.

Maximum dose:

≤60 kg: 50 mg 3 times/day

>60 kg: 100 mg 3 times/day

**Dosage Forms** Tablet: 25 mg, 50 mg, 100 mg

**A-Caro-25®** *see* beta-carotene *on page 76*

**Accolate®** *see* zafirlukast *on page 636*

**AccuNeb™** *see* albuterol *on page 16*

**Accupril®** *see* quinapril *on page 513*

**Accuretic® (Can)** *see* quinapril and hydrochlorothiazide *(Canada only)* *on page 513*

**Accutane®** *see* isotretinoin *on page 329*

**Accuzyme™** *see* papain and urea *on page 450*

## acebutolol (a se BYOO toe lole)

**U.S./Canadian Brand Names** Gen-Acebutolol (Can); Monitan® (Can); Novo-Acebutolol (Can); Rhotral (Can); Sectral®

**Therapeutic Category** Antiarrhythmic Agent, Class II; Beta-Adrenergic Blocker

**Use** Treatment of hypertension; ventricular arrhythmias; angina

**Usual Dosage** Adults: Oral: 400-800 mg/day in 2 divided doses

**Dosage Forms** Capsule, as hydrochloride: 200 mg, 400 mg

**Acel-Imune®** *see* diphtheria, tetanus toxoids, and acellular pertussis vaccine *on page 193*

**Aceon®** *see* perindopril erbumine *on page 461*

**Acephen® [OTC]** *see* acetaminophen *on this page*

**Aceta® [OTC]** *see* acetaminophen *on this page*

**Aceta® Children's [OTC]** *see* acetaminophen *on this page*

**Aceta-Gesic® [OTC]** *see* acetaminophen and phenyltoloxamine *on page 5*

**Acetagesic® [OTC]** *see* acetaminophen and phenyltoloxamine *on page 5*

## acetaminophen (a seet a MIN oh fen)

**Synonyms** APAP; n-acetyl-p-aminophenol; paracetamol

**U.S./Canadian Brand Names** Abenol® (Can); Acephen® [OTC]; Aceta® [OTC]; Aceta® Children's [OTC]; Actamin® [OTC]; Altenol® [OTC]; Amdol 500® [OTC]; Amdol 650®

(Continued)

## acetaminophen *(Continued)*

[OTC]; Amdoplus® [OTC]; Aminofen® [OTC]; Aminofen Plus® [OTC]; Apapedyn® Children's [OTC]; Apapedyn® Extra Strength [OTC]; Cetafen® [OTC]; Cetafen® Extra [OTC]; Dolono® [OTC]; Dolono® Infants [OTC]; Febrol® [OTC]; Feverall™ [OTC]; Genapap® [OTC]; Genapap® Children [OTC]; Genapap® Extra Strength [OTC]; Genapap® Infant [OTC]; Genebs® [OTC]; Genebs® Extra Strength [OTC]; Halenol® [OTC]; Infantaire® [OTC]; Mapap® [OTC]; Mapap® Children's [OTC]; Mapap® Extra Strength [OTC]; Mapap® Infants' [OTC]; Mardol® [OTC]; Meda-Cap® [OTC]; Oraphen PD® [OTC]; Pain-Eze® [OTC]; Pediatrix (Can); Pyrecot® [OTC]; Pyregesic® [OTC]; Q-Pap® [OTC]; Q-Pap® Children's [OTC]; Redutemp® [OTC]; Silapap® Children's [OTC]; Silapap® Infant's [OTC]; Tactinal® [OTC]; Tactinal® Children's [OTC]; Tactinal® Extra Strength [OTC]; Tempra® 1 [OTC]; Tempra® 2 [OTC]; T-Painol® [OTC]; T-Painol® Extra Strength [OTC]; Tycolene® [OTC]; Tylenol® [OTC]; Tylenol® Arthritis [OTC]; Tylenol® Children's [OTC]; Tylenol® Extra Strength [OTC]; Tylenol® Infants [OTC]; Tylenol® Infants Original [OTC]; Tylenol® Junior Strength [OTC]; Tylenol® Sore Throat [OTC]; Tylex® [OTC]; Tylex® Extra Strength [OTC]; Tylophen® [OTC]; Tyltabs® [OTC]; Tyltabs® Children's [OTC]; Tyltabs® Extra Strength [OTC]; Valorin® [OTC]; Valorin® Extra [OTC]

**Therapeutic Category** Analgesic, Non-narcotic; Antipyretic

**Use** Treatment of mild to moderate pain and fever; does not have antirheumatic or systemic anti-inflammatory effects

**Usual Dosage** Oral, rectal (if fever not controlled with acetaminophen alone, administer with full doses of aspirin on an every 4- to 6-hour schedule, if aspirin is not otherwise contraindicated):

Children <12 years: 10-15 mg/kg/dose every 4-6 hours as needed; do **not** exceed 5 doses (2.6 g) in 24 hours

Adults: 325-650 mg every 4-6 hours or 1000 mg 3-4 times/day; do **not** exceed 4 g/day

**Dosage Forms**

Caplet: 160 mg, 325 mg, 500 mg
Caplet, extended: 650 mg
Capsule: 80 mg
Drops: 48 mg/mL (15 mL); 60 mg/0.6 mL (15 mL); 80 mg/0.8 mL (15 mL); 100 mg/mL (15 mL, 30 mL)
Elixir: 80 mg/5 mL, 120 mg/5 mL, 160 mg/5 mL, 167 mg/5 mL, 325 mg/5 mL
Liquid, oral: 160 mg/5 mL, 500 mg/15 mL
Solution: 100 mg/mL (15 mL); 120 mg/2.5 mL
Suppository, rectal: 80 mg, 120 mg, 125 mg, 300 mg, 325 mg, 650 mg
Suspension, oral: 160 mg/5 mL
Suspension, oral drops: 80 mg/0.8 mL
Tablet: 325 mg, 500 mg, 650 mg
Tablet, chewable: 80 mg, 160 mg

## acetaminophen and codeine (a seet a MIN oh fen & KOE deen)

**Synonyms** codeine and acetaminophen

**U.S./Canadian Brand Names** Capital® and Codeine; Lenoltec No 1, 2, 3, 4 (Can); Phenaphen® With Codeine #3; Pyregesic-C®; Triatec-8® (Can); Triatec-8® Strong (Can); Triatec-30® (Can); Tylenol® With Codeine

**Therapeutic Category** Analgesic, Narcotic

**Controlled Substance** C-III; C-V

**Use** Relief of mild to moderate pain

**Usual Dosage** Doses should be adjusted according to severity of pain and response of the patient. Adult doses ≥60 mg codeine fail to give commensurate relief of pain but merely prolong analgesia and are associated with an appreciably increased incidence of side effects. Oral:

Children:

Analgesic: 0.5-1 mg codeine/kg/dose every 4-6 hours

Acetaminophen: 10-15 mg/kg/dose every 4 hours up to a maximum of 2.6 g/24 hours for children <12 years

3-6 years: 5 mL 3-4 times/day as needed of elixir
7-12 years: 10 mL 3-4 times/day as needed of elixir
>12 years: 15 mL every 4 hours as needed of elixir

Adults:
Antitussive: Based on codeine (15-30 mg/dose) every 4-6 hours
Analgesic: Based on codeine (30-60 mg/dose) every 4-6 hours
1-2 tablets every 4 hours to a maximum of 12 tablets/24 hours

**Dosage Forms**
Capsule:
#3: Acetaminophen 325 mg and codeine phosphate 30 mg (C-III)
#4: Acetaminophen 325 mg and codeine phosphate 60 mg (C-III)
Elixir: Acetaminophen 120 mg and codeine phosphate 12 mg per 5 mL with alcohol 7% (C-V)
Solution, oral: Acetaminophen 120 mg and codeine phosphate 12 mg per 5 mL with alcohol 7% (C-V)
Suspension, oral, alcohol free: Acetaminophen 120 mg and codeine phosphate 12 mg per 5 mL (C-V)
Tablet:
#2: Acetaminophen 300 mg and codeine phosphate 15 mg (C-III)
#3: Acetaminophen 300 mg and codeine phosphate 30 mg (C-III)
#4: Acetaminophen 300 mg and codeine phosphate 60 mg (C-III)

## acetaminophen and diphenhydramine

(a seet a MIN oh fen & dye fen HYE dra meen)

**U.S./Canadian Brand Names** Anacin® P.M. Aspirin Free [OTC]; Excedrin® P.M. [OTC]; Headache Formula PM® [OTC]; Headache Relief PM® [OTC]; Legatrin® PM Advanced Formula [OTC]; Leg Cramp Relief PM® [OTC]; Mapap-PM® [OTC]; Midol® PM [OTC]; Night-Time Cramp Relief® [OTC]; Night-Time Pain Reliever/Sleep [OTC]; Sominex® Pain Relief Formula [OTC]; Tylenol® PM Strength [OTC]; Tylenol® Severe Allergy [OTC]; Tyltabs® PM [OTC]; Unison® w/Pain Relief [OTC]

**Therapeutic Category** Analgesic, Non-narcotic

**Use** Relief of mild to moderate pain or sinus headache

**Usual Dosage** Oral:
Children <12 years: Not recommended
Adults: 2 caplets or 5 mL of liquid at bedtime or as directed by physician; do not exceed recommended dosage

**Dosage Forms** Tablet: Acetaminophen 500 mg and diphenhydramine 12.5 mg; acetaminophen 500 mg and diphenhydramine 25 mg; acetaminophen 500 mg and diphenhydramine 50 mg; acetaminophen 650 mg and diphenhydramine 50 mg

**acetaminophen and hydrocodone** *see* hydrocodone and acetaminophen *on page 300*

## acetaminophen and phenyltoloxamine

(a seet a MIN oh fen & fen il to LOKS a meen)

**U.S./Canadian Brand Names** Aceta-Gesic® [OTC]; Acetagesic® [OTC]; Anagesic® [OTC]; Apaphen® [OTC]; Eckogesic® [OTC]; Flextra-DS® [OTC]; Genasec® [OTC]; Major-Gesic® [OTC]; Novagesic® [OTC]; Ohmni-Gesic® [OTC]; Pain-Gesic® [OTC]; Percogesic® [OTC]; Phenylgesic® [OTC]; Q-Gesic® [OTC]; Relagesic® [OTC]; Staflex® [OTC]; Tension® [OTC]; UniPerr® [OTC]; Vitoxapap® [OTC]

**Therapeutic Category** Analgesic, Non-narcotic

**Use** Relief of mild to moderate pain

**Usual Dosage** Adults: Oral: 1-2 tablets every 4 hours

**Dosage Forms** Tablet: Acetaminophen 325 mg and phenyltoloxamine citrate 30 mg; acetaminophen 500 mg and phenyltoloxamine citrate 30 mg; acetaminophen 500 mg and phenyltoloxamine citrate 50 mg; acetaminophen 650 mg and phenyltoloxamine citrate 50 mg

## acetaminophen and pseudoephedrine

(a seet a MIN oh fen & soo doe e FED rin)

**Synonyms** pseudoephedrine and acetaminophen

**U.S./Canadian Brand Names** Allerest® No Drowsiness [OTC]; Coldrine® [OTC]; Dristan® Cold Maximum Strength [OTC]; Genapap Sinus® Maximum Strength [OTC]; Mapap Sinus® Maximum Strength [OTC]; Oranyl Plus® [OTC]; Ornex® [OTC]; Ornex® Maximum Strength [OTC]; Phenapap® [OTC]; Sine-Aid®, Maximum Strength [OTC]; Sine-Off® Maximum Strength [OTC]; Sinus Maximum Strength [OTC]; Sinus-Relief® Maximum Relief [OTC]; Sinustab® [OTC]; Sinutab® Regular Strength [OTC]; Sudafed® Sinus [OTC]; Sudogest® Sinus Maximum Strength [OTC]; Suphedrin® Sinus Maximum Strength [OTC]; Tylenol® Cold Infants [OTC]; Tylenol® Sinus Children's [OTC]; Tylenol® Sinus, Maximum Strength [OTC]

**Therapeutic Category** Decongestant/Analgesic

**Use** Symptomatic relief of congestion, fever, and aches/pain of colds/flu

**Usual Dosage** Adults: Oral: 2 tablets every 4-6 hours

**Dosage Forms**

Liquid: Acetaminophen 80 mg and pseudoephedrine hydrochloride 7.5 mg per 0.8 mL (15 mL); acetaminophen 80 mg and pseudoephedrine hydrochloride 15 mg per 5 mL (118 mL)

Tablet: Acetaminophen 325 mg and pseudoephedrine hydrochloride 30 mg; acetaminophen 500 mg and pseudoephedrine hydrochloride 30 mg

Tablet, chewable: Acetaminophen 80 mg and pseudoephedrine hydrochloride 7.5 mg

## acetaminophen, aspirin, and caffeine

(a seet a MIN oh fen, AS pir in, & KAF een)

**U.S./Canadian Brand Names** Double-Action Pain Relief® [OTC]; Excedrin®, Extra Strength [OTC]; Extraprin® [OTC]; Fem-Prin® [OTC]; Gelpirin® [OTC]; Goody's® Fast Pain Relief® [OTC]; Goody's® Headache Powders [OTC]; Headrin® Plus Pain Relief [OTC]; Pain-Off® [OTC]; Supac® [OTC]; Vanquish® [OTC]

**Therapeutic Category** Analgesic, Non-narcotic

**Use** Relief of mild to moderate pain or fever

**Usual Dosage** Adults: Oral: 1-2 tablets or powders every 2-6 hours as needed for pain

**Dosage Forms**

Powder: Acetaminophen 260 mg, aspirin 520 mg, and caffeine 32.5 mg per dose

Tablet: Acetaminophen 125 mg, aspirin 240 mg, and caffeine 32 mg; acetaminophen 160 mg, aspirin 230 mg, and caffeine 33 mg; acetaminophen 194 mg, aspirin 227 mg, and caffeine 33 mg; acetaminophen 250 mg, aspirin 250 mg, and caffeine 65 mg

## acetaminophen, chlorpheniramine, and pseudoephedrine

(a seet a MIN oh fen, klor fen IR a meen, & soo doe e FED rin)

**U.S./Canadian Brand Names** Allergy Sinus® Maximum Strength [OTC]; Allergy Sinus® Pain Relief [OTC]; Comtrex® Allergy-Sinus [OTC]; Comtrex® Allergy-Sinus Day & Night [OTC]; Drinex® [OTC]; Flu & Cold® Medicine [OTC]; Kolephrin® [OTC]; Lorsin® [OTC]; Simplet® [OTC]; Sinarest® Sinus [OTC]; Sine-Off® [OTC]; Singlet® [OTC]; Sinumed® [OTC]; Sinus® [OTC]; Sinutab® Maximum Strength [OTC]; Theraflu® Flu & Cold [OTC]; Tylenol® Allergy Sinus [OTC]; Tylenol® Allergy Sinus (Can); Tylenol® Cold (Can); Tylenol® Cold Children's [OTC]; Tyltabs® Allergy Sinus [OTC]

**Therapeutic Category** Antihistamine/Decongestant/Analgesic

**Use** Temporary relief of sinus symptoms

**Usual Dosage** Adults: Oral: 2 caplets/capsules/tablets every 6 hours

**Dosage Forms**

Capsule: Acetaminophen 250 mg, chlorpheniramine maleate 2 mg, and pseudoephedrine hydrochloride 30 mg

Liquid: Acetaminophen 160 mg, chlorpheniramine maleate 1 mg, and pseudoephedrine hydrochloride 15 mg per 5 mL (120 mL)

Powder: Acetaminophen 650 mg, chlorpheniramine maleate 4 mg, and pseudoephedrine hydrochloride 60 mg

Tablet: Acetaminophen 325 mg, chlorpheniramine maleate 2 mg, and pseudoephedrine hydrochloride 30 mg; acetaminophen 500 mg, chlorpheniramine maleate 2 mg, and pseudoephedrine hydrochloride 30 mg

Tablet, chewable: Acetaminophen 80 mg, chlorpheniramine maleate 0.5 mg, and pseudoephedrine hydrochloride 7.5 mg

## acetaminophen, dextromethorphan, and pseudoephedrine

(a seet a MIN oh fen, deks troe meth OR fan, & soo doe e FED rin)

**U.S./Canadian Brand Names** Comtrex® Non-Drowsy [OTC]; Contac® Severe Cold & Flu/Non-Drowsy [OTC]; Day-Time® Multi-Symptom Cold/Flu [OTC]; Mapap® Multi-Symptom Cold [OTC]; Medi-Phedrine® Severe Cold Formula [OTC]; Polyminic® Sore Throat Formula [OTC]; Sudafed® Severe Cold Formula [OTC]; Suphedrine® Severe Cold [OTC]; Theraflu® [OTC]; Theraflu® Flu Cold & Cough [OTC]; Triacting® Sore Throat Formula [OTC]; Tylenol® Cold [OTC]; Tylenol® Cold Plus Cough Infants' [OTC]; Tylenol® Flu Maximum Strength [OTC]; Vicks® Dayquil® [OTC]; Vicks® Dayquil® Multi-Symptom [OTC]

**Therapeutic Category** Cold Preparation

**Use** Symptomatic relief of congestion, fever, cough, and aches/pain of colds/flu

**Usual Dosage** Oral:

Analgesic: Based on acetaminophen component:

- Children: 10-15 mg/kg/dose every 4-6 hours as needed; do **not** exceed 5 doses/24 hours
- Adults: 325-650 mg every 4-7 hours as needed; do **not** exceed 4 g/day

Cough suppressant: Based on dextromethorphan component:

- Children 6-12 years: 15 mg every 6-8 hours; do **not** exceed 60 mg/24 hours
- Children >12 years and Adults: 10-20 mg every 4-8 hours **or** 30 mg every 8 hours; do **not** exceed 120 mg/24 hours

Decongestant: Based on pseudoephedrine component:

- Children:
  - 2-6 years: 15 mg every 4 hours (maximum: 90 mg/24 hours)
  - 6-12 years: 30 mg every 4 hours (maximum: 180 mg/24 hours)
- Children >12 years and Adults: 60 mg every 4 hours (maximum: 360 mg/24 hours)

**Product labeling:**

Infants' Tylenol® Cold Plus Cough Concentrated Drops: Children 2-3 years (24-55 lbs): 2 dropperfuls every 4-6 hours (maximum: 4 doses/24 hours)

Sudafed® Severe Cold, Thera-Flu® Non-Drowsy Maximum Strength (gelcap), Tylenol® Flu Non-Drowsy Maximum Strength: Children >12 years and Adults: 2 doses every 6 hours (maximum: 8 doses/24 hours)

Tylenol® Cold Non-Drowsy:

- Children 6-11 years: 1 dose every 6 hours (maximum: 4 doses/24 hours)
- Children ≥12 years and Adults: 2 doses every 6 hours (maximum: 8 doses/24 hours)

Thera-Flu® Non-Drowsy Maximum Strength: Children >12 years and Adults: 1 packet dissolved in hot water every 6 hours (maximum: 4 packets/24 hours)

**Dosage Forms**

Liquid:

- Acetaminophen 160 mg, dextromethorphan hydrobromide 7.5 mg, and pseudoephedrine hydrochloride 15 mg per 5 mL
- Acetaminophen 325 mg, dextromethorphan hydrobromide 10 mg, and pseudoephedrine hydrochloride 30 mg per 5 mL
- Acetaminophen 650 mg, dextromethorphan hydrobromide 20 mg, and pseudoephedrine hydrochloride 30 mg per 5 mL

Powder: Acetaminophen 1000 mg, dextromethorphan hydrobromide 30 mg, and pseudoephedrine hydrochloride 60 mg

Tablet:

- Acetaminophen 500 mg, dextromethorphan hydrobromide 10 mg, and pseudoephedrine hydrochloride 30 mg
- Acetaminophen 500 mg, dextromethorphan hydrobromide 15 mg, and pseudoephedrine hydrochloride 30 mg

(Continued)

## acetaminophen, dextromethorphan, and pseudoephedrine *(Continued)*

Acetaminophen 325 mg, dextromethorphan hydrobromide 15 mg, and pseudoephedrine hydrochloride 30 mg

## acetaminophen, isometheptene, and dichloralphenazone

(a seet a MIN oh fen, eye soe me THEP teen, & dye KLOR al FEN a zone)

**U.S./Canadian Brand Names** Amidrine®; Duradrin®; I.D.A.®; Midrin®; Migquin®; Migraine®; Migrapap®; Migratine®; Migrazone®; Va-Zone®

**Therapeutic Category** Analgesic, Non-narcotic

**Use** Relief of migraine and tension headache

**Usual Dosage** Adults: Oral: 2 capsules at first sign of headache, followed by 1 capsule every 60 minutes until relieved, up to 5 capsules in a 12-hour period

**Dosage Forms** Capsule: Acetaminophen 325 mg, isometheptene mucate 65 mg, dichloralphenazone 100 mg

**Acetasol® HC Otic** *see* acetic acid, propylene glycol diacetate, and hydrocortisone *on next page*

**Acetasol® Otic** *see* acetic acid *on this page*

## acetazolamide (a set a ZOLE a mide)

**U.S./Canadian Brand Names** Apo®-Acetazolamide (Can); Diamox®; Diamox Sequels®

**Therapeutic Category** Anticonvulsant; Carbonic Anhydrase Inhibitor

**Use** Reduce elevated intraocular pressure in glaucoma, a diuretic, an adjunct to the treatment of refractory seizures and acute altitude sickness; centrencephalic epilepsies

**Usual Dosage**

Children:
- Glaucoma:
  - Oral: 8-30 mg/kg/day divided every 6-8 hours
  - I.M., I.V.: 20-40 mg/kg/day divided every 6 hours
- Edema: Oral, I.M., I.V.: 5 mg/kg or 150 mg/m$^2$ once every day or every other day
- Epilepsy: Oral: 8-30 mg/kg/day in 2-4 divided doses, not to exceed 1 g/day

Adults:
- Glaucoma:
  - Oral: 250 mg 1-4 times/day or 500 mg sustained release capsule twice daily
  - I.M., I.V.: 250-500 mg, may repeat in 2-4 hours
- Edema: Oral, I.M., I.V.: 250-375 mg once daily
- Epilepsy: Oral: 8-30 mg/kg/day in 1-4 divided doses
- Altitude sickness: Oral: 250 mg every 8-12 hours

**Dosage Forms**

Capsule, sustained release: 500 mg
Injection, as sodium: 500 mg
Tablet: 125 mg, 250 mg

## acetic acid (a SEE tik AS id)

**Synonyms** ethanoic acid

**U.S./Canadian Brand Names** Acetasol® Otic; Aci-jel® Vaginal; Vasotate® Otic; VōSol® Otic

**Therapeutic Category** Antibacterial, Otic; Antibacterial, Topical

**Use** Continuous or intermittent irrigation of the bladder; treatment of superficial bacterial infections of the external auditory canal and vagina

**Usual Dosage**

Irrigation: For continuous irrigation of the urinary bladder with 0.25% acetic acid irrigation, the rate of administration will approximate the rate of urine flow; usually 500-1500 mL/24 hours; for periodic irrigation of an indwelling urinary catheter to maintain patency, approximately 50 mL of 0.25% acetic acid irrigation is required. (Note:

Dosage of an irrigating solution depends on the capacity or surface area of the structure being irrigated.)

Otic: Insert saturated wick, keep moist 24 hours; remove wick and instill 5 drops 3-4 times/day

Vaginal: One applicatorful morning and evening

**Dosage Forms**

Jelly, vaginal (Aci-jel®): 0.921% with oxyquinolone sulfate 0.025%, ricinoleic acid 0.7%, and glycerin 5% (85 g)

Liquid: 36% (500 mL, 2500 mL)

Solution: 3% (500 mL, 1000 mL); 5% (500 mL, 4000 mL); 36% (500 mL)

Irrigation: 0.25% (1000 mL)

Otic: Acetic acid 2% in propylene glycol (15 mL, 30 mL, 60 mL)

**acetic acid and aluminum acetate otic** *see* aluminum acetate and acetic acid *on page 25*

## acetic acid, propylene glycol diacetate, and hydrocortisone

(a SEE tik AS id, PRO pa leen GLY kole dye AS e tate, & hye droe KOR ti sone)

**U.S./Canadian Brand Names** Acetasol® HC Otic; Oticort® HC Otic; VōSol® HC Otic

**Therapeutic Category** Antibiotic/Corticosteroid, Otic

**Use** Treatment of superficial infections of the external auditory canal caused by organisms susceptible to the action of the antimicrobial, complicated by inflammation

**Usual Dosage** Adults: Otic: Instill 4 drops in ear(s) 3-4 times/day

**Dosage Forms** Solution, otic: Acetic acid 2%, propylene glycol diacetate 3%, and hydrocortisone 1% (10 mL)

## acetohexamide (a set oh HEKS a mide)

**Therapeutic Category** Antidiabetic Agent, Oral

**Use** Adjunct to diet for the management of mild to moderately severe, stable, noninsulin-dependent (type 2) diabetes mellitus

**Usual Dosage** Adults: Oral: 250 mg to 1.5 g/day in 1-2 divided doses

**Dosage Forms** Tablet: 250 mg, 500 mg

## acetohydroxamic acid (a SEE toe hye droks am ik AS id)

**Synonyms** AHA

**U.S./Canadian Brand Names** Lithostat®

**Therapeutic Category** Urinary Tract Product

**Use** Adjunctive therapy in chronic urea-splitting urinary infection

**Usual Dosage** Oral:

Children: Initial: 10 mg/kg/day

Adults: 250 mg 3-4 times/day for a total daily dose of 10-15 mg/kg/day

**Dosage Forms** Tablet: 250 mg

**Acetoxyl (Can)** *see* benzoyl peroxide *on page 74*

**acetoxymethylprogesterone** *see* medroxyprogesterone acetate *on page 369*

## acetylcholine (a se teel KOE leen)

**U.S./Canadian Brand Names** Miochol-E®

**Therapeutic Category** Cholinergic Agent

**Use** Produces complete miosis in cataract surgery, keratoplasty, iridectomy and other anterior segment surgery where rapid miosis is required

**Usual Dosage** Adults: Intraocular: 0.5-2 mL of 1% injection (5-20 mg) instilled into anterior chamber before or after securing one or more sutures

**Dosage Forms** Powder, intraocular, as chloride: 1:100 [10 mg/mL] (2 mL)

**acetylcysteine** (a se teel SIS teen)

**Synonyms** mercapturic acid; NAC; *N*-acetylcysteine; *N*-acetyl-L-cysteine

**U.S./Canadian Brand Names** Acys-5®; Mucomyst®; Parvolex® (Can)

**Therapeutic Category** Mucolytic Agent

**Use** Adjunctive therapy in patients with abnormal or viscid mucous secretions in bronchopulmonary diseases, pulmonary complications of surgery, and cystic fibrosis; diagnostic bronchial studies; antidote for acute acetaminophen toxicity; enema to treat bowel obstruction due to meconium ileus or its equivalent

**Usual Dosage**

Acetaminophen poisoning: Children and Adults: Oral: 140 mg/kg; followed by 17 doses of 70 mg/kg every 4 hours; repeat dose if emesis occurs within 1 hour of administration; therapy should continue until all doses are administered even though the acetaminophen plasma level has dropped below the toxic range

Inhalation: Acetylcysteine 10% and 20% solution (Mucomyst®) (dilute 20% solution with sodium chloride or sterile water for inhalation); 10% solution may be used undiluted

Infants: 1-2 mL of 20% solution or 2-4 mL 10% solution until nebulized administered 3-4 times/day

Children: 3-5 mL of 20% solution or 6-10 mL of 10% solution until nebulized administered 3-4 times/day

Adolescents: 5-10 mL of 10% to 20% solution until nebulized administered 3-4 times/day

**Note:** Patients should receive an aerosolized bronchodilator 10-15 minutes prior to acetylcysteine

Meconium ileus equivalent: Children and Adults: 100-300 mL of 4% to 10% solution by irrigation or orally

**Dosage Forms** Solution, as sodium: 10% [100 mg/mL] (4 mL, 10 mL, 30 mL); 20% [200 mg/mL] (4 mL, 10 mL, 30 mL, 100 mL)

**acetylsalicylic acid** *see* aspirin *on page 55*

**Aches-N-Pain® [OTC]** *see* ibuprofen *on page 311*

**Achromycin® Parenteral *(Discontinued)*** *see page 750*

**Achromycin® V Capsule *(Discontinued)*** *see page 750*

**Achromycin® V Oral Suspension *(Discontinued)*** *see page 750*

**aciclovir** *see* acyclovir *on page 12*

**Aci-jel® Vaginal** *see* acetic acid *on page 8*

**Acilac (Can)** *see* lactulose *on page 338*

**AcipHex™** *see* rabeprazole *on page 515*

**acitretin** (a si TRE tin)

**U.S./Canadian Brand Names** Soriatane®

**Therapeutic Category** Retinoid-like Compound

**Use** Treatment of severe psoriasis (includes erythrodermic and pustular types) and other disorders of keratinization

**Usual Dosage** Adults: Oral: Individualization of dosage is required to achieve maximum therapeutic response while minimizing side effects

Initial: Therapy should be initiated at 25 mg/day, given as a single dose with the main meal; if by 4 weeks the response is unsatisfactory, and in the absence of toxicity, the daily dose may be gradually increased to a maximum of 75 mg/day; the dose may be reduced if necessary to minimize side effects

Maintenance: Doses of 25 to 50 mg/day may be given after initial response to treatment; the maintenance dose should be based on clinical efficacy and tolerability; it may be necessary in some cases to increase the dose to a maximum of 75 mg/day

**Dosage Forms** Capsule: 10 mg, 25 mg

**Aclovate® Topical** *see* alclometasone *on page 18*

**Acne-5®** *see* benzoyl peroxide *on page 74*

**Acne-10®** *see* benzoyl peroxide *on page 74*

**Acne-Aid®** *see* benzoyl peroxide *on page 74*

## acrivastine and pseudoephedrine (AK ri vas teen & soo doe e FED rin)

**Synonyms** pseudoephedrine and acrivastine

**U.S./Canadian Brand Names** Semprex®-D

**Therapeutic Category** Antihistamine/Decongestant Combination

**Use** Temporary relief of nasal congestion, decongest sinus openings, running nose, itching of nose or throat, and itchy, watery eyes due to hay fever or other upper respiratory allergies

**Usual Dosage** Adults: 1 capsule 3-4 times/day

**Dosage Forms** Capsule: Acrivastine 8 mg and pseudoephedrine hydrochloride 60 mg

**ACT** *see* dactinomycin *on page 164*

**ACT® [OTC]** *see* fluoride *on page 255*

**Actagen-C® *(Discontinued)*** *see page 750*

**Actagen® Syrup *(Discontinued)*** *see page 750*

**Actagen® Tablet *(Discontinued)*** *see page 750*

**Act-A-Med® [OTC]** *see* triprolidine and pseudoephedrine *on page 609*

**Actamin® [OTC]** *see* acetaminophen *on page 3*

**Actanol® [OTC]** *see* triprolidine and pseudoephedrine *on page 609*

**Actedril® [OTC]** *see* triprolidine and pseudoephedrine *on page 609*

**ACTH** *see* corticotropin *on page 154*

**ACTH-40® *(Discontinued)*** *see page 750*

**Acthar®** *see* corticotropin *on page 154*

**ActHIB®** *see* *Haemophilus* B conjugate vaccine *on page 287*

**Actibine®** *see* yohimbine *on page 636*

**Acticin® Cream** *see* permethrin *on page 462*

**Acticort® Topical** *see* hydrocortisone (topical) *on page 304*

**Actidil® *(Discontinued)*** *see page 750*

**Actidose-Aqua® [OTC]** *see* charcoal *on page 123*

**Actidose® With Sorbitol [OTC]** *see* charcoal *on page 123*

**Actifed® Allergy Tablet (Day) [OTC]** *see* pseudoephedrine *on page 507*

**Actifed® Allergy Tablet (Night) [OTC]** *see* diphenhydramine and pseudoephedrine *on page 191*

**Actifed® Syrup *(Discontinued)*** *see page 750*

**Actifed® Tablet [OTC]** *see* triprolidine and pseudoephedrine *on page 609*

**Actifed® With Codeine *(Discontinued)*** *see page 750*

**Actigall™** *see* ursodiol *on page 619*

**Actimmune®** *see* interferon gamma-1b *on page 323*

**Actinex® *(Discontinued)*** *see page 750*

**actinomycin D** *see* dactinomycin *on page 164*

**Actiq® Oral Transmucosal** *see* fentanyl *on page 244*

**Activase®** *see* alteplase *on page 24*

**activated carbon** *see* charcoal *on page 123*

**activated dimethicone** *see* simethicone *on page 544*

**activated ergosterol** *see* ergocalciferol *on page 220*

**activated methylpolysiloxane** *see* simethicone *on page 544*

**activated recombinant human blood coagulation factor VII** *see* eptacog alfa (activated) *(Canada only) on page 219*

**Activelle™** *see* estradiol and norethindrone *on page 226*

**Actonel™** *see* risedronate *on page 528*

**Actos™** *see* pioglitazone *on page 472*

**Actron® [OTC]** *see* ketoprofen *on page 334*

**ACU-dyne® [OTC]** *see* povidone-iodine *on page 489*

**Acular® Ophthalmic** *see* ketorolac tromethamine *on page 334*

**Acutrim® 16 Hours *(Discontinued)*** *see page 750*

**Acutrim® II, Maximum Strength *(Discontinued)*** *see page 750*

**Acutrim® Late Day *(Discontinued)*** *see page 750*

**ACV** *see* acyclovir *on this page*

**acycloguanosine** *see* acyclovir *on this page*

## acyclovir (ay SYE kloe veer)

**Synonyms** aciclovir; ACV; acycloguanosine

**U.S./Canadian Brand Names** Apo®-Acyclovir (Can); Avirax™ (Can); Nu-Acyclovir (Can); Zovirax®

**Therapeutic Category** Antiviral Agent

**Use** Treatment of initial and prophylaxis of recurrent mucosal and cutaneous herpes simplex (HSV-1 and HSV-2) infections; herpes simplex encephalitis; herpes zoster infections; varicella-zoster infections in healthy, nonpregnant persons >13 years of age, children >12 months of age who have a chronic skin or lung disorder or are receiving long-term aspirin therapy, and immunocompromised patients

**Usual Dosage**

Children and Adults: I.V.:

Mucocutaneous HSV infection: 750 mg/m²/day divided every 8 hours or 15 mg/kg/day divided every 8 hours for 5-10 days

HSV encephalitis: 1500 mg/m²/day divided every 8 hours or 30 mg/kg/day divided every 8 hours for 10 days

Varicella-zoster virus infection: 1500 mg/m²/day divided every 8 hours or 30 mg/kg/day divided every 8 hours for 5-10 days

Adults:

Oral: Initial: 200 mg every 4 hours while awake (5 times/day); prophylaxis: 200 mg 3-4 times/day or 400 mg twice daily. Prophylaxis of varicella or herpes zoster in HIV positive patients: 400 mg 5 times/day

Topical: ½" ribbon of ointment every 3 hours (6 times/day)

Herpes zoster in immunocompromised patients:

Children: Oral: 250-600 mg/m²/dose 4-5 times/day

Adults: Oral: 800 mg every 4 hours (5 times/day) for 7-10 days

Children and Adults: I.V.: 7.5 mg/kg/dose every 8 hours

Varicella-zoster infections: Oral:

Children: 10-20 mg/kg/dose (up to 800 mg) 4 times/day

Adults: 600-800 mg/dose 5 times/day for 7-10 days or 1000 mg every 6 hours for 5 days

Prophylaxis of bone marrow transplant recipients: Children and Adults: I.V.:

Autologous patients who are HSV seropositive: 150 mg/m²/dose every 12 hours; with clinical symptoms of herpes simplex: 150 mg/m²/dose every 8 hours

Autologous patients who are CMV seropositive: 500 mg/m²/dose every 8 hours; for clinically symptomatic CMV infection, ganciclovir should be used in place of acyclovir

**Dosage Forms**

Capsule: 200 mg

Injection, as sodium: 25 mg/mL (20 mL, 40 mL); 50 mg/mL (10 mL, 20 mL)
Ointment, topical: 5% [50 mg/g] (3 g, 15 g)
Powder for Injection, as sodium: 500 mg (10 mL); 1000 mg (20 mL)
Suspension, oral (banana flavor): 200 mg/5 mL (5 mL, 480 mL)
Tablet: 400 mg, 800 mg

**Acys-5®** *see* acetylcysteine *on page 10*

**Adagen™** *see* pegademase (bovine) *on page 453*

**Adalat® *(Discontinued)*** *see page 750*

**Adalat® CC** *see* nifedipine *on page 420*

**Adalat PA® (Can)** *see* nifedipine *on page 420*

**adamantanamine** *see* amantadine *on page 28*

## adapalene (a DAP a leen)

**U.S./Canadian Brand Names** Differin®

**Therapeutic Category** Acne Products

**Use** Treatment of acne vulgaris

**Usual Dosage** Adults: Topical: Apply once daily, before retiring, in a thin film to affected areas after washing; not recommended in children

**Dosage Forms**
Cream, topical: 0.1% (15 g, 45 g)
Gel, topical (alcohol free): 0.1% (15 g, 45 g)
Solution, topical: 0.1% (30 mL)
Swab (pledget): 0.1% (60s)

**Adderall®** *see* amphetamine mixture *on page 36*

**Adeflor®** *see* vitamin (multiple/pediatric) *on page 632*

**ADEKs® Pediatric Drops** *see* vitamin (multiple/pediatric) *on page 632*

**adenine arabinoside** *see* vidarabine *on page 627*

**Adenocard®** *see* adenosine *on this page*

## adenosine (a DEN oh seen)

**Synonyms** 9-beta-D-ribofuranosyladenine

**U.S./Canadian Brand Names** Adenocard®

**Therapeutic Category** Antiarrhythmic Agent, Miscellaneous

**Use** Treatment of paroxysmal supraventricular tachycardia (PSVT)

**Usual Dosage**
Children: Initial: Rapid I.V.: 0.05 mg/kg; if not effective within 2 minutes, increase dose in 0.05 mg/kg increments every 2 minutes to a maximum dose of 0.25 mg/kg or until termination of PSVT; median dose required: 0.15 mg/kg; do not exceed adult doses
Adults: Rapid I.V. push: 6 mg, if the dose is not effective within 1-2 minutes, a rapid I.V. dose of 12 mg may be administered; may repeat 12 mg bolus if needed

**Dosage Forms** Injection, preservative free: 3 mg/mL (2 mL, 5 mL, 20 mL, 30 mL)

**Adipex-P®** *see* phentermine *on page 466*

**Adipost® *(Discontinued)*** *see page 750*

**Adlone® Injection** *see* methylprednisolone *on page 385*

**Adphen® *(Discontinued)*** *see page 750*

**ADR** *see* doxorubicin *on page 203*

**Adrenalin® Chloride** *see* epinephrine *on page 216*

**adrenaline** *see* epinephrine *on page 216*

**adrenocorticotropic hormone** *see* corticotropin *on page 154*

**Adriamycin PFS®** *see* doxorubicin *on page 203*

**Adriamycin RDF®** *see* doxorubicin *on page 203*

**Adrin®** ***(Discontinued)*** *see page 750*

**Adrucil® Injection** *see* fluorouracil *on page 256*

**Adsorbocarpine® Ophthalmic** ***(Discontinued)*** *see page 750*

**Adsorbonac® Ophthalmic [OTC]** *see* sodium chloride *on page 549*

**Adsorbotear® Ophthalmic Solution [OTC]** *see* artificial tears *on page 53*

**Advair™ Diskus®** *see* fluticasone and salmeterol *on page 259*

**Advantage 24™ (Can)** *see* nonoxynol 9 *on page 424*

**Advil® [OTC]** *see* ibuprofen *on page 311*

**Advil® Cold & Sinus Caplets [OTC]** *see* pseudoephedrine and ibuprofen *on page 508*

**Aeroaid®** ***(Discontinued)*** *see page 750*

**AeroBid®-M Oral Aerosol Inhaler** *see* flunisolide *on page 253*

**AeroBid® Oral Aerosol Inhaler** *see* flunisolide *on page 253*

**Aerodine®** ***(Discontinued)*** *see page 750*

**Aerolate III®** *see* theophylline *on page 581*

**Aerolate JR®** *see* theophylline *on page 581*

**Aerolate® Oral Solution** ***(Discontinued)*** *see page 750*

**Aerolate SR®** *see* theophylline *on page 581*

**Aeroseb-Dex®** *see* dexamethasone (topical) *on page 175*

**Aeroseb-HC® Topical** *see* hydrocortisone (topical) *on page 304*

**Aerosporin® Injection** ***(Discontinued)*** *see page 750*

**AeroZoin® [OTC]** *see* benzoin *on page 74*

**Afrin® Children's Nose Drops [OTC]** *see* oxymetazoline *on page 444*

**Afrin® Nasal Solution [OTC]** *see* oxymetazoline *on page 444*

**Afrinol® [OTC]** *see* pseudoephedrine *on page 507*

**Afrin® Saline Mist [OTC]** *see* sodium chloride *on page 549*

**Aftate® [OTC]** *see* tolnaftate *on page 595*

**Agenerase™** *see* amprenavir *on page 39*

**Aggrastat®** *see* tirofiban *on page 592*

**Aggrenox®** *see* dipyridamole and aspirin *on page 195*

**$AgNO_3$** *see* silver nitrate *on page 544*

**Agoral® Plain** ***(Discontinued)*** *see page 750*

**Agrylin®** *see* anagrelide *on page 40*

**AHA** *see* acetohydroxamic acid *on page 9*

**AHF** *see* antihemophilic factor (human) *on page 43*

**A-hydroCort®** *see* hydrocortisone (systemic) *on page 303*

**Airet®** *see* albuterol *on page 16*

**Ak-Chlor® Ophthalmic** ***(Discontinued)*** *see page 750*

**AK-Cide® Ophthalmic** *see* sulfacetamide and prednisolone *on page 563*

**AK-Con® Ophthalmic** *see* naphazoline *on page 409*

**AK-Dex® Ophthalmic** *see* dexamethasone (ophthalmic) *on page 174*

**AK-Dilate® Ophthalmic Solution** *see* phenylephrine *on page 467*

**AK-Fluor Injection** *see* fluorescein sodium *on page 254*

**Ak-Homatropine® Ophthalmic** ***(Discontinued)*** *see page 750*

**Akineton®** *see* biperiden *on page 80*

**AK-Mycin®** *see* erythromycin (systemic) *on page 222*

**AK-NaCl® [OTC]** *see* sodium chloride *on page 549*

**AK-Nefrin® Ophthalmic Solution** *see* phenylephrine *on page 467*

**Akne-Mycin® Topical** *see* erythromycin (ophthalmic/topical) *on page 222*

**Akoline® C.B. Tablet *(Discontinued)*** *see page 750*

**AK-Poly-Bac® Ophthalmic** *see* bacitracin and polymyxin B *on page 64*

**AK-Pred® Ophthalmic** *see* prednisolone (ophthalmic) *on page 492*

**AK-Spore® H.C. Ophthalmic Ointment** *see* bacitracin, neomycin, polymyxin B, and hydrocortisone *on page 65*

**AK-Spore® H.C. Ophthalmic Suspension** *see* neomycin, polymyxin B, and hydrocortisone *on page 415*

**AK-Spore® H.C. Otic** *see* neomycin, polymyxin B, and hydrocortisone *on page 415*

**AK-Spore® Ophthalmic Ointment** *see* bacitracin, neomycin, and polymyxin B *on page 65*

**AK-Spore® Ophthalmic Solution** *see* neomycin, polymyxin B, and gramicidin *on page 414*

**AK-Sulf®** *see* sulfacetamide *on page 562*

**AK-Taine®** *see* proparacaine *on page 502*

**AKTob® Ophthalmic** *see* tobramycin *on page 593*

**AK-Tracin® Ophthalmic** *see* bacitracin *on page 64*

**AK-Trol®** *see* neomycin, polymyxin B, and dexamethasone *on page 414*

**Akwa Tears® Solution [OTC]** *see* artificial tears *on page 53*

**AK-Zol® *(Discontinued)*** *see page 750*

**Ala-Cort® Topical** *see* hydrocortisone (topical) *on page 304*

**Alamast™** *see* pemirolast *on page 454*

**Ala-Quin®** *see* clioquinol and hydrocortisone *on page 143*

**Ala-Scalp® Topical** *see* hydrocortisone (topical) *on page 304*

**Ala-Tet® *(Discontinued)*** *see page 750*

**alatrofloxacin** *see* trovafloxacin *on page 611*

**Alazide® *(Discontinued)*** *see page 750*

**Albalon-A® Ophthalmic** *see* naphazoline and antazoline *on page 409*

**Albalon® Liquifilm® Ophthalmic** *see* naphazoline *on page 409*

## albendazole (al BEN da zole)

**U.S./Canadian Brand Names** Albenza®

**Therapeutic Category** Anthelmintic

**Use** Treatment of parenchymal neurocysticercosis and cystic hydatid disease of the liver, lung, and peritoneum; albendazole may also be useful in the treatment of ascariasis, trichuriasis, enterobiasis, hook worm, strongyloidiasis, giardiasis, and microsporidiosis in AIDS

**Usual Dosage** Oral:

Children ≤2 years:

Neurocysticercosis: 15 mg/kg for 8 days; repeat as necessary

Children >2 years and Adults:

Hydatid cyst: 400 mg twice daily with meals for 3 cycles (each cycle consists of 28 days of dosing followed by a 14-day albendazole-free interval)

Neurocysticercosis: 400 mg twice daily for 8-30 days

(Continued)

## albendazole *(Continued)*

Roundworm, pinworm, hookworm: 400 mg as a single dose; treatment may be repeated in 3 weeks

Giardiasis: Strongyloidiasis and tapeworm: 400 mg/day for 3 days; treatment may be repeated in 3 weeks (giardiasis is a single course)

**Dosage Forms** Tablet: 200 mg

**Albenza®** *see* albendazole *on previous page*

**Albert® Glyburide (Can)** *see* glyburide *on page 276*

**Albert® Oxybutynin (Can)** *see* oxybutynin *on page 443*

**Albert® Pentoxifylline (Can)** *see* pentoxifylline *on page 460*

**Albert® Tiafen (Can)** *see* tiaprofenic acid *(Canada only)* *on page 589*

## albumin (al BYOO min)

**Synonyms** albumin (human)

**U.S./Canadian Brand Names** Albuminar®; Albumisol®; Albunex®; Albutein®; Buminate®; Plasbumin®

**Therapeutic Category** Blood Product Derivative

**Use** Treatment of hypovolemia; plasma volume expansion and maintenance of cardiac output in the treatment of certain types of shock or impending shock; hypoproteinemia resulting in generalized edema or decreased intravascular volume (eg, hypoproteinemia associated with acute nephrotic syndrome, premature infants)

**Usual Dosage** 5% should be used in hypovolemic patients; 25% should be used in patients in whom fluid and sodium intake must be minimized

Children:

Emergency initial dose: 25 g

Nonemergencies: 25% to 50% of the adult dose

Adults: Dosage depends on the condition of patient, usual adult dose is 25 g; no more than 250 g should be administered within 48 hours

Hypoproteinemia: I.V.: 0.5-1 g/kg/dose; repeat every 1-2 days as calculated to replace ongoing losses

Hypovolemia: I.V.: 0.5-1 g/kg/dose; repeat as needed; maximum dose: 6 g/kg/day

**Dosage Forms** Injection, as human: 5% [50 mg/mL] (50 mL, 250 mL, 500 mL, 1000 mL); 25% [250 mg/mL] (10 mL, 20 mL, 50 mL, 100 mL)

**Albuminar®** *see* albumin *on this page*

**albumin (human)** *see* albumin *on this page*

**Albumisol®** *see* albumin *on this page*

**Albunex®** *see* albumin *on this page*

**Albutein®** *see* albumin *on this page*

## albuterol (al BYOO ter ole)

**Synonyms** salbutamol

**U.S./Canadian Brand Names** AccuNeb™; Airet®; Alti-Salbutamol (Can); Apo®-Salvent (Can); Novo-Salmol (Can); Proventil®; Proventil® HFA; Proventil® Repetabs®; Ventolin®; Ventolin® HFA; Ventolin Rotacaps®; Volmax®

**Therapeutic Category** Adrenergic Agonist Agent

**Use** Bronchodilator in reversible airway obstruction due to asthma or COPD; prevention of exercise-induced bronchospasm

**Usual Dosage**

Oral:

Children: Bronchospasm (treatment):

2-6 years: 0.1-0.2 mg/kg/dose 3 times/day; maximum dose not to exceed 12 mg/day (divided doses)

6-12 years: 2 mg/dose 3-4 times/day; maximum dose not to exceed 24 mg/day (divided doses)

Extended release: 4 mg every 12 hours; maximum dose not to exceed 24 mg/day (divided doses)

Children >12 years and Adults: Bronchospasm (treatment): 2-4 mg/dose 3-4 times/day; maximum dose not to exceed 32 mg/day (divided doses)

Extended release: 8 mg every 12 hours; maximum dose not to exceed 32 mg/day (divided doses). A 4 mg dose every 12 hours may be sufficient in some patients, such as adults of low body weight.

Elderly: Bronchospasm (treatment): 2 mg 3-4 times/day; maximum: 8 mg 4 times/day

Inhalation: Children ≥4 years and Adults:

Bronchospasm (treatment):

MDI: 90 mcg/spray: 1-2 inhalations every 4-6 hours; maximum: 12 inhalations/day

Capsule: 200-400 mcg every 4-6 hours

Exercise-induced bronchospasm (prophylaxis):

MDI-CFC aerosol: 2 inhalations 15 minutes before exercising

MDI-HFA aerosol: 2 inhalations 15-30 minutes before exercise

Capsule: 200 mcg 15 minutes before exercise

Nebulization:

Children:

Bronchospasm (treatment): 0.01-0.05 mL/kg of 0.5% solution every 4-6 hours

2-12 years: AccuNeb™: 0.63 mg or 1.25 mg 3-4 times/day, as needed, delivered over 5-15 minutes

Children >40 kg, patients with more severe asthma, or children 11-12 years: May respond better with a 1.25 mg dose

Bronchospasm (acute): 0.01-0.05 mL/kg of 0.5% solution every 4-6 hours; intensive care patients may require more frequent administration; minimum dose: 0.1 mL; maximum dose: 1 mL diluted in 1-2 mL normal saline; continuous nebulized albuterol at 0.3 mg/kg/hour has been used safely in the treatment of severe status asthmaticus in children; continuous nebulized doses of 3 mg/kg/hour ± 2.2 mg/kg/hour in children whose mean age was 20.7 months resulted in no cardiac toxicity; the optimal dosage for continuous nebulization remains to be determined.

Adults:

Bronchospasm (treatment): 2.5 mg, diluted to a total of 3 mL, 3-4 times/day over 5-15 minutes

Bronchospasm (acute) in intensive care patients: 2.5-5 mg every 20 minutes for 3 doses, then 2.5-10 mg every 1-4 hours as needed, **or** 10-15 mg/hour continuously

## Dosage Forms

Aerosol, as sulfate:

Proventil® HFA: 90 mcg/dose (3.7 g, 6.7 g) [chlorofluorocarbon free]

Ventolin® HFA: 90 mcg/dose (18 g) [200 doses] [chlorofluorocarbon free]

Aerosol: 90 mcg/dose (17 g) [200 doses]

Proventil®: 90 mcg/dose (17 g) [200 doses]

Ventolin®: 90 mcg/dose (6.8 g) [80 doses]; (17 g) [200 doses]

Powder for oral inhalation, as sulfate [capsule] (Ventolin Rotacaps®): 200 mcg [to be used with Rotahaler® inhalation device] [contains 25 mg lactose]

Solution for oral inhalation, as sulfate: 0.083% (3 mL); 0.5% (20 mL)

Airet®: 0.083%

Proventil®, Ventolin®: 0.083% (3 mL); 0.5% (20 mL)

AccuNeb™ 0.63 mg/3 mL (5 vials/pouch); 1.25 mg/3 mL (5 vials/pouch)

Syrup, as sulfate: 2 mg/5 mL (480 mL)

Proventil®, Ventolin®: 2 mg/5 mL (480 mL) [strawberry flavor]

Tablet, as sulfate: 2 mg, 4 mg

Proventil®, Ventolin®: 2 mg, 4 mg

Tablet, extended release, as sulfate:

Proventil® Repetabs®: 4 mg

Volmax®: 4 mg, 8 mg

**Alcaine®** *see* proparacaine *on page 502*

## alclometasone (al kloe MET a sone)

**U.S./Canadian Brand Names** Aclovate® Topical

**Therapeutic Category** Corticosteroid, Topical

**Use** Inflammation of corticosteroid-responsive dermatosis

**Usual Dosage** Topical: Apply a thin film to the affected area 2-3 times/day. Therapy should be discontinued when control is achieved. If no improvement is seen, reassessment of diagnosis may be necessary.

**Dosage Forms**

Cream, as dipropionate: 0.05% (15 g, 45 g, 60 g)

Ointment, topical, as dipropionate: 0.05% (15 g, 45 g, 60 g)

## alcohol (ethyl) (AL koe hol ETH il)

**Synonyms** ethanol

**U.S./Canadian Brand Names** Lavacol® [OTC]

**Therapeutic Category** Intravenous Nutritional Therapy; Pharmaceutical Aid

**Use** Topical anti-infective; pharmaceutical aid; an antidote for ethylene glycol overdose; an antidote for methanol overdose

**Usual Dosage**

I.V.: Doses of 100-125 mg/kg/hour to maintain blood levels of 100 mg/dL are recommended after a loading dose of 0.6 g/kg; maximum dose: 400 mL of a 5% solution within 1 hour

Topical: Use as needed

**Dosage Forms**

Injection, absolute: 2 mL

Liquid, topical, denatured: 70% (473 mL)

Solution, inhalation: 20%, 40%

**Alcomicin® (Can)** *see* gentamicin *on page 273*

**Alconefrin® Nasal Solution [OTC]** *see* phenylephrine *on page 467*

**Aldactazide®** *see* hydrochlorothiazide and spironolactone *on page 299*

**Aldactone®** *see* spironolactone *on page 556*

**Aldara™** *see* imiquimod *on page 315*

## aldesleukin (al des LOO kin)

**Synonyms** interleukin-2

**U.S./Canadian Brand Names** Proleukin®

**Therapeutic Category** Biological Response Modulator

**Use** Primarily investigated in tumors known to have a response to immunotherapy, such as melanoma and renal cell carcinoma; has been used in conjunction with LAK cells, TIL cells, IL-1, and interferon

**Usual Dosage** All orders should be written in million International units (million int. units) (refer to individual protocols)

Adults: Metastatic renal cell carcinoma:

Treatment consists of two 5-day treatment cycles separated by a rest period. 600,000 int. units/kg (0.037 mg/kg)/dose administered every 8 hours by a 15-minute I.V. infusion for a total of 14 doses; following 9 days of rest, the schedule is repeated for another 14 doses, for a maximum of 28 doses per course.

**Investigational regimen:** I.V. continuous infusion: 4.5 million int. units/m$^2$/day in 250-1000 mL of $D_5W$ for 5 days

**Dose modification:** Hold or interrupt a dose rather than reducing dose; refer to protocol

**Retreatment:** Patients should be evaluated for response ~4 weeks after completion of a course of therapy and again immediately prior to the scheduled start of the next treatment course. Additional courses of treatment may be administered to patients only if there is some tumor shrinkage following the last course and retreatment is not contraindicated. Each treatment course should be separated by a rest period of at least

7 weeks from the date of hospital discharge. Tumors have continued to regress up to 12 months following the initiation of therapy.

**Dosage Forms** Powder for injection, lyophilized: 22 x $10^6$ int. units [18 million int. units/mL = 1.1 mg/mL when reconstituted]

**Aldoclor®** ***(Discontinued)*** *see page 750*

**Aldomet®** *see* methyldopa *on page 383*

**Aldoril®** *see* methyldopa and hydrochlorothiazide *on page 384*

## alemtuzumab (ay lem TU zoo mab)

**Synonyms** campath-1H; DNA-derived humanized monoclonal antibody; humanized IgG1 anti-CD52 monoclonal antibody

**U.S./Canadian Brand Names** Campath®

**Therapeutic Category** Antineoplastic Agent

**Use** Treatment of B-cell chronic lymphocytic leukemia (B-CLL) in patients treated with alkylating agents and who have failed fludarabine therapy

**Usual Dosage** Note: **Dose escalation is required;** usually accomplished in 3-7 days. Do not exceed single doses >30 mg or cumulative doses >90 mg/week. Premedicate with diphenhydramine and acetaminophen 30 minutes before initiation of infusion. Start anti-infective prophylaxis. Discontinue therapy during serious infection, serious hematologic or other serious toxicity until the event resolves. Permanently discontinue if evidence of autoimmune anemia or autoimmune thrombocytopenia occurs.

I.V. infusion: Adults: B-CLL:

Initial: 3 mg/day as a 2-hour infusion; when daily dose is tolerated (eg, infusion-related toxicities at or below Grade 2) increase to 10 mg/day and continue until tolerated; when 10 mg dose tolerated, increase to 30 mg/day

Maintenance: 30 mg/day 3 times/week on alternate days (ie, Monday, Wednesday, Friday) for up to 12 weeks

**Dosage Forms** Injection: 10 mg/mL (3 mL)

## alendronate (a LEN droe nate)

**U.S./Canadian Brand Names** Fosamax®

**Therapeutic Category** Bisphosphonate Derivative

**Use** Treatment of osteoporosis in postmenopausal women, Paget's disease of the bone; treatment of glucocorticoid-induced osteoporosis in males and females with low bone mineral density who are receiving a daily dosage ≥7.5 mg of prednisone (or equivalent)

**Usual Dosage** Oral:

Adults: Patients with osteoporosis or Paget's disease should receive supplemental calcium and vitamin D if dietary intake is inadequate

**Osteoporosis in postmenopausal women:** 10 mg once daily. Safety of treatment for >4 years has not been studied (extension studies are ongoing).

**Paget's disease of bone:** 40 mg once daily for 6 months

Retreatment: Relapses during the 12 months following therapy occurred in 9% of patients who responded to treatment. Specific retreatment data are not available. Retreatment with alendronate may be considered, following a 6-month post-treatment evaluation period, in patients who have relapsed based on increases in serum alkaline phosphatase, which should be measured periodically. Retreatment may also be considered in those who failed to normalize their serum alkaline phosphatase.

Treatment of glucocorticoid-induced osteoporosis: 5 mg once daily. A dose of 10 mg once daily should be used in postmenopausal women who are not receiving estrogen. Patients treated with glucocorticoids should receive adequate amounts of calcium and vitamin D.

Elderly: No dosage adjustment is necessary

**Dosage Forms** Tablet, as sodium: 5 mg, 10 mg, 40 mg

**Alertec® (Can)** *see* modafinil *on page 397*

**Alesse™** *see* ethinyl estradiol and levonorgestrel *on page 232*

**Aleve® [OTC]** *see* naproxen *on page 409*

**Alfenta®** *see* alfentanil *on this page*

## alfentanil (al FEN ta nil)

**U.S./Canadian Brand Names** Alfenta®

**Therapeutic Category** Analgesic, Narcotic; General Anesthetic

**Controlled Substance** C-II

**Use** Analgesia; analgesia adjunct; anesthetic agent

**Usual Dosage** Doses should be titrated to appropriate effects; wide range of doses is dependent upon desired degree of analgesia/anesthesia

Children <12 years: Dose not established

Adults: Anesthesia of ≤30 minutes: Initial (induction): 8-20 mcg/kg, then 3-5 mcg/kg/dose or 0.5-1 mcg/kg/minute for maintenance; total dose: 8-40 mcg/kg; higher doses used for longer anesthesia required procedures

**Dosage Forms** Injection, preservative free, as hydrochloride: 500 mcg/mL (2 mL, 5 mL, 10 mL, 20 mL)

**Alferon® N** *see* interferon alfa-n3 *on page 323*

## alglucerase (al GLOO ser ase)

**Synonyms** glucocerebrosidase

**U.S./Canadian Brand Names** Ceredase®

**Therapeutic Category** Enzyme

**Use** Long-term enzyme replacement in patients with confirmed Type I Gaucher's disease who exhibit one or more of the following conditions: Moderate to severe anemia; thrombocytopenia and bleeding tendencies; bone disease; hepatomegaly or splenomegaly

**Usual Dosage** I.V. infusion: Administer 20-60 units/kg with a frequency ranging from 3 times/week to once every 2 weeks

**Dosage Forms** Injection: 10 units/mL (5 mL); 80 units/mL (5 mL)

## alitretinoin (a li TRET i noyn)

**U.S./Canadian Brand Names** Panretin™

**Therapeutic Category** Antineoplastic Agent; Retinoic Acid Derivative

**Use** Topical treatment of cutaneous lesions in AIDS-related Kaposi's sarcoma; not indicated when systemic therapy for Kaposi's sarcoma is indicated

**Usual Dosage** Topical: Apply gel twice daily to cutaneous Kaposi's sarcoma lesions

**Dosage Forms** Gel: 0.1% (60 g)

**Alkaban-AQ®** *see* vinblastine *on page 627*

**Alka-Mints® [OTC]** *see* calcium carbonate *on page 97*

**Alkeran®** *see* melphalan *on page 370*

**Allbee® With C [OTC]** *see* vitamin B complex with vitamin C *on page 630*

**Allegra®** *see* fexofenadine *on page 248*

**Allegra-D®** *see* fexofenadine and pseudoephedrine *on page 248*

**Aller-Chlor® [OTC]** *see* chlorpheniramine *on page 129*

**Allercon® Tablet *(Discontinued)*** *see page 750*

**Allerdryl® (Can)** *see* diphenhydramine *on page 191*

**Allerest® 12 Hour Capsule *(Discontinued)*** *see page 750*

**Allerest® 12 Hour Nasal Solution [OTC]** *see* oxymetazoline *on page 444*

**Allerest® Eye Drops [OTC]** *see* naphazoline *on page 409*

**Allerest® Maximum Strength [OTC]** *see* chlorpheniramine and pseudoephedrine *on page 130*

**Allerest® No Drowsiness [OTC]** *see* acetaminophen and pseudoephedrine *on page 6*

**Allerfed® [OTC]** *see* triprolidine and pseudoephedrine *on page 609*

**Allerfrim® [OTC]** *see* triprolidine and pseudoephedrine *on page 609*

**Allerfrin® Syrup *(Discontinued)*** *see page 750*

**Allerfrin® Tablet *(Discontinued)*** *see page 750*

**Allerfrin® w/Codeine *(Discontinued)*** *see page 750*

**Allergan® Ear Drops** *see* antipyrine and benzocaine *on page 44*

**Allergy Sinus® Maximum Strength [OTC]** *see* acetaminophen, chlorpheniramine, and pseudoephedrine *on page 6*

**Allergy Sinus® Pain Relief [OTC]** *see* acetaminophen, chlorpheniramine, and pseudoephedrine *on page 6*

**Allerhist-1®** *see* clemastine *on page 141*

**AllerMax® Oral [OTC]** *see* diphenhydramine *on page 191*

**Allernix® (Can)** *see* diphenhydramine *on page 191*

**Allerphed® Syrup [OTC]** *see* triprolidine and pseudoephedrine *on page 609*

## allopurinol (al oh PURE i nole)

**U.S./Canadian Brand Names** Aloprim™ Injection; Apo®-Allopurinol (Can); Zyloprim®

**Therapeutic Category** Xanthine Oxidase Inhibitor

**Use** Prevention of attacks of gouty arthritis and nephropathy; also used to treat secondary hyperuricemia which may occur during treatment of tumors or leukemia; prevent recurrent calcium oxalate calculi

**Usual Dosage**

Oral:

Children: 10 mg/kg/day in 2-3 divided doses or 200-300 mg/m$^2$/day in 2-4 divided doses, maximum: 600 mg/24 hours

Alternative:

<6 years: 150 mg/day in 3 divided doses

6-10 years: 300 mg/day in 2-3 divided doses

Children >10 years and Adults: Daily doses >300 mg should be administered in divided doses

Myeloproliferative neoplastic disorders: 600-800 mg/day in 2-3 divided doses for prevention of acute uric acid nephropathy for 2-3 days starting 1-2 days before chemotherapy

Gout: 200-300 mg/day (mild); 400-600 mg/day (severe)

Maximum dose: 800 mg/day

I.V.: Intravenous daily dose can be given as a single infusion or in equally divided doses at 6-, 8-, or 12-hour intervals. A fluid intake sufficient to yield a daily urinary output of at least 2 L in adults and the maintenance of a neutral or, preferably, slightly alkaline urine are desirable.

Children: Starting dose: 200 mg/m$^2$/day

Adults: 200-400 mg/m$^2$/day (max: 600 mg/day)

**Dosing adjustment in renal impairment: I.V.:**

$Cl_{cr}$ 10-20 mL/minute: 200 mg/day

$Cl_{cr}$ 3-10 mL/minute: 100 mg/day

$Cl_{cr}$ <3 mL/minute: 100 mg/day at extended intervals

**Dosage Forms**

Injection, as sodium: 500 mg

Tablet: 100 mg, 300 mg

**all-*trans*-retinoic acid** *see* tretinoin (oral) *on page 600*

**almotriptan** (al moh TRIP tan)

**U.S./Canadian Brand Names** Axert™

**Therapeutic Category** Serotonin 5-$HT_{1D}$ Receptor Agonist

**Use** Acute treatment of migraine with or without aura

**Usual Dosage** Oral: Adults: Migraine: Initial: 6.25-12.5 mg in a single dose; if the headache returns, repeat the dose after 2 hours; no more than 2 doses in 24-hour period

**Note:** If the first dose is ineffective, diagnosis needs to be re-evaluated. Safety of treating more than 4 migraines/month has not been established.

**Dosage adjustment in renal impairment:** Initial: 6.25 mg in a single dose; maximum daily dose: ≤12.5 mg

**Dosage adjustment in hepatic impairment:** Initial: 6.25 mg in a single dose; maximum daily dose: ≤12.5 mg

**Dosage Forms** Tablet, as malate: 6.25 mg, 12.5 mg

**Alocril™** *see* nedocromil (ophthalmic) *on page 412*

**Alomide® Ophthalmic** *see* lodoxamide tromethamine *on page 354*

**Aloprim™ Injection** *see* allopurinol *on previous page*

**Alor® 5/500 *(Discontinued)*** *see page 750*

**Alora® Transdermal** *see* estradiol *on page 224*

**$alpha_1$-PI** *see* $alpha_1$-proteinase inhibitor *on this page*

**$alpha_1$-proteinase inhibitor** (al fa won PRO tee in ase in HI bi tor)

**Synonyms** $alpha_1$-PI

**U.S./Canadian Brand Names** Prolastin®

**Therapeutic Category** Antitrypsin Deficiency Agent

**Use** Congenital $alpha_1$-antitrypsin deficiency

**Usual Dosage** Adults: I.V.: 60 mg/kg once weekly

**Dosage Forms** Injection (human): 500 mg $alpha_1$-PI (20 mL diluent); 1000 mg $alpha_1$-PI (40 mL diluent)

**Alphagan®** *see* brimonidine *on page 85*

**Alphamul® [OTC]** *see* castor oil *on page 112*

**Alphanate®** *see* antihemophilic factor (human) *on page 43*

**AlphaNine® SD** *see* factor IX complex (human) *on page 238*

**Alphatrex® Topical** *see* betamethasone (topical) *on page 78*

**alprazolam** (al PRAY zoe lam)

**U.S./Canadian Brand Names** Alti-Alprazolam (Can); Apo®-Alpraz (Can); Gen-Alprazolam (Can); Novo-Alprazol (Can); Nu-Alpraz (Can); Xanax®

**Therapeutic Category** Benzodiazepine

**Controlled Substance** C-IV

**Use** Treatment of anxiety; adjunct in the treatment of depression; management of panic attacks

**Usual Dosage** Oral:

Children <18 years: Dose not established

Adults: 0.25-0.5 mg 2-3 times/day, titrate dose upward; maximum: 4 mg/day (anxiety); 10 mg/day (panic attacks)

**Dosage Forms**

Solution, oral: 1 mg/mL (30 mL)

Tablet: 0.25 mg, 0.5 mg, 1 mg, 2 mg

## alprostadil (al PROS ta dill)

**Synonyms** $PGE_1$; prostaglandin $E_1$

**U.S./Canadian Brand Names** Caverject® Injection; Edex® Injection; Muse® Pellet; Prostin VR Pediatric® Injection

**Therapeutic Category** Prostaglandin

**Use** Temporary maintenance of patency of ductus arteriosus in neonates with ductal-dependent congenital cyanotic or acyanotic heart disease until surgery can be performed; these defects include cyanotic (eg, pulmonary atresia, pulmonary stenosis, tricuspid atresia, Fallot's tetralogy, transposition of the great vessels) and acyanotic (eg, interruption of aortic arch, coarctation of aorta, hypoplastic left ventricle) heart disease. Alprostadil has also been used investigationally for the treatment of pulmonary hypertension in infants and children with congenital heart defects with left-to-right shunts and primary graft nonfunction following liver transplant. Used in penile erectile dysfunction

**Usual Dosage**

**Patent ductus arteriosus** (Prostin VR Pediatric®):

I.V. continuous infusion into a large vein, or alternatively through an umbilical artery catheter placed at the ductal opening: 0.05-0.1 mcg/kg/minute with therapeutic response, rate is reduced to lowest effective dosage; with unsatisfactory response, rate is increased gradually; maintenance: 0.01-0.4 mcg/kg/minute

$PGE_1$ is usually given at an infusion rate of 0.1 mcg/kg/minute, but it is often possible to reduce the dosage to 1/2 or even 1/10 without losing the therapeutic effect. The mixing schedule is shown in the table.

**Alprostadil**

| Add 1 Ampul (500 mcg) to: | Concentration (mcg/mL) | Infusion Rate | |
|---|---|---|---|
| | | mL/min/kg Needed to Infuse 0.1 mcg/kg/min | mL/kg/24 h |
| 250 mL | 2 | 0.05 | 72 |
| 100 mL | 5 | 0.02 | 28.8 |
| 50 mL | 10 | 0.01 | 14.4 |
| 25 mL | 20 | 0.005 | 7.2 |

Therapeutic response is indicated by increased pH in those with acidosis or by an increase in oxygenation ($pO_2$) usually evident within 30 minutes

**Erectile dysfunction**:

Caverject®:

Vasculogenic, psychogenic, or mixed etiology: Individualize dose by careful titration; usual dose: 2.5-60 mcg (doses >60 mcg are not recommended); initiate dosage titration at 2.5 mcg, increasing by 2.5 mcg to a dose of 5 mcg and then in increments of 5-10 mcg depending on the erectile response until the dose produces an erection suitable for intercourse, not lasting >1 hour; if there is absolutely no response to initial 2.5 mcg dose, the second dose may increased to 7.5 mcg, followed by increments of 5-10 mcg

Neurogenic etiology (eg, spinal cord injury): Initiate dosage titration at 1.25 mcg, increasing to a doses of 2.5 mcg and then 5 mcg; increase further in increments 5 mcg until the dose is reached that produces an erection suitable for intercourse, not lasting >1 hour

**Note:** Patient must stay in the physician's office until complete detumescence occurs; if there is no response, then the next higher dose may be given within 1 hour; if there is still no response, a 1-day interval before giving the next dose is recommended; increasing the dose or concentration in the treatment of impotence results in increasing pain and discomfort

Muse® Pellet: Intraurethral: Administer as needed to achieve an erection; duration of action: ~30-60 minutes; use only two systems per 24-hour period

**Dosage Forms**

Injection:

Caverject®: 5 mcg, 10 mcg, 20 mcg

(Continued)

## alprostadil *(Continued)*

Edex® Injection: 10 mcg, 20 mcg, 40 mcg
Prostin VR Pediatric®: 500 mcg/mL (1 mL)
Pellet, urethral (Muse®): 125 mcg, 250 mcg, 500 mcg, 1000 mcg

**Alrex™** *see* loteprednol *on page 357*

**Altace™** *see* ramipril *on page 518*

**Altafed® [OTC]** *see* triprolidine and pseudoephedrine *on page 609*

**Altenol® [OTC]** *see* acetaminophen *on page 3*

## alteplase (AL te plase)

**Synonyms** alteplase, recombinant; tissue plasminogen activator, recombinant; t-PA

**U.S./Canadian Brand Names** Activase®

**Therapeutic Category** Fibrinolytic Agent

**Use** Management of acute myocardial infarction for the lysis of thrombi in coronary arteries; management of acute massive pulmonary embolism (PE) in adults

**Usual Dosage**

Coronary artery thrombi: I.V.: Front loading dose: Total dose is 100 mg over 1.5 hours (for patients who weigh <67 kg, use 1.25 mg/kg/total dose). Add this dose to a 100 mL bag of 0.9% sodium chloride for a total volume of 200 mL. Infuse 15 mg (30 mL) over 1-2 minutes; infuse 50 mg (100 mL) over 30 minutes. Begin heparin 5000-10,000 unit bolus followed by continuous infusion of 1000 units/hour. Infuse the remaining 35 mg (70 mL) of alteplase over the next hour. For ≤67 kg: 15 mg I.V. bolus over 1-2 minutes. Infuse 0.75 mg/kg (not to exceed 50 mg) over next 30 minutes and then 0.5 mg/kg over next 60 minutes (not to exceed 35 mg).

**Dosage Forms** Powder for injection, lyophilized (recombinant): 50 mg [29 million units] (50 mL); 100 mg [58 million units] (100 mL)

**alteplase, recombinant** *see* alteplase *on this page*

**ALternaGel® [OTC]** *see* aluminum hydroxide *on page 26*

**Alti-Alprazolam (Can)** *see* alprazolam *on page 22*

**Alti-Amiloride HCTZ (Can)** *see* amiloride and hydrochlorothiazide *on page 30*

**Alti-Amiodarone (Can)** *see* amiodarone *on page 32*

**Alti-Azathioprine (Can)** *see* azathioprine *on page 61*

**Alti-Beclomethasone (Can)** *see* beclomethasone *on page 68*

**Alti-Benzydamine (Can)** *see* benzydamine *(Canada only) on page 75*

**Alti-Bromazepam (Can)** *see* bromazepam *(Canada only) on page 86*

**Alti-Captopril (Can)** *see* captopril *on page 104*

**Alti-Clindamycin (Can)** *see* clindamycin *on page 142*

**Alti-Clobazam (Can)** *see* clobazam *(Canada only) on page 143*

**Alti-Clonazepam (Can)** *see* clonazepam *on page 145*

**Alti-CPA (Can)** *see* cyproterone *(Canada only) on page 161*

**Alti-Desipramine (Can)** *see* desipramine *on page 172*

**Alti-Diltiazem (Can)** *see* diltiazem *on page 187*

**Alti-Domperidone (Can)** *see* domperidone *(Canada only) on page 200*

**Alti-Doxepin (Can)** *see* doxepin *on page 202*

**Alti-Famotidine (Can)** *see* famotidine *on page 240*

**Alti-Flunisoline (Can)** *see* flunisolide *on page 253*

**Alti-Fluoxetine (Can)** *see* fluoxetine *on page 256*

**Alti-Flurbiprofen (Can)** *see* flurbiprofen *on page 259*

**Alti-Fluvoxamine (Can)** *see* fluvoxamine *on page 262*

**Alti-Ipratropium (Can)** *see* ipratropium *on page 325*

**Alti-Minocycline (Can)** *see* minocycline *on page 394*

**Alti-Moclobemide (Can)** *see* moclobemide *(Canada only) on page 397*

**Alti-MPA (Can)** *see* medroxyprogesterone acetate *on page 369*

**Altinac™ Cream** *see* tretinoin (topical) *on page 600*

**Alti-Nadolol (Can)** *see* nadolol *on page 405*

**Alti-Piroxicam (Can)** *see* piroxicam *on page 474*

**Alti-Prazosin (Can)** *see* prazosin *on page 491*

**Alti-Ranitidine (Can)** *see* ranitidine hydrochloride *on page 519*

**Alti-Salbutamol (Can)** *see* albuterol *on page 16*

**Alti-Sotalol (Can)** *see* sotalol *on page 555*

**Alti-Sulfasalazine (Can)** *see* sulfasalazine *on page 565*

**Alti-Terazosin (Can)** *see* terazosin *on page 574*

**Alti-Ticlopidine (Can)** *see* ticlopidine *on page 590*

**Alti-Trazodone (Can)** *see* trazodone *on page 600*

**Alti-Valproic (Can)** *see* valproic acid and derivatives *on page 620*

**Alti-Verapamil (Can)** *see* verapamil *on page 625*

## altretamine (al TRET a meen)

**Synonyms** hexamethylmelamine

**U.S./Canadian Brand Names** Hexalen®

**Therapeutic Category** Antineoplastic Agent

**Use** Palliative treatment of persistent or recurrent ovarian cancer

**Usual Dosage** Adults: Oral (refer to protocol): 4-12 mg/kg/day in 3-4 divided doses for 21-90 days

Alternatively: 240-320 mg/m$^2$/day in 3-4 divided doses for 21 days, repeated every 6 weeks

Alternatively: 260 mg/m$^2$/day for 14-21 days of a 28-day cycle in 4 divided doses

**Dosage Forms** Capsule: 50 mg

**Alu-Cap® [OTC]** *see* aluminum hydroxide *on next page*

**Aludrox® [OTC]** *see* aluminum hydroxide and magnesium hydroxide *on page 27*

## aluminum acetate and acetic acid

(a LOO mi num AS e tate & a SEE tik AS id)

**Synonyms** acetic acid and aluminum acetate otic; Burow's otic

**U.S./Canadian Brand Names** Otic Domeboro®

**Therapeutic Category** Otic Agent, Anti-infective

**Use** Treatment of superficial infections of the external auditory canal

**Usual Dosage** Otic: Instill 4-6 drops in ear(s) every 2-3 hours

**Dosage Forms** Solution, otic: Aluminum acetate 10% and acetic acid 2% (60 mL)

## aluminum carbonate (a LOO mi num KAR bun ate)

**U.S./Canadian Brand Names** Basaljel® [OTC]

**Therapeutic Category** Antacid

**Use** Hyperacidity; hyperphosphatemia

**Usual Dosage** Adults: Oral:

Antacid: 2 tablets/capsules or 10 mL of suspension every 2 hours, up to 12 times/day

Hyperphosphatemia: 2 tablets/capsules or 12 mL of suspension with meals

(Continued)

## aluminum carbonate *(Continued)*

**Dosage Forms**

Capsule: Equivalent to 500 mg aluminum hydroxide

Suspension: Equivalent to 400 mg/5 mL aluminum hydroxide

Tablet: Equivalent to 500 mg aluminum hydroxide

## aluminum chloride hexahydrate

(a LOO mi num KLOR ide heks a HYE drate)

**U.S./Canadian Brand Names** Drysol™

**Therapeutic Category** Topical Skin Product

**Use** Astringent in the management of hyperhidrosis

**Usual Dosage** Adults: Topical: Apply at bedtime

**Dosage Forms** Solution, topical: 20% in SD alcohol 40 (35 mL, 37.5 mL)

## aluminum hydroxide (a LOO mi num hye DROKS ide)

**U.S./Canadian Brand Names** ALternaGel® [OTC]; Alu-Cap® [OTC]; Alu-Tab® [OTC]; Amphojel® [OTC]; Dialume® [OTC]; Nephrox Suspension [OTC]

**Therapeutic Category** Antacid

**Use** Hyperacidity; hyperphosphatemia

**Usual Dosage** Oral:

Peptic ulcer disease:

Children: 5-15 mL/dose every 3-6 hours or 1 and 3 hours after meals and at bedtime

Adults: 15-45 mL every 3-6 hours or 1 and 3 hours after meals and at bedtime

Prophylaxis against gastrointestinal bleeding:

Infants: 2-5 mL/dose every 1-2 hours

Children: 5-15 mL/dose every 1-2 hours

Adults: 30-60 mL/dose every hour

Titrate to maintain the gastric pH >5

Hyperphosphatemia:

Children: 50 mg to 150 mg/kg/24 hours in divided doses every 4-6 hours, titrate dosage to maintain serum phosphorus within normal range

Adults: 500-1800 mg, 3-6 times/day, between meals and at bedtime

Antacid: Adults: 30 mL 1 and 3 hours postprandial and at bedtime

**Dosage Forms**

Capsule:

Alu-Cap®: 400 mg

Dialume®: 500 mg

Liquid: 600 mg/5 mL

ALternaGel®: 600 mg/5 mL

Suspension, oral: 320 mg/5 mL; 450 mg/5 mL; 675 mg/5 mL

Amphojel®: 320 mg/5 mL

Tablet:

Amphojel®: 300 mg, 600 mg

Alu-Tab®: 500 mg

## aluminum hydroxide and magnesium carbonate

(a LOO mi num hye DROKS ide & mag NEE zhum KAR bun nate)

**U.S./Canadian Brand Names** Gaviscon® Liquid [OTC]

**Therapeutic Category** Antacid

**Use** Temporary relief of symptoms associated with gastric acidity

**Usual Dosage** Adults: Oral: 15-30 mL 4 times/day after meals and at bedtime

**Dosage Forms** Liquid: Aluminum hydroxide 95 mg and magnesium carbonate 358 mg per 15 mL

## aluminum hydroxide and magnesium hydroxide

(a LOO mi num hye DROKS ide & mag NEE zhum hye DROK side)

**U.S./Canadian Brand Names** Aludrox® [OTC]; Diovol® (Can); Diovol® EX (Can); Gelusil® Tablet (Can); Maalox® [OTC]; Maalox® Therapeutic Concentrate [OTC]; Univol® (Can)

**Therapeutic Category** Antacid

**Use** Antacid, hyperphosphatemia in renal failure

**Usual Dosage** Adults: Oral: 5-10 mL or 1-2 tablets 4-6 times/day, between meals and at bedtime; may be used every hour for severe symptoms

**Dosage Forms**

Suspension:

Aludrox®: Aluminum hydroxide 307 mg and magnesium hydroxide 103 mg per 5 mL

Maalox®: Aluminum hydroxide 225 mg and magnesium hydroxide 200 mg per 5 mL

High potency (Maalox® TC): Aluminum hydroxide 600 mg and magnesium hydroxide 300 mg per 5 mL

Tablet, chewable (Maalox®): Aluminum hydroxide 600 mg and magnesium hydroxide 300 mg

## aluminum hydroxide and magnesium trisilicate

(a LOO mi num hye DROKS ide & mag NEE zhum trye SIL i kate)

**U.S./Canadian Brand Names** Gaviscon®-2 Tablet [OTC]; Gaviscon® Tablet [OTC]

**Therapeutic Category** Antacid

**Use** Temporary relief of hyperacidity

**Usual Dosage** Adults: Oral: Chew 2-4 tablets 4 times/day or as directed by physician

**Dosage Forms** Tablet, chewable:

Gaviscon®: Aluminum hydroxide 80 mg and magnesium trisilicate 20 mg

Gaviscon®-2: Aluminum hydroxide 160 mg and magnesium trisilicate 40 mg

## aluminum hydroxide, magnesium hydroxide, and simethicone

(a LOO mi num hye DROKS ide, mag NEE zhum hye DROKS ide, & sye METH i kone)

**U.S./Canadian Brand Names** Di-Gel® [OTC]; Gas-Ban DS® [OTC]; Maalox® Plus [OTC]; Magalox Plus® [OTC]; Mylanta® [OTC]; Mylanta®-II [OTC]

**Therapeutic Category** Antacid; Antiflatulent

**Use** Temporary relief of hyperacidity associated with gas; may also be used for indications associated with other antacids

**Usual Dosage** Adults: Oral: 15-30 mL or 2-4 tablets 4-6 times/day between meals and at bedtime; may be used every hour for severe symptoms

**Dosage Forms**

Liquid:

Mylanta®: Aluminum hydroxide 200 mg, magnesium hydroxide, 200 mg, and simethicone 20 mg per 5 mL

Maalox® Plus: Aluminum hydroxide 225 mg, magnesium hydroxide 200 mg, and simethicone 25 mg per 5 mL (30 mL, 180 mL)

Mylanta®-II: Aluminum hydroxide 400 mg, magnesium hydroxide 400 mg, and simethicone 40 mg per 5 mL (150 mL, 360 mL)

Tablet, chewable:

Magalox Plus®: Aluminum hydroxide 200 mg, magnesium hydroxide 200 mg, and simethicone 25 mg

Mylanta®: Aluminum hydroxide 200 mg, magnesium hydroxide 200 mg, and simethicone 20 mg

Gas-Ban DS®, Mylanta®-II: Aluminum hydroxide 400 mg, magnesium hydroxide 400 mg, and simethicone 40 mg

**aluminum sucrose sulfate, basic** *see* sucralfate *on page 561*

## aluminum sulfate and calcium acetate

(a LOO mi num SUL fate & KAL see um AS e tate)

**U.S./Canadian Brand Names** Bluboro® [OTC]; Boropak® [OTC]; Domeboro® Topical [OTC]; Pedi-Boro® [OTC]

**Therapeutic Category** Topical Skin Product

**Use** Astringent wet dressing for relief of inflammatory conditions of the skin and to reduce weeping that may occur in dermatitis

**Usual Dosage** Topical: Soak affected area in the solution 2-4 times/day for 15-30 minutes or apply wet dressing soaked in the solution 2-4 times/day for 30-minute treatment periods; rewet dressing with solution every few minutes to keep it moist

**Dosage Forms**

Powder, to make topical solution: 1 packet/pint of water [1:40 solution]

Tablet, effervescent: 1 tablet/pint [1:40 dilution]

**Alupent®** *see* metaproterenol *on page 376*

**Alu-Tab® [OTC]** *see* aluminum hydroxide *on page 26*

## amantadine (a MAN ta deen)

**Synonyms** adamantanamine

**U.S./Canadian Brand Names** Endantadine® (Can); Gen-Amantadine (Can); Symmetrel® Syrup; Symmetrel® Tablet

**Therapeutic Category** Anti-Parkinson's Agent; Antiviral Agent

**Use** Prophylaxis and treatment of influenza A viral infection; symptomatic and adjunct treatment of parkinsonism

**Usual Dosage** Oral:

Children:

1-9 years: 4.4-8.8 mg/kg/day in 1-2 divided doses to a maximum of 150 mg/day

9-12 years: 100-200 mg/day in 1-2 divided doses

After first influenza A virus vaccine dose, amantadine prophylaxis may be administered for up to 6 weeks or until 2 weeks after the second dose of vaccine

Adults:

Parkinson's disease: 100 mg twice daily

Influenza A viral infection: 200 mg/day in 1-2 divided doses

Prophylaxis: Minimum 10-day course of therapy following exposure or continue for 2-3 weeks after influenza A virus vaccine is administered

Elderly patients should administer the drug in 2 daily doses rather than a single dose to avoid adverse neurologic reactions

**Dosage Forms**

Capsule, as hydrochloride: 100 mg

Syrup, as hydrochloride: 50 mg/5 mL (120 mL, 480 mL)

Tablet, as hydrochloride: 100 mg

**Amaphen®** *see* butalbital compound and acetaminophen *on page 93*

**Amaryl®** *see* glimepiride *on page 275*

**Amatine® (Can)** *see* midodrine *on page 392*

## ambenonium (am be NOE nee um)

**U.S./Canadian Brand Names** Mytelase® Caplets®

**Therapeutic Category** Cholinergic Agent

**Use** Treatment of myasthenia gravis

**Usual Dosage** Adults: Oral: 5-25 mg 3-4 times/day

**Dosage Forms** Tablet, as chloride: 10 mg

**Ambenyl® Cough Syrup** *see* bromodiphenhydramine and codeine *on page 87*

**Ambien™** *see* zolpidem *on page 641*

**Ambi® Skin Tone [OTC]** *see* hydroquinone *on page 305*

**AmBisome®** *see* amphotericin B liposomal *on page 38*

## amcinonide (am SIN oh nide)

**U.S./Canadian Brand Names** Cyclocort® Topical

**Therapeutic Category** Corticosteroid, Topical

**Use** Relief of the inflammatory and pruritic manifestations of corticosteroid-responsive dermatoses

**Usual Dosage** Adults: Topical: Apply in a thin film 2-3 times/day. Therapy should be discontinued when control is achieved. If no improvement is seen, reassessment of diagnosis may be necessary.

**Dosage Forms**

Cream: 0.1% (15 g, 30 g, 60 g)
Lotion: 0.1% (20 mL, 60 mL)
Ointment, topical: 0.1% (15 g, 30 g, 60 g)

**Amcort® Injection** *see* triamcinolone (systemic) *on page 602*

**Amdol 500® [OTC]** *see* acetaminophen *on page 3*

**Amdol 650® [OTC]** *see* acetaminophen *on page 3*

**Amdoplus® [OTC]** *see* acetaminophen *on page 3*

**Amen® *(Discontinued)*** *see page 750*

**Amerge®** *see* naratriptan *on page 410*

**Americaine® [OTC]** *see* benzocaine *on page 72*

**A-methaPred® Injection** *see* methylprednisolone *on page 385*

**amethocaine** *see* tetracaine *on page 578*

**amethopterin** *see* methotrexate *on page 380*

**Ametop™ (Can)** *see* tetracaine *on page 578*

**amfepramone** *see* diethylpropion *on page 184*

**Amgenal® Cough Syrup** *see* bromodiphenhydramine and codeine *on page 87*

**Amicar®** *see* aminocaproic acid *on next page*

**Amidate®** *see* etomidate *on page 236*

**Amidrine®** *see* acetaminophen, isometheptene, and dichloralphenazone *on page 8*

## amifostine (am i FOS teen)

**Synonyms** ethiofos; gammaphos

**U.S./Canadian Brand Names** Ethyol®

**Therapeutic Category** Antidote

**Use** Reduce the incidence of moderate to severe xerostomia in patients undergoing postoperative radiation treatment for head and neck cancer, where the radiation port includes a substantial portion of the parotid glands. Protection against cisplatin-induced nephrotoxicity in advanced ovarian cancer patients; it may also provide protection from cisplatin-induced peripheral neuropathy

**Usual Dosage** I.V.: 910 mg/m$^2$ beginning 30 minutes before starting chemotherapy; reduction of xerostomia from head and neck radiation: 200 mg/m$^2$ I.V. (as a 3-minute infusion) once daily, starting 15-30 minutes before standard fraction radiation therapy; dose adjustment is recommended for subsequent doses if the previous dose was interrupted, and not able to be resumed; secondary to hypotension, the recommended dose for subsequent administration is 740 mg/m$^2$

**Dosage Forms** Injection: 500 mg

**Amigesic®** *see* salsalate *on page 536*

## amikacin (am i KAY sin)

**U.S./Canadian Brand Names** Amikin®

**Therapeutic Category** Aminoglycoside (Antibiotic)

**Use** Treatment of documented gram-negative enteric infection resistant to gentamicin and tobramycin; documented infection of mycobacterial organisms susceptible to amikacin

**Usual Dosage** I.M., I.V.:

Infants and Children: 15-20 mg/kg/day divided every 8 hours

Adults: 15 mg/kg/day divided every 8-12 hours

**Dosage Forms** Injection, as sulfate: 5 mg/mL (100 mL); 50 mg/mL (2 mL); 62.5 mg/mL (8 mL); 250 mg/mL (2 mL, 3 mL, 4 mL, 50 mL)

**Amikin®** *see* amikacin *on this page*

## amiloride (a MIL oh ride)

**U.S./Canadian Brand Names** Midamor®

**Therapeutic Category** Diuretic, Potassium Sparing

**Use** Counteract potassium loss induced by other diuretics in the treatment of hypertension or edematous conditions including CHF, hepatic cirrhosis and hypoaldosteronism; usually used in conjunction with a more potent diuretic such as thiazides or loop diuretics

**Usual Dosage** Oral:

Children: Although safety and efficacy have not been established by the FDA in children, a dosage of 0.625 mg/kg/day has been used in children weighing 6-20 kg

Adults: 5-10 mg/day (up to 20 mg)

**Dosage Forms** Tablet, as hydrochloride: 5 mg

## amiloride and hydrochlorothiazide

(a MIL oh ride & hye droe klor oh THYE a zide)

**U.S./Canadian Brand Names** Alti-Amiloride HCTZ (Can); Apo®-Amilzide (Can); Moduret® (Can); Moduretic®; Novamilor (Can); Nu-Amilzide (Can)

**Therapeutic Category** Diuretic, Combination

**Use** Antikaliuretic diuretic, antihypertensive

**Usual Dosage** Adults: Oral: Start with 1 tablet/day, then may be increased to 2 tablets/day if needed; usually administered in a single dose

**Dosage Forms** Tablet: Amiloride hydrochloride 5 mg and hydrochlorothiazide 50 mg

**Amin-Aid®** ***(Discontinued)*** *see page 750*

**2-amino-6-mercaptopurine** *see* thioguanine *on page 585*

**2-amino-6-trifluoromethoxy-benzothiazole** *see* riluzole *on page 527*

**aminobenzylpenicillin** *see* ampicillin *on page 39*

## aminocaproic acid (a mee noe ka PROE ik AS id)

**U.S./Canadian Brand Names** Amicar®

**Therapeutic Category** Hemostatic Agent

**Use** Treatment of excessive bleeding resulting from systemic hyperfibrinolysis and urinary fibrinolysis

**Usual Dosage** In the management of acute bleeding syndromes, oral dosage regimens are the same as the I.V. dosage regimens in adults and children

Chronic bleeding: Oral, I.V.: 5-30 g/day in divided doses at 3- to 6-hour intervals

Acute bleeding syndrome:

Children: Oral, I.V.: 100 mg/kg or 3 g/m$^2$ during the first hour, followed by continuous infusion at the rate of 33.3 mg/kg/hour or 1 g/m$^2$/hour; total dosage should not exceed 18 g/m$^2$/24 hours

Adults:

Oral: For elevated fibrinolytic activity, administer 5 g during first hour, followed by 1-1.25 g/hour for approximately 8 hours or until bleeding stops

I.V.: Administer 4-5 g in 250 mL of diluent during first hour followed by continuous infusion at the rate of 1-1.25 g/hour in 50 mL of diluent, continue for 8 hours or until bleeding stops

**Dosage Forms**

Injection: 250 mg/mL (20 mL)

Syrup: 1.25 g/5 mL (480 mL)

Tablet: 500 mg

**Amino-Cerv™ Vaginal Cream** *see* urea *on page 617*

**Aminofen® [OTC]** *see* acetaminophen *on page 3*

**Aminofen Plus® [OTC]** *see* acetaminophen *on page 3*

## aminoglutethimide (a mee noe gloo TETH i mide)

**U.S./Canadian Brand Names** Cytadren®

**Therapeutic Category** Antineoplastic Agent

**Use** Suppression of adrenal function in selected patients with Cushing's syndrome; also used successfully in postmenopausal patients with advanced breast carcinoma and in patients with metastatic prostate carcinoma

**Usual Dosage** Adults: Oral: 250 mg every 6 hours, may be increased at 1- to 2-week intervals to a total of 2 g/day; administer in divided doses 2-3 times/day to reduce incidence of nausea and vomiting

**Dosage Forms** Tablet, scored: 250 mg

## aminolevulinic acid (a MEE noh lev yoo lin ik AS id)

**U.S./Canadian Brand Names** Levulan® Kerastick™

**Therapeutic Category** Photosensitizing Agent, Topical; Porphyrin Agent, Topical

**Use** Treatment of non-hyperkeratotic actinic keratoses of the face or scalp; to be used in conjunction with blue light illumination

**Usual Dosage** Adults: Topical: Apply to actinic keratoses (**not** perilesional skin) followed 14-18 hours later by blue light illumination. Application/treatment may be repeated at a treatment site after 8 weeks.

**Dosage Forms** Solution, topical: 20% (with applicator)

**Amino-Opti-E® [OTC]** *see* vitamin E *on page 631*

## aminophylline (am in OFF i lin)

**Synonyms** theophylline ethylenediamine

**Therapeutic Category** Theophylline Derivative

**Use** Bronchodilator in reversible airway obstruction due to asthma or COPD; increase diaphragmatic contractility; neonatal idiopathic apnea of prematurity

**Usual Dosage**

Neonates: Apnea of prematurity:

Loading dose: 5 mg/kg for one dose

Maintenance: I.V.:

0-24 days: Begin at 2 mg/kg/day divided every 12 hours and titrate to desired levels and effects

>24 days: 3 mg/kg/day divided every 12 hours; increased dosages may be indicated as liver metabolism matures (usually >30 days of life); monitor serum levels to determine appropriate dosages

Theophylline levels should be initially drawn after 3 days of therapy; repeat levels are indicated 3 days after each increase in dosage or weekly if on a stabilized dosage

(Continued)

## aminophylline *(Continued)*

Treatment of acute bronchospasm:

Loading dose (in patients not currently receiving aminophylline or theophylline): 6 mg/kg (based on aminophylline) administered I.V. over 20-30 minutes; administration rate should not exceed 25 mg/minute (aminophylline)

Approximate I.V. maintenance dosages are based upon **continuous infusions**; bolus dosing (often used in children <6 months of age) may be determined by multiplying the hourly infusion rate by 24 hours and dividing by the desired number of doses/day

6 weeks to 6 months: 0.5 mg/kg/hour
6 months to 1 year: 0.6-0.7 mg/kg/hour
1-9 years: 1-1.2 mg/kg/hour
9-12 years and young adult smokers: 0.9 mg/kg/hour
12-16 years: 0.7 mg/kg/hour
Adults (healthy, nonsmoking): 0.7 mg/kg/hour
Older patients and patients with cor pulmonale, patients with congestive heart failure or liver failure: 0.25 mg/kg/hour
Dosage should be adjusted according to serum level measurements during the first 12- to 24-hour period; avoid using suppositories due to erratic, unreliable absorption.

Rectal: Adults: 500 mg 3 times/day

**Dosage Forms**
Injection: 25 mg/mL (10 mL, 20 mL)
Liquid, oral: 105 mg/5 mL (10 mL, 240 mL, 500 mL)
Suppository, rectal: 250 mg, 500 mg
Tablet: 100 mg, 200 mg

## aminosalicylate sodium (a MEE noe sa LIS i late SOW dee um)

**Synonyms** PAS
**U.S./Canadian Brand Names** Nemasol® (Can)
**Therapeutic Category** Nonsteroidal Anti-inflammatory Drug (NSAID)
**Use** Treatment of tuberculosis with combination drugs
**Usual Dosage** Oral:
Children: 150-300 mg/kg/day in 3-4 equally divided doses
Adults: 150 mg/kg/day in 2-3 equally divided doses (usually 12-14 g/day)
**Dosage Forms** Tablet: 500 mg

**5-aminosalicylic acid** *see* mesalamine *on page 374*

## amiodarone (a MEE oh da rone)

**U.S./Canadian Brand Names** Alti-Amiodarone (Can); Cordarone®; Gen-Amiodarone (Can); Novo-Amiodarone (Can); Pacerone®
**Therapeutic Category** Antiarrhythmic Agent, Class III
**Use** Management of resistant, life-threatening ventricular arrhythmias unresponsive to conventional therapy with less toxic agents; also used for treatment of supraventricular arrhythmias unresponsive to conventional therapy; injectable available from manufacturer via orphan drug status or compassionate use for acute treatment and prophylaxis of life-threatening ventricular tachycardia or ventricular fibrillation (see Dosage Forms)
**Usual Dosage** Children <1 year should be dosed as calculated by body surface area
Children: Loading dose: 10-15 mg/kg/day or 600-800 mg/1.73 $m^2$/day for 4-14 days or until adequate control of arrhythmia or prominent adverse effects occur (this loading dose may be administered in 1-2 divided doses/day); dosage should then be reduced to 5 mg/kg/day or 200-400 mg/1.73 $m^2$/day administered once daily for several weeks; if arrhythmia does not recur reduce to lowest effective dosage possible; usual daily minimal dose: 2.5 mg/kg; maintenance doses may be administered for 5 of 7 days/week
Adults: Ventricular arrhythmias: 800-1600 mg/day in 1-2 doses for 1-3 weeks, then 600-800 mg/day in 1-2 doses for 1 month; maintenance: 400 mg/day; lower doses are recommended for supraventricular arrhythmias, usually 100-400 mg/day

**Dosage Forms**
Injection, as hydrochloride: 50 mg/mL with benzyl alcohol (3 mL)
Tablet, scored, as hydrochloride: 200 mg

**Amipaque®** *see* radiological/contrast media (non-ionic) *on page 518*

**Ami-Tex LA®** ***(Discontinued)*** *see page 750*

**Amitone® [OTC]** *see* calcium carbonate *on page 97*

## amitriptyline (a mee TRIP ti leen)

**U.S./Canadian Brand Names** Apo®-Amitriptyline (Can); Elavil®; Vanatrip®
**Therapeutic Category** Antidepressant, Tricyclic (Tertiary Amine)
**Use** Treatment of various forms of depression, often in conjunction with psychotherapy; analgesic for certain chronic and neuropathic pain; migraine prophylaxis
**Usual Dosage**
Children <12 years: Not recommended
Adolescents: Oral: Initial: 25-50 mg/day; may administer in divided doses; increase gradually to 100 mg/day in divided doses
Adults:
Oral: 30-100 mg/day single dose at bedtime or in divided doses; dose may be gradually increased up to 300 mg/day; once symptoms are controlled, decrease gradually to lowest effective dose
I.M.: 20-30 mg 4 times/day
**Dosage Forms**
Injection, as hydrochloride: 10 mg/mL (10 mL)
Tablet, as hydrochloride: 10 mg, 25 mg, 50 mg, 75 mg, 100 mg, 150 mg

## amitriptyline and chlordiazepoxide
(a mee TRIP ti leen & klor dye az e POKS ide)

**U.S./Canadian Brand Names** Limbitrol® DS 10-25
**Therapeutic Category** Antidepressant, Tricyclic (Tertiary Amine)
**Controlled Substance** C-IV
**Use** Treatment of moderate to severe anxiety and/or agitation and depression
**Usual Dosage** Oral: Initial: 3-4 tablets in divided doses; this may be increased to 6 tablets/day as required; some patients respond to smaller doses and can be maintained on 2 tablets
**Dosage Forms** Tablet:
5-12.5: Amitriptyline hydrochloride 12.5 mg and chlordiazepoxide 5 mg
10-25: Amitriptyline hydrochloride 25 mg and chlordiazepoxide 10 mg

## amitriptyline and perphenazine (a mee TRIP ti leen & per FEN a zeen)

**U.S./Canadian Brand Names** Etrafon®; Triavil®
**Therapeutic Category** Antidepressant/Phenothiazine
**Use** Treatment of patients with moderate to severe anxiety and depression
**Usual Dosage** Oral: 1 tablet 2-4 times/day
**Dosage Forms** Tablet:
2-10: Amitriptyline hydrochloride 10 mg and perphenazine 2 mg
4-10: Amitriptyline hydrochloride 10 mg and perphenazine 4 mg
2-25: Amitriptyline hydrochloride 25 mg and perphenazine 2 mg
4-25: Amitriptyline hydrochloride 25 mg and perphenazine 4 mg
4-50: Amitriptyline hydrochloride 50 mg and perphenazine 4 mg

## amlexanox (am LEKS an oks)

**U.S./Canadian Brand Names** Aphthasol™
**Therapeutic Category** Anti-inflammatory Agent, Locally Applied
**Use** Treating signs and symptoms of canker sores (minor aphthous ulcers)
**Usual Dosage** Administer directly on ulcers 4 times/day following oral hygiene, after meals, and before going to bed
(Continued)

## amlexanox *(Continued)*

**Dosage Forms** Cream: 5% (5 g)

## amlodipine (am LOE di peen)

**U.S./Canadian Brand Names** Norvasc®

**Therapeutic Category** Calcium Channel Blocker

**Use** Treatment of hypertension alone or in combination with antihypertensives; chronic stable angina alone or with other antianginal agents; vasospastic angina alone or in combination with other agents

**Usual Dosage** Oral:

Adults: 2.5-10 mg once daily

Elderly: 2.5 mg once daily; increase by 2.5 mg increments at 7- to 14-day intervals; maximum recommended dose: 10 mg/day

**Dosage Forms** Tablet: 2.5 mg, 5 mg, 10 mg

## amlodipine and benazepril (am LOE di peen & ben AY ze pril)

**U.S./Canadian Brand Names** Lotrel®

**Therapeutic Category** Antihypertensive Agent, Combination

**Use** Treatment of hypertension

**Usual Dosage** Adults: Oral: 1 capsule daily

**Dosage Forms** Capsule:

Amlodipine 2.5 mg and benazepril hydrochloride 10 mg
Amlodipine 5 mg and benazepril hydrochloride 10 mg
Amlodipine 5 mg and benazepril hydrochloride 20 mg

**ammonapse** *see* sodium phenylbutyrate *on page 551*

## ammonia spirit (aromatic) (a MOE nee ah SPEAR it air oh MAT ik)

**Synonyms** smelling salts

**U.S./Canadian Brand Names** Aromatic Ammonia Aspirols®

**Therapeutic Category** Respiratory Stimulant

**Use** Respiratory and circulatory stimulant; treatment of fainting

**Usual Dosage** "Smelling salts" to treat or prevent fainting

**Dosage Forms**

Inhalant, crushable glass perles: 0.33 mL, 0.4 mL
Solution: 30 mL, 60 mL, 120 mL

## ammonium chloride (a MOE nee um KLOR ide)

**Therapeutic Category** Electrolyte Supplement, Oral

**Use** Diuretic or systemic and urinary acidifying agent; treatment of hypochloremic states

**Usual Dosage**

Children: Oral, I.V.: 75 mg/kg/day in 4 divided doses for urinary acidification; maximum daily dose: 6 g

Adults:

Oral: 2-3 g every 6 hours
I.V.: 1.5 g/dose every 6 hours

**Dosage Forms** Injection: 26.75% [5 mEq/mL] (20 mL)

**ammonium lactate** *see* lactic acid with ammonium hydroxide *on page 337*

## amobarbital (am oh BAR bi tal)

**Synonyms** amylobarbitone

**U.S./Canadian Brand Names** Amytal®

**Therapeutic Category** Barbiturate

**Controlled Substance** C-II

**Use** Used to control status epilepticus or acute seizure episodes; also used in catatonic, negativistic, or manic reactions and in "Amytal® Interviewing" for narcoanalysis

**Usual Dosage** Hypnotic: Adults:

I.M.: 65-500 mg, should not exceed 500 mg

I.V.: 65-500 mg, should not exceed 1000 mg

**Dosage Forms** Injection, as sodium: 500 mg

## amobarbital and secobarbital (am oh BAR bi tal & see koe BAR bi tal)

**U.S./Canadian Brand Names** Tuinal®

**Therapeutic Category** Barbiturate

**Controlled Substance** C-II

**Use** Short-term treatment of insomnia

**Usual Dosage** Adults: Oral: 1-2 capsules at bedtime

**Dosage Forms** Capsule: 100: Amobarbital 50 mg and secobarbital 50 mg

**Amonidrin® Tablet *(Discontinued)*** *see page 750*

**AMO Vitrax® *(Discontinued)*** *see page 750*

## amoxapine (a MOKS a peen)

**U.S./Canadian Brand Names** Asendin® (Can)

**Therapeutic Category** Antidepressant, Tricyclic (Secondary Amine)

**Use** Treatment of neurotic and endogenous depression and mixed symptoms of anxiety and depression

**Usual Dosage** Oral (once symptoms are controlled, decrease gradually to lowest effective dose):

Children <16 years: Dose not established

Adolescents: Initial: 25-50 mg/day; increase gradually to 100 mg/day; may administer as divided doses or as a single dose at bedtime

Adults: Initial: 25 mg 2-3 times/day, if tolerated, dosage may be increased to 100 mg 2-3 times/day; may be administered in a single bedtime dose when dosage <300 mg/day

Maximum daily dose:

Outpatient: 400 mg

Inpatient: 600 mg

**Dosage Forms** Tablet: 25 mg, 50 mg, 100 mg, 150 mg

## amoxicillin (a moks i SIL in)

**Synonyms** amoxycillin; *p*-hydroxyampicillin

**U.S./Canadian Brand Names** Amoxil®; Apo®-Amoxi (Can); Gen-Amoxicillin (Can); Lin-Amox (Can); Novamoxin® (Can); Nu-Amoxi (Can); Scheinpharm™ Amoxicillin (Can); Trimox®; Wymox®

**Therapeutic Category** Penicillin

**Use** Treatment of otitis media, sinusitis, and infections involving the respiratory tract, skin, and urinary tract due to susceptible *H. influenzae, N. gonorrhoeae, E. coli, P. mirabilis, E. faecalis*, streptococci, and nonpenicillinase-producing staphylococci; prophylaxis of bacterial endocarditis

**Usual Dosage** Oral:

Children: 25-50 mg/kg/day in divided doses every 8 hours

Uncomplicated gonorrhea: ≥2 years: 50 mg/kg plus probenecid 25 mg/kg in a single dose; do not use this regimen in children <2 years of age, probenecid is contraindicated in this age group

SBE prophylaxis: 50 mg/kg 1 hour before procedure and 25 mg/kg 6 hours later; not to exceed adult dosage

Adults: 250-500 mg every 8 hours or 500-875 mg twice daily; maximum dose: 2-3 g/day

Uncomplicated gonorrhea: 3 g plus probenecid 1 g in a single dose

Endocarditis prophylaxis: 3 g 1 hour before procedure and 1.5 g 6 hours later

**Dosage Forms**

Capsule, as trihydrate: 250 mg, 500 mg

(Continued)

## amoxicillin *(Continued)*

Powder for oral suspension, as trihydrate: 125 mg/5 mL (80 mL, 100 mL, 150 mL); 200 mg/5 mL (50 mL, 75 mL, 100 mL); 250 mg/5 mL (80 mL, 100 mL, 150 mL); 400 mg/5 mL (80 50 mL, 75 mL, 100 mL)

Powder for oral suspension, drops, as trihydrate: 50 mg/mL (15 mL, 30 mL)

Tablet, chewable, as trihydrate: 125 mg, 200 mg, 250 mg, 400 mg

Tablet, film coated: 500 mg, 875 mg

## amoxicillin and clavulanate potassium

(a moks i SIL in & klav yoo LAN ate poe TASS ee um)

**Synonyms** amoxicillin and clavulanic acid

**U.S./Canadian Brand Names** Augmentin®; Clavulin® (Can)

**Therapeutic Category** Penicillin

**Use** Infections caused by susceptible organisms involving the lower respiratory tract, otitis media, sinusitis, skin and skin structure, and urinary tract; spectrum same as amoxicillin in addition to beta-lactamase-producing *B. catarrhalis*, *H. influenzae*, *N. gonorrhoeae*, and *S. aureus* (not MRSA)

**Usual Dosage** Oral:

Children ≤40 kg: 20-40 mg (amoxicillin)/kg/day in divided doses every 8 hours

Children >40 kg and Adults: 250-500 mg every 8 hours or 875 mg every 12 hours

**Dosage Forms**

Suspension, oral:

125 (banana flavor): Amoxicillin trihydrate 125 mg and clavulanate potassium 31.25 mg per 5 mL (75 mL, 100 mL, 150 mL)

200: Amoxicillin 200 mg and clavulanate potassium 28.5 mg per 5 mL (50 mL, 75 mL, 100 mL, 150 mL)

250 (orange flavor): Amoxicillin trihydrate 250 mg and clavulanate potassium 62.5 mg per 5 mL (75 mL, 100 mL, 150 mL)

400: Amoxicillin 400 mg and clavulanate potassium 57 mg per 5 mL (50 mL, 75 mL, 100 mL)

Tablet:

250: Amoxicillin trihydrate 250 mg and clavulanate potassium 125 mg

500: Amoxicillin trihydrate 500 mg and clavulanate potassium 125 mg

875: Amoxicillin trihydrate 875 mg and clavulanate potassium 125 mg

Tablet, chewable:

125: Amoxicillin trihydrate 125 mg and clavulanate potassium 31.25 mg

200: Amoxicillin trihydrate 200 mg and clavulanate potassium 28.5 mg

250: Amoxicillin trihydrate 250 mg and clavulanate potassium 62.5 mg

400: Amoxicillin trihydrate 400 mg and clavulanate potassium 57 mg

**amoxicillin and clavulanic acid** *see* amoxicillin and clavulanate potassium *on this page*

**Amoxil®** *see* amoxicillin *on previous page*

**amoxycillin** *see* amoxicillin *on previous page*

## amphetamine mixture (am FET a meen MIKS chur)

**Synonyms** dextroamphetamine sulfate, dextroamphetamine saccharate, amphetamine aspartate, and amphetamine sulfate

**U.S./Canadian Brand Names** Adderall®

**Therapeutic Category** Amphetamine

**Controlled Substance** C-II

**Use** Treatment of attention deficit disorders (ADD) and narcolepsy

**Usual Dosage** Oral:

Narcolepsy: 5-60 mg/day in divided doses

Children >12 years, Geriatrics, and Adults: Initial: 10 mg/day; increase by 10 mg increments weekly

Children 6-12 years: Initial: 5 mg/day; increase in increments of 5 mg at weekly intervals until optimum response is obtained

ADD: Children:

3-5 years: 2.5 mg/day; increase by 2.5 mg/day at weekly intervals until optimal response; usual range: 0.1-0.5 mg/kg/dose every morning

>6 years: 5 mg/day or twice daily; increase by 5 mg/day at weekly intervals until optimal response; usual range: 0.1-0.5 mg/kg/dose every morning

**Dosage Forms** Tablet:

5 mg: Dextroamphetamine sulfate 1.25 mg, dextroamphetamine saccharate 1.25 mg, amphetamine aspartate 1.25 mg, amphetamine sulfate 1.25 mg

7.5 mg: Dextroamphetamine sulfate 1.875 mg, dextroamphetamine saccharate 1.875 mg, amphetamine aspartate 1.875 mg, amphetamine sulfate 1.875 mg

10 mg: Dextroamphetamine sulfate 2.5 mg, dextroamphetamine saccharate 2.5 mg, amphetamine aspartate 2.5 mg, amphetamine sulfate 2.5 mg

12.5 mg: Dextroamphetamine sulfate 3.125 mg, dextroamphetamine saccharate 3.125 mg, amphetamine aspartate 3.125 mg, amphetamine sulfate 3.125 mg

15 mg: Dextroamphetamine sulfate 3.75 mg, dextroamphetamine saccharate 3.75 mg, amphetamine aspartate 3.75 mg, amphetamine sulfate 3.75 mg

20 mg: Dextroamphetamine sulfate 5 mg, dextroamphetamine saccharate 5 mg, amphetamine aspartate 5 mg, amphetamine sulfate 5 mg

30 mg: Dextroamphetamine sulfate 7.5 mg, dextroamphetamine saccharate 7.5 mg, amphetamine aspartate 7.5 mg, amphetamine sulfate 7.5 mg

**Amphojel® [OTC]** *see* aluminum hydroxide *on page 26*

**Amphotec®** *see* amphotericin B cholesteryl sulfate complex *on this page*

## amphotericin B cholesteryl sulfate complex

(am foe TER i sin bee kole LES te ril SUL fate KOM plecks)

**Synonyms** ABCD; amphotericin B colloidal dispersion

**U.S./Canadian Brand Names** Amphotec®

**Therapeutic Category** Antifungal Agent

**Use** Effective in the treatment of invasive mycoses in patient refractory to or intolerant of conventional amphotericin B

**Usual Dosage** Children and Adults: 3-4 mg/kg/day I.V. (infusion of 1 mg/kg/hour); maximum: 7.5 mg/kg/day; duration of therapy is often <6 weeks

**Dosage Forms** Suspension for injection: 50 mg, 100 mg

**amphotericin B colloidal dispersion** *see* amphotericin B cholesteryl sulfate complex *on this page*

## amphotericin B (conventional) (am foe TER i sin bee con VEN sha nal)

**U.S./Canadian Brand Names** Fungizone®

**Therapeutic Category** Antifungal Agent

**Use** Treatment of severe systemic infections and meningitis caused by susceptible fungi such as *Candida* species, *Histoplasma capsulatum*, *Cryptococcus neoformans*, *Aspergillus* species, *Blastomyces dermatitidis*, *Torulopsis glabrata*, and *Coccidioides immitis*; fungal peritonitis; irrigant for bladder fungal infections; and topically for cutaneous and mucocutaneous candidal infections

**Usual Dosage**

I.V.:

Infants and Children:

Test dose (not required): I.V.: 0.1 mg/kg/dose to a maximum of 1 mg; infuse over 30-60 minutes

Initial therapeutic dose: 0.25 mg/kg gradually increased, usually in 0.25 mg/kg increments on each subsequent day, until the desired daily dose is reached

Maintenance dose: 0.25-1 mg/kg/day given once daily; infuse over 2-6 hours. Once therapy has been established, amphotericin B can be administered on an every other day basis at 1-1.5 mg/kg/dose; cumulative dose: 1.5-2 g over 6-10 weeks

(Continued)

## amphotericin B (conventional) *(Continued)*

Adults:

Test dose (not required): 1 mg infused over 20-30 minutes

Initial dose: 0.25 mg/kg administered over 2-6 hours, gradually increased on subsequent days to the desired level by 0.25 mg/kg increments per day; in critically ill patients, may initiate with 1-1.5 mg/kg/day with close observation

Maintenance dose: 0.25-1 mg/kg/day or 1.5 mg/kg over 4-6 hours every other day; do not exceed 1.5 mg/kg/day; cumulative dose: 1-4 g over 4-10 weeks

Duration of therapy varies with nature of infection: histoplasmosis, *Cryptococcus*, or blastomycosis may be treated with total dose of 2-4 g

I.T.:

Children.: 25-100 mcg every 48-72 hours; increase to 500 mcg as tolerated

Adults: 25-300 mcg every 48-72 hours; increase to 500 mcg to 1 mg as tolerated

Oral: 1 mL (100 mg) 4 times daily

Topical: Apply to affected areas 2-4 times/day for 1-4 weeks of therapy depending on nature and severity of infection

Administration in dialysate: Children and Adults: 1-2 mg/L of peritoneal dialysis fluid either with or without low-dose I.V. amphotericin B (a total dose of 2-10 mg/kg given over 7-14 days)

Administration via bladder irrigation: Children and Adults: 50 mg/day in 1 L of sterile water irrigation solution instilled over 24 hours for 2-7 days or until cultures are clear

**Dosage Forms**

Cream: 3% (20 g)

Lotion: 3% (30 mL)

Powder for injection, lyophilized, as deoxycholate: 50 mg

Suspension, oral: 100 mg/mL (24 mL with dropper)

## amphotericin B lipid complex (am foe TER i sin bee LIP id KOM pleks)

**Synonyms** ABLC

**U.S./Canadian Brand Names** Abelcet®

**Therapeutic Category** Antifungal Agent

**Use** Treatment of aspergillosis in patients who are refractory to or intolerant of conventional amphotericin B therapy. This indication is based on results obtained primarily from emergency use studies for the treatment of aspergillosis; orphan drug status for cryptococcal meningitis

**Usual Dosage** Children and Adults: I.V.: 2.5-5 mg/kg/day as a single infusion **Note:** Significantly higher dose of ABLC are tolerated; it appears that attaining higher doses with ABLC produce more rapid fungicidal activity *in vivo* than standard amphotericin B preparations

**Dosage Forms** Injection: 5 mg/mL (10 mL, 20 mL)

## amphotericin B liposomal (am foe TER i sin bee lye po SO mal)

**Synonyms** L-AmB

**U.S./Canadian Brand Names** AmBisome®

**Therapeutic Category** Antifungal Agent

**Use** Empirical therapy for presumed fungal infection in febrile, neutropenic patients. Treatment of patients with *Aspergillus* species, *Candida* species and/or *Cryptococcus* species infections refractory to amphotericin B deoxycholate, or in patients where renal impairment or unacceptable toxicity precludes the use of amphotericin B deoxycholate. Treatment of visceral leishmaniasis. In immunocompromised patients with visceral leishmaniasis treated with AmBisome, relapse rates were high following initial clearance of parasites

**Usual Dosage** Children and Adults: I.V.:

Empirical therapy: Recommended initial dose of 3 mg/kg/day

Systemic fungal infections (*Aspergillus*, *Candida*, *Cryptococcus*): Recommended initial dose of 3-5 mg/kg/day

Treatment of visceral leishmaniasis: AmBisome® achieved high rates of acute parasite clearance in immunocompetent patients when total doses of 12-30 mg/kg were administered. Most of these immunocompetent patients remained relapse-free during follow-up periods of 6 months or longer. While acute parasite clearance was achieved in most of the immunocompromised patients who received total doses of 30-40 mg/kg, the majority of these patients were observed to relapse in the 6 months following the completion of therapy.

**Dosage Forms** Injection: 50 mg

## ampicillin (am pi SIL in)

**Synonyms** aminobenzylpenicillin

**U.S./Canadian Brand Names** Marcillin®; Principen®

**Therapeutic Category** Penicillin

**Use** Treatment of susceptible bacterial infections caused by streptococci, pneumococci, nonpenicillinase-producing staphylococci, *Listeria*, meningococci; some strains of *H. influenzae*, *Salmonella*, *Shigella*, *E. coli*, *Enterobacter*, and *Klebsiella*

**Usual Dosage**

Infants and Children:

Oral: 50-100 mg/kg/day divided every 6 hours; maximum dose: 2-3 g/day

I.M., I.V.: 100-200 mg/kg/day in 4-6 divided doses; meningitis: 200-400 mg/kg/day in 4-6 divided doses; maximum dose: 12 g/day

Adults:

Oral: 250-500 mg every 6 hours

I.M., I.V.: 8-12 g/day in 4-6 divided doses

**Dosage Forms**

Capsule, as anhydrous: 250 mg, 500 mg

Capsule, as trihydrate: 250 mg, 500 mg

Powder for injection, as sodium: 125 mg, 250 mg, 500 mg, 1 g, 2 g, 10 g

Powder for oral suspension, as trihydrate: 125 mg/5 mL (100 mL, 150 mL, 200 mL); 250 mg/5 mL (100 mL, 150 mL, 200 mL)

## ampicillin and sulbactam (am pi SIL in & SUL bak tam)

**Synonyms** sulbactam and ampicillin

**U.S./Canadian Brand Names** Unasyn®

**Therapeutic Category** Penicillin

**Use** Treatment of susceptible bacterial infections involved with skin and skin structure, intra-abdominal infections, gynecological infections; spectrum is that of ampicillin plus organisms producing beta-lactamases such as *S. aureus*, *H. influenzae*, *E. coli*, *Klebsiella*, *Acinetobacter*, *Enterobacter* and anaerobes

**Usual Dosage** Unasyn® (ampicillin/sulbactam) is a combination product. Each 3 g vial contains 2 g of ampicillin and 1 g of sulbactam. Sulbactam has very little antibacterial activity by itself, but effectively extends the spectrum of ampicillin to include beta-lactamase producing strains that are resistant to ampicillin alone. Therefore, dosage recommendations for Unasyn® are based on the ampicillin component.

I.M., I.V.:

Children: 100-200 mg ampicillin/kg/day (150-300 mg Unasyn®) divided every 6 hours; maximum dose: 8 g ampicillin/day (12 g Unasyn®)

Adults: 1-2 g ampicillin (1.5-3 g Unasyn®) every 6-8 hours; maximum dose: 8 g ampicillin/day (12 g Unasyn®)

**Dosage Forms** Powder for injection: 1.5 g [ampicillin sodium 1 g and sulbactam sodium 0.5 g]; 3 g [ampicillin sodium 2 g and sulbactam sodium 1 g]; 15 g [ampicillin sodium 10 g and sulbactam sodium 5 g]

## amprenavir (am PRE na veer)

**U.S./Canadian Brand Names** Agenerase™

**Therapeutic Category** Protease Inhibitor

(Continued)

## amprenavir *(Continued)*

**Use** Treatment of HIV infections in combination with at least two other antiretroviral agents

**Usual Dosage** Adults: Oral: 1200 mg twice daily

**Dosage Forms**

Capsule: 50 mg, 150 mg

Solution, oral: 15 mg/mL (240 mL)

**AMPT** *see* metyrosine *on page 389*

**amrinone** *see* inamrinone *on page 316*

**Amvisc® *(Discontinued)*** *see page 750*

**Amvisc® Plus *(Discontinued)*** *see page 750*

## amyl nitrite (AM il NYE trite)

**Synonyms** isoamyl nitrite

**Therapeutic Category** Vasodilator

**Use** Coronary vasodilator in angina pectoris; an adjunct in treatment of cyanide poisoning; also used to produce changes in the intensity of heart murmurs

**Usual Dosage** 1-6 inhalations from 1 capsule are usually sufficient to produce the desired effect

**Dosage Forms** Inhalant, crushable glass perles: 0.3 mL

**amylobarbitone** *see* amobarbital *on page 34*

**Amytal®** *see* amobarbital *on page 34*

**Anabolin® *(Discontinued)*** *see page 750*

**Anacin® [OTC]** *see* aspirin *on page 55*

**Anacin-3® (all products) *(Discontinued)*** *see page 750*

**Anacin® P.M. Aspirin Free [OTC]** *see* acetaminophen and diphenhydramine *on page 5*

**Anadrol®** *see* oxymetholone *on page 445*

**Anafranil®** *see* clomipramine *on page 145*

**Anagesic® [OTC]** *see* acetaminophen and phenyltoloxamine *on page 5*

## anagrelide (an AG gre lide)

**U.S./Canadian Brand Names** Agrylin®

**Therapeutic Category** Platelet Reducing Agent

**Use** Agent for essential thrombocythemia (ET)

**Usual Dosage** Adults: Oral: 0.5 mg 4 times/day or 1 mg twice daily, maintain for ≥1 week, then adjust to the lowest effective dose to reduce and maintain platelet count <600,000 µL ideally to the normal range

**Dosage Forms** Capsule, as hydrochloride: 0.5 mg

**Anaids® Tablet *(Discontinued)*** *see page 750*

**Ana-Kit®** *see* insect sting kit *on page 319*

**Anamine® Syrup [OTC]** *see* chlorpheniramine and pseudoephedrine *on page 130*

**Anandron® (Can)** *see* nilutamide *on page 420*

**Anaplex® Liquid [OTC]** *see* chlorpheniramine and pseudoephedrine *on page 130*

**Anaprox®** *see* naproxen *on page 409*

**Anaspaz®** *see* hyoscyamine *on page 309*

**anastrozole** (an AS troe zole)

**U.S./Canadian Brand Names** Arimidex®

**Therapeutic Category** Antineoplastic Agent

**Use** Treatment of locally-advanced or metastatic breast cancer (ER-positive or hormone receptor unknown) in postmenopausal women; treatment of advanced breast cancer in postmenopausal women with disease progression following tamoxifen therapy; patients with ER-negative disease and patients who did not respond to tamoxifen therapy rarely responded to anastrozole

**Usual Dosage** Breast cancer: Adults: Oral (refer to individual protocols): 1 mg once daily

**Dosage Forms** Tablet: 1 mg

**Anatrast®** *see* radiological/contrast media (ionic) *on page 516*

**Anatuss® *(Discontinued)*** *see page 750*

**Anatuss® DM [OTC]** *see* guaifenesin, pseudoephedrine, and dextromethorphan *on page 285*

**Anbesol® [OTC]** *see* benzocaine *on page 72*

**Anbesol® Baby (Can)** *see* benzocaine *on page 72*

**Anbesol® Maximum Strength [OTC]** *see* benzocaine *on page 72*

**Ancef®** *see* cefazolin *on page 114*

**Ancobon®** *see* flucytosine *on page 252*

**Andehist® Drops** *see* carbinoxamine and pseudoephedrine *on page 107*

**Androcur® (Can)** *see* cyproterone *(Canada only)* *on page 161*

**Androcur® Depot (Can)** *see* cyproterone *(Canada only)* *on page 161*

**Androderm® Transdermal System** *see* testosterone *on page 576*

**Andro/Fem®** *see* estradiol and testosterone *on page 226*

**AndroGel®** *see* testosterone *on page 576*

**Android®** *see* methyltestosterone *on page 386*

**Andro-L.A.® Injection** *see* testosterone *on page 576*

**Androlone® *(Discontinued)*** *see page 750*

**Androlone®-D *(Discontinued)*** *see page 750*

**Andropository® Injection** *see* testosterone *on page 576*

**Anectine® Chloride** *see* succinylcholine *on page 560*

**Anectine® Flo-Pack®** *see* succinylcholine *on page 560*

**Anergan® 25 Injection *(Discontinued)*** *see page 750*

**Anestacon® Topical Solution** *see* lidocaine *on page 348*

**aneurine** *see* thiamine *on page 584*

**Anexate® (Can)** *see* flumazenil *on page 252*

**Anexsia®** *see* hydrocodone and acetaminophen *on page 300*

**Angio Conray®** *see* radiological/contrast media (ionic) *on page 516*

**Angiomax™** *see* bivalirudin *on page 83*

**Angiovist®** *see* radiological/contrast media (ionic) *on page 516*

**anisoylated plasminogen streptokinase activator complex** *see* anistreplase *on this page*

**anistreplase** (a NISS tre plase)

**Synonyms** anisoylated plasminogen streptokinase activator complex; APSAC

**U.S./Canadian Brand Names** Eminase®

**Therapeutic Category** Fibrinolytic Agent

(Continued)

## anistreplase *(Continued)*

**Use** Management of acute myocardial infarction (AMI) in adults; lysis of thrombi obstructing coronary arteries, reduction of infarct size; and reduction of mortality associated with AMI

**Usual Dosage** Adults: I.V.: 30 units injected over 2-5 minutes as soon as possible after onset of symptoms

**Dosage Forms** Powder for injection, lyophilized: 30 units

**Anodynos-DHC®** *see* hydrocodone and acetaminophen *on page 300*

**Anolor 300®** *see* butalbital compound and acetaminophen *on page 93*

**Anoquan®** *see* butalbital compound and acetaminophen *on page 93*

**Ansaid® Oral** *see* flurbiprofen *on page 259*

**ansamycin** *see* rifabutin *on page 526*

**Antabuse®** *see* disulfiram *on page 196*

**Antagon® *(Discontinued)*** *see page 750*

**Antazoline-V® Ophthalmic** *see* naphazoline and antazoline *on page 409*

**Anthra-Derm®** *see* anthralin *on this page*

**Anthraforte® (Can)** *see* anthralin *on this page*

## anthralin (AN thra lin)

**Synonyms** dithranol

**U.S./Canadian Brand Names** Anthra-Derm®; Anthraforte® (Can); Anthranol® (Can); Anthrascalp® (Can); Drithocreme®; Drithocreme® HP 1%; Dritho-Scalp®; Micanol® Cream

**Therapeutic Category** Keratolytic Agent

**Use** Treatment of psoriasis

**Usual Dosage** Adults: Topical: Generally, apply once daily or as directed. The irritant potential of anthralin is directly related to the strength being used and each patient's individual tolerance. Always commence treatment for at least one week using the lowest strength possible.

Skin application: Apply sparingly only to psoriatic lesions and rub gently and carefully into the skin until absorbed. Avoid applying an excessive quantity which may cause unnecessary soiling and staining of the clothing or bed linen.

Scalp application: Comb hair to remove scalar debris and, after suitably parting, rub cream well into the lesions, taking care to prevent the cream from spreading onto the forehead

Remove by washing or showering; optimal period of contact will vary according to the strength used and the patient's response to treatment. Continue treatment until the skin is entirely clear (ie, when there is nothing to feel with the fingers and the texture is normal)

**Dosage Forms** Cream: 0.1% (50 g); 0.5% (50 g); 1% (50 g)

**Anthranol® (Can)** *see* anthralin *on this page*

**Anthrascalp® (Can)** *see* anthralin *on this page*

## anthrax vaccine, adsorbed (AN thraks vak SEEN ad SORBED)

**Therapeutic Category** Vaccine

**Use** Recommended for individuals who may come in contact with animal products which come from anthrax endemic areas and may be contaminated with *Bacillus anthracis* spores; recommended for high-risk persons such as veterinarians and other handling potentially infected animals. Routine immunization for the general population is not recommended.

The Department of Defense is implementing an anthrax vaccination program against the biological warfare agent anthrax, which will be administered to all active duty and reserve personnel.

**Usual Dosage**

Primary immunization: S.C.: Three injections of 0.5 mL each given 2 weeks apart followed by three additional S.C. injections given at 6, 12, and 18 months

Subsequent booster injections: 0.5 mL at 1-year intervals are recommended for immunity to be maintained

**Dosage Forms** Injection: 5 mL (10 doses each)

**Antiben® *(Discontinued)*** *see page 750*

**AntibiOtic® Otic** *see* neomycin, polymyxin B, and hydrocortisone *on page 415*

**anti-CD20 monoclonal antibodies** *see* rituximab *on page 529*

**antidigoxin Fab fragments** *see* digoxin immune Fab *on page 186*

**antidiuretic hormone (ADH)** *see* vasopressin *on page 623*

**Antiflex®** *see* orphenadrine *on page 438*

**Anti-Gas® [OTC]** *see* simethicone *on page 544*

## antihemophilic factor (human) (an tee hee moe FIL ik FAK tor HYU man)

**Synonyms** AHF; factor VIII

**U.S./Canadian Brand Names** Alphanate®; Hemofil® M; Koāte®-DVI; Koāte®-HP; Monarc-M®

**Therapeutic Category** Blood Product Derivative

**Use** Management of hemophilia A in patients whom a deficiency in factor VIII has been demonstrated

**Usual Dosage** I.V.: Individualize dosage based on coagulation studies performed prior to and during treatment at regular intervals. One AHF unit is the activity present in 1 mL of normal pooled human plasma; dosage should be adjusted to actual vial size currently stocked in the pharmacy.

Hospitalized patients: 20-50 units/kg/dose; may be higher for special circumstances; dose can be administered every 12-24 hours and more frequently in special circumstances

**Dosage Forms** Injection: Dried concentrate of factor VIII: 1 unit

## antihemophilic factor (porcine) (an tee hee moe FIL ik FAK ter POR seen)

**U.S./Canadian Brand Names** Hyate®:C

**Therapeutic Category** Antihemophilic Agent

**Use** Treatment of congenital hemophiliacs with antibodies to human factor VIII:C and also for previously nonhemophiliac patients with spontaneously acquired inhibitors to human factor VIII:C; patients with inhibitors who are bleeding or who are to undergo surgery

**Usual Dosage** Clinical response should be used to assess efficacy rather than relying upon a particular laboratory value for recovery of factor VIII:C.

Initial dose:

Antibody level to human factor VIII:C <50 Bethesda units/mL: 100-150 porcine units/kg (body weight) is recommended

Antibody level to human factor VIII:C >50 Bethesda units/mL: Activity of the antibody to porcine factor VIII:C should be determined; **an antiporcine antibody level** >20 Bethesda units/mL indicates that the patient is unlikely to benefit from treatment; for lower titers, a dose of 100-150 porcine units/kg is recommended

If a patient has previously been treated with Hyate®:C, this may provide a guide to his likely response and, therefore, assist in estimation of the preliminary dose

Subsequent doses: Following administration of the initial dose, if the recovery of factor VIII:C in the patient's plasma is not sufficient, a further higher dose should be administered; if recovery after the second dose is still insufficient, a third and higher dose may prove effective

(Continued)

## antihemophilic factor (porcine) *(Continued)*

**Dosage Forms** Powder for injection, lyophilized: 400-700 porcine units to be reconstituted with 20 mL sterile water

## antihemophilic factor (recombinant)

(an tee hee moe FIL ik FAK tor ree KOM be nant)

**Synonyms** factor VIII recombinant

**U.S./Canadian Brand Names** Bioclate™; Helixate®; Kogenate®; Kogenate® FS; Recombinate™; ReFacto®

**Therapeutic Category** Blood Product Derivative

**Use** Management of hemophilia A in patients whom a deficiency in factor VIII has been demonstrated

**Usual Dosage** I.V.: Individualize dosage based on coagulation studies performed prior to and during treatment at regular intervals. One AHF unit is the activity present in 1 mL of normal pooled human plasma; dosage should be adjusted to actual vial size currently stocked in the pharmacy.

Hospitalized patients: 20-50 units/kg/dose; may be higher for special circumstances; dose can be administered every 12-24 hours and more frequently in special circumstances

**Dosage Forms** Injection, recombinant: 250 int. units/vial, 500 int. units/vial, 1000 int. units/vial

**Antihist-1®** ***(Discontinued)*** *see page 750*

**Antihist-D®** ***(Discontinued)*** *see page 750*

## anti-inhibitor coagulant complex

(an tee-in HI bi tor coe AG yoo lant KOM pleks)

**Synonyms** coagulant complex inhibitor

**U.S./Canadian Brand Names** Autoplex® T; Feiba VH Immuno®

**Therapeutic Category** Hemophilic Agent

**Use** Patients with factor VIII inhibitors who are to undergo surgery or those who are bleeding

**Usual Dosage** Dosage range: I.V.: 25-100 factor VIII correctional units per kg depending on the severity of hemorrhage

**Dosage Forms** Injection:

Autoplex® T, with heparin 2 units: Each bottle is labeled with correctional units of factor VIII

Feiba VH Immuno®, heparin free: Each bottle is labeled with correctional units of factor VIII

**Antilirium®** ***(Discontinued)*** *see page 750*

**Antiminth®** ***(Discontinued)*** *see page 750*

**Antinea® Cream** ***(Discontinued)*** *see page 750*

**Antiphlogistine Rub A-535 No Odour (Can)** *see* triethanolamine salicylate *on page 605*

## antipyrine and benzocaine (an tee PYE reen & BEN zoe kane)

**U.S./Canadian Brand Names** Allergan® Ear Drops; Auralgan®; Aurodex®; Auroto®; Dolotic®

**Therapeutic Category** Otic Agent, Analgesic; Otic Agent, Cerumenolytic

**Use** Temporary relief of pain and reduction of inflammation associated with acute congestive and serous otitis media, swimmer's ear, otitis externa; facilitates ear wax removal

**Usual Dosage** Otic: Fill ear canal; moisten cotton pledget, place in external ear, repeat every 1-2 hours until pain and congestion is relieved; for ear wax removal instill drops 3-4 times/day for 2-3 days

**Dosage Forms** Solution, otic: Antipyrine 5.4% and benzocaine 1.4% (10 mL, 15 mL)

## antirabies serum (equine) (an tee RAY beez SEER um EE kwine)

**Synonyms** ARS

**Therapeutic Category** Serum

**Use** Rabies prophylaxis

**Usual Dosage** I.M.: 1000 units/55 lb in a single dose, infiltrate up to 50% of dose around the wound

**Dosage Forms** Injection: 125 units/mL (8 mL)

**Antispas® Injection** *see* dicyclomine *on page 183*

## antithrombin III (an tee THROM bin three)

**Synonyms** ATIII; heparin cofactor I

**U.S./Canadian Brand Names** Thrombate III™

**Therapeutic Category** Blood Product Derivative

**Use** Agent for hereditary antithrombin III deficiency

**Usual Dosage** After first dose of antithrombin III, level should increase to 120% of normal; thereafter maintain at levels >80%. Generally, achieved by administration of maintenance doses once every 24 hours; initially and until patient is stabilized, measure antithrombin III level at least twice daily, thereafter once daily and always immediately before next infusion.

Initial dosage (units) = [desired AT-III level % - baseline AT-III level %] x body weight (kg) divided by 1%/units/kg

Measure antithrombin III preceding and 30 minutes after dose to calculate *in vivo* recovery rate; maintain level within normal range for 2-8 days depending on type of surgery or procedure

**Dosage Forms** Powder for injection: 500 units (50 mL)

**antithymocyte globulin (equine)** *see* lymphocyte immune globulin *on page 359*

## antithymocyte globulin (rabbit) (an te THY moe site GLOB yu lin RAB bit)

**U.S./Canadian Brand Names** Thymoglobulin®

**Therapeutic Category** Immunosuppressant Agent

**Use** Treatment of acute moderate-to-severe renal allograft rejection

**Usual Dosage** Adults: I.V.: Treatment of acute renal allograft rejection: 1.5 mg/kg/day for 7-14 days.

**Dosage Forms** Each package contains two 7 mL vials:

Vial 1: antithymocyte globulin (rabbit) 25 mg
Vial 2: Diluent (sterile water for injection) >5 mL

**Anti-Tuss® Expectorant [OTC]** *see* guaifenesin *on page 281*

## antivenin (*Crotalidae*) polyvalent

(an tee VEN in (kroe TAL ih die) pol i VAY lent)

**Synonyms** crotaline antivenin, polyvalent; North and South American antisnake-bite serum; pit vipers antivenin; snake (pit vipers) antivenin

**Therapeutic Category** Antivenin

**Use** Neutralization of venoms of North and South American crotalids: rattlesnake, copperhead, cottonmouth, tropical moccasins, fer-de-lance, bushmaster

**Usual Dosage** Initial intradermal sensitivity test. The entire initial dose of antivenin should be administered as soon as possible to be most effective (within 4 hours after the bite).

Children and Adults: I.V.: Minimal envenomation: 20-40 mL; moderate envenomation: 50-90 mL; severe envenomation: 100-150 mL

(Continued)

## antivenin (*Crotalidae*) polyvalent *(Continued)*

Additional doses of antivenin is based on clinical response to the initial dose. If swelling continues to progress, symptoms increase in severity, hypotension occurs, or decrease in hematocrit appears, an additional 10-50 mL should be administered.

For I.V. infusion: 1:1-1:10 dilution of reconstituted antivenin in normal saline or $D_5W$ should be prepared. Infuse the initial 5-10 mL of diluted antivenin over 3-5 minutes monitoring closely for signs of sensitivity reactions.

**Dosage Forms** Injection: Lyophilized serum, diluent (10 mL); one vacuum vial to yield 10 mL of serum

## antivenin (*Latrodectus mactans*) (an tee VEN in lak tro DUK tus MAK tans)

**Synonyms** black widow spider antivenin (*Latrodectus mactans*); *Latrodectus mactans* antivenin

**Therapeutic Category** Antivenin

**Use** Treat patients with symptoms of black widow spider bites

**Usual Dosage**

Children <12 years (severe or shock): I.V.: 2.5 mL in 10-50 mL over 15 minutes

Children and Adults: I.M.: 2.5 mL

**Dosage Forms** Powder for injection: 6000 antivenin units (2.5 mL)

## antivenin (*Micrurus fulvius*) (an tee VEN in mye KRU rus FUL vee us)

**Synonyms** North American coral snake antivenin

**Therapeutic Category** Antivenin

**Use** Neutralize the venom of Eastern coral snake and Texas coral snake but does not neutralize venom of Arizona or Sonoran coral snake

**Usual Dosage** I.V.: 3-5 vials by slow injection

**Dosage Forms** Injection: One vial antivenin and one vial diluent

**Antivert®** *see* meclizine *on page 367*

**Antivert® Chewable Tablet *(Discontinued)*** *see page 750*

**Antizol®** *see* fomepizole *on page 264*

**Antrizine®** *see* meclizine *on page 367*

**Antrocol® Capsule & Tablet *(Discontinued)*** *see page 750*

**Anturane®** *see* sulfinpyrazone *on page 566*

**Anusol® HC-1 Topical [OTC]** *see* hydrocortisone (topical) *on page 304*

**Anusol® HC-2.5% Topical [OTC]** *see* hydrocortisone (topical) *on page 304*

**Anusol-HC® Suppository** *see* hydrocortisone (rectal) *on page 302*

**Anusol® Ointment [OTC]** *see* pramoxine *on page 490*

**Anxanil® Oral *(Discontinued)*** *see page 750*

**Anzemet®** *see* dolasetron *on page 198*

**APAP** *see* acetaminophen *on page 3*

**Apapedyn® Children's [OTC]** *see* acetaminophen *on page 3*

**Apapedyn® Extra Strength [OTC]** *see* acetaminophen *on page 3*

**Apaphen® [OTC]** *see* acetaminophen and phenyltoloxamine *on page 5*

**Apatate® [OTC]** *see* vitamin B complex *on page 630*

**Aphedrid™ [OTC]** *see* triprolidine and pseudoephedrine *on page 609*

**Aphrodyne™** *see* yohimbine *on page 636*

**Aphthasol™** *see* amlexanox *on page 33*

**A.P.L.®** *see* chorionic gonadotropin *on page 136*

**Aplisol®** *see* tuberculin tests *on page 612*

**Apo®-Doxepin (Can)** *see* doxepin *on page 202*

**Apo®-Doxy Tabs (Can)** *see* doxycycline *on page 204*

**Apo®-Enalapril (Can)** *see* enalapril *on page 213*

**Apo®-Erythro E-C (Can)** *see* erythromycin (systemic) *on page 222*

**Apo®-Erythro-S (Can)** *see* erythromycin (systemic) *on page 222*

**Apo®-Etodolac (Can)** *see* etodolac *on page 236*

**Apo®-Famotidine (Can)** *see* famotidine *on page 240*

**Apo®-Fenofibrate (Can)** *see* fenofibrate *on page 243*

**Apo®-Ferrous Gluconate (Can)** *see* ferrous gluconate *on page 246*

**Apo®-Ferrous Sulfate (Can)** *see* ferrous sulfate *on page 247*

**Apo®-Fluconazole (Can)** *see* fluconazole *on page 251*

**Apo®-Flunisolide (Can)** *see* flunisolide *on page 253*

**Apo®-Fluoxetine (Can)** *see* fluoxetine *on page 256*

**Apo®-Flurazepam (Can)** *see* flurazepam *on page 259*

**Apo®-Flurbiprofen (Can)** *see* flurbiprofen *on page 259*

**Apo®-Flutamide (Can)** *see* flutamide *on page 259*

**Apo®-Fluvoxamine (Can)** *see* fluvoxamine *on page 262*

**Apo®-Folic (Can)** *see* folic acid *on page 262*

**Apo®-Furosemide (Can)** *see* furosemide *on page 267*

**Apo®-Gain (Can)** *see* minoxidil *on page 394*

**Apo®-Gemfibrozil (Can)** *see* gemfibrozil *on page 271*

**Apo®-Glyburide (Can)** *see* glyburide *on page 276*

**Apo®-Guanethidine (Can)** *see* guanethidine *on page 286*

**Apo®-Haloperidol (Can)** *see* haloperidol *on page 288*

**Apo®-Hydralazine (Can)** *see* hydralazine *on page 297*

**Apo®-Hydro (Can)** *see* hydrochlorothiazide *on page 299*

**Apo®-Hydroxyzine (Can)** *see* hydroxyzine *on page 308*

**Apo®-Ibuprofen (Can)** *see* ibuprofen *on page 311*

**Apo®-Imipramine (Can)** *see* imipramine *on page 314*

**Apo®-Indapadmide (Can)** *see* indapamide *on page 316*

**Apo®-Indomethacin (Can)** *see* indomethacin *on page 317*

**Apo®-Ipravent (Can)** *see* ipratropium *on page 325*

**Apo®-ISDN (Can)** *see* isosorbide dinitrate *on page 328*

**Apo®-K (Can)** *see* potassium chloride *on page 485*

**Apo®-Keto (Can)** *see* ketoprofen *on page 334*

**Apo®-Ketoconazole (Can)** *see* ketoconazole *on page 333*

**Apo®-Keto-E (Can)** *see* ketoprofen *on page 334*

**Apo®-Ketorolac (Can)** *see* ketorolac tromethamine *on page 334*

**Apo®-Ketotifen (Can)** *see* ketotifen *on page 335*

**Apo®-Levocarb (Can)** *see* carbidopa and levodopa *on page 107*

**Apo®-Lisinopril (Can)** *see* lisinopril *on page 352*

**Apo®-Loperamide (Can)** *see* loperamide *on page 354*

**Apo®-Lorazepam (Can)** *see* lorazepam *on page 356*

**Apo®-Lovastatin (Can)** *see* lovastatin *on page 358*

**Apo®-Sulfinpyraz (Can)** *see* sulfinpyrazone *on page 566*
**Apo®-Sulin (Can)** *see* sulindac *on page 567*
**Apo®-Tamox (Can)** *see* tamoxifen *on page 570*
**Apo®-Temazepam (Can)** *see* temazepam *on page 572*
**Apo®-Terazosin (Can)** *see* terazosin *on page 574*
**Apo®-Tetra® (Can)** *see* tetracycline *on page 579*
**Apo®-Theo LA (Can)** *see* theophylline *on page 581*
**Apo®-Thioridazine (Can)** *see* thioridazine *on page 586*
**Apo®-Tiaprofenic (Can)** *see* tiaprofenic acid *(Canada only) on page 589*
**Apo®-Ticlopidine (Can)** *see* ticlopidine *on page 590*
**Apo®-Timol (Can)** *see* timolol *on page 591*
**Apo®-Timop (Can)** *see* timolol *on page 591*
**Apo®-Tolbutamide (Can)** *see* tolbutamide *on page 594*
**Apo®-Trazodone (Can)** *see* trazodone *on page 600*
**Apo®-Triazide (Can)** *see* hydrochlorothiazide and triamterene *on page 299*
**Apo®-Triazo (Can)** *see* triazolam *on page 603*
**Apo®-Trifluoperazine (Can)** *see* trifluoperazine *on page 605*
**Apo®-Trihex (Can)** *see* trihexyphenidyl *on page 606*
**Apo®-Trimip (Can)** *see* trimipramine *on page 608*
**Apo®-Valproic (Can)** *see* valproic acid and derivatives *on page 620*
**Apo®-Verap (Can)** *see* verapamil *on page 625*
**Apo®-Zidovudine (Can)** *see* zidovudine *on page 638*
**Apo®-Zopiclone (Can)** *see* zopiclone *(Canada only) on page 641*
**APPG** *see* penicillin G procaine *on page 457*

## apraclonidine (a pra KLOE ni deen)

**U.S./Canadian Brand Names** Iopidine®
**Therapeutic Category** Alpha$_2$-Adrenergic Agonist Agent, Ophthalmic
**Use** 1%: Prevention and treatment of postsurgical intraocular pressure elevation; 0.5%: Short-term adjunctive therapy in patients on maximally tolerated medical therapy who require additional redirection of intraocular pressure
**Usual Dosage** Adults: Ophthalmic: Instill 1 drop in operative eye 1 hour prior to laser surgery, second drop in eye upon completion of procedure
**Dosage Forms** Solution, ophthalmic, as hydrochloride: 0.5% (5 mL, 10 mL); 1% (0.1 mL)

**Apresazide® *(Discontinued)*** *see page 750*
**Apresoline®** *see* hydralazine *on page 297*
**Apri®** *see* ethinyl estradiol and desogestrel *on page 230*
**Aprodine® Syrup [OTC]** *see* triprolidine and pseudoephedrine *on page 609*
**Aprodine® Tablet [OTC]** *see* triprolidine and pseudoephedrine *on page 609*
**Aprodine® w/C** *see* triprolidine, pseudoephedrine, and codeine *on page 609*

## aprotinin (a proe TYE nin)

**U.S./Canadian Brand Names** Trasylol®
**Therapeutic Category** Hemostatic Agent
**Use** Reduction or prevention of blood loss in patients undergoing coronary artery bypass surgery when a high index of suspicion of excessive bleeding potential exists; this includes open heart reoperation, pre-existing coagulopathy, operations on the great vessels, and patients whose religious beliefs prohibit blood transfusions

**Usual Dosage** Test dose: **All** patients should receive a 1 mL I.V. test dose at least 10 minutes prior to the loading dose to assess the potential for allergic reactions

Regimen A (standard dose):
2 million units (280 mg) loading dose I.V. over 20-30 minutes
2 million units (280 mg) into pump prime volume
500,000 units/hour (70 mg/hour) I.V. during operation

Regimen B (low dose):
1 million units (140 mg) loading dose I.V. over 20-30 minutes
1 million units (140 mg) into pump prime volume
250,000 units/hour (35 mg/hour) I.V. during operation

**Dosage Forms** Injection: 1.4 mg/mL [10,000 units/mL] (100 mL, 200 mL)

**APSAC** *see* anistreplase *on page 41*

**Aquacare® Topical [OTC]** *see* urea *on page 617*

**Aquachloral® Supprettes®** *see* chloral hydrate *on page 124*

**Aquacort® (Can)** *see* hydrocortisone (topical) *on page 304*

**Aquacot®** *see* trichlormethiazide *on page 604*

**AquaMEPHYTON® Injection** *see* phytonadione *on page 470*

**Aquaphyllin® *(Discontinued)*** *see page 750*

**AquaSite® Ophthalmic Solution [OTC]** *see* artificial tears *on page 53*

**Aquasol A®** *see* vitamin A *on page 629*

**Aquasol E® [OTC]** *see* vitamin E *on page 631*

**AquaTar® [OTC]** *see* coal tar *on page 149*

**Aquatensen®** *see* methyclothiazide *on page 383*

**Aquazide H®** *see* hydrochlorothiazide *on page 299*

**aqueous procaine penicillin G** *see* penicillin G procaine *on page 457*

**aqueous testosterone** *see* testosterone *on page 576*

**Aquest®** *see* estrone *on page 228*

**ARA-A** *see* vidarabine *on page 627*

**arabinofuranosyladenine** *see* vidarabine *on page 627*

**arabinosylcytosine** *see* cytarabine *on page 162*

**ARA-C** *see* cytarabine *on page 162*

**Aralen® Phosphate** *see* chloroquine phosphate *on page 127*

**Aralen® Phosphate With Primaquine Phosphate *(Discontinued)*** *see page 750*

**Aramine®** *see* metaraminol *on page 376*

**Arava™** *see* leflunomide *on page 341*

**Arcet®** *see* butalbital compound and acetaminophen *on page 93*

**Arcotinic® Tablet *(Discontinued)*** *see page 750*

**Arduan®** *see* pipecuronium *on page 472*

**Aredia™** *see* pamidronate *on page 447*

## argatroban (ar GA troh ban)

**Therapeutic Category** Anticoagulant, Thrombin Inhibitor

**Use** Prophylaxis or treatment of thrombosis in adults with heparin-induced thrombocytopenia

**Usual Dosage** I.V.: Adults:
Initial dose: 2 mcg/kg/minute
(Continued)

## argatroban *(Continued)*

Maintenance dose: Measure aPTT after 2 hours, adjust dose until the steady-state aPTT is 1.5-3.0 times the initial baseline value, not exceeding 100 seconds; dosage should not exceed 10 mcg/kg/minute

Conversion to oral anticoagulant: Because there may be a combined effect on the INR when argatroban is combined with warfarin, loading doses of warfarin should not be used. Warfarin therapy should be started at the expected daily dose.

Patients receiving ≤2 mcg/kg/minute of argatroban: Argatroban therapy can be stopped when the combined INR on warfarin and argatroban is >4; repeat INR measurement in 4-6 hours; if INR is below therapeutic level, argatroban therapy may be restarted. Repeat procedure daily until desired INR on warfarin alone is obtained.

Patients receiving >2 mcg/kg/minute of argatroban: Reduce dose of argatroban to 2 mcg/kg/minute; measure INR for argatroban and warfarin 4-6 hours after dose reduction; argatroban therapy can be stopped when the combined INR on warfarin and argatroban is >4. Repeat INR measurement in 4-6 hours; if INR is below therapeutic level, argatroban therapy may be restarted. Repeat procedure daily until desired INR on warfarin alone is obtained.

**Dosage Forms** Solution for injection: 100 mg/mL (2.5 mL)

**Argesic®-SA** *see* salsalate *on page 536*

## arginine (AR ji neen)

**U.S./Canadian Brand Names** R-Gene®

**Therapeutic Category** Diagnostic Agent

**Use** Pituitary function test (growth hormone); management of severe, uncompensated, metabolic alkalosis (pH ≥7.55) **after** optimizing therapy with sodium, potassium, or ammonium chloride supplements

**Usual Dosage** I.V.:

Growth hormone (pituitary function) reserve test:

Children: 500 mg (5 mL) kg/dose administered over 30 minutes

Adults: 30 g (300 mL) administered over 30 minutes

Metabolic alkalosis: Children and Adults: Usual dose: 10 g/hour

Acid required (mEq) =

[1] 0.2 (L/kg) x wt (kg) x [103 - serum chloride] (mEq/L) **or**

[2] 0.3 (L/kg) x wt (kg) x base excess (mEq/L) **or**

[3] 0.5 (L/kg) x wt (kg) x [serum $HCO_3$ - 24] (mEq/L)

Administer $1/2$ to $2/3$ of calculated dose and re-evaluate

**Note:** Arginine hydrochloride should never be used as an alternative to chloride supplementation but used in the patient who is unresponsive to sodium chloride or potassium chloride supplementation

**Dosage Forms** Injection, as hydrochloride: 10% [100 mg/mL = 950 mOsm/L] (500 mL)

**8-arginine vasopressin** *see* vasopressin *on page 623*

**Argyrol® S.S. *(Discontinued)*** *see page 750*

**Aricept®** *see* donepezil *on page 200*

**Arimidex®** *see* anastrozole *on page 41*

**Aristocort® A Topical** *see* triamcinolone (topical) *on page 602*

**Aristocort® Forte Injection** *see* triamcinolone (systemic) *on page 602*

**Aristocort® Intralesional Injection** *see* triamcinolone (systemic) *on page 602*

**Aristocort® Oral** *see* triamcinolone (systemic) *on page 602*

**Aristocort® Topical** *see* triamcinolone (topical) *on page 602*

**Aristospan® Intra-articular Injection** *see* triamcinolone (systemic) *on page 602*

**Aristospan® Intralesional Injection** *see* triamcinolone (systemic) *on page 602*

**Arlex®** *see* sorbitol *on page 554*

**Arlidin®** ***(Discontinued)*** *see page 750*

**Arm-a-Med® Isoetharine** ***(Discontinued)*** *see page 750*

**Arm-a-Med® Isoproterenol** ***(Discontinued)*** *see page 750*

**Arm-a-Med® Metaproterenol** ***(Discontinued)*** *see page 750*

**A.R.M.® Caplet** ***(Discontinued)*** *see page 750*

**Armour® Thyroid** *see* thyroid *on page 588*

**Aromasin®** *see* exemestane *on page 238*

**Aromatic Ammonia Aspirols®** *see* ammonia spirit (aromatic) *on page 34*

**Arrestin®** ***(Discontinued)*** *see page 750*

**ARS** *see* antirabies serum (equine) *on page 45*

## arsenic trioxide (AR se nik tri OKS id)

**U.S./Canadian Brand Names** Trisenox™

**Therapeutic Category** Antineoplastic Agent

**Use** Induction of remission and consolidation in patients with acute promyelocytic leukemia (APL) which is specifically characterized by t(15;17) translocation or PML/RAR-alpha gene expression. Should be used only in those patients who have relapsed or are refractory to retinoid and anthracycline chemotherapy.

**Usual Dosage** I.V.: Children >5 years and Adults:

Induction: 0.15 mg/kg/day; administer daily until bone marrow remission; maximum induction: 60 doses

Consolidation: 0.15 mg/kg/day starting 3-6 weeks after completion of induction therapy; maximum consolidation: 25 doses over 5 weeks

**Dosage Forms** Solution for injection: 1 mg/mL (10 mL)

**Artane®** *see* trihexyphenidyl *on page 606*

**Artha-G®** ***(Discontinued)*** *see page 750*

**Arth Dr®** *see* capsaicin *on page 104*

**Arthricare Hand & Body®** *see* capsaicin *on page 104*

**Arthritis Foundation® Ibuprofen** ***(Discontinued)*** *see page 750*

**Arthritis Foundation® Nighttime** ***(Discontinued)*** *see page 750*

**Arthritis Foundation® Pain Reliever [OTC]** *see* aspirin *on page 55*

**Arthritis Foundation® Pain Reliever, Aspirin Free** ***(Discontinued)*** *see page 750*

**Arthritis Strength Bufferin®** ***(Discontinued)*** *see page 750*

**Arthropan® [OTC]** *see* choline salicylate *on page 135*

**Arthrotec®** *see* diclofenac and misoprostol *on page 182*

**Articulose-50® Injection** ***(Discontinued)*** *see page 750*

## artificial tears (ar ti FISH il tears)

**Synonyms** polyvinyl alcohol

**U.S./Canadian Brand Names** Adsorbotear® Ophthalmic Solution [OTC]; Akwa Tears® Solution [OTC]; AquaSite® Ophthalmic Solution [OTC]; Bion® Tears Solution [OTC]; Comfort® Tears Solution [OTC]; Dakrina® Ophthalmic Solution [OTC]; Dry Eyes® Solution [OTC]; Dry Eye® Therapy Solution [OTC]; Dwelle® Ophthalmic Solution [OTC]; Eye-Lube-A® Solution [OTC]; HypoTears PF Solution [OTC]; HypoTears Solution [OTC]; Isopto® Plain Solution [OTC]; Isopto® Tears Solution [OTC]; Just Tears® Solution [OTC]; Lacril® Ophthalmic Solution [OTC]; Liquifilm® Forte Solution [OTC]; Liquifilm® Tears Solution [OTC]; LubriTears® Solution [OTC]; Moisture® Ophthalmic Drops [OTC]; Murine® Solution [OTC]; Murocel® Ophthalmic Solution [OTC]; Nature's Tears® Solution [OTC]; Nu-Tears® II Solution [OTC]; Nu-Tears® Solution [OTC]; OcuCoat® Ophthalmic Solution [OTC]; OcuCoat® PF Ophthalmic Solution [OTC]; Puralube® Tears Solution

(Continued)

## artificial tears *(Continued)*

[OTC]; Refresh® Ophthalmic Solution [OTC]; Refresh® Plus Ophthalmic Solution [OTC]; Tear Drop® Solution [OTC]; TearGard® Ophthalmic Solution [OTC]; Teargen® Ophthalmic Solution [OTC]; Tearisol® Solution [OTC]; Tears Naturale® Free Solution [OTC]; Tears Naturale® II Solution [OTC]; Tears Naturale® Solution [OTC]; Tears Plus® Solution [OTC]; Tears Renewed® Solution [OTC]; Ultra Tears® Solution [OTC]; Viva-Drops® Solution [OTC]

**Therapeutic Category** Ophthalmic Agent, Miscellaneous

**Use** Ophthalmic lubricant; relief of dry eyes and eye irritation

**Usual Dosage** Ophthalmic: Use as needed to relieve symptoms, 1-2 drops into eye(s) 3-4 times/day

**Dosage Forms** Solution, ophthalmic: 15 mL and 30 mL with dropper

**ASA** *see* aspirin *on next page*

**5-ASA** *see* mesalamine *on page 374*

**Asacol® Oral** *see* mesalamine *on page 374*

**Asbron-G® Elixir *(Discontinued)*** *see page 750*

**Asbron-G® Tablet *(Discontinued)*** *see page 750*

**Ascarel® [OTC]** *see* pyrantel pamoate *on page 509*

## ascorbic acid (a SKOR bik AS id)

**Synonyms** vitamin C

**U.S./Canadian Brand Names** Apo®-C (Can); Ascorbicap® [OTC]; C-Crystals® [OTC]; Cebid®; Cecon® [OTC]; Cevalin® [OTC]; Cevi-bid® [OTC]; Ce-Vi-Sol® [OTC]; Dull-C® [OTC]; Flavorcee® [OTC]; N'ice®; Proflavanol C™; Revitalose-C-1000® (Can); Timecelles® [OTC]; Vita-C® [OTC]; Vitamin C Drops [OTC]

**Therapeutic Category** Vitamin, Water Soluble

**Use** Prevention and treatment of scurvy; urinary acidification; dietary supplementation; prevention and reduction in the severity of colds

**Usual Dosage** Oral, I.M., I.V., S.C.:

Recommended daily allowance (RDA):
- <6 months: 30 mg
- 6 months to 1 year: 35 mg
- 1-3 years: 40 mg
- 4-10 years: 45 mg
- 11-14 years: 50 mg
- >14 years and Adults: 60 mg

Children:
- Scurvy: 100-300 mg/day in divided doses for at least 2 weeks
- Urinary acidification: 500 mg every 6-8 hours
- Dietary supplement: 35-100 mg/day

Adults:
- Scurvy: 100-250 mg 1-2 times/day for at least 2 weeks
- Urinary acidification: 4-12 g/day in 3-4 divided doses
- Prevention and treatment of colds: 1-3 g/day
- Dietary supplement: 50-200 mg/day

**Dosage Forms**

Capsule, timed release: 500 mg
Crystals: 4 g/teaspoonful (100 g, 500 g); 5 g/teaspoonful (180 g)
Injection: 250 mg/mL (2 mL, 30 mL); 500 mg/mL (2 mL, 50 mL)
Liquid, oral: 35 mg/0.6 mL (50 mL)
Lozenges: 60 mg
Powder: 4 g/teaspoonful (100 g, 500 g)
Solution, oral: 100 mg/mL (50 mL)
Syrup: 500 mg/5 mL (5 mL, 10 mL, 120 mL, 480 mL)
Tablet: 25 mg, 50 mg, 100 mg, 250 mg, 500 mg, 1000 mg

Tablet:
  Chewable: 100 mg, 250 mg, 500 mg
  Timed release: 500 mg, 1000 mg, 1500 mg

**Ascorbicap® [OTC]** *see* ascorbic acid *on previous page*

**Ascriptin® [OTC]** *see* aspirin *on this page*

**Asendin® (Can)** *see* amoxapine *on page 35*

**Asmalix® *(Discontinued)*** *see page 750*

## asparaginase (a SPIR a ji nase)

**Synonyms** colaspase

**U.S./Canadian Brand Names** Elspar®; Kidrolase (Can)

**Therapeutic Category** Antineoplastic Agent

**Use** Treatment of acute lymphocytic leukemia, lymphoma; used for induction therapy

**Usual Dosage** Refer to individual protocols; the manufacturer recommends performing intradermal sensitivity testing before the initial dose

Children and Adults:
  I.M. (preferred route): 6000 units/$m^2$ 3 times/week for 3 weeks for combination therapy
  I.V.: 1000 units/kg/day for 10 days for combination therapy or 200 units/kg/day for 28 days if combination therapy is inappropriate

**Dosage Forms** Injection: 10,000 units/vial

**A-Spas® S/L** *see* hyoscyamine *on page 309*

**Aspergum® [OTC]** *see* aspirin *on this page*

## aspirin (AS pir in)

**Synonyms** acetylsalicylic acid; ASA

**U.S./Canadian Brand Names** Anacin® [OTC]; Arthritis Foundation® Pain Reliever [OTC]; Ascriptin® [OTC]; Aspergum® [OTC]; Asprimox® [OTC]; Bayer® Aspirin [OTC]; Bayer® Buffered Aspirin [OTC]; Bayer® Low Adult Strength [OTC]; Bufferin® [OTC]; Buffex® [OTC]; Cama® Arthritis Pain Reliever [OTC]; Easprin®; Ecotrin® [OTC]; Ecotrin® Low Adult Strength [OTC]; Empirin® [OTC]; Extra Strength Adprin-B® [OTC]; Extra Strength Bayer® Enteric 500 Aspirin [OTC]; Extra Strength Bayer® Plus [OTC]; Halfprin® 81® [OTC]; Heartline® [OTC]; Regular Strength Bayer® Enteric 500 Aspirin [OTC]; St Joseph® Adult Chewable Aspirin [OTC]; ZORprin®

**Therapeutic Category** Analgesic, Non-narcotic; Antiplatelet Agent; Antipyretic; Nonsteroidal Anti-inflammatory Drug (NSAID)

**Use** Treatment of mild to moderate pain, inflammation and fever; adjunctive treatment of Kawasaki disease; may be used for prophylaxis of myocardial infarction and transient ischemic attacks (TIA)

**Usual Dosage**

Children:
  Analgesic and antipyretic: Oral, rectal: 10-15 mg/kg/dose every 4-6 hours
  Anti-inflammatory: Oral: Initial: 60-90 mg/kg/day in divided doses; usual maintenance: 80-100 mg/kg/day divided every 6-8 hours; monitor serum concentrations
  Kawasaki disease: Oral: 100 mg/kg/day divided every 6 hours; after fever resolves: 8-10 mg/kg/day once daily; monitor serum concentrations

Adults:
  Analgesic and antipyretic: Oral, rectal: 325-1000 mg every 4-6 hours up to 4 g/day
  Anti-inflammatory: Oral: Initial: 2.4-3.6 g/day in divided doses; usual maintenance: 3.6-5.4 g/day; monitor serum concentrations
  Transient ischemic attack: Oral: 1.3 g/day in 2-4 divided doses
  Myocardial infarction prophylaxis: 160-325 mg/day

**Dosage Forms**

Capsule: 356.4 mg and caffeine 30 mg
Suppository, rectal: 60 mg, 120 mg, 125 mg, 130 mg, 195 mg, 200 mg, 300 mg, 325 mg, 600 mg, 650 mg, 1.2 g
(Continued)

## aspirin *(Continued)*

Tablet: 65 mg, 75 mg, 81 mg, 325 mg, 500 mg
Tablet: 400 mg and caffeine 32 mg
Tablet:
Buffered: 325 mg and magnesium-aluminum hydroxide 150 mg; 325 mg, magnesium hydroxide 75 mg, aluminum hydroxide 75 mg, buffered with calcium carbonate; 325 mg and magnesium-aluminum hydroxide 75 mg
Chewable: 81 mg
Controlled release: 800 mg
Delayed release: 81 mg
Enteric coated: 81 mg, 325 mg, 500 mg, 650 mg, 975 mg
Gum: 227.5 mg
Timed release: 650 mg

## aspirin and codeine (AS pir in & KOE deen)

**U.S./Canadian Brand Names** Coryphen® Codeine (Can); Empirin® With Codeine; 222® Tablets (Can); 282® Tablets (Can); 292® Tablets (Can)
**Therapeutic Category** Analgesic, Narcotic
**Controlled Substance** C-III
**Use** Relief of mild to moderate pain
**Usual Dosage** Oral:
Children:
Aspirin: 10 mg/kg/dose every 4 hours
Codeine: 0.5-1 mg/kg/dose every 4 hours
Adults: 1-2 tablets every 4-6 hours as needed for pain
**Dosage Forms** Tablet:
#2: Aspirin 325 mg and codeine phosphate 15 mg
#3: Aspirin 325 mg and codeine phosphate 30 mg
#4: Aspirin 325 mg and codeine phosphate 60 mg

## aspirin and meprobamate (AS pir in & me proe BA mate)

**U.S./Canadian Brand Names** Equagesic®
**Therapeutic Category** Skeletal Muscle Relaxant
**Controlled Substance** C-IV
**Use** Adjunct to treatment of skeletal muscular disease in patients exhibiting tension and/or anxiety
**Usual Dosage** Oral: 1 tablet 3-4 times/day
**Dosage Forms** Tablet: Aspirin 325 mg and meprobamate 200 mg

**Aspirin® Backache (Can)** *see* methocarbamol and aspirin *on page 380*

**Asprimox® [OTC]** *see* aspirin *on previous page*

**Asproject® *(Discontinued)*** *see page 750*

**Astelin® Nasal Spray** *see* azelastine *on page 62*

**AsthmaHaler® Mist [OTC]** *see* epinephrine *on page 216*

**AsthmaNefrin® [OTC]** *see* epinephrine *on page 216*

**Atabrine® Tablet *(Discontinued)*** *see page 750*

**Atacand®** *see* candesartan *on page 102*

**Atacand HCT™** *see* candesartan and hydrochlorothiazide *on page 102*

**Atapryl®** *see* selegiline *on page 540*

**Atarax®** *see* hydroxyzine *on page 308*

## atenolol (a TEN oh lole)

**U.S./Canadian Brand Names** Apo®-Atenol (Can); Gen-Atenolol (Can); Nu-Atenol (Can); Taro-Atenol® (Can); Tenolin (Can); Tenormin®

**Therapeutic Category** Beta-Adrenergic Blocker

**Use** Treatment of hypertension, alone or in combination with other agents; management of angina pectoris; antiarrhythmic; postmyocardial infarction patients; acute alcohol withdrawal

**Usual Dosage**

Oral:

Children: 1-2 mg/kg/dose administered daily

Adults:

Hypertension: 50 mg once daily, may increase to 100 mg/day; doses >100 mg are unlikely to produce any further benefit

Angina pectoris: 50 mg once daily, may increase to 100 mg/day; some patients may require 200 mg/day

Postmyocardial infarction: Follow I.V. dose with 100 mg/day or 50 mg twice daily for 6-9 days postmyocardial infarction

I.V.: Postmyocardial infarction: Early treatment: 5 mg slow I.V. over 5 minutes; may repeat in 10 minutes; if both doses are tolerated, may start oral atenolol 50 mg every 12 hours or 100 mg/day for 6-9 days postmyocardial infarction

**Dosage Forms**

Injection: 0.5 mg/mL (10 mL)

Tablet: 25 mg, 50 mg, 100 mg

## atenolol and chlorthalidone (a TEN oh lole & klor THAL i done)

**U.S./Canadian Brand Names** Tenoretic®

**Therapeutic Category** Antihypertensive Agent, Combination

**Use** Treatment of hypertension with a cardioselective beta-blocker and a diuretic

**Usual Dosage** Adults: Oral: Initial: 1 tablet (50) once daily, then individualize dose until optimal dose is achieved

**Dosage Forms** Tablet:

50: Atenolol 50 mg and chlorthalidone 25 mg

100: Atenolol 100 mg and chlorthalidone 25 mg

**ATG** *see* lymphocyte immune globulin *on page 359*

**Atgam®** *see* lymphocyte immune globulin *on page 359*

**ATIII** *see* antithrombin III *on page 45*

**Ativan®** *see* lorazepam *on page 356*

**Atolone® Oral** *see* triamcinolone (systemic) *on page 602*

## atorvastatin (a TORE va sta tin)

**U.S./Canadian Brand Names** Lipitor®

**Therapeutic Category** HMG-CoA Reductase Inhibitor

**Use** Adjunct to diet for the reduction of elevated total and LDL-cholesterol levels in patients with hypercholesterolemia (Type IIa, IIb, and IIc); used in hypercholesterolemic patients without clinically evident heart disease to reduce the risk of myocardial infarction, to reduce the risk for revascularization, and reduce the risk of death due to cardiovascular causes with no increase in death from noncardiovascular diseases

**Usual Dosage** Adults: Oral: Initial: 10 mg/day, with a range of 10-80 mg/day, administered as a single dose at any time of day, with or without food

**Dosage Forms** Tablet: 10 mg, 20 mg, 40 mg

## atovaquone (a TOE va kwone)

**U.S./Canadian Brand Names** Mepron™

**Therapeutic Category** Antiprotozoal

**Use** Acute oral treatment of mild to moderate *Pneumocystis carinii* pneumonia (PCP) in patients who are intolerant to co-trimoxazole

**Usual Dosage** Adults: Oral: 750 mg twice daily with food for 21 days

**Dosage Forms** Suspension, oral (citrus flavor): 750 mg/5 mL (5 mL, 210 mL)

**atovaquone and proguanil** (a TOE va kwone & pro GWA nil)

**U.S./Canadian Brand Names** Malarone™

**Therapeutic Category** Antimalarial Agent

**Use** Prevention or treatment of acute, uncomplicated *P. falciparum* malaria

**Usual Dosage** Oral (doses given in mg of atovaquone and proguanil):

Adults:

Prevention of malaria: Atovaquone/proguanil 250 mg/100 mg once daily. Start 1-2 days prior to entering a malaria-endemic area, continue throughout the stay and for 7 days after returning.

Treatment of acute malaria: Atovaquone/proguanil 1 g/400 mg as a single dose, once daily for 3 consecutive days

Children (dosage based on body weight):

Prevention of malaria: Start 1-2 days prior to entering a malaria-endemic area, continue throughout the stay and for 7 days after returning. Take as a single dose, once daily.

11-20 kg: Atovaquone/proguanil 62.5 mg/25 mg
21-30 kg: Atovaquone/proguanil 125 mg/50 mg
31-40 kg: Atovaquone/proguanil 187.5 mg/75 mg
>40 kg: Atovaquone/proguanil 250 mg/100mg

Treatment of acute malaria: Take as a single dose, once daily for 3 consecutive days.

11-20 kg: Atovaquone/proguanil 250 mg/100 mg
21-30 kg: Atovaquone/proguanil 500 mg/200mg
31-40 kg: Atovaquone/proguanil 750 mg/300mg
>40 kg: Atovaquone/proguanil 1 g/400 mg

**Dosage Forms**

Tablet: Atovaquone 250 mg and proguanil hydrochloride 100 mg

Tablet, pediatric: Atovaquone 62.5 mg and proguanil hydrochloride 25 mg

**Atozine® Oral *(Discontinued)*** *see page 750*

**atracurium** (a tra KYOO ree um)

**U.S./Canadian Brand Names** Tracrium®

**Therapeutic Category** Skeletal Muscle Relaxant

**Use** Eases endotracheal intubation as an adjunct to general anesthesia and relaxes skeletal muscle during surgery or mechanical ventilation

**Usual Dosage** I.V.:

Children 1 month to 2 years: Initial: 0.3-0.4 mg/kg followed by maintenance doses of 0.08-0.1 mg/kg as needed to maintain neuromuscular blockade

Children >2 years to Adults: Initial: 0.4-0.5 mg/kg then 0.08-0.1 mg/kg every 20-45 minutes after initial dose to maintain neuromuscular block

Continuous infusion: 0.4-0.8 mg/kg/hour

**Dosage Forms**

Injection, as besylate: 10 mg/mL (5 mL, 10 mL)

Injection, preservative-free, as besylate: 10 mg/mL (5 mL)

**Atrohist® Plus *(Discontinued)*** *see page 750*

**Atromid-S®** *see* clofibrate *on page 145*

**Atropair®** *see* atropine *on this page*

**atropine** (A troe peen)

**U.S./Canadian Brand Names** Atropair®; Atropine-Care®; Atropisol®; Isopto® Atropine; I-Tropine®; Sal-Tropine™ Oral

**Therapeutic Category** Anticholinergic Agent

**Use** Preoperative medication to inhibit salivation and secretions; treatment of sinus bradycardia; management of peptic ulcer; treatment of exercise-induced bronchospasm; antidote for organophosphate pesticide poisoning; used to produce mydriasis and cycloplegia for examination of the retina and optic disk and accurate measurement of refractive errors; treatment of uveitis

**Usual Dosage Note**: Doses <0.1 mg have been associated with paradoxical bradycardia.

Neonates, Infants, and Children:

Preanesthetic: Oral, I.M., I.V., S.C.:

<5 kg: 0.02 mg/kg/dose 30-60 minutes preop then every 4-6 hours as needed. Use of a minimum dosage of 0.1 mg in neonates <5 kg will result in dosages >0.02 mg/kg. There is no documented minimum dosage in this age group.

>5 kg: 0.01-0.02 mg/kg/dose to a maximum 0.4 mg/dose 30-60 minutes preop; minimum dose: 0.1 mg

Bradycardia: I.V., intratracheal: 0.02 mg/kg, minimum dose 0.1 mg, maximum single dose: 0.5 mg in children and 1 mg in adolescents; may repeat in 5-minute intervals to a maximum total dose of 1 mg in children or 2 mg in adolescents. (**Note:** For intratracheal administration, the dosage must be diluted with normal saline to a total volume of 1-2 mL). When treating bradycardia in neonates, reserve use for those patients unresponsive to improved oxygenation and epinephrine.

Children:

Bronchospasm: Inhalation: 0.03-0.05 mg/kg/dose 3-4 times/day

Preprocedure: Ophthalmic: 0.5% solution: Instill 1-2 drops twice daily for 1-3 days before the procedure

Uveitis: Ophthalmic: 0.5% solution: Instill 1-2 drops up to 3 times/day

Adults (doses <0.5 mg have been associated with paradoxical bradycardia):

Asystole: I.V.: 1 mg; may repeat every 3-5 minutes as needed

Preanesthetic: I.M., I.V., S.C.: 0.4-0.6 mg 30-60 minutes preop and repeat every 4-6 hours as needed

Bradycardia: I.V.: 0.5-1 mg every 5 minutes, not to exceed a total of 2 mg or 0.04 mg/kg; may give intratracheal in 1 mg/10 mL dilution only, intratracheal dose should be 2-2.5 times the I.V. dose

Neuromuscular blockade reversal: I.V.: 25-30 mcg/kg 30 seconds before neostigmine or 10 mcg/kg 30 seconds before edrophonium

Organophosphate or carbamate poisoning: I.V.: 1-2 mg/dose every 10-20 minutes until atropine effect (dry flushed skin, tachycardia, mydriasis, fever) is observed, then every 1-4 hours for at least 24 hours; up to 50 mg in first 24 hours and 2 g over several days may be given in cases of severe intoxication

Bronchospasm: Inhalation: 0.025-0.05 mg/kg/dose every 4-6 hours as needed (maximum: 5 mg/dose)

Ophthalmic solution: 1%:

Preprocedure: Instill 1-2 drops 1 hour before the procedure.

Uveitis: Instill 1-2 drops 4 times/day.

Ophthalmic ointment: Apply a small amount in the conjunctival sac up to 3 times/day. Compress the lacrimal sac by digital pressure for 1-3 minutes after instillation.

**Dosage Forms**

Injection, as sulfate: 0.05 mg/mL (5 mL); 0.1 mg/mL (5 mL, 10 mL); 0.3 mg/mL (1 mL, 30 mL); 0.4 mg/mL (1 mL, 20 mL, 30 mL); 0.5 mg/mL (1 mL, 5 mL, 30 mL); 0.8 mg/mL (0.5 mL, 1 mL); 1 mg/mL (1 mL, 10 mL)

Ointment, ophthalmic, as sulfate: 1% (3.5 g)

Solution, ophthalmic, as sulfate: 0.5% (1 mL, 5 mL); 1% (1 mL, 2 mL, 5 mL, 15 mL); 2% (1 mL, 2 mL)

Tablet, as sulfate: 0.4 mg

**Atropine-Care**® *see* atropine *on previous page*

**atropine soluble tablet *(Discontinued)*** *see page 750*

**Atropisol**® *see* atropine *on previous page*

**Atrosept**® *see* methenamine, phenyl salicylate, atropine, hyoscyamine, benzoic acid, and methylene blue *on page 379*

**Atrovent**® *see* ipratropium *on page 325*

**A/T/S® Topical** *see* erythromycin (ophthalmic/topical) *on page 222*

## attapulgite (at a PULL gite)

**U.S./Canadian Brand Names** Children's Kaopectate® [OTC]; Diasorb® [OTC]; Kaopectate® Advanced Formula [OTC]; Kaopectate® Maximum Strength Caplets; Rheaban® [OTC]

**Therapeutic Category** Antidiarrheal

**Use** Treatment of uncomplicated diarrhea

**Usual Dosage** Oral:

Children:

<3 years: Not recommended

3-6 years: 750 mg/dose up to 2250 mg/24 hours

6-12 years: 1200-1500 mg/dose up to 4500 mg/24 hours

Adults: 1200-1500 mg after each loose bowel movement or every 2 hours; 15-30 mL up to 8 times/day, up to 9000 mg/24 hours

**Dosage Forms**

Liquid, oral concentrate: 600 mg/15 mL (180 mL, 240 mL, 360 mL, 480 mL); 750 mg/15 mL (120 mL)

Tablet: 750 mg

Tablet, chewable: 300 mg, 600 mg

**Attenuvax®** *see* measles virus vaccine (live) *on page 367*

**Augmentin®** *see* amoxicillin and clavulanate potassium *on page 36*

**Auralgan®** *see* antipyrine and benzocaine *on page 44*

## auranofin (au RANE oh fin)

**U.S./Canadian Brand Names** Ridaura®

**Therapeutic Category** Gold Compound

**Use** Management of active stage of classic or definite rheumatoid or psoriatic arthritis in patients that do not respond to or tolerate other agents

**Usual Dosage** Oral:

Children: Initial: 0.1 mg/kg/day divided daily; usual maintenance: 0.15 mg/kg/day in 1-2 divided doses; maximum: 0.2 mg/kg/day in 1-2 divided doses

Adults: 6 mg/day in 1-2 divided doses; after 3 months may be increased to 9 mg/day in 3 divided doses; if still no response after 3 months at 9 mg/day, discontinue drug

**Dosage Forms** Capsule: 3 mg [gold 29%]

**Aureomycin®** ***(Discontinued)*** *see page 750*

**Aurodex®** *see* antipyrine and benzocaine *on page 44*

**Auro® Ear Drops [OTC]** *see* carbamide peroxide *on page 106*

**Aurolate®** *see* gold sodium thiomalate *on page 279*

## aurothioglucose (aur oh thye oh GLOO kose)

**U.S./Canadian Brand Names** Solganal®

**Therapeutic Category** Gold Compound

**Use** Management of active stage of classic or definite rheumatoid or psoriatic arthritis in patients that do not respond to or tolerate other agents

**Usual Dosage** I.M. (doses should initially be administered at weekly intervals):

Children 6-12 years: Initial: 0.25 mg/kg/dose first week; increment at 0.25 mg/kg/dose increasing with each weekly dose; maintenance: 0.75-1 mg/kg/dose weekly not to exceed 25 mg/dose to a total of 20 doses, then every 2-4 weeks

Adults: 10 mg first week; 25 mg second and third week; then 50 mg/week until 800 mg to 1 g cumulative dose has been administered - if improvement occurs without adverse reactions, administer 25-50 mg every 2-3 weeks, then every 3-4 weeks

**Dosage Forms** Injection, suspension: 50 mg/mL [gold 50%] (10 mL)

**Auroto®** *see* antipyrine and benzocaine *on page 44*

**Autoplex® T** *see* anti-inhibitor coagulant complex *on page 44*

**Avalide®** *see* irbesartan and hydrochlorothiazide *on page 325*

**Avandia®** *see* rosiglitazone *on page 532*

**Avapro®** *see* irbesartan *on page 325*

**AVC™ Cream** *see* sulfanilamide *on page 565*

**AVC™ Suppository** *see* sulfanilamide *on page 565*

**Aveeno® Cleansing Bar [OTC]** *see* sulfur and salicylic acid *on page 566*

**Avelox™** *see* moxifloxacin *on page 401*

**Aventyl® Hydrochloride** *see* nortriptyline *on page 426*

**Avirax™ (Can)** *see* acyclovir *on page 12*

**Avita®** *see* tretinoin (topical) *on page 600*

**Avitene®** *see* microfibrillar collagen hemostat *on page 391*

**Avlosulfon® *(Discontinued)*** *see page 750*

**Avlosulfon® (Can)** *see* dapsone *on page 166*

**Avonex™** *see* interferon beta-1a *on page 323*

**Axert™** *see* almotriptan *on page 22*

**Axid®** *see* nizatidine *on page 424*

**Axid® AR [OTC]** *see* nizatidine *on page 424*

**Axocet®** *see* butalbital compound and acetaminophen *on page 93*

**Axotal® *(Discontinued)*** *see page 750*

**Ayercillin® (Can)** *see* penicillin G procaine *on page 457*

**Aygestin®** *see* norethindrone *on page 425*

**Ayr® Nasal [OTC]** *see* sodium chloride *on page 549*

**Azactam®** *see* aztreonam *on page 63*

## azatadine (a ZA ta deen)

**U.S./Canadian Brand Names** Optimine®

**Therapeutic Category** Antihistamine

**Use** Treatment of perennial and seasonal allergic rhinitis and chronic urticaria

**Usual Dosage** Children >12 years and Adults: Oral: 1-2 mg twice daily

**Dosage Forms** Tablet, as maleate: 1 mg

## azatadine and pseudoephedrine (a ZA ta deen & soo doe e FED rin)

**U.S./Canadian Brand Names** Rynatan® Extended Release; Trinalin® Repetabs®

**Therapeutic Category** Antihistamine/Decongestant Combination

**Use** Perennial and seasonal allergic rhinitis and other allergic symptoms including urticaria

**Usual Dosage** Adults: 1 tablet twice daily

**Dosage Forms** Tablet, extended release: Azatadine maleate 1 mg and pseudoephedrine sulfate 120 mg

## azathioprine (ay za THYE oh preen)

**U.S./Canadian Brand Names** Alti-Azathioprine (Can); Imuran®

**Therapeutic Category** Immunosuppressant Agent

**Use** Adjunct with other agents in prevention of transplant rejection; also used as an immunosuppressant in a variety of autoimmune diseases such as systemic lupus erythematosus, severe rheumatoid arthritis unresponsive to other agents, and nephrotic syndrome

(Continued)

## azathioprine *(Continued)*

**Usual Dosage**

Children and Adults: Renal transplantation: Oral, I.V.: Initial: 3-5 mg/kg/day; maintenance: 1-3 mg/kg/day

Adults: Rheumatoid arthritis: Oral: 1 mg/kg/day for 6-8 weeks; increase by 0.5 mg/kg every 4 weeks until response or up to 2.5 mg/kg/day I.V. dose is equivalent to oral dose

**Dosage Forms**

Injection, as sodium: 100 mg (20 mL)

Tablet (scored): 50 mg

**Azdone® *(Discontinued)*** *see page 750*

## azelaic acid (a zeh LAY ik AS id)

**U.S./Canadian Brand Names** Azelex®

**Therapeutic Category** Topical Skin Product

**Use** Treatment of mild to moderate acne vulgaris

**Usual Dosage** Adults: Topical: After skin is thoroughly washed and patted dry, gently but thoroughly massage a thin film of azelaic acid cream into the affected areas twice daily, in the morning and evening. The duration of use can vary and depends on the severity of the acne. In the majority of patients with inflammatory lesions, improvement of the condition occurs within 4 weeks.

**Dosage Forms** Cream: 20% (30 g, 50 g)

## azelastine (a ZEL as teen)

**U.S./Canadian Brand Names** Astelin® Nasal Spray; Optivar™ Ophthalmic Solution

**Therapeutic Category** Antihistamine; Antihistamine, Ophthalmic

**Use**

Nasal spray: Treatment of the symptoms of seasonal allergic rhinitis such as rhinorrhea, sneezing, and nasal pruritus in adults and children ≥5 years of age

Ophthalmic: Treatment of itching of the eye associated with seasonal allergic conjunctivitis

**Usual Dosage**

Nasal spray: Children ≥5 years and Adults: 2 sprays (137 mcg/spray) each nostril twice daily. Before initial use, the delivery system should be primed with 4 sprays or until a fine mist appears. If 3 or more days have elapsed since last use, the delivery system should be reprimed.

Ophthalmic: Instill 1 drop into affected eye(s) twice daily

**Dosage Forms**

Solution, nasal: 1 mg/mL (137 mcg/spray) (17 mL)

Solution, ophthalmic: 0.05% (10 mL)

**Azelex®** *see* azelaic acid *on this page*

**azidothymidine** *see* zidovudine *on page 638*

## azithromycin (az ith roe MYE sin)

**U.S./Canadian Brand Names** Zithromax®; Zithromax® Z-PAK®

**Therapeutic Category** Macrolide (Antibiotic)

**Use**

Children: Treatment of acute otitis media due to *H. influenzae*, *M. catarrhalis*, or *S. pneumoniae*; pharyngitis/tonsillitis due to *S. pyogenes*

Adults:

Treatment of mild to moderate upper and lower respiratory tract infections, infections of the skin and skin structure, and sexually transmitted diseases due to susceptible strains of *C. trachomatis*, *M. catarrhalis*, *H. influenzae*, *S. aureus*, *S. pneumoniae*, *Mycoplasma pneumoniae*, and *C. psittaci*; community-acquired pneumonia, pelvic inflammatory disease (PID)

Prevention of (or to delay onset of) infection with *Mycobacterium avium* complex (MAC)

Prevention or (or to delay onset of) or treatment of MAC in patients with advanced HIV infection

Prophylaxis of bacterial endocarditis in patients who are allergic to penicillin and undergoing surgical or dental procedures

**Usual Dosage** Oral:

Children:

Acute otitis media: 10 mg/kg on day 1 (not to exceed 500 mg/day) followed by 5 mg/kg/day once daily on days 2-5 (not to exceed 250 mg/day)

Pharyngitis/tonsillitis: 12 mg/kg/day for 5 days (not to exceed 500 mg/day)

Adolescents ≥16 years and Adults:

Mild to moderate respiratory tract, skin, and soft tissue infections: 500 mg in a single dose on day 1; 250 mg in a single dose on days 2-5

Nongonococcal urethritis and cervicitis: 1 g in a single dose

Chancroid and *Chlamydia*: 1 g in a single dose

I.V.: Adults:

Community-acquired pneumonia: 500 mg as a single dose for at least 2 days, follow I.V. therapy by the oral route with a single daily dose of 500 mg to complete a 7- to 10-day course of therapy

Pelvic inflammatory disease (PID): 500 mg as a single dose for 1-2 days, follow I.V. therapy by the oral route with a single daily dose of 250 mg to complete a 7-day course of therapy

**Dosage Forms**

Capsule, as dihydrate: 250 mg

Capsule, as dihydrate, dose pack (Zithromax® Z-PAK®): 250 mg (3 cards of 6 capsules each)

Powder for injection: 500 mg

Powder for oral suspension, as dihydrate [single-dose packet]: 100 mg/5 mL (15 mL); 200 mg/5 mL (15 mL, 22.5 mL, 30 mL); 1 g

Tablet, as dihydrate: 250 mg, 600 mg

Tablet, as dihydrate, dose pack (Zithromax® Z-PAK®): 250 mg (3 cards of 6 tablets each)

**Azlin® Injection *(Discontinued)*** *see page 750*

**Azmacort® Oral Inhaler** *see* triamcinolone (inhalation, oral) *on page 601*

**Azo-Dine® [OTC]** *see* phenazopyridine *on page 463*

**Azo Gantanol® *(Discontinued)*** *see page 750*

**Azo Gantrisin® *(Discontinued)*** *see page 750*

**Azo-Gesic® [OTC]** *see* phenazopyridine *on page 463*

**Azopt®** *see* brinzolamide *on page 86*

**Azo-Standard®** *see* phenazopyridine *on page 463*

**AZT** *see* zidovudine *on page 638*

**AZT + 3TC** *see* zidovudine and lamivudine *on page 638*

**azthreonam** *see* aztreonam *on this page*

## aztreonam (AZ tree oh nam)

**Synonyms** azthreonam

**U.S./Canadian Brand Names** Azactam®

**Therapeutic Category** Antibiotic, Miscellaneous

**Use** Treatment of patients with documented multidrug resistant aerobic gram-negative infection in which beta-lactam therapy is contraindicated; used for urinary tract infection, lower respiratory tract infections, septicemia, skin/skin structure infections, intra-abdominal infections and gynecological infections caused by susceptible Enterobacteriaceae, *H. influenzae*, and *P. aeruginosa*

**Usual Dosage**

Children >1 month: I.M., I.V.: 90-120 mg/kg/day divided every 6-8 hours

(Continued)

## aztreonam *(Continued)*

Cystic fibrosis: 50 mg/kg/dose every 6-8 hours (ie, up to 200 mg/kg/day); maximum: 6-8 g/day

Adults:

Urinary tract infection: I.M., I.V.: 500 mg to 1 g every 8-12 hours

Moderately severe systemic infections: 1 g I.V. or I.M. or 2 g I.V. every 8-12 hours

Severe systemic or life-threatening infections (especially caused by *Pseudomonas aeruginosa*): I.V.: 2 g every 6-8 hours; maximum: 8 g/day

**Dosage Forms**

Infusion, premixed: 1 g (50 mL); 2 g (50 mL)

Powder for injection: 500 mg (15 mL); 1 g (15 mL); 2 g (30 mL)

**Azulfidine®** *see* sulfasalazine *on page 565*

**Azulfidine® EN-tabs®** *see* sulfasalazine *on page 565*

**Azulfidine® Suspension *(Discontinued)*** *see page 750*

**Babee® Teething® [OTC]** *see* benzocaine *on page 72*

**BAC** *see* benzalkonium chloride *on page 72*

**B-A-C® *(Discontinued)*** *see page 750*

**Bacid® [OTC]** *see* Lactobacillus *on page 338*

**Baciguent® Topical [OTC]** *see* bacitracin *on this page*

**Baci-IM® Injection** *see* bacitracin *on this page*

**Bacillus Calmette-Guérin (BCG) Live** *see* BCG vaccine *on page 68*

## bacitracin (bas i TRAY sin)

**U.S./Canadian Brand Names** AK-Tracin® Ophthalmic; Baciguent® Topical [OTC]; Baci-IM® Injection

**Therapeutic Category** Antibiotic, Ophthalmic; Antibiotic, Topical; Antibiotic, Miscellaneous

**Use** Treatment of pneumonia and emphysema caused by susceptible staphylococci; prevention or treatment of superficial skin infections or infections of the eye caused by susceptible organisms; due to its toxicity, use of bacitracin systemically or as an irrigant should be limited to situations where less toxic alternatives would not be effective; treatment of antibiotic-associated colitis

**Usual Dosage** I.M. recommended; **do not administer I.V.**:

Infants:

<2.5 kg: 900 units/kg/day in 2-3 divided doses

>2.5 kg: 1000 units/kg/day in 2-3 divided doses

Children: 800-1200 units/kg/day divided every 8 hours

Adults: 10,000-25,000 units/dose every 6 hours; not to exceed 100,000 units/day

Topical: Apply 1-5 times/day

Ophthalmic ointment: 1/4" to 1/2" ribbon every 3-4 hours to conjunctival sac for acute infections or 2-3 times/day for mild to moderate infections for 7-10 days

Irrigation, solution: 50-100 units/mL in normal saline, lactated Ringer's, or sterile water for irrigation; soak sponges in solution for topical compresses 1-5 times/day or as needed during surgical procedures

**Dosage Forms**

Injection: 50,000 units

Ointment:

Ophthalmic: 500 units/g (3.5 g, 3.75 g)

AK-Tracin®: 500 units/g (3.5 g)

Topical: 500 units/g (1.5 g, 3.75 g, 15 g, 30 g, 120 g, 454 g)

## bacitracin and polymyxin B (bas i TRAY sin & pol i MIKS in bee)

**U.S./Canadian Brand Names** AK-Poly-Bac® Ophthalmic; Betadine® First Aid Antibiotics + Moisturizer [OTC]; Polysporin® Ophthalmic; Polysporin® Topical

**Therapeutic Category** Antibiotic, Ophthalmic; Antibiotic, Topical

**Use** Treatment of superficial infections involving the conjunctiva and/or cornea caused by susceptible organisms; prevent infection in minor cuts, scrapes and burns

**Usual Dosage**

Ophthalmic: Apply 1/2" ribbon to the affected eye(s) every 3-4 hours

Topical: Apply to affected area 1-3 times/day; may cover with sterile bandage if needed

**Dosage Forms**

Ointment:

Ophthalmic: Bacitracin 500 units and polymyxin B sulfate 10,000 units per g (3.5 g)

Topical: Bacitracin 500 units and polymyxin B sulfate 10,000 units per g in white petrolatum (15 g, 30 g)

Powder: Bacitracin 500 units and polymyxin B sulfate 10,000 units per g (10 g)

## bacitracin, neomycin, and polymyxin B

(bas i TRAY sin, nee oh MYE sin, & pol i MIKS in bee)

**U.S./Canadian Brand Names** AK-Spore® Ophthalmic Ointment; Medi-Quick® Topical Ointment [OTC]; Mycitracin® Topical [OTC]; Neomixin® Topical; Neosporin® Ophthalmic Ointment; Neosporin® Topical Ointment [OTC]; Neotopic (Can); Ocutricin® Topical Ointment; Septa® Topical Ointment [OTC]; Triple Antibiotic® Topical

**Therapeutic Category** Antibiotic, Ophthalmic; Antibiotic, Topical

**Use** Help prevent infection in minor cuts, scrapes and burns; short-term treatment of superficial external ocular infections caused by susceptible organisms

**Usual Dosage** Children and Adults:

Ophthalmic ointment: Instill into the conjunctival sac one or more times/day every 3-4 hours for 7-10 days

Topical: Apply 1-3 times/day

**Dosage Forms** Ointment:

Ophthalmic: Bacitracin 400 units, neomycin sulfate 3.5 mg, and polymyxin B sulfate 10,000 units and per g

Topical: Bacitracin 400 units, neomycin sulfate 3.5 mg, and polymyxin B sulfate 5000 units per g

## bacitracin, neomycin, polymyxin B, and hydrocortisone

(bas i TRAY sin, nee oh MYE sin, pol i MIKS in bee, & hye droe KOR ti sone)

**U.S./Canadian Brand Names** AK-Spore® H.C. Ophthalmic Ointment; Cortisporin® Ophthalmic Ointment; Cortisporin® Topical Ointment; Neotricin HC® Ophthalmic Ointment

**Therapeutic Category** Antibiotic/Corticosteroid, Ophthalmic; Antibiotic/Corticosteroid, Topical

**Use** Prevention and treatment of susceptible superficial topical infections

**Usual Dosage**

Ophthalmic ointment: Apply 1/2" ribbon to inside of lower lid every 3-4 hours until improvement occurs

Topical: Apply sparingly 2-4 times/day. Therapy should be discontinued when control is achieved. If no improvement is seen, reassessment of diagnosis may be necessary.

**Dosage Forms** Ointment:

Ophthalmic: Bacitracin 400 units, neomycin sulfate 3.5 mg, polymyxin B sulfate 10,000 units, and hydrocortisone 10 mg per g (3.5 g)

Topical: Bacitracin 400 units, neomycin sulfate 3.5 mg, polymyxin B sulfate 10,000 units, and hydrocortisone 10 mg per g (15 g)

## bacitracin, neomycin, polymyxin B, and lidocaine

(bas i TRAY sin, nee oh MYE sin, pol i MIKS in bee, & LYE doe kane)

**U.S./Canadian Brand Names** Clomycin® [OTC]

**Therapeutic Category** Antibiotic, Topical

**Use** Prevention and treatment of susceptible superficial topical infections

**Usual Dosage** Adults: Topical: Apply 1-4 times/day to infected areas; cover with sterile bandage if needed

(Continued)

## bacitracin, neomycin, polymyxin B, and lidocaine *(Continued)*

**Dosage Forms** Ointment, topical: Bacitracin 500 units, neomycin base 3.5 g, polymyxin B sulfate 5000 units, and lidocaine 40 mg per g (28.35 g)

**Back-Ese M (Can)** *see* magnesium salicylate *on page 362*

## baclofen (BAK loe fen)

**U.S./Canadian Brand Names** Apo®-Baclofen (Can); Gen-Baclofen (Can); Lioresal®; Liotec (Can); Novo-Baclofen (Can); Nu-Baclo (Can); PMS-Baclofen (Can)

**Therapeutic Category** Skeletal Muscle Relaxant

**Use** Treatment of reversible spasticity associated with multiple sclerosis or spinal cord lesions; intrathecal use for the management of spasticity in patients who are unresponsive to oral baclofen or experience intolerable CNS side effects; treatment of trigeminal neuralgia; adjunctive treatment of tardive dyskinesia

**Usual Dosage**

Oral:

Children:

2-7 years: Initial: 10-15 mg/24 hours divided every 8 hours; titrate dose every 3 days in increments of 5-15 mg/day to a maximum of 40 mg/day

≥8 years: Maximum: 60 mg/day in 3 divided doses

Adults: 5 mg 3 times/day, may increase 5 mg/dose every 3 days to a maximum of 80 mg/day

Intrathecal:

Test dose: 50-100 mcg, doses >50 mcg should be administered in 25 mcg increments, separated by 24 hours

Maintenance: After positive response to test dose, a maintenance intrathecal infusion can be administered via an implanted intrathecal pump. Initial dose via pump: Infusion at a 24-hourly rate dosed at twice the test dose.

**Dosage Forms**

Injection, intrathecal, preservative free: 500 mcg/mL (20 mL); 2000 mcg/mL (5 mL)

Tablet: 10 mg, 20 mg

**Bactine® Hydrocortisone [OTC]** *see* hydrocortisone (topical) *on page 304*

**Bactocill® *(Discontinued)*** *see page 750*

**BactoShield® [OTC]** *see* chlorhexidine gluconate *on page 126*

**Bactramycin®** *see* lincomycin *on page 350*

**Bactrim™** *see* sulfamethoxazole and trimethoprim *on page 564*

**Bactrim™ DS** *see* sulfamethoxazole and trimethoprim *on page 564*

**Bactroban®** *see* mupirocin *on page 402*

**Bactroban® Nasal** *see* mupirocin *on page 402*

**Baker's P&S Topical [OTC]** *see* phenol *on page 465*

**baking soda** *see* sodium bicarbonate *on page 548*

**BAL** *see* dimercaprol *on page 189*

## balanced salt solution (BAL anced salt soe LOO shun)

**U.S./Canadian Brand Names** BSS® Ophthalmic

**Therapeutic Category** Ophthalmic Agent, Miscellaneous

**Use** Intraocular irrigating solution; also used to soothe and cleanse the eye in conjunction with hard contact lenses

**Usual Dosage** Use as needed for foreign body removal, gonioscopy, and other general ophthalmic office procedures

**Dosage Forms** Ophthalmic:

Drops: 15 mL

Solution, sterile: 500 mL

**Baldex®** *see* dexamethasone (ophthalmic) *on page 174*

**BAL in Oil®** *see* dimercaprol *on page 189*

**Balminil® Decongestant (Can)** *see* pseudoephedrine *on page 507*

**Balminil DM D (Can)** *see* pseudoephedrine and dextromethorphan *on page 508*

**Balminil DM + Expectorant (Can)** *see* guaifenesin and dextromethorphan *on page 282*

**Balminil® Expectorant (Can)** *see* guaifenesin *on page 281*

**Balnetar® [OTC]** *see* coal tar, lanolin, and mineral oil *on page 149*

## balsalazide (bal SAL a zide)

**U.S./Canadian Brand Names** Colazal™

**Therapeutic Category** 5-Aminosalicylic Acid Derivative; Anti-inflammatory Agent

**Use** Treatment of mild to moderate active ulcerative colitis

**Usual Dosage** Oral: Adults: 2.25 g (three 750 mg capsules) 3 times/day for 8-12 weeks

**Dosage Forms** Capsule, as disodium: 750 mg

**Bancap®** ***(Discontinued)*** *see page 750*

**Bancap HC®** *see* hydrocodone and acetaminophen *on page 300*

**Banesin®** ***(Discontinued)*** *see page 750*

**Banophen® Decongestant Capsule [OTC]** *see* diphenhydramine and pseudoephedrine *on page 191*

**Banophen® Oral [OTC]** *see* diphenhydramine *on page 191*

**Banthine®** ***(Discontinued)*** *see page 750*

**Bantron®** ***(Discontinued)*** *see page 750*

**Barbidonna®** *see* hyoscyamine, atropine, scopolamine, and phenobarbital *on page 310*

**Barbita®** ***(Discontinued)*** *see page 750*

**Barc™ Liquid [OTC]** *see* pyrethrins *on page 510*

**Baricon®** *see* radiological/contrast media (ionic) *on page 516*

**Baridium®** *see* phenazopyridine *on page 463*

**Barobag®** *see* radiological/contrast media (ionic) *on page 516*

**Baro-CAT®** *see* radiological/contrast media (ionic) *on page 516*

**Baroflave®** *see* radiological/contrast media (ionic) *on page 516*

**Barosperse®** *see* radiological/contrast media (ionic) *on page 516*

**Bar-Test®** *see* radiological/contrast media (ionic) *on page 516*

**Basaljel® [OTC]** *see* aluminum carbonate *on page 25*

## basiliximab (ba si LIKS i mab)

**U.S./Canadian Brand Names** Simulect®

**Therapeutic Category** Immunosuppressant Agent

**Use** Prophylaxis of acute organ rejection in renal transplantation

**Usual Dosage** I.V.:

Children: 12 mg/m$^2$ (maximum: 20 mg) within 2 hours prior to transplant surgery, followed by a second dose of 12 mg/m$^2$ (maximum: 20 mg) 4 days after transplantation

Adults: 20 mg within 2 hours prior to transplant surgery, followed by a second 20 mg dose 4 days after transplantation

**Dosage Forms** Powder for injection: 20 mg

**Baycol®** ***(Discontinued)*** *see page 750*

**Bayer® Aspirin [OTC]** *see* aspirin *on page 55*

**Bayer® Buffered Aspirin [OTC]** *see* aspirin *on page 55*

**Bayer® Low Adult Strength [OTC]** *see* aspirin *on page 55*

**Bayhep B®** *see* hepatitis B immune globulin *on page 292*

**Baypress® *(Discontinued)*** *see page 750*

**Bayrab®** *see* rabies immune globulin (human) *on page 515*

**BayRho-D®** *see* $Rh_0$(D) immune globulin (intramuscular) *on page 523*

**BayTet™** *see* tetanus immune globulin (human) *on page 577*

**B-Caro-T®** *see* beta-carotene *on page 76*

## BCG vaccine (bee see jee vak SEEN)

**Synonyms** Bacillus Calmette-Guérin (BCG) Live

**U.S./Canadian Brand Names** ImmuCyst® (Can); OncoTICE™ (Can); PACIS™ (Can); TheraCys®; TICE® BCG

**Therapeutic Category** Biological Response Modulator

**Use** BCG vaccine is no longer recommended for adults at high risk for tuberculosis in the United States. BCG vaccination may be considered for infants and children who are skin test-negative to 5 tuberculin units of tuberculin and who cannot be given isoniazid preventive therapy but have close contact with untreated or ineffectively treated active tuberculosis patients or who belong to groups which other control measures have not been successful.

In the United States, tuberculosis control efforts are directed toward early identification, treatment of cases, and preventive therapy with isoniazid.

**Usual Dosage** Intravesical treatment and prophylaxis for carcinoma *in situ* of the urinary bladder: Begin between 7-14 days after biopsy or transurethral resection. Administer a dose of 3 vials of BCG live intravesically under aseptic conditions once weekly for 6 weeks (induction therapy). Each dose (3 reconstituted vials) is further diluted in an additional 50 mL sterile, preservative free saline for a total of 53 mL. A urethral catheter is inserted into the bladder under aseptic conditions, the bladder is drained, and then the 53 mL suspension is instilled slowly by gravity, following which the catheter is withdrawn. If the bladder catheterization has been traumatic, BCG live should not be administered, and there must be a treatment delay of at least 1 week. Resume subsequent treatment; follow the induction therapy by one treatment administered 3, 6, 12, 18 and 24 months following the initial treatment.

**Dosage Forms** Freeze-dried suspension for reconstitution
Injection: 50 mg (2 mL)
Injection, intravesical: 27 mg (3 vials)

**BCNU** *see* carmustine *on page 110*

**B-D Glucose® [OTC]** *see* glucose (instant) *on page 276*

## becaplermin (be KAP ler min)

**U.S./Canadian Brand Names** Regranex®

**Therapeutic Category** Topical Skin Product

**Use** Treatment of diabetic ulcers that occur on the lower limbs and feet

**Usual Dosage** Adults: Topical: Apply once daily; applied with a cotton swab or similar tool, as a coating over the ulcer

**Dosage Forms** Gel, topical: 0.01%

**Because® [OTC]** *see* nonoxynol 9 *on page 424*

**Beclodisk® (Can)** *see* beclomethasone *on this page*

**Becloforte® (Can)** *see* beclomethasone *on this page*

## beclomethasone (be kloe METH a sone)

**U.S./Canadian Brand Names** Alti-Beclomethasone (Can); Apo®-Beclomethasone (Can); Beclodisk® (Can); Becloforte® (Can); Beclovent® Oral Inhaler; Beconase AQ®

Nasal Inhaler; Beconase® Nasal Inhaler; Gen-Beclo (Can); Nu-Beclomethasone (Can); Propaderm® (Can); QVAR™; Rivanase AQ (Can); Vancenase® AQ 84 mcg; Vancenase® AQ Inhaler; Vancenase® Nasal Inhaler; Vanceril® 84 mcg Double Strength; Vanceril® Oral Inhaler

**Therapeutic Category** Adrenal Corticosteroid

**Use**

Oral inhalation: Treatment of bronchial asthma in patients who require chronic administration of corticosteroids

Nasal aerosol: Symptomatic treatment of seasonal or perennial rhinitis and nasal polyposis

**Usual Dosage**

Inhalation:

Children 6-12 years: 1-2 inhalations 3-4 times/day, not to exceed 10 inhalations/day

Adults: 2-4 inhalations twice daily, not to exceed 20 inhalations/day

Aerosol inhalation (nasal):

Children 6-12 years: 1 spray each nostril 3 times/day

Adults: 2-4 sprays each nostril twice daily

Aqueous inhalation (nasal): 1-2 sprays each nostril twice daily

**Dosage Forms**

Aerosol for oral inhalation, as dipropionate:

Beclovent®, Vanceril®: 42 mcg/inhalation [200 metered doses] (16.8 g)

QVAR™: 40 mcg/inhalation [100 metered doses] (7.3 g); 80 mcg/inhalation [100 metered doses] (7.3 g)

Vanceril® Double Strength: 84 mcg/inhalation [40 metered doses] (5.4 g), 84 mcg/inhalation [120 metered doses] (12.2 g)

Aerosol, intranasal, as dipropionate (Beconase®, Vancenase®): 42 mcg/inhalation: [80 metered doses] (6.7 g); [200 metered doses] (16.8 g)

Suspension, intranasal, aqueous, as dipropionate [spray]:

Beconase® AQ, Vancenase® AQ 0.042%: 42 mcg/inhalation [≥200 metered doses] (25 g)

Vancenase® AQ 0.084%: 84 mcg per inhalation [120 actuations] (19 g)

**Beclovent® Oral Inhaler** *see* beclomethasone *on previous page*

**Becomject-100®** ***(Discontinued)*** *see page 750*

**Beconase AQ® Nasal Inhaler** *see* beclomethasone *on previous page*

**Beconase® Nasal Inhaler** *see* beclomethasone *on previous page*

**Becotin® Pulvules®** *see* vitamin (multiple/oral) *on page 632*

**Beepen-VK®** ***(Discontinued)*** *see page 750*

**Beesix®** ***(Discontinued)*** *see page 750*

**Belix® Oral [OTC]** *see* diphenhydramine *on page 191*

## belladonna (bel a DON a)

**Therapeutic Category** Anticholinergic Agent

**Use** Decrease gastrointestinal activity in functional bowel disorders and to delay gastric emptying as well as decrease gastric secretion

**Usual Dosage** Tincture: Oral:

Children: 0.03 mL/kg 3 times/day

Adults: 0.6-1 mL 3-4 times/day

**Dosage Forms** Tincture: Belladonna alkaloids (principally hyoscyamine and atropine) 0.3 mg/mL with alcohol 65% to 70% (120 mL, 480 mL, 3780 mL)

## belladonna and opium (bel a DON a & OH pee um)

**U.S./Canadian Brand Names** B&O Supprettes®

**Therapeutic Category** Analgesic, Narcotic

**Controlled Substance** C-II

(Continued)

## belladonna and opium *(Continued)*

**Use** Relief of moderate to severe pain associated with rectal or bladder tenesmus that may occur in postoperative states and neoplastic situations; pain associated with ureteral spasms not responsive to non-narcotic analgesics and to space intervals between injections of opiates

**Usual Dosage** Rectal:

Children: Dose not established

Adults: 1 suppository 1-2 times/day, up to 4 doses/day

**Dosage Forms** Suppository:

#15 A: Belladonna extract 15 mg and opium 30 mg

#16 A: Belladonna extract 15 mg and opium 60 mg

## belladonna, phenobarbital, and ergotamine tartrate

(bel a DON a, fee noe BAR bi tal, & er GOT a meen TAR trate)

**U.S./Canadian Brand Names** Bellergal-S®; Bel-Phen-Ergot S®

**Therapeutic Category** Ergot Alkaloid and Derivative

**Use** Management and treatment of menopausal disorders, gastrointestinal disorders and recurrent throbbing headache

**Usual Dosage** Oral: 1 tablet each morning and evening

**Dosage Forms** Tablet, sustained release: l-alkaloids of belladonna 0.2 mg, phenobarbital 40 mg, and ergotamine tartrate 0.6 mg

**Bellafoline® *(Discontinued)*** *see page 750*

**Bellatal®** *see* hyoscyamine, atropine, scopolamine, and phenobarbital *on page 310*

**Bellergal-S®** *see* belladonna, phenobarbital, and ergotamine tartrate *on this page*

**Bel-Phen-Ergot S®** *see* belladonna, phenobarbital, and ergotamine tartrate *on this page*

**Bemote® *(Discontinued)*** *see page 750*

**Bena-D® *(Discontinued)*** *see page 750*

**Benadryl® 50 mg Capsule *(Discontinued)*** *see page 750*

**Benadryl® Cold/Flu *(Discontinued)*** *see page 750*

**Benadryl® Decongestant Allergy Tablet [OTC]** *see* diphenhydramine and pseudoephedrine *on page 191*

**Benadryl® Injection** *see* diphenhydramine *on page 191*

**Benadryl® Oral [OTC]** *see* diphenhydramine *on page 191*

**Benadryl® Topical** *see* diphenhydramine *on page 191*

**Benahist® Injection *(Discontinued)*** *see page 750*

**Ben-Allergin-50® Injection** *see* diphenhydramine *on page 191*

## benazepril (ben AY ze pril)

**U.S./Canadian Brand Names** Lotensin®

**Therapeutic Category** Angiotensin-Converting Enzyme (ACE) Inhibitor

**Use** Treatment of hypertension, either alone or in combination with other antihypertensive agents

**Usual Dosage** Adults: Oral: 20-40 mg/day as a single dose or 2 divided doses

**Dosage Forms** Tablet, as hydrochloride: 5 mg, 10 mg, 20 mg, 40 mg

## benazepril and hydrochlorothiazide

(ben AY ze pril & hye droe klor oh THYE a zide)

**U.S./Canadian Brand Names** Lotensin® HCT

**Therapeutic Category** Antihypertensive Agent, Combination

**Use** Treatment of hypertension

**Usual Dosage** Dose is individualized

**Dosage Forms** Tablet: Benazepril 5 mg and hydrochlorothiazide 6.25 mg; benazepril 10 mg and hydrochlorothiazide 12.5 mg; benazepril 20 mg and hydrochlorothiazide 12.5 mg; benazepril 20 mg and hydrochlorothiazide 25 mg

## bendroflumethiazide (ben droe floo meth EYE a zide)

**U.S./Canadian Brand Names** Naturetin®

**Therapeutic Category** Diuretic, Thiazide

**Use** Management of mild to moderate hypertension, edema associated with congestive heart failure, pregnancy, or nephrotic syndrome; reportedly does not alter serum electrolyte concentrations appreciably at recommended doses

**Usual Dosage** Oral:

Children: Initial: 0.1-0.4 mg/kg in 1-2 doses; maintenance dose: 0.05-0.1 mg/kg/day in 1-2 doses

Adults: 2.5-20 mg/day or twice daily in divided doses

**Dosage Forms** Tablet: 5 mg, 10 mg

**BeneFix™** *see* factor IX complex (human) *on page 238*

**Benoject® *(Discontinued)*** *see page 750*

**Benoquin®** *see* monobenzone *on page 399*

**Benoxyl®** *see* benzoyl peroxide *on page 74*

## bentoquatam (ben to KWA tam)

**U.S./Canadian Brand Names** IvyBlock®

**Therapeutic Category** Protectant, Topical

**Use** To protect the skin from rash due to exposure to poison sumac, poison ivy or poison oak

**Usual Dosage** Topical: Apply to exposed skin at least 15 minutes before potential contact and reapply every 4 hours

**Dosage Forms** Lotion: 5% (120 mL)

**Bentyl® Hydrochloride Injection** *see* dicyclomine *on page 183*

**Bentyl® Hydrochloride Oral** *see* dicyclomine *on page 183*

**Bentylol® (Can)** *see* dicyclomine *on page 183*

**Benuryl™ (Can)** *see* probenecid *on page 496*

**Benylin® Codeine (Can)** *see* guaifenesin, pseudoephedrine, and codeine *on page 284*

**Benylin® Cough Syrup [OTC]** *see* diphenhydramine *on page 191*

**Benylin DM® [OTC]** *see* dextromethorphan *on page 178*

**Benylin DM-D** *see* pseudoephedrine and dextromethorphan *on page 508*

**Benylin® DM-D-E (Can)** *see* guaifenesin, pseudoephedrine, and dextromethorphan *on page 285*

**Benylin® DM-E (Can)** *see* guaifenesin and dextromethorphan *on page 282*

**Benylin-E (Can)** *see* guaifenesin *on page 281*

**Benylin® Expectorant [OTC]** *see* guaifenesin and dextromethorphan *on page 282*

**Benylin® Pediatric [OTC]** *see* dextromethorphan *on page 178*

**Benza® [OTC]** *see* benzalkonium chloride *on next page*

**Benzac AC® Gel** *see* benzoyl peroxide *on page 74*

**Benzac AC® Wash** *see* benzoyl peroxide *on page 74*

**BenzaClin™** *see* clindamycin and benzoyl peroxide *on page 143*

**Benzacot®** *see* trimethobenzamide *on page 607*

**Benzac W® Gel** *see* benzoyl peroxide *on page 74*

**Benzac W® Wash** *see* benzoyl peroxide *on page 74*

**Benzagel-5®** *see* benzoyl peroxide *on page 74*

**Benzagel-10®** *see* benzoyl peroxide *on page 74*

**Benzagel® Wash** *see* benzoyl peroxide *on page 74*

## benzalkonium chloride (benz al KOE nee um KLOR ide)

**Synonyms** BAC

**U.S./Canadian Brand Names** Benza® [OTC]; Ony-Clear® [OTC]; Zephiran® [OTC]

**Therapeutic Category** Antibacterial, Topical

**Use** Surface antiseptic and germicidal preservative

**Usual Dosage** Thoroughly rinse anionic detergents and soaps from the skin or other areas prior to use of solutions because they reduce the antibacterial activity of BAC; to protect metal instruments stored in BAC solution, add crushed Anti-Rust Tablets, 4 tablets per quart, to antiseptic solution, change solution at least once weekly; not to be used for storage of aluminum or zinc instruments, instruments with lenses fastened by cement, lacquered catheters or some synthetic rubber goods

**Dosage Forms**

Concentrate, topical: 17% (500 mL, 4000 mL)
Solution, aqueous: 1:750 (60 mL, 120 mL, 240 mL)
Solution, topical: 1% (30 mL)
Tincture: 1:750 (30 mL, 960 mL)
Tincture, spray: 1:750 (30 g, 180 g)
Tissue: 1:750 (packets)

**Benzamycin®** *see* erythromycin and benzoyl peroxide *on page 221*

**Benzashave® Cream** *see* benzoyl peroxide *on page 74*

**benzathine benzylpenicillin** *see* penicillin G benzathine *on page 455*

**benzathine penicillin G** *see* penicillin G benzathine *on page 455*

**benzazoline** *see* tolazoline *on page 594*

**Benzedrex® [OTC]** *see* propylhexedrine *on page 505*

**benzene hexachloride** *see* lindane *on page 350*

**benzhexol** *see* trihexyphenidyl *on page 606*

## benzocaine (BEN zoe kane)

**Synonyms** ethyl aminobenzoate

**U.S./Canadian Brand Names** Americaine® [OTC]; Anbesol® [OTC]; Anbesol® Baby (Can); Anbesol® Maximum Strength [OTC]; Babee® Teething® [OTC]; Benzocol® [OTC]; Benzodent® [OTC]; Chiggertox® [OTC]; Cylex® [OTC]; Dermoplast® [OTC]; Foille® [OTC]; Foille® Medicated First Aid [OTC]; Hurricaine®; Lanacane® [OTC]; Maximum Strength Anbesol® [OTC]; Maximum Strength Orajel® [OTC]; Mycinettes® [OTC]; Numzitdent® [OTC]; Numzit Teething® [OTC]; Orabase®-B [OTC]; Orabase®-O [OTC]; Orajel® Brace-Aid Oral Anesthetic [OTC]; Orajel® Maximum Strength [OTC]; Orajel® Mouth-Aid [OTC]; Orasept® [OTC]; Orasol® [OTC]; Rhulicaine® [OTC]; Rid-A-Pain® Dental [OTC]; Slim-Mint® [OTC]; Solarcaine® [OTC]; Spec-T® [OTC]; Tanac® [OTC]; Trocaine® [OTC]; Unguentine® [OTC]; Vicks® Children's Chloraseptic® [OTC]; Vicks® Chloraseptic® Sore Throat [OTC]; Zilactin®-B Medicated [OTC]

**Therapeutic Category** Local Anesthetic

**Use** Temporary relief of pain associated with pruritic dermatosis, pruritus, minor burns, toothache, minor sore throat pain, canker sores, hemorrhoids, rectal fissures; anesthetic lubricant for passage of catheters and endoscopic tubes

**Usual Dosage**

Children and Adults:

Mucous membranes: Dosage varies depending on area to be anesthetized and vascularity of tissues

Oral mouth/throat preparations: Do not administer for >2 days or in children <2 years of age, unless directed by a physician; refer to specific package labeling
Topical: Apply to affected area as needed
Adults: Nonprescription diet aid: 6-15 mg just prior to food consumption, not to exceed 45 mg/day

**Dosage Forms**
Mouth/throat preparations:
Cream: 5% (10 g)
Gel: 6.3% (7.5 g); 7.5% (7.2 g, 9.45 g, 14.1 g); 10% (6 g, 9.45 g, 10 g, 15 g); 15% (10.5 g); 20% (9.45 g, 14.1 g)
Liquid: (3.7 mL); 5% (8.8 mL); 6.3% (9 mL, 22 mL, 14.79 mL); 10% (13 mL); 20% (13.3 mL)
Lotion: 0.2% (15 mL); 2.5% (15 mL)
Lozenges: 5 mg, 6 mg, 10 mg, 15 mg
Ointment: 20% (30 g)
Paste: 20% (5 g, 15 g)
Nonprescription diet aid:
Candy: 6 mg
Gum: 6 mg
Topical for mucous membranes:
Gel: 6% (7.5 g); 20% (2.5 g, 3.75 g, 7.5 g, 30 g)
Liquid: 20% (3.75 mL, 9 mL, 13.3 mL, 30 mL)
Topical for skin disorders:
Aerosol, external use: 5% (92 mL, 105 g); 20% (82.5 mL, 90 mL, 92 mL, 150 mL)
Cream: (30 g, 60 g); 5% (30 g, 1 lb); 6% (28.4 g)
Lotion: (120 mL); 8% (90 mL)
Ointment: 5% (3.5 g, 28 g)
Spray: 5% (97.5 mL); 20% (20 g, 60 g, 120 g, 13.3 mL, 120 mL)

## benzocaine, butyl aminobenzoate, tetracaine, and benzalkonium chloride

(BEN zoe kane, BYOO til a meen oh BENZ oh ate, TET ra kane, & benz al KOE nee um KLOR ide)

**U.S./Canadian Brand Names** Cetacaine®

**Therapeutic Category** Local Anesthetic

**Use** Topical anesthetic to control pain or gagging

**Usual Dosage** Topical: Apply to affected area for approximately 1 second or less

**Dosage Forms** Aerosol: Benzocaine 14%, butyl aminobenzoate 2%, tetracaine 2%, and benzalkonium chloride 0.5% (56 g)

## benzocaine, gelatin, pectin, and sodium carboxymethylcellulose

(BEN zoe kane, JEL a tin, PEK tin, & SOW dee um kar box ee meth il SEL yoo lose)

**U.S./Canadian Brand Names** Orabase® With Benzocaine [OTC]

**Therapeutic Category** Local Anesthetic

**Use** Topical anesthetic and emollient for oral lesions

**Usual Dosage** Topical: Apply 2-4 times/day

**Dosage Forms** Paste: Benzocaine 20%, gelatin, pectin, and sodium carboxymethylcellulose (15 g, 5 g)

**Benzocol® [OTC]** *see* benzocaine *on previous page*

**Benzodent® [OTC]** *see* benzocaine *on previous page*

## benzoic acid and salicylic acid (ben ZOE ik AS id & sal i SIL ik AS id)

**U.S./Canadian Brand Names** Whitfield's Ointment [OTC]

**Therapeutic Category** Antifungal Agent

**Use** Treatment of athlete's foot and ringworm of the scalp

(Continued)

## benzoic acid and salicylic acid *(Continued)*

**Usual Dosage** Topical: Apply 1-4 times/day

**Dosage Forms**

Lotion, topical:

Full strength: Benzoic acid 12% and salicylic acid 6% with isopropyl alcohol 70% (240 mL)

Half strength: Benzoic acid 6% and salicylic acid 3% with isopropyl alcohol 70% (240 mL)

Ointment, topical: Benzoic acid 12% and salicylic acid 6% in anhydrous lanolin and petrolatum (30 g, 454 g)

## benzoin (BEN zoyn)

**Synonyms** gum benjamin

**U.S./Canadian Brand Names** AeroZoin® [OTC]; TinBen® [OTC]; TinCoBen® [OTC]

**Therapeutic Category** Pharmaceutical Aid; Protectant, Topical

**Use** Protective application for irritations of the skin; sometimes used in boiling water as steam inhalants for their expectorant and soothing action

**Usual Dosage** Topical: Apply 1-2 times/day

**Dosage Forms**

Spray, as compound tincture: 40% (105 mL)

Tincture: 79% (480 mL)

Tincture, as compound tincture: 20% (60 mL); 25% (120 mL)

## benzonatate (ben ZOE na tate)

**U.S./Canadian Brand Names** Tessalon® Perles

**Therapeutic Category** Antitussive

**Use** Symptomatic relief of nonproductive cough

**Usual Dosage** Oral:

Children <10 years: 8 mg/kg in 3-6 divided doses

Children >10 years and Adults: 100 mg 3 times/day up to 600 mg/day

**Dosage Forms** Capsule: 100 mg, 200 mg

## benzoyl peroxide (BEN zoe il peer OKS ide)

**U.S./Canadian Brand Names** Acetoxyl (Can); Acne-5®; Acne-10®; Acne-Aid®; Benoxyl®; Benzac AC® Gel; Benzac AC® Wash; Benzac W® Gel; Benzac W® Wash; Benzagel-5®; Benzagel-10®; Benzagel® Wash; Benzashave® Cream; Brevoxyl-4®; Brevoxyl-8®; Clearplex®; Clinac®; Del-Aqua-5® Gel; Del Aqua-10® Gel; Desquam-E™ Gel; Desquam-X® Gel; Desquam-X® Wash; Exact® Cream [OTC]; Fostex® 10% BPO Gel [OTC]; Fostex® 10% Wash [OTC]; $H_2$Oxyl (Can); Loroxide® [OTC]; Neutrogena® Acne Mask [OTC]; Neutrogena® On-The-Spot [OTC]; Oxy-10® Balance Spot Treatment [OTC]; PanOxyl®-AQ 2.5; PanOxyl®-AQ 5; PanOxyl®-AQ 10; PanOxyl® Bar 5 [OTC]; PanOxyl® Bar 10 [OTC]; Seba-Gel®; Solugel® (Can); Triaz®; ZapZyt® [OTC]

**Therapeutic Category** Acne Products

**Use** Adjunctive treatment of mild to moderate acne vulgaris

**Usual Dosage** Children and Adults:

Cleansers: Wash once or twice daily; control amount of drying or peeling by modifying dose frequency or concentration

Topical: Apply sparingly once daily; gradually increase to 2-3 times/day if needed. If excessive dryness or peeling occurs, reduce dose frequency or concentration; if excessive stinging or burning occurs, remove with mild soap and water; resume use the next day.

**Dosage Forms**

Bar: 5% (113 g); 10% (106 g, 113 g)

Cream: 5% (18 g, 113.4 g); 10% (18 g, 28 g, 113.4 g)

Gel: 2.5% (30 g, 42.5 g, 45 g, 57 g, 60 g, 90 g, 113 g); 5% (42.5 g, 45 g, 60 g, 80 g, 90 g, 113.4 g); 10% (30 g, 42.5 g, 45 g, 56.7 g, 60 g, 90 g, 113.4 g, 120 g); 20% (30 g, 60 g)

Liquid: 5% (120 mL, 150 mL, 240 mL); 10% (120 mL, 150 mL, 240 mL)
Lotion: 5% (25 mL, 30 mL); 5.5% (25 mL); 10% (12 mL, 29 mL, 30 mL, 60 mL)
Mask: 5% (30 mL, 60 mL, 60 g)

## benzoyl peroxide and hydrocortisone

(BEN zoe il peer OKS ide & hye droe KOR ti sone)

**U.S./Canadian Brand Names** Vanoxide-HC®

**Therapeutic Category** Acne Products

**Use** Treatment of acne vulgaris and oily skin

**Usual Dosage** Topical: Shake well; apply thin film 1-3 times/day, gently massage into skin

**Dosage Forms** Lotion: Benzoyl peroxide 5% and hydrocortisone acetate 0.5% (25 mL)

## benzphetamine (benz FET a meen)

**U.S./Canadian Brand Names** Didrex®

**Therapeutic Category** Anorexiant

**Controlled Substance** C-III

**Use** Short-term adjunct in exogenous obesity

**Usual Dosage** Adults: Oral: 25-50 mg 2-3 times/day, preferably twice daily, midmorning and midafternoon

**Dosage Forms** Tablet, as hydrochloride: 25 mg, 50 mg

## benztropine (BENZ troe peen)

**U.S./Canadian Brand Names** Apo®-Benztropine (Can); Cogentin®

**Therapeutic Category** Anticholinergic Agent; Anti-Parkinson's Agent

**Use** Adjunctive treatment of parkinsonism; also used in treatment of drug-induced extrapyramidal effects (except tardive dyskinesia) and acute dystonic reactions

**Usual Dosage** Titrate dose in 0.5 mg increments at 5- to 6-day intervals

Extrapyramidal reaction, drug induced: Oral, I.M., I.V.:
- Children >3 years: 0.02-0.05 mg/kg/dose 1-2 times/day
- Adults: 1-4 mg/dose 1-2 times/day

Parkinsonism: Oral: 0.5-6 mg/day in 1-2 divided doses; if one dose is greater, administer at bedtime

**Dosage Forms**

Injection, as mesylate: 1 mg/mL (2 mL)
Tablet, as mesylate: 0.5 mg, 1 mg, 2 mg

## benzydamine *(Canada only)* (ben ZID a meen)

**U.S./Canadian Brand Names** Alti-Benzydamine (Can); Apo®-Benzydamine (Can); Novo-Benzydamine (Can); PMS-Benzydamine (Can); Sun-Benz (Can); Tantum™ (Can)

**Therapeutic Category** Analgesic, Topical

**Use** Local analgesic

**Dosage Forms** Solution: 0.15% (100 mL, 250 mL)

**benzylpenicillin** *see* penicillin G (parenteral/aqueous) *on page 456*

**benzylpenicillin benzathine** *see* penicillin G benzathine *on page 455*

## benzylpenicilloyl-polylysine (BEN zil pen i SIL oyl-pol i LIE seen)

**Synonyms** penicilloyl-polylysine; PPL

**U.S./Canadian Brand Names** Pre-Pen®

**Therapeutic Category** Diagnostic Agent

**Use** As an adjunct in assessing the risk of administering penicillin (penicillin or benzylpenicillin) in patients with a history of clinical penicillin hypersensitivity

**Usual Dosage**

Use scratch technique with a 20-gauge needle to make 3-5 mm scratch on epidermis, apply a small drop of solution to scratch, rub in gently with applicator or toothpick

(Continued)

## benzylpenicilloyl-polylysine *(Continued)*

A positive reaction consists of a pale wheal surrounding the scratch site which develops within 10 minutes and ranges from 5-15 mm or more in diameter

If the scratch test is negative an intradermal test may be performed

Intradermal test: Use intradermal test with a tuberculin syringe with a 26- to 30-gauge short bevel needle; a dose of 0.01-0.02 mL is injected intradermally. A control of 0.9% sodium chloride should be injected at least 1½" from the PPL test site. Most skin responses to the intradermal test will develop within 5-15 minutes.

(-) = no reaction or increase in size compared to control

(±) = wheal slightly larger with or without erythematous flare and larger than control site

(+) = itching and increase in size of original bleb may exceed 20 mm in diameter

**Dosage Forms** Solution: 0.25 mL

## bepridil (BE pri dil)

**U.S./Canadian Brand Names** Vascor®

**Therapeutic Category** Calcium Channel Blocker

**Use** Treatment of chronic stable angina; only approved indication is hypertension, but may be used for congestive heart failure; doses should not be adjusted for at least 10 days after beginning therapy

**Usual Dosage** Adults: Oral: Initial: 200 mg/day, then adjust dose until optimal response is achieved; maximum daily dose: 400 mg

**Dosage Forms** Tablet, as hydrochloride: 200 mg, 300 mg, 400 mg

## beractant (ber AKT ant)

**Synonyms** bovine lung surfactant; natural lung surfactant

**U.S./Canadian Brand Names** Survanta®

**Therapeutic Category** Lung Surfactant

**Use** Prevention and treatment of respiratory distress syndrome (RDS) in premature infants

Prophylactic therapy: Infants with body weight <1250 g who are at risk for developing or with evidence of surfactant deficiency

Rescue therapy: Treatment of infants with RDS confirmed by x-ray and requiring mechanical ventilation

**Usual Dosage** Intratracheal:

Prophylactic treatment: Administer 4 mL/kg as soon as possible; as many as 4 doses may be administered during the first 48 hours of life, no more frequently than 6 hours apart. The need for additional doses is determined by evidence of continuing respiratory distress; if the infant is still intubated and requiring at least 30% inspired oxygen to maintain a $PaO_2 \leq 80$ torr.

Rescue treatment: Administer 4 mL/kg as soon as the diagnosis of RDS is made

**Dosage Forms** Suspension: 200 mg (4 mL, 8 mL)

**Berocca®** *see* vitamin B complex with vitamin C and folic acid *on page 631*

**Berotec® (Can)** *see* fenoterol *(Canada only)* *on page 243*

**Berubigen®** *see* cyanocobalamin *on page 158*

**Beta-2® *(Discontinued)*** *see page 750*

## beta-carotene (BAY tah-KARE oh teen)

**U.S./Canadian Brand Names** A-Caro-25®; B-Caro-T®; Biotene®; Caroguard®; Eye Bright®; Lumitene™

**Therapeutic Category** Vitamin, Fat Soluble

**Use** Reduce the severity of photosensitivity reactions in patients with erythropoietic protoporphyria (EPP)

**Usual Dosage** Oral:

Children <14 years: 30-150 mg/day

Adults: 30-300 mg/day

**Dosage Forms** Capsule: 3 mg, 6 mg, 15 mg, 30 mg, 60 mg

**Betachron® *(Discontinued)*** *see page 750*

**Betadine® [OTC]** *see* povidone-iodine *on page 489*

**Betadine® 5% Sterile Ophthalmic Prep Solution** *see* povidone-iodine *on page 489*

**Betadine® First Aid Antibiotics + Moisturizer [OTC]** *see* bacitracin and polymyxin B *on page 64*

**9-beta-D-ribofuranosyladenine** *see* adenosine *on page 13*

**Betagan® [OTC]** *see* povidone-iodine *on page 489*

**Betagan® Liquifilm® Ophthalmic** *see* levobunolol *on page 344*

## betahistine *(Canada only)* (bay ta HISS teen)

**U.S./Canadian Brand Names** Serc® (Can)

**Therapeutic Category** Antihistamine

**Use** May be of value in the treatment of Ménière's disease

**Usual Dosage** Adult: Oral: 4-8 mg 3 times/day

**Dosage Forms** Tablet, as hydrochloride: 4 mg

## betaine anhydrous (BAY tayne an HY drus)

**U.S./Canadian Brand Names** Cystadane®

**Therapeutic Category** Urinary Tract Product

**Use** Treatment of homocystinuria

**Usual Dosage** Oral: 6 g/day, usually given in two 3 g doses

**Dosage Forms** Powder: 1 g/1.7 mL (180 g)

**Betalene® Topical** *see* betamethasone (topical) *on next page*

**Betalin® S *(Discontinued)*** *see page 750*

**Betaloc® (Can)** *see* metoprolol *on page 388*

## betamethasone and clotrimazole

(bay ta METH a sone & kloe TRIM a zole)

**U.S./Canadian Brand Names** Lotriderm® (Can); Lotrisone®

**Therapeutic Category** Antifungal/Corticosteroid

**Use** Topical treatment of various dermal fungal infections

**Usual Dosage** Topical: Apply twice daily

**Dosage Forms** Cream: Betamethasone dipropionate 0.05% and clotrimazole 1% (15 g, 45 g)

## betamethasone (systemic) (bay ta METH a sone sis TEM ik)

**U.S./Canadian Brand Names** Celestone® Oral; Celestone® Phosphate Injection; Celestone® Soluspan®; Cel-U-Jec® Injection

**Therapeutic Category** Adrenal Corticosteroid

**Use** Anti-inflammatory; immunosuppressant agent; corticosteroid replacement therapy

**Usual Dosage** Children and Adults:

I.M.: Betamethasone sodium phosphate and betamethasone acetate: 0.5-9 mg/day ($^1/_3$ to $^1/_2$ of oral dose)

Intrabursal, intra-articular: 0.5-2 mL

Oral: 0.6-7.2 mg/day

**Dosage Forms**

Base (Celestone®), Oral:

Syrup: 0.6 mg/5 mL (118 mL)

Tablet: 0.6 mg

(Continued)

## betamethasone (systemic) *(Continued)*

Injection: Sodium phosphate (Celestone Phosphate®, Cel-U-Jec®): 4 mg betamethasone phosphate/mL (equivalent to 3 mg betamethasone/mL) (5 mL)
Injection, suspension: Sodium phosphate and acetate (Celestone® Soluspan®): 6 mg/mL (3 mg of betamethasone sodium phosphate and 3 mg of betamethasone acetate per mL) (5 mL)

## betamethasone (topical) (bay ta METH a sone TOP i kal)

**Synonyms** flubenisolone

**U.S./Canadian Brand Names** Alphatrex® Topical; Betalene® Topical; Betatrex® Topical; Beta-Val® Cream; Beta-Val® Lotion; Diprolene® AF Topical; Diprolene® Topical; Diprosone® Topical; Maxivate® Topical; Psorion® Topical; Teladar® Topical; Valisone® Topical

**Therapeutic Category** Corticosteroid, Topical

**Use** Inflammatory dermatoses such as psoriasis, seborrheic or atopic dermatitis, neurodermatitis, inflammatory phase of xerosis, late phase of allergic dermatitis or irritant dermatitis

**Usual Dosage** Topical: Adults: Apply thin film 2-4 times/day. Therapy should be discontinued when control is achieved. If no improvement is seen, reassessment of diagnosis may be necessary.

**Dosage Forms**

Betamethasone dipropionate:
- Aerosol: 0.1% (85 g)
- Cream: 0.05% (15 g, 45 g)
- Lotion: 0.05% (20 mL, 30 mL, 60 mL)
- Ointment: 0.05% (15 g, 45 g)

Betamethasone dipropionate augmented:
- Cream: 0.05% (15 g, 45 g)
- Gel: 0.05% (15 g, 45 g)
- Lotion: 0.05% (30 mL, 60 mL)
- Ointment, topical: 0.05% (15 g, 45 g)

Betamethasone valerate:
- Cream: 0.01% (15 g, 60 g); 0.1% (15 g, 45 g, 110 g, 430 g)
- Lotion: 0.1% (20 mL, 60 mL)
- Ointment: 0.1% (15 g, 45 g)

**Betapace®** *see* sotalol *on page 555*

**Betapen®-VK *(Discontinued)*** *see page 750*

**Betasept® [OTC]** *see* chlorhexidine gluconate *on page 126*

**Betaseron®** *see* interferon beta-1b *on page 323*

**Betatrex® Topical** *see* betamethasone (topical) *on this page*

**Beta-Val® Cream** *see* betamethasone (topical) *on this page*

**Beta-Val® Lotion** *see* betamethasone (topical) *on this page*

**Beta-Val® Ointment *(Discontinued)*** *see page 750*

**Betaxin® (Can)** *see* thiamine *on page 584*

## betaxolol (be TAKS oh lol)

**U.S./Canadian Brand Names** Betoptic® S Ophthalmic; Kerlone® Oral

**Therapeutic Category** Beta-Adrenergic Blocker

**Use** Treatment of chronic open-angle glaucoma, ocular hypertension; management of hypertension

**Usual Dosage** Adults:

Ophthalmic: Instill 1 drop twice daily

Oral: 10 mg/day; may increase dose to 20 mg/day after 7-14 days if desired response is not achieved; initial dose in elderly patients: 5 mg/day

**Dosage Forms**
Solution, ophthalmic, as hydrochloride: 0.5% (2.5 mL, 5 mL, 10 mL)
Suspension, ophthalmic, as hydrochloride (Betoptic® S): 0.25% (2.5 mL, 5 mL, 10 mL, 15 mL)
Tablet, as hydrochloride (Kerlone®): 10 mg, 20 mg

**Betaxon®** *see* levobetaxolol *on page 344*

## bethanechol (be THAN e kole)

**U.S./Canadian Brand Names** Urecholine®
**Therapeutic Category** Cholinergic Agent
**Use** Treatment of nonobstructive urinary retention and retention due to neurogenic bladder; gastroesophageal reflux
**Usual Dosage**
Children:
Oral:
Abdominal distention or urinary retention: 0.6 mg/kg/day divided 3-4 times/day
Gastroesophageal reflux: 0.1-0.2 mg/kg/dose administered 30 minutes to 1 hour before each meal to a maximum of 4 times/day
S.C.: 0.15-0.2 mg/kg/day divided 3-4 times/day
Adults:
Oral: 10-50 mg 2-4 times/day
S.C.: 2.5-5 mg 3-4 times/day, up to 7.5-10 mg every 4 hours for neurogenic bladder
**Dosage Forms**
Injection, as chloride: 5 mg/mL (1 mL)
Tablet, as chloride: 5 mg, 10 mg, 25 mg, 50 mg

**Betoptic®** ***(Discontinued)*** *see page 750*

**Betoptic® S Ophthalmic** *see* betaxolol *on previous page*

## bexarotene (beks AIR oh teen)

**U.S./Canadian Brand Names** Targretin®
**Therapeutic Category** Retinoic Acid Derivative; Vitamin A Derivative; Vitamin, Fat Soluble
**Use** Treat cutaneous manifestations of cutaneous T-cell lymphoma in patients who are refractory to at least one prior systemic therapy.
**Usual Dosage**
Adult: Oral: 300 mg/m$^2$/day taken as a single daily dose. If there is no tumor response after 8 weeks and the initial dose was well tolerated, then an increase to 400 mg/m$^2$/day can be made with careful monitoring. Maintain as long as the patient is deriving benefit.
If the initial dose is not tolerated, then it may be adjusted to 200 mg/m$^2$/day, then to 100 mg/m$^2$/day or temporarily suspended if necessary to manage toxicity.
**Dosage Forms** Capsule: 75 mg

**Bexophene®** ***(Discontinued)*** *see page 750*

## bezafibrate *(Canada only)* (be za FYE brate)

**U.S./Canadian Brand Names** Bezalip® (Can); PMS-Bezafibrate (Can)
**Therapeutic Category** Antilipemic Agent
**Use** Adjunct to dietary therapy in the management of hyperlipidemias associated with high triglyceride levels (types III, IV, V); primarily lowers triglycerides and very low density lipoprotein
**Usual Dosage** Adult: Oral: 200 mg 3 times/day
**Dosage Forms** Tablet: 200 mg, 400 mg

**Bezalip® (Can)** *see* bezafibrate *(Canada only) on this page*

**Biamine® Injection** ***(Discontinued)*** *see page 750*

**Biavax® II** *see* rubella and mumps vaccines, combined *on page 533*

**Biaxin®** *see* clarithromycin *on page 141*

**Biaxin® XL** *see* clarithromycin *on page 141*

## bicalutamide (bye ka LOO ta mide)

**U.S./Canadian Brand Names** Casodex®

**Therapeutic Category** Androgen

**Use** Combination therapy with a luteinizing hormone-releasing hormone (LHRH) analog for the treatment of advanced prostate cancer

**Usual Dosage** Adults: Oral: 50 mg once daily (morning or evening), with or without food, in combination with a LHRH analog

**Dosage Forms** Tablet: 50 mg

**Bicillin® C-R** *see* penicillin G benzathine and procaine combined *on page 456*

**Bicillin® C-R 900/300** *see* penicillin G benzathine and procaine combined *on page 456*

**Bicillin® L-A** *see* penicillin G benzathine *on page 455*

**BiCNU®** *see* carmustine *on page 110*

**Bilezyme® Tablet *(Discontinued)*** *see page 750*

**Bilopaque®** *see* radiological/contrast media (ionic) *on page 516*

**Biltricide®** *see* praziquantel *on page 491*

## bimatoprost (bi MAT oh prost)

**U.S./Canadian Brand Names** Lumigan™

**Therapeutic Category** Ophthalmic Agent, Miscellaneous

**Use** Reduction of intraocular pressure (IOP) in patients with open-angle glaucoma or ocular hypertension; should be used in patients who are intolerant of other IOP-lowering medications or failed treatment with another IOP-lowering medication

**Usual Dosage** Ophthalmic: Adult: Open-angle glaucoma or ocular hypertension: Instill 1 drop into affected eye(s) once daily in the evening; do not exceed once-daily dosing (may decrease IOP-lowering effect). If used with other topical ophthalmic agents, separate administration by at least 5 minutes.

**Dosage Forms** Solution, ophthalmic: 0.03% [with benzalkonium chloride 0.05 mg] (2.5 mL, 5 mL)

**Biocef®** *see* cephalexin *on page 120*

**Bioclate™** *see* antihemophilic factor (recombinant) *on page 44*

**Biodine *(Discontinued)*** *see page 750*

**Biofed-PE® [OTC]** *see* triprolidine and pseudoephedrine *on page 609*

**Biohist® LA** *see* carbinoxamine and pseudoephedrine *on page 107*

**Biolon®** *see* sodium hyaluronate *on page 550*

**Biomox® *(Discontinued)*** *see page 750*

**Bion® Tears Solution [OTC]** *see* artificial tears *on page 53*

**Bio-Statin®** *see* nystatin *on page 432*

**Biotene®** *see* beta-carotene *on page 76*

**Biozyme-C® *(Discontinued)*** *see page 750*

## biperiden (bye PER i den)

**U.S./Canadian Brand Names** Akineton®

**Therapeutic Category** Anticholinergic Agent; Anti-Parkinson's Agent

**Use** Treatment of all forms of Parkinsonism including drug-induced type (extrapyramidal symptoms)

**Usual Dosage** Adults:
Parkinsonism: Oral: 2 mg 3-4 times/day
Extrapyramidal:
Oral: 2-6 mg 2-3 times/day
I.M., I.V.: 2 mg every 30 minutes up to 4 doses or 8 mg/day

**Dosage Forms**
Injection, as lactate: 5 mg/mL (1 mL)
Tablet, as hydrochloride: 2 mg

**Biphetamine® *(Discontinued)*** *see page 750*

**Biquin Durules® (Can)** *see* quinidine *on page 514*

**Bisac-Evac® [OTC]** *see* bisacodyl *on this page*

## bisacodyl (bis a KOE dil)

**U.S./Canadian Brand Names** Apo®-Bisacodyl (Can); Bisac-Evac® [OTC]; Bisacodyl Uniserts®; Bisco-Lax® [OTC]; Carter's Little Pills® [OTC]; Clysodrast®; Dacodyl® [OTC]; Deficol® [OTC]; Dulcolax® [OTC]; Fleet® Bisacodyl [OTC]; Fleet® Laxative [OTC]

**Therapeutic Category** Laxative

**Use** Treatment of constipation; colonic evacuation prior to procedures or examination

**Usual Dosage**
Children:
Oral: >6 years: 5-10 mg (0.3 mg/kg) at bedtime or before breakfast
Rectal suppository:
<2 years: 5 mg as a single dose
>2 years: 10 mg
Adults:
Oral: 5-15 mg as single dose (up to 30 mg when complete evacuation of bowel is required)
Rectal suppository: 10 mg as single dose
Tannex:
Enema: 2.5 g in 1000 mL warm water
Barium enema: 2.5-5 g in 1000 mL barium suspension
Do not administer >10 g within a 72-hour period

**Dosage Forms**
Enema: 0.333 mg/mL (37 mL)
Powder, as tannex: 2.5 g packets (50 packet/box)
Suppository, rectal: 5 mg, 10 mg
Tablet, enteric coated: 5 mg

**Bisacodyl Uniserts®** *see* bisacodyl *on this page*

**Bisco-Lax® [OTC]** *see* bisacodyl *on this page*

**bishydroxycoumarin** *see* dicumarol *on page 182*

**Bismatrol® [OTC]** *see* bismuth subsalicylate *on this page*

## bismuth subgallate (BIZ muth sub GAL ate)

**U.S./Canadian Brand Names** Devrom® [OTC]

**Therapeutic Category** Gastrointestinal Agent, Miscellaneous

**Use** Symptomatic treatment of mild, nonspecific diarrhea

**Usual Dosage** Oral: 1-2 tablets 3 times/day with meals

**Dosage Forms** Tablet, chewable: 200 mg

## bismuth subsalicylate (BIZ muth sub sa LIS i late)

**Synonyms** pink bismuth

**U.S./Canadian Brand Names** Bismatrol® [OTC]; Diotame® [OTC]; Pepto-Bismol® [OTC]

**Therapeutic Category** Gastrointestinal Agent, Miscellaneous

(Continued)

## bismuth subsalicylate *(Continued)*

**Use** Symptomatic treatment of mild, nonspecific diarrhea including traveler's diarrhea; chronic infantile diarrhea

**Usual Dosage** Oral:

Nonspecific diarrhea:

Children: Up to 8 doses/24 hours:

3-6 years: 1/3 tablet or 5 mL every 30 minutes to 1 hour as needed

6-9 years: 2/3 tablet or 10 mL every 30 minutes to 1 hour as needed

9-12 years: 1 tablet or 15 mL every 30 minutes to 1 hour as needed

Adults: 2 tablets or 30 mL every 30 minutes to 1 hour as needed up to 8 doses/24 hours

Prevention of traveler's diarrhea: 2.1 g/day or 2 tablets 4 times/day before meals and at bedtime

**Dosage Forms**

Caplet, swallowable: 262 mg

Liquid: 262 mg/15 mL (120 mL, 240 mL, 360 mL, 480 mL); 524 mg/15 mL (120 mL, 240 mL, 360 mL)

Tablet, chewable: 262 mg

## bismuth subsalicylate, metronidazole, and tetracycline

(BIZ muth sub sa LIS i late, me troe NI da zole, & tet ra SYE kleen)

**U.S./Canadian Brand Names** Helidac™

**Therapeutic Category** Antidiarrheal

**Use** In combination with an $H_2$ antagonist, used to treat and decrease rate of recurrence of active duodenal ulcer associated with *H. pylori* infection

**Usual Dosage** Adults: Chew 2 bismuth subsalicylate 262.4 mg tablets, swallow 1 metronidazole 250 mg tablet, and swallow 1 tetracycline 500 mg capsule plus an $H_2$ antagonist 4 times/day at meals and bedtime for 14 days; follow with 8 oz of water

**Dosage Forms**

Capsule: Tetracycline: 500 mg

Tablet:

Bismuth subsalicylate: Chewable: 262.4 mg

Metronidazole: 250 mg

## bisoprolol (bis OH proe lol)

**U.S./Canadian Brand Names** Monocor® (Can); Zebeta®

**Therapeutic Category** Beta-Adrenergic Blocker

**Use** Treatment of hypertension, alone or in combination with other agents

**Usual Dosage** Adults: Oral: 5 mg once daily, may be increased to 10 mg, and then up to 20 mg once daily, if necessary

**Dosage Forms** Tablet, as fumarate: 5 mg, 10 mg

## bisoprolol and hydrochlorothiazide

(bis OH proe lol & hye droe klor oh THYE a zide)

**U.S./Canadian Brand Names** Ziac™

**Therapeutic Category** Antihypertensive Agent, Combination

**Use** Treatment of hypertension

**Usual Dosage** Adults: Oral: Dose is individualized, administered once daily

**Dosage Forms** Tablet: Bisoprolol fumarate 2.5 mg and hydrochlorothiazide 6.25 mg; bisoprolol fumarate 5 mg and hydrochlorothiazide 6.25 mg; bisoprolol fumarate 10 mg and hydrochlorothiazide 6.25 mg

**bistropamide** *see* tropicamide *on page 611*

## bitolterol (bye TOLE ter ole)

**U.S./Canadian Brand Names** Tornalate®

**Therapeutic Category** Adrenergic Agonist Agent

**Use** Prevent and treat bronchial asthma and bronchospasm

**Usual Dosage** Children >12 years and Adults:

Bronchospasm: 2 inhalations at an interval of at least 1-3 minutes, followed by a third inhalation if needed

Prevention of bronchospasm: 2 inhalations every 8 hours

**Dosage Forms**

Aerosol, oral, as mesylate: 0.8% [370 mcg/metered spray, 300 inhalations] (15 mL)

Solution, inhalation, as mesylate: 0.2% (10 mL, 30 mL, 60 mL)

## bivalirudin (bye VAL i roo din)

**Synonyms** hirulog

**U.S./Canadian Brand Names** Angiomax™

**Therapeutic Category** Anticoagulant

**Use** Anticoagulant used in conjunction with aspirin for patients with unstable angina undergoing percutaneous transluminal coronary angioplasty (PTCA)

**Usual Dosage** Adults: Anticoagulant in patients with unstable angina undergoing PTCA (treatment should be started just prior to PTCA): I.V.: Initial: Bolus: 1 mg/kg, followed by continuous infusion: 2.5 mg/kg/hour over 4 hours; if needed, infusion may be continued at 0.2 mg/kg/hour for up to 20 hours; patients should also receive aspirin 300-325 mg/day

**Dosage Forms** Powder for injection: 250 mg

**Black Draught® [OTC]** *see* senna *on page 541*

**black widow spider antivenin (*Latrodectus mactans*)** *see* antivenin (*Latrodectus mactans*) *on page 46*

**Blanex® Capsule *(Discontinued)*** *see page 750*

**Blenoxane®** *see* bleomycin *on this page*

## bleomycin (blee oh MYE sin)

**Synonyms** BLM

**U.S./Canadian Brand Names** Blenoxane®

**Therapeutic Category** Antineoplastic Agent

**Use** Palliative treatment of squamous cell carcinoma, testicular carcinoma, germ cell tumors, and the following lymphomas: Hodgkin's, lymphosarcoma and reticulum cell sarcoma; sclerosing agent to control malignant effusions

**Usual Dosage** Refer to individual protocol

Children and Adults:

Test dose for lymphoma patients: I.M., I.V., S.C.: 1-2 units of bleomycin for the first 2 doses; monitor vital signs every 15 minutes; wait a minimum of 1 hour before administering remainder of dose

I.M., I.V., S.C.: 10-20 units/$m^2$ (0.25-0.5 units/kg) 1-2 times/week in combination regimens

I.V. continuous infusion: 15-20 units/$m^2$/day for 4-5 days

Adults: Intracavitary injection for pleural effusion: 15-240 units have been administered

**Dosage Forms** Powder for injection, as sulfate: 15 units

**Bleph®-10** *see* sulfacetamide *on page 562*

**Blephamide® Ophthalmic** *see* sulfacetamide and prednisolone *on page 563*

**Blis-To-Sol® [OTC]** *see* tolnaftate *on page 595*

**BLM** *see* bleomycin *on this page*

**Blocadren® Oral** *see* timolol *on page 591*

**Bluboro® [OTC]** *see* aluminum sulfate and calcium acetate *on page 28*

**Bonamine™ (Can)** *see* meclizine *on page 367*

**Bonefos® (Can)** *see* clodronate disodium *(Canada only) on page 144*

**Bonine® [OTC]** *see* meclizine *on page 367*

**Bontril PDM®** *see* phendimetrazine *on page 463*

**Bontril® Slow-Release** *see* phendimetrazine *on page 463*

## boric acid (BOR ik AS id)

**U.S./Canadian Brand Names** Borofax® Topical [OTC]; Dri-Ear® Otic [OTC]; Swim-Ear® Otic [OTC]

**Therapeutic Category** Pharmaceutical Aid

**Use**

Ophthalmic: Mild antiseptic used for inflamed eyelids

Otic: Prophylaxis of swimmer's ear

Topical ointment: Temporary relief of chapped, chafed, or dry skin, diaper rash, abrasions, minor burns, sunburn, insect bites, and other skin irritations

**Usual Dosage**

Ophthalmic: Apply to lower eyelid 1-2 times/day

Otic: Place 2-4 drops in ears

Topical: Apply as needed

**Dosage Forms**

Ointment:

Ophthalmic: 5% (3.5 g); 10% (3.5 g)

Topical: 5% (52.5 g); 10% (28 g)

Topical (Borofax®): 5% boric acid and lanolin (1¾ oz)

Solution, otic: 2.75% with isopropyl alcohol (30 mL)

**Born Again Super Pain Relieving®** *see* capsaicin *on page 104*

**Borofax® Topical [OTC]** *see* boric acid *on this page*

**Boropak® [OTC]** *see* aluminum sulfate and calcium acetate *on page 28*

**B&O Supprettes®** *see* belladonna and opium *on page 69*

**Botox®** *see* botulinum toxin type A *on this page*

## botulinum toxin type A (BOT yoo lin num TOKS in type aye)

**U.S./Canadian Brand Names** Botox®

**Therapeutic Category** Ophthalmic Agent, Toxin

**Use** Treatment of strabismus and blepharospasm

**Usual Dosage**

Strabismus: 1.25-5 units (0.05-0.15 mL) injected into any one muscle

Subsequent doses for residual/recurrent strabismus: Re-examine patients 7-14 days after each injection to assess the effect of that dose. Subsequent doses for patients experiencing incomplete paralysis of the target may be increased up to twofold the previously administered dose. Maximum recommended dose as a single injection for any one muscle is 25 units.

Blepharospasm: 1.25-2.5 units (0.05-0.10 mL) injected into the orbicularis oculi muscle

Subsequent doses: Each treatment lasts approximately 3 months. At repeat treatment sessions, the dose may be increased up to twofold if the response from the initial treatment is considered insufficient (usually defined as an effect that does not last >2 months). There appears to be little benefit obtainable from injecting >5 units per site. Some tolerance may be found if treatments are administered any more frequently than every 3 months.

The cumulative dose should not exceed 200 units in a 30-day period

**Dosage Forms** Injection: 100 units *Clostridium botulinum* toxin type A

## botulinum toxin type B (BOT yoo lin num TOKS in type bee)

**U.S./Canadian Brand Names** Myobloc®

**Therapeutic Category** Neuromuscular Blocker Agent, Toxin

**Use** Treatment of cervical dystonia (spasmodic torticollis)

**Usual Dosage**

Children: Not established in pediatric patients

Adults: Cervical dystonia: I.M.: Initial: 2500-5000 units divided among the affected muscles in patients **previously treated** with botulinum toxin; initial dose in **previously untreated** patients should be lower. Subsequent dosing should be optimized according to patient's response.

**Dosage Forms** Injection [single-dose vial]: 2500 units (0.5 mL); 5000 units (1 mL); 10,000 units (2 mL)

**bovine lung surfactant** *see* beractant *on page 76*

**Breathe Free® [OTC]** *see* sodium chloride *on page 549*

**Breezee® Mist Antifungal [OTC]** *see* miconazole *on page 390*

**Breonesin® [OTC]** *see* guaifenesin *on page 281*

**Brethaire®** ***(Discontinued)*** *see page 750*

**Brethine®** *see* terbutaline *on page 574*

## bretylium (bre TIL ee um)

**Therapeutic Category** Antiarrhythmic Agent, Class III

**Use** Ventricular tachycardia or ventricular fibrillation; other serious ventricular arrhythmias resistant to lidocaine

**Usual Dosage**

Children:

I.M.: 2-5 mg/kg as a single dose

I.V.: Initial: 5 mg/kg, then attempt electrical defibrillation; repeat with 10 mg/kg if ventricular fibrillation persists

Maintenance dose: I.M., I.V.: 5 mg/kg every 6-8 hours

Adults:

Immediate life-threatening ventricular arrhythmias; ventricular fibrillation; unstable ventricular tachycardia. **Note**: Patients should undergo defibrillation/cardioversion before and after bretylium doses as necessary:

Initial dose: I.V.: 5 mg/kg (undiluted) over 1 minute; if arrhythmia persists, administer 10 mg/kg (undiluted) over 1 minute and repeat as necessary (usually at 15- to 30-minute intervals) up to a total dose of 30 mg/kg

Other life-threatening ventricular arrhythmias:

Initial dose: I.M., I.V.: 5-10 mg/kg, may repeat every 1-2 hours if arrhythmia persist; administer I.V. dose (diluted) over 10-30 minutes

Maintenance dose: I.M.: 5-10 mg/kg every 6-8 hours; I.V. (diluted): 5-10 mg/kg every 6 hours; I.V. infusion (diluted): 1-2 mg/minute (little experience with doses >40 mg/kg/day)

**Dosage Forms**

Injection, as tosylate: 50 mg/mL (10 mL, 20 mL)

Injection, as tosylate, premixed in $D_5W$: 1 mg/mL (500 mL); 2 mg/mL (250 mL); 4 mg/mL (250 mL, 500 mL)

**Bretylol®** ***(Discontinued)*** *see page 750*

**Brevibloc®** *see* esmolol *on page 223*

**Brevicon®** *see* ethinyl estradiol and norethindrone *on page 232*

**Brevital® Sodium** *see* methohexital *on page 380*

**Brevoxyl-4®** *see* benzoyl peroxide *on page 74*

**Brevoxyl-8®** *see* benzoyl peroxide *on page 74*

**Bricanyl®** ***(Discontinued)*** *see page 750*

**Brietal Sodium® (Can)** *see* methohexital *on page 380*

## brimonidine (bri MOE ni deen)

**U.S./Canadian Brand Names** Alphagan®

**Therapeutic Category** $Alpha_2$-Adrenergic Agonist Agent, Ophthalmic

(Continued)

## brimonidine *(Continued)*

**Use** Lowering of intraocular pressure in patients with open-angle glaucoma or ocular hypertension

**Usual Dosage** Adults: Ophthalmic: 1 drop in affected eye(s) 3 times/day (approximately every 8 hours)

**Dosage Forms** Solution, ophthalmic, as tartrate: 0.2% (5 mL, 10 mL)

## brinzolamide (brin ZOH la mide)

**U.S./Canadian Brand Names** Azopt®

**Therapeutic Category** Carbonic Anhydrase Inhibitor

**Use** Lowers intraocular pressure to treat glaucoma in patients with ocular hypertension or open-angle glaucoma

**Usual Dosage** Adults: Ophthalmic: Instill 1 drop in eye(s) 3 times/day

**Dosage Forms** Suspension, ophthalmic: 1% (2.5 mL, 5 mL, 10 mL, 15 mL)

**British anti-lewisite** *see* dimercaprol *on page 189*

**BrodSpec®** *see* tetracycline *on page 579*

**Brofed® [OTC]** *see* brompheniramine and pseudoephedrine *on page 88*

**Bromaline® Elixir *(Discontinued)*** *see page 750*

**Bromanate® DC *(Discontinued)*** *see page 750*

**Bromanate® Elixir *(Discontinued)*** *see page 750*

**Bromanyl® Cough Syrup** *see* bromodiphenhydramine and codeine *on next page*

**Bromarest® [OTC]** *see* brompheniramine *on next page*

**Bromatapp® *(Discontinued)*** *see page 750*

## bromazepam *(Canada only)* (broe MA ze pam)

**U.S./Canadian Brand Names** Alti-Bromazepam (Can); Apo®-Bromazepam (Can); Gen-Bromazepam (Can); Lectopam® (Can); Novo-Bromazepam (Can); Nu-Bromazepam (Can)

**Therapeutic Category** Benzodiazepine; Sedative

**Use** Short-term, symptomatic relief of manifestations of excessive anxiety in patients with anxiety neurosis

**Usual Dosage** Adults: Oral: 6-18 mg/day in equally divided doses. depending on the severity of symptoms and response of the patient

**Dosage Forms** Tablet: 1.5 mg, 3 mg, 6 mg

**Brombay® [OTC]** *see* brompheniramine *on next page*

**Bromfed® [OTC]** *see* brompheniramine and pseudoephedrine *on page 88*

**Bromfed-PD® [OTC]** *see* brompheniramine and pseudoephedrine *on page 88*

**Bromfenex®** *see* brompheniramine and pseudoephedrine *on page 88*

**Bromfenex® PD** *see* brompheniramine and pseudoephedrine *on page 88*

## bromocriptine (broe moe KRIP teen)

**U.S./Canadian Brand Names** Apo®-Bromocriptine (Can); Parlodel®; PMS-Bromocriptine (Can)

**Therapeutic Category** Anti-Parkinson's Agent; Ergot Alkaloid and Derivative

**Use** Treatment of parkinsonism in patients unresponsive or allergic to levodopa; also used in conditions associated with hyperprolactinemia and to suppress lactation

**Usual Dosage** Oral:

Parkinsonism: 1.25 mg twice daily, increased by 2.5 mg/day in 2- to 4-week intervals (usual dose range: 30-90 mg/day in 3 divided doses)

Hyperprolactinemia and postpartum lactation: 2.5 mg 2-3 times/day

**Dosage Forms**
Capsule, as mesylate: 5 mg
Tablet, as mesylate: 2.5 mg

## bromodiphenhydramine and codeine

(brome oh dye fen HYE dra meen & KOE deen)

**U.S./Canadian Brand Names** Ambenyl® Cough Syrup; Amgenal® Cough Syrup; Bromanyl® Cough Syrup; Bromotuss® w/Codeine Cough Syrup

**Therapeutic Category** Antihistamine/Antitussive

**Controlled Substance** C-V

**Use** Relief of upper respiratory symptoms and cough associated with allergies or common cold

**Usual Dosage** Oral: 5-10 mL every 4-6 hours

**Dosage Forms** Liquid: Bromodiphenhydramine hydrochloride 12.5 mg and codeine phosphate 10 mg per 5 mL

**Bromotuss® w/Codeine Cough Syrup** *see* bromodiphenhydramine and codeine *on this page*

**Bromphen® [OTC]** *see* brompheniramine *on this page*

**Bromphen® DC With Codeine *(Discontinued)*** *see page 750*

## brompheniramine (brome fen IR a meen)

**Synonyms** parabromdylamine

**U.S./Canadian Brand Names** Bromarest® [OTC]; Brombay® [OTC]; Bromphen® [OTC]; Brotane® [OTC]; Chlorphed® [OTC]; Cophene-B®; Diamine T.D.® [OTC]; Dimetane® Extentabs® [OTC]; Nasahist B®; ND-Stat®

**Therapeutic Category** Antihistamine

**Use** Perennial and seasonal allergic rhinitis and other allergic symptoms including urticaria

**Usual Dosage**
Oral:
- Children:
  - <6 years: 0.125 mg/kg/dose administered every 6 hours; maximum: 6-8 mg/day
  - 6-12 years: 2-4 mg every 6-8 hours; maximum: 12-16 mg/day
- Adults: 4 mg every 4-6 hours or 8 mg of sustained release form every 8-12 hours or 12 mg of sustained release every 12 hours; maximum: 24 mg/day

I.M., I.V., S.C.:
- Children <12 years: 0.5 mg/kg/24 hours divided every 6-8 hours
- Adults: 5-50 mg every 4-12 hours, maximum: 40 mg/24 hours

**Dosage Forms**
Elixir, as maleate: 2 mg/5 mL with 3% alcohol (120 mL, 480 mL, 4000 mL)
Injection, as maleate: 10 mg/mL (10 mL)
Tablet, as maleate: 4 mg, 8 mg, 12 mg
Tablet, sustained release, as maleate: 8 mg, 12 mg

## brompheniramine and phenylephrine

(brome fen IR a meen & fen il EF rin)

**U.S./Canadian Brand Names** Dimetane® Decongestant Elixir [OTC]

**Therapeutic Category** Antihistamine/Decongestant Combination

**Use** Temporary relief of symptoms of seasonal and perennial allergic rhinitis, and vasomotor rhinitis, including nasal obstruction

**Usual Dosage** Children >12 years and Adults: Oral: 10 mL every 4 hours

**Dosage Forms** Elixir: Brompheniramine maleate 4 mg and phenylephrine hydrochloride 5 mg per 5 mL

## brompheniramine and pseudoephedrine

(brome fen IR a meen & soo doe e FED rin)

**U.S./Canadian Brand Names** Brofed® [OTC]; Bromfed® [OTC]; Bromfed-PD® [OTC]; Bromfenex®; Bromfenex® PD; Dimetapp® Elixir [New Formula]; Drixoral® Syrup [OTC]; Iofed®; Iofed® PD

**Therapeutic Category** Antihistamine/Decongestant Combination

**Use** Temporary relief of symptoms of seasonal and perennial allergic rhinitis, and vasomotor rhinitis, including nasal obstruction

**Usual Dosage** Oral:

Capsule, sustained release:

Based on 60 mg pseudoephedrine:

Children 6-12 years: 1 capsule every 12 hours

Children ≥12 years and Adults: 1-2 capsules every 12 hours

Based on 120 mg pseudoephedrine: Children ≥12 years and Adults: 1 capsule every 12 hours

Elixir: Children >12 years and Adults:

Brompheniramine 2 mg/pseudoephedrine 30 mg per 5 mL: 10 mL every 4-6 hours, up to 40 mL/day

Brompheniramine 4 mg/pseudoephedrine 30 mg per 5 mL: 10 mL 3 times/day

Tablet: Based on 60 mg pseudoephedrine: Children >12 years and Adults: 1 tablet every 4 hours

Brompheniramine 4 mg/pseudoephedrine 60 mg per 5 mL: 5 mL 4 times/day

Syrup:

Children 2-6 years of age: 2.5 mL 4 times/day

Children ≥6 years of age and Adults: 5 mL 4 times/day

**Dosage Forms**

Capsule, extended release:

Bromfed-PD®, Bromfenex® PD, Iofed® PD: Brompheniramine maleate 6 mg and pseudoephedrine hydrochloride 60 mg

Bromfed®, Bromfenex®, Iofed®: Brompheniramine maleate 12 mg and pseudoephedrine hydrochloride 120 mg

Elixir:

Brofed®: Brompheniramine maleate 4 mg and pseudoephedrine hydrochloride 30 mg per 5 mL

Bromfed®: Brompheniramine maleate 2 mg and pseudoephedrine hydrochloride 30 mg per 5 mL

Dimetapp®: Brompheniramine maleate 1 mg and pseudoephedrine hydrochloride 15 mg per 5 mL

Drixoral®: Brompheniramine maleate 2 mg and pseudoephedrine sulfate 30 mg per 5 mL

Tablet (Bromfed®): Brompheniramine maleate 4 mg and pseudoephedrine hydrochloride 60 mg

**Bromphen® Tablet *(Discontinued)*** *see page 750*

**Bronchial® *(Discontinued)*** *see page 750*

**Bronitin® Mist [OTC]** *see* epinephrine *on page 216*

**Bronkaid® Mist [OTC]** *see* epinephrine *on page 216*

**Bronkephrine® *(Discontinued)*** *see page 750*

**Bronkometer® *(Discontinued)*** *see page 750*

**Bronkosol® *(Discontinued)*** *see page 750*

**Brontex® Liquid** *see* guaifenesin and codeine *on page 282*

**Brontex® Tablet** *see* guaifenesin and codeine *on page 282*

**Brotane® [OTC]** *see* brompheniramine *on previous page*

**BSS® Ophthalmic** *see* balanced salt solution *on page 66*

**B-type natriuretic peptide (Human)** *see* nesiritide *on page 417*

**Bucladin®-S Softab®** ***(Discontinued)*** *see page 750*

## budesonide (byoo DES oh nide)

**U.S./Canadian Brand Names** Entocort® Capsule; Gen-Budesonide AQ (Can); Pulmicort Respules™; Pulmicort® Turbuhaler®; Rhinocort®; Rhinocort® Aqua™

**Therapeutic Category** Adrenal Corticosteroid

**Use**

Intranasal: Children and Adults: Management of symptoms of seasonal or perennial rhinitis

Nebulization: Children 12 months to 8 years: Maintenance and prophylactic treatment of asthma

Oral: For the induction and maintenance of remission in patients with mild to moderate Crohn's disease affecting the ileum and/or ascending colon.

Oral inhalation: Maintenance and prophylactic treatment of asthma; includes patients who require corticosteroids and those who may benefit from systemic dose reduction/elimination

**Usual Dosage**

Children ≥6 years and Adults: 256 mcg/day, administered as either 2 sprays in each nostril in the morning and evening or as 4 sprays in each nostril in the morning

Rhinocort® Aqua™: 64 mcg/day as a single 32 mcg spray in each nostril. Some patients who do not achieve adequate control may benefit from increased dosage. A reduced dosage may be effective after initial control is achieved.

Maximum dose: Children <12 years: 129 mcg/day; Adults: 256 mcg/day

Capsule:

Active Disease: The recommended daily dose for induction of remission is 9 mg, administered once daily in the morning, for up to 8 weeks. The dose should be taken before meals.

Maintenance of Remission: The recommended daily starting dose for the maintenance of remission is 6 mg, administered once daily in the morning before breakfast. The maintenance dose should be kept as low as necessary for control of disease symptoms. During prolonged treatment, dosing may have to be adjusted depending on the disease activity.

Treatment with budesonide capsules should be tapered before cessation. It is recommended that the dose be reduced for the last 2 to 4 weeks of therapy. The rate of tapering should be patient-specific and the patient should be monitored by the treating physician during this period. The capsules should be swallowed whole with water, and not chewed, broken or crushed before being swallowed.

**Dosage Forms**

Capsule: 3 mg

Powder for oral inhalation (Pulmicort® Turbuhaler): ~160 mcg delivered (200 mcg released) with each actuation (200 doses/inhaler)

Suspension for oral inhalation (Pulmicort Respules™): 0.25 mg/2 mL, 0.5 mg/2 mL

Suspension, intranasal [spray]:

Rhinocort® Aqua™: 32 mcg (60, 120 metered sprays); 64 mcg (120 metered sprays)

Rhinocort® Nasal Aerosol: 50 mcg released per actuation to deliver ~32 mcg to patient via nasal adapter [200 metered doses] (7 g)

**Buffered®, Tri-buffered** ***(Discontinued)*** *see page 750*

**Bufferin® [OTC]** *see* aspirin *on page 55*

**Bufferin® Arthritis Strength** ***(Discontinued)*** *see page 750*

**Bufferin® Extra Strength** ***(Discontinued)*** *see page 750*

**Buffex® [OTC]** *see* aspirin *on page 55*

**Buf-Puf® Acne Cleansing Bar** ***(Discontinued)*** *see page 750*

## bumetanide (byoo MET a nide)

**U.S./Canadian Brand Names** Bumex®; Burinex® (Can)

**Therapeutic Category** Diuretic, Loop

**Use** Management of edema secondary to congestive heart failure or hepatic or renal disease including nephrotic syndrome; may also be used alone or in combination with antihypertensives in the treatment of hypertension

**Usual Dosage**

Children:

<6 months: Dose not established

>6 months:

Oral: Initial: 0.015 mg/kg/dose once daily or every other day; maximum dose: 0.1 mg/kg/day

I.M., I.V.: Dose not established

Adults:

Oral: 0.5-2 mg/dose (maximum: 10 mg/day) 1-2 times/day

I.M., I.V.: 0.5-1 mg/dose (maximum: 10 mg/day)

**Dosage Forms**

Injection: 0.25 mg/mL (2 mL, 4 mL, 10 mL)

Tablet: 0.5 mg, 1 mg, 2 mg

**Bumex®** *see* bumetanide *on this page*

**Buminate®** *see* albumin *on page 16*

**Bupap®** *see* butalbital compound and acetaminophen *on page 93*

**Buphenyl®** *see* sodium phenylbutyrate *on page 551*

## bupivacaine (byoo PIV a kane)

**U.S./Canadian Brand Names** Marcaine®; Sensorcaine®; Sensorcaine®-MPF

**Therapeutic Category** Local Anesthetic

**Use** Local anesthetic (injectable) for peripheral nerve block, infiltration, sympathetic block, caudal or epidural block, retrobulbar block

**Usual Dosage** Dose varies with procedure, depth of anesthesia, vascularity of tissues, duration of anesthesia and condition of patient

Caudal block (with or without epinephrine):

Children: 1-3.7 mg/kg

Adults: 15-30 mL of 0.25% or 0.5%

Epidural block (other than caudal block):

Children: 1.25 mg/kg/dose

Adults: 10-20 mL of 0.25% or 0.5%

Peripheral nerve block: 5 mL dose of 0.25% or 0.5% (12.5-25 mg); maximum: 2.5 mg/kg (plain); 3 mg/kg (with epinephrine); up to a maximum of 400 mg/day

Sympathetic nerve block: 20-50 mL of 0.25% (no epinephrine) solution

**Dosage Forms**

Injection, as hydrochloride: 0.25% (10 mL, 20 mL, 30 mL, 50 mL); 0.5% (10 mL, 20 mL, 30 mL, 50 mL); 0.75% (2 mL, 10 mL, 20 mL, 30 mL)

Injection, as hydrochloride, with epinephrine (1:200,000): 0.25% (10 mL, 30 mL, 50 mL); 0.5% (1.8 mL, 3 mL, 5 mL, 10 mL, 30 mL, 50 mL); 0.75% (30 mL)

**Buprenex®** *see* buprenorphine *on this page*

## buprenorphine (byoo pre NOR feen)

**U.S./Canadian Brand Names** Buprenex®

**Therapeutic Category** Analgesic, Narcotic

**Controlled Substance** C-V

**Use** Management of moderate to severe pain

**Usual Dosage** Adults: I.M., slow I.V.: 0.3-0.6 mg every 6 hours as needed

**Dosage Forms** Injection, as hydrochloride: 0.3 mg/mL (1 mL)

## bupropion (byoo PROE pee on)

**U.S./Canadian Brand Names** Wellbutrin®; Wellbutrin® SR; Zyban™

**Therapeutic Category** Antidepressant, Aminoketone

**Use** Treatment of depression; as an aid to smoking cessation treatment

**Usual Dosage** Oral:

Adults:

Depression: 100 mg 3 times/day; begin at 100 mg twice daily; may increase to a maximum dose of 450 mg/day

Smoking cessation: Initiate with 150 mg once daily for 3 days; increase to 150 mg twice daily; treatment should continue for 7-12 weeks

Elderly: Depression: 50-100 mg/day, increase by 50-100 mg every 3-4 days as tolerated; there is evidence that the elderly respond at 150 mg/day in divided doses, but some may require a higher dose

**Dosage Forms**

Tablet: 75 mg, 100 mg

Wellbutrin®: 75 mg, 100 mg

Tablet, sustained release (Wellbutrin® SR, Zyban™): 100 mg, 150 mg

**Burinex® (Can)** *see* bumetanide *on previous page*

**Burow's otic** *see* aluminum acetate and acetic acid *on page 25*

**Buscopan® (Can)** *see* scopolamine *on page 539*

## buserelin (BYOO se rel in)

**U.S./Canadian Brand Names** Suprefact® (Can); Suprefact® Depot (Can)

**Therapeutic Category** Luteinizing Hormone-Releasing Hormone Analog

**Use** For the palliative treatment of patients with hormone-dependent advanced carcinoma of the prostate gland (Stage D). Buserelin is also indicated for the treatment of endometriosis in patients who do not require surgery as primary therapy. The duration of treatment is usually 6 months and should not exceed 9 months. Experience with buserelin for the management of endometriosis has been limited to women 18 years of age and older.

**Usual Dosage** Buserelin should be administered at approximately equal time intervals to ensure that the desired therapeutic effect is maintained.

Prostatic Cancer: Initial Treatment: For the first 7 days of treatment give buserelin 500 mcg (0.5 mL) every 8 hours by S.C. injection. For patient comfort, vary the injection site.

Maintenance Treatment: Depending upon patient preference, or physician recommendation, maintenance treatment may be by daily S.C. injection or by intranasal administration 3 times daily. During maintenance dosing by the S.C. route, the buserelin dose is 200 mcg (0.2 mL) daily. For patient comfort, vary the site of injection.

During maintenance dosing by the intranasal administration route, the buserelin dose is 400 mcg (200 mcg into each nostril) 3 times daily using the metered-dose pump (nebulizer) provided. Each pump action delivers 100 mcg buserelin acetate or 0.1mL solution.

Endometriosis: The dose of buserelin in patients with endometriosis is 400 mcg (200 mcg into each nostril) 3 times daily using the metered-dose pump (nebulizer) provided. Each pump action delivers 100 mcg or 0.1 mL solution. The treatment duration is usually 6 months and should not exceed 9 months.

**Dosage Forms** Injection, depot, as acetate: 6.6 mg [2 month]; 9.9 mg [3 month]

**BuSpar®** *see* buspirone *on this page*

## buspirone (byoo SPYE rone)

**U.S./Canadian Brand Names** BuSpar®

**Therapeutic Category** Antianxiety Agent

**Use** Management of anxiety

(Continued)

## buspirone *(Continued)*

**Usual Dosage** Adults: Oral: 15 mg/day (5 mg 3 times/day); may increase to a maximum of 60 mg/day

**Dosage Forms** Tablet, as hydrochloride: 5 mg, 10 mg, 15 mg, 30 mg

## busulfan (byoo SUL fan)

**U.S./Canadian Brand Names** Busulfex®; Myleran®

**Therapeutic Category** Antineoplastic Agent

**Use**

Injection: Use in combination with cyclophosphamide as a conditioning regimen prior to allogeneic hematopoietic progenitor cell transplantation for chronic myelogenous leukemia

Oral: Chronic myelogenous leukemia and bone marrow disorders, such as polycythemia vera and myeloid metaplasia, conditioning regimens for bone marrow transplantation

**Usual Dosage**

I.V.: Adult: As a component of a conditioning regimen prior to bone marrow or peripheral blood progenitor cell replacement support is 0.8 mg/kg of ideal body weight or actual body weight, whichever is lower, administered every 6 hours for 4 days (a total of 16 doses)

Oral (**refer to individual protocols**):

Children:

For remission induction of CML: 0.06-0.12 mg/kg/day **or** 1.8-4.6 mg/m$^2$/day; titrate dosage to maintain leukocyte count above 40,000/mm$^3$; reduce dosage by 50% if the leukocyte count reaches 30,000-40,000/mm$^3$; discontinue drug if counts fall to ≤20,000/mm$^3$

BMT marrow-ablative conditioning regimen: 1 mg/kg/dose (ideal body weight) every 6 hours for 16 doses

Adults:

BMT marrow-ablative conditioning regimen: 1 mg/kg/dose (ideal body weight) every 6 hours for 16 doses

**Dosage Forms**

Injection: 6 mg/mL (10 mL)

Tablet: 2 mg

**Busulfex®** *see* busulfan *on this page*

## butabarbital sodium (byoo ta BAR bi tal SOW dee um)

**U.S./Canadian Brand Names** Butalan®; Buticaps®; Butisol Sodium®

**Therapeutic Category** Barbiturate

**Controlled Substance** C-III

**Use** Sedative, hypnotic

**Usual Dosage**

Children: Preop: 2-6 mg/kg/dose; maximum: 100 mg

Adults:

Sedative: 15-30 mg 3-4 times/day

Hypnotic: 50-100 mg

Preop: 50-100 mg 1-1½ hours before surgery

**Dosage Forms**

Capsule: 15 mg, 30 mg

Elixir, with alcohol 7%: 30 mg/5 mL (480 mL, 3780 mL); 33.3 mg/5 mL (480 mL, 3780 mL)

Tablet: 15 mg, 30 mg, 50 mg, 100 mg

**Butace®** ***(Discontinued)*** *see page 750*

**Butalan®** *see* butabarbital sodium *on this page*

## butalbital compound and acetaminophen

(byoo TAL bi tal KOM pound & a seet a MIN oh fen)

**U.S./Canadian Brand Names** Amaphen®; Anolor 300®; Anoquan®; Arcet®; Axocet®; Bupap®; Endolor®; Esgic®; Esgic-Plus™; Ezol®; Femcet®; Fioricet®; G-1®; Geone®; Margesic®; Medigesic®; Phrenilin®; Phrenilin Forte®; Repan®; Sedapap-10®; Triad®; Triapin®; Two-Dyne®; Zebutal®

**Therapeutic Category** Barbiturate/Analgesic

**Controlled Substance** C-III

**Use** Relief of the symptomatic complex of tension or muscle contraction headache

**Usual Dosage** Adults: Oral: 1-2 tablets or capsules every 4 hours; not to exceed 6/day

**Dosage Forms**

Capsule:

Amaphen®, Anolor 300®; Anoquan®, Arcet®, Butace®, Endolor®, Esgic®, Ezol®, Femcet®, Geone®, G-1®, Margesic®, Medigesic®, Repan®, Triad®, Two-Dyne®: Butalbital 50 mg, caffeine 40 mg, and acetaminophen 325 mg

Zebutal®: Butalbital 50 mg, caffeine 40 mg, and acetaminophen 500 mg

Axocet®, Phrenilin Forte®: Butalbital 50 mg and acetaminophen 650 mg

Triapin®: Butalbital 50 mg and acetaminophen 325 mg

Tablet:

Bupap®: Butalbital 50 mg and acetaminophen 650 mg

Esgic®, Fioricet®, Repan®: Butalbital 50 mg, caffeine 40 mg, and acetaminophen 325 mg

Phrenilin®: Butalbital 50 mg and acetaminophen 325 mg

Sedapap-10®: Butalbital 50 mg and acetaminophen 650 mg

## butalbital compound and aspirin (byoo TAL bi tal KOM pound & AS pir in)

**U.S./Canadian Brand Names** Farbital®; Fiorgen PF®; Fiorinal®; Fortabs®; Laniroif®; Tecnal (Can)

**Therapeutic Category** Barbiturate/Analgesic

**Controlled Substance** C-III (Fiorinal®)

**Use** Relief of the symptomatic complex of tension or muscle contraction headache

**Usual Dosage** Adults: Oral: 1-2 tablets or capsules every 4 hours; not to exceed 6/day

**Dosage Forms**

Capsule: (Fiorgen PF®, Fiorinal®, Isollyl® Improved, Marnal®): Butalbital 50 mg, caffeine 40 mg, and aspirin 325 mg

Tablet: (Fiorinal®, Isollyl® Improved, Marnal®): Butalbital 50 mg, caffeine 40 mg, and aspirin 325 mg

## butalbital compound and codeine

(byoo TAL bi tal KOM pound & KOE deen)

**U.S./Canadian Brand Names** Fiorinal®-C (Can); Fiorinal® With Codeine; Tecnal C (Can)

**Therapeutic Category** Analgesic, Narcotic; Barbiturate

**Controlled Substance** C-III

**Use** Mild to moderate pain when sedation is needed

**Usual Dosage** Adults: Oral: 1-2 capsules every 4 hours as needed for pain; up to 6/day

**Dosage Forms** Capsule: Butalbital 50 mg, caffeine 40 mg, aspirin 325 mg and codeine phosphate 30 mg

## butenafine (byoo TEN a fine)

**U.S./Canadian Brand Names** Mentax®

**Therapeutic Category** Antifungal Agent

**Use** Topical treatment of interdigital tinea pedis (athlete's foot) due to *Epidermophyton floccosum*, *Trichophyton mentagrophytes*, or *Trichophyton rubrum*

**Usual Dosage** Adults: Topical: Apply cream to the affected area and surrounding skin once daily for 4 weeks

**Dosage Forms** Cream, as hydrochloride: 1% (2 g, 15 g, 30 g)

**Buticaps®** *see* butabarbital sodium *on page 92*

**Butisol Sodium®** *see* butabarbital sodium *on page 92*

## butoconazole (byoo toe KOE na zole)

**U.S./Canadian Brand Names** Gynazole•1®

**Therapeutic Category** Antifungal Agent

**Use** Local treatment of vulvovaginal candidiasis

**Usual Dosage** Adults:

Nonpregnant: Insert 1 applicatorful (~5 g) intravaginally at bedtime for 3 days, may extend for up to 6 days if necessary

Pregnant: **Use only during second or third trimesters**

**Dosage Forms** Cream, vaginal, as nitrate: 2% with applicator (28 g)

## butorphanol (byoo TOR fa nole)

**U.S./Canadian Brand Names** Stadol®; Stadol® NS

**Therapeutic Category** Analgesic, Narcotic

**Controlled Substance** C-IV

**Use** Management of moderate to severe pain

**Usual Dosage** Adults:

I.M.: 1-4 mg every 3-4 hours as needed

I.V.: 0.5-2 mg every 3-4 hours as needed

Nasal: Initial: 1 mg (1 spray in one nostril), allow 60-90 minutes to elapse before deciding whether a second 1 mg dose is needed; this 2-dose sequence may be repeated in 3-4 hours if needed

**Dosage Forms**

Injection, as tartrate: 1 mg/mL (1 mL); 2 mg/mL (1 mL, 2 mL, 10 mL)

Spray, nasal, as tartrate: 10 mg/mL [14-15 doses] (2.5 mL)

**Byclomine® Injection** *see* dicyclomine *on page 183*

**Bydramine® Cough Syrup [OTC]** *see* diphenhydramine *on page 191*

**C2B8 monoclonal antibody** *see* rituximab *on page 529*

**c7E3** *see* abciximab *on page 2*

**C8-CCK** *see* sincalide *on page 545*

**311C90** *see* zolmitriptan *on page 640*

## cabergoline (ca BER go leen)

**U.S./Canadian Brand Names** Dostinex®

**Therapeutic Category** Ergot-like Derivative

**Use** Treatment of hyperprolactinemia

**Usual Dosage** Adults: Oral: 0.25 mg twice weekly; dosage may be increased by 0.25 mg twice weekly to a dose of up to 1 mg twice weekly (according to the patient's prolactin level)

**Dosage Forms** Tablet: 0.5 mg

**Caelyx® (Can)** *see* doxorubicin *on page 203*

**Cafatine-PB®** *see* ergotamine *on page 221*

**Cafcit®** *see* caffeine (citrated) *on next page*

**Cafergot®** *see* ergotamine *on page 221*

**Cafetrate®** *see* ergotamine *on page 221*

## caffeine and sodium benzoate (KAF een & SOW dee um BEN zoe ate)

**Therapeutic Category** Diuretic, Miscellaneous

**Use** Emergency stimulant in acute circulatory failure; as a diuretic; and to relieve spinal puncture headache

**Usual Dosage**
Children: I.M., I.V., S.C.: 8 mg/kg every 4 hours as needed
Adults: I.M., I.V.: 500 mg, maximum single dose: 1 g

**Dosage Forms** Injection: Caffeine 125 mg and sodium benzoate 125 mg per mL (2 mL)

## caffeine (citrated) (KAF een SIT rated)

**U.S./Canadian Brand Names** Cafcit®

**Therapeutic Category** Respiratory Stimulant; Stimulant

**Use** Central nervous system stimulant; used in the treatment of apnea of prematurity (28 to <33 weeks gestational age). Has several advantages over theophylline in the treatment of neonatal apnea, its half-life is about 3 times as long, allowing once daily dosing, drug levels do not need to be drawn at peak and trough; has a wider therapeutic window, allowing more room between an effective concentration and toxicity.

**Usual Dosage** Apnea of prematurity: Neonates:
Loading dose (usually administered I.V.): 10-20 mg/kg as caffeine citrate (5-10 mg/kg as caffeine base). If theophylline has been administered to the patient within the previous 3 days, a full or modified loading dose (50% to 75% of a loading dose) may be given (caffeine is a significant metabolite of theophylline in the newborn.
Maintenance dose: Oral, I.V.: 5 mg/kg/day as caffeine citrate (2.5 mg/kg/day as caffeine base) once daily starting 24 hours after the loading dose. Maintenance dose is adjusted based on patient's response (efficacy and adverse effects), and serum caffeine concentrations.

**Dosage Forms**
Injection: 20 mg/mL as caffeine citrate [equivalent to 10 mg/mL caffeine base] (3 mL)
Solution, oral: 20 mg/mL as caffeine citrate [equivalent to 10 mg/mL caffeine base] (3 mL)

**Caladryl® Lotion** *see* pramoxine *on page 490*
**Caladryl® Spray *(Discontinued)*** *see page 750*
**Calan®** *see* verapamil *on page 625*
**Calan® SR** *see* verapamil *on page 625*
**Calbon®** *see* calcium lactate *on page 100*
**Cal Carb-HD® [OTC]** *see* calcium carbonate *on page 97*
**Calcibind®** *see* cellulose sodium phosphate *on page 119*
**Calci-Chew™ [OTC]** *see* calcium carbonate *on page 97*
**Calciday-667® [OTC]** *see* calcium carbonate *on page 97*

## calcifediol (kal si fe DYE ole)

**Synonyms** 25-$D_3$; 25-hydroxycholecalciferol; 25-hydroxyvitamin $D_3$

**U.S./Canadian Brand Names** Calderol®

**Therapeutic Category** Vitamin D Analog

**Use** Treatment and management of metabolic bone disease associated with chronic renal failure

**Usual Dosage** Hepatic osteodystrophy: Oral:
Infants: 5-7 mcg/kg/day
Children and Adults: 20-100 mcg/day or every other day; titrate to obtain normal serum calcium/phosphate levels

**Dosage Forms** Capsule: 20 mcg, 50 mcg

**Calciferol™** *see* ergocalciferol *on page 220*
**Calcijex™** *see* calcitriol *on next page*
**Calcimar® *(Discontinued)*** *see page 750*
**Calci-Mix™ [OTC]** *see* calcium carbonate *on page 97*
**Calcionate®** *see* calcium glubionate *on page 99*

**Calciparine® Injection *(Discontinued)*** *see page 750*

## calcipotriene (kal si POE try een)

**U.S./Canadian Brand Names** Dovonex®

**Therapeutic Category** Antipsoriatic Agent

**Use** Treatment of plaque psoriasis

**Usual Dosage** Topical: Apply to skin lesions twice daily

**Dosage Forms**

Cream: 0.005% (30 g, 60 g, 100 g)

Ointment, topical: 0.005% (30 g, 60 g, 100 g)

Solution, topical: 0.005%

**Calciquid®** *see* calcium glubionate *on page 99*

**Calcite 500 (Can)** *see* calcium carbonate *on next page*

## calcitonin (kal si TOE nin)

**Synonyms** calcitonin (salmon)

**U.S./Canadian Brand Names** Caltine® (Can); Miacalcin®

**Therapeutic Category** Polypeptide Hormone

**Use**

Calcitonin (salmon): Treatment of Paget's disease of bone and as adjunctive therapy for hypercalcemia; also used in postmenopausal osteoporosis and osteogenesis imperfecta

Calcitonin (human): Treatment of Paget's disease of bone

**Usual Dosage**

Children: Dosage not established

Adults:

Paget's disease: I.M., S.C.: Initial: 100 units/day; maintenance: 50 units/day or 50-100 units every 1-3 days

Hypercalcemia: Initial: I.M., S.C.: 4 units/kg every 12 hours; may increase up to 8 units/kg every 12 hours to a maximum of every 6 hours

Osteogenesis imperfecta: I.M., S.C.: 2 units/kg 3 times/week

Postmenopausal osteoporosis:

I.M., S.C.: 100 units/day

Intranasal: 200 units (1 spray)/day

**Dosage Forms**

Injection: 200 units/mL (2 mL)

Solution, intranasal [spray]: 200 units/activation (0.09 mL/dose) (2 mL glass bottle with pump)

**calcitonin (salmon)** *see* calcitonin *on this page*

## calcitriol (kal si TRYE ole)

**Synonyms** 1,25 dihydroxycholecalciferol

**U.S./Canadian Brand Names** Calcijex™; Rocaltrol®

**Therapeutic Category** Vitamin D Analog

**Use** Management of hypocalcemia in patients on chronic renal dialysis; reduce elevated parathyroid hormone levels

**Usual Dosage** Individualize dosage to maintain calcium levels of 9-10 mg/dL

Renal failure: Oral:

Children: Initial: 15 ng/kg/day; maintenance: 30-60 ng/kg/day

Adults: 0.25 mcg/day or every other day (may require 0.5-1 mcg/day)

**Unlabeled dose**:

Renal failure: I.V.: Adults: 0.5 mcg (0.01 mcg/kg) 3 times/week; most doses in the range of 0.5-3 mcg (0.01-0.05 mcg/kg) 3 times/week

Hypoparathyroidism/pseudohypoparathyroidism: Oral:

Children 1-5 years: 0.25-0.75 mcg/day

Children >6 years and Adults: 0.5-2 mcg/day

**Dosage Forms**
Capsule: 0.25 mcg, 0.5 mcg
Injection: 1 mcg/mL (1 mL); 2 mcg/mL (1 mL)

## calcium acetate (KAL see um AS e tate)

**U.S./Canadian Brand Names** Calphron®; PhosLo®

**Therapeutic Category** Electrolyte Supplement, Oral

**Use** Control of hyperphosphatemia in end-stage renal failure and does not promote aluminum absorption

**Usual Dosage** Adults: Oral: 2 tablets with each meal; dosage may be increased to bring serum phosphate value to <6 mg/dL; most patients require 3-4 tablets with each meal

**Dosage Forms** Elemental calcium listed in brackets
Injection: 0.5 mEq/mL
Tablet:
Calphron®: 667 mg [169 mg]
PhosLo®: 667 mg [169 mg]

## calcium carbonate (KAL see um KAR bun ate)

**U.S./Canadian Brand Names** Alka-Mints® [OTC]; Amitone® [OTC]; Apo®-Cal® (Can); Cal Carb-HD® [OTC]; Calci-Chew™ [OTC]; Calciday-667® [OTC]; Calci-Mix™ [OTC]; Calcite 500 (Can); Cal-Plus® [OTC]; Caltrate® 600 [OTC]; Caltrate, Jr.® [OTC]; Chooz® [OTC]; Dicarbosil® [OTC]; Equilet® [OTC]; Florical® [OTC]; Gencalc® 600 [OTC]; Mallamint® [OTC]; Nephro-Calci® [OTC]; Os-Cal® 500 [OTC]; Oyst-Cal 500 [OTC]; Oystercal® 500; Rolaids® Calcium Rich [OTC]; Tums® [OTC]; Tums® E-X Extra Strength Tablet [OTC]; Tums® Extra Strength Liquid [OTC]

**Therapeutic Category** Antacid; Electrolyte Supplement, Oral

**Use** Treatment and prevention of calcium depletion; relief of acid indigestion, heartburn

**Usual Dosage** Dosage is in terms of elemental calcium
Recommended daily allowance (RDA): Oral:
<6 months: 360 mg/day
6-12 months: 540 mg/day
1-10 years: 800 mg/day
10-18 years: 1200 mg/day
Adults: 800 mg/day
Hypocalcemia (dose depends on clinical condition and serum calcium level):
Children: 20-65 mg/kg/day in 4 divided doses
Adults: 1-2 g or more per day

**Dosage Forms** Elemental calcium listed in brackets
Capsule: 1500 mg [600 mg]
Calci-Mix™: 1250 mg [500 mg]
Florical®: 364 mg [145.6 mg] with sodium fluoride 8.3 mg
Liquid (Tums® Extra Strength): 1000 mg/5 mL (360 mL)
Lozenge (Mylanta® Soothing Antacids): 600 mg [240 mg]
Powder (Cal Carb-HD®): 6.5 g/packet [2.6 g]
Suspension, oral: 1250 mg/5 mL [500 mg]
Tablet: 650 mg [260 mg], 1500 mg [600 mg]
Calciday-667®: 667 mg [267 mg]
Os-Cal® 500, Oyst-Cal 500, Oystercal® 500: 1250 mg [500 mg]
Cal-Plus®, Caltrate® 600, Gencalc® 600, Nephro-Calci®: 1500 mg [600 mg]
Chewable:
Alka-Mints®: 850 mg [340 mg]
Amitone®: 350 mg [140 mg]
Caltrate, Jr.®: 750 mg [300 mg]
Calci-Chew™, Os-Cal®: 750 mg [300 mg]
Chooz®, Dicarbosil®, Equilet®, Tums®: 500 mg [200 mg]
Mallamint®: 420 mg [168 mg]
Rolaids® Calcium Rich: 550 mg [220 mg]
Tums® E-X Extra Strength: 750 mg [300 mg]

(Continued)

## calcium carbonate *(Continued)*

Tums® Ultra®: 1000 mg [400 mg]
Florical®: 364 mg [145.6 mg]with sodium fluoride 8.3 mg

## Calcium Carbonate and Magnesium Hydroxide

(KAL see um KAR bun ate & mag NEE zhum hye DROKS ide)

**U.S./Canadian Brand Names** Mylanta® Gelcaps® [OTC]; Mylanta® Tablets [OTC]; Mylanta® Ultra Tablet [OTC]

**Therapeutic Category** Antacid

**Use** Hyperacidity

**Usual Dosage** Adults: Oral: 2-4 Gelcaps® as needed

**Dosage Forms**

Gelcap: Calcium carbonate 550 mg and magnesium hydroxide 125 mg
Tablet, chewable:
Mylanta®: Calcium carbonate 350 mg and magnesium hydroxide 150 mg
Mylanta® Ultra: Calcium carbonate 700 mg and magnesium hydroxide 300 mg

## calcium carbonate and simethicone

(KAL see um KAR bun ate & sye METH i kone)

**U.S./Canadian Brand Names** Titralac® Plus Liquid [OTC]

**Therapeutic Category** Antacid; Antiflatulent

**Use** Relief of acid indigestion, heartburn, peptic esophagitis, hiatal hernia, and gas

**Usual Dosage** Oral: 0.5-2 g 4-6 times/day

**Dosage Forms** Elemental calcium listed in brackets

Liquid: Calcium carbonate 500 mg [200 mg] and simethicone 20 mg per 5 mL

## calcium chloride (KAL see um KLOR ide)

**Therapeutic Category** Electrolyte Supplement, Oral

**Use** Emergency treatment of hypocalcemic tetany; treatment of hypermagnesemia; cardiac disturbances of hyperkalemia, hypocalcemia or calcium channel blocking agent toxicity

**Usual Dosage** I.V.:

Cardiac arrest in the presence of hyperkalemia or hypocalcemia, magnesium toxicity, or calcium antagonist toxicity:
Infants and Children: 10-20 mg/kg; may repeat in 10 minutes if necessary
Adults: 1.5-4 mg/kg/dose or 2.5-5 mL/dose every 10 minutes
Hypocalcemia:
Infants and Children: 10-20 mg/kg/dose, repeat every 4-6 hours if needed
Adults: 500 mg to 1 g at 1- to 3-day intervals
Exchange transfusion: 0.45 mEq after each 100 mL of blood exchanged I.V.
Hypocalcemia secondary to citrated blood transfusion: Administer 0.45 mEq **elemental** calcium for each 100 mL citrated blood infused
Tetany:
Infants and Children: 10 mg/kg over 5-10 minutes; may repeat after 6 hours or follow with an infusion with a maximum dose of 200 mg/kg/day
Adults: 1 g over 10-30 minutes; may repeat after 6 hours

**Dosage Forms** Elemental calcium listed in brackets

Injection: 10% = 100 mg/mL [27.2 mg/mL] (10 mL)

## calcium citrate (KAL see um SIT rate)

**U.S./Canadian Brand Names** Citracal® [OTC]

**Therapeutic Category** Electrolyte Supplement, Oral

**Use** Adjunct in prevention of postmenopausal osteoporosis, treatment and prevention of calcium depletion

**Usual Dosage** Oral (dosage is in terms of elemental calcium): Adults: Oral: 1-2 g/day

Recommended daily allowance (RDA):
<6 months: 360 mg/day
6-12 months: 540 mg/day
1-10 years: 800 mg/day
10-18 years: 1200 mg/day
Adults: 800 mg/day

**Dosage Forms** Elemental calcium listed in brackets
Tablet: 950 mg [200 mg]
Effervescent: 2376 mg [500 mg]

**Calcium Disodium Versenate®** *see* edetate calcium disodium *on page 209*

**calcium edta** *see* edetate calcium disodium *on page 209*

## calcium glubionate (KAL see um gloo BYE oh nate)

**U.S./Canadian Brand Names** Calcionate®; Calciquid®; Neo-Calglucon® [OTC]

**Therapeutic Category** Electrolyte Supplement, Oral

**Use** Treatment and prevention of calcium depletion

**Usual Dosage** Oral (syrup is a hyperosmolar solution; dosage is in terms of calcium glubionate):

Neonatal hypocalcemia: 1200 mg/kg/day in 4-6 divided doses
Maintenance: Infants and Children: 600-2000 mg/kg/day in 4 divided doses up to a maximum of 9 g/day
Adults: 6-18 g/day in divided doses

Recommended daily allowance (RDA):
<6 months: 360 mg/day
6-12 months: 540 mg/day
1-10 years: 800 mg/day
10-18 years: 1200 mg/day
Adults: 800 mg/day

**Dosage Forms** Elemental calcium listed in brackets
Syrup: 1.8 g/5 mL [115 mg/5 mL] (480 mL)

## calcium gluceptate (KAL see um gloo SEP tate)

**Therapeutic Category** Electrolyte Supplement, Oral

**Use** Emergency treatment of hypocalcemia; treatment of hypermagnesemia; cardiac disturbances of hyperkalemia, hypocalcemia, or calcium channel blocker toxicity

**Usual Dosage** I.V.:
Cardiac resuscitation in the presence of hypocalcemia, hyperkalemia, or calcium channel blocker toxicity:
Children: 110 mg/kg/dose or 0.5 mL/kg/dose every 10 minutes
Adults: 5 mL every 10 minutes
Hypocalcemia:
Children: 200-500 mg/kg/day divided every 6 hours
Adults: 500 mg to 1.1 g/dose as needed
Exchange transfusion: 0.45 mEq (0.5 mL) after each 100 mL of blood exchanged
After citrated blood administration: Children and Adults: 0.4 mEq/100 mL blood infused

**Dosage Forms** Elemental calcium listed in brackets
Injection: 220 mg/mL [18 mg/mL] (5 mL, 50 mL)

## calcium gluconate (KAL see um GLOO koe nate)

**U.S./Canadian Brand Names** Calfort®; Cal-G®

**Therapeutic Category** Electrolyte Supplement, Oral

**Use** Treatment and prevention of hypocalcemia, hypermagnesemia, cardiac disturbances of hyperkalemia, hypocalcemia, or calcium channel blocker toxicity

**Usual Dosage** Dosage is in terms of elemental calcium
Recommended daily allowance (RDA):
<6 months: 360 mg/day
(Continued)

## calcium gluconate *(Continued)*

6-12 months: 540 mg/day
1-10 years: 800 mg/day
10-18 years: 1200 mg/day
Adults: 800 mg/day

Calcium gluconate electrolyte requirement in newborn period:
Premature: 200-1000 mg/kg/24 hours
Term:
0-24 hours: 0-500 mg/kg/24 hours
24-48 hours: 200-500 mg/kg/24 hours
48-72 hours: 200-600 mg/kg/24 hours
>3 days: 200-800 mg/kg/24 hours

Hypocalcemia:
I.V.:
Infants and Children: 200-1000 mg/kg/day as a continuous infusion or in 4 divided doses
Adults: 2-15 g/24 hours as a continuous infusion or in divided doses
Oral:
Children: 200-500 mg/kg/day divided every 6 hours
Adults: 500 mg to 2 g 2-4 times/day

Calcium antagonist toxicity, magnesium intoxication; cardiac arrest in the presence of hyperkalemia or hypocalcemia: I.V.:
Infants and Children: 100 mg/kg/dose
Adults: 1-3 g

Tetany: I.V.: doses or as an infusion
Infants and Children: 100-200 mg/kg/dose over 5-10 minutes; may repeat after 6 hours or follow with an infusion of 500 mg/kg/day
Adults: 1-3 g may be administered until therapeutic response occurs

Cardiac resuscitation: I.V.:
Infants and Children: 100 mg/kg/dose (1 mL/kg/dose) every 10 minutes
Adults: 500-800 mg/dose (5-8 mL) every 10 minutes

Hypocalcemia secondary to citrated blood infusion; administer 0.45 mEq **elemental** calcium for each 100 mL citrated blood infused

Exchange transfusion:
Adults: 300 mg/100 mL of citrated blood exchanged

Maintenance electrolyte requirements for total parenteral nutrition: I.V.: Daily requirements: Adults: 10-20 mEq/1000 kcals/24 hours

**Dosage Forms** Elemental calcium listed in brackets
Injection: 10% = 100 mg/mL [9 mg/mL] (10 mL, 50 mL, 100 mL, 200 mL)
Tablet: 500 mg [45 mg], 650 mg [58.5 mg], 975 mg [87.75 mg], 1 g [90 mg]

## calcium lactate (KAL see um LAK tate)

**U.S./Canadian Brand Names** Calbon®; Cal-Lac®; Ridactate®
**Therapeutic Category** Electrolyte Supplement, Oral
**Use** Treatment and prevention of calcium depletion
**Usual Dosage** Oral:
Infants: 400-500 mg/kg/day divided every 4-6 hours
Children: 500 mg/kg/day divided every 6-8 hours; maximum daily dose: 9 g
Adults: 1.5-3 g divided every 8 hours
**Dosage Forms** Elemental calcium listed in brackets
Tablet: 325 mg [42.25 mg], 650 mg [84.5 mg]

**calcium pantothenate** *see* pantothenic acid *on page 450*

## calcium phosphate (dibasic) (KAL see um FOS fate dye BAY sik)

**Synonyms** dicalcium phosphate
**U.S./Canadian Brand Names** Posture® [OTC]
**Therapeutic Category** Electrolyte Supplement, Oral

**Use** Adjunct in prevention of postmenopausal osteoporosis, treatment and prevention of calcium depletion

**Usual Dosage** Oral:

Children: 45-65 mg/kg/day

Adults: 1-2 g/day (doses in g of elemental calcium)

**Dosage Forms** Elemental calcium listed in brackets

Tablet, sugar free: 1565.2 mg [600 mg]

## calcium polycarbophil (KAL see um pol i KAR boe fil)

**U.S./Canadian Brand Names** Equalactin® Chewable Tablet [OTC]; Fiberall® Chewable Tablet [OTC]; FiberCon® Tablet [OTC]; Fiber-Lax® Tablet [OTC]; Mitrolan® Chewable Tablet [OTC]

**Therapeutic Category** Gastrointestinal Agent, Miscellaneous; Laxative

**Use** Treatment of constipation or diarrhea by restoring a more normal moisture level and providing bulk in the patient's intestinal tract; calcium polycarbophil is supplied as the approved substitute whenever a bulk-forming laxative is ordered in a tablet, capsule, wafer, or other oral solid dosage form

**Usual Dosage** Oral:

Children:

2-6 years: 500 mg 1-2 times/day, up to 1.5 g/day

6-12 years: 500 mg 1-3 times/day, up to 3 g/day

Adults: 1 g 4 times/day, up to 6 g/day

**Dosage Forms** Tablet:

Chewable:

Equalactin®, Mitrolan®: 500 mg

Equalactin®: 650 mg

Fiberall®: 1250 mg

Sodium free:

Fiber-Lax®: 625 mg

FiberCon®: 500 mg

**CaldeCORT® Anti-Itch Topical Spray** *see* hydrocortisone (topical) *on page 304*

**CaldeCORT® Topical [OTC]** *see* hydrocortisone (topical) *on page 304*

**Calderol®** *see* calcifediol *on page 95*

## calfactant (cal FAC tant)

**U.S./Canadian Brand Names** Infasurf®

**Therapeutic Category** Lung Surfactant

**Use** Prevention of respiratory distress syndrome (RDS) in premature infants at high risk for RDS and for the treatment ("rescue") of premature infants who develop RDS; decreases the incidence of RDS, mortality due to RDS, and air leaks associated with RDS

**Usual Dosage** Should be administered intratracheally through a side-port adapter into the endotracheal tube; two attendants, one to instill the suspension, the other to monitor the patient and assist in positioning, facilitate the dosing; the dose (3 mL/kg) should be administered in two aliquots of 1.5 mL/kg each; after each aliquot is instilled, the infant should be positioned with either the right or the left side dependent; administration is made while ventilation is continued over 20-30 breaths for each aliquot, with small bursts timed only during the inspiratory cycles; a pause followed by evaluation of the respiratory status and repositioning should separate the two aliquots

**Dosage Forms** Suspension, intratracheal: 6 mL

**Calfort®** *see* calcium gluconate *on page 99*

**Cal-G®** *see* calcium gluconate *on page 99*

**Cal-Lac®** *see* calcium lactate *on previous page*

**Calm-X® Oral [OTC]** *see* dimenhydrinate *on page 188*

**Calmylin #3 (Can)** *see* guaifenesin, pseudoephedrine, and dextromethorphan *on page 285*

**Calmylin with Codeine® (Can)** *see* guaifenesin, pseudoephedrine, and codeine *on page 284*

**Calphron®** *see* calcium acetate *on page 97*

**Cal-Plus® [OTC]** *see* calcium carbonate *on page 97*

**Caltine® (Can)** *see* calcitonin *on page 96*

**Caltrate® 600 [OTC]** *see* calcium carbonate *on page 97*

**Caltrate, Jr.® [OTC]** *see* calcium carbonate *on page 97*

**Cama® Arthritis Pain Reliever [OTC]** *see* aspirin *on page 55*

**Camalox® Suspension & Tablet *(Discontinued)*** *see page 750*

**Campath®** *see* alemtuzumab *on page 19*

**campath-1H** *see* alemtuzumab *on page 19*

**Campho-Phenique® [OTC]** *see* camphor and phenol *on this page*

## camphor and phenol (KAM for & FEE nole)

**U.S./Canadian Brand Names** Campho-Phenique® [OTC]
**Therapeutic Category** Topical Skin Product
**Use** Relief of pain and for minor infections
**Usual Dosage** Topical: Apply as needed
**Dosage Forms** Liquid: Camphor 10.8% and phenol 4.7%

**camphorated tincture of opium** *see* paregoric *on page 451*

## camphor, menthol, and phenol (KAM for, MEN thol, & FEE nole)

**U.S./Canadian Brand Names** Sarna [OTC]
**Therapeutic Category** Topical Skin Product
**Use** Relief of dry, itching skin
**Usual Dosage** Topical: Apply as needed for dry skin
**Dosage Forms** Lotion, topical: Camphor 0.5%, menthol 0.5%, and phenol 0.5% in emollient base (240 mL)

**Camptosar®** *see* irinotecan *on page 326*

**Canasa® Rectal** *see* mesalamine *on page 374*

**Cancidas®** *see* caspofungin *on page 112*

## candesartan (kan de SAR tan)

**U.S./Canadian Brand Names** Atacand®
**Therapeutic Category** Angiotensin II Antagonist
**Use** Treatment of hypertension; may be used alone or in combination with other antihypertensive agents
**Usual Dosage** Adults: Oral: Dosage must be individualized; blood pressure response is dose-related over the range of 2-32 mg; the usual recommended starting dose of 16 mg once daily when it is used as monotherapy in patients who are not volume depleted; it can be administered once or twice daily with total daily doses ranging from 8-32 mg; larger doses do not appear to have a greater effect and there is relatively little experience with such doses; most of the antihypertensive effect is present within 2 weeks and maximal blood pressure reduction is generally obtained within 4-6 weeks of treatment
**Dosage Forms** Tablet, as cilexetil: 4 mg, 8 mg, 16 mg, 32 mg

## candesartan and hydrochlorothiazide
(kan de SAR tan & hye droe klor oh THYE a zide)

**U.S./Canadian Brand Names** Atacand HCT™
**Therapeutic Category** Angiotensin II Antagonist Combination

**Use** Treatment of hypertension; combination product should not be used for initial therapy

**Usual Dosage** Adults: Oral: Replacement therapy: Combination product can be substituted for individual agents; maximum therapeutic effect would be expected within 4 weeks

Usual dosage range:

Candesartan: 8-32 mg/day, given once daily or twice daily in divided doses

Hydrochlorothiazide: 12.5-50 mg once daily

**Dosage Forms** Tablet:

Atacand HCT™ 16-12.5: Candesartan 16 mg and hydrochlorothiazide 12.5 mg

Atacand HCT™ 32-12.5: Candesartan 32 mg and hydrochlorothiazide 12.5 mg

## *Candida albicans* (*Monilia*) (KAN dee da AL bi kans mo NIL ya)

**Synonyms** *Monilia* skin test

**U.S./Canadian Brand Names** Dermatophytin-O

**Therapeutic Category** Diagnostic Agent

**Use** Screen for detection of nonresponsiveness to antigens in immunocompromised individuals

**Usual Dosage** Intradermal: 0.1 mL, examine reaction site in 24-48 hours; induration of ≥5 mm in diameter is a positive reaction

**Dosage Forms** Injection:

Intradermal: 1:100 (5 mL)

Scratch: 1:10 (5 mL)

**Candistatin® (Can)** *see* nystatin *on page 432*

**Canesten® (Can)** *see* clotrimazole *on page 147*

**Cantharone® *(Discontinued)*** *see page 750*

**Cantharone Plus® *(Discontinued)*** *see page 750*

**Cantil®** *see* mepenzolate *on page 371*

**Capastat® Sulfate** *see* capreomycin *on next page*

## capecitabine (kap eh SITE a bean)

**U.S./Canadian Brand Names** Xeloda®

**Therapeutic Category** Antineoplastic Agent

**Use** Treatment of patients with metastatic colorectal cancer. Treatment of patients with metastatic breast cancer resistant to both paclitaxel and an anthracycline-containing chemotherapy regimen or resistant to paclitaxel and for whom further anthracycline therapy is not indicated (eg, patients who have received cumulative doses of 400 mg/m$^2$ of doxorubicin or doxorubicin equivalents). Resistance is defined as progressive disease while on treatment, with or without an initial response, or relapse within 6 months of completing treatment with an anthracycline-containing adjuvant regimen.

**Usual Dosage** Refer to individual protocols.

2510 mg/m$^2$ days 1-14 every 3 weeks

1657 mg/m$^2$ days 1-14 every 3 weeks

1331 mg/m$^2$/day

**Dosage Forms** Tablet: 150 mg, 500 mg

**Capex® Shampoo** *see* fluocinolone *on page 253*

**Capital® and Codeine** *see* acetaminophen and codeine *on page 4*

**Capitrol®** *see* chloroxine *on page 128*

**Capoten®** *see* captopril *on next page*

**Capozide®** *see* captopril and hydrochlorothiazide *on page 105*

## capreomycin (kap ree oh MYE sin)

**U.S./Canadian Brand Names** Capastat® Sulfate

**Therapeutic Category** Antibiotic, Miscellaneous

**Use** In conjunction with at least one other antituberculosis agent in the treatment of tuberculosis

**Usual Dosage** Adults: I.M.: 15 mg/kg/day up to 1 g/day for 60-120 days

**Dosage Forms** Injection, as sulfate: 100 mg/mL (10 mL)

**Caprex®** *see* capsaicin *on this page*

**Caprex Plus®** *see* capsaicin *on this page*

**Capsagel®** *see* capsaicin *on this page*

**Capsagel Extra Strength®** *see* capsaicin *on this page*

**Capsagel Maximum Strength®** *see* capsaicin *on this page*

**Capsagesic-HP Arthritis Relief®** *see* capsaicin *on this page*

## capsaicin (kap SAY sin)

**U.S./Canadian Brand Names** Arth Dr®; Arthricare Hand & Body®; Born Again Super Pain Relieving®; Caprex®; Caprex Plus®; Capsagel®; Capsagel Extra Strength®; Capsagel Maximum Strength®; Capsagesic-HP Arthritis Relief®; Capsin® [OTC]; Capzasin-P® [OTC]; D-Care Circulation Stimulator®; Dolorex®; Double Cap®; Icy Hot Arthritis Therapy®; Pain Enz®; Pharmacist's Capsaicin®; Rid-A-Pain®; Rid-A-Pain-HP®; Sloan's Liniment®; Sportsmed®; Theragen®; Theragen HP®; Therapatch Warm®; Trixaicin®; Trixaicin HP®; Zostrix® [OTC]; Zostrix High Potency®; Zostrix®-HP [OTC]; Zostrix Sports®

**Therapeutic Category** Analgesic, Topical

**Use** FDA approved for the topical treatment of pain associated with postherpetic neuralgia, rheumatoid arthritis, osteoarthritis, diabetic neuropathy, and postsurgical pain

**Unlabeled uses:** Treatment of pain associated with psoriasis, chronic neuralgias unresponsive to other forms of therapy, and intractable pruritus

**Usual Dosage** Children >2 years and Adults: Topical: Apply to area up to 3-4 times/day only

**Dosage Forms**

Cream:

- Capzasin-P®, Zostrix®: 0.025% (45 g, 90 g)
- Dolorac™: 0.25% (28 g)
- Rid-A-Pain-HP®: 0.075% (45 g)
- Zostrix®-HP: 0.075% (30 g, 60 g)

Gel (R-Gel®): 0.025% (15 g, 30 g)

Lotion (Capsin®): 0.025% (59 mL); 0.075% (59 mL)

Roll-on (No Pain-HP®): 0.075% (60 mL)

**Capsin® [OTC]** *see* capsaicin *on this page*

## captopril (KAP toe pril)

**U.S./Canadian Brand Names** Alti-Captopril (Can); Apo®-Capto (Can); Capoten®; Novo-Captopril (Can); Nu-Capto (Can); PMS-Captopril (Can)

**Therapeutic Category** Angiotensin-Converting Enzyme (ACE) Inhibitor

**Use** Management of hypertension and treatment of congestive heart failure; in postmyocardial infarction, improves survival in clinically stable patients with left ventricular dysfunction

**Usual Dosage Note:** Dosage must be titrated according to patient's response; use lowest effective dose. Oral:

Infants: Initial: 0.15-0.3 mg/kg/dose; titrate dose upward to maximum of 6 mg/kg/day in 1-4 divided doses; usual required dose: 2.5-6 mg/kg/day

Children: Initial: 0.5 mg/kg/dose; titrate upward to maximum of 6 mg/kg/day in 2-4 divided doses

Older Children: Initial: 6.25-12.5 mg/dose every 12-24 hours; titrate upward to maximum of 6 mg/kg/day

Adolescents and Adults: Initial: 12.5-25 mg/dose administered every 8-12 hours; increase by 25 mg/dose to maximum of 450 mg/day

**Note:** Smaller dosages administered every 8-12 hours are indicated in patients with renal dysfunction. Renal function and leukocyte count should be carefully monitored during therapy.

**Dosage Forms** Tablet: 12.5 mg, 25 mg, 50 mg, 100 mg

## captopril and hydrochlorothiazide

(KAP toe pril & hye droe klor oh THYE a zide)

**U.S./Canadian Brand Names** Capozide®

**Therapeutic Category** Antihypertensive Agent, Combination

**Use** Management of hypertension and treatment of congestive heart failure

**Usual Dosage** Adults: Oral:

Hypertension: Initial: 25 mg 2-3 times/day; may increase at 1- to 2-week intervals up to 150 mg 3 times/day (captopril dosages)

Congestive heart failure: 6.25-25 mg 3 times/day (maximum: 450 mg/day) (captopril dosages)

**Dosage Forms** Tablet:

25/15: Captopril 25 mg and hydrochlorothiazide 15 mg
25/25: Captopril 25 mg and hydrochlorothiazide 25 mg
50/15: Captopril 50 mg and hydrochlorothiazide 15 mg
50/25: Captopril 50 mg and hydrochlorothiazide 25 mg

**Capzasin-P® [OTC]** *see* capsaicin *on previous page*

**Carac™ Topical** *see* fluorouracil *on page 256*

**Carafate®** *see* sucralfate *on page 561*

## carbachol (KAR ba kole)

**Synonyms** carbacholine; carbamylcholine chloride

**U.S./Canadian Brand Names** Carbastat® Ophthalmic; Carboptic® Ophthalmic; Isopto® Carbachol Ophthalmic; Miostat® Intraocular

**Therapeutic Category** Cholinergic Agent

**Use** Lower intraocular pressure in the treatment of glaucoma; to cause miosis during surgery

**Usual Dosage** Adults:

Intraocular: 0.5 mL instilled into anterior chamber before or after securing sutures

Ophthalmic: Instill 1-2 drops up to 4 times/day

**Dosage Forms** Solution:

Intraocular (Carbastat®, Miostat®): 0.01% (1.5 mL);

Topical, ophthalmic:

Carboptic®: 3% (15 mL)

Isopto® Carbachol: 0.75% (15 mL, 30 mL); 1.5% (15 mL, 30 mL); 2.25% (15 mL); 3% (15 mL, 30 mL)

**carbacholine** *see* carbachol *on this page*

## carbamazepine (kar ba MAZ e peen)

**U.S./Canadian Brand Names** Apo®-Carbamazepine (Can); Carbatrol®; Epitol®; Gen-Carbamazepine CR (Can); Novo-Carbamaz (Can); Nu-Carbamazepine (Can); PMS-Carbamazepine (Can); Taro-Carbamazepine (Can); Tegretol®; Tegretol®-XR

**Therapeutic Category** Anticonvulsant

**Use** Prophylaxis of generalized tonic-clonic, partial (especially complex partial), and mixed partial or generalized seizure disorder; may be used to relieve pain in trigeminal neuralgia or diabetic neuropathy; has been used to treat bipolar disorders

(Continued)

## carbamazepine *(Continued)*

**Usual Dosage** Oral (dosage must be adjusted according to patient's response and serum concentrations):

Children:

<6 years: Initial: 5 mg/kg/day; dosage may be increased every 5-7 days to 10 mg/kg/day; then up to 20 mg/kg/day if necessary; administer in 2-4 divided doses/day

6-12 years: Initial: 100 mg twice daily or 10 mg/kg/day in 2 divided doses; increase by 100 mg/day depending upon response; usual maintenance: 15-30 mg/kg/day in 2-4 divided doses/day; maximum: 1000 mg/24 hours

Children >12 years and Adults: 200 mg twice daily to start, increase by 200 mg/day at weekly intervals until therapeutic levels achieved; usual dose: 800-1200 mg/day in 3-4 divided doses; some patients have required up to 1.6-2.4 g/day

**Dosage Forms**

Capsule, extended release: 200 mg, 300 mg

Suspension, oral (citrus-vanilla flavor): 100 mg/5 mL (450 mL)

Tablet: 200 mg

Tablet, chewable: 100 mg

Tablet, extended release: 100 mg, 200 mg, 400 mg

**carbamide** *see* urea *on page 617*

## carbamide peroxide (KAR ba mide per OKS ide)

**Synonyms** urea peroxide

**U.S./Canadian Brand Names** Auro® Ear Drops [OTC]; Debrox® Otic [OTC]; E•R•O Ear [OTC]; Gly-Oxide® Oral [OTC]; Mollifene® Ear Wax Removing Formula [OTC]; Murine® Ear Drops [OTC]; Orajel® Perioseptic® [OTC]; Proxigel® Oral [OTC]

**Therapeutic Category** Anti-infective Agent, Oral; Otic Agent, Cerumenolytic

**Use**

Oral: Relief of minor inflammation of gums, oral mucosal surfaces and lips including canker sores and dental irritation; adjunct in oral hygiene

Otic: Emulsify and disperse ear wax

**Usual Dosage** Children >12 years and Adults:

Oral: Apply several drops undiluted to affected area of the mouth 4 times/day and at bedtime for up to 7 days, expectorate after 2-3 minutes; as an adjunct to oral hygiene after brushing, swish 10 drops for 2-3 minutes, then expectorate; gel: massage on affected area 4 times/day

Otic: Instill 5-10 drops twice daily for up to 4 days; keep drops in ear for several minutes by keeping head tilted or placing cotton in ear

**Dosage Forms**

Gel, oral (Proxigel®): 10% (34 g)

Solution:

Oral:

Gly-Oxide®: 10% in glycerin (15 mL, 60 mL)

Orajel® Perioseptic®: 15% in glycerin (13.3 mL)

Otic (Auro® Ear Drops, Debrox®, Mollifene® Ear Wax Removing, Murine® Ear Drops): 6.5% in glycerin (15 mL, 30 mL)

**carbamylcholine chloride** *see* carbachol *on previous page*

**Carbastat® Ophthalmic** *see* carbachol *on previous page*

**Carbatrol®** *see* carbamazepine *on previous page*

## carbenicillin (kar ben i SIL in)

**Synonyms** carindacillin

**U.S./Canadian Brand Names** Geocillin®

**Therapeutic Category** Penicillin

**Use** Treatment of urinary tract infections, asymptomatic bacteriuria, or prostatitis caused by susceptible strains of *Pseudomonas aeruginosa*, *E. coli*, indole-positive *Proteus*, and *Enterobacter*

**Usual Dosage** Oral:

Children: 30-50 mg/kg/day divided every 6 hours; maximum dose: 2-3 g/day

Adults: 1-2 tablets every 6 hours

**Dosage Forms** Tablet, film coated, as indanyl sodium ester: 382 mg [base]

## carbetocin *(Canada only)* (kar BE toe sin)

**U.S./Canadian Brand Names** Duratocin™ (Can)

**Therapeutic Category** Uteronic Agent

**Use** For the prevention of uterine atony and postpartum hemorrhage following elective cesarean section under epidural or spinal anesthesia.

**Usual Dosage** A single I.V. dose of 100 mcg (1 mL) is administered by bolus injection, over 1 minute, only when delivery of the infant has been completed by cesarean section under epidural anesthetic. Carbetocin can be administered either before or after delivery of the placenta

**Dosage Forms** Injection: 1 mcg/mL (1 mL)

## carbidopa (kar bi DOE pa)

**U.S./Canadian Brand Names** Lodosyn®

**Therapeutic Category** Anti-Parkinson's Agent; Dopaminergic Agent (Anti-Parkinson's)

**Use** With levodopa in the treatment of parkinsonism to enable a lower dosage of the latter to be used and a more rapid response to be obtained, and to decrease side-effects; for details of administration and dosage

**Usual Dosage** Adults: Oral: 70-100 mg/day; maximum daily dose: 200 mg

**Dosage Forms** Tablet: 25 mg

## carbidopa and levodopa (kar bi DOE pa & lee voe DOE pa)

**Synonyms** levodopa and carbidopa

**U.S./Canadian Brand Names** Apo®-Levocarb (Can); Endo® Levodopa/Carbidopa (Can); Nu-Levocarb (Can); Sinemet®

**Therapeutic Category** Anti-Parkinson's Agent; Dopaminergic Agent (Anti-Parkinson's)

**Use** Treatment of Parkinsonian's syndrome

**Usual Dosage** Adults: Oral (carbidopa/levodopa): 75/300 to 150/1500 mg/day in 3-4 divided doses; can increase up to 200/2000 mg/day

**Dosage Forms** Tablet:

10/100: Carbidopa 10 mg and levodopa 100 mg

25/100: Carbidopa 25 mg and levodopa 100 mg

25/250: Carbidopa 25 mg and levodopa 250 mg

Sustained release: Carbidopa 25 mg and levodopa 100 mg; carbidopa 50 mg and levodopa 200 mg

## carbinoxamine and pseudoephedrine

(kar bi NOKS a meen & soo doe e FED rin)

**U.S./Canadian Brand Names** Andehist® Drops; Biohist® LA; Carbiset® Tablet; Carbiset-TR® Tablet; Carbodec® Syrup; Carbodec® Tablet; Carbodec® TR Tablet; Cardec-S® Syrup; Rondec® Drops; Rondec® Filmtab®; Rondec® Syrup; Rondec-TR®

**Therapeutic Category** Antihistamine/Decongestant Combination

**Use** Temporary relief of nasal congestion, running nose, sneezing, itching of nose or throat, and itchy, watery eyes due to the common cold, hay fever, or other respiratory allergies

**Usual Dosage** Oral:

Children:

Drops: 1-18 months: 0.25-1 mL 4 times/day

Syrup:

18 months to 6 years: 2.5 mL 3-4 times/day

(Continued)

## carbinoxamine and pseudoephedrine *(Continued)*

>6 years: 5 mL 2-4 times/day
Adults:
Liquid: 5 mL 4 times/day
Tablet: 1 tablet 4 times/day

**Dosage Forms**
Drops:
Andehist®: Carbinoxamine maleate 2 mg and pseudoephedrine hydrochloride 15 mg per mL (30 mL with dropper)
Rondec®: Carbinoxamine maleate 2 mg and pseudoephedrine hydrochloride 25 mg per mL (30 mL with dropper)
Syrup: Carbinoxamine maleate 4 mg and pseudoephedrine hydrochloride 60 mg per 5 mL (120 mL, 480 mL)
Tablet:
Film-coated: Carbinoxamine maleate 4 mg and pseudoephedrine hydrochloride 60 mg
Sustained release: Carbinoxamine maleate 8 mg and pseudoephedrine hydrochloride 120 mg

## carbinoxamine, pseudoephedrine, and dextromethorphan

(kar bi NOKS a meen, soo doe e FED rin, & deks troe meth OR fan)

**U.S./Canadian Brand Names** Carbodec DM®; Cardec DM®; Pseudo-Car® DM; Rondamine-DM® Drops; Rondec®-DM; Tussafed® Drops

**Therapeutic Category** Antihistamine/Decongestant/Antitussive

**Use** Relief of coughs and upper respiratory symptoms, including nasal congestion, associated with allergy or the common cold

**Usual Dosage**
Infants: Drops:
1-3 months: 1/4 mL 4 times/day
3-6 months: 1/2 mL 4 times/day
6-9 months: 3/4 mL 4 times/day
9-18 months: 1 mL 4 times/day
Children 1 1/2 to 6 years: Syrup: 2.5 mL 4 times/day
Children >6 years and Adults: Syrup: 5 mL 4 times/day

**Dosage Forms**
Drops: Carbinoxamine maleate 2 mg, pseudoephedrine hydrochloride 25 mg, and dextromethorphan hydrobromide 4 mg per mL (30 mL)
Syrup: Carbinoxamine maleate 4 mg, pseudoephedrine hydrochloride 60 mg, and dextromethorphan hydrobromide 15 mg per 5 mL (120 mL, 480 mL, 4000 mL)

**Carbiset® Tablet** *see* carbinoxamine and pseudoephedrine *on previous page*

**Carbiset-TR® Tablet** *see* carbinoxamine and pseudoephedrine *on previous page*

**Carbocaine®** *see* mepivacaine *on page 373*

**Carbodec DM®** *see* carbinoxamine, pseudoephedrine, and dextromethorphan *on this page*

**Carbodec® Syrup** *see* carbinoxamine and pseudoephedrine *on previous page*

**Carbodec® Tablet** *see* carbinoxamine and pseudoephedrine *on previous page*

**Carbodec® TR Tablet** *see* carbinoxamine and pseudoephedrine *on previous page*

## carbol-fuchsin solution (kar bol-FOOK sin soe LOO shun)

**Synonyms** Castellani paint

**Therapeutic Category** Antifungal Agent

**Use** Treatment of superficial mycotic infections

**Usual Dosage** Topical: Apply to affected area 2-4 times/day

**Dosage Forms** Solution: Basic fuchsin 0.3%, boric acid 1%, phenol 4.5%, resorcinol 10%, acetone 5%, and alcohol 10%

**carbolic acid** *see* phenol *on page 465*

**Carbolith™ (Can)** *see* lithium *on page 353*

## carboplatin (KAR boe pla tin)

**Synonyms** CBDCA

**U.S./Canadian Brand Names** Paraplatin®

**Therapeutic Category** Antineoplastic Agent

**Use** Palliative treatment of ovarian carcinoma; also used in the treatment of small cell lung cancer, squamous cell carcinoma of the esophagus; solid tumors of the bladder, cervix and testes; pediatric brain tumor, neuroblastoma

**Usual Dosage** I.V. (refer to individual protocols):

Children:

Solid tumor: 560 mg/m$^2$ once every 4 weeks

Brain tumor: 175 mg/m$^2$ once weekly for 4 weeks with a 2-week recovery period between courses; dose is then adjusted on platelet count and neutrophil count values

Adults: Single agent: 360 mg/m$^2$ once every 4 weeks; dose is then adjusted on platelet count and neutrophil count values

**Dosage Forms** Powder for injection, lyophilized: 50 mg, 150 mg, 450 mg

## carbopol 940 *(Canada only)* (KAR boe pol nine forty)

**U.S./Canadian Brand Names** Lacrinorm (Can)

**Therapeutic Category** Ophthalmic Agent, Miscellaneous

**Use** Artificial tear

**Dosage Forms** Gel, ophthalmic: 20 mg (10 g)

## carboprost tromethamine (KAR boe prost tro METH a meen)

**U.S./Canadian Brand Names** Hemabate™

**Therapeutic Category** Prostaglandin

**Use** Termination of pregnancy

**Usual Dosage** I.M.: Initial: 250 mcg, then 250 mcg at 1½-hour to 3½-hour intervals depending on uterine response; a 500 mcg dose may be administered if uterine response is not adequate after several 250 mcg doses

**Dosage Forms** Injection: Carboprost 250 mcg and tromethamine 83 mcg per mL (1 mL)

**Carboptic® Ophthalmic** *see* carbachol *on page 105*

**carbose d** *see* carboxymethylcellulose *on this page*

## carboxymethylcellulose (kar boks ee meth il SEL yoo lose)

**Synonyms** carbose d; carboxymethylcellulose sodium

**U.S./Canadian Brand Names** Celluvisc® [OTC]

**Therapeutic Category** Ophthalmic Agent, Miscellaneous

**Use** Preservative-free artificial tear substitute

**Usual Dosage** Adults: Ophthalmic: Instill 1-2 drops into eye(s) 3-4 times/day

**Dosage Forms** Solution, ophthalmic, as sodium, preservative free: 0.5% (0.3 mL); 1% (0.3 mL)

**carboxymethylcellulose sodium** *see* carboxymethylcellulose *on this page*

**Cardec DM®** *see* carbinoxamine, pseudoephedrine, and dextromethorphan *on previous page*

**Cardec-S® Syrup** *see* carbinoxamine and pseudoephedrine *on page 107*

**Cardem® *(Discontinued)*** *see page 750*

**Cardene®** *see* nicardipine *on page 418*

**Cardene® SR** *see* nicardipine *on page 418*

**Cardilate® *(Discontinued)*** *see page 750*

**Cardio-Green® *(Discontinued)*** *see page 750*

**Cardizem® CD** *see* diltiazem *on page 187*

**Cardizem® Injectable** *see* diltiazem *on page 187*

**Cardizem® SR** *see* diltiazem *on page 187*

**Cardizem® Tablet** *see* diltiazem *on page 187*

**Cardura®** *see* doxazosin *on page 202*

**carindacillin** *see* carbenicillin *on page 106*

**carisoprodate** *see* carisoprodol *on this page*

## carisoprodol (kar i soe PROE dole)

**Synonyms** carisoprodate; isobamate

**U.S./Canadian Brand Names** Soma®

**Therapeutic Category** Skeletal Muscle Relaxant

**Use** Skeletal muscle relaxant

**Usual Dosage** Adults: Oral: 350 mg 3-4 times/day; administer last dose at bedtime; compound: 1-2 tablets 4 times/day

**Dosage Forms** Tablet: 350 mg

## carisoprodol and aspirin (kar i soe PROE dole & AS pir in)

**U.S./Canadian Brand Names** Soma® Compound

**Therapeutic Category** Skeletal Muscle Relaxant

**Use** Skeletal muscle relaxant

**Usual Dosage** Adults: Oral: 1-2 tablets 4 times/day

**Dosage Forms** Tablet: Carisoprodol 200 mg and aspirin 325 mg

## carisoprodol, aspirin, and codeine

(kar i soe PROE dole, AS pir in, & KOE deen)

**U.S./Canadian Brand Names** Soma® Compound w/Codeine

**Therapeutic Category** Skeletal Muscle Relaxant

**Controlled Substance** C-III

**Use** Skeletal muscle relaxant

**Usual Dosage** Adults: Oral: 1-2 tablets 4 times/day

**Dosage Forms** Tablet: Carisoprodol 200 mg, aspirin 325 mg, and codeine phosphate 16 mg

**Carmol-HC® Topical** *see* urea and hydrocortisone *on page 617*

**Carmol® Scalp** *see* sulfacetamide *on page 562*

**Carmol® Topical [OTC]** *see* urea *on page 617*

## carmustine (kar MUS teen)

**Synonyms** BCNU

**U.S./Canadian Brand Names** BiCNU®

**Therapeutic Category** Antineoplastic Agent

**Use** Brain tumors, multiple myeloma, Hodgkin's disease, and non-Hodgkin's lymphomas; some activity in malignant melanoma; glioblastoma multiforme (wafer)

**Usual Dosage** Children and Adults:

I.V. infusion (refer to individual protocols): 75-100 mg/m$^2$/day for 2 days or 150-200 mg/m$^2$ every 6 weeks as a single dose or divided into daily injections on 2 successive days; next dose is to be determined based on hematologic response to the previous dose

Wafer: Implant 8 wafer in resected brain cavity, if size and shape allow

**Dosage Forms**

Powder for injection: 100 mg/vial packaged with 3 mL of absolute alcohol for use as a sterile diluent

Wafer: 7.7 mg

**Carnation Instant Breakfast® [OTC]** *see* nutritional formula, enteral/oral *on page 432*

**Carnitor® Injection** *see* levocarnitine *on page 345*

**Carnitor® Oral** *see* levocarnitine *on page 345*

**Caroguard®** *see* beta-carotene *on page 76*

**Caroid® *(Discontinued)*** *see page 750*

## carteolol (KAR tee oh lole)

**U.S./Canadian Brand Names** Cartrol® Oral; Ocupress® Ophthalmic

**Therapeutic Category** Beta-Adrenergic Blocker

**Use** Management of hypertension; treatment of increased intraocular pressure

**Usual Dosage** Adults:

Oral: 2.5 mg as a single daily dose, maintenance dose: 2.5-5 mg once daily

Ophthalmic: 1 drop in eye(s) twice daily

**Dosage Forms** Carteolol hydrochloride:

Solution, ophthalmic (Ocupress®): 1% (5 mL, 10 mL)

Tablet (Cartrol®): 2.5 mg, 5 mg

**Carter's Little Pills® [OTC]** *see* bisacodyl *on page 81*

**Cartia® XT** *see* diltiazem *on page 187*

**Cartrol® Oral** *see* carteolol *on this page*

## carvedilol (KAR ve dil ole)

**U.S./Canadian Brand Names** Coreg®

**Therapeutic Category** Beta-Adrenergic Blocker

**Use** Management of hypertension, congestive heart failure; can be used alone or in combination with other agents, especially thiazide-type diuretics

**Usual Dosage** Adults: Oral:

Hypertension: 6.25 mg twice daily; if tolerated, dose should be maintained for 1-2 weeks, then increased to 12.5 mg twice daily; dosage may be increased to a maximum of 25 mg twice daily after 1-2 weeks; reduce dosage if heart rate drops to <55 beats/minute

Congestive heart failure: 3.125 mg twice daily for 2 weeks; if this dose is tolerated, may increase to 6.25 mg twice daily. Double the dose every 2 weeks to the highest dose tolerated by patient. (Prior to initiating therapy, other heart failure medications should be stabilized.)

Maximum recommended dose:

<85 kg: 25 mg twice daily

>85 kg: 50 mg twice daily

Angina pectoris (unlabeled use): 25-50 mg twice daily

Idiopathic cardiomyopathy (unlabeled use): 6.25-25 mg twice daily

**Dosage Forms** Tablet: 3.125 mg, 6.25 mg, 12.5 mg, 25 mg

## cascara sagrada (kas KAR a sah GRAH dah)

**Therapeutic Category** Laxative

**Use** Temporary relief of constipation; sometimes used with milk of magnesia ("black and white" mixture)

**Usual Dosage Note:** Cascara sagrada fluid extract is 5 times more potent than cascara sagrada aromatic fluid extract

Oral (aromatic fluid extract):

Infants: 1.25 mL/day (range: 0.5-1.5 mL) as needed

Children 2-11 years: 2.5 mL/day (range: 1-3 mL) as needed

Children ≥12 years and Adults: 5 mL/day (range: 2-6 mL) as needed at bedtime (1 tablet as needed at bedtime)

**Dosage Forms**

Aromatic fluid extract: 120 mL, 473 mL

(Continued)

## cascara sagrada *(Continued)*

Tablet: 325 mg

**Casodex®** *see* bicalutamide *on page 80*

## caspofungin (kas poe FUN jin)

**U.S./Canadian Brand Names** Cancidas®

**Therapeutic Category** Antifungal Agent

**Use** Treatment of invasive *Aspergillus* infection in patients who do not tolerate or do not respond to other antifungal therapies (including amphotericin B, lipid formulations of amphotericin B, or itraconazole); has not been studied as initial therapy for aspergillosis

**Usual Dosage** I.V.:

Children: Safety and efficacy in pediatric patients have not been established

Adults: *Aspergillus* infection (invasive):

Initial dose: 70 mg infused slowly (over 1 hour)

Subsequent dosing: 50 mg/day (infused over 1 hour)

Duration of treatment should be determined by patient status and clinical response (limited experience beyond 2 weeks of therapy); efficacy of 70 mg/day dose (in patients not responding to 50 mg/day) has not been adequately studied, although this dose appears to be well tolerated

Patients receiving carbamazepine, dexamethasone, efavirenz, nelfinavir, nevirapine, phenytoin, and rifampin (and possibly other enzyme inducers) may require an increased daily dose of caspofungin (70 mg/day) if response to 50 mg/day is inadequate.

**Dosage Forms** Powder for injection, as acetate: 50 mg, 70 mg

**Castellani paint** *see* carbol-fuchsin solution *on page 108*

## castor oil (KAS tor oyl)

**Synonyms** oleum ricini

**U.S./Canadian Brand Names** Alphamul® [OTC]; Emulsoil® [OTC]; Fleet® Flavored Castor Oil [OTC]; Neoloid® [OTC]; Purge® [OTC]

**Therapeutic Category** Laxative

**Use** Preparation for rectal or bowel examination or surgery; rarely used to relieve constipation; also applied to skin as emollient and protectant

**Usual Dosage** Oral:

Castor oil:

Infants <2 years: 1-5 mL or 15 mL/m$^2$/dose as a single dose

Children 2-11 years: 5-15 mL as a single dose

Children ≥12 years and Adults: 15-60 mL as a single dose

Emulsified castor oil:

Infants: 2.5-7.5 mL/dose

Children <2 years: 5-15 mL/dose

Children 2-11 years: 7.5-30 mL/dose

Children ≥12 years and Adults: 30-60 mL/dose

**Dosage Forms**

Emulsion, oral:

Alphamul®: 60% (90 mL, 3780 mL)

Emulsoil®: 95% (63 mL)

Fleet® Flavored Castor Oil: 67% (45 mL, 90 mL)

Neoloid®: 36.4% (118 mL)

Liquid, oral:

100% (60 mL, 120 mL, 480 mL)

Purge®: 95% (30 mL, 60 mL)

**Cataflam® Oral** *see* diclofenac *on page 181*

**Catapres® Oral** *see* clonidine *on page 146*

**Catapres-TTS® Transdermal** *see* clonidine *on page 146*

**Catarase® 1:5000 *(Discontinued)*** *see page 750*

**Caverject® Injection** *see* alprostadil *on page 23*

**CBDCA** *see* carboplatin *on page 109*

**CCNU** *see* lomustine *on page 354*

**C-Crystals® [OTC]** *see* ascorbic acid *on page 54*

**2-CdA** *see* cladribine *on page 140*

**CDDP** *see* cisplatin *on page 139*

**Cebid®** *see* ascorbic acid *on page 54*

**Ceclor®** *see* cefaclor *on this page*

**Ceclor® CD** *see* cefaclor *on this page*

**Cecon® [OTC]** *see* ascorbic acid *on page 54*

**Cedax®** *see* ceftibuten *on page 117*

**Cedilanid-D® Injection *(Discontinued)*** *see page 750*

**Cedocard®-SR (Can)** *see* isosorbide dinitrate *on page 328*

**CeeNU®** *see* lomustine *on page 354*

**Ceepryn® [OTC]** *see* cetylpyridinium *on page 122*

## cefaclor (SEF a klor)

**U.S./Canadian Brand Names** Apo®-Cefaclor (Can); Ceclor®; Ceclor® CD; Novo-Cefaclor (Can); Nu-Cefaclor (Can); PMS-Cefaclor (Can); Scheinpharm Cefaclor (Can)

**Therapeutic Category** Cephalosporin (Second Generation)

**Use** Infections caused by susceptible organisms including *Staphylococcus aureus*, *S. pneumoniae*, and *H. influenzae*; treatment of otitis media, sinusitis, and infections involving the respiratory tract, skin and skin structure, bone and joint, and urinary tract

**Usual Dosage** Oral:

Children >1 month: 20-40 mg/kg/day divided every 8-12 hours; maximum dose: 2 g/day (twice daily option is for treatment of otitis media or pharyngitis)

Adults: 250-500 mg every 8 hours or daily dose can be administered in 2 divided doses

**Dosage Forms**

Capsule: 250 mg, 500 mg

Powder for oral suspension (strawberry flavor): 125 mg/5 mL (75 mL, 150 mL); 187 mg/5 mL (100 mL); 250 mg/5 mL (75 mL, 150 mL); 375 mg/5 mL (100 mL)

Tablet, extended release: 375 mg, 500 mg

## cefadroxil (sef a DROKS il)

**U.S./Canadian Brand Names** Duricef®; Novo-Cefadroxil (Can)

**Therapeutic Category** Cephalosporin (First Generation)

**Use** Treatment of susceptible bacterial infections including group A beta-hemolytic streptococcal pharyngitis or tonsillitis; skin and soft tissue infections caused by streptococci or staphylococci; urinary tract infections caused by *Klebsiella*, *E. coli*, and *Proteus mirabilis*

**Usual Dosage** Oral:

Children: 30 mg/kg/day divided twice daily up to a maximum of 2 g/day

Adults: 1-2 g/day in 2 divided doses

**Dosage Forms**

Capsule, as monohydrate: 500 mg

Suspension, oral, as monohydrate: 125 mg/5 mL, 250 mg/5 mL, 500 mg/5 mL (50 mL, 100 mL)

Tablet, as monohydrate: 1 g

**Cefadyl®** *see* cephapirin *on page 120*

## cefamandole (sef a MAN dole)

**U.S./Canadian Brand Names** Mandol®

**Therapeutic Category** Cephalosporin (Second Generation)

**Use** Treatment of susceptible bacterial infection; mainly respiratory tract, skin and skin structure, bone and joint, urinary tract and gynecologic as well as septicemia, perioperative prophylaxis

**Usual Dosage** I.M., I.V.:

Children: 100-150 mg/kg/day in divided doses every 4-6 hours

Adults: 4-12 g/24 hours divided every 4-6 hours 500-1000 mg every 4-8 hours

**Dosage Forms** Powder for injection, as nafate: 500 mg (10 mL); 1 g (10 mL, 100 mL); 2 g (20 mL, 100 mL); 10 g (100 mL)

**Cefanex**® *see* cephalexin *on page 120*

## cefazolin (sef A zoe lin)

**U.S./Canadian Brand Names** Ancef®; Kefzol®; Zolicef®

**Therapeutic Category** Cephalosporin (First Generation)

**Use** Treatment of respiratory tract, skin and skin structure, urinary tract, biliary tract, bone and joint infections and septicemia due to susceptible gram-positive cocci (except enterococcus); some gram-negative bacilli including *E. coli*, *Proteus*, and *Klebsiella* may be susceptible; perioperative prophylaxis

**Usual Dosage** I.M., I.V.:

Infants and Children: 50-100 mg/kg/day in 3 divided doses; maximum dose: 6 g/day

Adults: 1-2 g every 8 hours

**Dosage Forms**

Infusion, premixed, as sodium, in $D_5W$ (frozen) (Ancef®): 500 mg (50 mL); 1 g (50 mL)

Injection, as sodium (Kefzol®): 500 mg, 1 g

Powder for injection, as sodium (Ancef®, Zolicef®): 250 mg, 500 mg, 1 g, 5 g, 10 g, 20 g

## cefdinir (SEF di ner)

**Synonyms** CFDN

**U.S./Canadian Brand Names** Omnicef®

**Therapeutic Category** Cephalosporin (Third Generation)

**Use** Treatment of community-acquired pneumonia, acute exacerbations of chronic bronchitis, acute bacterial otitis media, acute maxillary sinusitis, pharyngitis/tonsillitis, and uncomplicated skin and skin structure infections.

**Usual Dosage** Oral:

Children (otitis media with effusion): 7 mg/kg orally twice daily or 14 mg/kg orally once daily

Adolescents and Adults: 300 mg orally twice daily; an oral dose of 600 mg once daily has been used in streptococcal pharyngitis

**Dosage Forms**

Capsule: 300 mg

Suspension, oral: 125 mg/5 mL (60 mL, 100 mL)

## cefepime (SEF e pim)

**U.S./Canadian Brand Names** Maxipime®

**Therapeutic Category** Cephalosporin (Fourth Generation)

**Use** Treatment of respiratory tract infections (including bronchitis and pneumonia), cellulitis and other skin and soft tissue infections, and urinary tract infections; considered a fourth generation cephalosporin because it has good gram-negative coverage similar to third generation cephalosporins, but better gram-positive coverage

**Usual Dosage** I.V.:

Children: Unlabeled: 50 mg/kg every 8 hours; maximum dose: 2 g

Adults:

Most infections: 1-2 g every 12 hours for 5-10 days; higher doses or more frequent administration may be required in pseudomonal infections

Urinary tract infections, uncomplicated: 500 mg every 12 hours

**Dosage Forms** Powder for injection, as hydrochloride: 500 mg, 1 g, 2 g

## cefixime (sef IKS eem)

**U.S./Canadian Brand Names** Suprax®

**Therapeutic Category** Cephalosporin (Third Generation)

**Use** Treatment of urinary tract infections, otitis media, respiratory infections due to susceptible organisms including *S. pneumoniae* and *pyogenes*, *H. influenzae*, *M. catarrhalis*, and many Enterobacteriaceae; documented poor compliance with other oral antimicrobials; outpatient therapy of serious soft tissue or skeletal infections due to susceptible organisms; single-dose oral treatment of uncomplicated cervical/urethral gonorrhea due to *N. gonorrhoeae*; treatment of shigellosis in areas with a high rate of resistance to TMP-SMX

**Usual Dosage** Oral:

Children: 8 mg/kg/day in 1-2 divided doses; maximum dose: 400 mg/day

Children >50 kg or >12 years and Adults: 400 mg/day in 1-2 divided doses

**Dosage Forms**

Powder for oral suspension (strawberry flavor): 100 mg/5 mL (50 mL, 100 mL)

Tablet, film coated: 200 mg, 400 mg

**Cefizox®** *see* ceftizoxime *on page 117*

**Cefobid®** *see* cefoperazone *on this page*

**Cefol® Filmtab®** *see* vitamin (multiple/oral) *on page 632*

## cefonicid (se FON i sid)

**U.S./Canadian Brand Names** Monocid®

**Therapeutic Category** Cephalosporin (Second Generation)

**Use** Treatment of susceptible bacterial infection; mainly respiratory tract, skin and skin structure, bone and joint, urinary tract and gynecologic as well as septicemia; second generation cephalosporin

**Usual Dosage** Adults: I.M., I.V.: 1 g every 24 hours

**Dosage Forms** Powder for injection, as sodium: 500 mg, 1 g, 10 g

## cefoperazone (sef oh PER a zone)

**U.S./Canadian Brand Names** Cefobid®

**Therapeutic Category** Cephalosporin (Third Generation)

**Use** Treatment of susceptible bacterial infections, mainly respiratory tract, skin and skin structure, urinary tract and sepsis; as a third generation cephalosporin, cefoperazone has activity against gram-negative bacilli (eg, *E. coli*, *Klebsiella*, and *Haemophilus*) but variable activity against *Streptococcus* and *Staphylococcus* species; it has activity against *Pseudomonas aeruginosa*, but less than ceftazidime

**Usual Dosage** I.M., I.V.:

Children: 100-150 mg/kg/day divided every 8-12 hours

Adults: 2-4 g/day in divided doses every 12 hours (up to 12 g/day)

**Dosage Forms**

Injection, as sodium, premixed (frozen): 1 g (50 mL); 2 g (50 mL)

Powder for injection, as sodium: 1 g, 2 g

**Cefotan®** *see* cefotetan *on next page*

## cefotaxime (sef oh TAKS eem)

**U.S./Canadian Brand Names** Claforan®

**Therapeutic Category** Cephalosporin (Third Generation)

**Use** Treatment of susceptible lower respiratory tract, skin and skin structure, bone and joint, intra-abdominal and genitourinary tract infections; treatment of a documented or suspected meningitis due to susceptible organisms such as *H. influenzae* and *N. meningitidis*; nonpseudomonal gram-negative rod infection in a patient at risk of developing

(Continued)

## cefotaxime *(Continued)*

aminoglycoside-induced nephrotoxicity and/or ototoxicity; infection due to an organism whose susceptibilities clearly favor cefotaxime over cefuroxime or an aminoglycoside

**Usual Dosage** I.M., I.V.:

Infants and Children 1 month to 12 years:

<50 kg: 100-200 mg/kg/day in 3-4 divided doses

Meningitis: 200 mg/kg/day in 4 divided doses

>50 kg: Moderate to severe infection: 1-2 g every 6-8 hours; life-threatening infection: 2 g/dose every 4 hours; maximum dose: 12 g/day

Children >12 years and Adults: 1-2 g every 6-8 hours (up to 12 g/day)

**Dosage Forms**

Infusion, as sodium, premixed, in $D_5W$ (frozen): 1 g (50 mL); 2 g (50 mL)

Powder for injection, as sodium: 500 mg, 1 g, 2 g, 10 g

## cefotetan (SEF oh tee tan)

**U.S./Canadian Brand Names** Cefotan®

**Therapeutic Category** Cephalosporin (Second Generation)

**Use** Treatment of susceptible lower respiratory tract, skin and skin structure, bone and joint, genitourinary tract, sepsis, gynecologic, and intra-abdominal infections; active against anaerobes including *Bacteroides* species of gastrointestinal tract, gram-negative enteric bacilli including *E. coli*, *Klebsiella*, and *Proteus*; active against many strains of *N. gonorrhoeae*; perioperative prophylaxis

**Usual Dosage** I.M., I.V.:

Children: 40-80 mg/kg/day divided every 12 hours

Adults: 1-6 g/day in divided doses every 12 hours, 1-2 g may be administered every 24 hours for urinary tract infection

**Dosage Forms** Powder for injection, as disodium: 1 g (10 mL, 100 mL); 2 g (20 mL, 100 mL); 10 g (100 mL)

## cefoxitin (se FOKS i tin)

**U.S./Canadian Brand Names** Mefoxin®

**Therapeutic Category** Cephalosporin (Second Generation)

**Use** Treatment of susceptible lower respiratory tract, skin and skin structure, bone and joint, genitourinary tract, sepsis, gynecologic, and intra-abdominal infections; active against anaerobes including *Bacteroides* species of the gastrointestinal tract, gram-negative enteric bacilli including *E. coli*, *Klebsiella*, and *Proteus*; active against many strains of *N. gonorrhoeae*; perioperative prophylaxis

**Usual Dosage** I.M., I.V.:

Infants >3 months and Children:

Mild-moderate infection: 80-100 mg/kg/day in divided doses every 4-6 hours

Severe infection: 100-160 mg/kg/day in divided doses every 4-6 hours

Maximum dose: 12 g/day

Adults: 1-2 g every 6-8 hours (I.M. injection is painful)

**Dosage Forms**

Infusion, as sodium, premixed, in $D_5W$ (frozen): 1 g (50 mL); 2 g (50 mL)

Powder for injection, as sodium: 1 g, 2 g, 10 g

## cefpodoxime (sef pode OKS eem)

**U.S./Canadian Brand Names** Vantin®

**Therapeutic Category** Cephalosporin (Second Generation)

**Use** Treatment of susceptible acute, community-acquired pneumonia caused by *S. pneumoniae* or nonbeta-lactamase producing *H. influenzae*; alternative regimen for acute uncomplicated gonorrhea caused by *N. gonorrhoeae*; uncomplicated skin and skin structure infections caused by *S. aureus* or *S. pyogenes*; acute otitis media caused by *S. pneumoniae*, *H. influenzae*, or *M. catarrhalis*; pharyngitis or tonsillitis; and uncomplicated urinary tract infections caused by *E. coli*, *Klebsiella*, and *Proteus*

**Usual Dosage** Oral:
Children >6 months to 12 years: 10 mg/kg/day divided every 12 hours for 10 days
Adults: 100-400 mg every 12 hours for 7-14 days

**Dosage Forms**
Granules for oral suspension, as proxetil (lemon creme flavor): 50 mg/5 mL (100 mL); 100 mg/5 mL (100 mL)
Tablet, film coated, as proxetil: 100 mg, 200 mg

## cefprozil (sef PROE zil)

**U.S./Canadian Brand Names** Cefzil®

**Therapeutic Category** Cephalosporin (Second Generation)

**Use** Infections caused by susceptible organisms including *S. pneumoniae*, *H. influenzae*, *M. catarrhalis*, *S. aureus*, *S. pyogenes*; treatment of infections involving the respiratory tract, skin and skin structure, and otitis media

**Usual Dosage** Oral:
Infants and Children >6 months to 12 years: 15 mg/kg every 12 hours for 10 days
Children >13 years and Adults: 250-500 mg every 12-24 hours for 10 days

**Dosage Forms**
Powder for oral suspension, as anhydrous: 125 mg/5 mL (50 mL, 75 mL, 100 mL); 250 mg/5 mL (50 mL, 75 mL, 100 mL)
Tablet, as anhydrous: 250 mg, 500 mg

## ceftazidime (SEF tay zi deem)

**U.S./Canadian Brand Names** Ceptaz™; Fortaz®; Tazicef®; Tazidime®

**Therapeutic Category** Cephalosporin (Third Generation)

**Use** Treatment of documented susceptible *Pseudomonas aeruginosa* infection and infections due to other susceptible aerobic gram-negative organisms; empiric therapy of a febrile, granulocytopenic patient

**Usual Dosage**
Infants and Children 1 month to 12 years: 30-50 mg/kg/dose every 8 hours; maximum dose: 6 g/day
Adults: 1-2 g every 8-12 hours (250-500 mg every 12 hours for urinary tract infections)

**Dosage Forms**
Infusion, premixed (frozen) (Fortaz®): 1 g (50 mL); 2 g (50 mL)
Powder for injection: 500 mg, 1 g, 2 g, 6 g

## ceftibuten (sef TYE byoo ten)

**U.S./Canadian Brand Names** Cedax®

**Therapeutic Category** Cephalosporin (Third Generation)

**Use** Oral cephalosporin for bronchitis, otitis media, and strep throat

**Usual Dosage** Oral:
Children: 9 mg/kg/day for 10 days; maximum daily dose: 400 mg
Children ≥12 years and Adults: 400 mg once daily for 10 days

**Dosage Forms**
Capsule: 400 mg
Powder for oral suspension (cherry flavor): 90 mg/5 mL (30 mL, 60 mL, 120 mL); 180 mg/5 mL (30 mL, 60 mL, 120 mL)

**Ceftin® Oral** *see* cefuroxime *on next page*

## ceftizoxime (sef ti ZOKS eem)

**U.S./Canadian Brand Names** Cefizox®

**Therapeutic Category** Cephalosporin (Third Generation)

**Use** Treatment of susceptible bacterial infections, mainly respiratory tract, skin and skin structure, bone and joint, urinary tract and sepsis; as a third generation cephalosporin, ceftizoxime has activity against gram-negative enteric bacilli (eg, *E. coli*, *Klebsiella*), and cocci (eg, *Neisseria*), and variable activity against gram-positive cocci (*Staphylococcus* and *Streptococcus*); it has some anaerobic coverage but is less active against *B. fragilis*
(Continued)

## ceftizoxime *(Continued)*

than cefoxitin; also indicated for *Neisseria gonorrhoeae* infections (including uncomplicated cervical and urethral gonorrhea and gonorrhea pelvic inflammatory disease), and *Haemophilus influenzae* meningitis

**Usual Dosage** I.M., I.V.:

Children ≥6 months: 50 mg/kg every 6-8 hours to 200 mg/kg/day to maximum of 12 g/24 hours

Adults: 1-2 g every 8-12 hours, up to 2 g every 4 hours or 4 g every 8 hours for life-threatening infections

**Dosage Forms**

Injection, as sodium, in $D_5W$ (frozen): 1 g (50 mL); 2 g (50 mL)

Powder for injection, as sodium: 500 mg, 1 g, 2 g, 10 g

## ceftriaxone (sef trye AKS one)

**U.S./Canadian Brand Names** Rocephin®

**Therapeutic Category** Cephalosporin (Third Generation)

**Use** Treatment of sepsis, meningitis, infections of the lower respiratory tract, skin and skin structure, bone and joint, intra-abdominal and urinary tract due to susceptible organisms as a third generation cephalosporin, ceftriaxone has activity against gram-negative aerobic bacteria (ie, *H. influenzae*, Enterobacteriaceae, *Neisseria*) and variable activity against gram-positive cocci; documented or suspected infection due to susceptible organisms in home care patients and patients without I.V. line access; treatment of documented or suspected gonococcal infection or chancroid; emergency room management of patients at high risk for bacteremia, periorbital or buccal cellulitis, salmonellosis or shigellosis and pneumonia of unestablished etiology (<5 years of age)

**Usual Dosage**

Gonococcal ophthalmia: 25-50 mg/kg/day administered every 24 hours

Infants and Children: 50-100 mg/kg/day in 1-2 divided doses

Meningitis: 100 mg/kg/day divided every 12 hours; loading dose of 75 mg/kg may be administered at the start of therapy

Chancroid, uncomplicated gonorrhea: I.M.:

<45 kg: 125 mg as a single dose

>45 kg: 250 mg as a single dose

Adults: 1-2 g every 12-24 hours depending on the type and severity of the infection; maximum dose: 4 g/day

**Dosage Forms**

Infusion, as sodium, premixed (frozen): 1 g in $D_{3.8}W$ (50 mL); 2 g in $D_{2.4}W$ (50 mL)

Injection, as sodium: 350 mg/mL

Powder for injection, as sodium: 250 mg, 500 mg, 1 g, 2 g, 10 g

## cefuroxime (se fyoor OKS eem)

**U.S./Canadian Brand Names** Ceftin® Oral; Kefurox® Injection; Zinacef® Injection

**Therapeutic Category** Cephalosporin (Second Generation)

**Use** Second generation cephalosporin useful in infections caused by susceptible staphylococci, group B streptococci, pneumococci, *H. influenzae* (type A and B), *E. coli*, *Enterobacter*, and *Klebsiella*; treatment of susceptible infections of the upper and lower respiratory tract, otitis media, urinary tract, skin and soft tissue, bone and joint, and sepsis

**Usual Dosage**

Children:

Oral:

<12 years: 125 mg twice daily

>12 years: 250 mg twice daily

I.M., I.V.: 75-150 mg/kg/day divided every 8 hours; maximum dose: 9 g/day

Adults:

Oral: 125-500 mg twice daily, depending on severity of infection

I.M., I.V.: 100-150 mg/kg/day in divided doses every 6-8 hours; maximum: 6 g/24 hours

**Dosage Forms**
Infusion, as sodium, premixed (frozen) (Zinacef®): 750 mg (50 mL); 1.5 g (50 mL)
Powder for injection, as sodium: 750 mg, 1.5 g, 7.5 g
Powder for injection, as sodium (Kefurox®, Zinacef®): 750 mg, 1.5 g, 7.5 g
Powder for oral suspension, as axetil (tutti-frutti flavor) (Ceftin®): 125 mg/5 mL (50 mL, 100 mL, 200 mL) 250 mg/5 mL (50 mL, 100 mL)
Tablet, as axetil (Ceftin®): 125 mg, 250 mg, 500 mg

**Cefzil®** *see* cefprozil *on page 117*

**Celebrex™** *see* celecoxib *on this page*

## celecoxib (ce le COX ib)

**U.S./Canadian Brand Names** Celebrex™
**Therapeutic Category** Nonsteroidal Anti-inflammatory Drug (NSAID), COX-2 Selective
**Use** Short-term efficacy in rheumatoid arthritis and osteoarthritis; oral adjunct to usual care for patients with familial adenomatous polyposis
**Usual Dosage** Adults: Oral:
Osteoarthritis: 200 mg once/day or 100 mg twice daily
Rheumatoid arthritis: 100-200 mg twice daily
**Dosage Forms** Capsule: 100 mg, 200 mg

**Celectol®** ***(Discontinued)*** *see page 750*

**Celestone® Oral** *see* betamethasone (systemic) *on page 77*

**Celestone® Phosphate Injection** *see* betamethasone (systemic) *on page 77*

**Celestone® Soluspan®** *see* betamethasone (systemic) *on page 77*

**Celexa™** *see* citalopram *on page 140*

**CellCept®** *see* mycophenolate *on page 404*

## cellulose, oxidized (SEL yoo lose, OKS i dyzed)

**Synonyms** absorbable cotton
**U.S./Canadian Brand Names** Oxycel®; Surgicel®
**Therapeutic Category** Hemostatic Agent
**Use** Temporary packing for the control of capillary, venous, or small arterial hemorrhage
**Usual Dosage** Minimal amounts of an appropriate size are laid on the bleeding site
**Dosage Forms**
Pad (Oxycel®): 3" x 3", 8 ply
Pledget (Oxycel®): 2" x 1" x 1"
Strip:
Oxycel®: 18" x 2", 4 ply; 5" x 1/2", 4 ply; 36" x 1/2", 4 ply
Surgicel®: 2" x 14"; 4" x 8"; 2" x 3"; 1/2" x 2"

## cellulose sodium phosphate (sel yoo lose SOW dee um FOS fate)

**Synonyms** CSP; sodium cellulose phosphate
**U.S./Canadian Brand Names** Calcibind®
**Therapeutic Category** Urinary Tract Product
**Use** Adjunct to dietary restriction to reduce renal calculi formation in absorptive hypercalciuria type I
**Usual Dosage** Adults: Oral: 5 g 3 times/day with meals; decrease dose to 5 g with main meal and 2.5 g with each of two other meals when urinary calcium declines to <150 mg/day
**Dosage Forms** Powder: 2.5 g packets (90s), 300 g bulk pack

**Celluvisc® [OTC]** *see* carboxymethylcellulose *on page 109*

**Celontin®** *see* methsuximide *on page 382*

**Cel-U-Jec® Injection** *see* betamethasone (systemic) *on page 77*

**Cenafed® [OTC]** *see* pseudoephedrine *on page 507*

**Cenafed® Plus Tablet [OTC]** *see* triprolidine and pseudoephedrine *on page 609*

**Cena-K®** *see* potassium chloride *on page 485*

**Cenestin™** *see* estrogens (conjugated A/synthetic) *on page 227*

**Cenocort® A-40 *(Discontinued)*** *see page 750*

**Cenocort® Forte *(Discontinued)*** *see page 750*

**Centrax® Capsule & Tablet *(Discontinued)*** *see page 750*

**Cēpacol® Anesthetic Troches [OTC]** *see* cetylpyridinium and benzocaine *on page 122*

**Cēpacol® Troches [OTC]** *see* cetylpyridinium *on page 122*

**Cēpastat® [OTC]** *see* phenol *on page 465*

## cephalexin (sef a LEKS in)

**U.S./Canadian Brand Names** Apo®-Cephalex (Can); Biocef®; Cefanex®; Keflex®; Keftab®; Novo-Lexin® (Can); Nu-Cephalex (Can); PMS-Cephalexin (Can)

**Therapeutic Category** Cephalosporin (First Generation)

**Use** Treatment of susceptible bacterial infections, including those caused by group A beta-hemolytic *Streptococcus*, *Staphylococcus*, *Klebsiella pneumoniae*, *E. coli*, and *Proteus mirabilis*; not active against enterococci; used to treat susceptible infections of the respiratory tract, skin and skin structure, bone, genitourinary tract, and otitis media

**Usual Dosage** Oral:

Children: 25-50 mg/kg/day every 6 hours; severe infections: 50-100 mg/kg/day in divided doses every 6 hours; maximum: 3 g/24 hours

Adults: 250-1000 mg every 6 hours

**Dosage Forms**

Capsule, as monohydrate: 250 mg, 500 mg

Powder for oral suspension, as monohydrate: 125 mg/5 mL (5 mL unit dose, 60 mL, 100 mL, 200 mL); 250 mg/5 mL (5 mL unit dose, 100 mL, 200 mL)

Suspension, oral, as monohydrate, pediatric: 100 mg/mL [5 mg/drop] (10 mL)

Tablet, as hydrochloride: 500 mg

Tablet, as monohydrate: 250 mg, 500 mg, 1 g

## cephalothin (sef A loe thin)

**U.S./Canadian Brand Names** Ceporacin® (Can)

**Therapeutic Category** Cephalosporin (First Generation)

**Use** Treatment of respiratory tract, skin and skin structure, urinary tract, bone and joint infections, endocarditis, and septicemia due to susceptible gram-positive cocci (except enterococcus); some gram-negative bacilli including *E. coli*, *Proteus*, and *Klebsiella* may be susceptible; perioperative prophylaxis

**Usual Dosage** I.M., I.V.:

Children: 75-125 mg/kg/day divided every 4-6 hours; maximum dose: 10 g in a 24-hour period

Adults: 500 mg to 2 g every 4-6 hours

**Dosage Forms**

Infusion, as sodium, in $D_5W$ (frozen): 1 g (50 mL); 2 g (50 mL)

Powder for injection, as sodium: 1 g, 2 g, 20 g

## cephapirin (sef a PYE rin)

**U.S./Canadian Brand Names** Cefadyl®

**Therapeutic Category** Cephalosporin (First Generation)

**Use** Treatment of respiratory tract, skin and skin structure, urinary tract, bone and joint infections, endocarditis and septicemia due to susceptible gram-positive cocci (except enterococcus); some gram-negative bacilli including *E. coli*, *Proteus*, and *Klebsiella*, may be susceptible; perioperative prophylaxis

**Usual Dosage** I.M., I.V.:
Children: 10-20 mg/kg every 6 hours up to 4 g/24 hours
Adults: 1 g every 6 hours up to 12 g/day
**Dosage Forms** Powder for injection, as sodium: 500 mg, 1 g, 2 g, 4 g, 20 g

## cephradine (SEF ra deen)

**U.S./Canadian Brand Names** Velosef®
**Therapeutic Category** Cephalosporin (First Generation)
**Use** Treatment of susceptible bacterial infections, including those caused by group A beta-hemolytic *Streptococcus*
**Usual Dosage** Oral:
Children ≥9 months: 25-100 mg/kg/day in equally divided doses every 6-12 hours up to 4 g/day
Adults: 2-4 g/day in 4 equally divided doses up to 8 g/day
**Dosage Forms**
Capsule: 250 mg, 500 mg
Powder for injection: 250 mg, 500 mg, 1 g, 2 g (in ready to use infusion bottles)
Powder for oral suspension: 125 mg/5 mL (5 mL, 100 mL, 200 mL); 250 mg/5 mL (5 mL, 100 mL, 200 mL)

**Cephulac®** *see* lactulose *on page 338*

**Ceporacin® (Can)** *see* cephalothin *on previous page*

**Ceptaz™** *see* ceftazidime *on page 117*

**Cerebyx®** *see* fosphenytoin *on page 265*

**Ceredase®** *see* alglucerase *on page 20*

**Cerespan®** ***(Discontinued)*** *see page 750*

**Cerezyme®** *see* imiglucerase *on page 314*

**Cerose-DM® [OTC]** *see* chlorpheniramine, phenylephrine, and dextromethorphan *on page 131*

**Certiva™** *see* diphtheria, tetanus toxoids, and acellular pertussis vaccine *on page 193*

**Cerubidine®** *see* daunorubicin hydrochloride *on page 167*

**Cerumenex® Otic** *see* triethanolamine polypeptide oleate-condensate *on page 604*

**Cervidil® Vaginal Insert** *see* dinoprostone *on page 189*

**CES** *see* estrogens (conjugated/equine) *on page 227*

**Cesamet®** ***(Discontinued)*** *see page 750*

**C.E.S.® (Can)** *see* estrogens (conjugated/equine) *on page 227*

**Cetacaine®** *see* benzocaine, butyl aminobenzoate, tetracaine, and benzalkonium chloride *on page 73*

**Cetacort® Topical** *see* hydrocortisone (topical) *on page 304*

**Cetafen® [OTC]** *see* acetaminophen *on page 3*

**Cetafen® Extra [OTC]** *see* acetaminophen *on page 3*

**Cetamide®** *see* sulfacetamide *on page 562*

**Cetane®** ***(Discontinued)*** *see page 750*

**Cetapred® Ophthalmic** *see* sulfacetamide and prednisolone *on page 563*

## cetirizine (se TI ra zeen)

**Synonyms** P-071; UCB-P071
**U.S./Canadian Brand Names** Apo®-Cetirizine (Can); Reactine™ (Can); Zyrtec®
**Therapeutic Category** Antihistamine
(Continued)

## cetirizine *(Continued)*

**Use** Perennial and seasonal allergic rhinitis and other allergic symptoms including urticaria

**Usual Dosage** Children ≥6 years and Adults: Oral: 5-10 mg once daily, depending upon symptom severity

**Dosage Forms**

Syrup, as hydrochloride: 5 mg/5 mL (120 mL)

Tablet, as hydrochloride: 5 mg, 10 mg

## cetirizine and pseudoephedrine (se TI ra zeen & soo doe e FED rin)

**U.S./Canadian Brand Names** Zyrtec-D 12 Hour™

**Therapeutic Category** Antihistamine/Decongestant Combination

**Use** Treatment of symptoms of seasonal or perennial allergic rhinitis

**Usual Dosage** Oral:

Children ≥12 years and Adults: Seasonal/perennial allergic rhinitis: 1 tablet twice daily

**Dosage Forms** Tablet, extended release: Cetirizine hydrochloride 5 mg and pseudoephedrine hydrochloride 120 mg

## cetrorelix (se troh REE liks)

**U.S./Canadian Brand Names** Cetrotide™

**Therapeutic Category** Antigonadotropic Agent

**Use** Inhibits premature luteinizing hormone (LH) surges in women undergoing controlled ovarian stimulation

**Usual Dosage** S.C.: Adults: Female: Used in conjunction with controlled ovarian stimulation therapy using gonadotropins (FSH, HMG):

Single dose regimen: 3 mg given when serum estradiol levels show appropriate stimulation response, usually stimulation day 7 (range days 5-9). If hCG is not administered within 4 days, continue cetrorelix at 0.25 mg/day until hCG is administered

Multiple dose regimen: 0.25 mg morning or evening of stimulation day 5, or morning of stimulation day 6; continue until hCG is administered.

**Dosage Forms** Injection, single-dose vial:

0.25 mg with 1 mL sterile water for injection in a prefilled glass syringe

3 mg with 3 mL sterile water for injection in a prefilled glass syringe

**Cetrotide™** *see* cetrorelix *on this page*

## cetylpyridinium (SEE til peer i DI nee um)

**U.S./Canadian Brand Names** Ceepryn® [OTC]; Cēpacol® Troches [OTC]

**Therapeutic Category** Local Anesthetic

**Use** Temporary relief of sore throat

**Usual Dosage** Children >6 years and Adults: Oral: Dissolve 1 lozenge in the mouth every 2 hours as needed

**Dosage Forms**

Mouthwash, as chloride: 0.05% and alcohol 14% (180 mL)

Troches, as chloride: 1:1500 (24s)

## cetylpyridinium and benzocaine

(SEE til peer i DI nee um & BEN zoe kane)

**U.S./Canadian Brand Names** Cēpacol® Anesthetic Troches [OTC]

**Therapeutic Category** Local Anesthetic

**Use** Symptomatic relief of sore throat

**Usual Dosage** Oral: Use as needed for sore throat

**Dosage Forms** Troche: Cetylpyridinium chloride 1:1500 and benzocaine 10 mg per troche (18s)

**Cevalin® [OTC]** *see* ascorbic acid *on page 54*

**Cevi-bid® [OTC]** *see* ascorbic acid *on page 54*

**cevimeline** (se vi ME leen)

**U.S./Canadian Brand Names** Evoxac™

**Therapeutic Category** Cholinergic Agent

**Use** Treatment of symptoms of dry mouth in patients with Sjögren's syndrome

**Usual Dosage** Adults: Oral: 30 mg 3 times/day

**Dosage Forms** Capsule: 30 mg

**Ce-Vi-Sol® [OTC]** *see* ascorbic acid *on page 54*

**CFDN** *see* cefdinir *on page 114*

**CG** *see* chorionic gonadotropin *on page 136*

**CGP-42446** *see* zoledronic acid *on page 640*

**CGP 57148B** *see* imatinib *on page 313*

**CharcoAid® [OTC]** *see* charcoal *on this page*

**charcoal** (CHAR kole)

**Synonyms** activated carbon; liquid antidote; medicinal carbon

**U.S./Canadian Brand Names** Actidose-Aqua® [OTC]; Actidose® With Sorbitol [OTC]; CharcoAid® [OTC]; Charcocaps® [OTC]; Charcodote Aqueous (Can); Liqui-Char® [OTC]

**Therapeutic Category** Antidote

**Use** Emergency treatment in poisoning by drugs and chemicals; repetitive doses for gastrointestinal dialysis in drug overdose to enhance the elimination of certain drugs (eg, theophylline, phenobarbital, and aspirin) and in uremia to adsorb various waste products

**Usual Dosage** Oral:

Acute poisoning: Single dose: Charcoal with sorbitol:

Children 1-12 years: 1-2 g/kg/dose or 15-30 g or approximately 5-10 times the weight of the ingested poison; 1 g adsorbs 100-1000 mg of poison; the use of repeat oral charcoal with sorbitol doses is not recommended. In young children sorbitol should be repeated no more than 1-2 times/day.

Adults: 30-100 g

Charcoal in water:

Single dose:

Infants <1 year: 1 g/kg

Children 1-12 years: 15-30 g or 1-2 g/kg

Adults: 30-100 g or 1-2 g/kg

Multiple dose:

Infants <1 year: 1 g/kg every 4-6 hours

Children 1-12 years: 20-60 g or 1-2 g/kg every 2-6 hours until clinical observations and serum drug concentration have returned to a subtherapeutic range

Adults: 20-60 g or 1-2 g/kg every 2-6 hours

Gastric dialysis: Adults: 20-50 g every 6 hours for 1-2 days

**Dosage Forms**

Capsule (Charcocaps®): 260 mg

Liquid, activated:

Actidose-Aqua®: 12.5 g (60 mL); 25 g (120 mL)

Liqui-Char®: 12.5 g (60 mL); 15 g (75 mL); 25 g (120 mL); 30 g (120 mL); 50 g (240 mL)

Liquid, activated, with propylene glycol: 12.5 g (60 mL); 25 g (120 mL)

Liquid, activated, with sorbitol:

Actidose® With Sorbitol: 25 g (120 mL); 50 g (240 mL)

CharcoAid®: 30 g (150 mL)

Powder for suspension, activated: 15 g, 30 g, 40 g, 120 g, 240 g

**Charcocaps® [OTC]** *see* charcoal *on this page*

**Charcodote Aqueous (Can)** *see* charcoal *on this page*

**Chealamide®** *see* edetate disodium *on page 210*

**Chemet**® *see* succimer *on page 560*

**Chenix**® **Tablet *(Discontinued)*** *see page 750*

**Cheracol**® *see* guaifenesin and codeine *on page 282*

**Cheracol**® **D [OTC]** *see* guaifenesin and dextromethorphan *on page 282*

**Chibroxin**™ **Ophthalmic** *see* norfloxacin *on page 425*

**chicken pox vaccine** *see* varicella virus vaccine *on page 622*

**Chiggertox**® **[OTC]** *see* benzocaine *on page 72*

**Children's Advil**® **Suspension** *see* ibuprofen *on page 311*

**Children's Hold**® **[OTC]** *see* dextromethorphan *on page 178*

**Children's Kaopectate**® **[OTC]** *see* attapulgite *on page 60*

**Children's Motrin**® **Suspension [OTC]** *see* ibuprofen *on page 311*

**Children's Silfedrine**® **[OTC]** *see* pseudoephedrine *on page 507*

**children's vitamins** *see* vitamin (multiple/pediatric) *on page 632*

**Chirocaine**® *see* levobupivacaine *on page 345*

**Chlo-Amine**® **[OTC]** *see* chlorpheniramine *on page 129*

**Chlorafed**® **Liquid [OTC]** *see* chlorpheniramine and pseudoephedrine *on page 130*

**chloral** *see* chloral hydrate *on this page*

## chloral hydrate (KLOR al HYE drate)

**Synonyms** chloral; trichloroacetaldehyde monohydrate

**U.S./Canadian Brand Names** Aquachloral® Supprettes®; PMS-Chloral Hydrate (Can)

**Therapeutic Category** Hypnotic, Nonbarbiturate

**Controlled Substance** C-IV

**Use** Short-term sedative and hypnotic (<2 weeks), sedative/hypnotic prior to nonpainful therapeutic or diagnostic procedures (eg, EEG, CT scan, MRI, ophthalmic exam, dental procedure)

**Usual Dosage**

Children:

Sedation, anxiety: Oral, rectal: 5-15 mg/kg/dose every 8 hours, maximum: 500 mg/dose

Prior to EEG: Oral, rectal: 20-25 mg/kg/dose, 30-60 minutes prior to EEG; may repeat in 30 minutes to maximum of 100 mg/kg or 2 g total

Hypnotic: Oral, rectal: 20-40 mg/kg/dose up to a maximum of 50 mg/kg/24 hours or 1 g/dose or 2 g/24 hours

Sedation, nonpainful procedure: Oral: 50-75 mg/kg/dose 30-60 minutes prior to procedure; may repeat 30 minutes after initial dose if needed, to a total maximum dose of 120 mg/kg or 1 g total

Adults: Oral, rectal:

Sedation, anxiety: 250 mg 3 times/day

Hypnotic: 500-1000 mg at bedtime or 30 minutes prior to procedure, not to exceed 2 g/24 hours

**Dosage Forms**

Capsule: 250 mg, 500 mg

Suppository, rectal: 324 mg, 500 mg, 648 mg

Syrup: 250 mg/5 mL (10 mL); 500 mg/5 mL (5 mL, 10 mL, 480 mL)

## chlorambucil (klor AM byoo sil)

**U.S./Canadian Brand Names** Leukeran®

**Therapeutic Category** Antineoplastic Agent

**Use** Management of chronic lymphocytic leukemia (CLL), Hodgkin's and non-Hodgkin's lymphoma; breast and ovarian carcinoma, testicular carcinoma, choriocarcinoma;

Waldenström's macroglobulinemia, and nephrotic syndrome unresponsive to conventional therapy

**Usual Dosage** Children and Adults: Oral (refer to individual protocols):

General short courses: 0.1-0.2 mg/kg/day or 4-8 mg/m²/day for 2-3 weeks for remission induction, then adjust dose on basis of blood counts; maintenance therapy: 0.03-0.1 mg/kg/day

Nephrotic syndrome: 0.1-0.2 mg/kg/day every day for 5-15 weeks with low-dose prednisone

Chronic lymphocytic leukemia:

Biweekly regimen: Initial: 0.4 mg/kg dose is increased by 0.1 mg/kg every 2 weeks until a response occurs and/or myelosuppression occurs

Monthly regimen: Initial: 0.4 mg/kg, increase dose by 0.2 mg/kg every 4 weeks until a response occurs and/or myelosuppression occurs

Malignant lymphomas:

Non-Hodgkins: 0.1 mg/kg/day

Hodgkins: 0.2 mg/kg/day

**Dosage Forms** Tablet, sugar coated: 2 mg

## chloramphenicol (klor am FEN i kole)

**U.S./Canadian Brand Names** Chloromycetin® Injection; Chloroptic® Ophthalmic; Diochloram® (Can); Ocu-Chlor®; Pentamycetin® (Can)

**Therapeutic Category** Antibiotic, Ophthalmic; Antibiotic, Otic; Antibiotic, Miscellaneous

**Use** Treatment of serious infections due to organisms resistant to other less toxic antibiotics or when its penetrability into the site of infection is clinically superior to other antibiotics to which the organism is sensitive; useful in infections caused by *Bacteroides*, *H. influenzae*, *Neisseria meningitidis*, *S. pneumoniae*, *Salmonella*, and *Rickettsia*

**Usual Dosage**

I.V.:

Infants and Children: 50-75 mg/kg/day divided every 6 hours; maximum daily dose: 4 g/day

Adults: 50 mg/kg/day in divided doses every 6 hours; maximum daily dose: 4 g/day

Ophthalmic: Children and Adults: Instill 1-2 drops or small amount of ointment every 3-6 hours; increase interval between applications after 48 hours

**Dosage Forms**

Capsule: 250 mg

Ointment, ophthalmic: 1% [10 mg/g] (3.5 g)

Powder for injection, as sodium succinate: 1 g

Solution: 0.5% [5 mg/mL] (7.5 mL, 15 mL)

Ophthalmic: 0.5% [5 mg/mL] (2.5 mL, 7.5 mL, 15 mL)

Otic: 0.5% (15 mL)

## chloramphenicol and prednisolone

(klor am FEN i kole & pred NIS oh lone)

**U.S./Canadian Brand Names** Chloroptic-P® Ophthalmic

**Therapeutic Category** Antibiotic/Corticosteroid, Ophthalmic

**Use** Topical anti-infective and corticosteroid for treatment of ocular infections

**Usual Dosage** Ophthalmic: Instill 1-2 drops in eye(s) 2-4 times/day

**Dosage Forms** Ointment, ophthalmic: Chloramphenicol 1% and prednisolone 0.5% (3.5 g)

**Chloraseptic® Oral [OTC]** *see* phenol *on page 465*

## chlordiazepoxide (klor dye az e POKS ide)

**Synonyms** methaminodiazepoxide

**U.S./Canadian Brand Names** Apo®-Chlordiazepoxide (Can); Librium®; Novo-Poxide (Can)

(Continued)

## chlordiazepoxide *(Continued)*

**Therapeutic Category** Benzodiazepine

**Controlled Substance** C-IV

**Use** Management of anxiety and as a preoperative sedative, symptoms of alcohol withdrawal

**Usual Dosage**

Children >6 years: Anxiety: Oral, I.M.: 0.5 mg/kg/24 hours divided every 6-8 hours

Adults:

Anxiety: Oral: 15-100 mg divided 3-4 times/day

Severe anxiety: 20-25 mg 3-4 times/day

Preoperative sedation:

Oral: 5-10 mg 3-4 times/day, 1-day preop

I.M.: 50-100 mg 1-hour preop

Alcohol withdrawal symptoms: Oral, I.V.: 50-100 mg to start, dose may be repeated in 2-4 hours as necessary to a maximum of 300 mg/24 hours

**Dosage Forms**

Capsule, as hydrochloride: 5 mg, 10 mg, 25 mg

Powder for injection, as hydrochloride: 100 mg

**Chloresium® [OTC]** *see* chlorophyll *on next page*

**Chlorgest-HD® Elixir *(Discontinued)*** *see page 750*

## chlorhexidine gluconate (klor HEKS i deen GLOO koe nate)

**U.S./Canadian Brand Names** BactoShield® [OTC]; Betasept® [OTC]; Dyna-Hex® [OTC]; Exidine® Scrub [OTC]; Hibiclens® [OTC]; Hibidil® (Can); Hibistat® [OTC]; Oro-Clense (Can); Peridex®; Periochip®; PerioGard®; Spectro Gram "2"™ (Can)

**Therapeutic Category** Antibiotic, Oral Rinse; Antibiotic, Topical

**Use**

Dental:

Antibacterial dental rinse; chlorhexidine is active against gram-positive and gram-negative organisms, facultative anaerobes, aerobes, and yeast

Chip, for periodontal pocket insertion; indicated as an adjunct to scaling and root planing procedures for reduction of pocket depth in patients with adult periodontitis; may be used as part of a periodontal maintenance program

Medical: Skin cleanser for surgical scrub, cleanser for skin wounds, germicidal hand rinse

**Usual Dosage** Oral rinse (Peridex®)

Precede use of solution by flossing and brushing teeth, completely rinse toothpaste from mouth; swish 15 mL undiluted oral rinse around in mouth for 30 seconds, then expectorate. Caution patient not to swallow the medicine; avoid eating for 2-3 hours after treatment. (The cap on bottle of oral rinse is a measure for 15 mL.)

When used as a treatment of gingivitis, the regimen begins with oral prophylaxis. Patient treats mouth with 15 mL chlorhexidine; swish for 30 seconds, then expectorate; this is repeated twice daily (morning and evening). Patient should have a re-evaluation followed by a dental prophylaxis every 6 months.

**Dosage Forms**

Chip, for periodontal pocket insertion (PerioChip®): 2.5 mg

Foam, topical, with isopropyl alcohol 4% (BactoShield®): 4% (180 mL)

Liquid, topical, with isopropyl alcohol 4%:

Dyna-Hex® Skin Cleanser: 2% (120 mL, 240 mL, 480 mL, 960 mL, 4000 mL); 4% (120 mL, 240 mL, 480 mL, 4000 mL)

BactoShield® 2: 2% (960 mL)

BactoShield®, Betasept®, Exidine® Skin Cleanser, Hibiclens® Skin Cleanser: 4% (15 mL, 120 mL, 240 mL, 480 mL, 960 mL, 4000 mL)

Rinse:

Oral (mint flavor) (Peridex®, PerioGard®): 0.12% with alcohol 11.6% (480 mL)

Topical (Hibistat® Hand Rinse): 0.5% with isopropyl alcohol 70% (120 mL, 240 mL)

Sponge/Brush (Hibiclens®): 4% with isopropyl alcohol 4% (22 mL)

Wipes (Hibistat®): 0.5% (50s)

**2-chlorodeoxyadenosine** *see* cladribine *on page 140*

**chloroethane** *see* ethyl chloride *on page 235*

**Chlorofon-A® Tablet *(Discontinued)*** *see page 750*

**Chloromag®** *see* magnesium chloride *on page 361*

**Chloromycetin® Cream *(Discontinued)*** *see page 750*

**Chloromycetin® Injection** *see* chloramphenicol *on page 125*

**Chloromycetin® Kapseals® *(Discontinued)*** *see page 750*

**Chloromycetin® Ophthalmic *(Discontinued)*** *see page 750*

**Chloromycetin® Otic *(Discontinued)*** *see page 750*

**Chloromycetin® Palmitate Oral Suspension *(Discontinued)*** *see page 750*

**chlorophylin** *see* chlorophyll *on this page*

## chlorophyll (KLOR oh fil)

**Synonyms** chlorophylin

**U.S./Canadian Brand Names** Chloresium® [OTC]; Derifil® [OTC]; Nullo® [OTC]; PALS® [OTC]

**Therapeutic Category** Gastrointestinal Agent, Miscellaneous

**Use** Topically promotes normal healing, relieves pain and inflammation, and reduces malodors in wounds, burns, surface ulcers, abrasions and skin irritations; used orally to control fecal and urinary odors in colostomy, ileostomy, or incontinence

**Usual Dosage**

Oral: 1-2 tablets/day

Topical: Apply generously and cover with gauze, linen, or other appropriate dressing; do not change dressings more often than every 48-72 hours

**Dosage Forms**

Ointment, topical (Chloresium®): Chlorophyllin copper complex 0.5% (30 g, 120 g)

Solution, topical, in isotonic saline (Chloresium®): Chlorophyllin copper complex 0.2% (240 mL, 946 mL)

Tablet:

Chloresium®: Chlorophyllin copper complex 14 mg

Derifil®: Water soluble chlorophyll: 100 mg

Nullo®: Chlorophyllin copper complex 33.3 mg

PALS®: Chlorophyllin copper complex 100 mg

Sodium free, sugar free: 20 mg

## chloroprocaine (klor oh PROE kane)

**U.S./Canadian Brand Names** Nesacaine®; Nesacaine®-MPF

**Therapeutic Category** Local Anesthetic

**Use** For infiltration anesthesia and for peripheral and epidural anesthesia

**Usual Dosage** Dosage varies with anesthetic procedure, the area to be anesthetized, the vascularity of the tissues, depth of anesthesia required, degree of muscle relaxation required, and duration of anesthesia

**Dosage Forms** Injection, as hydrochloride:

Preservative free (Nesacaine®-MPF): 2% (20 mL); 3% (20 mL)

With preservative (Nesacaine®): 1% (30 mL); 2% (20 mL, 30 mL)

**Chloroptic® Ophthalmic** *see* chloramphenicol *on page 125*

**Chloroptic-P® Ophthalmic** *see* chloramphenicol and prednisolone *on page 125*

## chloroquine phosphate (KLOR oh kwin FOS fate)

**U.S./Canadian Brand Names** Aralen® Phosphate

**Therapeutic Category** Aminoquinoline (Antimalarial)

(Continued)

## chloroquine phosphate *(Continued)*

**Use** Suppression or chemoprophylaxis of malaria; treatment of uncomplicated or mild-moderate malaria; extraintestinal amebiasis; rheumatoid arthritis; discoid lupus erythematosus, scleroderma, pemphigus

**Usual Dosage** Oral:

Malaria (excluding resistant *P. falciparum*):

Suppression or prophylaxis in endemic areas (begin 1-2 weeks prior to, and continue for 6-8 weeks after the period of potential exposure):

Children: 5 mg base/kg/dose weekly, up to a maximum of 300 mg/dose

Adults: 300 mg/dose weekly

Treatment:

Children: 10 mg base/kg/dose, up to a maximum of 600 mg base/dose one time, followed by 5 mg base/kg/dose one time after 6 hours, and then daily for 2 days (total dose of 25 mg base/kg)

Adults: 600 mg base/dose one time, followed by 300 mg base/dose one time after 6 hours, and then daily for 2 days

Extraintestinal amebiasis: Dosage expressed in mg base:

Children: 10 mg/kg once daily for 2-3 weeks (up to 300 mg base/day)

Adults: 600 mg base/day for 2 days followed by 300 mg base/day for at least 2-3 weeks

Rheumatoid arthritis: Adults: 150 mg base once daily

Melanoma treatment: Children: 10 mg/kg base/dose (maximum: 600 mg) as a single dose followed by 5 mg/kg base one time after 6 hours, then daily for 2 days

**Dosage Forms** Tablet: 250 mg [150 mg base]; 500 mg [300 mg base]

**Chloroserpine®** ***(Discontinued)*** *see page 750*

## chlorothiazide (klor oh THYE a zide)

**U.S./Canadian Brand Names** Diuril®

**Therapeutic Category** Diuretic, Thiazide

**Use** Management of mild to moderate hypertension; edema associated with congestive heart failure, pregnancy, or nephrotic syndrome

**Usual Dosage** I.V. has been limited in infants and children and is generally not recommended

Infants <6 months and patients with pulmonary interstitial edema:

Oral: 20-40 mg/kg/day in 2 divided doses

I.V.: 2-8 mg/kg/day in 2 divided doses

Infants >6 months and Children:

Oral: 20 mg/kg/day in 2 divided doses

I.V.: 4 mg/kg/day

Adults:

Oral: 500 mg to 2 g/day divided in 1-2 doses

I.V.: 100-500 mg/day

**Dosage Forms**

Powder for injection, lyophilized, as sodium: 500 mg

Suspension, oral: 250 mg/5 mL (237 mL)

Tablet: 250 mg, 500 mg

## chloroxine (klor OKS een)

**U.S./Canadian Brand Names** Capitrol®

**Therapeutic Category** Antiseborrheic Agent, Topical

**Use** Treatment of dandruff or seborrheic dermatitis of the scalp

**Usual Dosage** Topical: Use twice weekly, massage into wet scalp, lather should remain on the scalp for approximately 3 minutes, then rinsed; application should be repeated and scalp rinsed thoroughly

**Dosage Forms** Shampoo: 2% (120 mL)

**Chlorphed® [OTC]** *see* brompheniramine *on page 87*

**Chlorphed®-LA Nasal Solution [OTC]** *see* oxymetazoline *on page 444*

## chlorphenesin *(Canada only)* (klor FEN e sin)

**U.S./Canadian Brand Names** Mycil® (Can)

**Therapeutic Category** Skeletal Muscle Relaxant

**Use** Adjunctive treatment of discomfort in short-term, acute, painful musculoskeletal conditions

**Usual Dosage** Adults: Oral: 800 mg 3 times/day, then adjusted to lowest effective dosage, usually 400 mg 4 times/day for up to a maximum of 2 months

**Dosage Forms** Tablet, as carbamate: 400 mg

## chlorpheniramine (klor fen IR a meen)

**U.S./Canadian Brand Names** Aller-Chlor® [OTC]; Chlo-Amine® [OTC]; Chlor-Trimeton® [OTC]; Chlor-Tripolon® (Can)

**Therapeutic Category** Antihistamine

**Use** Perennial and seasonal allergic rhinitis and other allergic symptoms including urticaria

**Usual Dosage**

Children: Oral: 0.35 mg/kg/day in divided doses every 4-6 hours

2-6 years: 1 mg every 4-6 hours, not to exceed 6 mg in 24 hours

6-12 years: 2 mg every 4-6 hours, not to exceed 12 mg/day or sustained release 8 mg at bedtime

Children >12 years and Adults: Oral: 4 mg every 4-6 hours, not to exceed 24 mg/day or sustained release 8-12 mg every 8-12 hours, not to exceed 24 mg/day

Adults: Allergic reactions: I.M., I.V., S.C.: 10-20 mg as a single dose; maximum recommended dose: 40 mg/24 hours

Elderly: 4 mg once or twice daily. **Note:** Duration of action may be 36 hours or more when serum concentrations are low.

**Dosage Forms**

Capsule, as maleate: 12 mg

Capsule, as maleate, timed release: 8 mg, 12 mg

Injection, as maleate: 10 mg/mL (1 mL, 30 mL); 100 mg/mL (2 mL)

Syrup, as maleate: 2 mg/5 mL (120 mL, 473 mL)

Tablet, as maleate: 4 mg, 8 mg, 12 mg

Tablet, as maleate:

Chewable: 2 mg

Timed release: 8 mg, 12 mg

## chlorpheniramine and acetaminophen

(klor fen IR a meen & a seet a MIN oh fen)

**U.S./Canadian Brand Names** Coricidin® [OTC]

**Therapeutic Category** Antihistamine/Analgesic

**Use** Symptomatic relief of congestion, headache, aches, and pains of colds and flu

**Usual Dosage** Adults: Oral: 2 tablets every 4 hours, up to 20 tablets/day

**Dosage Forms** Tablet: Chlorpheniramine maleate 2 mg and acetaminophen 325 mg

## chlorpheniramine and phenylephrine (klor fen IR a meen & fen il EF rin)

**U.S./Canadian Brand Names** Dallergy-D® Syrup; Ed A-Hist® Liquid; Histatab® Plus Tablet [OTC]; Histor-D® Syrup; Rolatuss® Plain Liquid

**Therapeutic Category** Antihistamine/Decongestant Combination

**Use** Temporary relief of nasal congestion and eustachian tube congestion as well as runny nose, sneezing, itching of nose or throat, itchy and watery eyes

**Usual Dosage** Oral:

Children:

2-5 years: 2.5 mL every 4 hours

6-12 years: 5 mL every 4 hours

(Continued)

## chlorpheniramine and phenylephrine *(Continued)*

Adults: 10 mL every 4 hours or 1-2 regular tablets 3-4 times daily or 1 sustained release capsule every 12 hours

**Dosage Forms**

Capsule, sustained release: Chlorpheniramine maleate 8 mg and phenylephrine hydrochloride 20 mg

Liquid:

Dallergy-D®, Histor-D®, Rolatuss® Plain: Chlorpheniramine maleate 2 mg and phenylephrine hydrochloride 5 mg per 5 mL

Ed A-Hist® Liquid: Chlorpheniramine maleate 4 mg and phenylephrine hydrochloride 10 mg per 5 mL

Tablet (Histatab® Plus): Chlorpheniramine maleate 2 mg and phenylephrine hydrochloride 5 mg

## chlorpheniramine and pseudoephedrine

(klor fen IR a meen & soo doe e FED rin)

**U.S./Canadian Brand Names** Allerest® Maximum Strength [OTC]; Anamine® Syrup [OTC]; Anaplex® Liquid [OTC]; Chlorafed® Liquid [OTC]; Chlor-Trimeton® 4 Hour Relief Tablet [OTC]; Chlor-Tripolon® Decongestant (Can); Co-Pyronil® 2 Pulvules® [OTC]; Deconamine® SR; Deconamine® Syrup [OTC]; Deconamine® Tablet [OTC]; Fedahist® Tablet [OTC]; Hayfebrol® Liquid [OTC]; Klerist-D® Tablet [OTC]; Pseudo-Gest Plus® Tablet [OTC]; Rhinosyn® Liquid [OTC]; Rhinosyn-PD® Liquid [OTC]; Ryna® Liquid [OTC]; Sudafed® Plus Tablet [OTC]

**Therapeutic Category** Antihistamine/Decongestant Combination

**Use** Relief of nasal congestion associated with the common cold, hay fever, and other allergies, sinusitis, eustachian tube blockage, and vasomotor and allergic rhinitis

**Usual Dosage** Oral:

Capsule: 1 capsule every 12 hours

Liquid: 5 mL 3-4 times/day

Tablet: 1 tablet 3-4 times/day

**Dosage Forms**

Capsule:

Co-Pyronil® 2 Pulvules®: Chlorpheniramine maleate 4 mg and pseudoephedrine hydrochloride 60 mg

Capsule, sustained release: Chlorpheniramine maleate 4 mg and pseudoephedrine hydrochloride 60 mg; chlorpheniramine maleate 8 mg and pseudoephedrine hydrochloride 120 mg

Liquid:

Anamine®, Anaplex®, Chlorafed®, Deconamine®, Hayfebrol®, Rhinosyn-PD®, Ryna®: Chlorpheniramine maleate 2 mg and pseudoephedrine sulfate 30 mg per 5 mL

Rhinosyn®: Chlorpheniramine maleate 2 mg and pseudoephedrine sulfate 60 mg per 5 mL

Tablet:

Allerest® Maximum Strength: Chlorpheniramine maleate 2 mg and pseudoephedrine hydrochloride 30 mg

Deconamine®, Fedahist®, Klerist-D®, Pseudo-Gest Plus®, Sudafed® Plus: Chlorpheniramine maleate 4 mg and pseudoephedrine hydrochloride 60 mg

Chlor-Trimeton® 4 Hour Relief: Chlorpheniramine maleate 4 mg and pseudoephedrine sulfate 60 mg

## chlorpheniramine, ephedrine, phenylephrine, and carbetapentane

(klor fen IR a meen, e FED rin, fen il EF rin, & kar bay ta PEN tane)

**U.S./Canadian Brand Names** Rentamine®; Rynatuss® Pediatric Suspension; Tri-Tannate Plus®

**Therapeutic Category** Antihistamine/Decongestant/Antitussive

**Use** Symptomatic relief of cough

**Usual Dosage** Children: Oral:

<2 years: Titrate dose individually

2-6 years: 2.5-5 mL every 12 hours

>6 years: 5-10 mL every 12 hours

**Dosage Forms** Liquid: Carbetapentane tannate 30 mg, ephedrine tannate 5 mg, phenylephrine tannate 5 mg, and chlorpheniramine tannate 4 mg per 5 mL

## chlorpheniramine, phenylephrine, and codeine

(klor fen IR a meen, fen il EF rin, & KOE deen)

**U.S./Canadian Brand Names** Pediacof®; Pedituss®

**Therapeutic Category** Antihistamine/Decongestant/Antitussive

**Controlled Substance** C-IV

**Use** Symptomatic relief of rhinitis, nasal congestion, and cough due to colds or allergy

**Usual Dosage** Children 6 months to 12 years: Oral: 1.25-10 mL every 4-6 hours

**Dosage Forms** Liquid: Chlorpheniramine maleate 0.75 mg, phenylephrine hydrochloride 2.5 mg, and codeine phosphate 5 mg with potassium iodide 75 mg per 5 mL

## chlorpheniramine, phenylephrine, and dextromethorphan

(klor fen IR a meen, fen il EF rin, & deks troe meth OR fan)

**U.S./Canadian Brand Names** Cerose-DM® [OTC]

**Therapeutic Category** Antihistamine/Decongestant/Antitussive

**Use** Temporary relief of cough due to minor throat and bronchial irritation; relief of nasal congestion, runny nose, and sneezing

**Usual Dosage** Adults: Oral: 5-10 mL 4 times/day

**Dosage Forms** Liquid: Chlorpheniramine maleate 4 mg, phenylephrine hydrochloride 10 mg, and dextromethorphan hydrobromide 15 mg per 5 mL

## chlorpheniramine, phenylephrine, and methscopolamine

(klor fen IR a meen, fen il EF rin, & meth skoe POL a meen)

**U.S./Canadian Brand Names** D.A.II® Tablet; Dallergy®; Dura-Vent/DA®; Extendryl® SR; Histor-D® Timecelles®

**Therapeutic Category** Antihistamine/Decongestant/Anticholinergic

**Use** Relief of nasal congestion, runny nose, and sneezing

**Usual Dosage** Adults: Oral: 1 capsule or caplet every 12 hours or 5 mL every 4-6 hours

**Dosage Forms**

Caplet, sustained release: Chlorpheniramine maleate 8 mg, phenylephrine hydrochloride 20 mg, and methscopolamine nitrate 2.5 mg

Capsule, sustained release: Chlorpheniramine maleate 8 mg, phenylephrine hydrochloride 10 mg, and methscopolamine nitrate 2.5 mg

Syrup: Chlorpheniramine maleate 2 mg, phenylephrine hydrochloride 10 mg, and methscopolamine nitrate 0.625 mg per 5 mL

Tablet: Chlorpheniramine maleate 4 mg, phenylephrine hydrochloride 10 mg, and methscopolamine nitrate 1.25 mg

## chlorpheniramine, phenylephrine, and phenyltoloxamine

(klor fen IR a meen, fen il EF rin, & fen il tole LOKS a meen)

**U.S./Canadian Brand Names** Comhist®; Comhist® LA

**Therapeutic Category** Antihistamine/Decongestant Combination

**Use** Symptomatic relief of rhinitis and nasal congestion due to colds or allergy

**Usual Dosage** Oral: 1 capsule every 8-12 hours or 1-2 tablets 3 times/day

**Dosage Forms**

Capsule, sustained release (Comhist® LA): Chlorpheniramine maleate 4 mg, phenylephrine hydrochloride 20 mg, and phenyltoloxamine citrate 50 mg

Tablet (Comhist®): Chlorpheniramine maleate 2 mg, phenylephrine hydrochloride 10 mg, and phenyltoloxamine citrate 25 mg

## chlorpheniramine, pseudoephedrine, and codeine

(klor fen IR a meen, soo doe e FED rin, & KOE deen)

**U.S./Canadian Brand Names** Codehist® DH; Decohistine® DH; Dihistine® DH; Novahistine® DH; Ryna-C® Liquid

**Therapeutic Category** Antihistamine/Decongestant/Antitussive

**Controlled Substance** C-V

**Use** Temporary relief of cough associated with minor throat or bronchial irritation; relief of nasal congestion due to common cold, allergic rhinitis, or sinusitis

**Usual Dosage** Oral:

Children:

25-50 lb: 1.25-2.50 mL every 4-6 hours, up to 4 doses in a 24-hour period

50-90 lb: 2.5-5 mL every 4-6 hours, up to 4 doses in a 24-hour period

Adults: 10 mL every 4-6 hours, up to 4 doses in a 24-hour period

**Dosage Forms** Liquid: Chlorpheniramine maleate 2 mg, pseudoephedrine hydrochloride 30 mg, and codeine phosphate 10 mg (120 mL, 480 mL)

## chlorpheniramine, pseudoephedrine, and methscopolamine

(klor fen IR a meen, soo doe e FED rin, & meth skoe POL a meen)

**U.S./Canadian Brand Names** Xiral®

**Therapeutic Category** Antihistamine/Decongestant/Anticholinergic

**Use** Treatment of upper respiratory symptoms such as respiratory congestion, allergic rhinitis, vasomotor rhinitis, sinusitis, and allergic skin reactions of urticaria and angioedema

**Usual Dosage** Oral:

Children 6-12 years: ½ tablet every 12 hours up to 1 tablet daily

Children ≥12 years and Adults: 1 tablet every 12 hours up to 2 tablets daily

**Dosage Forms** Tablet, sustained release: Chlorpheniramine maleate 8 mg, pseudoephedrine hydrochloride 120 mg, and methscopolamine nitrate 2.5 mg

## chlorpheniramine, pyrilamine, and phenylephrine

(klor fen IR a meen, pye RIL a meen, & fen il EF rin)

**U.S./Canadian Brand Names** Rhinatate® Tablet; R-Tannamine® Tablet; R-Tannate® Tablet; Rynatan® Pediatric Suspension; Rynatan® Tablet; Tanoral® Tablet; Triotann® Tablet; Tri-Tannate® Tablet

**Therapeutic Category** Antihistamine/Decongestant Combination

**Use** Symptomatic relief of nasal congestion associated with upper respiratory tract condition

**Usual Dosage** Oral:

Children:

<2 years: Titrate dose individually

2-6 years: 2.5-5 mL every 12 hours

Children >6 years and Adults: 5-10 mL every 12 hours

**Dosage Forms**

Liquid: Chlorpheniramine tannate 2 mg, pyrilamine tannate 12.5 mg, and phenylephrine tannate 5 mg per 5 mL

Tablet: Chlorpheniramine tannate 8 mg, pyrilamine maleate 12.5 mg, and phenylephrine tannate 25 mg

**Chlorpromanyl (Can)** *see* chlorpromazine *on this page*

## chlorpromazine (klor PROE ma zeen)

**U.S./Canadian Brand Names** Chlorpromanyl (Can); Largactil® (Can); Thorazine®

**Therapeutic Category** Phenothiazine Derivative

**Use** Treatment of nausea and vomiting; psychoses; Tourette's syndrome; mania; intractable hiccups (adults); behavioral problems (children)

**Usual Dosage**

Children >6 months:

Psychosis:

Oral: 0.5-1 mg/kg/dose every 4-6 hours; older children may require 200 mg/day or higher

I.M., I.V.: 0.5-1 mg/kg/dose every 6-8 hours; maximum I.M./I.V. dose for <5 years (22.7 kg): 40 mg/day; maximum I.M./I.V. for 5-12 years (22.7-45.5 kg): 75 mg/day

Nausea and vomiting:

Oral: 0.5-1 mg/kg/dose every 4-6 hours as needed

I.M., I.V.: 0.5-1 mg/kg/dose every 6-8 hours; maximum dose: Same as psychoses

Rectal: 1 mg/kg/dose every 6-8 hours as needed

Adults:

Psychosis:

Oral: Range: 30-800 mg/day in 1-4 divided doses, initiate at lower doses and titrate as needed; usual dose is 200 mg/day; some patients may require 1-2 g/day

I.M., I.V.: Initial: 25 mg, may repeat (25-50 mg) in 1-4 hours, gradually increase to a maximum of 400 mg/dose every 4-6 hours until patient controlled; usual dose: 300-800 mg/day

Nausea and vomiting:

Oral: 10-25 mg every 4-6 hours

I.M., I.V.: 25-50 mg every 4-6 hours

Rectal: 50-100 mg every 6-8 hours

Intractable hiccups: Oral, I.M.: 25-50 mg 3-4 times/day

**Dosage Forms**

Chlorpromazine hydrochloride:

Capsule, sustained action: 30 mg, 75 mg, 150 mg, 200 mg, 300 mg

Concentrate, oral: 30 mg/mL (120 mL); 100 mg/mL (60 mL, 240 mL)

Injection: 25 mg/mL (1 mL, 2 mL, 10 mL)

Syrup: 10 mg/5 mL (120 mL)

Tablet: 10 mg, 25 mg, 50 mg, 100 mg, 200 mg

Suppository, rectal, as base: 25 mg, 100 mg

## chlorpropamide (klor PROE pa mide)

**U.S./Canadian Brand Names** Apo®-Chlorpropamide (Can); Diabinese®

**Therapeutic Category** Antidiabetic Agent, Oral

**Use** Control blood sugar in adult onset, noninsulin-dependent diabetes (type 2)

**Usual Dosage** The dosage of chlorpropamide is variable and should be individualized based upon the patient's response

Adults: Oral: 250 mg once daily; initial dose in elderly patients: 100 mg once daily; subsequent dosages may be increased or decreased by 50-125 mg/day at 3- to 5-day intervals; maximum daily dose: 750 mg

**Dosage Forms** Tablet: 100 mg, 250 mg

**Chlor-Rest® Tablet *(Discontinued)*** *see page 750*

**Chlortab® *(Discontinued)*** *see page 750*

## chlorthalidone (klor THAL i done)

**U.S./Canadian Brand Names** Apo®-Chlorthalidone (Can); Thalitone®

**Therapeutic Category** Diuretic, Miscellaneous

**Use** Management of mild to moderate hypertension, used alone or in combination with other agents; treatment of edema associated with congestive heart failure, nephrotic syndrome, or pregnancy

**Usual Dosage** Oral:

Children: 2 mg/kg 3 times/week

Adults: 25-100 mg/day or 100 mg 3 times/week

**Dosage Forms**

Tablet: 25 mg, 50 mg, 100 mg

Thalitone®: 15 mg, 25 mg

**Chlor-Trimeton® [OTC]** *see* chlorpheniramine *on page 129*

**Chlor-Trimeton® 4 Hour Relief Tablet [OTC]** *see* chlorpheniramine and pseudoephedrine *on page 130*

**Chlor-Tripolon® (Can)** *see* chlorpheniramine *on page 129*

**Chlor-Tripolon® Decongestant (Can)** *see* chlorpheniramine and pseudoephedrine *on page 130*

**Chlor-Tripolon® N.D. (Can)** *see* loratadine and pseudoephedrine *on page 356*

## chlorzoxazone (klor ZOKS a zone)

**U.S./Canadian Brand Names** Parafon Forte™ DSC

**Therapeutic Category** Skeletal Muscle Relaxant

**Use** Symptomatic treatment of muscle spasm and pain associated with acute musculoskeletal conditions

**Usual Dosage** Oral:

Children: 20 mg/kg/day or 600 mg/$m^2$/day in 3-4 divided doses

Adults: 250-500 mg 3-4 times/day up to 750 mg 3-4 times/day

**Dosage Forms**

Caplet (Parafon Forte™ DSC): 500 mg

Capsule (Flexaphen®, Mus-Lax®): 250 mg with acetaminophen 300 mg

Tablet: Paraflex®: 250 mg

**Cholac®** *see* lactulose *on page 338*

**Cholan-HMB®** *see* dehydrocholic acid *on page 168*

**Cholebrine®** *see* radiological/contrast media (ionic) *on page 516*

## cholecalciferol (kole e kal SI fer ole)

**Synonyms** $D_3$

**U.S./Canadian Brand Names** Delta-D®; D-Vi-Sol®

**Therapeutic Category** Vitamin D Analog

**Use** Dietary supplement, treatment of vitamin D deficiency or prophylaxis of deficiency

**Usual Dosage** Adults: Oral: 400-1000 units/day

**Dosage Forms** Tablet: 400 units, 1000 units

**Choledyl®** ***(Discontinued)*** *see page 750*

**Choledyl SA®** *see* oxtriphylline *on page 442*

## cholera vaccine (KOL er a vak SEEN)

**Therapeutic Category** Vaccine, Inactivated Bacteria

**Use** Primary immunization for cholera prophylaxis

**Usual Dosage** I.M., S.C.:

Children:

6 months to 4 years: 0.2 mL with same dosage schedule

5-10 years: 0.3 mL with same dosage schedule

Children >10 years and Adults: 0.5 mL in 2 doses 1 week to 1 month or more apart

**Dosage Forms** Injection: Suspension of killed *Vibrio cholerae* (Inaba and Ogawa types) 8 units of each serotype per mL (1.5 mL, 20 mL)

## cholestyramine resin (koe LES tir a meen REZ in)

**U.S./Canadian Brand Names** LoCHOLEST®; LoCHOLEST® Light; Novo-Cholamine (Can); PMS-Cholestyramine (Can); Prevalite®; Questran®; Questran® Light

**Therapeutic Category** Bile Acid Sequestrant

**Use** Adjunct in the management of primary hypercholesterolemia; pruritus associated with elevated levels of bile acids; diarrhea associated with excess fecal bile acids; pseudomembraneous colitis

**Usual Dosage** Dosages are expressed in terms of anhydrous resin. Oral:
Children: 240 mg/kg/day in 3 divided doses; need to titrate dose depending on indication
Adults: 3-4 g 3-4 times/day to a maximum of 16-32 g/day in 2-4 divided doses

**Dosage Forms**
Powder: 4 g of resin/9 g of powder (9 g, 378 g)
For oral suspension:
With aspartame: 4 g of resin/5 g of powder (5 g, 210 g)
With phenylalanine: 4 g of resin/5.5 g of powder (60s)

## choline magnesium trisalicylate

(KOE leen mag NEE zhum trye sa LIS i late)

**U.S./Canadian Brand Names** Tricosal®; Trilisate®

**Therapeutic Category** Analgesic, Non-narcotic; Nonsteroidal Anti-inflammatory Drug (NSAID)

**Use** Management of osteoarthritis, rheumatoid arthritis, and other arthritides

**Usual Dosage** Oral (based on total salicylate content):
Children: 30-60 mg/kg/day administered in 3-4 divided doses
Adults: 500 mg to 1.5 g 1-3 times/day

**Dosage Forms**
Liquid: 500 mg/5 mL [choline salicylate 293 mg and magnesium salicylate 362 mg per 5 mL] (237 mL)
Tablet:
500 mg: Choline salicylate 293 mg and magnesium salicylate 362 mg
750 mg: Choline salicylate 440 mg and magnesium salicylate 544 mg
1000 mg: Choline salicylate 587 mg and magnesium salicylate 725 mg

## choline salicylate (KOE leen sa LIS i late)

**U.S./Canadian Brand Names** Arthropan® [OTC]; Teejel® (Can)

**Therapeutic Category** Analgesic, Non-narcotic; Nonsteroidal Anti-inflammatory Drug (NSAID)

**Use** Temporary relief of pain of rheumatoid arthritis, rheumatic fever, osteoarthritis, and other conditions for which oral salicylates are recommended; useful in patients in which there is difficulty in administering doses in a tablet or capsule dosage form, because of the liquid dosage form

**Usual Dosage** Adults: Oral: 5 mL every 3-4 hours, if necessary, but not more than 6 doses in 24 hours

**Dosage Forms** Liquid (mint flavor): 870 mg/5 mL (240 mL, 480 mL)

**choline theophyllinate** *see* oxtriphylline *on page 442*

**Cholografin® Meglumine** *see* radiological/contrast media (ionic) *on page 516*

**Choloxin® *(Discontinued)*** *see page 750*

## chondroitin sulfate-sodium hyaluronate

(kon DROY tin SUL fate-SOW de um hye a loo ROE nate)

**Synonyms** sodium hyaluronate-chrondroitin sulfate

**U.S./Canadian Brand Names** Duovisc®; Viscoat®

**Therapeutic Category** Ophthalmic Agent, Viscoelastic

**Use** Surgical aid in anterior segment procedures, protects corneal endothelium and coats intraocular lens thus protecting it

**Usual Dosage** Ophthalmic: Carefully introduce into anterior chamber after thoroughly cleaning the chamber with a balanced salt solution

**Dosage Forms**
Solution:
Duovisc®: Sodium chondroitin 40 mg and sodium hyaluronate 30 (Viscoat®) 0.5 mL and sodium hyaluronate 10 mg/mL (Provisc®) 0.55 mL
Viscoat®: Sodium chondroitin 40 mg and sodium hyaluronate 30 mg (0.25 mL, 0.5 mL)

**Chooz® [OTC]** *see* calcium carbonate *on page 97*

**Chorex®** *see* chorionic gonadotropin *on this page*

**choriogonadotropin alfa** *see* chorionic gonadotropin (recombinant) *on this page*

## chorionic gonadotropin (kor ee ON ik goe NAD oh troe pin)

**Synonyms** CG; HCG

**U.S./Canadian Brand Names** A.P.L.®; Chorex®; Choron®; Novarel™; Pregnyl®; Profasi® HP

**Therapeutic Category** Gonadotropin

**Use** Treatment of hypogonadotropic hypogonadism, prepubertal cryptorchidism; induce ovulation

**Usual Dosage** Children: I.M.:

Prepubertal cryptorchidism: 1000-2000 units/m$^2$/dose 3 times/week for 3 weeks

Hypogonadotropic hypogonadism: 500-1000 USP units 3 times/week for 3 weeks, followed by the same dose twice weekly for 3 weeks

**Dosage Forms** Powder for injection: 200 units/mL (10 mL, 25 mL); 500 units/mL (10 mL); 1000 units/mL (10 mL); 2000 units/mL (10 mL)

## chorionic gonadotropin (recombinant)

(kor ee ON ik goe NAD oh troe pin ree KOM be nant)

**Synonyms** choriogonadotropin alfa; r-hCG

**U.S./Canadian Brand Names** Ovidrel®

**Therapeutic Category** Gonadotropin; Ovulation Stimulator

**Use** As part of an assisted reproductive technology (ART) program, induces ovulation in infertile females who have been pretreated with follicle stimulating hormones (FSH); induces ovulation and pregnancy in infertile females when the cause of infertility is functional

**Usual Dosage** S.C.:

Adults: Female:

Assisted reproductive technologies (ART) and ovulation induction: 250 mcg given 1 day following the last dose of follicle stimulating agent. Use only after adequate follicular development has been determined. Hold treatment when there is an excessive ovarian response.

**Dosage Forms** Injection, single-dose vial: 285 mcg r-hCG per vial with 1 mL sterile water for injection (delivers 250 mcg r-hCG following reconstitution)

**Choron®** *see* chorionic gonadotropin *on this page*

**Chromagen® OB [OTC]** *see* vitamin (multiple/prenatal) *on page 632*

**Chroma-Pak®** *see* trace metals *on page 598*

**chromium injection** *see* trace metals *on page 598*

**Chronovera® (Can)** *see* verapamil *on page 625*

**Chronulac®** *see* lactulose *on page 338*

**Chymex®** ***(Discontinued)*** *see page 750*

**Cibacalcin®** ***(Discontinued)*** *see page 750*

## ciclopirox (sye kloe PEER oks)

**U.S./Canadian Brand Names** Loprox®; Penlac™

**Therapeutic Category** Antifungal Agent

**Use** Treatment of tinea pedis, tinea cruris, tinea corporis, cutaneous candidiasis, tinea versicolor

**Usual Dosage** Children >10 years and Adults: Topical: Apply twice daily, gently massage into affected areas; safety and efficacy in children <10 years have not been established

**Dosage Forms**
Cream, topical, as olamine: 1% (15 g, 30 g, 90 g)
Lotion, as olamine: 1% (30 mL)
Solution, topical: 8% (3.3 mL)

## cidofovir (si DOF o veer)

**U.S./Canadian Brand Names** Vistide®

**Therapeutic Category** Antiviral Agent

**Use** Treatment of CMV retinitis in patients with acquired immunodeficiency syndrome (AIDS)

**Usual Dosage**
Induction treatment: 5 mg/kg once weekly for 2 consecutive weeks
Maintenance treatment: 5 mg/kg administered once every 2 weeks
**Probenecid must be administered orally with each dose of cidofovir**
Probenecid dose: 2 g 3 hours prior to cidofovir dose, 1 g 2 hours and 8 hours after completion of the infusion; patients should also receive 1 L of normal saline intravenously prior to each infusion of cidofovir; saline should be infused over 1-2 hours

**Dosage Forms** Injection: 75 mg/mL (5 mL)

## cilazapril *(Canada only)* (sye LAY za pril)

**U.S./Canadian Brand Names** Inhibace® (Can)

**Therapeutic Category** Angiotensin-Converting Enzyme (ACE) Inhibitor

**Use** Management of hypertension and treatment of congestive heart failure

**Usual Dosage** Adults: Oral:
Congestive heart failure: Recommended starting dose is 0.5 mg once daily, usual maintenance dose: 1-2.5 mg/day
Hypertension: 2.5-5 mg once daily

**Dosage Forms** Tablet: 1 mg, 2.5 mg, 5 mg

## cilostazol (sil OH sta zol)

**U.S./Canadian Brand Names** Pletal®

**Therapeutic Category** Platelet Aggregation Inhibitor

**Use** Symptomatic management of peripheral vascular disease, primarily intermittent claudication

**Usual Dosage** Adults: Oral: 100 mg twice daily taken at least 30 minutes before or 2 hours after breakfast and dinner; dosage should be reduced to 50 mg twice daily during concurrent therapy with inhibitors of CYP3A4 or CYP2C19

**Dosage Forms** Tablet: 50 mg, 100 mg

**Ciloxan™ Ophthalmic** *see* ciprofloxacin *on next page*

## cimetidine (sye MET i deen)

**U.S./Canadian Brand Names** Apo®-Cimetidine (Can); Gen-Cimetidine (Can); Novo-Cimetine (Can); Nu-Cimet (Can); PMS-Cimetidine (Can); Tagamet®; Tagamet-HB® [OTC]

**Therapeutic Category** Histamine $H_2$ Antagonist

**Use** Short-term treatment of active duodenal ulcers and benign gastric ulcers; long-term prophylaxis of duodenal ulcer; gastric hypersecretory states; gastroesophageal reflux

**Usual Dosage** Oral, I.M., I.V.:
Infants: 10-20 mg/kg/day divided every 6-12 hours
Children: 20-30 mg/kg/day in divided doses every 6 hours

Patients with an active bleed: Administer cimetidine as a continuous infusion

Adults:
Short-term treatment of active ulcers:
Oral: 300 mg 4 times/day or 800 mg at bedtime or 400 mg twice daily for up to 8 weeks

(Continued)

## cimetidine *(Continued)*

I.M., I.V.: 300 mg every 6 hours or 37.5 mg/hour by continuous infusion; I.V. dosage should be adjusted to maintain an intragastric pH of 5 or greater

Duodenal ulcer prophylaxis: Oral: 400-800 mg at bedtime

Gastric hypersecretory conditions: Oral, I.M., I.V.: 300-600 mg every 6 hours; dosage not to exceed 2.4 g/day

**Dosage Forms**

Infusion, as hydrochloride, in NS: 300 mg (50 mL)

Injection, as hydrochloride: 150 mg/mL (2 mL, 8 mL)

Liquid, oral, as hydrochloride (mint-peach flavor): 300 mg/5 mL with alcohol 2.8% (5 mL, 240 mL)

Tablet: 200 mg, 300 mg, 400 mg, 800 mg

**Cinobac® Pulvules®** *see* cinoxacin *on this page*

## cinoxacin (sin OKS a sin)

**U.S./Canadian Brand Names** Cinobac® Pulvules®

**Therapeutic Category** Quinolone

**Use** Urinary tract infections

**Usual Dosage** Children >12 years and Adults: Oral: 1 g/day in 2-4 doses

**Dosage Forms** Capsule: 250 mg, 500 mg

**Cipro®** *see* ciprofloxacin *on this page*

## ciprofloxacin (sip roe FLOKS a sin)

**U.S./Canadian Brand Names** Ciloxan™ Ophthalmic; Cipro®

**Therapeutic Category** Antibiotic, Ophthalmic; Quinolone

**Use** Treatment of documented or suspected infections of the lower respiratory tract, sinuses, skin and skin structure, bone/joints, and urinary tract (including prostatitis) due to susceptible bacterial strains; especially indicated for pseudomonal infections and those due to multidrug-resistant gram-negative organisms, chronic bacterial prostatitis, infectious diarrhea, complicated gram-negative and anaerobic intra-abdominal infections (with metronidazole) due to *E. coli* (enteropathic strains), *B. fragilis*, *P. mirabilis*, *K. pneumoniae*, *P. aeruginosa*, *Campylobacter jejuni* or *Shigella*; approved for acute sinusitis caused by *H. influenzae* or *M. catarrhalis*; also used in treatment of typhoid fever due to *Salmonella typhi* (although eradication of the chronic typhoid carrier state has not been proven), osteomyelitis when parenteral therapy is not feasible, acute uncomplicated cystitis in females, to reduce incidence or progression of disease following exposure to aerolized *Bacillus anthracis*, and sexually-transmitted diseases such as uncomplicated cervical and urethral gonorrhea due to *Neisseria gonorrhoeae*; used ophthalmologically for superficial ocular infections (corneal ulcers, conjunctivitis) due to susceptible strains

**Usual Dosage**

Children: Oral: 20-30 mg/kg/day in 2 divided doses; maximum dose: 1.5 g/day

Adults:

Oral: 250-750 mg every 12 hours, depending on severity of infection and susceptibility

Ophthalmic: Instill 1-2 drops in eye(s) every 2 hours while awake for 2 days and 1-2 drops every 4 hours while awake for the next 5 days

I.V.: 200-400 mg every 12 hours depending on severity of infection

**Dosage Forms**

Infusion, as hydrochloride, in $D_5W$: 400 mg (200 mL)

Infusion, as hydrochloride, in NS or $D_5W$: 200 mg (100 mL)

Injection, as hydrochloride: 200 mg (20 mL); 400 mg (40 mL)

Solution, ophthalmic, as hydrochloride: 3.5 mg/mL (2.5 mL, 5 mL)

Suspension, oral: 250 mg/5 mL (100 mL); 500 mg/5 mL (100 mL)

Tablet, as hydrochloride: 100 mg, 250 mg, 500 mg, 750 mg

## ciprofloxacin and hydrocortisone

(sip roe FLOKS a sin & hye droe KOR ti sone)

**U.S./Canadian Brand Names** Cipro® HC Otic

**Therapeutic Category** Antibiotic/Corticosteroid, Otic

**Use** Treatment of acute otitis externa, sometimes known as "swimmer's ear"

**Usual Dosage** Children >1 year of age and Adults: Otic: The recommended dosage for all patients is three drops of the suspension in the affected ear twice daily for seven day; twice-daily dosing schedule is more convenient for patients than that of existing treatments with hydrocortisone, which are typically administered three or four times a day; a twice-daily dosage schedule may be especially helpful for parents and caregivers of young children

**Dosage Forms** Suspension, otic: Ciprofloxacin hydrochloride 0.2% and hydrocortisone 1%

**Cipro® HC Otic** *see* ciprofloxacin and hydrocortisone *on this page*

## cisapride (SIS a pride)

**U.S./Canadian Brand Names** Propulsid®

**Therapeutic Category** Gastrointestinal Agent, Prokinetic

**Use** Treatment of nocturnal symptoms of gastroesophageal reflux disease (GERD), also demonstrated effectiveness for gastroparesis, refractory constipation, and nonulcer dyspepsia

**Usual Dosage** Adults: Oral: 10 mg 4 times/day at least 15 minutes before meals and at bedtime; in some patients the dosage will need to be increased to 20 mg to obtain a satisfactory result

**Dosage Forms**

Suspension, oral (cherry cream flavor): 1 mg/mL (450 mL)

Tablet, scored: 10 mg, 20 mg

## cisatracurium (sis a tra KYOO ree um)

**U.S./Canadian Brand Names** Nimbex®

**Therapeutic Category** Skeletal Muscle Relaxant

**Use** As an adjunct to general anesthesia to facilitate endotracheal intubation and to relax skeletal muscles during surgery; to facilitate mechanical ventilation in ICU patients; does not relieve pain or produce sedation

**Usual Dosage** I.V.: Dose to effect; doses will vary due to interpatient variability; use ideal body weight for obese patients

Surgery:

Children 2-12 years: 0.1 mg/kg, produces clinically effective block for 28 minutes

Adults: 0.15-0.2 mg/kg, then 0.03 mg/kg 40-60 minutes after initial dose to maintain neuromuscular block, followed by repeat doses of 0.03 mg/kg at 20-minute intervals; initial dose after succinylcholine for intubation: 0.1 mg/kg

Continuous infusion: At initial signs of recovery from bolus dose, begin at 3 mcg/kg/minute, block usually maintained by a rate of 1-2 mcg/kg/minute

Pretreatment/priming: 10% of intubating dose given 3-5 minutes before initial dose

ICU: Adults: 0.1 mg/kg bolus; at initial signs of recovery begin at rate of 3 mcg/kg/minute and adjust accordingly (rates of 0.5-10 mcg/kg/minute reported)

**Dosage Forms** Injection, as besylate: 2 mg/mL (5 mL, 10 mL); 10 mg/mL (20 mL)

## cisplatin (SIS pla tin)

**Synonyms** CDDP

**U.S./Canadian Brand Names** Platinol®; Platinol®-AQ

**Therapeutic Category** Antineoplastic Agent

**Use** Management of metastatic testicular or ovarian carcinoma, advanced bladder cancer, osteosarcoma, Hodgkin's and non-Hodgkin's lymphoma, head or neck cancer, cervical cancer, lung cancer, brain tumors, neuroblastoma; used alone or in combination with other agents

(Continued)

## cisplatin *(Continued)*

**Usual Dosage** Children and Adults (refer to individual protocols): I.V.:
Intermittent dosing schedule: 37-75 mg/m$^2$ once every 2-3 weeks or 50-120 mg/m$^2$ once every 3-4 weeks
Daily dosing schedule: 15-20 mg/m$^2$/day for 5 days every 3-4 weeks

**Dosage Forms**
Injection, aqueous: 1 mg/mL (50 mL, 100 mL, 200 mL)
Powder for injection: 10 mg, 50 mg

**13-*cis*-retinoic acid** *see* isotretinoin *on page 329*

## citalopram (sye TAL oh pram)

**Synonyms** nitalapram
**U.S./Canadian Brand Names** Celexa™
**Therapeutic Category** Antidepressant
**Use** Depression
**Usual Dosage** Oral: 20-60 mg/day; reduce dosage in elderly or those with hepatic impairment
**Dosage Forms** Tablet, as hydrobromide: 20 mg, 40 mg

**Citanest® Forte** *see* prilocaine *on page 495*

**Citanest® Plain** *see* prilocaine *on page 495*

**Cithalith-S® Syrup *(Discontinued)*** *see page 750*

**Citracal® [OTC]** *see* calcium citrate *on page 98*

**citrate of magnesia** *see* magnesium citrate *on page 361*

**citric acid and d-gluconic acid irrigant** *see* citric acid bladder mixture *on this page*

## citric acid bladder mixture (SI trik AS id BLAD dur MIKS chur)

**Synonyms** citric acid and d-gluconic acid irrigant; hemiacidrin
**U.S./Canadian Brand Names** Renacidin®
**Therapeutic Category** Irrigating Solution
**Use** Preparing solutions for irrigating indwelling urethral catheters; to dissolve or prevent formation of calcifications
**Usual Dosage** 30-60 mL of 10% (sterile) solution 2-3 times/day by means of a rubber syringe

**Dosage Forms**
Powder for solution: Citric acid 156-171 g, magnesium hydroxycarbonate 75-87 g, D-gluconic acid 21-30 g, magnesium acid citrate 9-15 g, calcium carbonate 2-6 g (150 g, 300 g)
Solution, irrigation: Citric acid 6.602 g, magnesium hydroxycarbonate 3.177 g, glucono-delta-lactone 0.198 g and benzoic acid 0.023 g per 100 mL (500 mL)

**Citro-Mag (Can)** *see* magnesium citrate *on page 361*

**Citro-Nesia™ Solution *(Discontinued)*** *see page 750*

**Citrotein® [OTC]** *see* nutritional formula, enteral/oral *on page 432*

**citrovorum factor** *see* leucovorin *on page 343*

**Citrucel® [OTC]** *see* methylcellulose *on page 383*

**CI-719** *see* gemfibrozil *on page 271*

## cladribine (KLA dri been)

**Synonyms** 2-CdA; 2-chlorodeoxyadenosine
**U.S./Canadian Brand Names** Leustatin™
**Therapeutic Category** Antineoplastic Agent
**Use** Hairy cell and chronic lymphocytic leukemias

**Usual Dosage** Adults: I.V. continuous infusion: 0.09 mg/kg/day
**Dosage Forms** Injection, preservative free: 1 mg/mL (10 mL)

**Claforan®** *see* cefotaxime *on page 115*

## clarithromycin (kla RITH roe mye sin)

**U.S./Canadian Brand Names** Biaxin®; Biaxin® XL
**Therapeutic Category** Macrolide (Antibiotic)
**Use** Treatment of upper and lower respiratory tract infections, acute otitis media, and infections of the skin and skin structure due to susceptible strains of *S. aureus*, *S. pyogenes*, *S. pneumoniae*, *H. influenzae*, *M. catarrhalis*, *Mycoplasma pneumoniae*, *C. trachomatis*, *Legionella* sp, and *M. avium*; prophylaxis of disseminated *M. avium* complex (MAC) infections in HIV-infected patients
**Usual Dosage** Oral: 250-500 mg every 12 hours for 7-14 days; Biaxin® XL: 2 x 500 mg once daily for 7-14 days
Upper respiratory tract: 250-500 mg every 12 hours for 10-14 days
Pharyngitis/tonsillitis: 250 mg every 12 hours for 10 days
Acute maxillary sinusitis: 500 mg every 12 hours for 14 days
Lower respiratory tract: 250-500 mg every 12 hours for 7-14 days
Acute exacerbation of chronic bronchitis due to:
*S. pneumoniae*: 250 mg every 12 hours for 7-14 days
*M. catarrhalis*: 250 mg every 12 hours for 7-14 days
*H. influenzae*: 500 mg every 12 hours for 7-14 days
Pneumonia due to:
*S. pneumoniae*: 250 mg every 12 hours for 7-14 days
*M. pneumoniae*: 250 mg every 12 hours for 7-14 days
Uncomplicated skin and skin structure: 250 mg every 12 hours for 7-14 days
**Dosage Forms**
Granules for oral suspension: 125 mg/5 mL (50 mL, 100 mL); 187.5 mg/5 mL (100 mL); 250 mg/5 mL (50 mL, 100 mL)
Tablet, film-coated: 250 mg, 500 mg
Tablet, film-coated, extended release: 500 mg

**Claritin®** *see* loratadine *on page 356*

**Claritin-D®** *see* loratadine and pseudoephedrine *on page 356*

**Claritin-D® 24-Hour** *see* loratadine and pseudoephedrine *on page 356*

**Claritin® Extra (Can)** *see* loratadine and pseudoephedrine *on page 356*

**Claritin® RediTab®** *see* loratadine *on page 356*

**Clavulin® (Can)** *see* amoxicillin and clavulanate potassium *on page 36*

**Clear Away® Disc [OTC]** *see* salicylic acid *on page 535*

**Clear Eyes® [OTC]** *see* naphazoline *on page 409*

**Clearplex®** *see* benzoyl peroxide *on page 74*

**Clear Tussin® 30** *see* guaifenesin and dextromethorphan *on page 282*

## clemastine (KLEM as teen)

**U.S./Canadian Brand Names** Allerhist-1®; Dayhist-1®; Tavist®; Tavist®-1 [OTC]
**Therapeutic Category** Antihistamine
**Use** Perennial and seasonal allergic rhinitis and other allergic symptoms including urticaria
**Usual Dosage** Oral:
Children:
<12 years: 0.67-1.34 mg every 8-12 hours as needed
>12 years: 1.34 mg twice daily to 2.68 mg 3 times/day; do not exceed 8.04 mg/day
Adults: 1.34 mg twice daily to 2.68 mg 3 times/day; do not exceed 8.04 mg/day
**Dosage Forms**
Syrup, as fumarate (citrus flavor): 0.67 mg/5 mL with alcohol 5.5% (120 mL)
(Continued)

## clemastine *(Continued)*

Tablet, as fumarate: 1.34 mg, 2.68 mg

**Cleocin HCl® Oral** *see* clindamycin *on this page*

**Cleocin Pediatric® Oral** *see* clindamycin *on this page*

**Cleocin Phosphate® Injection** *see* clindamycin *on this page*

**Cleocin T® Topical** *see* clindamycin *on this page*

**Cleocin® Vaginal** *see* clindamycin *on this page*

## clidinium and chlordiazepoxide (kli DI nee um & klor dye az e POKS ide)

**U.S./Canadian Brand Names** Apo®-Chlorax (Can); Librax®

**Therapeutic Category** Anticholinergic Agent

**Use** Adjunct treatment of peptic ulcer, treatment of irritable bowel syndrome

**Usual Dosage** Oral: 1-2 capsules 3-4 times/day, before meals or food and at bedtime

**Dosage Forms** Capsule: Clidinium bromide 2.5 mg and chlordiazepoxide hydrochloride 5 mg

**Climara® Transdermal** *see* estradiol *on page 224*

**Clinac®** *see* benzoyl peroxide *on page 74*

**Clinda-Derm® Topical** *see* clindamycin *on this page*

## clindamycin (klin da MYE sin)

**U.S./Canadian Brand Names** Alti-Clindamycin (Can); Cleocin HCl® Oral; Cleocin Pediatric® Oral; Cleocin Phosphate® Injection; Cleocin T® Topical; Cleocin® Vaginal; Clinda-Derm® Topical; Dalacin® C (Can)

**Therapeutic Category** Acne Products; Antibiotic, Miscellaneous

**Use** Useful agent against most aerobic gram-positive staphylococci and streptococci (except enterococci); also useful against *Fusobacterium*, *Bacteroides* sp. and *Actinomyces* for treatment of respiratory tract infections, skin and soft tissue infections, sepsis, intra-abdominal infections, and infections of the female pelvis and genital tract; used topically in treatment of severe acne

**Usual Dosage** Avoid in neonates (contains benzyl alcohol)

Infants and Children:

Oral: 10-30 mg/kg/day in 3-4 divided doses

I.M., I.V.: 25-40 mg/kg/day in 3-4 divided doses

Children and Adults: Topical: Apply twice daily

Adults:

Oral: 150-450 mg/dose every 6-8 hours; maximum dose: 1.8 g/day

I.M., I.V.: 1.2-1.8 g/day in 2-4 divided doses; maximum dose: 4.8 g/day

Vaginal: 1 full applicator (100 mg) inserted intravaginally once daily before bedtime for 7 consecutive days

**Dosage Forms**

Capsule, as hydrochloride: 75 mg, 150 mg, 300 mg

Cream, vaginal: 2% (40 g)

Gel, topical, as phosphate: 1% [10 mg/g] (7.5 g, 30 g)

Granules for oral solution, as palmitate: 75 mg/5 mL (100 mL)

Infusion, as phosphate, in $D_5W$: 300 mg (50 mL); 600 mg (50 mL)

Injection, as phosphate: 150 mg/mL (2 mL, 4 mL, 6 mL, 50 mL, 60 mL)

Lotion: 1% [10 mg/mL] (60 mL)

Pledgets: 1%

Solution, topical, as phosphate: 1% [10 mg/mL] (30 mL, 60 mL, 480 mL)

Suppository, vaginal: 100 mg

## clindamycin and benzoyl peroxide

(klin da MYE sin & BEN zoe il peer OKS ide)

**U.S./Canadian Brand Names** BenzaClin™

**Therapeutic Category** Topical Skin Product; Topical Skin Product, Acne

**Use** Topical treatment of acne vulgaris

**Usual Dosage** Topical: Children ≥12 years and Adults: Acne: Apply twice daily (morning and evening) to affected areas after skin has been cleansed and dried

**Dosage Forms** Gel, topical: Clindamycin 1% and benzol peroxide 5% (25 g)

**Clindex® *(Discontinued)*** *see page 750*

**Clinoril®** *see* sulindac *on page 567*

## clioquinol (klye oh KWIN ole)

**Therapeutic Category** Antifungal Agent

**Use** Treatment of tinea pedis, tinea cruris, and skin infections caused by dermatophytic fungi (ring worm)

**Usual Dosage** Children and Adults: Topical: Apply 2-4 times/day; do not use for >7 days

**Dosage Forms**

Cream: 3% (30 g)

Ointment, topical: 3% (30 g)

## clioquinol and hydrocortisone (klye oh KWIN ole & hye droe KOR ti sone)

**Synonyms** iodochlorhydroxyquin and hydrocortisone

**U.S./Canadian Brand Names** Ala-Quin®; Dek-Quin®; Vioform® Hydrocortisone (Can)

**Therapeutic Category** Antifungal/Corticosteroid

**Use** Contact or atopic dermatitis; eczema; neurodermatitis; anogenital pruritus; mycotic dermatoses; moniliasis

**Usual Dosage** Topical: Apply in a thin film 3-4 times/day

**Dosage Forms** Cream: Clioquinol 3% and hydrocortisone 0.5% (15 g, 30 g); clioquinol 3% and hydrocortisone 1% (20 g, 30 g, 454 g)

**Clistin® Tablet *(Discontinued)*** *see page 750*

## clobazam *(Canada only)* (KLOE ba zam)

**U.S./Canadian Brand Names** Alti-Clobazam (Can); Frisium® (Can); Novo-Clobazam (Can)

**Therapeutic Category** Anticonvulsant; Antidepressant

**Use** Antianxiety, anticonvulsant, and sedative agent

**Usual Dosage** Adults: 20-30 mg/day in divided doses or at night; maximum daily dose: 60 mg

**Dosage Forms** Tablet: 10 mg

## clobetasol (kloe BAY ta sol)

**U.S./Canadian Brand Names** Clobevate®; Cormax® Ointment; Dermovate® (Can); Embeline E®; Eumovate® (Can); Gen-Clobetasol (Can); Novo-Clobetasol (Can); Olux™; Temovate®; Temovate E®

**Therapeutic Category** Corticosteroid, Topical

**Use** Short-term relief of inflammation of moderate to severe corticosteroid-responsive dermatosis

**Usual Dosage** Topical: Apply twice daily for up to 2 weeks with no more than 50 g/week. Therapy should be discontinued when control is achieved. If no improvement is seen, reassessment of diagnosis may be necessary.

**Dosage Forms**

Cream, as propionate: 0.05% (15 g, 30 g, 45 g)

Cream, as propionate, in emollient base: 0.05% (15 g, 30 g, 60 g)

Gel, as propionate: 0.05% (15 g, 30 g, 45 g)

Ointment, topical, as propionate: 0.05% (15 g, 30 g, 45 g)

(Continued)

## clobetasol *(Continued)*

Scalp application, as propionate: 0.05% (25 mL, 50 mL)
Solution, topical: 0.05%

**Clobevate®** *see* clobetasol *on previous page*

**Clocort® Maximum Strength [OTC]** *see* hydrocortisone (topical) *on page 304*

## clocortolone (kloe KOR toe lone)

**U.S./Canadian Brand Names** Cloderm® Topical

**Therapeutic Category** Corticosteroid, Topical

**Use** Inflammation of corticosteroid-responsive dermatoses

**Usual Dosage** Topical: Apply sparingly and gently rub into affected area 1-4 times/day. Therapy should be discontinued when control is achieved. If no improvement is seen, reassessment of diagnosis may be necessary.

**Dosage Forms** Cream, as pivalate: 0.1% (15 g, 45 g)

**Cloderm® Topical** *see* clocortolone *on this page*

## clodronate disodium *(Canada only)* (KLOE droh nate dy SOW de um)

**U.S./Canadian Brand Names** Bonefos® (Can); Ostac® (Can)

**Therapeutic Category** Bisphosphonate Derivative

**Use** For the management of hypercalcemia of malignancy. Prior to treatment with clodronate renal excretion of excess calcium should be promoted by restoration and maintenance of adequate fluid balance and urine output. In responsive patients I.V. infusion of clodronate decreases the flux of calcium from the bones by inhibiting the osteoclastic activity and bone resorption, thus reducing the calcium level in blood. Treatment with oral clodronate following I.V. infusion has been found to prolong the duration of action.

**Usual Dosage**

I.V. Infusion: The recommended adult dose is 300 mg/day (one 5 mL ampul). The contents of the ampul must be diluted in 500 mL of sodium chloride 0.9% injection or dextrose 5% injection and administered by infusion lasting at least 2 hours. Treatment should be continued until plasma calcium returns to normal, this generally being achieved after 2 to 5 days of treatment. Treatment should not be prolonged beyond 7 days.

Capsule: The oral recommended daily maintenance dose following I.V. therapy is in the range of 1600 mg (4 capsules) to 2400 mg (6 capsules) given in single or 2 divided doses. Maximal recommended daily dose is 3200 mg (8 capsules). The drug should be taken at least 2 hours before or after food, because food may decrease the amount of clodronate absorbed by the body.

**Dosage Forms**

Injection: 30 mg, 60 mg
Capsule: 400 mg

## clofazimine (kloe FA zi meen)

**U.S./Canadian Brand Names** Lamprene®

**Therapeutic Category** Leprostatic Agent

**Use** Treatment of dapsone-resistant lepromatous leprosy (*Mycobacterium leprae*); multibacillary dapsone-sensitive leprosy; erythema nodosum leprosum; *Mycobacterium avium-intracellulare* (MAI) infections

**Usual Dosage** Oral:

Children: Leprosy: 1 mg/kg/day every 24 hours in combination with dapsone and rifampin

Adults:

Dapsone-resistant leprosy: 50-100 mg/day in combination with one or more antileprosy drugs for 2 years; then alone 50-100 mg/day

Dapsone-sensitive multibacillary leprosy: 50-100 mg/day in combination with two or more antileprosy drugs for at least 2 years and continue until negative skin smears are obtained, then institute single drug therapy with appropriate agent

Erythema nodosum leprosum: 100-200 mg/day for up to 3 months or longer then taper dose to 100 mg/day when possible

MAI: Combination therapy using clofazimine 100 mg 1 or 3 times/day in combination with other antimycobacterial agents

**Dosage Forms** Capsule, as palmitate: 50 mg

## clofibrate (kloe FYE brate)

**U.S./Canadian Brand Names** Atromid-S®

**Therapeutic Category** Antihyperlipidemic Agent, Miscellaneous

**Use** Adjunct to dietary therapy in the management of hyperlipidemias associated with high triglyceride levels

**Usual Dosage** Adults: Oral: 500 mg 4 times/day

**Dosage Forms** Capsule: 500 mg

**Clomid®** *see* clomiphene *on this page*

## clomiphene (KLOE mi feen)

**U.S./Canadian Brand Names** Clomid®; Serophene®

**Therapeutic Category** Ovulation Stimulator

**Use** Treatment of ovulatory failure in patients desiring pregnancy

**Usual Dosage** Oral: 50 mg/day for 5 days (first course); start the regimen on or about the fifth day of cycle; if ovulation occurs do not increase dosage; if not, increase next course to 100 mg/day for 5 days

**Dosage Forms** Tablet, as citrate: 50 mg

## clomipramine (kloe MI pra meen)

**U.S./Canadian Brand Names** Anafranil®; Apo®-Clomipramine (Can); Gen-Clomipramine (Can); Novo-Clopamine (Can)

**Therapeutic Category** Antidepressant, Tricyclic (Tertiary Amine)

**Use** Treatment of obsessive-compulsive disorder (OCD)

**Usual Dosage** Oral:

Children: Initial: 25 mg/day and gradually increase, as tolerated to a maximum of 3 mg/kg or 100 mg, whichever is smaller

Adults: Initial: 25 mg/day and gradually increase, as tolerated to 100 mg/day the first 2 weeks, may then be increased to a total of 250 mg/day

**Dosage Forms** Capsule, as hydrochloride: 25 mg, 50 mg, 75 mg

**Clomycin® [OTC]** *see* bacitracin, neomycin, polymyxin B, and lidocaine *on page 65*

**Clonapam (Can)** *see* clonazepam *on this page*

## clonazepam (kloe NA ze pam)

**U.S./Canadian Brand Names** Alti-Clonazepam (Can); Apo®-Clonazepam (Can); Clonapam (Can); Gen-Clonazepam (Can); Klonopin™; Novo-Clonazepam (Can); Nu-Clonazepam (Can); PMS-Clonazepam (Can); Rho®-Clonazepam (Can); Rivotril® (Can)

**Therapeutic Category** Benzodiazepine

**Controlled Substance** C-IV

**Use** Prophylaxis of absence (petit mal), petit mal variant (Lennox-Gastaut), akinetic, and myoclonic seizures

**Usual Dosage** Oral:

Children <10 years or 30 kg:

Initial daily dose: 0.01-0.03 mg/kg/day (maximum: 0.05 mg/kg/day) administered in 2-3 divided doses; increase by no more than 0.5 mg every third day until seizures are controlled or adverse effects are seen

(Continued)

## clonazepam *(Continued)*

Maintenance dose: 0.1-0.2 mg/kg/day divided 3 times/day; not to exceed 0.2 mg/kg/day

Adults:

Initial daily dose not to exceed 1.5 mg administered in 3 divided doses; may increase by 0.5-1 mg every third day until seizures are controlled or adverse effects seen

Maintenance dose: 0.05-0.2 mg/kg; do not exceed 20 mg/day

**Dosage Forms** Tablet: 0.5 mg, 1 mg, 2 mg

## clonidine (KLOE ni deen)

**U.S./Canadian Brand Names** Apo®-Clonidine (Can); Catapres® Oral; Catapres-TTS® Transdermal; Dixarit® (Can); Duraclon™ Injection; Novo-Clonidine (Can); Nu-Clonidine (Can)

**Therapeutic Category** Alpha-Adrenergic Agonist

**Use** Management of hypertension; aid in the diagnosis of pheochromocytoma and growth hormone deficiency; has orphan drug status for epidural use for pain control; used for heroin withdrawal and smoking cessation therapy in adults

**Investigational use:** Alternate agent for the treatment of attention-deficit/hyperactivity disorder (ADHD)

**Usual Dosage**

Epidural infusion (continuous): 30 mcg/hour, titrated up or down depending on pain relief

Oral:

Children: Initial: 5-10 mcg/kg/day in divided doses every 8-12 hours; increase gradually at 5- to 7-day intervals to 25 mcg/kg/day in divided doses every 6 hours; maximum: 0.9 mg/day

Clonidine tolerance test (test of growth hormone release from pituitary): 0.15 mg/m$^2$ or 4 mcg/kg as single dose

Adults: Initial dose: 0.1 mg twice daily, usual maintenance dose: 0.2-1.2 mg/day in 2-4 divided doses; maximum recommended dose: 2.4 mg/day

Nicotine withdrawal symptoms: 0.1 mg twice daily to maximum of 0.4 mg/day for 3-4 weeks

Elderly: Initial: 0.1 mg once daily at bedtime, increase gradually as needed

Transdermal: Apply once every 7 days; for initial therapy start with 0.1 mg and increase by 0.1 mg at 1- to 2-week intervals; dosages >0.6 mg do not improve efficacy

**Dosage Forms**

Injection, preservative free, as hydrochloride: 100 mcg/mL (10 mL); 500 mcg/mL (10 mL)

Patch, transdermal, as hydrochloride: 1, 2, and 3 (0.1, 0.2, 0.3 mg/day, 7-day duration)

Tablet, as hydrochloride: 0.1 mg, 0.2 mg, 0.3 mg

## clonidine and chlorthalidone (KLOE ni deen & klor THAL i done)

**U.S./Canadian Brand Names** Combipres®

**Therapeutic Category** Antihypertensive Agent, Combination

**Use** Management of mild to moderate hypertension

**Usual Dosage** Oral: 1 tablet 1-2 times/day

**Dosage Forms** Tablet:

0.1: Clonidine 0.1 mg and chlorthalidone 15 mg

0.2: Clonidine 0.2 mg and chlorthalidone 15 mg

0.3: Clonidine 0.3 mg and chlorthalidone 15 mg

## clopidogrel (kloh PID oh grel)

**U.S./Canadian Brand Names** Plavix®

**Therapeutic Category** Antiplatelet Agent

**Use** The reduction of atherosclerotic events (myocardial infarction, stroke, vascular deaths) in patients with atherosclerosis documented by recent myocardial infarctions, recent stroke or established peripheral arterial disease

**Usual Dosage** Adults: Oral: 75 mg once daily
**Dosage Forms** Tablet, as bisulfate: 75 mg

**Clopixol-Acuphase® (Can)** *see* zuclopenthixol *(Canada only)* *on page 641*

**Clopixol® (Can)** *see* zuclopenthixol *(Canada only)* *on page 641*

**Clopixol® Depot (Can)** *see* zuclopenthixol *(Canada only)* *on page 641*

**Clopra® *(Discontinued)*** *see page 750*

## clorazepate (klor AZ e pate)

**U.S./Canadian Brand Names** Apo®-Clorazepate (Can); Gen-XENE®; Novo-Clopate (Can); Tranxene®

**Therapeutic Category** Anticonvulsant; Benzodiazepine

**Controlled Substance** C-IV

**Use** Treatment of generalized anxiety and panic disorders; management of alcohol withdrawal; adjunct anticonvulsant in management of partial seizures

**Usual Dosage** Oral:

Anticonvulsant:

Children:

<9 years: Dose not established

9-12 years: Initial: 3.75-7.5 mg/dose twice daily; increase dose by 3.75 mg at weekly intervals, not to exceed 60 mg/day in 2-3 divided doses

Children >12 years and Adults: Initial: Up to 7.5 mg/dose 2-3 times/day; increase dose by 7.5 mg at weekly intervals; usual dose: 0.5-1 mg/kg/day; not to exceed 90 mg/day (up to 3 mg/kg/day has been used)

Anxiety: Adults: 7.5-15 mg 2-4 times/day, or administered as single dose of 15-22.5 mg at bedtime

Alcohol withdrawal: Adults: Initial: 30 mg, then 15 mg 2-4 times/day on first day; maximum daily dose: 90 mg; gradually decrease dose over subsequent days

**Dosage Forms**

Capsule, as dipotassium: 3.75 mg, 7.5 mg, 15 mg

Tablet, as dipotassium: 3.75 mg, 7.5 mg, 15 mg

Tablet, as dipotassium, single dose: 11.25 mg, 22.5 mg

**Clorpactin® WCS-90** *see* oxychlorosene *on page 443*

**Clorpactin® XCB Powder *(Discontinued)*** *see page 750*

**Clotrimaderm (Can)** *see* clotrimazole *on this page*

## clotrimazole (kloe TRIM a zole)

**U.S./Canadian Brand Names** Canesten® (Can); Clotrimaderm (Can); Fungoid® Solution; Gyne-Lotrimin® [OTC]; Gyne-Lotrimin® 3 [OTC]; Lotrimin®; Lotrimin® AF Cream [OTC]; Lotrimin® AF Lotion [OTC]; Lotrimin® AF Solution [OTC]; Mycelex®; Mycelex®-7; Mycelex®-G; Trivagizole 3™ [OTC]

**Therapeutic Category** Antifungal Agent

**Use** Treatment of susceptible fungal infections, including oropharyngeal candidiasis, dermatophytoses, superficial mycoses, cutaneous candidiasis, as well as vulvovaginal candidiasis; limited data suggests that the use of clotrimazole troches may be effective for prophylaxis against oropharyngeal candidiasis in neutropenic patients

**Usual Dosage**

Children >3 years and Adults:

Oral:

Prophylaxis: 10 mg troche dissolved 3 times/day for the duration of chemotherapy or until steroids are reduced to maintenance levels

Treatment: 10 mg troche dissolved slowly 5 times/day for 14 consecutive days

Topical: Apply twice daily; if no improvement occurs after 4 weeks of therapy, reevaluate diagnosis

(Continued)

## clotrimazole *(Continued)*

Children >12 years and Adults:
Vaginal:
Cream:
1%: Insert 1 applicatorful vaginal cream daily (preferably at bedtime) for 7 consecutive days
2%: Insert 1 applicatorful vaginal cream daily (preferably at bedtime) for 3 consecutive days
Tablet: Insert 100 mg/day for 7 days or 500 mg single dose
Topical: Apply to affected area twice daily (morning and evening) for 7 consecutive days

**Dosage Forms**
Combination pack:
Gyne-Lotrimin®, Mycelex®-7: Vaginal tablet 100 mg (7s) and vaginal cream 1% (7 g)
Gyne-Lotrimin® 3: Vaginal tablet 200 mg and vaginal cream 1%
Cream:
Topical (Lotrimin®, Lotrimin® AF, Mycelex®, Mycelex® OTC): 1% (15 g, 30 g, 45 g, 90 g)
Vaginal:
Gyne-Lotrimin®, Mycelex®-7: 1% (45 g, 90 g)
Gyne-Lotrimin® 3, Trivagizole 3™: 2% (25 g)
Lotion (Lotrimin®): 1% (30 mL)
Solution, topical (Fungoid®, Lotrimin®, Lotrimin® AF, Mycelex®, Mycelex® OTC): 1% (10 mL, 30 mL)
Tablet, vaginal:
Gyne-Lotrimin®, Gynix®, Mycelex®-7: 100 mg (7s)
Mycelex®-G: 500 mg (1s)
Troche (Mycelex®): 10 mg
Twin pack (Mycelex®): Vaginal tablet 500 mg (1s) and vaginal cream 1% (7 g)

## cloxacillin (kloks a SIL in)

**U.S./Canadian Brand Names** Apo®-Cloxi (Can); Novo-Cloxin (Can); Nu-Cloxi (Can)
**Therapeutic Category** Penicillin
**Use** Treatment of susceptible bacterial infections of the respiratory tract, skin and skin structure, bone and joint caused by penicillinase-producing staphylococci
**Usual Dosage** Oral:
Children >1 month: 50-100 mg/kg/day in divided doses every 6 hours; up to a maximum of 4 g/day
Adults: 250-500 mg every 6 hours
**Dosage Forms**
Capsule, as sodium: 250 mg, 500 mg
Powder for oral suspension, as sodium: 125 mg/5 mL (100 mL, 200 mL)

**Cloxapen®** ***(Discontinued)*** *see page 750*

## clozapine (KLOE za peen)

**U.S./Canadian Brand Names** Clozaril®
**Therapeutic Category** Antipsychotic Agent, Dibenzodiazepine
**Use** Management of schizophrenic patients
**Usual Dosage** Adults: Oral: Initial: 25 mg once or twice daily, increase as tolerated to a target dose of 300-450 mg/day, may require doses as high as 600-900 mg/day
**Dosage Forms** Tablet: 25 mg, 100 mg

**Clozaril®** *see* clozapine *on this page*

**Clysodrast®** *see* bisacodyl *on page 81*

**CMV-IGIV** *see* cytomegalovirus immune globulin (intravenous-human) *on page 163*

**CoActifed® (Can)** *see* triprolidine, pseudoephedrine, and codeine *on page 609*

**coagulant complex inhibitor** *see* anti-inhibitor coagulant complex *on page 44*

**coagulation factor VIIa** *see* factor VIIa (recombinant) *on page 239*

## coal tar (KOLE tar)

**Synonyms** crude coal tar; LCD; pix carbonis

**U.S./Canadian Brand Names** AquaTar® [OTC]; Denorex® [OTC]; DHS® Tar [OTC]; Duplex® T [OTC]; Estar® [OTC]; Fototar® [OTC]; Neutrogena® T/Derm; Pentrax® [OTC]; Polytar® [OTC]; psoriGel® [OTC]; T/Gel® [OTC]; Zetar® [OTC]

**Therapeutic Category** Antipsoriatic Agent; Antiseborrheic Agent, Topical

**Use** Topically for controlling dandruff, seborrheic dermatitis, or psoriasis

**Usual Dosage**

Bath: Add appropriate amount to bath water, for adults usually 60-90 mL of a 5% to 20% solution or 15-25 mL of 30% lotion; soak 5-20 minutes, then pat dry; use once daily for 3 days

Shampoo: Rub shampoo onto wet hair and scalp, rinse thoroughly; repeat; leave on 5 minutes; rinse thoroughly; apply twice weekly for the first 2 weeks then once weekly or more often if needed

Skin: Apply to the affected area 1-4 times/day; decrease frequency to 2-3 times/week once condition has been controlled

Scalp psoriasis: Tar oil bath or coal tar solution may be painted sparingly to the lesions 3-12 hours before each shampoo

Psoriasis of the body, arms, legs: Apply at bedtime; if thick scales are present, use product with salicylic acid and apply several times during the day

**Dosage Forms**

Cream: 1% to 5%

Gel: Coal tar 5%

Lotion: 2.5% to 30%

Lotion: 2%; 5%; 25%

Shampoo: Coal tar extract 2% with salicylic acid 2% (60 mL)

Shampoo, topical: Coal tar: 0.5% to 5%

Solution:

Coal tar: 2.5%, 5%, 20%

Coal tar extract: 5%

Suspension, coal tar: 30% to 33.3%

## coal tar and salicylic acid (KOLE tar & sal i SIL ik AS id)

**U.S./Canadian Brand Names** X-Seb® T [OTC]

**Therapeutic Category** Antipsoriatic Agent; Antiseborrheic Agent, Topical

**Use** Treatment of seborrheal dermatitis, dandruff

**Usual Dosage** Topical: Shampoo twice weekly

**Dosage Forms** Shampoo: Coal tar solution 10% and salicylic acid 4% (120 mL)

## coal tar, lanolin, and mineral oil (KOLE tar, LAN oh lin, & MIN er al oyl)

**U.S./Canadian Brand Names** Balnetar® [OTC]

**Therapeutic Category** Antipsoriatic Agent; Antiseborrheic Agent, Topical

**Use** Treatment of psoriasis, seborrheal dermatitis, atopic dermatitis, eczematoid dermatitis

**Usual Dosage** Add to bath water, soak for 5-20 minutes then pat dry

**Dosage Forms** Oil, bath: Water-dispersible emollient tar 2.5%, lanolin fraction, and mineral oil (240 mL)

**Cobalasine® Injection *(Discontinued)*** *see page 750*

**Cobex®** *see* cyanocobalamin *on page 158*

## cocaine (koe KANE)

**Therapeutic Category** Local Anesthetic

**Controlled Substance** C-II

**Use** Topical anesthesia for mucous membranes

**Usual Dosage** Topical: Use lowest effective dose; do not exceed 1 mg/kg; patient tolerance, anesthetic technique, vascularity of tissue and area to be anesthetized will determine dose needed

**Dosage Forms**

Powder, as hydrochloride: 5 g, 25 g

Solution, topical, as hydrochloride: 4% [40 mg/mL] (2 mL, 4 mL, 10 mL); 10% [100 mg/mL] (4 mL, 10 mL)

Solution, topical, viscous, as hydrochloride: 4% [40 mg/mL] (4 mL, 10 mL); 10% [100 mg/mL] (4 mL, 10 mL)

Tablet, soluble, for topical solution, as hydrochloride: 135 mg

## coccidioidin skin test (koks i dee OH i din skin test)

**U.S./Canadian Brand Names** Spherulin®

**Therapeutic Category** Diagnostic Agent

**Use** Intradermal skin test in diagnosis of coccidioidomycosis; differential diagnosis of this disease from histoplasmosis, sarcoidosis and other mycotic and bacterial infections. The skin test may be negative in severe forms of disease (anergy) or when prolonged periods of time have passed since infection.

**Usual Dosage** Children and Adults: Intradermally: 0.1 mL of 1:100 or flexor surface of forearm

Positive reaction: Induration of 5 mm or more; erythema without induration is considered negative; read the test at 24 and 48 hours, since some reactions may not be noticeable after 36 hours. A positive reaction indicates present or past infection with *Coccidioides immitis.*

Negative reaction: A negative test means the individual has not been sensitized to coccidioidin or has lost sensitivity

**Dosage Forms** Injection: 1:10 (0.5 mL); 1:100 (1 mL)

**Codafed® Expectorant** *see* guaifenesin, pseudoephedrine, and codeine *on page 284*

**Codamine® *(Discontinued)*** *see page 750*

**Codamine® Pediatric *(Discontinued)*** *see page 750*

**Codehist® DH** *see* chlorpheniramine, pseudoephedrine, and codeine *on page 132*

## codeine (KOE deen)

**Synonyms** methylmorphine

**U.S./Canadian Brand Names** Codeine Contin® (Can)

**Therapeutic Category** Analgesic, Narcotic; Antitussive

**Controlled Substance** C-II

**Use** Treatment of mild to moderate pain; antitussive in lower doses

**Usual Dosage** Doses should be titrated to appropriate analgesic effect; when changing routes of administration, note that oral dose is $^2/_3$ as effective as parenteral dose

Analgesic: Oral, I.M., S.C.:

- Children: 0.5-1 mg/kg/dose every 4-6 hours as needed; maximum: 60 mg/dose
- Adults: 30 mg/dose; range: 15-60 mg every 4-6 hours as needed

Antitussive: Oral (for nonproductive cough):

- Children: 1-1.5 mg/kg/day in divided doses every 4-6 hours as needed: Alternatively dose according to age:
  - 2-6 years: 2.5-5 mg every 4-6 hours as needed; maximum: 30 mg/day
  - 6-12 years: 5-10 mg every 4-6 hours as needed; maximum: 60 mg/day
- Adults: 10-20 mg/dose every 4-6 hours as needed; maximum: 120 mg/day

**Dosage Forms**
Injection, as phosphate: 30 mg (1 mL, 2 mL); 60 mg (1 mL, 2 mL)
Solution, oral: 15 mg/5 mL
Tablet, as phosphate, soluble: 30 mg, 60 mg
Tablet, as sulfate: 15 mg, 30 mg, 60 mg
Tablet, as sulfate, soluble: 15 mg, 30 mg, 60 mg

**codeine and acetaminophen** *see* acetaminophen and codeine *on page 4*

**Codeine Contin® (Can)** *see* codeine *on previous page*

**Codiclear® DH** *see* hydrocodone and guaifenesin *on page 301*

**Codimal-A® Injection *(Discontinued)*** *see page 750*

**Codimal® Expectorant *(Discontinued)*** *see page 750*

**cod liver oil** *see* vitamin A and vitamin D *on page 630*

**Cogentin®** *see* benztropine *on page 75*

**Co-Gesic®** *see* hydrocodone and acetaminophen *on page 300*

**Cognex®** *see* tacrine *on page 569*

**Colace® [OTC]** *see* docusate *on page 197*

**colaspase** *see* asparaginase *on page 55*

**Colazal™** *see* balsalazide *on page 67*

## colchicine (KOL chi seen)

**Therapeutic Category** Antigout Agent

**Use** Treat acute gouty arthritis attacks and to prevent recurrences of such attacks; management of familial Mediterranean fever

**Usual Dosage**
Acute gouty arthritis:
Oral: Initial: 0.5-1.2 mg, then 0.5-0.6 mg every 1-2 hours or 1-1.2 mg every 2 hours until relief or GI side effects occur to a maximum total dose of 8 mg, wait 3 days before initiating a second course
I.V.: Initial: 1-3 mg, then 0.5 mg every 6 hours until response, not to exceed 4 mg/day; following a full course of colchicine (4 mg), wait 7 days before initiating another course of colchicine (by any route)
Prophylaxis of recurrent attacks: Oral:
<1 attack/year: 0.5 or 0.6 mg/day/dose for 3-4 days/week
>1 attack/year: 0.5 or 0.6 mg/day/dose
Severe cases: 1-1.8 mg/day

**Dosage Forms**
Injection: 0.5 mg/mL (2 mL)
Tablet: 0.5 mg, 0.6 mg

## colchicine and probenecid (KOL chi seen & proe BEN e sid)

**Therapeutic Category** Antigout Agent

**Use** Treatment of chronic gouty arthritis when complicated by frequent, recurrent acute attacks of gout

**Usual Dosage** Adults: Oral: 1 tablet daily for 1 week, then 1 tablet twice daily thereafter

**Dosage Forms** Tablet: Colchicine 0.5 mg and probenecid 0.5 g

**Cold & Allergy® Elixir *(Discontinued)*** *see page 750*

**Coldlac-LA® *(Discontinued)*** *see page 750*

**Coldloc® *(Discontinued)*** *see page 750*

**Coldrine® [OTC]** *see* acetaminophen and pseudoephedrine *on page 6*

## colesevelam (koh le SEV a lam)

**U.S./Canadian Brand Names** Welchol™

**Therapeutic Category** Antilipemic Agent; Bile Acid Sequestrant

**Use** Adjunctive therapy to diet and exercise in the management of elevated LDL in primary hypercholesterolemia (Fredrickson Type IIa) when used alone or in combination with an HMG-CoA reductase inhibitor.

**Usual Dosage**

Adults: Oral: Monotherapy: 3 tablets twice daily with meals or 6 tablets once daily with a meal; maximum dose: 7 tablets/day

Combination therapy with an HMG-CoA reductase inhibitor: 4-6 tablets daily; maximum dose: 6 tablets/day

**Dosage Forms** Tablet: 625 mg

**Colestid®** *see* colestipol *on this page*

## colestipol (koe LES ti pole)

**U.S./Canadian Brand Names** Colestid®

**Therapeutic Category** Antihyperlipidemic Agent, Miscellaneous

**Use** Adjunct in the management of primary hypercholesterolemia; to relieve pruritus associated with elevated levels of bile acids, possibly used to decrease plasma half-life of digoxin as an adjunct in the treatment of toxicity

**Usual Dosage** Oral: 15-30 g/day in divided doses 2-4 times/day

**Dosage Forms**

Granules, as hydrochloride: 5 g packet, 300 g, 500 g

Tablet, as hydrochloride: 1 g

## colfosceril palmitate (kole FOS er il PALM i tate)

**Synonyms** dipalmitoylphosphatidylcholine; DPPC; synthetic lung surfactant

**U.S./Canadian Brand Names** Exosurf® Neonatal™

**Therapeutic Category** Lung Surfactant

**Use** Neonatal respiratory distress syndrome (RDS):

Prophylactic therapy: Infants at risk for developing RDS with body weight <1350 g; infants with evidence of pulmonary immaturity with body weight >1350 g

Rescue therapy: Treatment of infants with RDS based on respiratory distress not attributable to any other causes and chest radiographic findings consistent with RDS

**Usual Dosage**

Prophylactic treatment: Administer 5 mL/kg as soon as possible; the second and third doses should be administered at 12 and 24 hours later to those infants remaining on ventilators

Rescue treatment: Administer 5 mL/kg as soon as the diagnosis of RDS is made; the second 5 mL/kg dose should be administered 12 hours later

**Dosage Forms** Powder for injection, lyophilized: 108 mg (10 mL)

## colistimethate (koe lis ti METH ate)

**U.S./Canadian Brand Names** Coly-Mycin® M Parenteral

**Therapeutic Category** Antibiotic, Miscellaneous

**Use** Treatment of infections due to sensitive strains of certain gram-negative bacilli

**Usual Dosage** Children and Adults: I.M., I.V.: 2.5-5 mg/kg/day in 2-4 divided doses

**Dosage Forms** Powder for injection, as sodium, lyophilized: 150 mg

## collagenase (KOL la je nase)

**U.S./Canadian Brand Names** Santyl®

**Therapeutic Category** Enzyme

**Use** Promote debridement of necrotic tissue in dermal ulcers and severe burns

**Usual Dosage** Topical: Apply daily or every other day

**Dosage Forms** Ointment, topical: 250 units/g (15 g, 30 g)

**collagen implants** (KOL a jen im PLANTS)
**Therapeutic Category** Ophthalmic Agent, Miscellaneous
**Use** Relief of dry eyes; enhance the effect of ocular medications
**Usual Dosage** Implants inserted by physician
**Dosage Forms** Implant: 0.2 mm, 0.3 mm, 0.4 mm, 0.5 mm, 0.6 mm

**Colocort™** *see* hydrocortisone (rectal) *on page 302*
**Coly-Mycin® M Parenteral** *see* colistimethate *on previous page*
**Coly-Mycin® S Oral *(Discontinued)*** *see page 750*
**Colyte®** *see* polyethylene glycol solution *on page 480*
**Combantrin™ (Can)** *see* pyrantel pamoate *on page 509*
**Combipres®** *see* clonidine and chlorthalidone *on page 146*
**Combivent®** *see* ipratropium and albuterol *on page 325*
**Combivir®** *see* zidovudine and lamivudine *on page 638*
**Comfort® Ophthalmic [OTC]** *see* naphazoline *on page 409*
**Comfort® Tears Solution [OTC]** *see* artificial tears *on page 53*
**Comhist®** *see* chlorpheniramine, phenylephrine, and phenyltoloxamine *on page 131*
**Comhist® LA** *see* chlorpheniramine, phenylephrine, and phenyltoloxamine *on page 131*
**Compazine®** *see* prochlorperazine *on page 497*
**compound E** *see* cortisone acetate *on page 155*
**compound F** *see* hydrocortisone (systemic) *on page 303*
**compound S** *see* zidovudine *on page 638*
**Compoz® Gel Caps [OTC]** *see* diphenhydramine *on page 191*
**Compoz® Nighttime Sleep Aid [OTC]** *see* diphenhydramine *on page 191*
**Comtan®** *see* entacapone *on page 215*
**Comtrex® Allergy-Sinus [OTC]** *see* acetaminophen, chlorpheniramine, and pseudoephedrine *on page 6*
**Comtrex® Allergy-Sinus Day & Night [OTC]** *see* acetaminophen, chlorpheniramine, and pseudoephedrine *on page 6*
**Comtrex® Non-Drowsy [OTC]** *see* acetaminophen, dextromethorphan, and pseudoephedrine *on page 7*
**Comvax®** *see* *Haemophilus* B conjugate and hepatitis B vaccine *on page 287*
**Concerta™** *see* methylphenidate *on page 384*
**Condyline™ (Can)** *see* podofilox *on page 479*
**Condylox®** *see* podofilox *on page 479*
**Conex® *(Discontinued)*** *see page 750*
**Congess® Jr** *see* guaifenesin and pseudoephedrine *on page 283*
**Congess® Sr** *see* guaifenesin and pseudoephedrine *on page 283*
**Congestac®** *see* guaifenesin and pseudoephedrine *on page 283*
**Congestant D® *(Discontinued)*** *see page 750*
**Congest (Can)** *see* estrogens (conjugated/equine) *on page 227*
**conjugated estrogens** *see* estrogens (conjugated/equine) *on page 227*
**Conray®** *see* radiological/contrast media (ionic) *on page 516*
**Constant-T® Tablet *(Discontinued)*** *see page 750*
**Constilac®** *see* lactulose *on page 338*

**Constulose®** *see* lactulose *on page 338*

**Contac® Cough Formula Liquid [OTC]** *see* guaifenesin and dextromethorphan *on page 282*

**Contac® Severe Cold & Flu/Non-Drowsy [OTC]** *see* acetaminophen, dextromethorphan, and pseudoephedrine *on page 7*

**Control® *(Discontinued)*** *see page 750*

**Control-L® *(Discontinued)*** *see page 750*

**Contuss® *(Discontinued)*** *see page 750*

**Contuss® XT *(Discontinued)*** *see page 750*

**Copaxone®** *see* glatiramer acetate *on page 274*

**Cophene-B®** *see* brompheniramine *on page 87*

**Cophene XP®** *see* hydrocodone, pseudoephedrine, and guaifenesin *on page 302*

**copolymer-1** *see* glatiramer acetate *on page 274*

**copper injection** *see* trace metals *on page 598*

**Co-Pyronil® 2 Pulvules® [OTC]** *see* chlorpheniramine and pseudoephedrine *on page 130*

**Cordarone®** *see* amiodarone *on page 32*

**Cordran®** *see* flurandrenolide *on page 258*

**Cordran® SP** *see* flurandrenolide *on page 258*

**Coreg®** *see* carvedilol *on page 111*

**Corgard®** *see* nadolol *on page 405*

**Corgonject® *(Discontinued)*** *see page 750*

**Coricidin® [OTC]** *see* chlorpheniramine and acetaminophen *on page 129*

**Corliprol® *(Discontinued)*** *see page 750*

**Corlopam®** *see* fenoldopam *on page 243*

**Cormax® Ointment** *see* clobetasol *on page 143*

**Correctol® [OTC]** *see* senna *on page 541*

**CortaGel® Topical [OTC]** *see* hydrocortisone (topical) *on page 304*

**Cortaid® Maximum Strength Topical [OTC]** *see* hydrocortisone (topical) *on page 304*

**Cortaid® Ointment *(Discontinued)*** *see page 750*

**Cortaid® with Aloe Topical [OTC]** *see* hydrocortisone (topical) *on page 304*

**Cortatrigen® Otic** *see* neomycin, polymyxin B, and hydrocortisone *on page 415*

**Cort-Dome® Topical** *see* hydrocortisone (topical) *on page 304*

**Cortef® Feminine Itch Topical** *see* hydrocortisone (topical) *on page 304*

**Cortenema® Rectal** *see* hydrocortisone (rectal) *on page 302*

**Corticaine® Topical** *see* dibucaine and hydrocortisone *on page 181*

## corticotropin (kor ti koe TROE pin)

**Synonyms** ACTH; adrenocorticotropic hormone

**U.S./Canadian Brand Names** Acthar®; H.P. Acthar® Gel

**Therapeutic Category** Adrenal Corticosteroid

**Use** Infantile spasms; diagnostic aid in adrenocortical insufficiency; acute exacerbations of multiple sclerosis; severe muscle weakness in myasthenia gravis

**Usual Dosage**

Acute exacerbation of multiple sclerosis: I.M.: 80-120 units/day for 2-3 weeks

Diagnostic purposes:

I.M., S.C.: 20 units 4 times/day

I.V.: 10-25 units in 500 mL 5% dextrose in water over 8 hours

**Dosage Forms**

Injection, repository (H.P. Acthar® Gel): 40 units/mL (1 mL, 5 mL); 80 units/mL (1 mL, 5 mL)

Powder for injection (Acthar®): 25 units, 40 units

**Cortifoam® Rectal** *see* hydrocortisone (rectal) *on page 302*

**Cortimyxin® (Can)** *see* neomycin, polymyxin B, and hydrocortisone *on page 415*

## cortisone acetate (KOR ti sone AS e tate)

**Synonyms** compound E

**Therapeutic Category** Adrenal Corticosteroid

**Use** Management of adrenocortical insufficiency

**Usual Dosage** Depends upon the condition being treated and the response of the patient

Children:

Anti-inflammatory or immunosuppressive:

Oral: 2.5-10 mg/kg/day or 20-300 mg/m²/day in divided doses every 6-8 hours

I.M.: 1-5 mg/kg/day or 14-375 mg/m²/day in divided doses every 12-24 hours

Physiologic replacement:

Oral: 0.5-0.75 mg/kg/day in divided doses every 8 hours

I.M.: 0.25-0.35 mg/kg/day once daily

Stress coverage for surgery: I.M.: 1 and 2 days before preanesthesia, and 1-3 days after surgery: 50-62.5 mg/m²/day; 4 days after surgery: 31-50 mg/m²/day

Adults: Oral, I.M.: 20-300 mg/day

**Dosage Forms**

Injection: 50 mg/mL (10 mL)

Tablet: 5 mg, 10 mg, 25 mg

**Cortisporin® Ophthalmic Ointment** *see* bacitracin, neomycin, polymyxin B, and hydrocortisone *on page 65*

**Cortisporin® Ophthalmic Suspension** *see* neomycin, polymyxin B, and hydrocortisone *on page 415*

**Cortisporin® Otic** *see* neomycin, polymyxin B, and hydrocortisone *on page 415*

**Cortisporin®-TC® Otic Suspension** *see* neomycin, colistin, hydrocortisone, and thonzonium *on page 414*

**Cortisporin® Topical Cream** *see* neomycin, polymyxin B, and hydrocortisone *on page 415*

**Cortisporin® Topical Ointment** *see* bacitracin, neomycin, polymyxin B, and hydrocortisone *on page 65*

**Cortizone®-5 Topical [OTC]** *see* hydrocortisone (topical) *on page 304*

**Cortizone®-10 Topical [OTC]** *see* hydrocortisone (topical) *on page 304*

**Cortoderm (Can)** *see* hydrocortisone (topical) *on page 304*

**Cortone® Acetate *(Discontinued)*** *see page 750*

**Cortrophin-Zinc® *(Discontinued)*** *see page 750*

**Cortrosyn®** *see* cosyntropin *on next page*

**Corvert®** *see* ibutilide *on page 312*

**Coryphen® Codeine (Can)** *see* aspirin and codeine *on page 56*

**Cosmegen®** *see* dactinomycin *on page 164*

**Cosopt®** *see* dorzolamide and timolol *on page 201*

## cosyntropin (koe sin TROE pin)

**Synonyms** synacthen; tetracosactide

**U.S./Canadian Brand Names** Cortrosyn®; Synacthen Depot (Can)

**Therapeutic Category** Diagnostic Agent

**Use** Diagnostic test to differentiate primary adrenal from secondary (pituitary) adrenocortical insufficiency

**Usual Dosage**

Adrenocortical insufficiency: I.M., I.V.:

Children <2 years: 0.125 mg injected over 2 minutes

Children >2 years and Adults: 0.25 mg injected over 2 minutes

When greater cortisol stimulation is needed, an I.V. infusion may be used: I.V. infusion: 0.25 mg administered over 4-8 hours

Congenital adrenal hyperplasia evaluation: 1 mg/m$^2$/dose up to a maximum of 1 mg

**Dosage Forms** Powder for injection: 0.25 mg

**Cotazym®** *see* pancrelipase *on page 448*

**Cotazym-S®** *see* pancrelipase *on page 448*

**Cotridin® (Can)** *see* triprolidine, pseudoephedrine, and codeine *on page 609*

**Cotrim® *(Discontinued)*** *see page 750*

**Cotrim® DS *(Discontinued)*** *see page 750*

**co-trimoxazole** *see* sulfamethoxazole and trimethoprim *on page 564*

**Coumadin®** *see* warfarin *on page 634*

**Covera-HS®** *see* verapamil *on page 625*

**Coversyl® (Can)** *see* perindopril erbumine *on page 461*

**Cozaar®** *see* losartan *on page 357*

**CP-99,219-27** *see* trovafloxacin *on page 611*

**CPM** *see* cyclophosphamide *on page 159*

**Creon®** *see* pancreatin *on page 447*

**Creon® 5** *see* pancrelipase *on page 448*

**Creon® 10** *see* pancrelipase *on page 448*

**Creon® 20** *see* pancrelipase *on page 448*

**Creo-Terpin® [OTC]** *see* dextromethorphan *on page 178*

**Cresylate®** *see* m-cresyl acetate *on page 366*

**Crinone®** *see* progesterone *on page 498*

**Criticare HN® [OTC]** *see* nutritional formula, enteral/oral *on page 432*

**Crixivan®** *see* indinavir *on page 317*

**Crolom®** *see* cromolyn sodium *on this page*

**cromoglicic acid** *see* cromolyn sodium *on this page*

## cromolyn sodium (KROE moe lin SOW dee um)

**Synonyms** cromoglicic acid; disodium cromoglycate; DSCG

**U.S./Canadian Brand Names** Crolom®; Gastrocrom®; Intal®; Nalcrom® (Can); Nasalcrom® [OTC]; Opticrom®

**Therapeutic Category** Mast Cell Stabilizer

**Use** Adjunct in the prophylaxis of allergic disorders, including rhinitis, conjunctivitis, and asthma; inhalation product may be used for prevention of exercise-induced bronchospasm

Ophthalmologic: Vernal conjunctivitis, vernal keratoconjunctivitis, and vernal keratitis
Systemic: Mastocytosis, food allergy, and treatment of inflammatory bowel disease

**Usual Dosage**
Children:
Inhalation: >2 years: 20 mg 4 times/day
Nebulization solution: >5 years: 2 inhalations 4 times/day by metered spray, or 20 mg 4 times/day (Spinhaler®); taper frequency to the lowest effective level
For prevention of exercise-induced bronchospasm: Single dose of 2 inhalations (aerosol) just prior to exercise
Nasal: >6 years: 1 spray in each nostril 3-4 times/day
Adults: Nasal: 1 spray in each nostril 3-4 times/day

Systemic mastocytosis: Oral:
Infants ≤2 years: 20 mg/kg/day in 4 divided doses, not to exceed 30 mg/kg/day
Children 2-12 years: 100 mg 4 times/day; not to exceed 40 mg/kg/day
Adults: 200 mg 4 times/day
Food allergy and inflammatory bowel disease: Oral:
Children: 100 mg 4 times/day 15-20 minutes before meals, not to exceed 40 mg/kg/day
Adults: 200 mg 4 times/day 15-20 minutes before meal, up to 400 mg 4 times/day

**Dosage Forms**
Capsule: Oral (Gastrocrom®): 100 mg
Solution:
For nebulization: 10 mg/mL (2 mL)
Intal®: 10 mg/mL (2 mL)
Nasal (Nasalcrom®): 40 mg/mL (13 mL)
Ophthalmic (Crolom®, Opticrom®): 4% (2.5 mL, 10 mL)

**crotaline antivenin, polyvalent** *see* antivenin (*Crotalidae*) polyvalent *on page 45*

## crotamiton (kroe TAM i tonn)

**U.S./Canadian Brand Names** Eurax® Topical
**Therapeutic Category** Scabicides/Pediculicides
**Use** Treatment of scabies (*Sarcoptes scabiei*) in infants and children
**Usual Dosage** Scabicide: Children and Adults: Topical: Wash thoroughly and scrub away loose scales, then towel dry; apply a thin layer and massage drug onto skin of the entire body from the neck to the toes (with special attention to skin folds, creases, and interdigital spaces). Repeat application in 24 hours; patient should take a cleansing bath 48 hours after the final application.
**Dosage Forms**
Cream: 10% (60 g)
Lotion: 10% (60 mL, 454 mL)

**crude coal tar** *see* coal tar *on page 149*

**crystalline penicillin** *see* penicillin G (parenteral/aqueous) *on page 456*

**Crystamine®** *see* cyanocobalamin *on next page*

**Crysticillin® 300 A.S.** ***(Discontinued)*** *see page 750*

**Crysticillin® 600 A.S.** ***(Discontinued)*** *see page 750*

**Crysticillin® A.S.** *see* penicillin G procaine *on page 457*

**Crystodigin®** ***(Discontinued)*** *see page 750*

**CSP** *see* cellulose sodium phosphate *on page 119*

**CTX** *see* cyclophosphamide *on page 159*

**Cuprimine®** *see* penicillamine *on page 455*

**Curosurf®** *see* poractant alfa *on page 483*

**Cutivate™** *see* fluticasone (topical) *on page 261*

**CYA** *see* cyclosporine *on page 160*

## cyanide antidote kit (SYE a nide AN tee dote kit)

**Therapeutic Category** Antidote

**Use** Treatment of cyanide poisoning

**Usual Dosage** Cyanide poisoning: 0.3 mL ampul of amyl nitrite is crushed every minute and vapor is inhaled for 15-30 seconds until an I.V. sodium nitrite infusion is available. Following administration of 300 mg I.V. sodium nitrite, inject 12.5 g sodium thiosulfate I.V. (over ~10 minutes), if needed; injection of both may be repeated at ½ the original dose.

**Dosage Forms** Kit: Sodium nitrite 300 mg/10 mL (#2); sodium thiosulfate 12.5 g/50 mL (#2); amyl nitrite 0.3 mL (#12); also disposable syringes, stomach tube, tourniquet and instructions

## cyanocobalamin (sye an oh koe BAL a min)

**Synonyms** vitamin $B_{12}$

**U.S./Canadian Brand Names** Berubigen®; Cobex®; Crystamine®; Cyanoject®; Cyomin®; Ener-B® [OTC]; Kaybovite-1000®; Redisol®; Rubramin-PC®; Sytobex®

**Therapeutic Category** Vitamin, Water Soluble

**Use** Pernicious anemia; vitamin $B_{12}$ deficiency; increased $B_{12}$ requirements due to pregnancy, thyrotoxicosis, hemorrhage, malignancy, liver or kidney disease

**Usual Dosage**

- Congenital pernicious anemia (if evidence of neurologic involvement): I.M.: 1000 mcg/day for at least 2 weeks; maintenance: 50 mcg/month
- Vitamin $B_{12}$ deficiency: I.M., S.C. (oral is not recommended due to poor absorption):
  - Children: 100 mcg/day for 10-15 days (total dose of 1-1.5 mg), then once or twice weekly for several months; may taper to 250-1000 mcg every month
  - Adults: 100 mcg/day for 6-7 days
  - Hematologic signs only:
    - Children: 10-50 mcg/day for 5-10 days, then maintenance: 100-250 mcg/dose every 2-4 weeks
    - Adults: 30 mcg/day for 5-10 days, followed by 100-200 mcg/month
- Methylmalonic aciduria: I.M.: 1 mg/day

**Dosage Forms**

- Gel, nasal:
  - Ener-B®: 400 mcg/0.1 mL
  - Nascobal®: 500 mcg/0.1 mL (5 mL)
- Injection: 30 mcg/mL (30 mL); 100 mcg/mL (1 mL, 10 mL, 30 mL); 1000 mcg/mL (1 mL, 10 mL, 30 mL)
- Tablet [OTC]: 25 mcg, 50 mcg, 100 mcg, 250 mcg, 500 mcg, 1000 mcg

**Cyanoject®** *see* cyanocobalamin *on this page*

## cyclandelate (sye KLAN de late)

**Therapeutic Category** Vasodilator, Peripheral

**Use** Considered as "possibly effective" for adjunctive therapy in peripheral vascular disease and possibly senility due to cerebrovascular disease or multi-infarct dementia; migraine prophylaxis, vertigo, tinnitus, and visual disturbances secondary to cerebrovascular insufficiency and diabetic peripheral polyneuropathy

**Usual Dosage** Adults: Oral: Initial: 1.2-1.6 g/day in divided doses before meals and at bedtime until response; maintenance therapy: 400-800 mg/day in 2-4 divided doses; start with lowest dose in elderly due to hypotensive potential; decrease dose by 200 mg decrements to achieve minimal maintenance dose; improvement can usually be seen over weeks of therapy and prolonged use; short courses of therapy are usually ineffective and not recommended

**Dosage Forms** Capsule: 200 mg, 400 mg

## cyclizine (SYE kli zeen)

**U.S./Canadian Brand Names** Marezine® Oral [OTC]

**Therapeutic Category** Antihistamine

**Use** Prevention and treatment of nausea, vomiting and vertigo associated with motion sickness; control of postoperative nausea and vomiting

**Usual Dosage** Oral:

Children 6-12 years: 25 mg up to 3 times/day

Adults: 50 mg taken 30 minutes before departure, may repeat in 4-6 hours if needed, up to 200 mg/day

**Dosage Forms** Tablet, as hydrochloride: 50 mg

## cyclobenzaprine (sye kloe BEN za preen)

**U.S./Canadian Brand Names** Apo®-Cyclobenzaprine (Can); Flexeril®; Flexitec (Can); Gen-Cyclobenzaprine (Can); Novo-Cycloprine (Can); Nu-Cyclobenzaprine (Can)

**Therapeutic Category** Skeletal Muscle Relaxant

**Use** Treatment of muscle spasm associated with acute painful musculoskeletal conditions; supportive therapy in tetanus

**Usual Dosage** Oral:

Children: Dosage has not been established

Adults: 20-40 mg/day in 2-4 divided doses; maximum dose: 60 mg/day

**Dosage Forms** Tablet, as hydrochloride: 10 mg

**Cyclocort® Topical** *see* amcinonide *on page 29*

**Cyclogyl®** *see* cyclopentolate *on this page*

**Cyclomen® (Can)** *see* danazol *on page 165*

**Cyclomydril® Ophthalmic** *see* cyclopentolate and phenylephrine *on this page*

## cyclopentolate (sye kloe PEN toe late)

**U.S./Canadian Brand Names** Cyclogyl®; Diopentolate® (Can); I-Pentolate®

**Therapeutic Category** Anticholinergic Agent

**Use** Diagnostic procedures requiring mydriasis and cycloplegia

**Usual Dosage** Ophthalmic:

Infants: Instill 1 drop of 0.5% into each eye 5-10 minutes before examination

Children: Instill 1 drop of 0.5%, 1%, or 2% in eye followed by 1 drop of 0.5% or 1% in 5 minutes, if necessary

Adults: Instill 1 drop of 1% followed by another drop in 5 minutes; 2% solution in heavily pigmented iris

**Dosage Forms** Solution, ophthalmic, as hydrochloride: 0.5% (2 mL, 5 mL, 15 mL); 1% (2 mL, 5 mL, 15 mL); 2% (2 mL, 5 mL, 15 mL)

## cyclopentolate and phenylephrine (sye kloe PEN toe late & fen il EF rin)

**U.S./Canadian Brand Names** Cyclomydril® Ophthalmic

**Therapeutic Category** Anticholinergic/Adrenergic Agonist

**Use** Induce mydriasis greater than that produced with cyclopentolate HCl alone

**Usual Dosage** Ophthalmic: Instill 1 drop every 5-10 minutes, not to exceed 3 instillations

**Dosage Forms** Solution, ophthalmic: Cyclopentolate hydrochloride 0.2% and phenylephrine hydrochloride 1% (2 mL, 5 mL)

## cyclophosphamide (sye kloe FOS fa mide)

**Synonyms** CPM; CTX; CYT

**U.S./Canadian Brand Names** Cytoxan®; Neosar®; Procytox® (Can)

**Therapeutic Category** Antineoplastic Agent

**Use** Management of Hodgkin's disease, malignant lymphomas, multiple myeloma, leukemias, sarcomas, mycosis fungoides, neuroblastoma, ovarian carcinoma, breast carcinoma, a variety of other tumors; nephrotic syndrome, lupus erythematosus, severe rheumatoid arthritis, and rheumatoid vasculitis

**Usual Dosage**

Patients with compromised bone marrow function may require a 33% to 50% reduction in initial loading dose

(Continued)

## cyclophosphamide *(Continued)*

Children:

SLE: I.V.: 500-750 mg/m$^2$ every month; maximum dose: 1 g/m$^2$

JRA/vasculitis: I.V.: 10 mg/kg every 2 weeks

Children and Adults:

Oral: 50-100 mg/m$^2$/day as continuous therapy or 400-1000 mg/m$^2$ in divided doses over 4-5 days as intermittent therapy

I.V.:

Single Doses: 400-1800 mg/m$^2$ (30-50 mg/kg) per treatment course (1-5 days) which can be repeated at 2-4 week intervals

**MAXIMUM SINGLE DOSE WITHOUT BMT is 7 g/m$^2$ (190 mg/kg) SINGLE AGENT THERAPY**

Continuous daily doses: 60-120 mg/m$^2$ (1-2.5 mg/kg) per day

Autologous BMT: IVPB: 50 mg/kg/dose x 4 days or 60 mg/kg/dose for 2 days; total dose is usually divided over 2-4 days

Nephrotic syndrome: Oral: 2-3 mg/kg/day every day for up to 12 weeks when corticosteroids are unsuccessful

**Dosage Forms**

Powder for injection: 100 mg, 200 mg, 500 mg, 1 g, 2 g

Powder for injection, lyophilized: 100 mg, 200 mg, 500 mg, 1 g, 2 g

Tablet: 25 mg, 50 mg

## cycloserine (sye kloe SER een)

**U.S./Canadian Brand Names** Seromycin® Pulvules®

**Therapeutic Category** Antibiotic, Miscellaneous

**Use** Adjunctive treatment in pulmonary or extrapulmonary tuberculosis; treatment of acute urinary tract infections caused by *E. coli* or *Enterobacter* sp. when less toxic conventional therapy has failed or is contraindicated

**Usual Dosage** Oral:

Tuberculosis:

Children: 10-20 mg/kg/day in 2 divided doses up to 1000 mg/day

Adults: Initial: 250 mg every 12 hours for 14 days, then administer 500 mg to 1 g/day in 2 divided doses

Urinary tract infection: Adults: 250 mg every 12 hours for 14 days

**Dosage Forms** Capsule: 250 mg

**Cyclospasmol®** ***(Discontinued)*** *see page 750*

**cyclosporin A** *see* cyclosporine *on this page*

## cyclosporine (SYE kloe spor een)

**Synonyms** CYA; cyclosporin A

**U.S./Canadian Brand Names** Gengraf™; Neoral®; Sandimmune®

**Therapeutic Category** Immunosuppressant Agent

**Use** Immunosuppressant used with corticosteroids to prevent graft vs host disease in patients with kidney, liver, heart, and bone marrow transplants; has been used in the treatment of nephrotic syndrome in patients with documented focal glomerulosclerosis when corticosteroids and cyclophosphamide were unsuccessful; monotherapy or in combination with methotrexate for treatment of severe active rheumatoid arthritis where the disease has not adequately responded to methotrexate

**Usual Dosage** Children and Adults:

Oral: Initial: 14-18 mg/kg/dose daily, beginning 4-12 hours prior to organ transplantation; maintenance: 5-10 mg/kg/day

I.V.: Initial: 5-6 mg/kg/day in divided doses every 12-24 hours; patients should be switched to oral cyclosporine as soon as possible

**Dosage Forms**

Capsule (Gengraf™, Sandimmune®): 25 mg, 100 mg

Capsule, soft gel: 25 mg, 100 mg

Capsule, soft gel (Sandimmune®): 50 mg
Capsule, soft gel for microemulsion (Neoral®): 25 mg, 100 mg
Injection (Sandimmune®): 50 mg/mL (5 mL)
Solution, oral (Sandimmune®): 100 mg/mL (50 mL)
Solution, oral for microemulsion (Neoral®): 100 mg/mL (50 mL)

**Cycofed® Pediatric** *see* guaifenesin, pseudoephedrine, and codeine *on page 284*

**Cycrin® 10 mg Tablet *(Discontinued)*** *see page 750*

**Cyklokapron®** *see* tranexamic acid *on page 599*

**Cylert®** *see* pemoline *on page 454*

**Cylex® [OTC]** *see* benzocaine *on page 72*

**Cyomin®** *see* cyanocobalamin *on page 158*

## cyproheptadine (si proe HEP ta deen)

**U.S./Canadian Brand Names** Periactin®

**Therapeutic Category** Antihistamine

**Use** Perennial and seasonal allergic rhinitis and other allergic symptoms including urticaria

**Usual Dosage** Oral:

Children: 0.25 mg/kg/day in 2-3 divided doses **or**
2-6 years: 2 mg every 8-12 hours (not to exceed 12 mg/day)
7-14 years: 4 mg every 8-12 hours (not to exceed 16 mg/day)
Adults: 12-16 mg/day every 8 hours (not to exceed 0.5 mg/kg/day)

**Dosage Forms**

Syrup, as hydrochloride: 2 mg/5 mL with alcohol 5% (473 mL)
Tablet, as hydrochloride: 4 mg

## cyproterone *(Canada only)* (sye PROE ter one)

**U.S./Canadian Brand Names** Alti-CPA (Can); Androcur® (Can); Androcur® Depot (Can); Gen-Cyproterone (Can); Novo-Cyproterone (Can)

**Therapeutic Category** Antiandrogen; Progestin

**Use** Palliative treatment of patients with advanced prostatic carcinoma

**Usual Dosage** Adults:

I.M.: 300 mg (3 mL) once a week
Oral: 200-300 mg divided into 2-3 doses and taken after meals

**Dosage Forms**

Injection, as acetate: 100 mg/mL (3 mL)
Tablet, as acetate: 50 mg

**Cystadane®** *see* betaine anhydrous *on page 77*

**Cystagon®** *see* cysteamine *on this page*

## cysteamine (sis TEE a meen)

**U.S./Canadian Brand Names** Cystagon®

**Therapeutic Category** Urinary Tract Product

**Use** Nephropathic cystinosis in children and adults

**Usual Dosage** Initiate therapy with $^1/_4$ to $^1/_8$ of maintenance dose; titrate slowly upward over 4-6 weeks

Children <12 years: Oral: Maintenance: 1.3 g/m$^2$/day divided into 4 doses
Children >12 years and Adults (>110 lbs): Oral: 2 g/day in 4 divided doses; dosage may in increased to 1.95 g/m$^2$/day if cystine levels are <1 nmol/$^1/_2$ cystine/mg protein, although intolerance and incidence of adverse events may be increased

**Dosage Forms** Capsule, as bitartrate: 50 mg, 150 mg

## cysteine (SIS teen)

**Therapeutic Category** Nutritional Supplement

**Use** Total parenteral nutrition of infants as an additive to meet the I.V. amino acid requirements

**Usual Dosage** Combine 500 mg of cysteine with 12.5 g of amino acid, then dilute with 50% dextrose

**Dosage Forms** Injection, as hydrochloride: 50 mg/mL (10 mL)

**Cystistat® (Can)** *see* sodium hyaluronate *on page 550*

**Cystografin®** *see* radiological/contrast media (ionic) *on page 516*

**Cystospaz®** *see* hyoscyamine *on page 309*

**Cystospaz-M®** *see* hyoscyamine *on page 309*

**CYT** *see* cyclophosphamide *on page 159*

**Cytadren®** *see* aminoglutethimide *on page 31*

## cytarabine (sye TARE a been)

**Synonyms** arabinosylcytosine; ARA-C; cytosine arabinosine

**U.S./Canadian Brand Names** Cytosar (Can); Cytosar-U®; Tarabine® PFS

**Therapeutic Category** Antineoplastic Agent

**Use** In combination regimens for the treatment of leukemias and non-Hodgkin's lymphomas

**Usual Dosage** Children and Adults (refer to individual protocols):

Induction remission:

I.T.: 5-75 mg/m$^2$ once daily for 4 days or 1 every 4 days until CNS

I.V.: 200 mg/m$^2$/day for 5 days at 2-week intervals; 100-200 mg/m$^2$/day for 5- to 10-day therapy course or every day until remission administered I.V. continuous drip, or in 2-3 divided doses findings normalize

Maintenance remission:

I.M., S.C.: 1-1.5 mg/kg single dose for maintenance at 1- to 4-week intervals

I.V.: 70-200 mg/m$^2$/day for 2-5 days at monthly intervals

High-dose therapies: Doses as high as 1-3 g/m$^2$ have been used for refractory or secondary leukemias or refractory non-Hodgkins lymphoma; dosages of 3 g/m$^2$ every 12 hours for up to 12 doses have been used

**Dosage Forms**

Powder for injection, as hydrochloride: 100 mg, 500 mg, 1 g, 2 g

Powder for injection, as hydrochloride (Cytosar-U®): 100 mg, 500 mg, 1 g, 2 g

## cytarabine (liposomal) (sye TARE a been lip po SOE mal)

**U.S./Canadian Brand Names** DepoCyt™

**Therapeutic Category** Antineoplastic Agent

**Use** Intrathecal treatment of lymphomatous meningitis

**Usual Dosage** Adults:

Induction: 50 mg intrathecally every 14 days for a total of 2 doses (weeks 1 and 3)

Consolidation: 50 mg intrathecally every 14 days for 3 doses (weeks 5, 7, and 9), followed by an additional dose at week 13

Maintenance: 50 mg intrathecally every 28 days for 4 doses (weeks 17, 21, 25, and 29)

If drug-related neurotoxicity develops, the dose should be reduced to 25 mg; if toxicity persists, treatment with liposomal cytarabine should be discontinued

**Note:** Patients should be started on dexamethasone 4 mg twice daily (oral or I.V.) for 5 days, beginning on the day of liposomal cytarabine injection

**Dosage Forms** Injection: 10 mg/mL (5 mL)

**CytoGam®** *see* cytomegalovirus immune globulin (intravenous-human) *on next page*

## cytomegalovirus immune globulin (intravenous-human)

(sye toe meg a low VYE rus i MYUN GLOB yoo lin in tra VEE nus-HYU man)

**Synonyms** CMV-IGIV

**U.S./Canadian Brand Names** CytoGam®

**Therapeutic Category** Immune Globulin

**Use** Attenuation of primary CMV disease associated with kidney transplantation

**Usual Dosage** I.V.: Adults:

Kidney transplant:

Initial dose (within 72 hours of transplant): 150 mg/kg/dose

2-, 4-, 6-, and 8 weeks after transplant: 100 mg/kg/dose

12 and 16 weeks after transplant: 50 mg/kg/dose

Liver, lung, pancreas, or heart transplant:

Initial dose (within 72 hours of transplant): 150 mg/kg/dose

2-, 4-, 6-, and 8 weeks after transplant: 150 mg/kg/dose

12 and 16 weeks after transplant: 100 mg/kg/dose

Severe CMV pneumonia: Various regimens have been used, including 400 mg/kg CMV-IGIV in combination with ganciclovir on days 1, 2, 7, or 8, followed by 200 mg/kg CMV-IGIV

**Dosage Forms** Injection, detergent treated: 50 mg ± 10 mg (20 mL, 50 mL)

**Cytomel® Oral** *see* liothyronine *on page 351*

**Cytosar (Can)** *see* cytarabine *on previous page*

**Cytosar-U®** *see* cytarabine *on previous page*

**cytosine arabinosine** *see* cytarabine *on previous page*

**Cytotec®** *see* misoprostol *on page 395*

**Cytovene®** *see* ganciclovir *on page 269*

**Cytoxan®** *see* cyclophosphamide *on page 159*

**$D_3$** *see* cholecalciferol *on page 134*

**25-$D_3$** *see* calcifediol *on page 95*

**d-3-mercaptovaline** *see* penicillamine *on page 455*

**d4T** *see* stavudine *on page 557*

## dacarbazine (da KAR ba zeen)

**Synonyms** DIC; imidazole carboxamide

**U.S./Canadian Brand Names** DTIC-Dome®

**Therapeutic Category** Antineoplastic Agent

**Use** Singly or in various combination therapy to treat malignant melanoma, Hodgkin's disease, soft-tissue sarcomas (fibrosarcomas, rhabdomyosarcoma), islet cell carcinoma, medullary carcinoma of the thyroid, and neuroblastoma

**Usual Dosage** Refer to individual protocols. I.V.:

Children:

Solid tumors: 200-470 mg/m$^2$/day over 5 days every 21-28 days

Neuroblastoma: 800-900 mg/m$^2$ as a single dose every 3-4 weeks in combination therapy

Adults:

Malignant melanoma: 2-4.5 mg/kg/day for 10 days, repeat in 4 weeks or may use 250 mg/m$^2$/day for 5 days, repeat in 3 weeks

Hodgkin's disease: 150 mg/m$^2$/day for 5 days, repeat every 4 weeks or 375 mg/m$^2$ on day 1, repeat in 15 days of each 28-day cycle in combination with other agents

**Dosage Forms** Injection: 100 mg (10 mL, 20 mL); 200 mg (20 mL, 30 mL); 500 mg (50 mL)

**daclizumab** (da KLIK si mab)

**U.S./Canadian Brand Names** Zenapax®

**Therapeutic Category** Immunosuppressant Agent

**Use** In combination with an immunosuppressive regimen, including cyclosporine and corticosteroids, for prophylaxis of acute organ rejection in patients receiving renal transplants

**Usual Dosage** Children and Adults: IVPB: 1 mg/kg, used as part of an immunosuppressive regimen that includes cyclosporine and corticosteroids for a total of 5 doses; give the first dose ≤24 hours before transplantation. The 4 remaining doses should be administered at intervals of 14 days.

**Dosage Forms** Injection: 5 mg/mL (5 mL)

**Dacodyl® [OTC]** *see* bisacodyl *on page 81*

**dactinomycin** (dak ti noe MYE sin)

**Synonyms** ACT; actinomycin D

**U.S./Canadian Brand Names** Cosmegen®

**Therapeutic Category** Antineoplastic Agent

**Use** Management, either alone or in combination with other treatment modalities of Wilms' tumor, rhabdomyosarcoma, neuroblastoma, retinoblastoma, Ewing's sarcoma, trophoblastic neoplasms, testicular carcinoma, and other malignancies

**Usual Dosage** Refer to individual protocols; dosage should be based on body surface area in obese or edematous patients

Children >6 months and Adults: I.V.: 15 mcg/kg/day or 400-600 mcg/$m^2$/day for 5 days, may repeat every 3-6 weeks; or 2.5 mg/$m^2$ administered in divided doses over 1 week; 0.75-2 mg/$m^2$ as a single dose administered at intervals of 1-4 weeks have been used

**Dosage Forms** Powder for injection, lyophilized: 0.5 mg

**D.A.II® Tablet** *see* chlorpheniramine, phenylephrine, and methscopolamine *on page 131*

**Dairyaid® (Can)** *see* lactase *on page 337*

**Dairy Ease® [OTC]** *see* lactase *on page 337*

**Dakin's solution** *see* sodium hypochlorite solution *on page 550*

**Dakrina® Ophthalmic Solution [OTC]** *see* artificial tears *on page 53*

**Dalacin® C (Can)** *see* clindamycin *on page 142*

**Dalgan® *(Discontinued)*** *see page 750*

**Dallergy®** *see* chlorpheniramine, phenylephrine, and methscopolamine *on page 131*

**Dallergy-D® Syrup** *see* chlorpheniramine and phenylephrine *on page 129*

**Dalmane®** *see* flurazepam *on page 259*

***d*-alpha tocopherol** *see* vitamin E *on page 631*

**dalteparin** (dal TE pa rin)

**U.S./Canadian Brand Names** Fragmin®

**Therapeutic Category** Anticoagulant

**Use** Prevent deep vein thrombosis following abdominal surgery

**Usual Dosage** Adults: S.C.: 2500 units 1-2 hours prior to surgery, then once daily for 5-10 days postoperatively

**Dosage Forms** Injection:

Prefilled syringe: Antifactor Xa 2500 int. units per 0.2 mL; antifactor Xa 5000 int. units per 0.2 mL

Multidose vial: 95,000 int. units (9.5 mL) [10,000 antifactor Xa int. units/mL]

**Damason-P®** *see* hydrocodone and aspirin *on page 300*

**D-Amp® *(Discontinued)*** *see page 750*

## danaparoid (da NAP a roid)

**U.S./Canadian Brand Names** Orgaran®

**Therapeutic Category** Anticoagulant

**Use** Prophylaxis of postoperative deep vein thrombosis (DVT)

**Usual Dosage** Adults: S.C.: 750 anti-Xa units twice daily beginning 1-4 hours preoperatively, and then not sooner than 2 hours hours after surgery

**Dosage Forms** Injection, as sodium: 750 anti-Xa units/0.6 mL

## danazol (DA na zole)

**U.S./Canadian Brand Names** Cyclomen® (Can); Danocrine®

**Therapeutic Category** Androgen

**Use** Treatment of endometriosis, fibrocystic breast disease, and hereditary angioedema

**Usual Dosage** Adults: Oral:

Endometriosis: 200-400 mg twice daily

Fibrocystic breast disease: 100-400 mg twice daily for 3-6 months (may extend to 9 months)

Hereditary angioedema: 400-600 mg/day in 2-3 divided doses

**Dosage Forms** Capsule: 50 mg, 100 mg, 200 mg

**Dandrex® [OTC]** *see* selenium sulfide *on page 540*

**Danex® Shampoo *(Discontinued)*** *see page 750*

**Danocrine®** *see* danazol *on this page*

**Dantrium®** *see* dantrolene *on this page*

## dantrolene (DAN troe leen)

**U.S./Canadian Brand Names** Dantrium®

**Therapeutic Category** Skeletal Muscle Relaxant

**Use** Treatment of spasticity associated with upper motor neuron disorders such as spinal cord injury, stroke, cerebral palsy, or multiple sclerosis; also used as treatment of malignant hyperthermia

**Usual Dosage**

Spasticity: Oral:

Children: Initial: 0.5 mg/kg/dose twice daily, increase frequency to 3-4 times/day at 4- to 7-day intervals, then increase dose by 0.5 mg/kg to a maximum of 3 mg/kg/dose 2-4 times/day up to 400 mg/day

Adults: 25 mg/day to start, increase frequency to 3-4 times/day, then increase dose by 25 mg every 4-7 days to a maximum of 100 mg 2-4 times/day or 400 mg/day

Hyperthermia: Children and Adults:

Oral: 4-8 mg/kg/day in 4 divided doses

I.V.: 1 mg/kg; may repeat dose up to cumulative dose of 10 mg/kg (mean effective dose: 2.5 mg/kg), then switch to oral dosage

**Dosage Forms**

Capsule, as sodium: 25 mg, 50 mg, 100 mg

Powder for injection, as sodium: 20 mg

**Dapacin® Cold Capsule *(Discontinued)*** *see page 750*

## dapiprazole (DA pi pray zole)

**U.S./Canadian Brand Names** Rēv-Eyes™

**Therapeutic Category** Alpha-Adrenergic Blocking Agent

**Use** Treatment of iatrogenically induced mydriasis produced by adrenergic or parasympatholytic agents

**Usual Dosage** Ophthalmic: Instill 2 drops followed 5 minutes later by an additional 2 drops applied to the conjunctiva

(Continued)

## dapiprazole *(Continued)*

**Dosage Forms** Powder, lyophilized, as hydrochloride: 25 mg [0.5% solution when mixed with supplied diluent]

## dapsone (DAP sone)

**Synonyms** DDS; diaminodiphenylsulfone

**U.S./Canadian Brand Names** Avlosulfon® (Can)

**Therapeutic Category** Sulfone

**Use** Treatment of leprosy due to susceptible strains of *M. leprae*; treatment of dermatitis herpetiformis; prophylaxis against *Pneumocystis carinii* in children who cannot tolerate sulfamethoxazole/trimethoprim or aerosolized pentamidine

**Usual Dosage** Oral:

Children: Leprosy: 1-2 mg/kg/24 hours; maximum: 100 mg/day

Adults:

Leprosy: 50-100 mg/day

Dermatitis herpetiformis: Start at 50 mg/day, increase to 300 mg/day, or higher to achieve full control, reduce dosage to minimum level as soon as possible

**Dosage Forms** Tablet: 25 mg, 100 mg

**Daranide®** *see* dichlorphenamide *on page 181*

**Daraprim®** *see* pyrimethamine *on page 511*

**Darbid® Tablet *(Discontinued)*** *see page 750*

**Daricon® *(Discontinued)*** *see page 750*

**Darvocet-N®** *see* propoxyphene and acetaminophen *on page 504*

**Darvocet-N® 100** *see* propoxyphene and acetaminophen *on page 504*

**Darvon®** *see* propoxyphene *on page 503*

**Darvon® 32 mg Capsule *(Discontinued)*** *see page 750*

**Darvon® Compound-65 Pulvules®** *see* propoxyphene and aspirin *on page 504*

**Darvon-N®** *see* propoxyphene *on page 503*

**Darvon-N® Oral Suspension *(Discontinued)*** *see page 750*

**Datril® Extra Strength *(Discontinued)*** *see page 750*

**daunomycin** *see* daunorubicin hydrochloride *on next page*

## daunorubicin citrate (liposomal)

(daw noe ROO bi sin SI trate lip po SOE mal)

**U.S./Canadian Brand Names** DaunoXome®

**Therapeutic Category** Antineoplastic Agent

**Use** Advanced HIV-associated Kaposi's sarcoma

**Usual Dosage** I.V. (refer to individual protocols):

Children:

ALL combination therapy: Remission induction: 25-45 mg/m$^2$ on day 1 every week for 4 cycles **or** 30-45 mg/m$^2$/day for 3 days

In children <2 years or <0.5 m$^2$, daunorubicin should be based on weight (mg/kg): 1 mg/kg per protocol with frequency dependent on regimen employed

Cumulative dose should not exceed 300 mg/m$^2$ in children >2 years or 10 mg/kg in children <2 years

Adults: 30-60 mg/m$^2$/day for 3-5 days, repeat dose in 3-4 weeks

Single agent induction for AML: 60 mg/m$^2$/day for 3 days; repeat every 3-4 weeks

Combination therapy induction for AML: 45 mg/m$^2$/day for 3 days of the first course of induction therapy; subsequent courses: Every day for 2 days

ALL combination therapy: 45 mg/m$^2$/day for 3 days

Cumulative dose should not exceed 400-600 mg/m$^2$

**Dosage Forms** Injection: 2 mg/mL equivalent to 50 mg daunorubicin base

**daunorubicin hydrochloride** (daw noe ROO bi sin hye droe KLOR ide)

**Synonyms** daunomycin; DNR; rubidomycin

**U.S./Canadian Brand Names** Cerubidine®

**Therapeutic Category** Antineoplastic Agent

**Use** In combination with other agents in the treatment of leukemias (ALL, AML)

**Usual Dosage** I.V.:

Children:

Combination therapy: Remission induction for ALL: 25-45 mg/m$^2$ on day 1 every week for 4 cycles

<2 years or <0.5 m$^2$: Manufacturer recommends that the dose is based on body weight rather than body surface area

Adults: 30-60 mg/m$^2$/day for 3-5 days, repeat dose in 3-4 weeks; total cumulative dose should not exceed 400-600 mg/m$^2$

Single agent induction for AML: 60 mg/m$^2$/day for 3 days; repeat every 3-4 weeks

Combination therapy induction for AML: 45 mg/m$^2$/day for 3 days; Subsequent courses: Every day for 2 days

Combination therapy: Remission induction for ALL: 45 mg/m$^2$ on days 1, 2, and 3

**Dosage Forms** Powder for injection, lyophilized: 20 mg

**DaunoXome®** *see* daunorubicin citrate (liposomal) *on previous page*

**Dayhist-1®** *see* clemastine *on page 141*

**Daypro™** *see* oxaprozin *on page 441*

**Day-Time® Multi-Symptom Cold/Flu [OTC]** *see* acetaminophen, dextromethorphan, and pseudoephedrine *on page 7*

**Dayto Himbin®** ***(Discontinued)*** *see page 750*

**DC 240® Softgel® [OTC]** *see* docusate *on page 197*

**D-Care® [OTC]** *see* tolnaftate *on page 595*

**D-Care Circulation Stimulator®** *see* capsaicin *on page 104*

**DCF** *see* pentostatin *on page 460*

**DDAVP®** *see* desmopressin acetate *on page 172*

**ddC** *see* zalcitabine *on page 637*

**ddI** *see* didanosine *on page 183*

**DDS** *see* dapsone *on previous page*

**1-deamino-8-d-arginine vasopressin** *see* desmopressin acetate *on page 172*

**Debrisan® [OTC]** *see* dextranomer *on page 177*

**Debrox® Otic [OTC]** *see* carbamide peroxide *on page 106*

**Decadron® 0.25 mg & 6 mg Tablets** ***(Discontinued)*** *see page 750*

**Decadron® Injection** *see* dexamethasone (systemic) *on page 174*

**Decadron®-LA** *see* dexamethasone (systemic) *on page 174*

**Decadron® Ophthalmic** *see* dexamethasone (ophthalmic) *on page 174*

**Decadron® Oral** *see* dexamethasone (systemic) *on page 174*

**Decadron® Phosphate** *see* dexamethasone (topical) *on page 175*

**Decadron® Phosphate Ophthalmic Ointment** ***(Discontinued)*** *see page 750*

**Deca-Durabolin®** *see* nandrolone *on page 408*

**Decaject®** *see* dexamethasone (systemic) *on page 174*

**Decaject-LA®** *see* dexamethasone (systemic) *on page 174*

**Decaspray®** ***(Discontinued)*** *see page 750*

**Decholin®** ***(Discontinued)*** *see page 750*

**Declomycin®** *see* demeclocycline *on page 169*

**Decofed® Syrup [OTC]** *see* pseudoephedrine *on page 507*

**Decohistine® DH** *see* chlorpheniramine, pseudoephedrine, and codeine *on page 132*

**Decohistine® Expectorant** *see* guaifenesin, pseudoephedrine, and codeine *on page 284*

**Deconamine® SR** *see* chlorpheniramine and pseudoephedrine *on page 130*

**Deconamine® Syrup [OTC]** *see* chlorpheniramine and pseudoephedrine *on page 130*

**Deconamine® Tablet [OTC]** *see* chlorpheniramine and pseudoephedrine *on page 130*

**Decongest (Can)** *see* xylometazoline *on page 636*

**Deconsal® II** *see* guaifenesin and pseudoephedrine *on page 283*

**Deconsal® Sprinkle®** *see* guaifenesin and phenylephrine *on page 283*

**Defen-LA®** *see* guaifenesin and pseudoephedrine *on page 283*

## deferoxamine (de fer OKS a meen)

**U.S./Canadian Brand Names** Desferal® Mesylate

**Therapeutic Category** Antidote

**Use** Acute iron intoxication; chronic iron overload secondary to multiple transfusions; diagnostic test for iron overload

**Investigational use:** Treatment of aluminum accumulation in renal failure

**Usual Dosage**

Children and Adults: Acute iron toxicity: I.V. route is used when severe toxicity is evidenced by systemic symptoms (coma, shock, metabolic acidosis, or severe gastrointestinal bleeding) or potentially severe intoxications (serum iron level >500 mcg/dL). When severe symptoms are not present, the I.M. route may be preferred; however, the use of deferoxamine in situations where the serum iron concentration is <500 mcg/dL or when severe toxicity is not evident is a subject of some clinical debate.

Dose: 15 mg/kg/hour (although rates up to 40-50 mg/kg/hour have been given in patients with massive iron intoxication); maximum recommended dose: 6 g/day (however, doses as high as 16-37 g have been administered)

Children:

Chronic iron overload:

I.V.: 15 mg/kg/hour

S.C.: 20-40 mg/kg/day over 8-12 hours

Aluminum-induced bone disease: 20-40 mg/kg every hemodialysis treatment, frequency dependent on clinical status of the patient

Adults:

Chronic iron overload:

I.M.: 0.5-1 g every day

S.C.: 1-2 g every day over 8-24 hours

**Dosage Forms** Powder for injection, as mesylate: 500 mg, 2 g

**Deficol® [OTC]** *see* bisacodyl *on page 81*

**Degest® 2 Ophthalmic [OTC]** *see* naphazoline *on page 409*

**Dehist®** ***(Discontinued)*** *see page 750*

**Dehydral® (Can)** *see* methenamine *on page 379*

## dehydrocholic acid (dee hye droe KOE lik AS id)

**U.S./Canadian Brand Names** Cholan-HMB®

**Therapeutic Category** Laxative

**Use** Relief of constipation; adjunct to various biliary tract conditions

**Usual Dosage** Children >12 years and Adults: Oral: 250-500 mg 2-3 times/day after meals up to 1.5 g/day

**Dosage Forms** Tablet: 250 mg

**Dek-Quin®** *see* clioquinol and hydrocortisone *on page 143*

**Deladumone®** *see* estradiol and testosterone *on page 226*

**Del-Aqua-5® Gel** *see* benzoyl peroxide *on page 74*

**Del Aqua-10® Gel** *see* benzoyl peroxide *on page 74*

**Delatest® Injection** *see* testosterone *on page 576*

**Delatestryl® Injection** *see* testosterone *on page 576*

## delavirdine (de la VIR deen)

**Synonyms** U-90152S

**U.S./Canadian Brand Names** Rescriptor®

**Therapeutic Category** Antiviral Agent

**Use** Treatment of HIV-1 infection in combination with appropriate antiretrovirals

**Usual Dosage** Adults: Oral: 400 mg 3 times/day

**Dosage Forms** Tablet: 100 mg, 200 mg

**Delcort® Topical** *see* hydrocortisone (topical) *on page 304*

**Delestrogen® (Can)** *see* estradiol *on page 224*

**Delfen® [OTC]** *see* nonoxynol 9 *on page 424*

**Del-Mycin® Topical** *see* erythromycin (ophthalmic/topical) *on page 222*

**Delsym® [OTC]** *see* dextromethorphan *on page 178*

**Delta-Cortef® Oral** *see* prednisolone (systemic) *on page 493*

**deltacortisone** *see* prednisone *on page 493*

**Delta-D®** *see* cholecalciferol *on page 134*

**deltadehydrocortisone** *see* prednisone *on page 493*

**deltahydrocortisone** *see* prednisolone (systemic) *on page 493*

**Deltalin® Capsule *(Discontinued)*** *see page 750*

**Deltasone®** *see* prednisone *on page 493*

**Delta-Tritex® Topical** *see* triamcinolone (topical) *on page 602*

**Del-Vi-A®** *see* vitamin A *on page 629*

**Demadex®** *see* torsemide *on page 597*

**Demazin® Syrup *(Discontinued)*** *see page 750*

## demecarium (dem e KARE ee um)

**U.S./Canadian Brand Names** Humorsol® Ophthalmic

**Therapeutic Category** Cholinesterase Inhibitor

**Use** Management of chronic simple glaucoma, chronic and acute angle-closure glaucoma; counter effects of cycloplegics

**Usual Dosage** Ophthalmic:

Children: Instill 1 drop into eyes twice weekly to a maximum dosage of 1 or 2 drops twice daily for up to 4 months

Adults: Instill 1-2 drops into eyes twice weekly to a maximum dosage of 1 or 2 drops twice daily for up to 4 months

**Dosage Forms** Solution, ophthalmic, as bromide: 0.125% (5 mL); 0.25% (5 mL)

## demeclocycline (dem e kloe SYE kleen)

**Synonyms** demethylchlortetracycline

**U.S./Canadian Brand Names** Declomycin®

**Therapeutic Category** Tetracycline Derivative

**Use** Treatment of susceptible bacterial infections (acne, gonorrhea, pertussis, chronic bronchitis, and urinary tract infections) caused by both gram-negative and gram-positive (Continued)

## demeclocycline *(Continued)*

organisms; treatment of chronic syndrome of inappropriate antidiuretic hormone (SIADH) secretion

**Usual Dosage** Oral:

Children ≥8 years: 8-12 mg/kg/day divided every 6-12 hours

Adults: 150 mg 4 times/day or 300 mg twice daily

Uncomplicated gonorrhea: 600 mg stat, 300 mg every 12 hours for 4 days (3 g total)

SIADH: Initial: 900-1200 mg/day or 13-15 mg/kg/day divided every 6-8 hours, then decrease to 0.6-0.9 g/day

**Dosage Forms**

Capsule, as hydrochloride: 150 mg

Tablet, as hydrochloride: 150 mg, 300 mg

**Demerol®** *see* meperidine *on page 372*

**4-demethoxydaunorubicin** *see* idarubicin *on page 312*

**demethylchlortetracycline** *see* demeclocycline *on previous page*

**Demser®** *see* metyrosine *on page 389*

**Demulen®** *see* ethinyl estradiol and ethynodiol diacetate *on page 232*

**Denavir™** *see* penciclovir *on page 455*

## denileukin diftitox (de ne LU kin DIFT e tox)

**U.S./Canadian Brand Names** Ontak®

**Therapeutic Category** Antineoplastic Agent

**Use** Treatment of patients with persistent or recurrent cutaneous T-cell lymphoma whose malignant cells express the CD25 component of the IL-2 receptor

**Usual Dosage** Adults: I.V.: A treatment cycle consists of 9 or 18 mcg/kg/day for 5 consecutive days administered every 21 days. The optimal duration of therapy has not been determined. Only 2% of patients who failed to demonstrate a response (at least a 25% decrease in tumor burden) prior to the fourth cycle responded to subsequent treatment.

**Dosage Forms** Injection: 150 mcg/mL (2 mL)

**Denorex® [OTC]** *see* coal tar *on page 149*

**deodorized opium tincture** *see* opium tincture *on page 436*

**2′-deoxycoformycin** *see* pentostatin *on page 460*

**Depacon™** *see* valproic acid and derivatives *on page 620*

**Depade®** *see* naltrexone *on page 408*

**Depakene®** *see* valproic acid and derivatives *on page 620*

**Depakote® Delayed Release** *see* valproic acid and derivatives *on page 620*

**Depakote® ER** *see* valproic acid and derivatives *on page 620*

**depAndrogyn®** *see* estradiol and testosterone *on page 226*

**depAndro® Injection** *see* testosterone *on page 576*

**Depen®** *see* penicillamine *on page 455*

**depGynogen® Injection** *see* estradiol *on page 224*

**depMedalone® Injection** *see* methylprednisolone *on page 385*

**DepoCyt™** *see* cytarabine (liposomal) *on page 162*

**Depo®-Estradiol Injection** *see* estradiol *on page 224*

**Depogen® Injection** *see* estradiol *on page 224*

**Depoject® Injection** *see* methylprednisolone *on page 385*

**Depo-Medrol® Injection** *see* methylprednisolone *on page 385*

**Deponit® Patch** *see* nitroglycerin *on page 422*

**Depopred® Injection** *see* methylprednisolone *on page 385*

**Depo-Provera® 100 mg/mL *(Discontinued)*** *see page 750*

**Depo-Provera® Injection** *see* medroxyprogesterone acetate *on page 369*

**Depo-Testadiol®** *see* estradiol and testosterone *on page 226*

**Depotest® Injection** *see* testosterone *on page 576*

**Depotestogen®** *see* estradiol and testosterone *on page 226*

**Depo®-Testosterone Injection** *see* testosterone *on page 576*

**deprenyl** *see* selegiline *on page 540*

**Deproic® (Can)** *see* valproic acid and derivatives *on page 620*

**Deproist® Expectorant With Codeine** *see* guaifenesin, pseudoephedrine, and codeine *on page 284*

**Deprol® *(Discontinued)*** *see page 750*

**Dequadin® (Can)** *see* dequalinium *(Canada only) on this page*

## dequalinium *(Canada only)* (de kwal LI ne um)

**U.S./Canadian Brand Names** Dequadin® (Can)

**Therapeutic Category** Antibacterial, Topical; Antifungal Agent

**Use** Treatment of mouth and throat infections

**Usual Dosage** Adults:

Lozenge: One lozenge sucked slowly every 2-3 hours

Oral paint: Apply freely to infected area, every 2-3 hours, or as directed by physician

**Dosage Forms**

Lozenge, as chloride: 0.25 mg (20s)

Oral paint, as chloride: 0.5% (25 mL)

**Derifil® [OTC]** *see* chlorophyll *on page 127*

**Dermacort® Topical** *see* hydrocortisone (topical) *on page 304*

**Dermarest Dricort® Topical** *see* hydrocortisone (topical) *on page 304*

**Derma-Smoothe/FS® Topical** *see* fluocinolone *on page 253*

**Dermatop®** *see* prednicarbate *on page 492*

**Dermatophytin®** *see Trichophyton* skin test *on page 604*

**Dermatophytin-O** *see Candida albicans* (*Monilia*) *on page 103*

**Dermazin™ (Can)** *see* silver sulfadiazine *on page 544*

**Dermolate® Topical [OTC]** *see* hydrocortisone (topical) *on page 304*

**Dermoplast® [OTC]** *see* benzocaine *on page 72*

**Dermovate® (Can)** *see* clobetasol *on page 143*

**Dermoxyl® Gel *(Discontinued)*** *see page 750*

**Dermtex® HC with Aloe Topical [OTC]** *see* hydrocortisone (topical) *on page 304*

**DES** *see* diethylstilbestrol *on page 184*

**Desenex® Foot & Sneaker [OTC]** *see* undecylenic acid and derivatives *on page 616*

**Desferal® Mesylate** *see* deferoxamine *on page 168*

## desflurane (des FLOO rane)

**U.S./Canadian Brand Names** Suprane®

**Therapeutic Category** General Anesthetic

**Use** Induction or maintenance of anesthesia for adults in outpatient and inpatient surgery

(Continued)

## desflurane *(Continued)*

**Usual Dosage**

Children: Maintenance: Surgical levels of anesthesia may be maintained with concentrations of 5.2% to 10% desflurane, with or without nitrous oxide

Adults: Titrate dose based on individual response

Induction: Frequent starting concentration 3%; increased in 0.5% to 1% increments every 2-3 breaths; end tidal concentrations of 4% to 11% desflurane with and without nitrous oxide produce anesthesia within 2-4 minutes

Maintenance: Surgical levels of anesthesia in adults may be maintained with concentrations of 2.5% to 8.5% desflurane, with or without nitrous oxide

**Note:** Because of the higher vapor pressure and higher MAC of desflurane, special vaporizer canisters must be used. Equipment is **not** interchangeable with that for isoflurane.

**Dosage Forms** Liquid: 240 mL

**desiccated thyroid** *see* thyroid *on page 588*

## desipramine (des IP ra meen)

**Synonyms** desmethylimipramine

**U.S./Canadian Brand Names** Alti-Desipramine (Can); Apo®-Desipramine (Can); Norpramin®; Novo-Desipramine (Can); Nu-Desipramine (Can); PMS-Desipramine (Can)

**Therapeutic Category** Antidepressant, Tricyclic (Secondary Amine)

**Use** Treatment of various forms of depression, often in conjunction with psychotherapy; analgesic in chronic pain, peripheral neuropathies

**Usual Dosage** Oral (not recommended for use in children <12 years):

Adolescents: Initial: 25-50 mg/day; gradually increase to 100 mg/day in single or divided doses; maximum: 150 mg/day

Adults: Initial: 75 mg/day in divided doses; increase gradually to 150-200 mg/day in divided or single dose; maximum: 300 mg/day

**Dosage Forms** Tablet, as hydrochloride: 10 mg, 25 mg, 50 mg, 75 mg, 100 mg, 150 mg

**Desitin® [OTC]** *see* zinc oxide, cod liver oil, and talc *on page 639*

**desmethylimipramine** *see* desipramine *on this page*

## desmopressin acetate (des moe PRES in AS e tate)

**Synonyms** 1-deamino-8-d-arginine vasopressin

**U.S./Canadian Brand Names** DDAVP®; Stimate™

**Therapeutic Category** Vasopressin Analog, Synthetic

**Use** Treatment of diabetes insipidus and controlling bleeding in certain types of hemophilia

**Usual Dosage**

Children:

Diabetes insipidus: 3 months to 12 years: Intranasal: Initial: 5 mcg/day divided 1-2 times/day; range: 5-30 mcg/day divided 1-2 times/day

Hemophilia: >3 months: I.V.: 0.3 mcg/kg by slow infusion; may repeat dose if needed

Nocturnal enuresis: ≥6 years: Intranasal: Initial: 20 mcg at bedtime; range: 10-40 mcg

Adults:

Diabetes insipidus: I.V., S.C.: 2-4 mcg/day in 2 divided doses or $^1/_{10}$ of the maintenance intranasal dose; intranasal: 5-40 mcg/day 1-3 times/day

Hemophilia: I.V.: 0.3 mcg/kg by slow infusion

**Dosage Forms**

Injection (DDAVP®): 4 mcg/mL (1 mL)

Solution, nasal:

DDAVP®: 100 mcg/mL (2.5 mL, 5 mL)

Stimate™: 1.5 mg/mL (2.5 mL)

Tablet (DDAVP®): 0.1 mg, 0.2 mg

**Desocort® (Can)** *see* desonide *on this page*

**Desogen®** *see* ethinyl estradiol and desogestrel *on page 230*

## desonide (DES oh nide)

**U.S./Canadian Brand Names** Desocort® (Can); DesOwen® Topical; Tridesilon® Topical

**Therapeutic Category** Corticosteroid, Topical

**Use** Adjunctive therapy for inflammation in acute and chronic corticosteroid responsive dermatosis

**Usual Dosage** Topical: Apply 2-4 times/day. Therapy should be discontinued when control is achieved. If no improvement is seen, reassessment of diagnosis may be necessary.

**Dosage Forms**

Cream, topical: 0.05% (15 g, 60 g)
Lotion: 0.05% (60 mL, 120 mL)
Ointment, topical: 0.05% (15 g, 60 g)

**DesOwen® Topical** *see* desonide *on this page*

## desoximetasone (des oks i MET a sone)

**U.S./Canadian Brand Names** Taro-Desoximetasone (Can); Topicort®; Topicort®-LP

**Therapeutic Category** Corticosteroid, Topical

**Use** Relief of inflammation and pruritic symptoms of corticosteroid-responsive dermatosis

**Usual Dosage** Topical:

Children: Apply sparingly in a very thin film to affected area 1-2 times/day
Adults: Apply sparingly in a thin film twice daily

**Note:** Therapy should be discontinued when control is achieved. If no improvement is seen, reassessment of diagnosis may be necessary.

**Dosage Forms**

Cream, topical:
Topicort®: 0.25% (15 g, 60 g, 120 g)
Topicort®-LP: 0.05% (15 g, 60 g)
Gel, topical: 0.05% (15 g, 60 g)
Ointment, topical (Topicort®): 0.25% (15 g, 60 g)

**desoxyephedrine** *see* methamphetamine *on page 378*

**Desoxyn®** *see* methamphetamine *on page 378*

**desoxyphenobarbital** *see* primidone *on page 495*

**Despec® Liquid *(Discontinued)*** *see page 750*

**Desquam-E™ Gel** *see* benzoyl peroxide *on page 74*

**Desquam-X® Gel** *see* benzoyl peroxide *on page 74*

**Desquam-X® Wash** *see* benzoyl peroxide *on page 74*

**Desyrel®** *see* trazodone *on page 600*

**Detrol™** *see* tolterodine *on page 595*

**Detrol® LA** *see* tolterodine *on page 595*

**Detussin® Expectorant** *see* hydrocodone, pseudoephedrine, and guaifenesin *on page 302*

**Detussin® Liquid** *see* hydrocodone and pseudoephedrine *on page 301*

**Devrom® [OTC]** *see* bismuth subgallate *on page 81*

**Dexacen-4® *(Discontinued)*** *see page 750*

**Dexacen® LA-8 *(Discontinued)*** *see page 750*

**Dexacidin®** *see* neomycin, polymyxin B, and dexamethasone *on page 414*

**Dexacort® Phosphate in Respihaler®** *see* dexamethasone (oral inhalation) *on this page*

**Dexacort® Phosphate Turbinaire®** *see* dexamethasone (nasal) *on this page*

**DexAlone® [OTC]** *see* dextromethorphan *on page 178*

## dexamethasone (nasal) (deks a METH a sone NAY sal)

**U.S./Canadian Brand Names** Dexacort® Phosphate Turbinaire®

**Therapeutic Category** Adrenal Corticosteroid

**Use** Chronic inflammation and/or allergic conditions

**Dosage Forms** Dexamethasone sodium phosphate: Aerosol, nasal 84 mcg/activation [170 metered doses] (12.6 g)

## dexamethasone (ophthalmic) (deks a METH a sone op THAL mik)

**U.S./Canadian Brand Names** AK-Dex® Ophthalmic; Baldex®; Decadron® Ophthalmic; Maxidex®

**Therapeutic Category** Adrenal Corticosteroid

**Use** Inflammatory or allergic conjunctivitis

**Usual Dosage** Ophthalmic: Instill 3-4 times/day

**Dosage Forms** Dexamethasone base:

Solution, ophthalmic: 0.1% (5 mL)

Suspension, ophthalmic: 0.1% (5 mL, 15 mL)

## dexamethasone (oral inhalation)

(deks a METH a sone OR al in hil LA shun)

**U.S./Canadian Brand Names** Dexacort® Phosphate in Respihaler®

**Therapeutic Category** Adrenal Corticosteroid

**Use** Chronic inflammation or allergic conditions

**Dosage Forms** Aerosol, oral: 84 mcg/activation [170 metered doses] (12.6 g)

## dexamethasone (systemic) (deks a METH a sone sis TEM ik)

**U.S./Canadian Brand Names** Decadron® Injection; Decadron®-LA; Decadron® Oral; Decaject®; Decaject-LA®; Dexasone®; Dexasone® L.A.; Dexone®; Dexone® LA; Hexadrol®; PMS-Dexamethasone (Can); Solurex L.A.®

**Therapeutic Category** Adrenal Corticosteroid

**Use** Systemically for chronic inflammation, allergic, hematologic, neoplastic, and autoimmune diseases; may be used in management of cerebral edema, septic shock, and as a diagnostic agent

**Usual Dosage**

Children:

Antiemetic (prior to chemotherapy): 10 mg/m$^2$/dose for first dose then 5 mg/m$^2$/dose every 6 hours as needed

Physiologic replacement: Oral, I.M., I.V.: 0.03-0.15 mg/kg/day or 0.6-0.75 mg/m$^2$/day in divided doses every 6-12 hours

Extubation or airway edema: Oral, I.M., I.V.: 0.5-1 mg/kg/day in divided doses every 6 hours beginning 24 hours prior to extubation and continuing for 4-6 doses afterwards

Anti-inflammatory: Oral, I.M., I.V.: 0.75-9 mg/day in divided doses every 6-12 hours

Cerebral edema: I.V. 10 mg stat, 4 mg I.M./I.V. every 6 hours until response is maximized, then switch to oral regimen, then taper off if appropriate

Diagnosis for Cushing's syndrome: Oral: 1 mg at 11 PM, draw blood at 8 AM

ANLL protocol: I.V.: 2 mg/m$^2$/dose every 8 hours for 12 doses

**Dosage Forms**

Dexamethasone acetate:

Injection:

Dalalone L.A.®, Decadron®-LA, Decaject-LA®, Dexasone® L.A., Dexone® LA, Solurex L.A.®: 8 mg/mL (1 mL, 5 mL)

Dalalone D.P.®: 16 mg/mL (1 mL, 5 mL)

Dexamethasone base:
Elixir (Decadron®, Hexadrol®): 0.5 mg/5 mL (5 mL, 20 mL, 100 mL, 120 mL, 240 mL, 500 mL)
Injection:
Dalalone®, Decadron® Phosphate, Decaject®, Dexasone®, Hexadrol® Phosphate, Solurex®: 4 mg/mL (1 mL, 2 mL, 2.5 mL, 5 mL, 10 mL, 30 mL)
Decadron® Phosphate: 24 mg/mL (5 mL, 10 mL)
Hexadrol® Phosphate: 10 mg/mL (1 mL, 10 mL); 20 mg/mL (5 mL)
Solution, oral: 0.5 mg/5 mL (5 mL, 20 mL, 500 mL)
Solution, oral concentrate: 0.5 mg/0.5 mL (30 mL)
Tablet (Decadron®, Dexone®, Hexadrol®): 0.25 mg, 0.5 mg, 0.75 mg, 1 mg, 1.5 mg, 2 mg, 4 mg, 6 mg
Therapeutic pack: Six 1.5 mg tablets and eight 0.75 mg tablets

## dexamethasone (topical) (deks a METH a sone TOP i kal)

**U.S./Canadian Brand Names** Aeroseb-Dex®; Decadron® Phosphate

**Therapeutic Category** Adrenal Corticosteroid

**Use** For chronic inflammation and/or allergic conditions

**Usual Dosage** Topical: Apply 2-4 times daily. Therapy should be discontinued when control is achieved. If no improvement is seen, reassessment of diagnosis may be necessary.

**Dosage Forms** Dexamethasone base:
Aerosol, topical: 0.01% (58 g)
Cream: 0.1% (15 g, 30 g)

**Dexasone®** *see* dexamethasone (systemic) *on previous page*

**Dexasone® L.A.** *see* dexamethasone (systemic) *on previous page*

**Dexasporin®** *see* neomycin, polymyxin B, and dexamethasone *on page 414*

**Dexatrim® Pre-Meal *(Discontinued)*** *see page 750*

## dexbrompheniramine and pseudoephedrine

(deks brom fen EER a meen & soo doe e FED rin)

**U.S./Canadian Brand Names** Disobrom® [OTC]; Disophrol® Chronotabs® [OTC]; Disophrol® Tablet [OTC]; Drixomed®; Drixoral® [OTC]

**Therapeutic Category** Antihistamine/Decongestant Combination

**Use** Relief of symptoms of upper respiratory mucosal congestion in seasonal and perennial nasal allergies, acute rhinitis, rhinosinusitis and eustachian tube blockage

**Usual Dosage** Children >12 years and Adults: Oral: 1 tablet every 12 hours, may require 1 tablet every 8 hours

**Dosage Forms**
Tablet (Disophrol®): Dexbrompheniramine maleate 2 mg and pseudoephedrine sulfate 60 mg
Timed release (Disobrom®, Disophrol® Chrontabs®, Drixomed®, Drixoral®, Histrodrix®, Resporal®): Dexbrompheniramine maleate 6 mg and pseudoephedrine sulfate 120 mg

**Dexchlor® *(Discontinued)*** *see page 750*

## dexchlorpheniramine (deks klor fen EER a meen)

**U.S./Canadian Brand Names** Polaramine®

**Therapeutic Category** Antihistamine

**Use** Perennial and seasonal allergic rhinitis and other allergic symptoms including urticaria

**Usual Dosage** Oral:
Children:
2-5 years: 0.5 mg every 4-6 hours
6-11 years: 1 mg every 4-6 hours or 4 mg timed release at bedtime
Adults: 2 mg every 4-6 hours or 4-6 mg timed release at bedtime or 8-10 hours

(Continued)

## dexchlorpheniramine *(Continued)*

**Dosage Forms** Dexchlorpheniramine maleate:
Syrup (orange flavor): 2 mg/5 mL with alcohol 6% (480 mL)
Tablet: 2 mg
Tablet, sustained action: 4 mg, 6 mg

**Dexedrine® Elixir *(Discontinued)*** *see page 750*

**Dexedrine® Spansule®** *see* dextroamphetamine *on next page*

**Dexedrine® Tablet** *see* dextroamphetamine *on next page*

**Dexferrum®** *see* iron dextran complex *on page 326*

**Dexiron™ (Can)** *see* iron dextran complex *on page 326*

## dexmedetomidine (deks MED e toe mi deen)

**U.S./Canadian Brand Names** Precedex™

**Therapeutic Category** Alpha-Adrenergic Blockers - Central-Acting (Alpha$_2$-Agonists); Sedative

**Use** Sedation of initially intubated and mechanically ventilated patients during treatment in an intensive care setting; duration of infusion should not exceed 24 hours.

**Usual Dosage** Adults: I.V.: Solution must be diluted prior to administration. Initial: Loading infusion 1 mcg/kg over 10 minutes, followed by a maintenance infusion of 0.2-0.7 mcg/kg/hour. Maintenance: Dosing should be individualized and titrated to the desired level of sedation. Not indicated for infusions lasting longer than 24 hours.

**Dosage Forms** Injection: 100 mcg/mL (2 mL vial, 2 mL ampul)

**Dexone®** *see* dexamethasone (systemic) *on page 174*

**Dexone® LA** *see* dexamethasone (systemic) *on page 174*

## dexpanthenol (deks PAN the nole)

**Synonyms** pantothenyl alcohol

**U.S./Canadian Brand Names** D-Pan®; Panthoderm® Cream [OTC]

**Therapeutic Category** Gastrointestinal Agent, Stimulant

**Use** Prophylactic use to minimize paralytic ileus, treatment of postoperative distention

**Usual Dosage**
Children and Adults: Relief of itching and aid in skin healing: Topical: Apply to affected area 1-2 times/day
Adults:
Relief of gas retention: Oral: 2-3 tablets 3 times/day
Prevention of postoperative ileus: I.M.: 250-500 mg stat, repeat in 2 hours, followed by doses every 6 hours until danger passes
Paralyzed ileus: I.M.: 500 mg stat, repeat in 2 hours, followed by doses every 6 hours, if needed

**Dosage Forms**
Cream: 2% (30 g, 60 g)
Injection: 250 mg/mL (2 mL, 10 mL, 30 mL)
Tablet: 50 mg with choline bitartrate 25 mg

## dexrazoxane (deks ray ZOKS ane)

**Synonyms** ICRF-187

**U.S./Canadian Brand Names** Zinecard®

**Therapeutic Category** Cardiovascular Agent, Other

**Use** Prevention of cardiomyopathy associated with doxorubicin administration

**Usual Dosage** I.V.: 1000 mg/m$^2$ 30 minutes before administration of doxorubicin; maximal doses in patients with and without prior treatment with nitrosoureas, respectively = 750 mg/m$^2$ and 120 mg/m$^2$; 3500 mg/m$^2$/day for 3 days has been maximally used in pediatric patients. The recommended dosage ratio of dexrazoxane:doxorubicin is 10:1.

**Dosage Forms** Powder for injection, lyophilized: 250 mg, 500 mg (10 mg/mL when reconstituted)

## dextran (DEKS tran)

**Synonyms** dextran, high molecular weight; dextran, low molecular weight

**U.S./Canadian Brand Names** Gentran®; LMD®; Macrodex®; Rheomacrodex®

**Therapeutic Category** Plasma Volume Expander

**Use** Fluid replacement and blood volume expander used in the treatment of hypovolemia, shock, or near shock states

**Usual Dosage** I.V.:

Children: Total dose should not be >20 mL/kg during first 24 hours

Adults: 500-1000 mL at rate of 20-40 mL/minute

**Dosage Forms** Injection:

High molecular weight:

6% dextran 75 in dextrose 5% (500 mL)

Gentran®: 6% dextran 75 in sodium chloride 0.9% (500 mL)

Gentran®, Macrodex®: 6% dextran 70 in sodium chloride 0.9% (500 mL)

Macrodex®: 6% dextran 70 in dextrose 5% (500 mL)

Low molecular weight: Gentran®, LMD®, Rheomacrodex®:

10% dextran 40 in dextrose 5% (500 mL)

10% dextran 40 in sodium chloride 0.9% (500 mL)

## dextran 1 (DEKS tran won)

**U.S./Canadian Brand Names** Promit®

**Therapeutic Category** Plasma Volume Expander

**Use** Prophylaxis of serious anaphylactic reactions to I.V. infusion of dextran

**Usual Dosage** I.V. (time between dextran 1 and dextran solution should not exceed 15 minutes):

Children: 0.3 mL/kg 1-2 minutes before I.V. infusion of dextran

Adults: 20 mL 1-2 minutes before I.V. infusion of dextran

**Dosage Forms** Injection: 150 mg/mL (20 mL)

**dextran, high molecular weight** *see* dextran *on this page*

**dextran, low molecular weight** *see* dextran *on this page*

## dextranomer (deks TRAN oh mer)

**U.S./Canadian Brand Names** Debrisan® [OTC]

**Therapeutic Category** Topical Skin Product

**Use** Clean exudative wounds; no controlled studies have found dextranomer to be more effective than conventional therapy

**Usual Dosage** Topical: Apply to affected area once or twice daily

**Dosage Forms**

Beads: 4 g, 25 g, 60 g, 120 g

Paste: 10 g foil packets

## dextroamphetamine (deks troe am FET a meen)

**U.S./Canadian Brand Names** Dexedrine® Spansule®; Dexedrine® Tablet; Dextrostat®

**Therapeutic Category** Amphetamine

**Controlled Substance** C-II

**Use** Adjunct in treatment of attention-deficit/hyperactivity disorder (ADHD) in children, narcolepsy, exogenous obesity

**Usual Dosage** Oral:

Children:

Narcolepsy: 6-12 years: Initial: 5 mg/day, may increase at 5 mg increments in weekly intervals until side effects appear; maximum dose: 60 mg/day

(Continued)

## dextroamphetamine *(Continued)*

Attention deficit disorder:

3-5 years: Initial: 2.5 mg/day administered every morning; increase by 2.5 mg/day in weekly intervals until optimal response is obtained, usual range is 0.1-0.5 mg/kg/dose every morning with maximum of 40 mg/day

≥6 years: 5 mg once or twice daily; increase in increments of 5 mg/day at weekly intervals until optimal response is reached, usual range is 0.1-0.5 mg/kg/dose every morning (5-20 mg/day) with maximum of 40 mg/day

Adults:

Narcolepsy: Initial: 10 mg/day, may increase at 10 mg increments in weekly intervals until side effects appear; maximum: 60 mg/day

Exogenous obesity: 5-30 mg/day in divided doses of 5-10 mg 30-60 minutes before meals

**Dosage Forms**

Capsule, as sulfate, sustained release: 5 mg, 10 mg, 15 mg

Tablet, as sulfate: 5 mg, 10 mg (5 mg tablets contain tartrazine)

**dextroamphetamine sulfate, dextroamphetamine saccharate, amphetamine aspartate, and amphetamine sulfate** *see* amphetamine mixture *on page 36*

## dextromethorphan (deks troe meth OR fan)

**U.S./Canadian Brand Names** Benylin DM® [OTC]; Benylin® Pediatric [OTC]; Children's Hold® [OTC]; Creo-Terpin® [OTC]; Delsym® [OTC]; DexAlone® [OTC]; Drixoral® Cough Liquid Caps [OTC]; Hold® DM [OTC]; Pertussin® CS [OTC]; Pertussin® ES [OTC]; Robitussin® Cough Calmers [OTC]; Robitussin® Pediatric [OTC]; Scot-Tussin DM® Cough Chasers [OTC]; Silphen DM® [OTC]; St. Joseph® Cough Suppressant [OTC]; Sucrets® Cough Calmers [OTC]; Suppress® [OTC]; Trocal® [OTC]; Vicks Formula 44® [OTC]; Vicks Formula 44® Pediatric Formula [OTC]

**Therapeutic Category** Antitussive

**Use** Symptomatic relief of coughs caused by minor viral upper respiratory tract infections or inhaled irritants; most effective for a chronic nonproductive cough

**Usual Dosage** Oral:

Children:

2-5 years: 2.5-5 mg every 4 hours or 7.5 mg every 6-8 hours; extended release is 50 mg twice daily

6-11 years: 5-10 mg every 4 hours or 15 mg every 6-8 hours; extended release is 30 mg twice daily

Adults: 10-20 mg every 4 hours or 30 mg every 6-8 hours; extended release is 60 mg twice daily

**Dosage Forms**

Capsule (Drixoral® Cough Liquid Caps): 30 mg

Gelcaps (DexAlone®): 30 mg

Liquid:

Creo-Terpin®: 10 mg/15 mL (120 mL)

Pertussin® CS: 3.5 mg/5 mL (120 mL)

Pertussin® ES, Vicks® Formula 44®: 15 mg/5 mL (120 mL, 240 mL)

Robitussin® Pediatric, St. Joseph® Cough Suppressant: 7.5 mg/5 mL (60 mL, 120 mL, 240 mL)

Liquid, sustained release, as polistirex (Delsym®): 30 mg/5 mL (89 mL)

Lozenges:

Children's Hold®, Hold® DM, Robitussin® Cough Calmers, Sucrets® Cough Calmers: 5 mg

Scot-Tussin DM® Cough Chasers: 2.5 mg

Suppress®, Trocal®: 7.5 mg

Syrup:

Benylin® Pediatric: 7.5 mg/mL (118 mL)

Benylin DM®, Silphen DM®: 10 mg/5 mL (120 mL, 3780 mL)

Vicks® Formula 44® Pediatric Formula: 15 mg/15 mL (120 mL)

**dextropropoxyphene** *see* propoxyphene *on page 503*

**Dextrostat®** *see* dextroamphetamine *on page 177*

**Dey-Dose® Isoproterenol *(Discontinued)*** *see page 750*

**Dey-Dose® Metaproterenol *(Discontinued)*** *see page 750*

**Dey-Lute® Isoetharine *(Discontinued)*** *see page 750*

**DFMO** *see* eflornithine *on page 211*

**DHAD** *see* mitoxantrone *on page 396*

**DHC Plus®** *see* dihydrocodeine compound *on page 186*

**D.H.E. 45® Injection** *see* dihydroergotamine *on page 186*

**DHPG sodium** *see* ganciclovir *on page 269*

**DHS® Tar [OTC]** *see* coal tar *on page 149*

**DHS Zinc® [OTC]** *see* pyrithione zinc *on page 512*

**DHT™** *see* dihydrotachysterol *on page 187*

**Diaβeta®** *see* glyburide *on page 276*

**Diabetic Tussin DM® [OTC]** *see* guaifenesin and dextromethorphan *on page 282*

**Diabetic Tussin® EX [OTC]** *see* guaifenesin *on page 281*

**Diabinese®** *see* chlorpropamide *on page 133*

**Dialose® Capsule *(Discontinued)*** *see page 750*

**Dialose® Plus Capsule [OTC]** *see* docusate and casanthranol *on page 198*

**Dialose® Tablet [OTC]** *see* docusate *on page 197*

**Dialume® [OTC]** *see* aluminum hydroxide *on page 26*

**Diamicron® (Can)** *see* gliclazide *(Canada only) on page 274*

**Diamine T.D.® [OTC]** *see* brompheniramine *on page 87*

**diaminodiphenylsulfone** *see* dapsone *on page 166*

**Diamode® [OTC]** *see* loperamide *on page 354*

**Diamox®** *see* acetazolamide *on page 8*

**Diamox Sequels®** *see* acetazolamide *on page 8*

**Diaparene® [OTC]** *see* methylbenzethonium chloride *on page 383*

**Diaparene® Cradol® *(Discontinued)*** *see page 750*

**Diapid® Nasal Spray *(Discontinued)*** *see page 750*

**Diar-aid® *(Discontinued)*** *see page 750*

**Diarr-Eze (Can)** *see* loperamide *on page 354*

**Diarrid® [OTC]** *see* loperamide *on page 354*

**Diasorb® [OTC]** *see* attapulgite *on page 60*

**Diastat® Rectal Delivery System** *see* diazepam *on this page*

**Diazemuls® Injection** *see* diazepam *on this page*

## diazepam (dye AZ e pam)

**U.S./Canadian Brand Names** Apo®-Diazepam (Can); Diastat® Rectal Delivery System; Diazemuls® Injection; Diazepam Intensol®; Dizac® Injectable Emulsion; Valium® Injection; Valium® Oral; Vivol® (Can)

**Therapeutic Category** Benzodiazepine

**Controlled Substance** C-IV

(Continued)

## diazepam *(Continued)*

**Use** Management of general anxiety disorders, panic disorders; to provide preoperative sedation, light anesthesia, and amnesia; treatment of status epilepticus, alcohol withdrawal symptoms; used as a skeletal muscle relaxant

**Usual Dosage**

Children:

Sedation or muscle relaxation or anxiety:

Oral: 0.12-0.8 mg/kg/day in divided doses every 6-8 hours

I.M., I.V.: 0.04-0.3 mg/kg/dose every 2-4 hours to a maximum of 0.6 mg/kg within an 8-hour period if needed

Status epilepticus: I.V.:

Infants 30 days to 5 years: 0.05-0.3 mg/kg/dose administered over 2-3 minutes, every 15-30 minutes to a maximum total dose of 5 mg; repeat in 2-4 hours as needed or 0.2-0.5 mg/dose every 2-5 minutes to a maximum total dose of 5 mg

>5 years: 0.05-0.3 mg/kg/dose administered over 2-3 minutes, every 15-30 minutes to a maximum total dose of 10 mg; repeat in 2-4 hours as needed or 1 mg/dose every 2-5 minutes to a maximum of 10 mg;

Adults:

Anxiety:

Oral: 2-10 mg 2-4 times/day

I.M., I.V.: 2-10 mg, may repeat in 3-4 hours if needed

Skeletal muscle relaxation:

Oral: 2-10 mg 2-4 times/day

I.M., I.V.: 5-10 mg, may repeat in 2-4 hours

Status epilepticus: I.V.: 0.2-0.5 mg/kg/dose every 15-30 minutes for 2-3 doses; maximum dose: 30 mg

**Dosage Forms**

Gel, rectal:

Adult: 10 mg, 15 mg, 20 mg

Pediatric: 2.5 mg, 5 mg, 10 mg

Injection: 5 mg/mL (1 mL, 2 mL, 5 mL, 10 mL)

Injection, emulsified (Dizac®): 5 mg/mL (3 mL)

Solution, oral (wintergreen-spice flavor): 5 mg/5 mL (5 mL, 10 mL, 500 mL)

Solution, oral concentrate: 5 mg/mL (30 mL)

Tablet: 2 mg, 5 mg, 10 mg

**Diazepam Intensol®** *see* diazepam *on previous page*

## diazoxide (dye az OKS ide)

**U.S./Canadian Brand Names** Hyperstat® I.V.; Proglycem® Oral

**Therapeutic Category** Antihypertensive Agent; Antihypoglycemic Agent

**Use** I.V.: Emergency lowering of blood pressure; Oral: Hypoglycemia related to hyperinsulinism secondary to islet cell adenoma, carcinoma, or hyperplasia; adenomatosis; nesidioblastosis (persistent hyperinsulinemic hypoglycemia of infancy); leucine sensitivity, or extrapancreatic malignancy

**Usual Dosage**

Hyperinsulinemic hypoglycemia: Oral:

Newborns and Infants: 8-15 mg/kg/day in divided doses every 8-12 hours

Children and Adults: 3-8 mg/kg/day in divided doses every 8-12 hours

Hypertension: Children and Adults: I.V.: 1-3 mg/kg (maximum: 150 mg in a single injection); repeat dose in 5-15 minutes until blood pressure adequately reduced; repeat administration every 4-24 hours; monitor blood pressure closely

**Dosage Forms**

Capsule (Proglycem®): 50 mg

Injection (Hyperstat®): 15 mg/mL (1 mL, 20 mL)

Suspension, oral (chocolate-mint flavor) (Proglycem®): 50 mg/mL (30 mL)

**Dibent® Injection** *see* dicyclomine *on page 183*

**Dibenzyline®** *see* phenoxybenzamine *on page 466*

## dibucaine (DYE byoo kane)

**U.S./Canadian Brand Names** Nupercainal® [OTC]

**Therapeutic Category** Local Anesthetic

**Use** Fast, temporary relief of pain and itching due to hemorrhoids, minor burns, other minor skin conditions

**Usual Dosage** Children and Adults:

Rectal: Hemorrhoids: Insert ointment into rectum using a rectal applicator; administer each morning,evening, and after each bowel movement

Topical: Apply gently to the affected areas; no more than 30 g for adults or 7.5 g for children should be used in any 24-hour period

**Dosage Forms**

Cream: 0.5% (45 g)

Ointment, topical: 1% (30 g, 60 g)

## dibucaine and hydrocortisone (DYE byoo kane & hye droe KOR ti sone)

**U.S./Canadian Brand Names** Corticaine® Topical

**Therapeutic Category** Anesthetic/Corticosteroid

**Use** Relief of the inflammatory and pruritic manifestations of corticosteroid-responsive dermatoses and for external anal itching

**Usual Dosage** Topical: Apply to affected areas 2-4 times/day

**Dosage Forms** Cream: Dibucaine 5% and hydrocortisone 5%

**DIC** *see* dacarbazine *on page 163*

**dicalcium phosphate** *see* calcium phosphate (dibasic) *on page 100*

**Dicarbosil® [OTC]** *see* calcium carbonate *on page 97*

**Dicetel® (Can)** *see* pinaverium *(Canada only) on page 472*

## dichlorodifluoromethane and trichloromonofluoromethane

(dye klor oh dye flor oh METH ane & tri klor oh mon oh flor oh METH ane)

**U.S./Canadian Brand Names** Fluori-Methane® Topical Spray

**Therapeutic Category** Analgesic, Topical

**Use** Management of myofascial pain, restricted motion, muscle pain; control of pain associated with injections

**Usual Dosage** Topical: Apply to area from approximately 12" away

**Dosage Forms** Spray, topical: Dichlorodifluoromethane 15% and trichloromonofluoromethane 85%

## dichlorphenamide (dye klor FEN a mide)

**Synonyms** diclofenamide

**U.S./Canadian Brand Names** Daranide®

**Therapeutic Category** Carbonic Anhydrase Inhibitor

**Use** Adjunct in treatment of open-angle glaucoma and perioperative treatment for angle-closure glaucoma

**Usual Dosage** Adults: Oral: 100-200 mg to start followed by 100 mg every 12 hours until desired response is obtained; maintenance dose: 25-50 mg 1-3 times/day

**Dosage Forms** Tablet: 50 mg

**dichysterol** *see* dihydrotachysterol *on page 187*

## diclofenac (dye KLOE fen ak)

**U.S./Canadian Brand Names** Apo®-Diclo (Can); Cataflam® Oral; Novo-Difenac-K (Can); Novo-Difenac®-SR (Can); Nu-Diclo (Can); PMS-Diclofenac (Can); Vofenal™ (Can); Voltaren® Ophthalmic; Voltaren® Oral; Voltaren Rapide® (Can); Voltaren®-XR Oral

(Continued)

## diclofenac *(Continued)*

**Therapeutic Category** Analgesic, Non-narcotic; Nonsteroidal Anti-inflammatory Drug (NSAID)

**Use** Acute treatment of mild to moderate pain; acute and chronic treatment of rheumatoid arthritis, ankylosing spondylitis, and osteoarthritis; used for juvenile rheumatoid arthritis, gout, dysmenorrhea; ophthalmic solution for postoperative inflammation after cataract extraction; temporary relief of pain and photophobia in patients undergoing corneal refractive surgery

**Usual Dosage** Adults:

Oral:

Rheumatoid arthritis: 150-200 mg/day in 2-4 divided doses

Osteoarthritis: 100-150 mg/day in 2-3 divided doses

Ankylosing spondylitis: 100-125 mg/day in 4-5 divided doses

Ophthalmic: Instill 1 drop into affected eye 4 times/day beginning 24 hours after cataract surgery and continuing for 2 weeks

**Dosage Forms**

Solution, ophthalmic, as sodium: 0.1% (5 mL)

Voltaren®: 0.1% (2.5 mL, 5 mL)

Tablet, enteric coated, as sodium: 25 mg, 50 mg, 75 mg

Voltaren®: 25 mg, 50 mg, 75 mg

Tablet, extended release, as sodium: 100 mg

Voltaren®-XR: 100 mg

Tablet, as potassium: 50 mg

Cataflam®: 50 mg

## diclofenac and misoprostol (dye KLOE fen ak & mye soe PROST ole)

**U.S./Canadian Brand Names** Arthrotec®

**Therapeutic Category** Analgesic, Non-narcotic; Prostaglandin

**Use** The diclofenac component is indicated for the treatment of osteoarthritis and rheumatoid arthritis; the misoprostol component is indicated for the prophylaxis of NSAID-induced gastric and duodenal ulceration

**Usual Dosage** Adults: Oral: 1 tablet 2-3 times/day with food; tablets should be swallowed whole, not chewed

**Dosage Forms** Tablet: Diclofenac 50 mg and misoprostol 200 mcg; diclofenac 75 mg and misoprostol 200 mcg

**diclofenamide** *see* dichlorphenamide *on previous page*

## dicloxacillin (dye kloks a SIL in)

**U.S./Canadian Brand Names** Dynapen®

**Therapeutic Category** Penicillin

**Use** Treatment of skin and soft tissue infections, pneumonia and follow-up therapy of osteomyelitis caused by susceptible penicillinase-producing staphylococci

**Usual Dosage** Oral:

Children <40 kg: 12.5-50 mg/kg/day divided every 6 hours; doses of 50-100 mg/kg/day in divided doses every 6 hours have been used for follow-up therapy of osteomyelitis

Children >40 kg and Adults: 125-500 mg every 6 hours

**Dosage Forms**

Capsule, as sodium: 125 mg, 250 mg, 500 mg

Powder for oral suspension, as sodium: 62.5 mg/5 mL (80 mL, 100 mL, 200 mL)

## dicumarol (dye KOO ma role)

**Synonyms** bishydroxycoumarin

**Therapeutic Category** Anticoagulant

**Use** Prophylaxis and treatment of thromboembolic disorders

**Usual Dosage** Adults: Oral: 25-200 mg/day based on prothrombin time (PT) determinations

**Dosage Forms** Tablet: 25 mg, 50 mg, 100 mg

## dicyclomine (dye SYE kloe meen)

**Synonyms** dicycloverine

**U.S./Canadian Brand Names** Antispas® Injection; Bentyl® Hydrochloride Injection; Bentyl® Hydrochloride Oral; Bentylol® (Can); Byclomine® Injection; Dibent® Injection; Dilomine® Injection; Di-Spaz® Injection; Di-Spaz® Oral; Formulex® (Can); Lomine (Can); Or-Tyl® Injection; Protylol (Can); Spasmoban (Can)

**Therapeutic Category** Anticholinergic Agent

**Use** Treatment of functional disturbances of GI motility such as irritable bowel syndrome

**Usual Dosage**

Oral:

Infants >6 months: 5 mg/dose 3-4 times/day

Children: 10 mg/dose 3-4 times/day

Adults: Begin with 80 mg/day in 4 equally divided doses, then increase up to 160 mg/day

I.M. **(should not be used I.V.)**: 80 mg/day in 4 divided doses (20 mg/dose)

**Dosage Forms**

Capsule, as hydrochloride: 10 mg, 20 mg

Injection, as hydrochloride: 10 mg/mL (2 mL, 10 mL)

Syrup, as hydrochloride: 10 mg/5 mL (118 mL, 473 mL, 946 mL)

Tablet, as hydrochloride: 20 mg

**dicycloverine** *see* dicyclomine *on this page*

## didanosine (dye DAN oh seen)

**Synonyms** ddI

**U.S./Canadian Brand Names** Videx®

**Therapeutic Category** Antiviral Agent

**Use** Treatment of patients with advanced HIV infection which is resistant to zidovudine therapy or in those patients with zidovudine intolerance; has been used in asymptomatic patients with very low $CD4^+$ lymphocyte counts (<200 cells/$mm^3$) with or without AIDS-related complex

**Usual Dosage** Administer on an empty stomach: Oral:

Children (dosing is based on body surface area ($m^2$)):

<0.4: 25 mg tablets twice daily or 31 mg powder twice daily

0.5-0.7: 50 mg tablets twice daily or 62 mg powder twice daily

0.8-1: 75 mg tablets twice daily or 94 mg powder twice daily

1.1-1.4: 100 mg tablets twice daily or 125 mg powder twice daily

Adults: Dosing is based on patient weight:

35-49 kg: 125 mg tablets twice daily or 167 mg buffered powder twice daily

50-74 kg: 200 mg tablets twice daily or 250 mg buffered powder twice daily

≥75 mg: 300 mg tablets twice daily or 375 mg buffered powder twice daily

**Note:** Children >1 year and Adults should receive 2 tablets per dose and children <1 year should receive 1 tablet per dose for adequate buffering and absorption; tablets should be chewed

**Dosage Forms**

Capsule, sustained release: 125 mg, 200 mg, 250 mg, 400 mg

Powder for oral solution:

Buffered (single-dose packet): 100 mg, 167 mg, 250 mg

Pediatric powder for reconstitution: 2 g, 4 g

Tablet, buffered, chewable/dispersible (mint flavor): 25 mg, 50 mg, 100 mg, 150 mg, 200 mg

**dideoxycytidine** *see* zalcitabine *on page 637*

**Didrex®** *see* benzphetamine *on page 75*

**Didronel®** *see* etidronate disodium *on page 235*

## dienestrol (dye en ES trole)

**U.S./Canadian Brand Names** DV® Vaginal Cream; Ortho®-Dienestrol Vaginal

**Therapeutic Category** Estrogen Derivative

**Use** Symptomatic management of atrophic vaginitis in postmenopausal women

**Usual Dosage** Adults: Vaginal: 1-2 applicatorfuls/day for 2 weeks and then ½ of that dose for 2 weeks; maintenance dose: 1 applicatorful 1-3 times/week for 3 weeks each month

**Dosage Forms** Cream, vaginal: 0.01% (30 g, 78 g)

**dietary supplements** *see* nutritional formula, enteral/oral *on page 432*

## diethylpropion (dye eth il PROE pee on)

**Synonyms** amfepramone

**U.S./Canadian Brand Names** Tenuate®; Tenuate® Dospan®

**Therapeutic Category** Anorexiant

**Controlled Substance** C-IV

**Use** Short-term adjunct in exogenous obesity

**Usual Dosage** Adults: Oral: 25 mg 3 times/day before meals or food or 75 mg controlled release tablet at midmorning

**Dosage Forms**

Tablet, as hydrochloride: 25 mg

Tablet, as hydrochloride, controlled release: 75 mg

## diethylstilbestrol (dye eth il stil BES trole)

**Synonyms** DES; stilbestrol

**U.S./Canadian Brand Names** Honvol® (Can); Stilphostrol®

**Therapeutic Category** Estrogen Derivative

**Use** Management of severe vasomotor symptoms of menopause, for estrogen replacement, and for palliative treatment of inoperable metastatic prostatic carcinoma

**Usual Dosage** Adults:

Hypogonadism and ovarian failure: Oral: 0.2-0.5 mg/day

Menopausal symptoms: Oral: 0.1-2 mg/day for 3 weeks and then off 1 week

Postmenopausal breast carcinoma: Oral: 15 mg/day

Prostate carcinoma: Oral: 1-3 mg/day

Prostatic cancer: I.V.: 0.5 g to start, then 1 g every 2-5 days followed by 0.25-0.5 g 1-2 times/week as maintenance

Diphosphate:

Oral: 50 mg 3 times/day; increase up to 200 mg or more 3 times/day

I.V.: Administer 0.5 g, dissolved in 250 mL of saline or $D_5W$, administer slowly the first 10-15 minutes then adjust rate so that the entire amount is administered in 1 hour

**Dosage Forms**

Injection, as diphosphate sodium (Stilphostrol®): 0.25 g (5 mL)

Tablet (Honvol®): 0.1 mg, 0.5 mg, 1 mg

## difenoxin and atropine (dye fen OKS in & A troe peen)

**U.S./Canadian Brand Names** Motofen®

**Therapeutic Category** Antidiarrheal

**Controlled Substance** C-IV

**Use** Treatment of diarrhea

**Usual Dosage** Adults: Oral: Initial: 2 tablets, then 1 tablet after each loose stool; 1 tablet every 3-4 hours, up to 8 tablets in a 24-hour period; if no improvement after 48 hours, continued administration is not indicated

**Dosage Forms** Tablet: Difenoxin hydrochloride 1 mg and atropine sulfate 0.025 mg

**Differin®** *see* adapalene *on page 13*

## diflorasone (dye FLOR a sone)

**U.S./Canadian Brand Names** Florone®; Florone E®; Flutone (Can); Maxiflor®; Psorcon™

**Therapeutic Category** Corticosteroid, Topical

**Use** Relief of inflammation and pruritic symptoms of corticosteroid-responsive dermatosis

**Usual Dosage** Topical:

Cream: Apply 2-4 times/day

Ointment: Apply sparingly 1-3 times/day

**Note:** Therapy should be discontinued when control is achieved. If no improvement is seen, reassessment of diagnosis may be necessary.

**Dosage Forms**

Cream, as diacetate: 0.05% (30 g, 60 g)

Ointment, topical, as diacetate: 0.05% (15 g, 30 g, 60 g)

**Diflucan®** *see* fluconazole *on page 251*

## diflunisal (dye FLOO ni sal)

**U.S./Canadian Brand Names** Apo®-Diflunisal (Can); Dolobid®; Novo-Diflunisal (Can); Nu-Diflunisal (Can)

**Therapeutic Category** Analgesic, Non-narcotic; Nonsteroidal Anti-inflammatory Drug (NSAID)

**Use** Management of inflammatory disorders usually including rheumatoid arthritis and osteoarthritis; can be used as an analgesic for treatment of mild to moderate pain

**Usual Dosage** Adults: Oral:

Pain: Initial: 500-1000 mg followed by 250-500 mg every 8-12 hours

Inflammatory condition: 500-1000 mg/day in 2 divided doses

**Dosage Forms** Tablet: 250 mg, 500 mg

**Di-Gel® [OTC]** *see* aluminum hydroxide, magnesium hydroxide, and simethicone *on page 27*

**Digepepsin®** *see* pancreatin *on page 447*

**Digibind®** *see* digoxin immune Fab *on next page*

**Digitek®** *see* digoxin *on this page*

## digoxin (di JOKS in)

**U.S./Canadian Brand Names** Digitek®; Lanoxicaps®; Lanoxin®

**Therapeutic Category** Antiarrhythmic Agent, Miscellaneous; Cardiac Glycoside

**Use** Treatment of congestive heart failure; slows the ventricular rate in tachyarrhythmias such as atrial fibrillation, atrial flutter, supraventricular tachycardia

**Usual Dosage** Adults (based on lean body weight and normal renal function for age. Decrease dose in patients with decreased renal function)

Total digitalizing dose: Administer $\frac{1}{2}$ as initial dose, then administer $\frac{1}{4}$ of the total digitalizing dose (TDD) in each of 2 subsequent doses at 8- to 12-hour intervals; obtain EKG 6 hours after each dose to assess potential toxicity

Oral: 0.75-1.5 mg

I.M., I.V.: 0.5-1 mg

Daily maintenance dose:

Oral: 0.125-0.5 mg

I.M., I.V.: 0.1-0.4 mg

**Dosage Forms**

Capsule: 50 mcg, 100 mcg, 200 mcg

Elixir: 50 mcg/mL with alcohol 10% (60 mL)

Injection: 250 mcg/mL (1 mL, 2 mL)

Injection, pediatric: 100 mcg/mL (1 mL)

Tablet: 125 mcg, 250 mcg, 500 mcg

## digoxin immune Fab (di JOKS in i MYUN fab)

**Synonyms** antidigoxin Fab fragments

**U.S./Canadian Brand Names** Digibind®

**Therapeutic Category** Antidote

**Use** Treatment of potentially life-threatening digoxin or digitoxin intoxication in carefully selected patients

**Usual Dosage** Each vial of Digibind® will bind approximately 0.5 mg of digoxin or digitoxin

I.V.: To determine the dose of digoxin immune Fab, first determine the total body load of digoxin (TBL using either an approximation of the amount ingested or a postdistribution serum digoxin concentration). If neither ingestion amount or serum level is known: Adult dosage is 20 vials (760 mg) I.V. infusion.

**Dosage Forms** Powder for injection, lyophilized: 38 mg

**Dihistine® DH** *see* chlorpheniramine, pseudoephedrine, and codeine *on page 132*

**Dihistine® Expectorant** *see* guaifenesin, pseudoephedrine, and codeine *on page 284*

## dihydrocodeine compound (dye hye droe KOE deen KOM pound)

**U.S./Canadian Brand Names** DHC Plus®; Synalgos®-DC

**Therapeutic Category** Analgesic, Narcotic

**Controlled Substance** C-III

**Use** Management of mild to moderate pain that requires relaxation

**Usual Dosage** Adults: Oral: 1-2 capsules every 4-6 hours as needed for pain

**Dosage Forms** Capsule:

DHC Plus®: Dihydrocodeine bitartrate 16 mg, acetaminophen 356.4 mg, and caffeine 30 mg

Synalgos®-DC: Dihydrocodeine bitartrate 16 mg, aspirin 356.4 mg, and caffeine 30 mg

## dihydroergotamine (dye hye droe er GOT a meen)

**U.S./Canadian Brand Names** D.H.E. 45® Injection; Migranal® Nasal Spray

**Therapeutic Category** Ergot Alkaloid and Derivative

**Use** Abort or prevent vascular headaches

**Usual Dosage** Adults:

I.M.: 1 mg at first sign of headache; repeat hourly to a maximum dose of 3 mg total

I.V.: Up to 2 mg maximum dose for faster effects; maximum dose: 6 mg/week

Intranasal: One spray (0.5 mg) of nasal spray should be administered into each nostril; if the condition has not sufficiently improved approximately fifteen minutes later, an additional spray should be administered to each nostril. The usual dosage required to obtain optimal efficacy is a total dosage of 4 sprays (2 mg); nasal spray is exclusively indicated for the symptomatic treatment of migraine attacks; no more than 4 sprays (2 mg) should be administered for any single migraine attack; an interval of at least 6-8 hours should be observed before treating another migraine attack with the nasal spray or any drug containing dihydroergotamine or ergotamine; no more than 8 sprays (4 mg) (corresponding to the use of 2 ampuls) should be administered during any 24-hour period; the maximum weekly dosage is 24 sprays (12 mg)

**Dosage Forms**

Injection, as mesylate: 1 mg/mL (1 mL)

Spray, nasal: 4 mg/mL [0.5 mg/spray] (1 mL)

**dihydroergotoxine** *see* ergoloid mesylates *on page 220*

**dihydrohydroxycodeinone** *see* oxycodone *on page 443*

**dihydromorphinone** *see* hydromorphone *on page 305*

## dihydrotachysterol (dye hye droe tak IS ter ole)

**Synonyms** dichysterol

**U.S./Canadian Brand Names** DHT™

**Therapeutic Category** Vitamin D Analog

**Use** Treatment of hypocalcemia associated with hypoparathyroidism; prophylaxis of hypocalcemic tetany following thyroid surgery; suppress hyperparathyroidism and treat renal osteodystrophy in patients with chronic renal failure

**Usual Dosage** Oral:

Hypoparathyroidism:

Infants and young Children: 0.1-0.5 mg/day

Older Children and Adults: 0.5-1 mg/day

Nutritional rickets: 0.5 mg as a single dose or 13-50 mcg/day until healing occurs

Renal osteodystrophy: 0.6-6 mg/24 hours; maintenance: 0.25-0.6 mg/24 hours adjusted as necessary to achieve normal serum calcium levels and promote bone healing

**Dosage Forms**

Capsule (Hytakerol®): 0.125 mg

Solution, oral concentrate (DHT™): 0.2 mg/mL (30 mL)

Tablet (DHT™): 0.125 mg, 0.2 mg, 0.4 mg

## dihydroxyaluminum sodium carbonate

(dye hye DROKS i a LOO mi num SOW dee um KAR bun ate)

**U.S./Canadian Brand Names** Rolaids® [OTC]

**Therapeutic Category** Antacid

**Use** Symptomatic relief of upset stomach associated with hyperacidity

**Usual Dosage** Oral: Chew 1-2 tablets as needed

**Dosage Forms** Tablet, chewable: 334 mg

**1,25 dihydroxycholecalciferol** *see* calcitriol *on page 96*

**dihydroxypropyl theophylline** *see* dyphylline *on page 208*

**Dihyrex® Injection** *see* diphenhydramine *on page 191*

**diiodohydroxyquin** *see* iodoquinol *on page 324*

**Dilacor XR®** *see* diltiazem *on this page*

**Dilantin®** *see* phenytoin *on page 468*

**Dilantin-30® Pediatric Suspension *(Discontinued)*** *see page 750*

**Dilantin® With Phenobarbital *(Discontinued)*** *see page 750*

**Dilatrate®-SR** *see* isosorbide dinitrate *on page 328*

**Dilaudid® 1 mg & 3 mg Tablet *(Discontinued)*** *see page 750*

**Dilaudid® Cough Syrup** *see* hydromorphone *on page 305*

**Dilaudid-HP® Injection** *see* hydromorphone *on page 305*

**Dilaudid® Injection** *see* hydromorphone *on page 305*

**Dilaudid® Oral** *see* hydromorphone *on page 305*

**Dilaudid® Suppository** *see* hydromorphone *on page 305*

**Dilocaine® Injection** *see* lidocaine *on page 348*

**Dilomine® Injection** *see* dicyclomine *on page 183*

**Dilor®** *see* dyphylline *on page 208*

**Diltia XT®** *see* diltiazem *on this page*

## diltiazem (dil TYE a zem)

**U.S./Canadian Brand Names** Alti-Diltiazem (Can); Apo®-Diltiaz (Can); Cardizem® CD; Cardizem® Injectable; Cardizem® SR; Cardizem® Tablet; Cartia® XT; Dilacor XR®; Diltia XT®; Gen-Diltiazem (Can); Novo-Diltazem (Can); Nu-Diltiaz (Can); Nu-Diltiaz-CD (Can); Tiamate®; Tiazac®

(Continued)

## diltiazem *(Continued)*

**Therapeutic Category** Calcium Channel Blocker

**Use**

Oral: Hypertension; chronic stable angina or angina from coronary artery spasm

Injection: Atrial fibrillation or atrial flutter; paroxysmal supraventricular tachycardias (PSVT)

**Usual Dosage** Adults:

Oral: 30-120 mg 3-4 times/day; dosage should be increased gradually, at 1- to 2-day intervals until optimum response is obtained; usual maintenance dose: 240-360 mg/day

Sustained-release capsules (SR): Initial dose of 60-120 mg twice daily

Sustained-release capsules (CD, XR): 180-300 mg once daily

I.V.: Initial: 0.25 mg/kg as a bolus over 2 minutes, then continuous infusion of 5-15 mg/hour for up to 24 hours

**Dosage Forms**

Capsule, sustained release, as hydrochloride: 60 mg, 90 mg, 120 mg, 180 mg, 240 mg, 300 mg

Cardizem® CD: 120 mg, 180 mg, 240 mg, 300 mg, 360 mg

Cardizem® SR: 60 mg, 90 mg, 120 mg

Cartia® XT: 120 mg, 180 mg, 240 mg, 300 mg

Dilacor® XR: 180 mg, 240 mg

Diltia XT®: 120 mg, 180 mg, 240 mg

Tiazac®: 120 mg, 180 mg, 240 mg, 300 mg, 360 mg, 420 mg

Injection, as hydrochloride: 5 mg/mL (5 mL, 10 mL)

Cardizem®: 5 mg/mL (5 mL, 10 mL, 25 mL)

Tablet, as hydrochloride (Cardizem®): 30 mg, 60 mg, 90 mg, 120 mg

Tablet, extended release, as hydrochloride (Tiamate®): 120 mg, 180 mg, 240 mg

**Dimacol® Caplets [OTC]** *see* guaifenesin, pseudoephedrine, and dextromethorphan *on page 285*

**Dimaphen® Elixir *(Discontinued)*** *see page 750*

**Dimaphen® Tablets *(Discontinued)*** *see page 750*

## dimenhydrinate (dye men HYE dri nate)

**U.S./Canadian Brand Names** Apo®-Dimenhydrinate (Can); Calm-X® Oral [OTC]; Dimetabs® Oral; Dinate® Injection; Dramamine® Oral [OTC]; Dramilin® Injection; Dymenate® Injection; Gravol® (Can); Hydrate® Injection; Marmine® Injection; Marmine® Oral [OTC]; Tega-Vert® Oral; TripTone® Caplets® [OTC]

**Therapeutic Category** Antihistamine

**Use** Treatment and prevention of nausea, vertigo, and vomiting associated with motion sickness

**Usual Dosage** Oral:

Children:

2-5 years: 12.5-25 mg every 6-8 hours, maximum: 75 mg/day

6-12 years: 25-50 mg every 6-8 hours, maximum: 75 mg/day

**or**

Alternately: 5 mg/kg/day in 4 divided doses, not to exceed 300 mg/day

Adults: 50-100 mg every 4-6 hours, not to exceed 400 mg/day

**Dosage Forms**

Capsule: 50 mg

Injection: 50 mg/mL (1 mL, 5 mL, 10 mL)

Liquid: 12.5 mg/4 mL (90 mL, 473 mL); 16.62 mg/5 mL (480 mL)

Tablet: 50 mg

Chewable: 50 mg

## dimercaprol (dye mer KAP role)

**Synonyms** BAL; British anti-lewisite; dithioglycerol

**U.S./Canadian Brand Names** BAL in Oil®

**Therapeutic Category** Chelating Agent

**Use** Antidote to gold, arsenic, and mercury poisoning; adjunct to edetate calcium disodium in lead poisoning

**Usual Dosage** Children and Adults: I.M.:

Mild arsenic and gold poisoning: 2.5 mg/kg/dose every 6 hours for 2 days, then every 12 hours on the third day, and once daily thereafter for 10 days

Severe arsenic and gold poisoning: 3 mg/kg/dose every 4 hours for 2 days then every 6 hours on the third day, then every 12 hours thereafter for 10 days

Mercury poisoning: Initial: 5 mg/kg followed by 2.5 mg/kg/dose 1-2 times/day for 10 days

Lead poisoning (use with edetate calcium disodium):

Mild: 3 mg/kg/dose every 4 hours for 5-7 days

Severe: 4 mg/kg/dose every 4 hours for 5-7 days

Acute encephalopathy: Initial: 4 mg/kg/dose, then every 4 hours

**Dosage Forms** Injection: 100 mg/mL (3 mL)

**Dimetabs® Oral** *see* dimenhydrinate *on previous page*

**Dimetane® *(Discontinued)*** *see page 750*

**Dimetane® DC *(Discontinued)*** *see page 750*

**Dimetane® Decongestant Elixir [OTC]** *see* brompheniramine and phenylephrine *on page 87*

**Dimetane® Extentabs® [OTC]** *see* brompheniramine *on page 87*

**Dimetapp® 4-Hour Liqui-Gel Capsule *(Discontinued)*** *see page 750*

**Dimetapp® Elixir *(Discontinued)*** *see page 750*

**Dimetapp® Elixir [New Formula]** *see* brompheniramine and pseudoephedrine *on page 88*

**Dimetapp® Extentabs® *(Discontinued)*** *see page 750*

**Dimetapp® Sinus Caplets [OTC]** *see* pseudoephedrine and ibuprofen *on page 508*

**Dimetapp® Tablet *(Discontinued)*** *see page 750*

**β,β-dimethylcysteine** *see* penicillamine *on page 455*

## dimethyl sulfoxide (dye meth il sul FOKS ide)

**Synonyms** DMSO

**U.S./Canadian Brand Names** Kemsol® (Can); Rimso®-50

**Therapeutic Category** Urinary Tract Product

**Use** Symptomatic relief of interstitial cystitis

**Usual Dosage** Instill 50 mL directly into bladder and allow to remain for 15 minutes; repeat every 2 weeks until maximum symptomatic relief is obtained

**Dosage Forms** Solution: 50% [500 mg/mL] (50 mL)

**Dinate® Injection** *see* dimenhydrinate *on previous page*

## dinoprostone (dye noe PROST one)

**Synonyms** $PGE_2$; prostaglandin $E_2$

**U.S./Canadian Brand Names** Cervidil® Vaginal Insert; Prepidil® Vaginal Gel; Prostin $E_2$® Vaginal Suppository

**Therapeutic Category** Prostaglandin

**Use** Terminate pregnancy from 12th through 28th week of gestation; evacuate uterus in cases of missed abortion or intrauterine fetal death; manage benign hydatidiform mole

**Usual Dosage** Vaginal: Insert 1 suppository high in vagina, repeat at 3- to 5-hour intervals until abortion occurs up to 240 mg (maximum dose)

(Continued)

## dinoprostone *(Continued)*

**Dosage Forms**

Insert, vaginal (Cervidil®): 10 mg

Gel, vaginal: 0.5 mg in 3 g syringes [each package contains a 10-mm and 20-mm shielded catheter]

Suppository, vaginal: 20 mg

## dinoprost tromethamine (DYE noe prost tro METH a meen)

**Synonyms** $PGF_{2\alpha}$; prostaglandin $F_2$ alpha

**U.S./Canadian Brand Names** Prostin $F_2$ Alpha®

**Therapeutic Category** Prostaglandin

**Use** Abort 2nd trimester pregnancy

**Usual Dosage** 40 mg (8 mL) via transabdominal tap; if abortion not completed in 24 hours, another 10-40 mg may be administered

**Dosage Forms** Injection: 5 mg/mL (4 mL, 8 mL)

**Diocaine® (Can)** *see* proparacaine *on page 502*

**Diocarpine (Can)** *see* pilocarpine *on page 471*

**Diochloram® (Can)** *see* chloramphenicol *on page 125*

**Diocto® [OTC]** *see* docusate *on page 197*

**Diocto C® [OTC]** *see* docusate and casanthranol *on page 198*

**Diocto-K® [OTC]** *see* docusate *on page 197*

**Diocto-K Plus® [OTC]** *see* docusate and casanthranol *on page 198*

**Dioctolose Plus® [OTC]** *see* docusate and casanthranol *on page 198*

**dioctyl calcium sulfosuccinate** *see* docusate *on page 197*

**dioctyl potassium sulfosuccinate** *see* docusate *on page 197*

**dioctyl sodium sulfosuccinate** *see* docusate *on page 197*

**Diodoquin® (Can)** *see* iodoquinol *on page 324*

**Dioeze® [OTC]** *see* docusate *on page 197*

**Diofluor™ (Can)** *see* fluorescein sodium *on page 254*

**Diogent® (Can)** *see* gentamicin *on page 273*

**Diomycin® (Can)** *see* erythromycin (systemic) *on page 222*

**Dionephrine® (Can)** *see* phenylephrine *on page 467*

**Dionosil Oily®** *see* radiological/contrast media (ionic) *on page 516*

**Diopentolate® (Can)** *see* cyclopentolate *on page 159*

**Dioptimyd® (Can)** *see* sulfacetamide and prednisolone *on page 563*

**Dioptrol® (Can)** *see* neomycin, polymyxin B, and dexamethasone *on page 414*

**Diosulf™ (Can)** *see* sulfacetamide *on page 562*

**Diotame® [OTC]** *see* bismuth subsalicylate *on page 81*

**Diotrope® (Can)** *see* tropicamide *on page 611*

**Dioval® Injection** *see* estradiol *on page 224*

**Diovan™** *see* valsartan *on page 621*

**Diovan HCT™** *see* valsartan and hydrochlorothiazide *on page 621*

**Diovol® (Can)** *see* aluminum hydroxide and magnesium hydroxide *on page 27*

**Diovol® EX (Can)** *see* aluminum hydroxide and magnesium hydroxide *on page 27*

**dipalmitoylphosphatidylcholine** *see* colfosceril palmitate *on page 152*

**Dipentum®** *see* olsalazine *on page 435*

**Diphenacen-50® Injection [OTC]** *see* diphenhydramine *on this page*

**Diphenatol®** *see* diphenoxylate and atropine *on next page*

**Diphen® Cough [OTC]** *see* diphenhydramine *on this page*

**Diphenhist [OTC]** *see* diphenhydramine *on this page*

## diphenhydramine (dye fen HYE dra meen)

**U.S./Canadian Brand Names** Allerdryl® (Can); AllerMax® Oral [OTC]; Allernix® (Can); Banophen® Oral [OTC]; Belix® Oral [OTC]; Benadryl® Injection; Benadryl® Oral [OTC]; Benadryl® Topical; Ben-Allergin-50® Injection; Benylin® Cough Syrup [OTC]; Bydramine® Cough Syrup [OTC]; Compoz® Gel Caps [OTC]; Compoz® Nighttime Sleep Aid [OTC]; Dihyrex® Injection; Diphenacen-50® Injection [OTC]; Diphen® Cough [OTC]; Diphenhist [OTC]; Dormarex® 2 Oral [OTC]; Dormin® Oral [OTC]; Genahist® Oral; Hydramyn® Syrup [OTC]; Hyrexin-50® Injection; Maximum Strength Nytol® [OTC]; Miles Nervine® Caplets [OTC]; Nordryl® Injection; Nordryl® Oral; Nytol® Oral [OTC]; Phendry® Oral [OTC]; PMS-Diphenhydramine (Can); Siladryl® Oral [OTC]; Silphen® Cough [OTC]; Sleep-eze 3® Oral [OTC]; Sleepinal® [OTC]; Sleepwell 2-nite® [OTC]; Sominex® Oral [OTC]; Tusstat® Syrup; Twilite® Oral [OTC]; Uni-Bent® Cough Syrup; Winks® [OTC]

**Therapeutic Category** Antihistamine

**Use** Symptomatic relief of allergic symptoms caused by histamine release which include nasal allergies and allergic dermatosis; mild nighttime sedation, prevention of motion sickness, as an antitussive; treatment of phenothiazine-induced dystonic reactions

**Usual Dosage**

Children: Oral, I.M., I.V.: 5 mg/kg/day or 150 mg/m$^2$/day in divided doses every 6-8 hours, not to exceed 300 mg/day

Adults:

Oral: 25-50 mg every 4-6 hours

I.M., I.V.: 10-50 mg in a single dose every 2-4 hours, not to exceed 400 mg/day

Topical: For external application, not longer than 7 days

**Dosage Forms**

Capsule, as hydrochloride: 25 mg, 50 mg

Cream, as hydrochloride: 1%, 2%

Elixir, as hydrochloride: 12.5 mg/5 mL (5 mL, 10 mL, 20 mL, 120 mL, 480 mL, 3780 mL)

Injection, as hydrochloride: 10 mg/mL (10 mL, 30 mL); 50 mg/mL (1 mL, 10 mL)

Lotion, as hydrochloride: 1% (75 mL)

Solution, topical spray, as hydrochloride: 1% (60 mL)

Syrup, as hydrochloride: 12.5 mg/5 mL (5 mL, 120 mL, 240 mL, 480 mL, 3780 mL)

Tablet, as hydrochloride: 25 mg, 50 mg

## diphenhydramine and pseudoephedrine

(dye fen HYE dra meen & soo doe e FED rin)

**U.S./Canadian Brand Names** Actifed® Allergy Tablet (Night) [OTC]; Banophen® Decongestant Capsule [OTC]; Benadryl® Decongestant Allergy Tablet [OTC]

**Therapeutic Category** Antihistamine/Decongestant Combination

**Use** Relief of symptoms of upper respiratory mucosal congestion in seasonal and perennial nasal allergies, acute rhinitis, rhinosinusitis, and eustachian tube blockage

**Usual Dosage** Adults: Oral: 1 capsule or tablet every 4-6 hours, up to 4/day

**Dosage Forms**

Capsule: Diphenhydramine hydrochloride 25 mg and pseudoephedrine hydrochloride 60 mg

Tablet:

Actifed® Allergy (Night): Diphenhydramine hydrochloride 25 mg and pseudoephedrine hydrochloride 30 mg

Benadryl® Decongestant Allergy: Diphenhydramine hydrochloride 25 mg and pseudoephedrine hydrochloride 60 mg

**diphenoxylate and atropine** (dye fen OKS i late & A troe peen)

**U.S./Canadian Brand Names** Diphenatol®; Lomocot®; Lomotil®; Lonox®

**Therapeutic Category** Antidiarrheal

**Controlled Substance** C-V

**Use** Treatment of diarrhea

**Usual Dosage** Oral (as diphenoxylate): Initial dose:

Children: 0.3-0.4 mg/kg/day in 2-4 divided doses

<2 years: Not recommended

2-5 years: 2 mg 3 times/day

5-8 years: 2 mg 4 times/day

8-12 years: 2 mg 5 times/day

Adults: 15-20 mg/day in 3-4 divided doses

Reduce dosage as soon as initial control of symptoms is achieved

**Dosage Forms**

Solution, oral: Diphenoxylate hydrochloride 2.5 mg and atropine sulfate 0.025 mg per 5 mL (4 mL, 10 mL, 60 mL)

Tablet: Diphenoxylate hydrochloride 2.5 mg and atropine sulfate 0.025 mg

**Diphenylan Sodium® *(Discontinued)*** *see page 750*

**diphenylhydantoin** *see* phenytoin *on page 468*

**diphtheria and tetanus toxoid** (dif THEER ee a & TET a nus TOKS oyd)

**Synonyms** DT; Td; tetanus and diphtheria toxoid

**Therapeutic Category** Toxoid

**Use** Active immunity against diphtheria and tetanus

**Usual Dosage** I.M.:

Infants and Children:

6 weeks to 1 year: Three 0.5 mL doses at least 4 weeks apart; administer a reinforcing dose 6-12 months after the third injection

1-6 years: Administer two 0.5 mL doses at least 4 weeks apart; reinforcing dose 6-12 months after second injection; if final dose is administered after seventh birthday, use adult preparation

4-6 years (booster immunization): 0.5 mL; not necessary if all 4 doses were administered after fourth birthday - routinely administer booster doses at 10-year intervals with the adult preparation

Children >7 years and Adults: 2 primary doses of 0.5 mL each, administered at an interval of 4-6 weeks; third (reinforcing) dose of 0.5 mL 6-12 months later; boosters every 10 years

**Dosage Forms** Injection:

Pediatric use:

Diphtheria 6.6 Lf units and tetanus 5 Lf units per 0.5 mL (5 mL)

Diphtheria 10 Lf units and tetanus 5 Lf units per 0.5 mL (0.5 mL, 5 mL)

Diphtheria 12.5 Lf units and tetanus 5 Lf units per 0.5 mL (5 mL)

Diphtheria 15 Lf units and tetanus 10 Lf units per 0.5 mL (5 mL)

Adult use:

Diphtheria 1.5 Lf units and tetanus 5 Lf units per 0.5 mL (0.5 mL, 5 mL)

Diphtheria 2 Lf units and tetanus 5 Lf units per 0.5 mL (5 mL)

Diphtheria 2 Lf units and tetanus 10 Lf units per 0.5 mL (5 mL)

**diphtheria antitoxin** (dif THEER ee a an tee TOKS in)

**Therapeutic Category** Antitoxin

**Use** Passive prevention and treatment of diphtheria

**Usual Dosage** I.M. or slow I.V. infusion: Dosage varies; range: 20,000-120,000 units

**Dosage Forms** Injection: 500 units/mL (20 mL, 40 mL)

**diphtheria $CRM_{197}$ protein** *see* pneumococcal conjugate vaccine (7-valent) *on page 477*

## diphtheria, tetanus toxoids, and acellular pertussis vaccine

(dif THEER ee a, TET a nus TOKS oyds, & ay CEL yoo lar per TUS sis vak SEEN)

**Synonyms** DTAP

**U.S./Canadian Brand Names** Acel-Imune®; Certiva™; Infanrix™; Tripedia®

**Therapeutic Category** Toxoid

**Use** Fourth or fifth immunization of children 15 months to 7 years of age (prior to seventh birthday) who have been previously immunized with 3 or 4 doses of whole-cell pertussis DTP vaccine

**Usual Dosage** I.M.: After at least 3 doses of whole-cell DTP, administer 0.5 mL at ~18 months (at least 6 months after third DTWP dose), then another dose at 4-5 years of age

**Dosage Forms** Injection:

Acel-Imune®: Diphtheria 7.5 Lf units, tetanus 5 Lf units, and acellular pertussis vaccine 40 mcg per 0.5 mL (7.5 mL)

Certiva™: Diphtheria 15 Lf units, tetanus 6 Lf units, and acellular pertussis vaccine 40 mcg per 0.5 mL (7.5 mL)

Infanrix™: Diphtheria 25 Lf units, tetanus 10 Lf units, and acellular pertussis vaccine 25 mcg per 0.5 mL (7.5 mL)

Tripedia®: Diphtheria 6.7 Lf units, tetanus 5 Lf units, and acellular pertussis vaccine 46.8 mcg per 0.5 mL (7.5 mL)

## diphtheria, tetanus toxoids, and acellular pertussis vaccine and *Haemophilus* b conjugate vaccine

(dif THEER ee a, TET a nus TOKS oyds, & ay CEL yoo lar per TUS sis vak SEEN, & hem OF fi lus bee KON joo gate vak SEEN)

**U.S./Canadian Brand Names** TriHIBit®

**Therapeutic Category** Toxoid; Vaccine, Inactivated Bacteria

**Use** Active immunization of children 15-18 months of age for prevention of diphtheria, tetanus, pertussis, and invasive disease caused by *H. influenzae* type b.

**Usual Dosage** Children >15 months of age: I.M.: 0.5 mL (as part of a general vaccination schedule; see individual vaccines). Vaccine should be used within 30 minutes of reconstitution.

**Dosage Forms** Injection: Tetanus toxoid 5 Lf units, diphtheria toxoid 6.7 Lf units, pertussis antigens 46.8 mcg, and *H. influenzae* type b purified capsular polysaccharide 10 mcg [Tripedia® vaccine used to reconstitute ActHIB®] (0.5 mL)

## diphtheria, tetanus toxoids, and whole-cell pertussis vaccine

(dif THEER ee a, TET a nus TOKS oyds, & hole-sel per TUS sis vak SEEN)

**Synonyms** DPT

**U.S./Canadian Brand Names** Tri-Immunol®

**Therapeutic Category** Toxoid

**Use** Active immunization of infants and children through 6 years of age (between 2 months and the seventh birthday) against diphtheria, tetanus, and pertussis; recommended for both primary immunization and routine recall; start immunization at once if whooping cough or diphtheria is present in the community

**Usual Dosage** The primary immunization for children 2 months to 6 years of age, ideally beginning at the age of 2-3 months or at 6-week check-up. Administer 0.5 mL I.M. on 3 occasions at 4- to 8-week intervals with a re-enforcing dose administered 1 year after the third injection. The booster doses (0.5 mL I.M.) are administered when the child is 4-6 years of age.

**Dosage Forms** Injection:

Diphtheria 6.7 Lf units, tetanus 5 Lf units, and pertussis 4 protective units per 0.5 mL (7.5 mL)

Tri-Immunol®: Diphtheria 12.5 Lf units, tetanus 5 Lf units, and pertussis 4 protective units per 0.5 mL (7.5 mL)

## diphtheria, tetanus toxoids, whole-cell pertussis, and *Haemophilus* B conjugate vaccine

(dif THEER ee a, TET a nus TOKS oyds, hole-sel per TUS sis, & hem OF fil us bee KON joo gate vak SEEN)

**Synonyms** DTwP-HIB

**U.S./Canadian Brand Names** Tetramune®

**Therapeutic Category** Toxoid

**Use** Active immunization of infants and children through 5 years of age (between 2 months and the sixth birthday) against diphtheria, tetanus, and pertussis and *Haemophilus* B disease when indications for immunization with DTP vaccine and HIB vaccine coincide

**Usual Dosage** The primary immunization for children 2 months to 5 years of age, ideally beginning at the age of 2-3 months or at 6-week check-up; administer 0.5 mL I.M. on 3 occasions at ~2 month intervals, followed by a fourth 0.5 mL dose at ~15 months of age

**Dosage Forms** Injection: Diphtheria toxoid 12.5 Lf units, tetanus toxoid 5 Lf units, and whole-cell pertussis vaccine 4 units, and *Haemophilus influenzae* type B oligosaccharide 10 mcg per 0.5 mL (5 mL)

**dipivalyl epinephrine** *see* dipivefrin *on this page*

## dipivefrin (dye PI ve frin)

**Synonyms** dipivalyl epinephrine; DPE

**U.S./Canadian Brand Names** Ophtho-Pipivefrin™ (Can); PMS-Dipivefrin (Can); Propine®

**Therapeutic Category** Adrenergic Agonist Agent

**Use** Reduces elevated intraocular pressure in chronic open-angle glaucoma; treatment of ocular hypertension

**Usual Dosage** Adults: Ophthalmic: Initial: 1 drop every 12 hours

**Dosage Forms** Solution, ophthalmic, as hydrochloride: 0.1% (5 mL, 10 mL, 15 mL)

**Diprivan®** *see* propofol *on page 503*

**Diprolene® AF Topical** *see* betamethasone (topical) *on page 78*

**Diprolene® Topical** *see* betamethasone (topical) *on page 78*

**dipropylacetic acid** *see* valproic acid and derivatives *on page 620*

**Diprosone® Topical** *see* betamethasone (topical) *on page 78*

## dipyridamole (dye peer ID a mole)

**U.S./Canadian Brand Names** Apo®-Dipyridamole FC (Can); Novo-Dipiradol (Can); Persantine®

**Therapeutic Category** Antiplatelet Agent; Vasodilator

**Use** Maintain patency after surgical grafting procedures including coronary artery bypass; with warfarin to decrease thrombosis in patients after artificial heart valve replacement; for chronic management of angina pectoris; with aspirin to prevent coronary artery thrombosis; in combination with aspirin or warfarin to prevent other thromboembolic disorders; dipyridamole may also be administered 2 days prior to open heart surgery to prevent platelet activation by extracorporeal bypass pump; diagnostic agent I.V. (dipyridamole stress test) for coronary artery disease

**Usual Dosage**

Children: Oral: 3-6 mg/kg/day in 3 divided doses

Dipyridamole stress test (for evaluation of myocardial perfusion): I.V.: 0.14 mg/kg/minute for a total of 4 minutes

Adults: Oral: 75-400 mg/day in 3-4 divided doses

**Dosage Forms**

Injection: 5 mg/mL (2 mL, 10 mL)

Tablet: 25 mg, 50 mg, 75 mg

## dipyridamole and aspirin (dye peer ID a mole & AS pir in)

**U.S./Canadian Brand Names** Aggrenox®

**Therapeutic Category** Antiplatelet Agent

**Use** Combined therapy with dipyridamole and aspirin is indicated in patients who are recovering from a myocardial infarction; the rate of reinfarction is significantly reduced by such therapy; combined treatment is also indicated for the prevention of occlusion of saphenous vein coronary artery bypass grafts

**Usual Dosage** Adults: Oral: 1 capsule (dipyridamole 200 mg, aspirin 25 mg) twice daily.

**Dosage Forms** Capsule: Dipyridamole (extended release) 200 mg and aspirin 25 mg

**Diquinol®** *see* iodoquinol *on page 324*

## dirithromycin (dye RITH roe mye sin)

**U.S./Canadian Brand Names** Dynabac®

**Therapeutic Category** Macrolide (Antibiotic)

**Use** Treatment of mild to moderate upper and lower respiratory tract infections, infections of the skin and skin structure, and sexually transmitted diseases due to susceptible strains

**Usual Dosage** Adults: Oral: 500 mg once daily for 7-14 days

**Dosage Forms** Tablet, enteric coated: 250 mg

**Disalcid®** *see* salsalate *on page 536*

**disalicylic acid** *see* salsalate *on page 536*

**Disanthrol® [OTC]** *see* docusate and casanthranol *on page 198*

**Disobrom® [OTC]** *see* dexbrompheniramine and pseudoephedrine *on page 175*

**disodium cromoglycate** *see* cromolyn sodium *on page 156*

***d*-isoephedrine** *see* pseudoephedrine *on page 507*

**Disonate® [OTC]** *see* docusate *on page 197*

**Disophrol® Chronotabs® [OTC]** *see* dexbrompheniramine and pseudoephedrine *on page 175*

**Disophrol® Tablet [OTC]** *see* dexbrompheniramine and pseudoephedrine *on page 175*

## disopyramide (dye soe PEER a mide)

**U.S./Canadian Brand Names** Norpace®; Norpace® CR; Rythmodan® (Can); Rythmodan®-LA (Can)

**Therapeutic Category** Antiarrhythmic Agent, Class I-A

**Use** Suppression and prevention of unifocal and multifocal ventricular premature complexes, coupled ventricular premature complexes, and/or paroxysmal ventricular tachycardia; also effective in the conversion and prevention of recurrence of atrial fibrillation, atrial flutter, and paroxysmal atrial tachycardia

**Usual Dosage** Oral:

Children:

- <1 year: 10-30 mg/kg/24 hours in 4 divided doses
- 1-4 years: 10-20 mg/kg/24 hours in 4 divided doses
- 4-12 years: 10-15 mg/kg/24 hours in 4 divided doses
- 12-18 years: 6-15 mg/kg/24 hours in 4 divided doses

Adults:

- <50 kg: 100 mg every 6 hours or 200 mg every 12 hours (controlled release)
- >50 kg: 150 mg every 6 hours or 300 mg every 12 hours (controlled release); if no response, may increase to 200 mg every 6 hours; maximum dose required for patients with severe refractory ventricular tachycardia is 400 mg every 6 hours

**Dosage Forms**

Capsule, as phosphate: 100 mg, 150 mg

(Continued)

## disopyramide *(Continued)*

Capsule, sustained action, as phosphate: 100 mg, 150 mg

**Disotate®** *see* edetate disodium *on page 210*

**Di-Spaz® Injection** *see* dicyclomine *on page 183*

**Di-Spaz® Oral** *see* dicyclomine *on page 183*

**Dispos-a-Med® Isoproterenol *(Discontinued)*** *see page 750*

## disulfiram (dye SUL fi ram)

**U.S./Canadian Brand Names** Antabuse®

**Therapeutic Category** Aldehyde Dehydrogenase Inhibitor Agent

**Use** Management of chronic alcoholics

**Usual Dosage** Oral:

Maximum daily dose: 500 mg/day in a single dose for 1-2 weeks

Average maintenance dose: 250 mg/day; range: 125-500 mg; duration of therapy is to continue until the patient is fully recovered socially and a basis for permanent self control has been established; maintenance therapy may be required for months or even years

**Dosage Forms**

Tablet: 250 mg, 500 mg

Antabuse®: 250 mg

**Dital® *(Discontinued)*** *see page 750*

**dithioglycerol** *see* dimercaprol *on page 189*

**dithranol** *see* anthralin *on page 42*

**Ditropan®** *see* oxybutynin *on page 443*

**Ditropan® XL** *see* oxybutynin *on page 443*

**Diucardin®** *see* hydroflumethiazide *on page 304*

**Diupress® *(Discontinued)*** *see page 750*

**Diurigen® *(Discontinued)*** *see page 750*

**Diuril®** *see* chlorothiazide *on page 128*

**Dixarit® (Can)** *see* clonidine *on page 146*

**Dizac® Injectable Emulsion** *see* diazepam *on page 179*

**Dizmiss® [OTC]** *see* meclizine *on page 367*

**Dizymes® Tablet *(Discontinued)*** *see page 750*

***dl*-alpha tocopherol** *see* vitamin E *on page 631*

***d*-mannitol** *see* mannitol *on page 364*

**4-dmdr** *see* idarubicin *on page 312*

**D-Med® Injection** *see* methylprednisolone *on page 385*

**DMSO** *see* dimethyl sulfoxide *on page 189*

**DNA-derived humanized monoclonal antibody** *see* alemtuzumab *on page 19*

**DNASE** *see* dornase alfa *on page 201*

**DNR** *see* daunorubicin hydrochloride *on page 167*

**Doan's Backache Pills (Can)** *see* magnesium salicylate *on page 362*

**Doan's®, Original [OTC]** *see* magnesium salicylate *on page 362*

## dobutamine (doe BYOO ta meen)

**U.S./Canadian Brand Names** Dobutrex®

**Therapeutic Category** Adrenergic Agonist Agent

**Use** Short-term management of patients with cardiac decompensation

**Usual Dosage** I.V. infusion:

Children: 2.5-15 mcg/kg/minute, titrate to desired response

Adults: 2.5-15 mcg/kg/minute; maximum: 40 mcg/kg/minute, titrate to desired response

**Dosage Forms** Injection, as hydrochloride: 12.5 mg/mL (20 mL)

**Dobutrex®** *see* dobutamine *on previous page*

## docetaxel (doe se TAKS el)

**U.S./Canadian Brand Names** Taxotere®

**Therapeutic Category** Antineoplastic Agent

**Use** Treatment of breast cancer; advanced or metastatic nonsmall-cell lung cancer in patients whose disease has progressed after platinum-based chemotherapy

**Usual Dosage** Adults: I.V.: 60-100 mg/m$^2$ administered over 1 hour every 3 weeks

**Dosage Forms** Injection: 40 mg/mL (0.5 mL, 2 mL)

## docosanol (doe KOE san ole)

**U.S./Canadian Brand Names** Abreva™ [OTC]

**Therapeutic Category** Antiviral Agent

**Use** Treatment of herpes simplex of the face or lips

**Usual Dosage** Children ≥12 years and Adults: Topical: Apply 5 times/day to affected area of face or lips. Start at first sign of cold sore or fever blister and continue until healed.

**Dosage Forms** Cream, topical: 10% (2 g)

## docusate (DOK yoo sate)

**Synonyms** dioctyl calcium sulfosuccinate; dioctyl potassium sulfosuccinate; dioctyl sodium sulfosuccinate; DOSS; DSS

**U.S./Canadian Brand Names** Colace® [OTC]; DC 240® Softgel® [OTC]; Dialose® Tablet [OTC]; Diocto® [OTC]; Diocto-K® [OTC]; Dioeze® [OTC]; Disonate® [OTC]; DOK® [OTC]; DOS® Softgel® [OTC]; Doxinate® Solution; D-S-S® [OTC]; Kasof® [OTC]; Modane® Soft [OTC]; Pro-Cal-Sof® [OTC]; Regulax SS® [OTC]; Selax® (Can); SoFlax™ (Can); Sulfalax® [OTC]; Surfak® [OTC]

**Therapeutic Category** Stool Softener

**Use** Stool softener in patients who should avoid straining during defecation and constipation associated with hard, dry stools

**Usual Dosage** Docusate salts are interchangeable; the amount of sodium, calcium, or potassium per dosage unit is clinically insignificant

Infants and Children <3 years: Oral: 10-40 mg/day in 1-4 divided doses

Children: Oral:

3-6 years: 20-60 mg/day in 1-4 divided doses

6-12 years: 40-150 mg/day in 1-4 divided doses

Adolescents and Adults: Oral: 50-500 mg/day in 1-4 divided doses

Older Children and Adults: Rectal: Add 50-100 mg of docusate liquid to enema fluid (saline or water); administer as retention or flushing enema

**Dosage Forms**

Capsule:

As calcium:

DC 240® Softgel®, Pro-Cal-Sof®, Sulfalax®: 240 mg

Surfak®: 50 mg, 240 mg

As potassium:

Diocto-K®: 100 mg

Kasof®: 240 mg

As sodium:

Colace®: 50 mg, 100 mg

Dioeze®: 250 mg

Disonate®: 100 mg, 240 mg

(Continued)

## docusate *(Continued)*

DOK®: 100 mg, 250 mg
DOS® Softgel®: 100 mg, 250 mg
D-S-S®: 100 mg
Modane® Soft: 100 mg
Regulax SS®: 100 mg, 250 mg

Liquid, as sodium (Diocto®, Colace®, Disonate®, DOK®): 150 mg/15 mL (30 mL, 60 mL, 480 mL)
Solution, oral, as sodium (Doxinate®): 50 mg/mL with alcohol 5% (60 mL, 3780 mL)
Syrup, as sodium:
50 mg/15 mL (15 mL, 30 mL)
Colace®, Diocto®, Disonate®, DOK®: 60 mg/15 mL (240 mL, 480 mL, 3780 mL)
Tablet, as sodium: 100 mg

## docusate and casanthranol (DOK yoo sate & ka SAN thra nole)

**U.S./Canadian Brand Names** Dialose® Plus Capsule [OTC]; Diocto C® [OTC]; Diocto-K Plus® [OTC]; Dioctolose Plus® [OTC]; Disanthrol® [OTC]; DSMC Plus® [OTC]; Genasoft® Plus [OTC]; Peri-Colace® [OTC]; Pro-Sof® Plus [OTC]; Regulace® [OTC]; Silace-C® [OTC]

**Therapeutic Category** Laxative/Stool Softner

**Use** Treatment of constipation generally associated with dry, hard stools and decreased intestinal motility

**Usual Dosage** Oral:

Children: 5-15 mL of syrup at bedtime or 1 capsule at bedtime

Adults: 1-2 capsules or 15-30 mL syrup at bedtime, may be increased to 2 capsules or 30 mL twice daily or 3 capsules at bedtime

**Dosage Forms**

Capsule:

Dialose® Plus, Diocto-K Plus®, Dioctolose Plus®, DSMC Plus®: Docusate potassium 100 mg and casanthranol 30 mg

Disanthrol®, Genasoft® Plus, Peri-Colace®, Pro-Sof® Plus, Regulace®: Docusate sodium 100 mg and casanthranol 30 mg

Syrup (Diocto C®, Peri-Colace®, Silace-C®): Docusate sodium 60 mg and casanthranol 30 mg per 15 mL with alcohol 10% (240 mL, 480 mL, 4000 mL)

## dofetilide (doe FET il ide)

**Synonyms** UK-68-798

**U.S./Canadian Brand Names** Tikosyn™

**Therapeutic Category** Antiarrhythmic Agent, Class III

**Use** Maintenance of normal sinus rhythm in patients with chronic atrial fibrillation/atrial flutter of longer than 1-week duration who have been converted to normal sinus rhythm; conversion of atrial fibrillation and atrial flutter to normal sinus rhythm

**Usual Dosage** Adults: Oral: Initial: 500 mcg orally twice daily.

**Dosage Forms** Capsule: 125 mcg, 250 mcg, 500 mcg

**DOK® [OTC]** *see* docusate *on previous page*

**Doktors® Nasal Solution [OTC]** *see* phenylephrine *on page 467*

**Dolacet®** *see* hydrocodone and acetaminophen *on page 300*

## dolasetron (dol A se tron)

**U.S./Canadian Brand Names** Anzemet®

**Therapeutic Category** Selective 5-$HT_3$ Receptor Antagonist

**Use** The prevention of nausea and vomiting associated with moderately emetogenic cancer chemotherapy, including initial and repeat courses; the prevention of postoperative nausea and vomiting.

### Usual Dosage

Oral:

Prevention of cancer chemotherapy-induced nausea and vomiting:

Children 2-16 years: 1.8 mg/kg given within 1 hour before chemotherapy, up to a maximum of 100 mg; safety and effectiveness in pediatric patients <2 years of age have not been established

Adults: 100 mg given within 1 hour before chemotherapy

Use in the elderly, renal failure patients, or hepatically impaired patients: No dosage adjustment is recommended

Prevention of postoperative nausea and vomiting:

Children 2-16 years: 1.2 mg/kg given within 2 hours before surgery, up to a maximum of 100 mg; safety and effectiveness in pediatric patients <2 years of age have not been established

Adults: 100 mg within 2 hours before surgery

Use in the elderly, renal failure patients, or hepatically impaired patients: No dosage adjustment is recommended

Parenteral (injection):

Prevention of cancer chemotherapy-induced nausea and vomiting:

Children 2-16 years: 1.8 mg/kg given as a single dose approximately 30 minutes before chemotherapy, up to a maximum of 100 mg; safety and effectiveness in pediatric patients <2 years of age have not been established. Injection mixed in apple or apple-grape juice may be used for oral dosing of pediatric patients. When injection is administered orally, the recommended dosage in pediatric patients 2-16 years of age is 1.8 mg/kg up to a maximum 100 mg dose given within 1 hour before chemotherapy. The diluted product may be kept up to 2 hours at room temperature before use.

Adults: From clinical trials, the dose is 1.8 mg/kg given as a single dose approximately 30 minutes before chemotherapy; alternatively, for most patients, a fixed dose of 100 mg can be administered over 30 seconds

Use in the elderly, renal failure patients, or hepatically impaired patients: No dosage adjustment is recommended

Prevention of postoperative nausea and/or vomiting:

Children 2-16 years: 0.35 mg/kg, with a maximum dose of 12.5 mg, given as a single dose approximately 15 minutes before the cessation of anesthesia or as soon as nausea or vomiting presents. Safety and effectiveness in pediatric patients <2 years of age have not been established. Injection mixed in apple or apple-grape juice may be used for oral dosing of pediatric patients; dosage in pediatric patients 2-16 years is 1.2 mg/kg up to a maximum 100 mg dose given before surgery.

Adults: 12.5 mg given as a single dose approximately 15 minutes before the cessation of anesthesia (prevention) or as soon as nausea or vomiting presents (treatment)

### Dosage Forms

Injection: 20 mg/mL (0.625 mL, 5 mL)

Tablet: 50 mg, 100 mg

**Dolene® *(Discontinued)*** *see page 750*

**Dolobid®** *see* diflunisal *on page 185*

**Dolono® [OTC]** *see* acetaminophen *on page 3*

**Dolono® Infants [OTC]** *see* acetaminophen *on page 3*

**Dolophine®** *see* methadone *on page 378*

**Dolorac™ *(Discontinued)*** *see page 750*

**Dolorex®** *see* capsaicin *on page 104*

**Dolotic®** *see* antipyrine and benzocaine *on page 44*

**Dolsed®** *see* methenamine, phenyl salicylate, atropine, hyoscyamine, benzoic acid, and methylene blue *on page 379*

**Domeboro® Topical [OTC]** *see* aluminum sulfate and calcium acetate *on page 28*

**Dommanate® Injection *(Discontinued)*** *see page 750*

## domperidone *(Canada only)* (dom PE ri done)

**U.S./Canadian Brand Names** Alti-Domperidone (Can); Apo®-Domperidone (Can); Motilium® (Can); Novo-Domperidone (Can); Nu-Domperidone (Can); PMS-Domperidone (Can)

**Therapeutic Category** Dopamine Antagonist

**Use** Symptomatic management of upper gastrointestinal motility disorders associated with chronic and subacute gastritis and diabetic gastroparesis; may also be used to prevent gastrointestinal symptoms associated with the use of dopamine agonist antiparkinsonian agents

**Usual Dosage** Adults: Oral:

Upper gastrointestinal motility disorders: Usual dosage in adults: 10 mg 3-4 times/day, 15-30 minutes before meals and at bedtime if required. In severe or resistant cases the dose may be increased to a maximum of 20 mg 3-4 times/day.

Nausea and vomiting associated with dopamine agonist antiparkinsonian agents: Usual dosage in adults: 20 mg 3-4 times/day. Higher doses may be required to achieve symptom control while titration of the antiparkinsonian medication is occurring.

**Dosage Forms** Tablet, as maleate: 12.72 mg [10 mg base]

## donepezil (don EH pa zil)

**Synonyms** E2020

**U.S./Canadian Brand Names** Aricept®

**Therapeutic Category** Acetylcholinesterase Inhibitor; Cholinergic Agent

**Use** Treatment of mild to moderate dementia of the Alzheimer's type

**Usual Dosage** Adults: Oral: Initial: 5 mg at bedtime; may be increased to 10 mg at bedtime after 4-6 weeks; a 10 mg dose may provide additional benefit for some patients

**Dosage Forms** Tablet: 5 mg, 10 mg

**Donnagel®-PG Suspension® (Can)** *see* kaolin and pectin with opium *on page 332*

**Donnamar®** *see* hyoscyamine *on page 309*

**Donnapectolin-PG®** *see* hyoscyamine, atropine, scopolamine, kaolin, pectin, and opium *on page 310*

**Donnatal®** *see* hyoscyamine, atropine, scopolamine, and phenobarbital *on page 310*

**Donnazyme®** *see* pancreatin *on page 447*

**Donphen® Tablet *(Discontinued)*** *see page 750*

## dopamine (DOE pa meen)

**Therapeutic Category** Adrenergic Agonist Agent

**Use** Adjunct in the treatment of shock which persists after adequate fluid volume replacement

**Usual Dosage** I.V. infusion:

Children: 1-20 mcg/kg/minute, maximum: 50 mcg/kg/minute continuous infusion, titrate to desired response

Adults: 1 mcg/kg/minute up to 50 mcg/kg/minute, titrate to desired response

If dosages >20-30 mcg/kg/minute are needed, a more direct acting pressor may be more beneficial (ie, epinephrine, norepinephrine)

Hemodynamic effects of dopamine are dose-dependent:

Low-dose: 1-5 mcg/kg/minute, increased renal blood flow and urine output

Intermediate-dose: 5-15 mcg/kg/minute, increased renal blood flow, heart rate, cardiac contractility, and cardiac output

High-dose: >15 mcg/kg/minute, alpha-adrenergic effects begin to predominate, vasoconstriction, increased blood pressure

**Dosage Forms**

Infusion, as hydrochloride, in $D_5W$: 0.8 mg/mL (250 mL, 500 mL); 1.6 mg/mL (250 mL, 500 mL); 3.2 mg/mL (250 mL, 500 mL)

Injection, as hydrochloride: 40 mg/mL (5 mL, 10 mL, 20 mL); 80 mg/mL (5 mL, 20 mL); 160 mg/mL (5 mL)

**Dopar® *(Discontinued)*** *see page 750*

**Dopastat® Injection *(Discontinued)*** *see page 750*

**Dopram®** *see* doxapram *on next page*

**Doral®** *see* quazepam *on page 512*

**Doriden® Tablet *(Discontinued)*** *see page 750*

**Dormarex® 2 Oral [OTC]** *see* diphenhydramine *on page 191*

**Dormin® Oral [OTC]** *see* diphenhydramine *on page 191*

## dornase alfa (DOOR nase AL fa)

**Synonyms** DNASE; recombinant human deoxyribonuclease

**U.S./Canadian Brand Names** Pulmozyme®

**Therapeutic Category** Enzyme

**Use** Management of cystic fibrosis patients to reduce the frequency of respiratory infections and to improve pulmonary function

**Usual Dosage** Children >5 years and Adults: Inhalation: 2.5 mg once daily through selected nebulizers in conjunction with a Pulmo-Aide® or a Pari-Proneb® compressor

**Dosage Forms** Solution, inhalation: 1 mg/mL (2.5 mL)

**Doryx®** *see* doxycycline *on page 204*

## dorzolamide (dor ZOLE a mide)

**U.S./Canadian Brand Names** Trusopt®

**Therapeutic Category** Carbonic Anhydrase Inhibitor

**Use** Lower intraocular pressure to treat glaucoma

**Usual Dosage** Adults: Ophthalmic: 1 drop in eye(s) 3 times/day

**Dosage Forms** Solution, ophthalmic, as hydrochloride: 2%

## dorzolamide and timolol (dor ZOLE a mide & TYE moe lole)

**U.S./Canadian Brand Names** Cosopt®

**Therapeutic Category** Beta-Adrenergic Blocker; Carbonic Anhydrase Inhibitor

**Use** Lowers intraocular pressure to treat glaucoma in patients with ocular hypertension or open-angle glaucoma

**Usual Dosage** Adults: ophthalmic: One drop in eye(s) twice daily

**Dosage Forms** Solution, ophthalmic: Dorzolamide 2% and timolol 0.5% (5 mL, 10 mL)

**DOSS** *see* docusate *on page 197*

**DOS® Softgel® [OTC]** *see* docusate *on page 197*

**Dostinex®** *see* cabergoline *on page 94*

**Double-Action Pain Relief® [OTC]** *see* acetaminophen, aspirin, and caffeine *on page 6*

**Double Cap®** *see* capsaicin *on page 104*

**Dovonex®** *see* calcipotriene *on page 96*

## doxacurium (doks a KYOO ri um)

**U.S./Canadian Brand Names** Nuromax®

**Therapeutic Category** Skeletal Muscle Relaxant

(Continued)

## doxacurium *(Continued)*

**Use** Doxacurium is indicated for use as an adjunct to general anesthesia. It provides skeletal muscle relaxation during surgery or endotracheal intubation; increases pulmonary compliance during mechanical ventilation

**Usual Dosage** I.V. (in obese patients, use ideal body weight to calculate dosage):

Children >2 years: Initial: 0.03-0.05 mg/kg followed by maintenance doses of 0.005-0.01 mg/kg after 30-45 minutes

Adults: Surgery: 0.05 mg/kg with thiopental/narcotic or 0.025 mg/kg with succinylcholine; maintenance dose: 0.005-0.01 mg/kg after 60-100 minutes

**Dosage Forms** Injection, as chloride: 1 mg/mL (5 mL)

## doxapram (DOKS a pram)

**U.S./Canadian Brand Names** Dopram®

**Therapeutic Category** Respiratory Stimulant

**Use** Respiratory and CNS stimulant; idiopathic apnea of prematurity refractory to xanthines

**Usual Dosage** I.V.:

Neonatal apnea (apnea of prematurity):

Initial: 0.5 mg/kg/hour

Maintenance: 0.5-2.5 mg/kg/hour, titrated to the lowest rate at which apnea is controlled

Adults: Respiratory depression following anesthesia:

Initial: 0.5-1 mg/kg; may repeat at 5-minute intervals; maximum total dose: 2 mg/kg; single doses should not exceed 1.5 mg/kg

I.V. infusion: Initial: 5 mg/minute until adequate response or adverse effects seen; decrease to 1-3 mg/minute; usual total dose: 0.5-4 mg/kg; maximum: 300 mg

**Dosage Forms** Injection, as hydrochloride: 20 mg/mL (20 mL)

## doxazosin (doks AYE zoe sin)

**U.S./Canadian Brand Names** Apo®-Doxazosin (Can); Cardura®; Gen-Doxazosin (Can)

**Therapeutic Category** Alpha-Adrenergic Blocking Agent

**Use** Alpha-adrenergic blocking agent for treatment of hypertension

**Usual Dosage** Adults: Oral: 1 mg once daily, may be increased to 2 mg once daily thereafter up to 16 mg if needed

**Dosage Forms** Tablet: 1 mg, 2 mg, 4 mg, 8 mg

## doxepin (DOKS e pin)

**U.S./Canadian Brand Names** Alti-Doxepin (Can); Apo®-Doxepin (Can); Novo-Doxepin (Can); Sinequan® Oral; Zonalon® Topical Cream

**Therapeutic Category** Antidepressant, Tricyclic (Tertiary Amine); Topical Skin Product

**Use**

Oral: Treatment of various forms of depression, usually in conjunction with psychotherapy; treatment of anxiety disorders; analgesic for certain chronic and neuropathic pain

Topical: Adults: Short-term (<8 days) therapy of moderate pruritus due to atopic dermatitis or lichen simplex chronicus

**Usual Dosage**

Oral:

Adolescents: Initial: 25-50 mg/day in single or divided doses; gradually increase to 100 mg/day

Adults: Initial: 30-150 mg/day at bedtime or in 2-3 divided doses; may increase up to 300 mg/day; single dose should not exceed 150 mg; select patients may respond to 25-50 mg/day

Topical: Apply in a thin film 4 times/day

**Dosage Forms**

Capsule, as hydrochloride: 10 mg, 25 mg, 50 mg, 75 mg, 100 mg, 150 mg

Concentrate, oral, as hydrochloride: 10 mg/mL (120 mL)

Cream: 5% (30 g)

**doxercalciferol** (dox er kal si fe FEER ole)

**U.S./Canadian Brand Names** Hectorol®

**Therapeutic Category** Vitamin D Analog

**Use** Reduction of elevated intact parathyroid hormone (iPTH) in the management of secondary hyperparathyroidism in patients on chronic hemodialysis.

**Usual Dosage** Adults: Oral: If the iPTH >400 pg/mL, then the initial dose is 10 mcg 3 times/week at dialysis. The dose is adjusted at 8-week intervals based upon the iPTH levels. If the iPTH level is decreased by 50% and above 300 pg/mL, then the dose can be increased to 12.5 mcg 3 times/week for 8 more weeks. This titration process can continue at 8-week intervals up to a maximum dose of 20 mcg 3 times/week. Each increase should be by 2.5 mcg/dose. If the iPTH is between 150-300 pg/mL, maintain the current dose. If the iPTH is <100 pg/mL, then suspend the drug for 1 week. Resume doxercalciferol at a reduced dose. Decrease each dose (not weekly dose) by at least 2.5 mcg.

**Dosage Forms** Capsule: 2.5 mcg

**Doxil®** *see* doxorubicin (liposomal) *on this page*

**Doxinate® Capsule *(Discontinued)*** *see page 750*

**Doxinate® Solution** *see* docusate *on page 197*

**doxorubicin** (doks oh ROO bi sin)

**Synonyms** ADR; hydroxydaunomycin

**U.S./Canadian Brand Names** Adriamycin PFS®; Adriamycin RDF®; Caelyx® (Can); Rubex®

**Therapeutic Category** Antineoplastic Agent

**Use** Treatment of various solid tumors including ovarian, breast, and bladder tumors; various lymphomas and leukemias (ANL, ALL), soft tissue sarcomas, neuroblastoma, osteosarcoma

**Usual Dosage** I.V. (refer to individual protocols; patient's ideal weight should be used to calculate body surface area):

Children: 35-75 mg/m$^2$ as a single dose, repeat every 21 days; or 20 mg/m$^2$ once weekly

Adults: 60-75 mg/m$^2$ as a single dose, repeat every 21 days or other dosage regimens like 20-30 mg/m$^2$/day for 2-3 days, repeat in 4 weeks or 20 mg/m$^2$ once weekly

The lower dose regimen should be administered to patients with decreased bone marrow reserve, prior therapy or marrow infiltration with malignant cells

**Dosage Forms**

Injection, as hydrochloride:

Aqueous, with NS: 2 mg/mL (5 mL, 10 mL, 25 mL)

Preservative free: 2 mg/mL (5 mL, 10 mL, 25 mL, 100 mL)

Powder for injection, as hydrochloride, lyophilized: 10 mg, 20 mg, 50 mg, 100 mg

Powder for injection, as hydrochloride, lyophilized, rapid dissolution formula: 10 mg, 20 mg, 50 mg, 150 mg

**doxorubicin (liposomal)** (doks oh ROO bi sin lip pah SOW mal)

**U.S./Canadian Brand Names** Doxil®

**Therapeutic Category** Antineoplastic Agent

**Use** Treatment of AIDS-related Kaposi's sarcoma in patients with disease that has progressed on prior combination chemotherapy or in patients who are intolerant to such therapy; treatment of metastatic carcinoma of the ovary in patients with disease that is refractory to both paclitaxel and platinum-based regimens

**Usual Dosage** Refer to individual protocols

I.V. (patient's ideal weight should be used to calculate body surface area): 20 mg/m$^2$ over 30 minutes, once every 3 weeks, for as long as patients respond satisfactorily and tolerate treatment.

(Continued)

## doxorubicin (liposomal) *(Continued)*

AIDS-KS patients: I.V.: 20 mg/m²/dose over 30 minutes once every 3 weeks for as long as patients respond satisfactorily and tolerate treatment

Breast cancer: I.V.: 20-80 mg/m²/dose has been studied in a limited number of phase I/II trials

Ovarian cancer: I.V.: 50 mg/m²/dose repeated every 4 weeks (minimum of 4 courses is recommended)

Solid tumors: I.V.: 50-60 mg/m²/dose repeated every 3-4 weeks has been studied in a limited number of phase I/II trials

**Dosage Forms** Injection, as hydrochloride: 2 mg/mL (10 mL)

**Doxy-100®** *see* doxycycline *on this page*

**Doxycin (Can)** *see* doxycycline *on this page*

## doxycycline (doks i SYE kleen)

**U.S./Canadian Brand Names** Apo®-Doxy Tabs (Can); Doryx®; Doxy-100®; Doxycin (Can); Doxytec (Can); Monodox®; Novo-Doxylin (Can); Nu-Doxycycline (Can); Vibramycin®; Vibra-Tabs®

**Therapeutic Category** Tetracycline Derivative

**Use**

Children, Adolescents, and Adults: Treatment of Rocky Mountain spotted fever caused by susceptible *Rickettsia* or brucellosis

Older Children, Adolescents, and Adults: Treatment of Lyme disease, mycoplasmal disease, or *Legionella*; management of malignant pleural effusions when intrapleural therapy is indicated

Adolescents and Adults: Treatment of nongonococcal pelvic inflammatory disease and urethritis due to *Chlamydia*; treatment for victims of sexual assault

Adults: Periostat® (20 mg capsule) is used as an adjunct to scaling and root planing to promote attachment level gain and to reduce pocket depth in patients with adult periodontitis

**Unapproved use:** Treatment for syphilis in penicillin-allergic patients; sclerosing agent for pleural effusions

**Usual Dosage** Oral, I.V.:

Children ≥8 years (<45 kg): 2-5 mg/kg/day in 1-2 divided doses, not to exceed 200 mg/day

Children >8 years (>45 kg) and Adults: 100-200 mg/day in 1-2 divided doses

Sclerosing agent for pleural effusion injection: 500 mg as a single dose in 30-50 mL of NS or SWI

Adults: Periodontitis: 20 mg twice/day for up to 9 months; safety beyond 12 months and efficacy beyond 9 months have not been established

**Dosage Forms**

Capsule, as hyclate:

Periostat®: 20 mg

Doxychel®, Vibramycin®: 50 mg

Doxy®, Doxychel®, Vibramycin®: 100 mg

Capsule, coated pellets, as hyclate (Doryx®): 100 mg

Gel, for subgingival application: Atridox™: 50 mg in each 500 mg of blended formulation; 2-syringe system contains doxycycline syringe (50 mg) and delivery system syringe (450 mg) along with a blunt cannula

Powder for injection, as hyclate (Doxy®, Doxychel®, Vibramycin® IV): 100 mg, 200 mg

Powder for oral suspension, as monohydrate (raspberry flavor) (Vibramycin®): 25 mg/5 mL (60 mL)

Syrup, as calcium (raspberry-apple flavor) (Vibramycin®): 50 mg/5 mL (30 mL, 473 mL)

Tablet, as hyclate (Vibra-Tabs®): 100 mg

**Doxytec (Can)** *see* doxycycline *on this page*

**DPA** *see* valproic acid and derivatives *on page 620*

## dronabinol (droe NAB i nol)

**Synonyms** tetrahydrocannabinol; THC

**U.S./Canadian Brand Names** Marinol®

**Therapeutic Category** Antiemetic

**Controlled Substance** C-III

**Use** Treatment of nausea and vomiting secondary to cancer chemotherapy in patients who have not responded to conventional antiemetics; treatment of anorexia associated with weight loss in AIDS patients

**Usual Dosage** Oral:

Children: NCI protocol recommends 5 mg/m$^2$ starting 6-8 hours before chemotherapy and every 4-6 hours after to be continued for 12 hours after chemotherapy is discontinued

Adults: 5 mg/m$^2$ 1-3 hours before chemotherapy, then administer 5 mg/m$^2$/dose every 2-4 hours after chemotherapy for a total of 4-6 doses/day; dose may be increased up to a

(Continued)

## dronabinol *(Continued)*

maximum of 15 mg/m$^2$/dose if needed (dosage may be increased by 2.5 mg/m$^2$ increments)

**Dosage Forms** Capsule: 2.5 mg, 5 mg, 10 mg

## droperidol (droe PER i dole)

**U.S./Canadian Brand Names** Inapsine®

**Therapeutic Category** Antiemetic; Antipsychotic Agent, Butyrophenone

**Use** Tranquilizer and antiemetic in surgical and diagnostic procedures; antiemetic for cancer chemotherapy; preoperative medication

**Usual Dosage** Titrate carefully to desired effect

Children 2-12 years:

Premedication: I.M.: 0.088-0.165 mg/kg; smaller doses may be sufficient for control of nausea or vomiting

Adjunct to general anesthesia: I.V. induction: 0.088-0.165 mg/kg

Nausea and vomiting: I.M., I.V.: 0.05-0.06 mg/kg/dose every 4-6 hours as needed

Adults:

Premedication: I.M., I.V.: 2.5-10 mg 30 minutes to 1 hour preoperatively

Adjunct to general anesthesia: I.V. induction: 0.22-0.275 mg/kg; maintenance: 1.25-2.5 mg/dose

Alone in diagnostic procedures: I.M.: Initial: 2.5-10 mg 30 minutes to 1 hour before; then 1.25-2.5 mg if needed

Nausea and vomiting: I.M., I.V.: 2.5-5 mg/dose every 3-4 hours as needed

**Dosage Forms** Injection: 2.5 mg/mL (1 mL, 2 mL, 5 mL, 10 mL)

## droperidol and fentanyl (droe PER i dole & FEN ta nil)

**U.S./Canadian Brand Names** Innovar®

**Therapeutic Category** Analgesic, Narcotic

**Use** Produce and maintain analgesia and sedation during diagnostic or surgical procedures (neuroleptanalgesia and neuroleptanesthesia); adjunct to general anesthesia

**Usual Dosage**

Children:

Premedication: I.M.: 0.03 mL/kg 30-60 minutes prior to surgery

Adjunct to general anesthesia: I.V.: Total dose: 0.05 mL/kg as slow infusion (1 mL/1-2 minutes) until sleep occurs

Adults:

Premedication: I.M.: 0.5-2 mL 30-60 minutes prior to surgery

Adjunct to general anesthesia: I.V.: 0.09-0.11 mL/kg as slow infusion (1 mL/1-2 minutes) until sleep occurs

**Dosage Forms** Injection: Droperidol 2.5 mg and fentanyl 50 mcg per mL (2 mL, 5 mL)

**Droxia**™ *see* hydroxyurea *on page 307*

**Drug Products No Longer Available** *see page 750*

**Dry Eyes® Solution [OTC]** *see* artificial tears *on page 53*

**Dry Eye® Therapy Solution [OTC]** *see* artificial tears *on page 53*

**Drysol**™ *see* aluminum chloride hexahydrate *on page 26*

**DSCG** *see* cromolyn sodium *on page 156*

**DSMC Plus® [OTC]** *see* docusate and casanthranol *on page 198*

**DSS** *see* docusate *on page 197*

**D-S-S® [OTC]** *see* docusate *on page 197*

**D-S-S Plus®** ***(Discontinued)*** *see page 750*

**DT** *see* diphtheria and tetanus toxoid *on page 192*

**DTAP** *see* diphtheria, tetanus toxoids, and acellular pertussis vaccine *on page 193*

**Dwelle® Ophthalmic Solution [OTC]** *see* artificial tears *on page 53*

## d-xylose (dee ZYE lose)

**Synonyms** wood sugar

**U.S./Canadian Brand Names** Xylo-Pfan® [OTC]

**Therapeutic Category** Diagnostic Agent

**Use** Evaluating intestinal absorption and diagnosing malabsorptive states

**Usual Dosage** Oral:

Infants and young Children: 500 mg/kg as a 5% to 10% aqueous solution

Children: 5 g is dissolved in 250 mL water; additional fluids are permitted and are encouraged for children

Adults: 25 g dissolved in 200-300 mL water followed with an additional 200-400 mL water **or** 5 g dissolved in 200-300 mL water followed by an additional 200-400 mL water

**Dosage Forms** Powder for oral solution: 25 g

**Dyazide®** *see* hydrochlorothiazide and triamterene *on page 299*

**Dycill®** ***(Discontinued)*** *see page 750*

**Dyclone®** *see* dyclonine *on this page*

## dyclonine (DYE kloe neen)

**U.S./Canadian Brand Names** Dyclone®; Sucrets® [OTC]

**Therapeutic Category** Local Anesthetic

**Use** Local anesthetic prior to laryngoscopy, bronchoscopy, or endotracheal intubation; used topically for temporary relief of pain associated with oral mucosa, skin, episiotomy, or anogenital lesions; the 0.5% topical solution may be used to block the gag reflex, and to relieve the pain of oral ulcers or stomatitis

**Usual Dosage**

Children and Adults: Topical solution:

Mouth sores: 5-10 mL of 0.5% or 1% to oral mucosa (swab or swish and then spit) 3-4 times/day as needed; maximum single dose: 200 mg (40 mL of 0.5% solution or 20 mL of 1% solution)

Bronchoscopy: Use 2 mL of the 1% solution or 4 mL of the 0.5% solution sprayed onto the larynx and trachea every 5 minutes until the reflex has been abolished

Children >3 years and Adults: Lozenge: Dissolve 1 in mouth slowly every 2 hours

**Dosage Forms**

Lozenges, as hydrochloride: 1.2 mg, 3 mg

Solution, topical, as hydrochloride: 0.5% (30 mL); 1% (30 mL)

**Dyflex-400® Tablet** ***(Discontinued)*** *see page 750*

**Dylix®** *see* dyphylline *on this page*

**Dymenate® Injection** *see* dimenhydrinate *on page 188*

**Dynabac®** *see* dirithromycin *on page 195*

**Dynacin® Oral** *see* minocycline *on page 394*

**DynaCirc®** *see* isradipine *on page 329*

**Dyna-Hex® [OTC]** *see* chlorhexidine gluconate *on page 126*

**Dynapen®** *see* dicloxacillin *on page 182*

## dyphylline (DYE fi lin)

**Synonyms** dihydroxypropyl theophylline

**U.S./Canadian Brand Names** Dilor®; Dylix®; Lufyllin®

**Therapeutic Category** Theophylline Derivative

**Use** Bronchodilator in reversible airway obstruction due to asthma or COPD

**Usual Dosage**

Children: I.M.: 4.4-6.6 mg/kg/day in divided doses

Adults:
Oral: Up to 15 mg/kg 4 times/day, individualize dosage
I.M.: 250-500 mg, do not exceed total dosage of 15 mg/kg every 6 hours

**Dosage Forms**
Elixir:
Dylix®, Lufyllin®: 100 mg/15 mL with alcohol 20% (473 mL, 3780 mL)
Dilor®: 160 mg/15 mL with alcohol 18% (473 mL)
Injection (Dilor®, Lufyllin®): 250 mg/mL (2 mL)
Tablet: 200 mg, 400 mg
Dilor®, Lufyllin®: 200 mg, 400 mg

**Dyrenium®** *see* triamterene *on page 603*

**E2020** *see* donepezil *on page 200*

**Easprin®** *see* aspirin *on page 55*

## echothiophate iodide (ek oh THYE oh fate EYE oh dide)

**U.S./Canadian Brand Names** Phospholine Iodide® Ophthalmic

**Therapeutic Category** Cholinesterase Inhibitor

**Use** Reverse toxic CNS effects caused by anticholinergic drugs; used as miotic in treatment of glaucoma

**Usual Dosage** Adults: Ophthalmic: Glaucoma: Instill 1 drop twice daily into eyes with one dose just prior to bedtime; some patients have been treated with 1 dose/day or every other day. Use lowest concentration and frequency which gives satisfactory response, with a maximum dose of 0.125% once daily, although more intensive therapy may be used for short periods of time

**Dosage Forms** Powder for reconstitution, ophthalmic: 1.5 mg [0.03%] (5 mL); 3 mg [0.06%] (5 mL); 6.25 mg [0.125%] (5 mL); 12.5 mg [0.25%] (5 mL)

**Eckogesic® [OTC]** *see* acetaminophen and phenyltoloxamine *on page 5*

**E-Complex-600® [OTC]** *see* vitamin E *on page 631*

## econazole (e KONE a zole)

**U.S./Canadian Brand Names** Ecostatin® (Can); Spectazole™

**Therapeutic Category** Antifungal Agent

**Use** Topical treatment of tinea pedis, tinea cruris, tinea corporis, tinea versicolor, and cutaneous candidiasis

**Usual Dosage** Children and Adults: Topical: Apply a sufficient amount to cover affected areas once daily; for cutaneous candidiasis: apply twice daily; candidal infections and tinea cruris, versicolor, and corporis should be treated for 2 weeks and tinea pedis for 1 month; occasionally, longer treatment periods may be required

**Dosage Forms** Cream, as nitrate: 1% (15 g, 30 g, 85 g)

**Econopred® Ophthalmic** *see* prednisolone (ophthalmic) *on page 492*

**Econopred® Plus Ophthalmic** *see* prednisolone (ophthalmic) *on page 492*

**Ecostatin® (Can)** *see* econazole *on this page*

**Ecotrin® [OTC]** *see* aspirin *on page 55*

**Ecotrin® Low Adult Strength [OTC]** *see* aspirin *on page 55*

**Ed A-Hist® Liquid** *see* chlorpheniramine and phenylephrine *on page 129*

**edathamil disodium** *see* edetate disodium *on next page*

**Edecrin®** *see* ethacrynic acid *on page 229*

## edetate calcium disodium (ED e tate KAL see um dye SOW dee um)

**Synonyms** calcium edta

**U.S./Canadian Brand Names** Calcium Disodium Versenate®

**Therapeutic Category** Chelating Agent

(Continued)

## edetate calcium disodium *(Continued)*

**Use** Treatment of acute and chronic lead poisoning; also used as an aid in the diagnosis of lead poisoning

**Usual Dosage**

Children:

Diagnosis of lead poisoning: Mobilization test: (Asymptomatic patients or lead levels <55 mcg/dL): (**Note:** Urine is collected for 24 hours after first EDTA dose and analyzed for lead content; if the ratio of mcg of lead in urine to mg calcium EDTA given is >1, then test is considered positive): Children: 500 mg/m$^2$ (maximum: 1 g/dose) I.M. or I.V. over 1 hour **or** 2 doses of 500 mg/m$^2$ at 12-hour intervals

Asymptomatic lead poisoning: (Blood lead concentration >55 mcg/dL or blood lead concentrations of 25-55 mcg/dL with blood erythrocyte protoporphyrin concentrations of ≥35 mcg/dL and positive mobilization test) or symptomatic lead poisoning without encephalopathy with lead level <100 mcg/dL: 1 g/m$^2$/day I.M./I.V. in divided doses every 8-12 hours for 3-5 days (usually 5 days); maximum: 1 g/24 hours or 50 mg/kg/day

Symptomatic lead poisoning with encephalopathy with lead level >100 mcg/dL (treatment with calcium EDTA and dimercaprol is preferred): 250 mg/m$^2$ I.M. or intermittent I.V. infusion 4 hours after dimercaprol, then at 4-hour intervals thereafter for 5 days (1.5 g/m$^2$/day); dose (1.5 g/m$^2$/day) can also be administered as a single I.V. continuous infusion over 12-24 hours/day for 5 days; maximum: 1 g/24 hours or 75 mg/kg/day

**Note:** Course of therapy may be repeated in 2-3 weeks until blood lead level is normal

Adults: I.M., I.V.:

Diagnosis of lead poisoning: 500 mg/m$^2$ (maximum: 1 g/dose) over 1 hour

Treatment: 2 g/day or 1.5 g/m$^2$/day in divided doses every 12-24 hours for 5 days; may repeat course one time after at least 2 days (usually after 2 weeks)

**Dosage Forms** Injection: 200 mg/mL (5 mL)

## edetate disodium (ED e tate dye SOW dee um)

**Synonyms** edathamil disodium; EDTA; sodium edetate

**U.S./Canadian Brand Names** Chealamide®; Disotate®; Endrate®

**Therapeutic Category** Chelating Agent

**Use** Emergency treatment of hypercalcemia; control digitalis-induced cardiac dysrhythmias (ventricular arrhythmias)

**Usual Dosage** I.V.:

Hypercalcemia:

Children: 40-70 mg/kg slow infusion over 3-4 hours

Adults: 50 mg/kg/day over 3 or more hours

Dysrhythmias: Children and Adults: 15 mg/kg/hour up to 60 mg/kg/day

**Dosage Forms** Injection: 150 mg/mL (20 mL)

**Edex® Injection** *see* alprostadil *on page 23*

## edrophonium (ed roe FOE nee um)

**U.S./Canadian Brand Names** Enlon®; Reversol®; Tensilon®

**Therapeutic Category** Cholinergic Agent

**Use** Diagnosis of myasthenia gravis; differentiation of cholinergic crises from myasthenia crises; reversal of nondepolarizing neuromuscular blockers; treatment of paroxysmal atrial tachycardia

**Usual Dosage**

Infants: I.V.: Initial: 0.1 mg, followed by 0.4 mg if no response; total dose: 0.5 mg

Children:

Diagnosis: Initial: 0.04 mg/kg followed by 0.16 mg/kg if no response, to a maximum total dose of 5 mg for children ≤34 kg, or 10 mg for children >34 kg

Titration of oral anticholinesterase therapy: 0.04 mg/kg once; if strength improves, an increase in neostigmine or pyridostigmine dose is indicated

Adults:

Diagnosis: I.V.: 2 mg test dose administered over 15-30 seconds; 8 mg administered 45 seconds later if no response is seen. Test dose may be repeated after 30 minutes.

Titration of oral anticholinesterase therapy: 1-2 mg administered 1 hour after oral dose of anticholinesterase; if strength improves, an increase in neostigmine or pyridostigmine dose is indicated

Differentiation of cholinergic from myasthenic crisis: I.V.: 1 mg, may repeat after 1 minute (**Note:** Intubation and controlled ventilation may be required if patient has cholinergic crises.)

Reversal of nondepolarizing neuromuscular blocking agents (neostigmine with atropine usually preferred): I.V.: 10 mg, may repeat every 5-10 minutes up to 40 mg

Termination of paroxysmal atrial tachycardia: I.V.: 5-10 mg

**Dosage Forms** Injection, as chloride: 10 mg/mL (1 mL, 10 mL, 15 mL)

**ED-SPAZ®** *see* hyoscyamine *on page 309*

**EDTA** *see* edetate disodium *on previous page*

**E.E.S.®** *see* erythromycin (systemic) *on page 222*

**E.E.S.® Chewable** *see* erythromycin (systemic) *on page 222*

**E.E.S.® Granules** *see* erythromycin (systemic) *on page 222*

## efavirenz (e FAV e renz)

**U.S./Canadian Brand Names** Sustiva™

**Therapeutic Category** Non-nucleoside Reverse Transcriptase Inhibitor (NNRTI)

**Use** Treatment of HIV-1 infections in combination with at least 2 other antiretroviral agents. Also has some activity against hepatitis B virus and herpes viruses.

**Usual Dosage** Dosing at bedtime is recommended to limit central nervous system effects; should not be used as single-agent therapy

Oral:

Adults: 600 mg once daily

Children: Dosage is based on body weight

10 to <15 kg: 200 mg

15 to <20 kg: 250 mg

20 to <25 kg: 300 mg

25 to <32.5 kg: 350 mg

32.5 to <40 kg: 400 mg

≥40 kg: 600 mg

**Dosage Forms** Capsule: 50 mg, 100 mg, 200 mg

**Effer-K™** *see* potassium bicarbonate and potassium citrate, effervescent *on page 485*

**Effer-Syllium® [OTC]** *see* psyllium *on page 509*

**Effexor®** *see* venlafaxine *on page 624*

**Effexor-XR®** *see* venlafaxine *on page 624*

**Efidac/24® [OTC]** *see* pseudoephedrine *on page 507*

## eflornithine (ee FLOR ni theen)

**Synonyms** DFMO

**U.S./Canadian Brand Names** Ornidyl® Injection; Vaniqa™ Cream

**Therapeutic Category** Antiprotozoal; Topical Skin Product

**Use**

Injection: Treatment of meningoencephalitic stage of *Trypanosoma brucei gambiense* infection (sleeping sickness)

Cream, females ≥12 years: Reduce unwanted hair from face and adjacent areas under the chin

(Continued)

## eflornithine *(Continued)*

### Usual Dosage

Children ≥12 years and Adults: Females: Topical: Apply thin layer of cream to affected areas of face and adjacent chin twice daily, at least 8 hours apart

Adults: I.V. infusion: 100 mg/kg/dose given every 6 hours (over at least 45 minutes) for 14 days

### Dosage Forms

Cream, as hydrochloride: 13.9% (30 g)

Injection, as hydrochloride: 200 mg/mL (100 mL)

**Efodine® *(Discontinued)*** *see page 750*

**Efudex® Topical** *see* fluorouracil *on page 256*

**EHDP** *see* etidronate disodium *on page 235*

**Elase®-Chloromycetin® Ointment *(Discontinued)*** *see page 750*

**Elase® Topical** *see* fibrinolysin and desoxyribonuclease *on page 248*

**Elavil®** *see* amitriptyline *on page 33*

**Eldecort® Topical** *see* hydrocortisone (topical) *on page 304*

**Eldepryl®** *see* selegiline *on page 540*

**Eldepryl® Tablet (only) *(Discontinued)*** *see page 750*

**Eldercaps® [OTC]** *see* vitamin (multiple/oral) *on page 632*

**Eldopaque® [OTC]** *see* hydroquinone *on page 305*

**Eldopaque Forte®** *see* hydroquinone *on page 305*

**Eldoquin® [OTC]** *see* hydroquinone *on page 305*

**Eldoquin® Forte®** *see* hydroquinone *on page 305*

**Eldoquin® Lotion *(Discontinued)*** *see page 750*

**Elimite™ Cream** *see* permethrin *on page 462*

**Elixomin® *(Discontinued)*** *see page 750*

**Elixophyllin®** *see* theophylline *on page 581*

**Elixophyllin-GG®** *see* theophylline and guaifenesin *on page 583*

**Elixophyllin SR® *(Discontinued)*** *see page 750*

**Ellence™** *see* epirubicin *on page 217*

**Elmiron®** *see* pentosan polysulfate sodium *on page 459*

**Elocom® (Can)** *see* mometasone furoate *on page 398*

**Elocon®** *see* mometasone furoate *on page 398*

**E-Lor® Tablet *(Discontinued)*** *see page 750*

**Elspar®** *see* asparaginase *on page 55*

**Eltor® 120 (Can)** *see* pseudoephedrine *on page 507*

**Eltor® (Can)** *see* pseudoephedrine *on page 507*

**Eltroxin® (Can)** *see* levothyroxine *on page 348*

**Embeline E®** *see* clobetasol *on page 143*

**Emcyt®** *see* estramustine *on page 226*

**Emecheck® [OTC]** *see* phosphorated carbohydrate solution *on page 469*

**Emete-Con® Injection *(Discontinued)*** *see page 750*

**emetine hydrochloride *(Discontinued)*** *see page 750*

**Emetrol® [OTC]** *see* phosphorated carbohydrate solution *on page 469*

**Emgel™ Topical** *see* erythromycin (ophthalmic/topical) *on page 222*

**Eminase®** *see* anistreplase *on page 41*

**Emitrip® *(Discontinued)*** *see page 750*

**Emko® [OTC]** *see* nonoxynol 9 *on page 424*

**EMLA®** *see* lidocaine and prilocaine *on page 350*

**Empirin® [OTC]** *see* aspirin *on page 55*

**Empirin® With Codeine** *see* aspirin and codeine *on page 56*

**EmTet-500®** *see* tetracycline *on page 579*

**Emulsoil® [OTC]** *see* castor oil *on page 112*

**E-Mycin®** *see* erythromycin (systemic) *on page 222*

**E-Mycin-E®** *see* erythromycin (systemic) *on page 222*

**ENA 713** *see* rivastigmine *on page 529*

## enalapril (e NAL a pril)

**U.S./Canadian Brand Names** Apo®-Enalapril (Can); Vasotec® I.V.; Vasotec® Oral

**Therapeutic Category** Angiotensin-Converting Enzyme (ACE) Inhibitor

**Use** Management of mild to severe hypertension, congestive heart failure, and asymptomatic left ventricular dysfunction

**Usual Dosage** Use lower listed initial dose in patients with hyponatremia, hypovolemia, severe congestive heart failure, decreased renal function, or in those receiving diuretics

Children:

Investigational initial oral doses of enalapril of 0.1 mg/kg/day increasing over 2 weeks to 0.12-0.43 mg/kg/day have been used to treat severe congestive heart failure in infants (n=8)

Investigational I.V. doses of enalaprilat of 5-10 mcg/kg/dose administered every 8-24 hours (as determined by blood pressure readings) have been used for the treatment of neonatal hypertension (n=10); monitor patients carefully; select patients may require higher doses

Adults:

Oral: **Enalapril**: 2.5-5 mg/day then increase as required, usually 10-40 mg/day in 1-2 divided doses

I.V.: **Enalaprilat**: 0.625-1.25 mg/dose, administered over 5 minutes every 6 hours

**Dosage Forms**

Injection, as enalaprilat: 1.25 mg/mL (1 mL, 2 mL)

Tablet, as maleate: 2.5 mg, 5 mg, 10 mg, 20 mg

## enalapril and diltiazem (e NAL a pril & dil TYE a zem)

**U.S./Canadian Brand Names** Teczem®

**Therapeutic Category** Antihypertensive Agent, Combination

**Use** Combination drug for treatment of hypertension

**Usual Dosage** Adults: Oral: One tablet daily, if further blood pressure control is required, increase dosage to two tablets daily

**Dosage Forms** Tablet, extended release: Enalapril maleate 5 mg and diltiazem maleate 180 mg

## enalapril and felodipine (e NAL a pril & fe LOE di peen)

**U.S./Canadian Brand Names** Lexxel™

**Therapeutic Category** Antihypertensive Agent, Combination

**Use** Treatment of hypertension

**Usual Dosage** Adults: Oral: The dose of this combination when given as a replacement to patients taking both components separately should be equal to the component doses previously used. Patients whose blood pressure is not sufficiently controlled on either component may be switched to one combination tablet (5 mg enalapril and 5 mg extended-release felodipine) daily. If control remains inadequate after 1 or 2 weeks, the dosage may be increased to two tablets daily, and if lack of control persists, a thiazide diuretic may be added

(Continued)

## enalapril and felodipine *(Continued)*

**Dosage Forms** Tablet, extended release: Enalapril maleate 5 mg and felodipine 5 mg

## enalapril and hydrochlorothiazide

(e NAL a pril & hye droe klor oh THYE a zide)

**U.S./Canadian Brand Names** Vaseretic® 10-25

**Therapeutic Category** Antihypertensive Agent, Combination

**Use** Treatment of hypertension

**Usual Dosage** Oral: Dose is individualized

**Dosage Forms** Tablet: Enalapril maleate 5 mg and hydrochlorothiazide 12.5 mg; enalapril maleate 10 mg and hydrochlorothiazide 25 mg

**Enbrel®** *see* etanercept *on page 229*

**Encare® [OTC]** *see* nonoxynol 9 *on page 424*

**Endal®** *see* guaifenesin and phenylephrine *on page 283*

**Endantadine® (Can)** *see* amantadine *on page 28*

**Endep® 25 mg, 50 mg, 100 mg *(Discontinued)*** *see page 750*

**End Lice® Liquid [OTC]** *see* pyrethrins *on page 510*

**Endocet®** *see* oxycodone and acetaminophen *on page 444*

**Endocodone®** *see* oxycodone *on page 443*

**Endodan®** *see* oxycodone and aspirin *on page 444*

**Endo® Levodopa/Carbidopa (Can)** *see* carbidopa and levodopa *on page 107*

**Endolor®** *see* butalbital compound and acetaminophen *on page 93*

**Endrate®** *see* edetate disodium *on page 210*

**Enduron®** *see* methyclothiazide *on page 383*

**Enduron® 2.5 mg Tablet *(Discontinued)*** *see page 750*

**Enduronyl®** *see* methyclothiazide and deserpidine *on page 383*

**Enduronyl® Forte** *see* methyclothiazide and deserpidine *on page 383*

**Enecat®** *see* radiological/contrast media (ionic) *on page 516*

**Ener-B® [OTC]** *see* cyanocobalamin *on page 158*

## enflurane (EN floo rane)

**U.S./Canadian Brand Names** Ethrane®

**Therapeutic Category** General Anesthetic

**Use** General induction and maintenance of anesthesia (inhalation)

**Usual Dosage** Inhalation: 0.5% to 3%

**Dosage Forms** Liquid: 125 mL, 250 mL

**Engerix-B®** *see* hepatitis B vaccine *on page 292*

**Enisyl® [OTC]** *see* l-lysine *on page 353*

**Enkaid® *(Discontinued)*** *see page 750*

**Enlon®** *see* edrophonium *on page 210*

**Enomine® *(Discontinued)*** *see page 750*

**Enovid® *(Discontinued)*** *see page 750*

**Enovil® *(Discontinued)*** *see page 750*

## enoxacin (en OKS a sin)

**U.S./Canadian Brand Names** Penetrex™

**Therapeutic Category** Quinolone

**Use** Complicated and uncomplicated urinary tract infections caused by susceptible gram-negative and gram-positive bacteria

**Usual Dosage** Adults: Oral: 400 mg twice daily

**Dosage Forms** Tablet: 200 mg, 400 mg

## enoxaparin (ee noks a PA rin)

**U.S./Canadian Brand Names** Lovenox®

**Therapeutic Category** Anticoagulant

**Use** Prophylaxis and treatment of thromboembolic disorders (deep vein thrombosis)

**Usual Dosage** Adults: S.C.: 30 mg twice daily

**Dosage Forms** Injection, as sodium, preservative free:

Prefilled syringes: 30 mg/0.3 mL, 40 mg/0.4 mL

Graduated prefilled syringe: 60 mg/0.6 mL, 80 mg/0.8 mL, 90 mg/0.6 mL, 100 mg/1 mL, 120 mg/0.8 mL, 150 mg/mL

Ampul: 30 mg/0.3 mL

**Ensure® [OTC]** *see* nutritional formula, enteral/oral *on page 432*

**Ensure Plus® [OTC]** *see* nutritional formula, enteral/oral *on page 432*

**E.N.T.® *(Discontinued)*** *see page 750*

## entacapone (en TA ka pone)

**U.S./Canadian Brand Names** Comtan®

**Therapeutic Category** Anti-Parkinson's Agent; Reverse COMT Inhibitor

**Controlled Substance** [EZ100,MG250]parkinsonism

**Use** Adjunct to levodopa/carbidopa therapy in patients with idiopathic Parkinson's disease who experience "wearing-off" symptoms at the end of a dosing interval

**Usual Dosage** Adults: Oral: 200 mg dose, up to a maximum of 8 times/day; maximum daily dose: 1600 mg/day. Always administer with levodopa/carbidopa. To optimize therapy the levodopa/carbidopa dosage must be reduced, usually by 25%. This reduction is usually necessary when the patient is taking more than 800 mg of levodopa daily.

**Dosage Forms** Tablet: 200 mg

**Entertainer's Secret® Spray [OTC]** *see* saliva substitute *on page 536*

**Entex® *(Discontinued)*** *see page 750*

**Entex® LA *(Discontinued)*** *see page 750*

**Entex® PSE** *see* guaifenesin and pseudoephedrine *on page 283*

**Entocort® Capsule** *see* budesonide *on page 89*

**Entozyme® *(Discontinued)*** *see page 750*

**Entrobar®** *see* radiological/contrast media (ionic) *on page 516*

**Entuss-D® Liquid** *see* hydrocodone and pseudoephedrine *on page 301*

**Enulose®** *see* lactulose *on page 338*

**Enzone®** *see* pramoxine and hydrocortisone *on page 490*

**EPEG** *see* etoposide *on page 236*

## ephedrine (e FED rin)

**U.S./Canadian Brand Names** Pretz-D® [OTC]

**Therapeutic Category** Adrenergic Agonist Agent

**Use** Bronchial asthma; nasal congestion; acute bronchospasm; acute hypotensive states

**Usual Dosage**

Children:

Oral, S.C.: 3 mg/kg/day or 25-100 mg/m$^2$/day in 4-6 divided doses every 4-6 hours

I.M., slow I.V. push: 0.2-0.3 mg/kg/dose every 4-6 hours

Adults:

Oral: 25-50 mg every 3-4 hours as needed

(Continued)

## ephedrine *(Continued)*

I.M., S.C.: 25-50 mg, parenteral adult dose should not exceed 150 mg in 24 hours
I.V.: 5-25 mg/dose slow I.V. push repeated after 5-10 minutes as needed, then every 3-4 hours not to exceed 150 mg/24 hours

**Dosage Forms**
Capsule, as sulfate: 25 mg, 50 mg
Injection, as sulfate: 25 mg/mL (1 mL); 50 mg/mL (1 mL, 10 mL)
Spray, as sulfate (Pretz-D®): 0.25% (15 mL)

**Epi-C®** *see* radiological/contrast media (ionic) *on page 516*

**Epifrin®** *see* epinephrine *on this page*

**E-Pilo-x® Ophthalmic** *see* pilocarpine and epinephrine *on page 471*

**Epinal®** *see* epinephryl borate *on next page*

## epinephrine (ep i NEF rin)

**Synonyms** adrenaline

**U.S./Canadian Brand Names** Adrenalin® Chloride; AsthmaHaler® Mist [OTC]; AsthmaNefrin® [OTC]; Bronitin® Mist [OTC]; Bronkaid® Mist [OTC]; Epifrin®; EpiPen®; EpiPen® Jr; Glaucon®; microNefrin® [OTC]; Primatene® Mist [OTC]; Sus-Phrine®; Vaponefrin® [OTC]

**Therapeutic Category** Adrenergic Agonist Agent

**Use** Treatment of bronchospasm, anaphylactic reactions, cardiac arrest, and management of open-angle (chronic simple) glaucoma

**Usual Dosage**

Bronchodilator:

Children: S.C.: 10 mcg/kg (0.01 mL/kg of 1:1000) (single doses not to exceed 0.5 mg); injection suspension (1:200): 0.005 mL/kg/dose (0.025 mg/kg/dose) to a maximum of 0.15 mL (0.75 mg for single dose) every 8-12 hours

Adults:
I.M., S.C. (1:1000): 0.1-0.5 mg every 10-15 minutes to 4 hours
Suspension (1:200) S.C.: 0.1-0.3 mL (0.5-1.5 mg)
I.V.: 0.1-0.25 mg (single dose maximum: 1 mg)

Cardiac arrest:

Neonates: I.V. or intratracheal: 0.01-0.03 mg/kg (0.1-0.3 mL/kg of 1:10,000 solution) every 3-5 minutes as needed; dilute intratracheal doses in 1-2 mL of normal saline

Infants and Children: Asystole or pulseless arrest:
I.V., intraosseous: First dose: 0.01 mg/kg (0.1 mL/kg of a 1:10,000 solution); subsequent doses: 0.1 mg/kg (0.1 mL/kg of a 1:1000 solution); doses as high as 0.2 mg/kg may be effective; repeat every 3-5 minutes
Intratracheal: 0.1 mg/kg (0.1 mL/kg of a 1:1000 solution); doses as high as 0.2 mg/kg may be effective

Adults: Asystole:
I.V.: 1 mg every 3-5 minutes; if this approach fails, alternative regimens include: Intermediate: 2-5 mg every 3-5 minutes; Escalating: 1 mg, 3 mg, 5 mg at 3-minute intervals; High: 0.1 mg/kg every 3-5 minutes
Intratracheal: Although optimal dose is unknown, doses of 2-2.5 times the I.V. dose may be needed

Bradycardia: Children:
I.V.: 0.01 mg/kg (0.1 mL/kg of 1:10,000 solution) every 3-5 minutes as needed (maximum: 1 mg/10 mL)
Intratracheal: 0.1 mg/kg (0.1 mL/kg of 1:1000 solution every 3-5 minutes); doses as high as 0.2 mg/kg may be effective

Refractory hypotension (refractory to dopamine/dobutamine): I.V. infusion administration requires the use of an infusion pump:
Children: Infusion rate 0.1-4 mcg/kg/minute
Adults: I.V. infusion: 1 mg in 250 mL NS/$D_5W$ at 0.1-1 mcg/kg/minute; titrate to desired effect

Hypersensitivity reaction:
Children: S.C.: 0.01 mg/kg every 15 minutes for 2 doses then every 4 hours as needed (single doses not to exceed 0.5 mg)
Adults: I.M., S.C.: 0.2-0.5 mg every 20 minutes to 4 hours (single dose maximum: 1 mg)

Nebulization:
Children <2 years: 0.25 mL of 1:1000 diluted in 3 mL NS with treatments ordered individually
Children >2 years and Adolescents: 0.5 mL of 1:1000 concentration diluted in 3 mL NS
Children >2 years and Adults (racemic epinephrine):
<10 kg: 2 mL of 1:8 dilution over 15 minutes every 1-4 hours
10-15 kg: 2 mL of 1:6 dilution over 15 minutes every 1-4 hours
15-20 kg: 2 mL of 1:4 dilution over 15 minutes every 1-4 hours
>20 kg: 2 mL of 1:3 dilution over 15 minutes every 1-4 hours
Adults: Instill 8-15 drops into nebulizer reservoirs; administer 1-3 inhalations 4-6 times/day
Ophthalmic: Instill 1-2 drops in eye(s) once or twice daily
Intranasal: Children ≥6 years and Adults: Apply locally as drops or spray or with sterile swab

**Dosage Forms**
Aerosol, oral:
Bitartrate (AsthmaHaler®, Bronitin®): 0.3 mg/spray [epinephrine base 0.16 mg/spray] (10 mL, 15 mL, 22.5 mL)
Bronkaid®: 0.5% (10 mL, 15 mL, 22.5 mL)
Primatene® Mist: 0.2 mg/spray (15 mL, 22.5 mL)
Auto-injector:
EpiPen®: 1 mg/mL [1:1000] (2 mL)
EpiPen® Jr.: 0.5 mg/mL [1:2000] (2 mL)
Solution:
Inhalation:
Adrenalin®: 1% [10 mg/mL, 1:100] (7.5 mL)
Injection:
Adrenalin®: 0.01 mg/mL [1:100,000] (5 mL); 0.1 mg/mL [1:10,000] (3 mL, 10 mL); 1 mg/mL [1:1000] (1 mL, 2 mL, 30 mL)
Suspension (Sus-Phrine®): 5 mg/mL [1:200] (0.3 mL, 5 mL)
Nasal (Adrenalin®): 0.1% [1 mg/mL, 1:1000] (30 mL)
Ophthalmic, as hydrochloride (Epifrin®, Glaucon®): 0.1% (1 mL, 30 mL); 0.5% (15 mL); 1% (1 mL, 10 mL, 15 mL); 2% (10 mL, 15 mL)
Topical (Adrenalin®): 0.1% [1 mg/mL, 1:1000] (10 mL, 30 mL)

## epinephryl borate (ep i NEF ril BOR ate)

**U.S./Canadian Brand Names** Epinal®
**Therapeutic Category** Adrenergic Agonist Agent
**Use** Reduces elevated intraocular pressure in chronic open-angle glaucoma
**Usual Dosage** Adults: Ophthalmic: Instill 1 drop into the eyes once or twice daily
**Dosage Forms** Solution, ophthalmic: 0.5% (7.5 mL); 1% (7.5 mL)

**EpiPen®** *see* epinephrine *on previous page*

**EpiPen® Jr** *see* epinephrine *on previous page*

## epirubicin (ep i ROO bi sin)

**U.S./Canadian Brand Names** Ellence™; Pharmorubicin® (Can)
**Therapeutic Category** Antineoplastic Agent
**Use** As a component of adjuvant therapy following primary resection of primary breast cancer in patients with evidence of axillary node tumor involvement
**Usual Dosage** Adults: I.V. (refer to individual protocols): 100-120 mg/m$^2$, repeated in 3- to 4-week cycles. The total dose of epirubicin may be given on Day 1 of each cycle or the dose may be divided equally and given on Day 1 and Day 8 of each cycle.
(Continued)

## epirubicin *(Continued)*

**Dosage Forms** Injection: 2 mg/mL (25 mL, 100 mL)

**Epitol®** *see* carbamazepine *on page 105*

**Epival® (Can)** *see* valproic acid and derivatives *on page 620*

**Epivir®** *see* lamivudine *on page 339*

**Epivir®-HBV™** *see* lamivudine *on page 339*

**E.P. Mycin® Capsule *(Discontinued)*** *see page 750*

**EPO** *see* epoetin alfa *on this page*

## epoetin alfa (e POE e tin AL fa)

**Synonyms** EPO; erythropoietin; RHUEPO-α

**U.S./Canadian Brand Names** Epogen®; Eprex® (Can); Procrit®

**Therapeutic Category** Colony-Stimulating Factor

**Use** Anemia associated with end-stage renal disease; anemia related to therapy with AZT-treated HIV-infected patients; anemia in cancer patients receiving chemotherapy; anemia of prematurity

**Usual Dosage**

In patients on dialysis, epoetin alfa usually has been administered as an I.V. bolus 3 times/week; while the administration is independent of the dialysis procedure, it may be administered into the venous line at the end of the dialysis procedure to obviate the need for additional venous access. In patients with CRF not on dialysis, epoetin alfa may be administered either as an I.V. or S.C. injection.

AZT-treated HIV-infected patients: I.V., S.C.: Initial: 100 units/kg/dose 3 times/week for 8 weeks; after 8 weeks of therapy the dose can be adjusted by 50-100 units/kg increments 3 times/week to a maximum dose of 300 units/kg 3 times/week; if the hematocrit exceeds 40%, the dose should be discontinued until the hematocrit drops to 36%

Anemia of prematurity: S.C.: 25-100 units/kg/dose 3 times/week

**Dosage Forms**

1 mL single-dose vials: Preservative-free solution
- 2000 units/mL
- 3000 units/mL
- 4000 units/mL
- 10,000 units/mL
- 20,000 units/mL
- 40,000 units/mL

2 mL multidose vials: Preserved solution: 10,000 units/mL

**Epogen®** *see* epoetin alfa *on this page*

## epoprostenol (e poe PROST en ole)

**U.S./Canadian Brand Names** Flolan®

**Therapeutic Category** Platelet Inhibitor

**Use** Long-term intravenous treatment of primary pulmonary hypertension (PPH)

**Usual Dosage** I.V. continuous infusion: 2 ng/kg/minute

**Dosage Forms** Injection, as sodium: 0.5 mg/vial and 1.5 mg/vial, each supplied with 50 mL of sterile diluent

**Eprex® (Can)** *see* epoetin alfa *on this page*

## eprosartan (ep roe SAR tan)

**U.S./Canadian Brand Names** Teveten®

**Therapeutic Category** Angiotensin II Antagonist

**Use** Treatment of hypertension; may be used alone or in combination with other antihypertensives

**Usual Dosage** Adults: Oral: Dosage must be individualized; can administer once or twice daily with total daily doses of 400-800 mg. Usual starting dose is 600 mg once daily as monotherapy in patients who are euvolemic. Limited clinical experience with doses >800 mg.

**Dosage Forms** Tablet: 400 mg (scored), 600 mg

**epsom salts** *see* magnesium sulfate *on page 363*

**EPT** *see* teniposide *on page 573*

## eptacog alfa (activated) *(Canada only)* (EP ta cog AL fa AK ti vay ted)

**Synonyms** activated recombinant human blood coagulation factor VII

**Therapeutic Category** Coagulation Factor

**Use** In hemophilia A/B patients with inhibitors to FVIII or FIX, respectively, for the treatment of bleeding episodes (including treatment and prevention of those occurring during and after surgery). Based on the data obtained so far with eptacog alfa (activated) in the treatment of hemophilia patients with inhibitors, the apparent lack of anamnestic response during and after exposure to eptacog alfa (activated) makes it suitable for use in all inhibitor patients.

**Usual Dosage** Eptacog alfa (activated) is intended for I.V. bolus administration only. The recommended dose range, dose, frequency, and duration of eptacog alfa (activated) administration as a single agent. Evaluation of hemostasis should be used to determine the effectiveness of eptacog alfa (activated) and to provide a basis for modification of the eptacog alfa (activated) treatment schedule. Coagulation parameters should not be used to evaluate eptacog alfa (activated) effectiveness.

**Dosage Forms** Injection: Each vial of sterile, white lyophilized powder for reconstitution, contains: Eptacog alfa (activated) 1.2 mg, 2.4 mg, 4.8 mg

## eptifibatide (ep TIF i ba tide)

**U.S./Canadian Brand Names** Integrilin®

**Therapeutic Category** Antiplatelet Agent

**Use** Treatment of patients with acute coronary syndrome (UA/NQMI), including patients who are to be managed medically and those undergoing percutaneous coronary intervention (PCI); it has been shown to decrease the rate of a combined endpoint of death or new myocardial infarction. For the treatment of patients undergoing PCI, it has been shown to decrease the rate of a combined endpoint of death, new myocardial infarction, or need for urgent intervention.

**Usual Dosage** Adults: I.V.:

Acute coronary syndrome: Bolus of 180 mcg/kg as soon as possible following diagnosis, followed by a continuous infusion of 2 mcg/kg/minute until hospital discharge or initiation of CABG surgery, up to 72 hours. If a patient is to undergo a percutaneous coronary intervention (PCI) while receiving eptifibatide, consideration can be given to decreasing the infusion rate to 0.5 mcg/kg/minute (the infusion rate in IMPACT II) at the time of the procedure. Infusion should be continued for an additional 20-24 hours after the procedure, allowing for up to 96 hours of therapy.

Percutaneous coronary intervention (PCI) in patients not presenting with an acute coronary syndrome: Bolus of 135 mcg/kg administered immediately before the initiation of PCI followed by a continuous infusion of 0.5 mcg/kg/minute for 20-24 hours. In the IMPACT II Study, there was little experience in patients weighing more than 143 kg.

**Dosage Forms** Injection: 0.75 mg/mL (100 mL); 2 mg/mL (10 mL)

**Equagesic®** *see* aspirin and meprobamate *on page 56*

**Equalactin® Chewable Tablet [OTC]** *see* calcium polycarbophil *on page 101*

**Equanil®** *see* meprobamate *on page 373*

**Equilet® [OTC]** *see* calcium carbonate *on page 97*

**Ercaf®** ***(Discontinued)*** *see page 750*

**Ergamisol®** *see* levamisole *on page 344*

## ergocalciferol (er goe kal SIF e role)

**Synonyms** activated ergosterol; viosterol; vitamin $D_2$

**U.S./Canadian Brand Names** Calciferol™; Drisdol®; Ostoforte® (Can)

**Therapeutic Category** Vitamin D Analog

**Use** Refractory rickets; hypophosphatemia; hypoparathyroidism

**Usual Dosage**

Dietary supplementation: Oral:

Premature infants: 10-20 mcg/day (400-800 units), up to 750 mcg/day (30,000 units)

Infants and healthy Children: 10 mcg/day (400 units)

Renal failure: Oral:

Children: 0.1-1 mg/day (4000-40,000 units)

Adults: 0.5 mg/day (20,000 units)

Hypoparathyroidism: Oral:

Children: 1.25-5 mg/day (50,000-200,000 units) and calcium supplements

Adults: 625 mcg to 5 mg/day (25,000-200,000 units) and calcium supplements

Vitamin D-dependent rickets: Oral:

Children: 75-125 mcg/day (3000-5000 units)

Adults: 250 mcg to 1.5 mg/day (10,000-60,000 units)

Nutritional rickets and osteomalacia:

Oral:

Children and Adults (with normal absorption): 25 mcg/day (1000 units)

Children with malabsorption: 250-625 mcg/day (10,000-25,000 units)

I.M.: Adults: 250 mcg/day

**Dosage Forms**

Capsule (Drisdol®): 50,000 units [1.25 mg]

Injection (Calciferol™): 500,000 units/mL [12.5 mg/mL] (1 mL)

Liquid (Calciferol™, Drisdol®): 8000 units/mL [200 mcg/mL] (60 mL)

Tablet (Calciferol™): 50,000 units [1.25 mg]

## ergoloid mesylates (ER goe loid MES i lates)

**Synonyms** dihydroergotoxine; hydrogenated ergot alkaloids

**U.S./Canadian Brand Names** Germinal®; Hydergine®; Hydergine® LC

**Therapeutic Category** Ergot Alkaloid and Derivative

**Use** Treatment of cerebrovascular insufficiency in primary progressive dementia, Alzheimer's dementia, and senile onset

**Usual Dosage** Adults: Oral: 1 mg 3 times/day up to 4.5-12 mg/day; up to 6 months of therapy may be necessary

**Dosage Forms**

Capsule, liquid (Hydergine® LC): 1 mg

Liquid (Hydergine®): 1 mg/mL (100 mL)

Tablet:

Oral: 0.5 mg

Gerimal®, Hydergine®: 1 mg

Sublingual: Gerimal®, Hydergine®: 0.5 mg, 1 mg

**Ergomar®** *see* ergotamine *on next page*

## ergonovine (er goe NOE veen)

**U.S./Canadian Brand Names** Ergotrate® Maleate Injection

**Therapeutic Category** Ergot Alkaloid and Derivative

**Use** Prevention and treatment of postpartum and postabortion hemorrhage caused by uterine atony or subinvolution

**Usual Dosage** Adults:

Oral: 1-2 tablets (0.2-0.4 mg) every 6-12 hours for up to 48 hours

I.M., I.V. (I.V. should be reserved for emergency use only): 0.2 mg, repeat dose in 2-4 hours as needed

**Dosage Forms**

Injection, as maleate: 0.2 mg/mL (1 mL)

Tablet, as maleate: 0.2 mg

**Ergostat® *(Discontinued)*** *see page 750*

## ergotamine (er GOT a meen)

**U.S./Canadian Brand Names** Cafatine-PB®; Cafergot®; Cafetrate®; Ergomar®; Ergotamine Tartrate and Caffeine Cafatine®; Wigraine®

**Therapeutic Category** Ergot Alkaloid and Derivative

**Use** Prevent or abort vascular headaches, such as migraine or cluster

**Usual Dosage**

Older Children and Adolescents: Oral: 1 tablet at onset of attack; then 1 tablet every 30 minutes as needed, up to a maximum of 3 tablets per attack

Adults:

Oral (Cafergot®): 2 tablets at onset of attack; then 1 tablet every 30 minutes as needed; maximum: 6 tablets per attack; do not exceed 10 tablets/week

Oral (Ergostat®): 1 tablet under tongue at first sign, then 1 tablet every 30 minutes, 3 tablets/24 hours, 5 tablets/week

Rectal (Cafergot® suppositories, Wigraine® suppositories, Cafatine-PB® suppositories): 1 at first sign of an attack; follow with second dose after 1 hour, if needed; maximum dose: 2 per attack; do not exceed 5/week

**Dosage Forms**

Suppository, rectal (Cafatine®, Cafergot®, Cafetrate®, Wigraine®): Ergotamine tartrate 2 mg and caffeine 100 mg (12s)

Tablet (Wigraine®): Ergotamine tartrate 1 mg and caffeine 100 mg

Sublingual (Ergomar®): Ergotamine tartrate 2 mg

**Ergotamine Tartrate and Caffeine Cafatine®** *see* ergotamine *on this page*

**Ergotrate® Maleate Injection** *see* ergonovine *on previous page*

**Eridium® *(Discontinued)*** *see page 750*

**E•R•O Ear [OTC]** *see* carbamide peroxide *on page 106*

**Erybid™ (Can)** *see* erythromycin (systemic) *on next page*

**Eryc®** *see* erythromycin (systemic) *on next page*

**EryDerm® Topical** *see* erythromycin (ophthalmic/topical) *on next page*

**Erygel® Topical** *see* erythromycin (ophthalmic/topical) *on next page*

**Erymax® Topical** *see* erythromycin (ophthalmic/topical) *on next page*

**Ery-Sol® Topical Solution *(Discontinued)*** *see page 750*

**Ery-Tab®** *see* erythromycin (systemic) *on next page*

**Erythrocin®** *see* erythromycin (systemic) *on next page*

**Erythromid® (Can)** *see* erythromycin (systemic) *on next page*

## erythromycin and benzoyl peroxide

(er ith roe MYE sin & BEN zoe il per OKS ide)

**U.S./Canadian Brand Names** Benzamycin®

**Therapeutic Category** Acne Products

**Use** Topical control of acne vulgaris

**Usual Dosage** Topical: Apply twice daily (morning and evening)

**Dosage Forms** Gel: Erythromycin 30 mg and benzoyl peroxide 50 mg per g

## erythromycin and sulfisoxazole (er ith roe MYE sin & sul fi SOKS a zole)

**U.S./Canadian Brand Names** Eryzole®; Pediazole®

**Therapeutic Category** Macrolide (Antibiotic); Sulfonamide

**Use** Treatment of susceptible bacterial infections of the upper and lower respiratory tract; otitis media in children caused by susceptible strains of *Haemophilus influenzae*; other infections in patients allergic to penicillin

(Continued)

## erythromycin and sulfisoxazole *(Continued)*

**Usual Dosage** Dosage recommendation is based on the product's erythromycin content; Oral:

Children ≥2 months: 40-50 mg/kg/day of erythromycin in divided doses every 6-8 hours; not to exceed 2 g erythromycin or 6 g sulfisoxazole/day or approximately 1.25 mL/kg/day divided every 6-8 hours

Adults: 400 mg erythromycin and 1200 mg sulfisoxazole every 6 hours

**Dosage Forms** Suspension, oral: Erythromycin ethylsuccinate 200 mg and sulfisoxazole acetyl 600 mg per 5 mL (100 mL, 150 mL, 200 mL, 250 mL)

## erythromycin (ophthalmic/topical)

(er ith roe MYE sin op THAL mik/TOP i kal)

**U.S./Canadian Brand Names** Akne-Mycin® Topical; A/T/S® Topical; Del-Mycin® Topical; Emgel™ Topical; EryDerm® Topical; Erygel® Topical; Erymax® Topical; E-Solve-2® Topical; ETS-2%® Topical; Staticin® Topical; T-Stat® Topical

**Therapeutic Category** Acne Products; Antibiotic, Ophthalmic; Antibiotic, Topical

**Use** Topical treatment of acne vulgaris

**Usual Dosage** Children and Adults:

Ophthalmic: Instill one or more times daily depending on the severity of the infection

Topical: Apply 2% solution over the affected area twice daily after the skin has been thoroughly washed and patted dry

**Dosage Forms**

Gel: 2% (30 g, 60 g)

Gel (A/T/S®, Emgel™, Erygel®): 2% (27 g, 30 g, 60 g)

Ointment:

Ophthalmic: 0.5% [5 mg/g] (3.5 g)

Topical (Akne-Mycin®): 2% (25 g)

Solution, topical:

Staticin®: 1.5% (60 mL)

Akne-Mycin®, A/T/S®, Del-Mycin®, EryDerm®, ETS-2%®, Romycin®, Theramycin Z®, T-Stat®: 2% (60 mL, 66 mL, 120 mL)

Pad (T-Stat®): 2% (60s)

Pledgets: 2% (60s)

Swab: 2% (60s)

## erythromycin (systemic) (er ith roe MYE sin sis TEM ik)

**U.S./Canadian Brand Names** AK-Mycin®; Apo®-Erythro E-C (Can); Apo®-Erythro-S (Can); Diomycin® (Can); E.E.S.®; E.E.S.® Chewable; E.E.S.® Granules; E-Mycin®; E-Mycin-E®; Erybid™ (Can); Eryc®; Ery-Tab®; Erythrocin®; Erythromid® (Can); Ilosone® Pulvules®; Novo-Rythro Encap (Can); PCE®; PMS-Erythromycin (Can)

**Therapeutic Category** Macrolide (Antibiotic)

**Use** Treatment of mild to moderately severe infections of the upper and lower respiratory tract, pharyngitis and skin infections due to susceptible streptococci and staphylococci; other susceptible bacterial infections including *Mycoplasma* pneumonia, *Legionella* pneumonia, diphtheria, pertussis, chancroid, *Chlamydia*, and *Campylobacter* gastroenteritis; used in conjunction with neomycin for decontaminating the bowel for surgery; dental procedure prophylaxis in penicillin allergic patients

**Usual Dosage**

Infants and Children:

Oral: Do not exceed 2 g/day

Base and ethylsuccinate: 30-50 mg/kg/day divided every 6-8 hours

Estolate: 30-50 mg/kg/day divided every 8-12 hours

Stearate: 20-40 mg/kg/day divided every 6 hours

Pre-op bowel preparation: 20 mg/kg erythromycin base at 1, 2, and 11 PM on the day before surgery combined with mechanical cleansing of the large intestine and oral neomycin

I.V.: Lactobionate: 20-40 mg/kg/day divided every 6 hours, not to exceed 4 g/day

Adults:
Oral:
Base: 333 mg every 8 hours
Estolate, stearate or base: 250-500 mg every 6-12 hours
Ethylsuccinate: 400-800 mg every 6-12 hours
Pre-op bowel preparation: 1 g erythromycin base at 1, 2, and 11 PM on the day before surgery combined with mechanical cleansing of the large intestine and oral neomycin
I.V.: 15-20 mg/kg/day divided every 6 hours or administered as a continuous infusion over 24 hours

**Dosage Forms**
Erythromycin base:
Capsule:
Delayed release: 250 mg
Delayed release, enteric coated pellets (Eryc®): 250 mg
Tablet:
Delayed release: 333 mg
Enteric coated (E-Mycin®, Ery-Tab®, E-Base®): 250 mg, 333 mg, 500 mg
Film coated: 250 mg, 500 mg
Polymer coated particles (PCE®): 333 mg, 500 mg
Erythromycin estolate:
Capsule: 250 mg
Suspension, oral: 125 mg/5 mL (480 mL); 250 mg/5 mL (480 mL)
Erythromycin ethylsuccinate:
Granules for oral suspension (EryPed®): 400 mg/5 mL (60 mL, 100 mL, 200 mL)
Powder for oral suspension (E.E.S.®): 200 mg/5 mL (100 mL, 200 mL)
Suspension:
Oral (E.E.S.®, EryPed®): 200 mg/5 mL (5 mL, 100 mL, 200 mL, 480 mL); 400 mg/5 mL (5 mL, 60 mL, 100 mL, 200 mL, 480 mL)
Oral [drops] (EryPed®): 100 mg/2.5 mL (50 mL)
Tablet (E.E.S.®): 400 mg
Tablet, chewable (EryPed®): 200 mg
Erythromycin gluceptate: Injection: 1000 mg (30 mL)
Erythromycin lactobionate: Powder for injection: 500 mg, 1000 mg
Erythromycin stearate: Tablet, film coated (Eramycin®, Erythrocin®): 250 mg, 500 mg

**erythropoietin** *see* epoetin alfa *on page 218*

**Eryzole®** *see* erythromycin and sulfisoxazole *on page 221*

**Esclim® Transdermal** *see* estradiol *on next page*

**Esgic®** *see* butalbital compound and acetaminophen *on page 93*

**Esgic-Plus™** *see* butalbital compound and acetaminophen *on page 93*

**Esidrix®** *see* hydrochlorothiazide *on page 299*

**Esidrix® 100 mg Tablet *(Discontinued)*** *see page 750*

**Eskalith®** *see* lithium *on page 353*

**Eskalith CR®** *see* lithium *on page 353*

## esmolol (ES moe lol)

**U.S./Canadian Brand Names** Brevibloc®

**Therapeutic Category** Antiarrhythmic Agent, Class II; Beta-Adrenergic Blocker

**Use** Supraventricular tachycardia (primarily to control ventricular rate) and hypertension (especially perioperatively)

**Usual Dosage** Must be adjusted to individual response and tolerance
Children: An extremely limited amount of information regarding esmolol use in pediatric patients is currently available. Some centers have utilized doses of 100-500 mcg/kg administered over 1 minute for control of supraventricular tachycardias. Loading doses of 500 mcg/kg/minute over 1 minute with maximal doses of 50-250 mcg/kg/minute (mean 173) have been used in addition to nitroprusside in a small number of patients

(Continued)

## esmolol *(Continued)*

(7 patients; 7-19 years of age; median 13 years) to treat postoperative hypertension after coarctation of aorta repair.

Adults: I.V.: Loading dose: 500 mcg/kg over 1 minute; follow with a 50 mcg/kg/minute infusion for 4 minutes; if response is inadequate, rebolus with another 500 mcg/kg loading dose over 1 minute, and increase the maintenance infusion to 100 mcg/kg/minute. Repeat this process until a therapeutic effect has been achieved or to a maximum recommended maintenance dose of 200 mcg/kg/minute. Usual dosage range: 50-200 mcg/kg/minute with average dose = 100 mcg/kg/minute.

**Dosage Forms** Injection, as hydrochloride: 10 mg/mL (10 mL); 250 mg/mL (10 mL)

**E-Solve-2® Topical** *see* erythromycin (ophthalmic/topical) *on page 222*

## esomeprazole (es oh ME pray zol)

**U.S./Canadian Brand Names** Nexium™

**Therapeutic Category** Proton Pump Inhibitor

**Use** Short-term (4-8 weeks) treatment of erosive esophagitis; maintaining symptom resolution and healing of erosive esophagitis; treatment of symptomatic gastroesophageal reflux disease; as part of a multidrug regimen for *Helicobacter pylori* eradication in patients with duodenal ulcer disease (active or history of within the past 5 years)

**Usual Dosage** Note: Delayed-release capsules should be swallowed whole and taken at least 1 hour before eating

Children: Safety and efficacy have not been established in pediatric patients

Adults: Oral:

Erosive esophagitis (healing): 20-40 mg once daily for 4-8 weeks; maintenance: 20 mg once daily

Symptomatic GERD: 20 mg once daily for 4 weeks

*H. pylori* eradication: 40 mg once daily **with** amoxicillin 1000 mg twice daily **and** clarithromycin 500 mg twice daily for a total of 10 days

**Dosage Forms** Capsule, delayed-release: 20 mg, 40 mg

**Esoterica® Facial [OTC]** *see* hydroquinone *on page 305*

**Esoterica® Regular [OTC]** *see* hydroquinone *on page 305*

**Esoterica® Sensitive Skin Formula [OTC]** *see* hydroquinone *on page 305*

**Esoterica® Sunscreen [OTC]** *see* hydroquinone *on page 305*

**Estar® [OTC]** *see* coal tar *on page 149*

## estazolam (es TA zoe lam)

**U.S./Canadian Brand Names** ProSom™

**Therapeutic Category** Benzodiazepine

**Controlled Substance** C-IV

**Use** Short-term management of insomnia

**Usual Dosage** Adults: Oral: 1 mg at bedtime, some patients may require 2 mg

**Dosage Forms** Tablet: 1 mg, 2 mg

**esterified estrogens** *see* estrogens (esterified) *on page 228*

**Estinyl®** *see* ethinyl estradiol *on page 230*

**Estivin® II Ophthalmic [OTC]** *see* naphazoline *on page 409*

**Estrace® Oral** *see* estradiol *on this page*

**Estracomb® (Can)** *see* estradiol and norethindrone *on page 226*

**Estraderm® Transdermal** *see* estradiol *on this page*

## estradiol (es tra DYE ole)

**U.S./Canadian Brand Names** Alora® Transdermal; Climara® Transdermal; Delestrogen® (Can); depGynogen® Injection; Depo®-Estradiol Injection; Depogen® Injection;

Dioval® Injection; Esclim® Transdermal; Estrace® Oral; Estraderm® Transdermal; Estra-L® Injection; Estring®; Estro-Cyp® Injection; Estrogel® (Can); Gynodiol™; Gynogen L.A.® Injection; Vagifem®; Vivelle™ Transdermal

**Therapeutic Category** Estrogen Derivative

**Use** Atrophic vaginitis, atrophic dystrophy of vulva, menopausal symptoms, female hypogonadism

**Usual Dosage** Adults (all dosage needs to be adjusted based upon the patient's response):

Male: Prostate cancer: Valerate:
- I.M.: ≥30 mg or more every 1-2 weeks
- Oral: 1-2 mg 3 times/day

Female:
- Hypogonadism:
  - Oral: 1-2 mg/day in a cyclic regimen for 3 weeks on drug, then 1 week off drug
  - I.M.: Cypionate: 1.5-2 mg/month; valerate: 10-20 mg/month
  - Transdermal: 0.05 mg patch initially (titrate dosage to response) applied twice weekly in a cyclic regimen, for 3 weeks on drug and 1 week off drug
- Atrophic vaginitis, kraurosis vulvae: Vaginal: Insert 2-4 g/day for 2 weeks then gradually reduce to 1/2 the initial dose for 2 weeks followed by a maintenance dose of 1 g 1-3 times/week
- Moderate to severe vasomotor symptoms: I.M.:
  - Cypionate: 1-5 mg every 3-4 weeks
  - Valerate: 10-20 mg every 4 weeks
- Postpartum breast engorgement: I.M.: Valerate: 10-25 mg at end of first stage of labor

**Dosage Forms**

Cream, vaginal (Estrace®): 0.1 mg/g (42.5 g)

Injection, as cypionate (depGynogen®, Depo®-Estradiol, Depogen®, Dura-Estrin®, Estra-D®, Estro-Cyp®, Estroject-L.A.®): 5 mg/mL (5 mL, 10 mL)

Injection, as valerate:
- Valergen®: 10 mg/mL (5 mL, 10 mL); 20 mg/mL (1 mL, 5 mL, 10 mL); 40 mg/mL (5 mL, 10 mL)
- Dioval®, Duragen®, Estra-L®, Gynogen L.A.®: 20 mg/mL (10 mL); 40 mg/mL (10 mL)

Tablet, micronized
- Estrace®: 1 mg, 2 mg
- Gynodiol™: 0.5 mg, 1 mg, 1.5 mg, 2 mg

Transdermal system
- Alora®:
  - 0.05 mg/24 hours [18 $cm^2$], total estradiol 1.5 mg
  - 0.075 mg/24 hours [27 $cm^2$], total estradiol 2.3 mg
  - 0.1 mg/24 hours [36 $cm^2$], total estradiol 3 mg
- Climara®:
  - 0.05 mg/24 hours [12.5 $cm^2$], total estradiol 3.9 mg
  - 0.075 mg/24 hours [18.75 $cm^2$], total estradiol 5.85 mg
  - 0.1 mg/24 hours [25 $cm^2$], total estradiol 7.8 mg
- Esclim®:
  - 0.025 mg/day
  - 0.0375 mg/day
  - 0.05 mg/day
  - 0.075 mg/day
  - 0.1 mg/day
- Estraderm®:
  - 0.05 mg/24 hours [10 $cm^2$], total estradiol 4 mg
  - 0.1 mg/24 hours [20 $cm^2$], total estradiol 8 mg
- Vivelle®:
  - 0.0375 mg/day
  - 0.05 mg/day
  - 0.075 mg/day

Vaginal ring (Estring®): 2 mg gradually released over 90 days

## estradiol and norethindrone (es tra DYE ole & nor eth IN drone)

**U.S./Canadian Brand Names** Activelle™; Estracomb® (Can)

**Therapeutic Category** Estrogen and Progestin Combination

**Use** Treatment of moderate to severe vasomotor symptoms associated with menopause; treatment of vulvar and vaginal atrophy

**Usual Dosage** Adults: Oral: Take one tablet daily

**Dosage Forms**

Tablet: Estradiol 1 mg and norethindrone acetate 0.5 mg (28s)

Transdermal system: Estradiol 0.05 mg and norethindrone acetate 0.14 mg per day; estradiol 0.05 mg and norethindrone acetate 0.25 mg per day

## estradiol and testosterone (es tra DYE ole & tes TOS ter one)

**U.S./Canadian Brand Names** Andro/Fem®; Deladumone®; depAndrogyn®; Depo-Testadiol®; Depotestogen®; Duo-Cyp®; Duratestrin®; Valertest No.1®

**Therapeutic Category** Estrogen and Androgen Combination

**Use** Vasomotor symptoms associated with menopause; postpartum breast engorgement

**Usual Dosage** Adults (all dosage needs to be adjusted based upon the patient's response)

**Dosage Forms** Injection:

Andro/Fem®, depAndrogyn®, Depo-Testadiol®, Depotestogen®, Duo-Cyp®, Duratestrin®: Estradiol cypionate 2 mg and testosterone cypionate 50 mg per mL in cottonseed oil (1 mL, 10 mL)

Androgyn L.A.®, Deladumone®, Estra-Testrin®, Valertest No.1®: Estradiol valerate 4 mg and testosterone enanthate 90 mg per mL in sesame oil (5 mL, 10 mL)

## estradiol cypionate and medroxyprogesterone acetate

(es tra DYE ole sip pe OH nate & me DROKS ee proe JES te rone AS e tate)

**U.S./Canadian Brand Names** Lunelle™

**Therapeutic Category** Contraceptive, Oral

**Use** Prevention of pregnancy

**Usual Dosage** Adults: Female: I.M.: 0.5 mL

First dose: Within first 5 days of menstrual period or within 5 days of a complete first trimester abortion; do not administer <4 weeks postpartum **if not breast-feeding** or <6 weeks postpartum **if breast-feeding**

Maintenance dose: Monthly, every 28-30 days following previous injection; do not exceed 33 days; pregnancy must be ruled out if >33 days have past between injections; bleeding episodes cannot be used to guide injection schedule; shortening schedule may lead to menstrual pattern changes

Switching from other forms of contraception: First injection should be given within 7 days of last active oral contraceptive pill; when switching from other methods, timing of injection should ensure continuous contraceptive coverage

**Dosage Forms** Injection, suspension: Estradiol cypionate 5 mg and medroxyprogesterone acetate 25 mg per 0.5 mL

**Estradurin® Injection *(Discontinued)*** *see page 750*

**Estra-L® Injection** *see* estradiol *on page 224*

## estramustine (es tra MUS teen)

**U.S./Canadian Brand Names** Emcyt®

**Therapeutic Category** Antineoplastic Agent

**Use** Palliative treatment of prostatic carcinoma

**Usual Dosage** Oral: 1 capsule for each 22 lb/day, in 3-4 divided doses

**Dosage Forms** Capsule, as phosphate sodium: 140 mg

**Estratab®** *see* estrogens (esterified) *on page 228*

**Estratest®** *see* estrogens and methyltestosterone *on next page*

**Estratest® H.S.** *see* estrogens and methyltestosterone *on next page*

**Estring®** *see* estradiol *on page 224*

**Estro-Cyp® Injection** *see* estradiol *on page 224*

**Estrogel® (Can)** *see* estradiol *on page 224*

**estrogenic substance aqueous** *see* estrone *on next page*

## estrogens and medroxyprogesterone

(ES troe jenz & me DROKS ee proe JES te rone)

**U.S./Canadian Brand Names** Premphase®; Prempro™

**Therapeutic Category** Estrogen and Progestin Combination

**Use** Women with an intact uterus for the treatment of moderate to severe vasomotor symptoms associated with the menopause; treatment of atrophic vaginitis; primary ovarian failure; osteoporosis prophylactic

**Usual Dosage** Adults: Oral:

Premphase®: Conjugated estrogen 0.625 mg [Premarin®] and taken orally for 28 days and medroxyprogesterone acetate [Cycrin®] 5 mg (14s) which are taken orally with a Premarin® tablet on days 15 through 28

Prempro™: Conjugated estrogen 0.625 mg [Premarin®] and medroxyprogesterone acetate [Cycrin®] 2.5 mg are taken continuously one each day

**Dosage Forms** Tablet:

Premphase®: Two separate tablets in therapy pack: Conjugated estrogens 0.625 mg [Premarin®] (28s) taken orally for 28 days and medroxyprogesterone acetate [Cycrin®] 5 mg (14s) which are taken orally with a Premarin® tablet on days 15 through 28

Prempro™: Conjugated estrogens 0.625 mg and medroxyprogesterone acetate 2.5 mg (14s)

## estrogens and methyltestosterone

(ES troe jenz & meth il tes TOS te rone)

**U.S./Canadian Brand Names** Estratest®; Estratest® H.S.; Premarin® With Methyltestosterone

**Therapeutic Category** Estrogen and Androgen Combination

**Use** Atrophic vaginitis; hypogonadism; primary ovarian failure; vasomotor symptoms of menopause; prostatic carcinoma; osteoporosis prophylactic

**Usual Dosage** Oral: Lowest dose that will control symptoms should be chosen, normally administered 3 weeks on and 1 week off

**Dosage Forms** Tablet:

Estratest®, Menogen®: Esterified estrogen 1.25 mg and methyltestosterone 2.5 mg

Estratest® H.S., Menogen H.S.®: Esterified estrogen 0.625 mg and methyltestosterone 1.25 mg

Premarin® With Methyltestosterone: Conjugated estrogen 0.625 mg and methyltestosterone 5 mg; conjugated estrogen 1.25 mg and methyltestosterone 10 mg

## estrogens (conjugated A/synthetic)

(ES troe jenz KON joo gate ed aye/sin THET ik)

**U.S./Canadian Brand Names** Cenestin™

**Therapeutic Category** Estrogen Derivative

**Use** Treatment of moderate to severe vasomotor symptoms of menopause

**Usual Dosage** Moderate to severe vasomotor symptoms: Oral: 0.625 mg/day; may be titrated up to 1.25 mg daily. Attempts to discontinue medication should be made at 3-6 month intervals.

**Dosage Forms** Tablet: 0.625 mg, 0.9 mg, 1.25 mg

## estrogens (conjugated/equine) (ES troe jenz KON joo gate ed/EE kwine)

**Synonyms** CES; conjugated estrogens

**U.S./Canadian Brand Names** C.E.S.® (Can); Congest (Can); PMS-Conjugated Estrogens (Can); Premarin®

**Therapeutic Category** Estrogen Derivative

(Continued)

## estrogens (conjugated/equine) *(Continued)*

**Use** Dysfunctional uterine bleeding, atrophic vaginitis, hypogonadism, vasomotor symptoms of menopause

**Usual Dosage** Adults:

Male: Prostate cancer: Oral: 1.25-2.5 mg 3 times/day

Female:

Hypogonadism: Oral: 2.5-7.5 mg/day for 20 days, off 10 days and repeat until menses occur

Abnormal uterine bleeding:

Oral: 2.5-5 mg/day for 7-10 days; then decrease to 1.25 mg/day for 2 weeks

I.V.: 25 mg every 6-12 hours until bleeding stops

Moderate to severe vasomotor symptoms: Oral: 0.625-1.25 mg/day

Postpartum breast engorgement: Oral: 3.75 mg every 4 hours for 5 doses, then 1.25 mg every 4 hours for 5 days

**Dosage Forms**

Cream, vaginal: 0.625 mg/g (42.5 g)

Injection: 25 mg (5 mL)

Tablet: 0.3 mg, 0.625 mg, 0.9 mg, 1.25 mg, 2.5 mg

## estrogens (esterified) (ES troe jenz es TER i fied)

**Synonyms** esterified estrogens

**U.S./Canadian Brand Names** Estratab®; Menest®

**Therapeutic Category** Estrogen Derivative

**Use** Atrophic vaginitis; hypogonadism; primary ovarian failure; vasomotor symptoms of menopause; prostatic carcinoma; osteoporosis prophylactic

**Usual Dosage** Adults: Oral:

Male: Prostate cancer: 1.25-2.5 mg 3 times/day

Female:

Hypogonadism: 2.5-7.5 mg/day for 20 days, off 10 days and repeat until menses occur

Moderate to severe vasomotor symptoms: 0.3-1.25 mg/day

**Dosage Forms** Tablet: 0.3 mg, 0.625 mg, 1.25 mg, 2.5 mg

**Estroject-2® Injection *(Discontinued)*** *see page 750*

**Estroject-L.A.® Injection *(Discontinued)*** *see page 750*

## estrone (ES trone)

**Synonyms** estrogenic substance aqueous

**U.S./Canadian Brand Names** Aquest®; Kestrone®; Oestrilin (Can)

**Therapeutic Category** Estrogen Derivative

**Use** Atrophic vaginitis; hypogonadism; primary ovarian failure; vasomotor symptoms of menopause; prostatic carcinoma; osteoporosis prophylactic

**Usual Dosage** Adults: I.M.:

Vasomotor symptoms, atrophic vaginitis: 0.1-0.5 mg 2-3 times/week

Primary ovarian failure, hypogonadism: 0.1-1 mg/week, up to 2 mg/week

Prostatic carcinoma: 2-4 mg 2-3 times/week

**Dosage Forms** Injection: 2 mg/mL (10 mL, 30 mL); 5 mg/mL (10 mL)

**Estronol® Injection *(Discontinued)*** *see page 750*

## estropipate (ES troe pih pate)

**Synonyms** piperazine estrone sulfate

**U.S./Canadian Brand Names** Ogen® Oral; Ogen® Vaginal; Ortho-Est® Oral

**Therapeutic Category** Estrogen Derivative

**Use** Atrophic vaginitis; hypogonadism; primary ovarian failure; vasomotor symptoms of menopause; prostatic carcinoma; osteoporosis prophylactic

**Usual Dosage** Adults: Female:

Moderate to severe vasomotor symptoms: Oral: 0.625-5 mg/day

Hypogonadism: Oral: 1.25-7.5 mg/day for 3 weeks followed by an 8- to 10-day rest period

Atrophic vaginitis or kraurosis vulvae: Vaginal: Instill 2-4 g/day 3 weeks on and 1 week off

**Dosage Forms**

Cream, vaginal: 0.15% [estropipate 1.5 mg/g] (42.5 g tube)

Tablet: 0.625 mg [estropipate 0.75 mg]; 1.25 mg [estropipate 1.5 mg]; 2.5 mg [estropipate 3 mg]; 5 mg [estropipate 6 mg]

**Estrostep® 21** *see* ethinyl estradiol and norethindrone *on page 232*

**Estrostep® Fe** *see* ethinyl estradiol and norethindrone *on page 232*

**Estrovis®** ***(Discontinued)*** *see page 750*

## etanercept (et a NER cept)

**U.S./Canadian Brand Names** Enbrel®

**Therapeutic Category** Antirheumatic, Disease Modifying

**Use** Reduction in signs and symptoms of moderately to severely active rheumatoid arthritis in patients who have had an inadequate response to one or more disease-modifying antirheumatic drugs (DMARDs).

**Usual Dosage** S.C.:

Children: 0.4 mg/kg (maximum: 25 mg dose)

Adult: 25 mg given twice weekly; if the physician determines that it is appropriate, patients may self-inject after proper training in injection technique

**Dosage Forms** Powder for injection: 25 mg

## ethacrynic acid (eth a KRIN ik AS id)

**Synonyms** sodium ethacrynate

**U.S./Canadian Brand Names** Edecrin®

**Therapeutic Category** Diuretic, Loop

**Use** Management of edema secondary to congestive heart failure; hepatic or renal disease, hypertension

**Usual Dosage**

Children:

Oral: 25 mg/day to start, increase by 25 mg/day at intervals of 2-3 days as needed, to a maximum of 3 mg/kg/day

I.V.: 1 mg/kg/dose, (maximum: 50 mg/dose); repeat doses not recommended

Adults:

Oral: 50-100 mg/day increased in increments of 25-50 mg at intervals of several days to a maximum of 400 mg/24 hours

I.V.: 0.5-1 mg/kg/dose (maximum: 50 mg/dose); repeat doses not recommended

**Dosage Forms**

Powder for injection, as ethacrynate sodium: 50 mg (50 mL)

Tablet: 25 mg, 50 mg

## ethambutol (e THAM byoo tole)

**U.S./Canadian Brand Names** Etibi® (Can); Myambutol®

**Therapeutic Category** Antimycobacterial Agent

**Use** Treatment of tuberculosis and other mycobacterial diseases in conjunction with other antimycobacterial agents

**Usual Dosage** Oral (not recommended in children <12 years of age):

Children >12 years: 15 mg/kg/day once daily

Adolescents and Adults: 15-25 mg/kg/day once daily, not to exceed 2.5 g/day

**Dosage Forms** Tablet, as hydrochloride: 100 mg, 400 mg

**Ethamolin®** *see* ethanolamine oleate *on next page*

**ethanoic acid** *see* acetic acid *on page 8*

**ethanol** *see* alcohol (ethyl) *on page 18*

**ethanolamine oleate** (ETH a nol a meen OH lee ate)

**U.S./Canadian Brand Names** Ethamolin®

**Therapeutic Category** Sclerosing Agent

**Use** Mild sclerosing agent used for bleeding esophageal varices

**Usual Dosage** Adults: 1.5-5 mL per varix, up to 20 mL total or 0.4 mL/kg; patients with severe hepatic dysfunction should receive less than recommended maximum dose

**Dosage Forms** Injection: 5% [50 mg/mL] (2 mL)

**Ethaquin®** ***(Discontinued)*** *see page 750*

**Ethatab®** ***(Discontinued)*** *see page 750*

**ethaverine** (eth AV er een)

**U.S./Canadian Brand Names** Ethavex-100®

**Therapeutic Category** Vasodilator

**Use** Peripheral and cerebral vascular insufficiency associated with arterial spasm

**Usual Dosage** Adults: Oral: 100 mg 3 times/day

**Dosage Forms** Tablet, as hydrochloride: 100 mg

**Ethavex-100®** *see* ethaverine *on this page*

**ethchlorvynol** (eth klor VI nole)

**U.S./Canadian Brand Names** Placidyl®

**Therapeutic Category** Hypnotic, Nonbarbiturate

**Controlled Substance** C-IV

**Use** Short-term management of insomnia

**Usual Dosage** Oral: 500-1000 mg at bedtime

**Dosage Forms** Capsule: 200 mg, 500 mg, 750 mg

**ethinyl estradiol** (ETH in il es tra DYE ole)

**U.S./Canadian Brand Names** Estinyl®

**Therapeutic Category** Estrogen Derivative

**Use** Atrophic vaginitis; hypogonadism; primary ovarian failure; vasomotor symptoms of menopause; prostatic carcinoma; osteoporosis prophylactic

**Usual Dosage** Adults: Oral:

Hypogonadism: 0.05 mg 1-3 times/day for 2 weeks

Prostatic carcinoma: 0.15-2 mg/day

Vasomotor symptoms: 0.02-0.05 mg for 21 days, off 7 days and repeat

**Dosage Forms** Tablet: 0.02 mg, 0.05 mg

**ethinyl estradiol and desogestrel**

(ETH in il es tra DYE ole & des oh JES trel)

**U.S./Canadian Brand Names** Apri®; Desogen®; Marvelon® (Can); Mircette®; Ortho-Cept®

**Therapeutic Category** Contraceptive, Oral

**Use** Prevention of pregnancy

**Usual Dosage** Oral: Adults: Female: Contraception:

Schedule 1 (Sunday starter): Dose begins on first Sunday after onset of menstruation; if the menstrual period starts on Sunday, take first tablet that very same day. **With a Sunday start, an additional method of contraception should be used until after the first 7 days of consecutive administration.**

For 21-tablet package: Dosage is 1 tablet daily for 21 consecutive days, followed by 7 days off of the medication; a new course begins on the 8th day after the last tablet is taken.

For 28-tablet package: Dosage is 1 tablet daily without interruption.

Schedule 2 (Day 1 starter): Dose starts on first day of menstrual cycle taking 1 tablet daily.

For 21-tablet package: Dosage is 1 tablet daily for 21 consecutive days, followed by 7 days off of the medication; a new course begins on the 8th day after the last tablet is taken.

For 28-tablet package: Dosage is 1 tablet daily without interruption.

If all doses have been taken on schedule and one menstrual period is missed, continue dosing cycle. If two consecutive menstrual periods are missed, pregnancy test is required before new dosing cycle is started.

**Missed doses monophasic formulations** (refer to package insert for complete information):

One dose missed: Take as soon as remembered or take 2 tablets next day

Two consecutive doses missed in the first 2 weeks: Take 2 tablets as soon as remembered or 2 tablets next 2 days. **An additional method of contraception should be used for 7 days after missed dose.**

Two consecutive doses missed in week 3 or three consecutive doses missed at any time: Schedule 1 (Sunday starter): Continue to take 1 tablet daily until Sunday, then discard the rest of the pack, and a new pack is started that same day. Schedule 2 (Day 1 starter): Current pack should be discarded, and a new pack started that same day. **An additional method of contraception should be used for 7 days after missed dose.**

**Dosage Forms** Tablet:

Apri®:

Day 1-21: Ethinyl estradiol 0.03 mg and desogestrel 0.15 mg

Day 22-28: Placebo

Desogen®, Ortho-Cept®: Ethinyl estradiol 0.03 mg and desogestrel 0.15 mg (21s, 28s)

Mircette®:

Day 1-21: Ethinyl estradiol 0.02 mg and desogestrel 0.15 mg

Day 22-23: Placebo

Day 24-28: Ethinyl estradiol 0.01 mg

## ethinyl estradiol and drospirenone

(ETH in il es tra DYE ole & droh SPYE re none)

**U.S./Canadian Brand Names** Yasmin®

**Therapeutic Category** Contraceptive, Oral

**Use** Prevention of pregnancy

**Usual Dosage** Oral: Adults: Female: Contraception: Dosage is 1 tablet daily for 28 consecutive days. Dose should be taken at the same time each day, either after the evening meal or at bedtime. Dosing may be started on the first day of menstrual period (Day 1 starter) or on the first Sunday after the onset of the menstrual period (Sunday starter).

Day 1 starter: Dose starts on first day of menstrual cycle taking 1 tablet daily.

Sunday starter: Dose begins on first Sunday after onset of menstruation; if the menstrual period starts on Sunday, take first tablet that very same day. **With a Sunday start, an additional method of contraception should be used until after the first 7 days of consecutive administration.**

If all doses have been taken on schedule and one menstrual period is missed, continue dosing cycle. If two consecutive menstrual periods are missed, pregnancy test is required before new dosing cycle is started.

If doses have been missed during the first 3 weeks and the menstrual period is missed, pregnancy should be ruled out prior to continuing treatment.

**Missed doses (monophasic formulations)** (refer to package insert for complete information):

One dose missed: Take as soon as remembered or take 2 tablets next day

Two consecutive doses missed in the first 2 weeks: Take 2 tablets as soon as remembered or 2 tablets next 2 days. **An additional method of contraception should be used for 7 days after missed dose.**

Two consecutive doses missed in week 3 or three consecutive doses missed at any time: **An additional method of contraception must be used for 7 days after a missed dose.**

(Continued)

## ethinyl estradiol and drospirenone *(Continued)*

Day 1 starter: Current pack should be discarded, and a new pack should be started that same day.

Sunday starter: Continue dose of 1 tablet daily until Sunday, then discard the rest of the pack, and a new pack should be started that same day.

Any number of doses missed in week 4: Continue taking one pill each day until pack is empty; no back-up method of contraception is needed

**Dosage adjustment in renal impairment:** Contraindicated in patients with renal dysfunction ($Cl_{cr}$ ≤50 mL/minute)

**Dosage adjustment in hepatic impairment:** Contraindicated in patients with hepatic dysfunction

**Dosage Forms** Tablet: Ethinyl estradiol 0.03 mg and drospirenone 3 mg [21 yellow round active tablets and 7 white inert round tablets] (28s)

## ethinyl estradiol and ethynodiol diacetate

(ETH in il es tra DYE ole & e thye noe DYE ole dye AS e tate)

**U.S./Canadian Brand Names** Demulen®; Zovia™

**Therapeutic Category** Contraceptive, Oral

**Use** Prevention of pregnancy; treatment of hypermenorrhea, endometriosis, female hypogonadism

**Usual Dosage** See ethinyl estradiol and desogestrel

**Dosage Forms** Tablet:

1/35: Ethinyl estradiol 0.035 mg and ethynodiol diacetate 1 mg (21s, 28s)

1/50: Ethinyl estradiol 0.05 mg and ethynodiol diacetate 1 mg (21s, 28s)

## ethinyl estradiol and levonorgestrel

(ETH in il es tra DYE ole & LEE voe nor jes trel)

**U.S./Canadian Brand Names** Alesse™; Levlen®; Levlite™; Levora®; Min-Ovral® (Can); Nordette®; Preven™; Tri-Levlen®; Triphasil®; Triquilar® (Can)

**Therapeutic Category** Contraceptive, Oral

**Use** Prevention of pregnancy; treatment of hypermenorrhea, endometriosis, female hypogonadism

**Usual Dosage** See ethinyl estradiol and desogestrel

**Dosage Forms** Tablet:

Alesse™, Levlite™: Ethinyl estradiol 0.02 mg and levonorgestrel 0.1 mg (21s, 28s)

Levlen®, Levora®, Nordette®: Ethinyl estradiol 0.03 mg and levonorgestrel 0.15 mg (21s, 28s)

Preven®: Ethinyl estradiol 0.05 mg and levonorgestrel 0.25 mg (4s)

Trivora®: Phase 1 (6 blue tablets): Ethinyl estradiol 0.03 mg and levonorgestrel 0.05 mg; Phase 2 (5 white tablets): Ethinyl estradiol 0.04 mg and levonorgestrel 0.075 mg; Phase 3 (10 pink tablets): Ethinyl estradiol 0.03 mg and levonorgestrel 0.125 mg (21s, 28s)

Tri-Levlen®, Triphasil®: Phase 1 (6 brown tablets): Ethinyl estradiol 0.03 mg and levonorgestrel 0.05 mg; Phase 2 (5 white tablets): Ethinyl estradiol 0.04 mg and levonorgestrel 0.075 mg; Phase 3 (10 yellow tablets): Ethinyl estradiol 0.03 mg and levonorgestrel 0.125 mg (21s, 28s)

## ethinyl estradiol and norethindrone

(ETH in il es tra DYE ole & nor eth IN drone)

**U.S./Canadian Brand Names** Brevicon®; Estrostep® 21; Estrostep® Fe; Femhrt™; Genora® 0.5/35; Genora® 1/35; Jenest-28™; Loestrin®; Minestrin™ (Can); Modicon™; Nelova™ 0.5/35E; Nelova™ 10/11; Norethin™ 1/35E; Norinyl® 1+35; Ortho® 0.5/35 (Can); Ortho-Novum® 1/35; Ortho-Novum® 7/7/7; Ortho-Novum® 10/11; Ovcon® 35; Ovcon® 50; Synphasic® (Can); Tri-Norinyl®

**Therapeutic Category** Contraceptive, Oral

**Use** Prevention of pregnancy; treatment of hypermenorrhea, endometriosis, female hypogonadism

**Usual Dosage** See ethinyl estradiol and desogestrel

**Dosage Forms** Tablet:

Brevicon®, Genora® 0.5/35, Modicon™, Nelova™ 0.5/35E: Ethinyl estradiol 0.035 mg and norethindrone 0.5 mg (21s, 28s)

Estrostep®:

Triangular tablet (white): Ethinyl estradiol 0.02 mg and norethindrone acetate 1 mg

Square tablet (white): Ethinyl estradiol 0.03 mg and norethindrone acetate 1 mg

Round tablet (white): Ethinyl estradiol 0.035 mg and norethindrone acetate 1 mg

Estrostep® Fe:

Triangular tablet (white): Ethinyl estradiol 0.02 mg and norethindrone acetate 1 mg

Square tablet (white): Ethinyl estradiol 0.03 mg and norethindrone acetate 1 mg

Round tablet (white): Ethinyl estradiol 0.035 mg and norethindrone acetate 1 mg

Brown tablet: Ferrous fumarate 75 mg

Femhrt™: Ethinyl estradiol 0.005 mg and norethindrone acetate 1 mg

Loestrin® 1.5/30: Ethinyl estradiol 0.03 mg and norethindrone acetate 1.5 mg (21s)

Loestrin® Fe 1.5/30: Ethinyl estradiol 0.03 mg and norethindrone acetate 1.5 mg with ferrous fumarate 75 mg in 7 inert tablets (28s)

Loestrin® 1/20: Ethinyl estradiol 0.02 mg and norethindrone acetate 1 mg (21s)

Loestrin® Fe 1/20: Ethinyl estradiol 0.02 mg and norethindrone acetate 1 mg with ferrous fumarate 75 mg in 7 inert tablets (28s)

Genora® 1/35, N.E.E.® 1/35, Nelova® 1/35E, Norethin™ 1/35E, Norinyl® 1+35, Ortho-Novum® 1/35: Ethinyl estradiol 0.035 mg and norethindrone 1 mg (21s, 28s)

Jenest-28™: Phase 1 (7 white tablets): Ethinyl estradiol 0.035 mg and norethindrone 0.5 mg; Phase 2 (14 peach tablets): Ethinyl estradiol 0.035 mg and norethindrone 1 mg and 7 green inert tablets (28s)

Ortho-Novum® 7/7/7: Phase 1 (7 white tablets): Ethinyl estradiol 0.035 mg and norethindrone 0.5 mg; Phase 2 (7 light peach tablets): Ethinyl estradiol 0.035 mg and norethindrone 0.75 mg; Phase 3 (7 peach tablets): Ethinyl estradiol 0.035 mg and norethindrone 1 mg (21s, 28s)

Ortho-Novum® 10/11: Phase 1 (10 white tablets): Ethinyl estradiol 0.035 mg and norethindrone 0.5 mg; Phase 2 (11 dark yellow tablets): Ethinyl estradiol 0.035 mg and norethindrone 1 mg (21s, 28s)

Ovcon® 35: Ethinyl estradiol 0.035 mg and norethindrone 0.4 mg (21s, 28s)

Ovcon® 50: Ethinyl estradiol 0.050 mg and norethindrone 1 mg (21s, 28s)

Tri-Norinyl®: Phase 1 (7 blue tablets): Ethinyl estradiol 0.035 mg and norethindrone 0.5 mg; Phase 2 (9 green tablets): Ethinyl estradiol 0.035 mg and norethindrone 1 mg; Phase 3 (5 blue tablets): Ethinyl estradiol 0.035 mg and norethindrone 0.5 mg (21s, 28s)

## ethinyl estradiol and norgestimate

(ETH in il es tra DYE ole & nor JES ti mate)

**U.S./Canadian Brand Names** Ortho-Cyclen®; Ortho-Prefest®; Ortho Tri-Cyclen®

**Therapeutic Category** Contraceptive, Oral

**Use** Prevention of pregnancy

**Usual Dosage** See ethinyl estradiol and desogestrel

**Dosage Forms** Tablet:

Ortho-Cyclen®: Ethinyl estradiol 0.035 mg and norgestimate 0.25 mg (21s, 28s)

Ortho Tri-Cyclen®: Phase 1 (7 white tablets): Ethinyl estradiol 0.035 mg and norgestimate 0.18 mg; Phase 2 (5 light blue tablets): Ethinyl estradiol 0.035 mg and norgestimate 0.215 mg; Phase 3 (10 blue tablets): Ethinyl estradiol 0.035 mg and norgestimate 0.25 mg (21s, 28s)

Ortho-Prefest®: Estradiol 1 mg (#15) and estradiol 1 mg and norgestimate 0.09 mg (#15)

## ethinyl estradiol and norgestrel (ETH in il es tra DYE ole & nor JES trel)

**U.S./Canadian Brand Names** Lo/Ovral®; Ovral®

**Therapeutic Category** Contraceptive, Oral

(Continued)

## ethinyl estradiol and norgestrel *(Continued)*

**Use** Prevention of pregnancy; treatment of hypermenorrhea, endometriosis, female hypogonadism

**Usual Dosage** See ethinyl estradiol and desogestrel

Postcoital contraception or "morning after" pill: Oral (ethinyl estradiol 0.05 mg and norgestrel 0.5 mg): 2 tablets at initial visit and 2 tablets 12 hours later

**Dosage Forms** Tablet:

Lo/Ovral®: Ethinyl estradiol 0.03 mg and norgestrel 0.3 mg (21s and 28s)

Ovral®: Ethinyl estradiol 0.05 mg and norgestrel 0.5 mg (21s and 28s)

**Ethiodol®** *see* radiological/contrast media (ionic) *on page 516*

**ethiofos** *see* amifostine *on page 29*

## ethionamide (e thye on AM ide)

**U.S./Canadian Brand Names** Trecator®-SC

**Therapeutic Category** Antimycobacterial Agent

**Use** In conjunction with other antituberculosis agents in the treatment of tuberculosis and other mycobacterial diseases

**Usual Dosage** Oral:

Children: 15-20 mg/kg/day in 2 divided doses, not to exceed 1 g/day

Adults: 500-1000 mg/day in 1-3 divided doses

**Dosage Forms** Tablet, sugar coated: 250 mg

**Ethmozine®** *see* moricizine *on page 399*

## ethopropazine *(Canada only)* (eth oh PROE pa zeen)

**U.S./Canadian Brand Names** Parsitan® (Can)

**Therapeutic Category** Anti-Parkinson's Agent

**Use** Symptomatic treatment of drug induced extrapyramidal manifestations and of Parkinson's disease of postencephalitic, arteriosclerotic or idiopathic etiology.

**Usual Dosage** Must be adapted to each individual. In drug induced extrapyramidal reactions 100 mg twice daily usually brings about good control of symptoms. In post encephalitic, arteriosclerotic or idiopathic parkinsonism, initiate treatment at a low dose of 50 mg 3 times a day and increase from 50 to 100 mg daily every 2 to 3 days until the optimum effect is obtained or the limit of tolerance is attained. Drowsiness and anticholinergic effects which may appear at the beginning of treatment generally subside after a few days. The normal daily dose usually ranges between 100 and 500 mg but it may reach 1 g or more per day in certain patients.

**Dosage Forms** Tablet, hydrochloride: 50 mg

## ethosuximide (eth oh SUKS i mide)

**U.S./Canadian Brand Names** Zarontin®

**Therapeutic Category** Anticonvulsant

**Use** Management of absence (petit mal) seizures, myoclonic seizures, and akinetic epilepsy

**Usual Dosage** Oral:

Children 3-6 years:

Initial: 250 mg

Increment: 250 mg/day at 4- to 7-day intervals

Maintenance: 20-40 mg/kg/day

Maximum: 1500 mg/day in 2 divided doses

Children >6 years and Adults:

Initial: 500 mg/day

Increment: 250 mg/day at 4- to 7-day intervals

Maintenance: 20-40 mg/kg/day

Maximum: 1500 mg/day in 2 divided doses

**Dosage Forms**
Capsule: 250 mg
Syrup (raspberry flavor): 250 mg/5 mL (473 mL)

## ethotoin (ETH oh toyn)

**Synonyms** ethylphenylhydantoin
**U.S./Canadian Brand Names** Peganone®
**Therapeutic Category** Hydantoin
**Use** Generalized tonic-clonic or complex-partial seizures
**Usual Dosage** Oral:
Children: 250 mg twice daily, up to 250 mg 4 times/day
Adults: 250 mg 4 times/day after meals, may be increased up to 3 g/day in divided doses 4 times/day
**Dosage Forms** Tablet: 250 mg

**ethoxynaphthamido penicillin sodium** *see* nafcillin *on page 406*

**Ethrane®** *see* enflurane *on page 214*

**ethyl aminobenzoate** *see* benzocaine *on page 72*

## ethyl chloride (ETH il KLOR ide)

**Synonyms** chloroethane
**Therapeutic Category** Local Anesthetic
**Use** Local anesthetic in minor operative procedures and to relieve pain caused by insect stings and burns, and irritation caused by myofascial and visceral pain syndromes
**Usual Dosage** Topical: Dosage varies with use
**Dosage Forms** Spray: 100 mL, 120 mL

## ethyl chloride and dichlorotetrafluoroethane

(ETH il KLOR ide & dye klor oh te tra floo or oh ETH ane)
**U.S./Canadian Brand Names** Fluro-Ethyl® Aerosol
**Therapeutic Category** Local Anesthetic
**Use** Topical refrigerant anesthetic to control pain associated with minor surgical procedures, dermabrasion, injections, contusions, and minor strains
**Usual Dosage** Topical: Press gently on side of spray valve allowing the liquid to emerge as a fine mist approximately 2" to 4" from site of application
**Dosage Forms** Aerosol: Ethyl chloride 25% and dichlorotetrafluoroethane 75% (225 g)

**ethylphenylhydantoin** *see* ethotoin *on this page*

**Ethyol®** *see* amifostine *on page 29*

**Etibi® (Can)** *see* ethambutol *on page 229*

## etidocaine (e TI doe kane)

**U.S./Canadian Brand Names** Duranest®
**Therapeutic Category** Local Anesthetic
**Use** Infiltration anesthesia; peripheral nerve blocks; central neural blocks
**Usual Dosage** Varies with procedure; use 1% for peripheral nerve block, central nerve block, lumbar peridural caudal; use 1.5% for maxillary infiltration or inferior alveolar nerve block; use 1% or 1.5% for intra-abdominal or pelvic surgery, lower limb surgery, or caesarean section
**Dosage Forms**
Injection, as hydrochloride: 1% [10 mg/mL] (30 mL)
With epinephrine 1:200,000: 1% [10 mg/mL] (30 mL); 1.5% [15 mg/mL] (20 mL)

## etidronate disodium (e ti DROE nate dye SOW dee um)

**Synonyms** EHDP
**U.S./Canadian Brand Names** Didronel®
(Continued)

## etidronate disodium *(Continued)*

**Therapeutic Category** Bisphosphonate Derivative

**Use** Symptomatic treatment of Paget's disease and heterotopic ossification due to spinal cord injury; hypercalcemia associated with malignancy

**Usual Dosage** Adults: Oral:

Paget's disease: 5 mg/kg/day administered every day for no more than 6 months; may administer 10 mg/kg/day for up to 3 months. Daily dose may be divided if adverse GI effects occur.

Heterotopic ossification with spinal cord injury: 20 mg/kg/day for 2 weeks, then 10 mg/kg/day for 10 weeks (this dosage has been used in children, however, treatment >1 year has been associated with a rachitic syndrome)

Hypercalcemia associated with malignancy: I.V.: 7.5 mg/kg/day for 3 days

**Dosage Forms**

Injection: 50 mg/mL (6 mL)

Tablet: 200 mg, 400 mg

## etodolac (ee toe DOE lak)

**Synonyms** etodolic acid

**U.S./Canadian Brand Names** Apo®-Etodolac (Can); Gen-Etodolac (Can); Lodine®; Lodine® XL; Ultradol™ (Can)

**Therapeutic Category** Analgesic, Non-narcotic; Nonsteroidal Anti-inflammatory Drug (NSAID)

**Use** Acute and long-term use in the management of signs and symptoms of osteoarthritis and management of pain

**Usual Dosage** Adults: Oral:

Acute pain: 200-400 mg every 6-8 hours, as needed, not to exceed total daily doses of 1200 mg

Osteoarthritis: Initial: 800-1200 mg/day administered in divided doses: 400 mg 2 or 3 times/day; 300 mg 2, 3 or 4 times/day; 200 mg 3 or 4 times/day; total daily dose should not exceed 1200 mg; for patients weighing <60 kg, total daily dose should not exceed 20 mg/kg; extended release dose: one tablet daily

**Dosage Forms**

Capsule: 200 mg, 300 mg

Lodine®: 200 mg, 300 mg

Tablet: 400 mg, 500 mg

Lodine®: 400 mg, 500 mg

Tablet, extended release (Lodine® XL): 400 mg, 500 mg, 600 mg

**etodolic acid** *see* etodolac *on this page*

## etomidate (e TOM i date)

**U.S./Canadian Brand Names** Amidate®

**Therapeutic Category** General Anesthetic

**Use** Induction of general anesthesia

**Usual Dosage** Children >10 years and Adults: I.V.: 0.2-0.6 mg/kg over period of 30-60 seconds

**Dosage Forms** Injection: 2 mg/mL (10 mL, 20 mL)

**Etopophos®** *see* etoposide phosphate *on next page*

## etoposide (e toe POE side)

**Synonyms** EPEG; VP-16

**U.S./Canadian Brand Names** Toposar® Injection; VePesid®

**Therapeutic Category** Antineoplastic Agent

**Use** Treatment of testicular and lung carcinomas, malignant lymphoma, Hodgkin's disease, leukemias (ALL, AML), neuroblastoma; also used in the treatment of Ewing's sarcoma, rhabdomyosarcoma, Wilms' tumor, brain tumors, and as a conditioning regimen for bone marrow transplantation in patients with advanced hematologic malignancies

**Usual Dosage** Refer to individual protocols

Pediatric solid tumors: I.V.: 60-120 mg/m$^2$/day for 3-5 days every 3-6 weeks

Leukemia in children: I.V.: 100-200 mg/m$^2$/day for 5 days

Testicular cancer: I.V.: 50-100 mg/m$^2$/day on days 1-5 or 100 mg/m$^2$/day on days 1, 3 and 5 every 3-4 weeks for 3-4 courses

Small cell lung cancer:

Oral: Twice the I.V. dose rounded to the nearest 50 mg administered once daily if total dose ≤400 mg or in divided doses if >400 mg

I.V.: 35 mg/m$^2$/day for 4 days or 50 mg/m$^2$/day for 5 days every 3-4 weeks

**Dosage Forms**

Capsule (VePesid®): 50 mg

Injection (VePesid®, Toposar®): 20 mg/mL (5 mL, 7.5 mL, 25 mL, 50 mL)

## etoposide phosphate (e toe POE side FOS fate)

**U.S./Canadian Brand Names** Etopophos®

**Therapeutic Category** Antineoplastic Agent

**Use** Treatment of refractory testicular tumors and small cell lung cancer

**Usual Dosage** Refer to individual protocols. Adults:

Small cell lung cancer:

I.V. (in combination with other approved chemotherapeutic drugs): **Equivalent doses of etoposide phosphate to an etoposide dosage** range of 35 mg/m$^2$/day for 4 days to 50 mg/m$^2$/day for 5 days. Courses are repeated at 3- to 4-week intervals after adequate recovery from any toxicity.

Testicular cancer:

I.V. (in combination with other approved chemotherapeutic agents): **Equivalent dose of etoposide phosphate to etoposide dosage** range of 50-100 mg/m$^2$/day on days 1-5 to 100 mg/m$^2$/day on days 1, 3, and 5. Courses are repeated at 3- to 4-week intervals after adequate recovery from any toxicity.

**Dosage Forms** Powder for injection, lyophilized: 119.3 mg (100 mg base)

**Etrafon®** *see* amitriptyline and perphenazine *on page 33*

## etretinate (e TRET i nate)

**U.S./Canadian Brand Names** Tegison®

**Therapeutic Category** Antipsoriatic Agent

**Use** Treatment of severe recalcitrant psoriasis in patients intolerant of or unresponsive to standard therapies

**Usual Dosage** Adults: Oral (individualized): Initial: 0.75-1 mg/kg/day in divided doses up to 1.5 mg/kg/day; maintenance dose established after 8-10 weeks of therapy 0.5-0.75 mg/kg/day

**Dosage Forms** Capsule: 10 mg, 25 mg

**ETS-2%® Topical** *see* erythromycin (ophthalmic/topical) *on page 222*

**Eudal®-SR** *see* guaifenesin and pseudoephedrine *on page 283*

**Euflex® (Can)** *see* flutamide *on page 259*

**Euglucon® (Can)** *see* glyburide *on page 276*

**Eulexin®** *see* flutamide *on page 259*

**Eumovate® (Can)** *see* clobetasol *on page 143*

**Eurax® Topical** *see* crotamiton *on page 157*

**Euthroid® Tablet *(Discontinued)*** *see page 750*

**Eutron® *(Discontinued)*** *see page 750*

**Evac-Q-Mag® *(Discontinued)*** *see page 750*

**Evalose®** *see* lactulose *on page 338*

**Everone® Injection** *see* testosterone *on page 576*

**Evista®** *see* raloxifene *on page 518*

**E-Vitamin® [OTC]** *see* vitamin E *on page 631*

**Evoxac™** *see* cevimeline *on page 123*

**Exact® Cream [OTC]** *see* benzoyl peroxide *on page 74*

**Excedrin®, Extra Strength [OTC]** *see* acetaminophen, aspirin, and caffeine *on page 6*

**Excedrin® IB [OTC]** *see* ibuprofen *on page 311*

**Excedrin® P.M. [OTC]** *see* acetaminophen and diphenhydramine *on page 5*

**Exelderm® Topical** *see* sulconazole *on page 562*

**Exelon®** *see* rivastigmine *on page 529*

## exemestane (ex e MES tane)

**U.S./Canadian Brand Names** Aromasin®

**Therapeutic Category** Antineoplastic Agent

**Controlled Substance** [EX196]cancer

**Use** Treatment of advanced breast cancer in postmenopausal women whose disease has progressed following tamoxifen therapy

**Dosage Forms** Tablet: 25 mg

**Exidine® Scrub [OTC]** *see* chlorhexidine gluconate *on page 126*

**Exna® *(Discontinued)*** *see page 750*

**Exosurf® Neonatal™** *see* colfosceril palmitate *on page 152*

**Exsel® Shampoo** *see* selenium sulfide *on page 540*

**Extendryl® SR** *see* chlorpheniramine, phenylephrine, and methscopolamine *on page 131*

**Extra Action Cough Syrup [OTC]** *see* guaifenesin and dextromethorphan *on page 282*

**Extraprin® [OTC]** *see* acetaminophen, aspirin, and caffeine *on page 6*

**Extra Strength Adprin-B® [OTC]** *see* aspirin *on page 55*

**Extra Strength Bayer® Enteric 500 Aspirin [OTC]** *see* aspirin *on page 55*

**Extra Strength Bayer® Plus [OTC]** *see* aspirin *on page 55*

**Extra Strength Doan's® [OTC]** *see* magnesium salicylate *on page 362*

**Eye Bright®** *see* beta-carotene *on page 76*

**Eye-Lube-A® Solution [OTC]** *see* artificial tears *on page 53*

**Eye-Sed® Ophthalmic [OTC]** *see* zinc sulfate *on page 639*

**Eyesine® Ophthalmic [OTC]** *see* tetrahydrozoline *on page 580*

**Eyestil® (Can)** *see* sodium hyaluronate *on page 550*

**Eye-Zine® [OTC]** *see* tetrahydrozoline *on page 580*

**Ezide®** *see* hydrochlorothiazide *on page 299*

**Ezol®** *see* butalbital compound and acetaminophen *on page 93*

**$f_3t$** *see* trifluridine *on page 605*

## factor IX complex (human) (FAK ter nyne KOM pleks HYU man)

**U.S./Canadian Brand Names** AlphaNine® SD; BeneFix™; Hemonyne®; Konȳne® 80; Profilnine® SD; Proplex® T

**Therapeutic Category** Antihemophilic Agent

**Use**

Control bleeding in patients with factor IX deficiency (hemophilia B or Christmas disease). **Note:** Factor IX concentrate containing ONLY factor IX is also available and preferable for this indication.

Prevention/control of bleeding in hemophilia A patients with inhibitors to factor VIII

Prevention/control of bleeding in patients with factor VII deficiency

Emergency correction of the coagulopathy of warfarin excess in critical situations

**Usual Dosage** Factor IX deficiency (1 unit/kg raises IX levels 1%)

Children and Adults: I.V.:

Hospitalized patients: 20-50 units/kg/dose; may be higher in special cases; may be administered every 24 hours or more often in special cases

Inhibitor patients: 75-100 units/kg/dose; may be administered every 6-12 hours

**Dosage Forms** Injection:

AlphaNine® SD: Single-dose vial

BeneFix™: 250 units, 500 units, 1000 units

Konÿne® 80: 20 mL, 40 mL

Hemonyne®: 20 mL, 40 mL

Profilnine® SD: Single-dose vial

Proplex® T: 30 mL vial

**factor IX purified** *see* factor IX (purified/human) *on this page*

## factor IX (purified/human) (FAK ter nyne PURE eh fide/HYU man)

**Synonyms** factor IX purified; monoclonal antibody purified

**U.S./Canadian Brand Names** Mononine®

**Therapeutic Category** Antihemophilic Agent

**Use**

Control bleeding in patients with factor IX deficiency (hemophilia B or Christmas disease)

Mononine® contains **nondetectable levels of factors II, VII, and X** (<0.0025 units per factor IX unit using standard coagulation assays) and is, therefore, **NOT INDICATED** for replacement therapy of any of these clotting factors

Mononine® is also **NOT INDICATED** in the treatment or reversal of coumarin-induced anticoagulation or in a hemorrhagic state caused by hepatitis-induced lack of production of liver dependent coagulation factors.

**Usual Dosage** Children and Adults: Dosage is expressed in units of factor IX activity and must be individualized. I.V. only:

**Formula for units required to raise blood level %:**

Number of factor IX Units Required = body weight (in kg) x desired factor IX level increase (% normal) x 1 unit/kg

For example, for a 100% level a patient who has an actual level of 20%: Number of factor IX Units needed = 70 kg x 80% x 1 Unit/kg = 5,600 Units

**Dosage Forms** Factor IX units listed per vial and per lot to lot variation *$0.72*/unit of factor IX

Injection: 250 units, 500 units, 1000 units

## factor VIIa (recombinant) (factor seven ay ree KOM be nant)

**Synonyms** coagulation factor VIIa; rFVIIa

**U.S./Canadian Brand Names** Novo-Seven®

**Therapeutic Category** Antihemophilic Agent; Blood Product Derivative

**Use** Treatment of bleeding episodes in patients with hemophilia A or B when inhibitors to factor VIII or factor IX are present

**Usual Dosage** Children and Adults: I.V. administration only: 90 mcg/kg every 2 hours until hemostasis is achieved or until the treatment is judged ineffective. The dose and interval may be adjusted based upon the severity of bleeding and the degree of hemostasis achieved. The duration of therapy following hemostasis has not been fully established; for patients experiencing severe bleeds, dosing should be continued at 3- to 6-

(Continued)

## factor VIIa (recombinant) *(Continued)*

hour intervals after hemostasis has been achieved and the duration of dosing should be minimized.

In clinical trials, dosages have ranged from 35-120 mcg/kg and a decision on the final therapeutic dosages was reached within 8 hours in the majority of patients

**Dosage Forms** Powder for injection: 1.2 mg, 2.4 mg, 4.8 mg

**factor VIII** *see* antihemophilic factor (human) *on page 43*

**factor VIII recombinant** *see* antihemophilic factor (recombinant) *on page 44*

**Factrel®** *see* gonadorelin *on page 279*

## famciclovir (fam SYE kloe veer)

**U.S./Canadian Brand Names** Famvir™

**Therapeutic Category** Antiviral Agent

**Use** Management of acute herpes zoster (shingles); treatment of recurrent herpes simplex in immunocompetent patients; treatment of recurrent mucocutaneous herpes simplex infections in HIV-infected patients

**Usual Dosage** Adults: Oral:

Acute herpes zoster: 500 mg every 8 hours for 7 days

Recurrent herpes simplex in immunocompetent patients: 125 mg twice daily for 5 days

Herpes simplex infections in HIV-infected patients: 500 mg twice daily

**Dosage Forms** Tablet: 125 mg, 250 mg, 500 mg

## famotidine (fa MOE ti deen)

**U.S./Canadian Brand Names** Alti-Famotidine (Can); Apo®-Famotidine (Can); Gen-Famotidine (Can); Mylanta AR®; Novo-Famotidine (Can); Nu-Famotidine (Can); Pepcid®; Pepcid® AC Acid Controller [OTC]; Pepcid RPD®; Rhoxal-famotidine (Can); Ulcidine® (Can)

**Therapeutic Category** Histamine $H_2$ Antagonist

**Use** Therapy and treatment of duodenal ulcer, gastric ulcer, control gastric pH in critically ill patients, symptomatic relief in gastritis, gastroesophageal reflux, active benign ulcer, and pathological hypersecretory conditions

**Usual Dosage**

Children: Oral, I.V.: Doses of 1-2 mg/kg/day have been used; maximum dose: 40 mg

Adults:

Oral:

Duodenal ulcer, gastric ulcer: 40 mg/day at bedtime for 4-8 weeks

Hypersecretory conditions: Initial: 20 mg every 6 hours, may increase up to 160 mg every 6 hours

GERD: 20 mg twice daily for 6 weeks

I.V.: 20 mg every 12 hours

**Dosage Forms**

Gelcap (Pepcid® AC): 10 mg

Infusion, premixed in NS: 20 mg (50 mL)

Injection: 10 mg/mL (2 mL, 4 mL)

Powder for oral suspension (cherry-banana-mint flavor): 40 mg/5 mL (50 mL)

Tablet (Mylanta AR®): 10 mg

Tablet, chewable (Pepcid® AC): 10 mg

Tablet, film coated: 20 mg, 40 mg

Tablet, orally disintegrating (Pepcid RPD™): 20 mg, 40 mg

Pepcid® AC Acid Controller: 10 mg

## famotidine, calcium carbonate, and magnesium hydroxide

(fa MOE ti deen, KAL see um KAR bun ate, & mag NEE zhum hye DROKS ide)

**U.S./Canadian Brand Names** Pepcid® Complete [OTC]

**Therapeutic Category** Antacid; Histamine $H_2$ Antagonist

**Use** Relief of heartburn due to acid indigestion

**Usual Dosage** Children ≥12 years and Adults: Relief of heartburn due to acid indigestion: Oral: Pepcid® Complete: 1 tablet as needed; no more than 2 tablets in 24 hours; do **not** swallow whole, chew tablet completely before swallowing; do not use for longer than 14 days

**Dosage Forms** Tablet, chewable: Famotidine 10 mg, calcium carbonate 800 mg, and magnesium hydroxide 165 mg

**Famvir™** *see* famciclovir *on previous page*

**Fansidar®** *see* sulfadoxine and pyrimethamine *on page 564*

**Farbital®** *see* butalbital compound and aspirin *on page 93*

**Fareston®** *see* toremifene *on page 597*

**Fastin®** ***(Discontinued)*** *see page 750*

## fat emulsion (fat e MUL shun)

**Synonyms** intravenous fat emulsion

**U.S./Canadian Brand Names** Intralipid®; Liposyn®; Nutrilipid®; Soyacal®

**Therapeutic Category** Intravenous Nutritional Therapy

**Use** Source of calories and essential fatty acids for patients requiring parenteral nutrition of extended duration

**Usual Dosage** Fat emulsion should not exceed 60% of the total daily calories

Initial dose:

Infants, premature: 0.25-0.5 g/kg/day, increase by 0.25-0.5 g/kg/day to a maximum of 3-4 g/kg/day; maximum rate of infusion: 0.15 g/kg/hour (0.75 mL/kg/hour of 20% solution)

Infants and Children: 0.5-1 g/kg/day, increase by 0.5 g/kg/day to a maximum of 3-4 g/kg/day; maximum rate of infusion: 0.25 g/kg/hour (1.25 mL/kg/hour of 20% solution)

Adolescents and Adults: 1 g/kg/day, increase by 0.5-1 g/kg/day to a maximum of 2.5 g/kg/day; maximum rate of infusion: 0.25 g/kg/hour (1.25 mL/kg/hour of 20% solution); do not exceed 50 mL/hour (20%) or 100 mL/hour (10%)

Fatty acid deficiency: Children and Adults: 8% to 10% of total caloric intake; infuse once or twice weekly

**Note:** At the onset of therapy, the patient should be observed for any immediate allergic reactions such as dyspnea, cyanosis, and fever. Slower initial rates of infusion may be used for the first 10-15 minutes of the infusion (eg, 0.1 mL/minute of 10% or 0.05 mL/minute of 20% solution).

**Dosage Forms** Injection: 10% [100 mg/mL] (50 mL, 100 mL, 200 mL, 250 mL, 500 mL); 20% [200 mg/mL] (50 mL, 100 mL, 200 mL, 250 mL, 500 mL)

**5-FC** *see* flucytosine *on page 252*

**FC1157a** *see* toremifene *on page 597*

**Febrol® [OTC]** *see* acetaminophen *on page 3*

**Fedahist® Expectorant [OTC]** *see* guaifenesin and pseudoephedrine *on page 283*

**Fedahist® Expectorant Pediatric [OTC]** *see* guaifenesin and pseudoephedrine *on page 283*

**Fedahist® Tablet [OTC]** *see* chlorpheniramine and pseudoephedrine *on page 130*

**Feiba VH Immuno®** *see* anti-inhibitor coagulant complex *on page 44*

## felbamate (FEL ba mate)

**U.S./Canadian Brand Names** Felbatol®

**Therapeutic Category** Anticonvulsant

**Use** Not a first-line agent; reserved for patients who do not adequately respond to alternative agents and whose epilepsy is so severe that benefit outweighs risk of liver

(Continued)

## felbamate *(Continued)*

failure or aplastic anemia; used as monotherapy and adjunctive therapy in patients ≥14 years of age with partial seizures with and without secondary generalization; adjunctive therapy in children ≥2 years of age who have partial and generalized seizures associated with Lennox-Gastaut syndrome

**Usual Dosage** Oral:

Monotherapy: 1200 mg/day in divided doses 3 or 4 times/day; titrate previously untreated patients under close clinical supervision, increasing the dosage in 600 mg increments every 2 weeks to 2400 mg/day based on clinical response and thereafter to 3600 mg/day in clinically indicated

Conversion to monotherapy: Initiate at 1200 mg/day in divided doses 3 or 4 times/day, reduce the dosage of the concomitant anticonvulsant(s) by 33% at the initiation of felbamate therapy; at week 2, increase the felbamate dosage to 2400 mg/day while reducing the dosage of the other anticonvulsant(s) up to an additional 33% of their original dosage; at week 3, increase the felbamate dosage up to 3600 mg/day and continue to reduce the dosage of the other anticonvulsant(s) as clinically indicated

Adjunctive therapy:

Week 1:

Felbamate: 1200 mg/day initial dose

Concomitant anticonvulsant(s): Reduce original dosage by 20% to 33%

Week 2:

Felbamate: 2400 mg/day (Therapeutic range)

Concomitant anticonvulsant(s): Reduce original dosage by up to an additional 33%

Week 3:

Felbamate: 3600 mg/day (Therapeutic range)

Concomitant anticonvulsant(s): Reduce original dosage as clinically indicated

**Dosage Forms**

Suspension, oral: 600 mg/5 mL (240 mL, 960 mL)

Tablet: 400 mg, 600 mg

**Felbatol®** *see* felbamate *on previous page*

**Feldene®** *see* piroxicam *on page 474*

## felodipine (fe LOE di peen)

**U.S./Canadian Brand Names** Plendil®; Renedil® (Can)

**Therapeutic Category** Calcium Channel Blocker

**Use** Management of angina pectoris due to coronary insufficiency, hypertension

**Usual Dosage** Oral:

Adults: Initial: 5 mg once daily; dosage range: 2.5-10 mg once daily; may increase dose up to a maximum of 10 mg

Elderly: Initial: 2.5 mg/day

**Dosage Forms** Tablet, extended release: 2.5 mg, 5 mg, 10 mg

**Femara®** *see* letrozole *on page 342*

**FemCare®** ***(Discontinued)*** *see page 750*

**Femcet®** *see* butalbital compound and acetaminophen *on page 93*

**Femguard®** ***(Discontinued)*** *see page 750*

**Femhrt™** *see* ethinyl estradiol and norethindrone *on page 232*

**Femiron® [OTC]** *see* ferrous fumarate *on page 246*

**Femizol-M® [OTC]** *see* miconazole *on page 390*

**Fem-Prin® [OTC]** *see* acetaminophen, aspirin, and caffeine *on page 6*

**Femstat®** ***(Discontinued)*** *see page 750*

**Fenesin™** *see* guaifenesin *on page 281*

**Fenesin™ DM** *see* guaifenesin and dextromethorphan *on page 282*

## fenofibrate (fen oh FYE brate)

**Synonyms** procetofene; proctofene

**U.S./Canadian Brand Names** Apo®-Fenofibrate (Can); Nu-Fenofibrate (Can); TriCor®

**Therapeutic Category** Antihyperlipidemic Agent, Miscellaneous

**Use** Adjunct to dietary therapy for the treatment of adults with very high elevations of serum triglyceride levels (types IV and V hyperlipidemia) who are at risk of pancreatitis and who do not respond adequately to a determined dietary effort; its efficacy can be enhanced by combination with other hypolipidemic agents that have a different mechanism of action; safety and efficacy may be greater than that of clofibrate

**Usual Dosage** Adults: Oral: Initial: 67 mg/day, up to 3 capsules (201 mg)

**Dosage Forms** Capsule: 67 mg, 134 mg, 200 mg

## fenoldopam (fe NOL doe pam)

**U.S./Canadian Brand Names** Corlopam®

**Therapeutic Category** Antihypertensive Agent

**Use** Patients presenting with emergency hypertension and those requiring blood pressure control during hospitalization pose a challenge due to the associated risk of renal failure and end-organ compromise

**Usual Dosage**

Oral: 100 mg 2-4 times/day

I.V.: Severe hypertension: Initial: 0.1 mcg/kg/minute; may be increased in increments of 0.05-0.2 mcg/kg/minute; maximal infusion rate: 1.6 mcg/kg/minute

**Dosage Forms** Injection, as mesylate: 10 mg/mL

## fenoprofen (fen oh PROE fen)

**U.S./Canadian Brand Names** Nalfon®

**Therapeutic Category** Analgesic, Non-narcotic; Nonsteroidal Anti-inflammatory Drug (NSAID)

**Use** Symptomatic treatment of acute and chronic rheumatoid arthritis and osteoarthritis; relief of mild to moderate pain

**Usual Dosage** Oral:

Children: Juvenile arthritis: 900 mg/m$^2$/day, then increase over 4 weeks to 1.8 g/m$^2$/day

Adults:

Arthritis: 300-600 mg 3-4 times/day up to 3.2 g/day

Pain: 200 mg every 4-6 hours as needed

**Dosage Forms**

Capsule, as calcium: 200 mg, 300 mg

Tablet, as calcium: 600 mg

## fenoterol *(Canada only)* (fen oh TER ole)

**U.S./Canadian Brand Names** Berotec® (Can)

**Therapeutic Category** Beta$_2$-Adrenergic Agonist Agent

**Use** For the symptomatic relief and acute prophylaxis of bronchial obstruction in asthma and other conditions in which reversible bronchospasm is a complicating factor, such as chronic bronchitis or emphysema.

**Usual Dosage** Adults:

MDI: Acute symptoms: One puff will usually be adequate to relieve bronchospasm in the majority of patients, however, if required, a second puff may be taken preferably after waiting 5 minutes for the effect of the first puff to be obtained. This delay allows better assessment of the effectiveness of 1 puff and deeper penetration of the second puff. If an attack has not been relieved by 2 puffs, further puffs may be required. In these cases, patients should immediately consult the physician or the nearest hospital. If, despite other adequate maintenance therapy, regular use of beta-agonists remains necessary for the control of bronchospasm, the recommended dose is 1-2 puffs of the 100 mcg inhaler 3-4 times/day. A maximum of 8 puffs/day should not be exceeded.

(Continued)

## fenoterol *(Canada only) (Continued)*

Solution: Dosage should be individualized, and patient response should be monitored by the prescribing physician on an ongoing basis. Should be used only under medical supervision.

Motorized, compressed air or ultrasonic nebulizers: These nebulizers generate low pressure, low velocity aerosols. The average single dose is 0.5 to 1 mg of fenoterol. In more refractory cases, up to 2.5 mg of fenoterol may be given. Fenoterol solution should be diluted to 5 mL with preservative-free sterile sodium chloride inhalation solution, USP 0.9% (normal saline) and the total volume should be nebulized over a period of 10 to 15 minutes. Optimal deposition in the lungs is achieved with the patient breathing quietly and slowly. Treatment may be repeated every 6 hours if necessary.

Intermittent positive pressure ventilation: Fenoterol solution may be used in conjunction with Intermittent Positive Pressure Ventilation (IPPV) when such therapy is indicated. The average single dose is 0.5 to 1 mg of fenoterol. In more refractory cases, up to 2.5 mg of fenoterol may be given. Fenoterol solution should be diluted to 5 mL with preservative-free sterile sodium chloride inhalation solution, USP 0.9% and the total volume should be nebulized over a period of 10-15 minutes. The inspiratory pressure is usually 10 to 20 cm H2O and optimal deposition of the drug in the lungs is achieved with the patient breathing quietly and slowly. Treatment may be repeated every 6 hours if necessary. If a previous effective dosage regimen fails to provide the usual relief, or the effects of a dose last for less than 3 hours, medical advice should be sought immediately; this is a sign of seriously worsening asthma that requires reassessment of therapy. In accordance with the present practice for asthma treatment, concomitant anti-inflammatory therapy should be part of the regimen if fenoterol inhalation solution needs to be used on a regular daily basis.

**Dosage Forms**

Metered dose inhalers: 100 mcg/actuation (200 doses; 200 mcg/actuation) (100 doses)

Solution, inhalation: 1 mg/mL (20 mL)

## fentanyl (FEN ta nil)

**U.S./Canadian Brand Names** Actiq® Oral Transmucosal; Duragesic® Transdermal; Fentanyl Oralet®; Sublimaze® Injection

**Therapeutic Category** Analgesic, Narcotic; General Anesthetic

**Controlled Substance** C-II

**Use** Sedation; relief of pain; preoperative medication; adjunct to general or regional anesthesia; management of chronic pain (transdermal product)

Oral transmucosal: Hospital setting use only as preoperative anesthetic agent or to induce conscious sedation before procedures

**Usual Dosage** Doses should be titrated to appropriate effects; wide range of doses, dependent upon desired degree of analgesia/anesthesia

Children:

Sedation for minor procedures/analgesia: I.M., I.V.:

1-3 years: 2-3 mcg/kg/dose; may repeat after 30-60 minutes as required

3-12 years: 1-2 mcg/kg/dose; may repeat at 30- to 60-minute intervals as required. **Note:** Children 18-36 months of age may require 2-3 mcg/kg/dose

Continuous sedation/analgesia: Initial I.V. bolus: 1-2 mcg/kg then 1 mcg/kg/hour; titrate upward; usual: 1-3 mcg/kg/hour

Transdermal: Not recommended

Children <12 years and Adults:

Sedation for minor procedures/analgesia: 0.5-1 mcg/kg/dose; higher doses are used for major procedures

Preoperative sedation, adjunct to regional anesthesia, postoperative pain: I.M., I.V.: 50-100 mcg/dose

Adjunct to general anesthesia: I.M., I.V.: 2-50 mcg/kg

General anesthesia without additional anesthetic agents: I.V. 50-100 mcg/kg with $O_2$ and skeletal muscle relaxant

Transdermal: Initial: 25 mcg/hour system; if currently receiving opiates, convert to fentanyl equivalent and administer equianalgesic dosage (see package insert for further information)

**Dosage Forms**

Injection, as citrate: 0.05 mg/mL (2 mL, 5 mL, 10 mL, 20 mL, 50 mL)

Lozenge, oral transmucosal:

Fentanyl Oralet® (raspberry flavored): 200 mcg, 300 mcg, 400 mcg

Actiq® Oral Transmucosal: 200 mcg, 400 mcg, 600 mcg, 800 mcg, 1200 mcg, 1600 mcg

Transdermal system: 25 mcg/hour [10 $cm^2$]; 50 mcg/hour [20 $cm^2$]; 75 mcg/hour [30 $cm^2$]; 100 mcg/hour [40 $cm^2$] (all available in 5s)

**Fentanyl Oralet®** *see* fentanyl *on previous page*

**Feosol® [OTC]** *see* ferrous sulfate *on page 247*

**Feostat® [OTC]** *see* ferrous fumarate *on next page*

**Feracid®** *see* glutamic acid *on page 276*

**Ferancee® [OTC]** *see* ferrous salt and ascorbic acid *on next page*

**Feratab® [OTC]** *see* ferrous sulfate *on page 247*

**Fergon® [OTC]** *see* ferrous gluconate *on next page*

**Fergon Plus® *(Discontinued)*** *see page 750*

**Feridex I.V.®** *see* ferumoxides *on page 248*

**Fer-in-Sol® Capsule *(Discontinued)*** *see page 750*

**Fer-In-Sol® Drops [OTC]** *see* ferrous sulfate *on page 247*

**Fer-Iron® [OTC]** *see* ferrous sulfate *on page 247*

**Fermalac (Can)** *see* Lactobacillus *on page 338*

**Fermalox® *(Discontinued)*** *see page 750*

**Ferndex® *(Discontinued)*** *see page 750*

**Ferodan™ (Can)** *see* ferrous sulfate *on page 247*

**Fero-Grad 500® [OTC]** *see* ferrous salt and ascorbic acid *on next page*

**Fero-Gradumet® [OTC]** *see* ferrous sulfate *on page 247*

**Ferospace® [OTC]** *see* ferrous sulfate *on page 247*

**Ferralet® [OTC]** *see* ferrous gluconate *on next page*

**Ferralyn® Lanacaps® [OTC]** *see* ferrous sulfate *on page 247*

**Ferra-TD® [OTC]** *see* ferrous sulfate *on page 247*

**Ferrex® 150 [OTC]** *see* polysaccharide-iron complex *on page 482*

## ferric gluconate (FER ik GLOO koe nate)

**U.S./Canadian Brand Names** Ferrlecit®

**Therapeutic Category** Iron Salt

**Use** Repletion of total body iron content in patients with iron deficiency anemia who are undergoing hemodialysis in conjunction with erythropoietin therapy

**Usual Dosage** Adults:

Test dose (recommended): 2 mL diluted in 50 mL 0.9% sodium chloride over 60 minutes

Repletion of iron in hemodialysis patients: I.V.: 125 mg (10 mL) in 100 mL 0.9% sodium chloride over 1 hour during hemodialysis. Most patients will require a cumulative dose of 1 g elemental iron over approximately 8 sequential dialysis treatments to achieve a favorable response.

**Dosage Forms** Injection: 12.5 mg/mL (5 mL)

**Ferrlecit®** *see* ferric gluconate *on this page*

**Ferro-Sequels® [OTC]** *see* ferrous fumarate *on this page*

## ferrous fumarate (FER us FYOO ma rate)

**U.S./Canadian Brand Names** Femiron® [OTC]; Feostat® [OTC]; Ferro-Sequels® [OTC]; Fumasorb® [OTC]; Fumerin® [OTC]; Hemocyte® [OTC]; Ircon® [OTC]; Nephro-Fer™ [OTC]; Palafer® (Can); Span-FF® [OTC]

**Therapeutic Category** Electrolyte Supplement, Oral; Iron Salt

**Use** Prevention and treatment of iron deficiency anemias

**Usual Dosage** Oral:

Children: 3 mg/kg 3 times/day

Adults: 200 mg 3-4 times/day

**Dosage Forms** Amount of elemental iron is listed in brackets

Capsule, controlled release (Span-FF®): 325 mg [106 mg]

Drops (Feostat®): 45 mg/0.6 mL [15 mg/0.6 mL] (60 mL)

Suspension, oral (Feostat®): 100 mg/5 mL [33 mg/5 mL] (240 mL)

Tablet: 325 mg [106 mg]

Chewable (chocolate flavor) (Feostat®): 100 mg [33 mg]

Femiron®: 63 mg [20 mg]

Fumerin®: 195 mg [64 mg]

Fumasorb®, Ircon®: 200 mg [66 mg]

Hemocyte®: 324 mg [106 mg]

Nephro-Fer™: 350 mg [115 mg]

Timed release (Ferro-Sequels®): Ferrous fumarate 150 mg [50 mg] and docusate sodium 100 mg

## ferrous gluconate (FER us GLOO koe nate)

**U.S./Canadian Brand Names** Apo®-Ferrous Gluconate (Can); Fergon® [OTC]; Ferralet® [OTC]; Simron® [OTC]

**Therapeutic Category** Electrolyte Supplement, Oral; Iron Salt

**Use** Prevention and treatment of iron deficiency anemias

**Usual Dosage** Oral (dose expressed in terms of elemental iron):

Iron deficiency anemia: 3-6 Fe mg/kg/day in 3 divided doses

Maintenance:

Preterm infants:

Birthweight <1000 g: 4 Fe mg/kg/day

Birthweight 1000-1500 g: 3 Fe mg/kg/day

Birthweight 1500-2500 g: 2 Fe mg/kg/day

Term Infants and Children: 1-2 Fe mg/kg/day in 3 divided doses, up to a maximum of 18 Fe mg/day

Adults: 60-100 Fe mg/day in 3 divided doses

**Dosage Forms** Amount of elemental iron is listed in brackets

Capsule, soft gelatin (Simron®): 86 mg [10 mg]

Elixir (Fergon®): 300 mg/5 mL [34 mg/5 mL] with alcohol 7% (480 mL)

Tablet: 300 mg [34 mg]; 325 mg [38 mg]

Fergon®, Ferralet®: 320 mg [37 mg]

Sustained release (Ferralet® Slow Release): 320 mg [37 mg]

## ferrous salt and ascorbic acid (FER us salt & a SKOR bik AS id)

**U.S./Canadian Brand Names** Ferancee® [OTC]; Fero-Grad 500® [OTC]

**Therapeutic Category** Iron Salt; Vitamin

**Use** Treatment of iron deficiency in nonpregnant adults; treatment and prevention of iron deficiency in pregnant adults

**Usual Dosage** Adults: Oral: 1 tablet daily

**Dosage Forms** Amount of elemental iron is listed in brackets

Caplet, sustained release (Ferromar®): Ferrous fumarate 201.5 mg [65 mg] and ascorbic acid 200 mg

Tablet (Fero-Grad 500®): Ferrous sulfate 525 mg [105 mg] and ascorbic acid 500 mg

Chewable (Ferancee®): Ferrous fumarate 205 mg [67 mg] and ascorbic acid 150 mg

## ferrous sulfate (FER us SUL fate)

**Synonyms** $FeSO_4$

**U.S./Canadian Brand Names** Apo®-Ferrous Sulfate (Can); Feosol® [OTC]; Feratab® [OTC]; Fer-In-Sol® Drops [OTC]; Fer-Iron® [OTC]; Ferodan™ (Can); Fero-Gradumet® [OTC]; Ferospace® [OTC]; Ferralyn® Lanacaps® [OTC]; Ferra-TD® [OTC]; Mol-Iron® [OTC]; Slow FE® [OTC]

**Therapeutic Category** Electrolyte Supplement, Oral; Iron Salt

**Use** Prevention and treatment of iron deficiency anemias

**Usual Dosage** Oral (dose expressed in terms of elemental iron):

Children:

Severe iron deficiency anemia: 4-6 mg Fe/kg/day in 3 divided doses

Mild to moderate iron deficiency anemia: 3 mg Fe/kg/day in 1-2 divided doses

Prophylaxis: 1-2 mg Fe/kg/day up to a maximum of 15 mg/day

Adults: Iron deficiency: 60-100 Fe/kg/day in divided doses

**Dosage Forms** Amount of elemental iron is listed in brackets

Capsule:

Exsiccated, timed release (Feosol®): 159 mg [50 mg]

Exsiccated, timed release (Ferralyn® Lanacaps®, Ferra-TD®): 250 mg [50 mg]

Ferospace®: 250 mg [50 mg]

Drops, oral:

Fer-In-Sol®: 75 mg/0.6 mL [15 mg/0.6 mL] (50 mL)

Fer-Iron®: 125 mg/mL [25 mg/mL] (50 mL)

Elixir (Feosol®): 220 mg/5 mL [44 mg/5 mL] with alcohol 5% (473 mL, 4000 mL)

Syrup (Fer-In-Sol®): 90 mg/5 mL [18 mg/5 mL] with alcohol 5% (480 mL)

Tablet: 324 mg [65 mg]

Exsiccated (Feosol®) 200 mg [65 mg]

Exsiccated, timed release (Slow FE®): 160 mg [50 mg]

Feratab®: 300 mg [60 mg]

Mol-Iron®: 195 mg [39 mg]

Timed release (Fero-Gradumet®): 525 mg [105 mg]

## ferrous sulfate, ascorbic acid, and vitamin B-complex

(FER us SUL fate, a SKOR bik AS id, & VYE ta min bee KOM pleks)

**U.S./Canadian Brand Names** Iberet®-Liquid [OTC]

**Therapeutic Category** Iron Salt; Vitamin

**Use** Treatment of conditions of iron deficiency with an increased need for B complex vitamins and vitamin C

**Usual Dosage** Oral:

Children 1-3 years: 5 mL twice daily after meals

Children >4 years and Adults: 10 mL 3 times/day after meals

**Dosage Forms** Liquid: Ferrous sulfate: 78.75 mg; Ascorbic acid: 375 mg; $B_1$: 4.5 mg; $B_2$: 4.5 mg; $B_3$: 22.5 mg; $B_5$: 7.5 mg; $B_6$: 3.75 mg; $B_{12}$: 18.75 mg all per 15 mL

## ferrous sulfate, ascorbic acid, vitamin B-complex, and folic acid

(FER us SUL fate, a SKOR bik AS id, VYE ta min bee KOM pleks, & FOE lik AS id)

**U.S./Canadian Brand Names** Iberet-Folic-500®

**Therapeutic Category** Iron Salt; Vitamin

**Use** Treatment of iron deficiency and prevention of concomitant folic acid deficiency where there is an associated deficient intake or increased need for B complex vitamins

**Usual Dosage** Adults: Oral: 1 tablet daily

**Dosage Forms** Tablet, controlled release: Ferrous sulfate: 105 mg; Ascorbic acid: 500 mg; $B_1$: 6 mg; $B_2$: 6 mg; $B_3$: 30 mg; $B_6$: 5 mg; $B_{12}$: 25 mcg; Folic acid: 800 mcg

**Fertinex®** *see* urofollitropin *on page 618*

**Fertinorm® HP (Can)** *see* urofollitropin *on page 618*

## ferumoxides (fer yoo MOX ides)

**U.S./Canadian Brand Names** Feridex I.V.®

**Therapeutic Category** Radiopaque Agents

**Use** For I.V. administration as an adjunct to MRI (in adult patients) to enhance the T2 weighted images used in the detection and evaluation of lesions of the liver

**Usual Dosage** Adults: 0.56 mg of iron (0.05 mL Feridex I.V.®)/kg body weight diluted in 100 mL of 5% dextrose and infused over 30 minutes; a 5-micron filter is recommended; do not administer undiluted

**Dosage Forms** Injection: Iron 11.2 mg and mannitol per mL (5 mL)

**$FeSO_4$** *see* ferrous sulfate *on previous page*

**Fe-Tinic® 150 [OTC]** *see* polysaccharide-iron complex *on page 482*

**Feverall™ [OTC]** *see* acetaminophen *on page 3*

**Fexicam (Can)** *see* piroxicam *on page 474*

## fexofenadine (feks oh FEN a deen)

**U.S./Canadian Brand Names** Allegra®

**Therapeutic Category** Antihistamine

**Use** Nonsedating antihistamine indicated for the relief of seasonal allergic rhinitis

**Usual Dosage** Children ≥12 years and Adults: Oral: 1 capsule (60 mg) twice daily

**Dosage Forms**

Capsule, as hydrochloride: 60 mg

Tablet, as hydrochloride: 30 mg, 60 mg, 180 mg

## fexofenadine and pseudoephedrine

(feks oh FEN a deen & soo doe e FED rin)

**U.S./Canadian Brand Names** Allegra-D®

**Therapeutic Category** Antihistamine/Decongestant Combination

**Use** Relief of symptoms associated with seasonal allergic rhinitis in adults and children ≥12 years. Symptoms treated effectively include sneezing, rhinorrhea, itchy nose/ palate/ and/or throat, itchy/watery/red eyes, and nasal congestion.

**Usual Dosage** Oral: Adults: 1 tablet twice daily for adults and children ≥12 years of age. It is recommended that the administration with food should be avoided. A dose of 1 tablet once daily is recommended as the starting dose in patients with decreased renal function.

**Dosage Forms** Tablet, extended release: Fexofenadine hydrochloride 60 mg and pseudoephedrine hydrochloride 120 mg

**Fiberall® Chewable Tablet [OTC]** *see* calcium polycarbophil *on page 101*

**Fiberall® Powder [OTC]** *see* psyllium *on page 509*

**Fiberall® Wafer [OTC]** *see* psyllium *on page 509*

**FiberCon® Tablet [OTC]** *see* calcium polycarbophil *on page 101*

**Fiber-Lax® Tablet [OTC]** *see* calcium polycarbophil *on page 101*

## fibrinolysin and desoxyribonuclease

(fye brin oh LYE sin & des oks i rye boe NOO klee ase)

**U.S./Canadian Brand Names** Elase® Topical

**Therapeutic Category** Enzyme

**Use** Debriding agent; cervicitis; and irrigating agent in infected wounds

**Dosage Forms** Ointment, topical: Fibrinolysin 1 unit and desoxyribonuclease 666.6 units per g (10 g, 30 g)

## fibrin sealant kit (FI brin SEEL ent kit)

**Synonyms** FS

**U.S./Canadian Brand Names** Tisseel® VH Fibrin Sealant Kit

**Therapeutic Category** Hemostatic Agent

**Use** Adjunct to hemostasis in cardiopulmonary bypass surgery and splenic injury (due to blunt or penetrating trauma to the abdomen) when the control of bleeding by conventional surgical techniques is ineffective or impractical; adjunctive sealant for closure of colostomies; hemostatic agent in heparinized patients undergoing cardiopulmonary bypass

**Usual Dosage** Adjunct to hemostasis: Adults: Apply topically; actual dose is based on size of surface to be covered:

Maximum area to be sealed: 4 $cm^2$
 Required size of Tisseel® VH kit: 0.5 mL
Maximum area to be sealed: 8 $cm^2$
 Required size of Tisseel® VH kit: 1 mL
Maximum area to be sealed: 16 $cm^2$
 Required size of Tisseel® VH kit: 2 mL
Maximum area to be sealed: 40 $cm^2$
 Required size of Tisseel® VH kit: 5 mL

Apply in thin layers to avoid excess formation of granulation tissue and slow absorption of the sealant. Following application, hold the sealed parts in the desired position for 3-5 minutes. To prevent sealant from adhering to gloves or surgical instruments, wet them with saline prior to contact.

**Dosage Forms** Tisseel® VH Kit: Fibrin Sealant, two-component fibrin sealant, vapor-heated, kit (0.5 mL, 1 mL, 2 mL, 5 mL)

## filgrastim (fil GRA stim)

**Synonyms** G-CSF; granulocyte colony-stimulating factor

**U.S./Canadian Brand Names** Neupogen®

**Therapeutic Category** Colony-Stimulating Factor

**Use** To reduce the duration of neutropenia and the associated risk of infection in patients with nonmyeloid malignancies receiving myelosuppressive chemotherapeutic regimens associated with a significant incidence of severe neutropenia with fever; it has also been used in AIDS patients on zidovudine and in patients with noncancer chemotherapy-induced neutropenia

**Usual Dosage** Children and Adults (refer to individual protocols): I.V., S.C.: 5-10 mcg/kg/day (~150-300 mcg/$m^2$/day) once daily for up to 14 days until ANC = 10,000/$mm^3$; dose escalations at 5 mcg/kg/day may be required in some individuals when response at 5 mcg/kg/day is not adequate; dosages of 0.6-120 mcg/kg/day have been used in children ranging in age from 3 months to 18 years

**Dosage Forms** Injection, preservative free: 300 mcg/mL (1 mL, 1.6 mL)

## finasteride (fi NAS teer ide)

**U.S./Canadian Brand Names** Proscar®

**Therapeutic Category** Antiandrogen

**Use** Early data indicate that finasteride is useful in the treatment of benign prostatic hyperplasia

**Usual Dosage** Benign prostatic hyperplasia: Adults: Oral: 5 mg/day as a single dose; clinical responses occur within 12 weeks to 6 months of initiation of therapy; long-term administration is recommended for maximal response

**Dosage Forms**

Tablet, film coated:
 Propecia®: 1 mg
 Proscar®: 5 mg

**Fiorgen PF®** *see* butalbital compound and aspirin *on page 93*

**Fioricet®** *see* butalbital compound and acetaminophen *on page 93*

**Fiorinal®** *see* butalbital compound and aspirin *on page 93*

**Fiorinal®-C (Can)** *see* butalbital compound and codeine *on page 93*

**Fiorinal® With Codeine** *see* butalbital compound and codeine *on page 93*

**Fiorital®** ***(Discontinued)*** *see page 750*

**fisalamine** *see* mesalamine *on page 374*

**FK506** *see* tacrolimus *on page 569*

**Flagyl® Oral** *see* metronidazole *on page 388*

**Flamazine® (Can)** *see* silver sulfadiazine *on page 544*

**Flarex®** *see* fluorometholone *on page 256*

**Flatulex® [OTC]** *see* simethicone *on page 544*

**Flavorcee® [OTC]** *see* ascorbic acid *on page 54*

## flavoxate (fla VOKS ate)

**U.S./Canadian Brand Names** Urispas®

**Therapeutic Category** Antispasmodic Agent, Urinary

**Use** Antispasmodic to provide symptomatic relief of dysuria, nocturia, suprapubic pain, urgency, and incontinence

**Usual Dosage** Children >12 years and Adults: Oral: 100-200 mg 3-4 times/day

**Dosage Forms** Tablet, film coated, as hydrochloride: 100 mg

**Flaxedil®** ***(Discontinued)*** *see page 750*

## flecainide (fle KAY nide)

**U.S./Canadian Brand Names** Tambocor™

**Therapeutic Category** Antiarrhythmic Agent, Class I-C

**Use** Prevention and suppression of documented life-threatening ventricular arrhythmias (ie, sustained ventricular tachycardia); prevention of symptomatic, disabling supraventricular tachycardias in patients without structural heart disease

**Usual Dosage** Oral:

Children: Initial: 3 mg/kg/day in 3 divided doses; usual 3-6 mg/kg/day in 3 divided doses; up to 11 mg/kg/day for uncontrolled patients with subtherapeutic levels

Adults: Initial: 100 mg every 12 hours, increase by 100 mg/day (administer in 2 doses/day) every 4 days to maximum of 400 mg/day; for patients receiving 400 mg/day who are not controlled and have trough concentrations <0.6 mcg/mL, dosage may be increased to 600 mg/day

**Dosage Forms** Tablet, as acetate: 50 mg, 100 mg, 150 mg

**Fleet® Babylax® Rectal [OTC]** *see* glycerin *on page 277*

**Fleet® Bisacodyl [OTC]** *see* bisacodyl *on page 81*

**Fleet® Enema [OTC]** *see* sodium phosphates *on page 551*

**Fleet® Flavored Castor Oil [OTC]** *see* castor oil *on page 112*

**Fleet® Laxative [OTC]** *see* bisacodyl *on page 81*

**Fleet® Pain Relief [OTC]** *see* pramoxine *on page 490*

**Fleet® Phospho®-Soda [OTC]** *see* sodium phosphates *on page 551*

**Fletcher's® Castoria® [OTC]** *see* senna *on page 541*

**Flexaphen®** ***(Discontinued)*** *see page 750*

**Flexeril®** *see* cyclobenzaprine *on page 159*

**Flexitec (Can)** *see* cyclobenzaprine *on page 159*

**Flextra-DS® [OTC]** *see* acetaminophen and phenyltoloxamine *on page 5*

**Flo-Coat®** *see* radiological/contrast media (ionic) *on page 516*

## floctafenine *(Canada only)* (flok ta FEN een)

**U.S./Canadian Brand Names** Idarac® (Can)

**Therapeutic Category** Nonsteroidal Anti-inflammatory Drug (NSAID), Oral

**Use** Short-term use in acute pain of mild and moderate severity

**Usual Dosage** Adults: Oral: 200-400 mg every 6-8 hours as required; maximum recommended daily dose: 1200 mg

**Dosage Forms** Tablet: 200 mg, 400 mg

**Flolan®** *see* epoprostenol *on page 218*

**Flomax®** *see* tamsulosin *on page 570*

**Flonase®** *see* fluticasone (nasal) *on page 260*

**Flonase® 9 g *(Discontinued)*** *see page 750*

**Florical® [OTC]** *see* calcium carbonate *on page 97*

**Florinef® Acetate** *see* fludrocortisone *on next page*

**Florone®** *see* diflorasone *on page 185*

**Florone E®** *see* diflorasone *on page 185*

**Floropryl® Ophthalmic *(Discontinued)*** *see page 750*

**Flovent®** *see* fluticasone (oral inhalation) *on page 261*

**Flovent® Rotadisk®** *see* fluticasone (oral inhalation) *on page 261*

**Floxin®** *see* ofloxacin *on page 434*

## floxuridine (floks YOOR i deen)

**Synonyms** fluorodeoxyuridine

**U.S./Canadian Brand Names** FUDR®

**Therapeutic Category** Antineoplastic Agent

**Use** Palliative management of carcinomas of head, neck, and brain as well as liver, gallbladder, and bile ducts

**Usual Dosage** Adults:

Intra-arterial infusion: 0.1-0.6 mg/kg/day for 14 days followed by heparinized saline for 14 days

Investigational: I.V.: 0.5-1 mg/kg/day for 6-15 days

**Dosage Forms**

Injection, preservative free: 100 mg/mL (5 mL)

Powder for injection: 500 mg (5 mL, 10 mL)

**Fluanxol® Depot (Can)** *see* flupenthixol *(Canada only) on page 257*

**Fluanxol® Tablet (Can)** *see* flupenthixol *(Canada only) on page 257*

**flubenisolone** *see* betamethasone (topical) *on page 78*

**Flu & Cold® Medicine [OTC]** *see* acetaminophen, chlorpheniramine, and pseudoephedrine *on page 6*

## fluconazole (floo KOE na zole)

**U.S./Canadian Brand Names** Apo®-Fluconazole (Can); Diflucan®

**Therapeutic Category** Antifungal Agent

**Use** Treatment of susceptible fungal infections including oropharyngeal, esophageal, and vaginal candidiasis; treatment of systemic candidal infections including urinary tract infection, peritonitis, cystitis, and pneumonia; treatment and suppression of cryptococcal meningitis; prophylaxis of candidiasis in patients undergoing bone marrow transplantation; alternative to amphotericin B in patients with pre-existing renal impairment or when requiring concomitant therapy with other potentially nephrotoxic drugs

**Usual Dosage** Daily dose of fluconazole is the same for oral and I.V. administration

Infants and Children: Oral, I.V.: Safety profile of fluconazole has been studied in 577 children, ages 1 day to 17 years; doses as high as 12 mg/kg/day once daily (equivalent to adult doses of 400 mg/day) have been used to treat candidiasis in immunocompromised children; 10-12 mg/kg/day doses once daily have been used prophylactically against fungal infections in pediatric bone marrow transplantation patients. Do not exceed 600 mg/day.

(Continued)

## fluconazole *(Continued)*

Adults:

Vaginal candidiasis: Oral: 150 mg single dose

Prophylaxis against fungal infections in bone marrow transplantation patients: Oral, I.V.: 400 mg/day once daily

**Dosage Forms**

Injection: 2 mg/mL (100 mL, 200 mL)

Powder for oral suspension: 10 mg/mL (35 mL); 40 mg/mL (35 mL)

Tablet: 50 mg, 100 mg, 150 mg, 200 mg

## flucytosine (floo SYE toe seen)

**Synonyms** 5-FC; 5-flurocytosine

**U.S./Canadian Brand Names** Ancobon®

**Therapeutic Category** Antifungal Agent

**Use** In combination with amphotericin B in the treatment of serious *Candida*, *Aspergillus*, *Cryptococcus*, and *Torulopsis* infections

**Usual Dosage** Children and Adults: Oral: 50-150 mg/kg/day in divided doses every 6 hours

**Dosage Forms** Capsule: 250 mg, 500 mg

**Fludara®** *see* fludarabine *on this page*

## fludarabine (floo DARE a been)

**U.S./Canadian Brand Names** Fludara®

**Therapeutic Category** Antineoplastic Agent

**Use** Treatment of B-cell chronic lymphocytic leukemia unresponsive to previous therapy with an alkylating agent containing regimen. Fludarabine has been tested in patients with refractory acute lymphocytic leukemia and acute nonlymphocytic leukemia, but required a highly toxic dose to achieve response.

**Usual Dosage** Adults: I.V.:

Chronic lymphocytic leukemia: 25 mg/m$^2$/day over a 30-minute period for 5 days

Non-Hodgkin's lymphoma: Loading dose: 20 mg/m$^2$ followed by 30 mg/m$^2$/day for 48 hours

**Dosage Forms** Powder for injection, as phosphate, lyophilized: 50 mg (6 mL)

## fludrocortisone (floo droe KOR ti sone)

**Synonyms** fluohydrocortisone; 9α-fluorohydrocortisone

**U.S./Canadian Brand Names** Florinef® Acetate

**Therapeutic Category** Adrenal Corticosteroid (Mineralocorticoid)

**Use** Addison's disease; partial replacement therapy for adrenal insufficiency; treatment of salt-losing forms of congenital adrenogenital syndrome; has been used with increased sodium intake for the treatment of idiopathic orthostatic hypotension

**Usual Dosage** Oral:

Infants and Children: 0.05-0.1 mg/day

Adults: 0.05-0.2 mg/day

**Dosage Forms** Tablet, as acetate: 0.1 mg

**Flumadine®** *see* rimantadine *on page 527*

## flumazenil (FLO may ze nil)

**U.S./Canadian Brand Names** Anexate® (Can); Romazicon®

**Therapeutic Category** Antidote

**Use** Benzodiazepine antagonist; reverses sedative effects of benzodiazepines used in general anesthesia or conscious sedation; management of benzodiazepine overdose; not indicated for ethanol, barbiturate, general anesthetic or narcotic overdose

**Usual Dosage** Reversal of conscious sedation or general anesthesia: 0.2 mg (2 mL) administered I.V. over 15 seconds; if desired effect is not achieved after 60 seconds, repeat in 0.2 mg (2 mL) increments every 60 seconds up to a total of 1 mg (10 mL); in event of resedation, repeat doses may be administered at 20-minute intervals with no more than 1 mg (10 mL) administered at any one time, with a maximum of 3 mg in any 1 hour

**Dosage Forms** Injection: 0.1 mg/mL (5 mL, 10 mL)

## flunarizine *(Canada only)* (floo NAR i zeen)

**U.S./Canadian Brand Names** Sibelium® (Can)

**Therapeutic Category** Calcium-entry Blocker (Selective)

**Use** Prophylaxis of migraine with and without aura; the safety of flunarizine in long-term use (ie, >4 months) has not been systematically evaluated in controlled clinical trials. Flunarizine is not indicated in the treatment of acute migraine attacks.

**Usual Dosage** The usual adult dosage is 10 mg/day administered in the evening. Patients who experience side effects may be maintained on 5 mg at bedtime.

Duration of therapy: Clinical experience indicates that the onset of effect of flunarizine is gradual and maximum benefits may not be seen before the patient has completed several weeks of continuous treatment. Therapy, therefore, should not be discontinued for lack of response before an adequate time period has elapsed (ie, 6-8 weeks).

**Dosage Forms** Capsule, as hydrochloride: 5 mg

## flunisolide (floo NIS oh lide)

**U.S./Canadian Brand Names** AeroBid®-M Oral Aerosol Inhaler; AeroBid® Oral Aerosol Inhaler; Alti-Flunisoline (Can); Apo®-Flunisolide (Can); Nasalide® Nasal Aerosol; Nasarel® Nasal Spray; Rhinalar® (Can)

**Therapeutic Category** Adrenal Corticosteroid

**Use** Steroid-dependent asthma; nasal solution is used for seasonal or perennial rhinitis

**Usual Dosage**

Children:

Oral inhalation: >6 years: 2 inhalations twice daily up to 4 inhalations/day

Nasal: 6-14 years: 1 spray each nostril 2-3 times/day, not to exceed 4 sprays/day each nostril

Adults:

Oral inhalation: 2 inhalations twice daily up to 8 inhalations/day

Nasal: 2 sprays each nostril twice daily; maximum dose: 8 sprays/day in each nostril

**Dosage Forms**

Inhalant:

Nasal (Nasalide®): 25 mcg/actuation [200 sprays] (25 mL)

Nasal (Nasarel®): 25 mcg/actuation [200 sprays] (25 mL)

Oral:

AeroBid®: 250 mcg/actuation [100 metered doses] (7 g)

AeroBid-M® (menthol flavor): 250 mcg/actuation [100 metered doses] (7 g)

Solution, spray: 0.025% [200 actuations] (25 mL)

## fluocinolone (floo oh SIN oh lone)

**U.S./Canadian Brand Names** Capex® Shampoo; Derma-Smoothe/FS® Topical; Fluoderm (Can); Synalar® Topical

**Therapeutic Category** Corticosteroid, Topical

**Use** Relief of susceptible inflammatory dermatosis

**Usual Dosage** Children and Adults: Topical: Apply 2-4 times/day. Therapy should be discontinued when control is achieved. If no improvement is seen, reassessment of diagnosis may be necessary.

**Dosage Forms**

Cream, as acetonide: 0.01% (15 g, 60 g); 0.025% (15 g, 60 g)

Flurosyn®, Synalar®: 0.01% (15 g, 30 g, 60 g, 425 g)

Flurosyn®, Synalar®, Synemol®: 0.025% (15 g, 60 g, 425 g)

Synalar-HP®: 0.2% (12 g)

Oil, as acetonide (Derma-Smoothe/FS®): 0.01% (120 mL)

Ointment, topical, as acetonide: 0.025% (15 g, 60 g)

(Continued)

## fluocinolone *(Continued)*

Flurosyn®, Synalar®: 0.025% (15 g, 30 g, 60 g, 425 g)
Shampoo, as acetonide (Capex®): 0.01% (180 mL)
Solution, topical, as acetonide: 0.01% (20 mL, 60 mL)
Fluonid®, Synalar®: 0.01% (20 mL, 60 mL)
Tablet: 20 mg

## fluocinonide (floo oh SIN oh nide)

**U.S./Canadian Brand Names** Lidemol® (Can); Lidex®; Lidex-E®; Lyderm (Can); Lydonide (Can); Tiamol® (Can); Topsyn® (Can)

**Therapeutic Category** Corticosteroid, Topical

**Use** Inflammation of corticosteroid-responsive dermatoses

**Usual Dosage** Children and Adults: Topical: Apply thin layer to affected area 2-4 times/day depending on the severity of the condition. Therapy should be discontinued when control is achieved. If no improvement is seen, reassessment of diagnosis may be necessary.

**Dosage Forms**

Cream: 0.05% (15 g, 30 g, 60 g, 120 g)
Anhydrous, emollient (Lidex®): 0.05% (15 g, 30 g, 60 g, 120 g)
Aqueous, emollient (Lidex-E®): 0.05% (15 g, 30 g, 60 g, 120 g)
Gel, topical: 0.05% (15 g, 60 g)
Lidex®: 0.05% (15 g, 30 g, 60 g, 120 g)
Ointment, topical: 0.05% (15 g, 30 g, 60 g)
Lidex®: 0.05% (15 g, 30 g, 60 g, 120 g)
Solution, topical: 0.05% (20 mL, 60 mL)
Lidex®: 0.05% (20 mL, 60 mL)

**Fluoderm (Can)** *see* fluocinolone *on previous page*

**Fluogen®** *see* influenza virus vaccine *on page 318*

**fluohydrocortisone** *see* fludrocortisone *on page 252*

**Fluonid® Topical *(Discontinued)*** *see page 750*

**Fluoracaine® Ophthalmic** *see* proparacaine and fluorescein *on page 503*

**Fluor-A-Day® (Can)** *see* fluoride *on next page*

**FluorCare® Neutral** *see* fluoride *on next page*

## fluorescein sodium (FLURE e seen SOW dee um)

**Synonyms** soluble fluorescein

**U.S./Canadian Brand Names** AK-Fluor Injection; Diofluor™ (Can); Fluorescite® Injection; Fluorets® Ophthalmic Strips; Fluor-I-Strip®; Fluor-I-Strip-AT®; Flurate® Ophthalmic Solution; Fluress® Ophthalmic Solution; Ful-Glo® Ophthalmic Strips; Funduscein® Injection

**Therapeutic Category** Diagnostic Agent

**Use** Demonstrates defects of corneal epithelium; diagnostic aid in ophthalmic angiography

**Usual Dosage**

Injection: Perform intradermal skin test before use to avoid possible allergic reaction
Children: 3.5 mg/lb (7.5 mg/kg) injected rapidly into antecubital vein
Adults: 500-750 mg injected rapidly into antecubital vein
Strips: Moisten with sterile water or irrigating solution, touch conjunctiva with moistened tip, blink several times after application
Topical solution: Instill 1-2 drops, allow a few seconds for staining, then wash out excess with sterile irrigation solution

**Dosage Forms**

Injection (AK-Fluor, Fluorescite®, Funduscein®, Ophthifluor®): 10% [100 mg/mL] (5 mL); 25% [250 mg/mL] (2 mL, 3 mL)

Ophthalmic:
Solution: 2% [20 mg/mL] (1 mL, 2 mL, 15 mL)
Flurate®, Fluress®: 0.25% [2.5 mg/mL] with benoxinate 0.4% (5 mL)
Strip:
Ful-Glo®: 0.6 mg
Fluorets®, Fluor-I-Strip-AT®: 1 mg
Fluor-I-Strip®: 9 mg

**Fluorescite® Injection** *see* fluorescein sodium *on previous page*

**Fluorets® Ophthalmic Strips** *see* fluorescein sodium *on previous page*

## fluoride (FLOR ide)

**U.S./Canadian Brand Names** ACT® [OTC]; Fluor-A-Day® (Can); FluorCare® Neutral; Fluorigard® [OTC]; Fluorinse®; Fluoritab®; Fluotic® (Can); Flura®; Flura-Drops®; Flura-Loz®; Gel-Kam®; Gel-Tin® [OTC]; Karidium®; Karigel®; Karigel®-N; Listermint® with Fluoride [OTC]; Lozi-Tab®; Luride®; Luride®-SF; Minute-Gel®; Pediaflor®; Pharmaflur®; Phos-Flur®; Point-Two®; PreviDent®; Stop® [OTC]; Thera-Flur®; Thera-Flur-N®

**Therapeutic Category** Mineral, Oral

**Use** Prevention of dental caries

**Usual Dosage** Oral: Dental rinse or gel:
Children 6-12 years: 5-10 mL rinse or apply to teeth and spit daily after brushing
Adults: 10 mL rinse or apply to teeth and spit daily after brushing

**Dosage Forms** Fluoride ion content listed in brackets
Acidulated phosphate fluoride: Rinse, topical:
Minute-Gel®: 1.23% (480 mL)

Sodium fluoride:
Drops, oral:
Fluoritab®, Flura-Drops®: 0.55 mg/drop [0.25 mg/drop] (22.8 mL, 24 mL)
Karidium®, Luride®: 0.275 mg/drop [0.125 mg/drop] (30 mL, 60 mL)
Pediaflor®: 1.1 mg/mL [0.5 mg/mL] (50 mL)
Gel, topical:
Karigel®, Karigel®-N, PreviDent®: 1.1% [0.5%] (24 g, 30 g, 60 g, 120 g, 130 g, 250 g)
Rinse, topical:
ACT®, Fluorigard®: 0.05% [0.02%] (90 mL, 180 mL, 300 mL, 360 mL, 480 mL)
Fluorinse®, Point-Two®: 0.2% [0.09%] (240 mL, 480 mL, 3780 mL)
Listermint® with Fluoride: 0.02% [0.01%] (180 mL, 300 mL, 360 mL, 480 mL, 540 mL, 720 mL, 960 mL, 1740 mL)
Solution, oral, as sodium (Phos-Flur®): 0.44 mg/mL [0.2 mg/mL] (250 mL, 500 mL, 3780 mL)
Tablet:
Chewable:
Fluoritab®, Luride® Lozi-Tab®, Pharmaflur®: 1.1 mg [0.5 mg]
Fluoritab®, Karidium®, Luride® Lozi-Tab®, Luride®-SF Lozi-Tab®, Pharmaflur®: 2.2 mg [1 mg]
Oral: Flura®, Karidium®: 2.2 mg [1 mg]

Stannous fluoride: Rinse, topical:
Gel-Kam®, Gel-Tin®, Stop®: 0.4% [0.1%] (60 g, 15 g, 105 g, 120 g)

**Fluorigard® [OTC]** *see* fluoride *on this page*

**Fluori-Methane® Topical Spray** *see* dichlorodifluoromethane and trichloromonofluoromethane *on page 181*

**Fluorinse®** *see* fluoride *on this page*

**Fluor-I-Strip®** *see* fluorescein sodium *on previous page*

**Fluor-I-Strip-AT®** *see* fluorescein sodium *on previous page*

**Fluoritab®** *see* fluoride *on this page*

**fluorodeoxyuridine** *see* floxuridine *on page 251*

**9α-fluorohydrocortisone** *see* fludrocortisone *on page 252*

## fluorometholone (flure oh METH oh lone)

**U.S./Canadian Brand Names** Flarex®; Fluor-Op®; FML®; FML® Forte

**Therapeutic Category** Adrenal Corticosteroid

**Use** Inflammatory conditions of the eye, including keratitis, iritis, cyclitis, and conjunctivitis

**Usual Dosage** Children >2 years and Adults: Ophthalmic: 1-2 drops into conjunctival sac every hour during day, every 2 hours at night until favorable response is obtained, then use 1 drop every 4 hours; in mild or moderate inflammation: 1-2 drops into conjunctival sac 2-4 times/day. Ointment may be applied every 4 hours in severe cases or 1-3 times/day in mild to moderate cases.

**Dosage Forms** Ophthalmic:

Ointment (FML®): 0.1% (3.5 g)

Suspension:

Flarex®, Fluor-Op®, FML®: 0.1% (2.5 mL, 5 mL, 10 mL)

FML® Forte: 0.25% (2 mL, 5 mL, 10 mL, 15 mL)

**Fluor-Op®** *see* fluorometholone *on this page*

**Fluoroplex® Topical** *see* fluorouracil *on this page*

## fluorouracil (flure oh YOOR a sil)

**Synonyms** 5-fluorouracil; 5-FU

**U.S./Canadian Brand Names** Adrucil® Injection; Carac™ Topical; Efudex® Topical; Fluoroplex® Topical

**Therapeutic Category** Antineoplastic Agent

**Use** Treatment of carcinoma of stomach, colon, rectum, breast, and pancreas; also used topically for management of multiple actinic keratoses and superficial basal cell carcinomas

**Usual Dosage** Children and Adults (refer to individual protocol):

I.V.: Initial: 12 mg/kg/day (maximum: 800 mg/day) for 4-5 days; maintenance: 6 mg/kg every other day for 4 doses

Single weekly bolus dose of 15 mg/kg can be administered depending on the patient's reaction to the previous course of treatment; maintenance dose of 5-15 mg/kg/week as a single dose not to exceed 1 g/week

I.V. infusion: 15 mg/kg/day (maximum daily dose: 1 g) has been administered by I.V. infusion over 4 hours for 5 days

Oral: 20 mg/kg/day for 5 days every 5 weeks for colorectal carcinoma; 15 mg/kg/week for hepatoma

Topical: 5% cream twice daily

**Dosage Forms**

Cream, topical:

Carac™: 0.5% (30 g)

Efudex®: 5% (25 g)

Fluoroplex®: 1% (30 g)

Injection (Adrucil®): 50 mg/mL (10 mL, 20 mL, 50 mL, 100 mL)

Solution, topical:

Efudex®: 2% (10 mL); 5% (10 mL)

Fluoroplex®: 1% (30 mL)

**5-fluorouracil** *see* fluorouracil *on this page*

**Fluothane® *(Discontinued)*** *see* *page 750*

**Fluotic® (Can)** *see* fluoride *on previous page*

## fluoxetine (floo OKS e teen)

**U.S./Canadian Brand Names** Alti-Fluoxetine (Can); Apo®-Fluoxetine (Can); Gen-Fluoxetine (Can); Novo-Fluoxetine (Can); Nu-Fluoxetine (Can); PMS-Fluoxetine (Can); Prozac®; Prozac® Weekly™; Sarafem™

**Therapeutic Category** Antidepressant, Selective Serotonin Reuptake Inhibitor

**Use** Treatment of major depression; treatment of binge-eating and vomiting in patients with moderate-to-severe bulimia nervosa; obsessive-compulsive disorder (OCD); premenstrual dysphoric disorder (PMDD)

**Usual Dosage** Oral:

Children <18 years: Dose and safety not established; preliminary experience in children 6-14 years using initial doses of 20 mg/day have been reported

Adults: 20 mg/day in the morning; may increase after several weeks by 20 mg/day increments; maximum: 80 mg/day; doses >20 mg should be divided into morning and noon doses

Usual dosage range:

Depression: 20-40 mg/day

OCD: 40-80 mg/day

PMDD (Sarafem™): 20 mg/day

Obesity: 20-60 mg/day

Bulimia nervosa: 60-80 mg/day

**Note:** Lower doses of 5 mg/day have been used for initial treatment

Elderly: Some patients may require an initial dose of 10 mg/day with dosage increases of 10 and 20 mg every several weeks as tolerated; should not be taken at night unless patient experiences sedation

**Dosage Forms**

Capsule, as hydrochloride:

Prozac®: 10 mg, 20 mg, 40 mg

Sarafem™: 10 mg, 20 mg

Capsule, sustained release, as hydrochloride (Prozac® Weekly™): 90 mg

Solution, oral, as hydrochloride (Prozac®): 20 mg/5 mL (120 mL) [contains 0.23% alcohol] [mint flavor]

Tablet, scored, as hydrochloride (Prozac®): 10 mg

## fluoxymesterone (floo oks i MES te rone)

**U.S./Canadian Brand Names** Halotestin®

**Therapeutic Category** Androgen

**Use** Replacement of endogenous testicular hormone; in female used as palliative treatment of breast cancer, postpartum breast engorgement

**Usual Dosage** Adults: Oral:

Male:

Hypogonadism: 5-20 mg/day

Delayed puberty: 2.5-20 mg/day for 4-6 months

Female:

Breast carcinoma: 10-40 mg/day in divided doses for 1-3 months

Breast engorgement: 2.5 mg after delivery, 5-10 mg/day in divided doses for 4-5 days

**Dosage Forms** Tablet: 2 mg, 5 mg, 10 mg

## flupenthixol *(Canada only)* (floo pen THIKS ol)

**U.S./Canadian Brand Names** Fluanxol® Depot (Can); Fluanxol® Tablet (Can)

**Therapeutic Category** Antipsychotic Agent; Thioxanthene Derivative

**Use** Maintenance therapy of chronic schizophrenic patients whose main manifestations do not include excitement, agitation, or hyperactivity

**Usual Dosage**

Injection: Flupenthixol is administered by deep I.M. injection, preferably in the gluteus maximus, NOT for I.V. use

Patients not previously treated with long-acting depot neuroleptics should be given an initial test dose of 5 mg (0.25 mL) to 20 mg (1 mL). An initial dose of 20 mg (1 mL) is usually well tolerated; however, a 5 mg (0.25 mL) test dose is recommended in elderly, frail and cachectic patients, and in patients whose individual or family history suggests a predisposition to extrapyramidal reactions. In the subsequent 5-10 days, the therapeutic response and the appearance of extrapyramidal symptoms should be carefully

(Continued)

## flupenthixol *(Canada only)* *(Continued)*

monitored. Oral neuroleptic drugs may be continued, but in diminishing dosage, during this period.

Tablets: The dosage should be individualized and adjusted according to the severity of symptoms and tolerance to the drug. Initial recommended dose: 1 mg, 3 times/day. This may be increased, if necessary by 1 mg every 2-3 days until there is effective control of psychotic symptoms. The usual maintenance dosage: 3-6 mg/day in divided doses, although doses of up to 12 mg/day or more have been used in some patients.

**Dosage Forms**

Injection, depot: 20 mg/mL (10 mL); 100 mg/mL (2 mL)
Tablet: 0.5 mg, 3 mg

## fluphenazine (floo FEN a zeen)

**U.S./Canadian Brand Names** Modecate® (Can); Permitil® Oral; PMS-Fluphenazine Decanoate (Can); Prolixin Decanoate® Injection; Prolixin Enanthate® Injection; Prolixin® Injection; Prolixin® Oral

**Therapeutic Category** Phenothiazine Derivative

**Use** Management of manifestations of psychotic disorders

**Usual Dosage** Adults:

Oral: 0.5-10 mg/day in divided doses every 6-8 hours; usual maximum dose 20 mg/day
I.M.: 2.5-10 mg/day in divided doses every 6-8 hours; usual maximum dose 10 mg/day
I.M., S.C. (Decanoate®): Oral to I.M., S.C. conversion ratio = 12.5 mg, I.M., S.C. every 3 weeks for every 10 mg of oral fluphenazine

**Dosage Forms**

Concentrate, as hydrochloride:
- Permitil®: 5 mg/mL with alcohol 1% (118 mL)
- Prolixin®: 5 mg/mL with alcohol 14% (120 mL)

Elixir, as hydrochloride (Prolixin®): 2.5 mg/5 mL with alcohol 14% (60 mL, 473 mL)
Injection, as decanoate (Prolixin Decanoate®): 25 mg/mL (1 mL, 5 mL)
Injection, as enanthate (Prolixin Enanthate®): 25 mg/mL (5 mL)
Injection, as hydrochloride (Prolixin®): 2.5 mg/mL (10 mL)
Tablet, as hydrochloride
- Permitil®: 2.5 mg, 5 mg, 10 mg
- Prolixin®: 1 mg, 2.5 mg, 5 mg, 10 mg

**Flura®** *see* fluoride *on page 255*

**Flura-Drops®** *see* fluoride *on page 255*

**Flura-Loz®** *see* fluoride *on page 255*

## flurandrenolide (flure an DREN oh lide)

**Synonyms** flurandrenolone

**U.S./Canadian Brand Names** Cordran®; Cordran® SP

**Therapeutic Category** Corticosteroid, Topical

**Use** Inflammation of corticosteroid-responsive dermatoses

**Usual Dosage** Topical:

Children:
- Ointment or cream: Apply 1-2 times/day
- Tape: Apply once daily

Adults: Cream, lotion, ointment: Apply 2-3 times/day; therapy should be discontinued when control is achieved. If no improvement is seen, reassessment of diagnosis may be necessary.

**Dosage Forms**

Cream, emulsified base (Cordran® SP): 0.025% (30 g, 60 g); 0.05% (15 g, 30 g, 60 g)
Lotion (Cordran®): 0.05% (15 mL, 60 mL)
Ointment, topical (Cordran®): 0.025% (30 g, 60 g); 0.05% (15 g, 30 g, 60 g)
Tape, topical (Cordran®): 4 mcg/cm$^2$ (7.5 cm x 60 cm, 7.5 cm x 200 cm rolls)

**flurandrenolone** *see* flurandrenolide *on previous page*

**Flurate® Ophthalmic Solution** *see* fluorescein sodium *on page 254*

## flurazepam (flure AZ e pam)

**U.S./Canadian Brand Names** Apo®-Flurazepam (Can); Dalmane®; Somnol® (Can)

**Therapeutic Category** Benzodiazepine

**Controlled Substance** C-IV

**Use** Short-term treatment of insomnia

**Usual Dosage** Oral:

Children:

<15 years: Dose not established

>15 years: 15 mg at bedtime

Adults: 15-30 mg at bedtime

**Dosage Forms** Capsule, as hydrochloride: 15 mg, 30 mg

## flurbiprofen (flure BI proe fen)

**U.S./Canadian Brand Names** Alti-Flurbiprofen (Can); Ansaid® Oral; Apo®-Flurbiprofen (Can); Froben® (Can); Novo-Flurprofen (Can); Nu-Flurprofen (Can); Ocufen® Ophthalmic

**Therapeutic Category** Analgesic, Non-narcotic; Nonsteroidal Anti-inflammatory Drug (NSAID)

**Use**

Ophthalmic: For inhibition of intraoperative trauma-induced miosis; the value of flurbiprofen for the prevention and management of postoperative ocular inflammation and postoperative cystoid macular edema remains to be determined

Systemic: Management of inflammatory disease and rheumatoid disorders; dysmenorrhea; pain

**Usual Dosage**

Oral: Rheumatoid arthritis and osteoarthritis: 200-300 mg/day in 2, 3, or 4 divided doses

Ophthalmic: Instill 1 drop every 30 minutes, 2 hours prior to surgery (total of 4 drops to each affected eye)

**Dosage Forms**

Solution, ophthalmic, as sodium (Ocufen®): 0.03% (2.5 mL, 5 mL, 10 mL)

Tablet, as sodium (Ansaid®): 50 mg, 100 mg

**Fluress® Ophthalmic Solution** *see* fluorescein sodium *on page 254*

**5-flurocytosine** *see* flucytosine *on page 252*

**Fluro-Ethyl® Aerosol** *see* ethyl chloride and dichlorotetrafluoroethane *on page 235*

**Flurosyn® Topical *(Discontinued)*** *see page 750*

## flutamide (FLOO ta mide)

**U.S./Canadian Brand Names** Apo®-Flutamide (Can); Euflex® (Can); Eulexin®; Novo-Flutamide (Can); PMS-Flutamide (Can)

**Therapeutic Category** Antiandrogen

**Use** In combination with LHRH agonistic analogs for the treatment of metastatic prostatic carcinoma

**Usual Dosage** Oral: 2 capsules every 8 hours

**Dosage Forms** Capsule: 125 mg

**Flutex® Topical** *see* triamcinolone (topical) *on page 602*

## fluticasone and salmeterol (floo TIK a sone & sal ME te role)

**U.S./Canadian Brand Names** Advair™ Diskus®

**Therapeutic Category** Beta$_2$-Adrenergic Agonist Agent; Corticosteroid, Inhalant

(Continued)

## fluticasone and salmeterol *(Continued)*

**Use** Maintenance treatment of asthma in adults and children ≥12 years; **not** for use for relief of acute bronchospasm

**Usual Dosage** Do not use to transfer patients from systemic corticosteroid therapy

Children ≥12 and Adults: Oral inhalation: One inhalation twice daily, morning and evening, 12 hours apart

Advair™ Diskus® is available in 3 strengths, initial dose prescribed should be based upon previous asthma therapy. Dose should be increased after 2 weeks if adequate response is not achieved. Patients should be titrated to lowest effective dose once stable. (Because each strength contains salmeterol 50 mcg/inhalation, dose adjustments should be made by changing inhaler strength. No more than 1 inhalation of any strength should be taken more than twice a day). Maximum dose: Fluticasone 500 mcg/salmeterol 50 mcg, one inhalation twice daily.

Patients not currently on inhaled corticosteroids: Fluticasone 100 mcg/salmeterol 50 mcg

Patients currently using inhaled beclomethasone dipropionate:
- ≤420 mcg/day: Fluticasone 100 mcg/salmeterol 50 mcg
- 462-840 mcg/day: Fluticasone 250 mcg/salmeterol 50 mcg

Patients currently using inhaled budesonide:
- ≤400 mcg/day: Fluticasone 100 mcg/salmeterol 50 mcg
- 800-1200 mcg/day: Fluticasone 250 mcg/salmeterol 50 mcg
- 1600 mcg/day: Fluticasone 500 mcg/salmeterol 50 mcg

Patients currently using inhaled flunisolide:
- ≤1000 mcg/day: Fluticasone 100 mcg/salmeterol 50 mcg
- 1250-2000 mcg/day: Fluticasone 250 mcg/salmeterol 50 mcg

Patients currently using inhaled fluticasone propionate aerosol:
- ≤176 mcg/day: Fluticasone 100 mcg/salmeterol 50 mcg
- 440 mcg/day: Fluticasone 250 mcg/salmeterol 50 mcg
- 660-880 mcg/day: Fluticasone 500 mcg/salmeterol 50 mcg

Patients currently using inhaled fluticasone propionate powder:
- ≤200 mcg/day: Fluticasone 100 mcg/salmeterol 50 mcg
- 500 mcg/day: Fluticasone 250 mcg/salmeterol 50 mcg
- 1000 mcg/day: Fluticasone 500 mcg/salmeterol 50 mcg

Patients currently using inhaled triamcinolone acetonide:
- ≤1000 mcg/day: Fluticasone 100 mcg/salmeterol 50 mcg
- 1100-1600 mcg/day: Fluticasone 250 mcg/salmeterol 50 mcg

**Dosage Forms** Powder for inhalation, oral:
- Fluticasone 100 mcg and salmeterol 50 mcg
- Fluticasone 250 mcg and salmeterol 50 mcg
- Fluticasone 500 mcg and salmeterol 50 mcg

## fluticasone (nasal) (floo TIK a sone NAY sal)

**U.S./Canadian Brand Names** Flonase®

**Therapeutic Category** Adrenal Corticosteroid

**Use** Management of seasonal and perennial allergic rhinitis in patients ≥12 years of age

**Usual Dosage**

Adolescents:

Intranasal: Initial: 1 spray (50 mcg/spray) per nostril once daily. Patients not adequately responding or patients with more severe symptoms may use 2 sprays (100 mcg) per nostril. Depending on response, dosage may be reduced to 100 mcg daily. Total daily dosage should not exceed 4 sprays (200 mcg)/day.

Adults:

Intranasal: Initial: 2 sprays (50 mcg/spray) per nostril once daily. After the first few days, dosage may be reduced to 1 spray per nostril once daily for maintenance therapy. Maximum total daily dose should not exceed 4 sprays (200 mcg)/day.

**Dosage Forms** Spray, intranasal: 50 mcg/actuation (16 g = 120 actuations)

## fluticasone (oral inhalation) (floo TIK a sone OR al in hil LA shun)

**U.S./Canadian Brand Names** Flovent®; Flovent® Rotadisk®

**Therapeutic Category** Adrenal Corticosteroid

**Use** Inhalation: Maintenance treatment of asthma as prophylactic therapy. It is also indicated for patients requiring oral corticosteroid therapy for asthma to assist in total discontinuation or reduction of total oral dose. NOT indicated for the relief of acute bronchospasm.

**Usual Dosage** Oral inhalation: If adequate response is not seen after 2 weeks of initial dosage, increase dosage; doses should be titrated to the lowest effective dose once asthma is controlled; Manufacturer recommendations:

Inhalation aerosol (Flovent®): Children ≥12 years and Adults:

Patients previously treated with bronchodilators only: Initial: 88 mcg twice daily; maximum dose: 440 mcg twice daily

Patients treated with an inhaled corticosteroid: Initial: 88-220 mcg twice daily; maximum dose: 440 mcg twice daily; may start doses above 88 mcg twice daily in poorly controlled patients or in those who previously required higher doses of inhaled corticosteroids

Patients previously treated with oral corticosteroids: Initial: 880 mcg twice daily; maximum dose: 880 mcg twice daily

Inhalation powder (Flovent® Rotadisk®):

Children 4-11 years: Patients previously treated with bronchodilators alone or inhaled corticosteroids: Initial: 50 mcg twice daily; maximum dose: 100 mcg twice daily; may start higher initial dose in poorly controlled patients or in those who previously required higher doses of inhaled corticosteroids

Adolescents and Adults:

Patients previously treated with bronchodilators alone: Initial: 100 mcg twice daily; maximum dose: 500 mcg twice daily

Patients previously treated with inhaled corticosteroids: Initial: 100-250 mcg twice daily; maximum dose: 500 mcg twice daily; may start doses above 100 mcg twice daily in poorly controlled patients or in those who previously required higher doses of inhaled corticosteroids

Patients previously treated with oral corticosteroids: Initial: 1000 mcg twice daily; maximum dose: 1000 mcg twice daily

**Dosage Forms**

Powder (in 4 blisters containing 15 Rotodisk® with inhalation device): 50 mcg, 100 mcg, 250 mcg

Spray, aerosol, oral inhalation (Flovent®): 44 mcg/actuation (7.9 g = 60 actuations or 13 g = 120 actuations), 110 mcg/actuation (13 g = 120 actuations); 220 mcg/actuation (13 g = 120 actuations)

## fluticasone (topical) (floo TIK a sone TOP i kal)

**U.S./Canadian Brand Names** Cutivate™

**Therapeutic Category** Adrenal Corticosteroid; Corticosteroid, Topical

**Use** Relief of inflammation and pruritus associated with corticosteroid-responsive dermatoses [medium potency topical corticosteroid]

**Usual Dosage** Topical:

Children: Cutivate™ approved for use in patients ≥3 months of age

Adolescents and Adults: Apply sparingly in a thin film twice daily

**Note:** Therapy should be discontinued when control is achieved. If no improvement is seen, reassessment of diagnosis may be necessary.

**Dosage Forms**

Cream: 0.05% (15 g, 30 g, 60 g)

Ointment: 0.005% (15 g, 60 g )

**Flutone (Can)** *see* diflorasone *on page 185*

## fluvastatin (FLOO va sta tin)

**U.S./Canadian Brand Names** Lescol®; Lescol® XL

**Therapeutic Category** HMG-CoA Reductase Inhibitor

**Use** Adjunct to dietary therapy to decrease elevated serum total and LDL cholesterol concentrations in primary hypercholesterolemia; slowing of progression of coronary atherosclerosis in patients with coronary heart disease as part of a treatment strategy to lower serum total and LDL cholesterol to target levels

**Usual Dosage** Adults: Oral:

Patients requiring ≥25% decrease in LDL-C: 40 mg capsule or 80 mg extended release tablet once daily in the evening; may also use 40 mg capsule twice daily

Patients requiring < 25% decrease in LDL-C: 20 mg capsule once daily in the evening

**Note:** Dosing range: 20-80 mg/day; adjust dose based on response to therapy; maximum response occurs within 4-6 weeks

**Dosage Forms**

Capsule: 20 mg, 40 mg

Tablet, extended release: 80 mg

**Fluviral® S/F (Can)** *see* influenza virus vaccine *on page 318*

## fluvoxamine (floo VOKS ah meen)

**U.S./Canadian Brand Names** Alti-Fluvoxamine (Can); Apo®-Fluvoxamine (Can); Luvox®; Novo-Fluvoxamine (Can); Nu-Fluvoxamine (Can); PMS-Fluvoxamine (Can)

**Therapeutic Category** Antidepressant, Selective Serotonin Reuptake Inhibitor

**Use** Treatment of major depression and obsessive-compulsive disorder (OCD)

**Usual Dosage** Adults: Initial: 50 mg at bedtime; adjust in 50 mg increments at 4- to 7-day intervals; usual dose range: 100-300 mg/day; divide total daily dose into 2 doses; administer larger portion at bedtime

**Dosage Forms** Tablet: 25 mg, 50 mg, 100 mg

**Fluzone®** *see* influenza virus vaccine *on page 318*

**FML®** *see* fluorometholone *on page 256*

**FML® Forte** *see* fluorometholone *on page 256*

**FML-S® Ophthalmic Suspension** *see* sulfacetamide sodium and fluorometholone *on page 563*

**Foille® [OTC]** *see* benzocaine *on page 72*

**Foille® Medicated First Aid [OTC]** *see* benzocaine *on page 72*

**folacin** *see* folic acid *on this page*

**folate** *see* folic acid *on this page*

**Folex® Injection *(Discontinued)*** *see page 750*

**Folex® PFS™ *(Discontinued)*** *see page 750*

## folic acid (FOE lik AS id)

**Synonyms** folacin; folate; pteroylglutamic acid

**U.S./Canadian Brand Names** Apo®-Folic (Can); Folvite®

**Therapeutic Category** Vitamin, Water Soluble

**Use** Treatment of megaloblastic and macrocytic anemias due to folate deficiency

**Usual Dosage** Folic acid deficiency:

Infants: 15 mcg/kg/dose daily or 50 mcg/day

Children: Oral, I.M., I.V., S.C.: 1 mg/day initial dosage; maintenance dose: 1-10 years: 0.1-0.3 mg/day

Children >11 years and Adults: Oral, I.M., I.V., S.C.: 1 mg/day initial dosage; maintenance dose: 0.5 mg/day

**Dosage Forms**

Injection, as sodium folate: 5 mg/mL (10 mL); 10 mg/mL (10 mL)

Folvite®: 5 mg/mL (10 mL)

Tablet: 0.1 mg, 0.4 mg, 0.8 mg, 1 mg
Folvite®: 1 mg

**folinic acid** *see* leucovorin *on page 343*

**Follistim®** *see* follitropin beta *on this page*

## follitropin alfa (foe li TRO pin AL fa)

**U.S./Canadian Brand Names** Gonal-F®

**Therapeutic Category** Ovulation Stimulator

**Use** Induction of ovulation in the anovulatory infertile patient in whom the cause of infertility is functional and not caused by primary ovarian failure

**Usual Dosage** Adults (women): S.C.: Initial: 75 units/day for the first cycle; an incremental dose adjustment of up to 37.5 units may be considered after 14 days; treatment duration should not exceed 35 days unless an E2 rise indicates follicular development

**Dosage Forms** Injection: 37.5 FSH units, 75 FSH units, 150 FSH units

## follitropin beta (foe li TRO pin BAY ta)

**U.S./Canadian Brand Names** Follistim®

**Therapeutic Category** Ovulation Stimulator

**Use** The development of multiple follicles in infertility patients treated in Assisted Reproductive Technology (ART) program and for the induction of ovulation

**Usual Dosage** Adults (female): I.M./S.C.:

Ovulation: In general, a sequential treatment scheme is recommended. This usually starts with daily administration of 75 int. units (International Units) FSH activity. The starting dose is maintained for at least seven days. If there is no ovarian response, the daily dose is then gradually increased until follicle growth and/or plasma estradiol levels indicate an adequate pharmacodynamic response. A daily increase in estradiol levels of 40% to 100% is considered to be optimal. The daily dose is then maintained until preovulatory conditions are reached. Preovulatory conditions are reached when there ultrasonographic evidence of a dominant follicle of at least 18 mm in diameter and/or when plasma estradiol levels of 300-900 picograms/mL (1000-3000 pmol/L) are attained; usually, 7-14 days of treatment are sufficient to reach this state. The administration is then discontinued and ovulation can be induced by administering human chorionic gonadotropin (hCG). If the number of responding follicles is too high or estradiol levels increase too rapidly (ie, more than a daily doubling of estradiol for 2-3 consecutive days), the daily dose should be decreased. Since follicles of >14 mm may lead to pregnancies, multiple preovulatory follicles exceeding 14 mm carry the risk of multiple gestations. In that case, hCG should be withheld and pregnancy should be avoided in order to prevent multiple gestations.

ART: Various stimulation protocols are applied; starting dose of 150-225 units is recommended for at least the first four days; thereafter, the dose may be adjusted individually, based upon ovarian response. In clinical studies, it was shown that maintenance dosages ranging from 75-375 units for 6-12 days are sufficient, although longer treatment may be necessary. May be given either alone, or in combination with a GnRH agonist to prevent premature luteinization; in the latter case, a higher total treatment dose of Follistim® may be required. Ovarian response is monitored by ultrasonography and measurement of plasma estradiol levels; when ultrasonographic evaluation indicates the presence of at least three follicles of 16-20 mm, and there is evidence of a good estradiol (plasma levels of about 300-400 picogram/mL (1000-1300 pmol/L) for each follicle with a diameter >18 mm), the final phase of maturation of the follicles is induced by administration of hCG. Oocyte retrieval is performed 34-35 hours later.

**Dosage Forms** Injection: 75 FSH units

**Follutein®** ***(Discontinued)*** *see page 750*

**Folvite®** *see* folic acid *on previous page*

## fomepizole (foe ME pi zole)

**Synonyms** 4-methylpyrazole; 4-MP

**U.S./Canadian Brand Names** Antizol®

**Therapeutic Category** Antidote

**Use** Ethylene glycol and methanol toxicity (antifreeze); may be useful in propylene glycol; unclear whether it is useful in disulfiram-ethanol reactions

**Usual Dosage** Oral: 15 mg/kg followed by 5 mg/kg in 12 hours and then 10 mg/kg every 12 hours until levels of toxin are not present

One other protocol (from France) suggests an infusion of 10-20 mg/kg before dialysis and intravenous infusion of 1-1.5 mg/kg/hour during hemodialysis

META (methylpyrazole for toxic alcohol) study in U.S. (investigational): Loading I.V. dose of 15 mg/kg followed by 10 mg/kg I.V. every 12 hours for 48 hours; continue treatment until methanol or ethylene glycol levels are <20 mg/dL; supplemental doses required during dialysis; contact your local poison center regarding this study

**Dosage Forms** Injection: 1 g/mL (1.5 mL)

## fomivirsen (foe MI vir sen)

**U.S./Canadian Brand Names** Vitravene™

**Therapeutic Category** Antiviral Agent

**Use** Treatment of cytomegalovirus (CMV); CMV can affect one or both eyes in patients with acquired immunodeficiency syndrome (AIDS) who cannot take other treatment(s) for CMV retinitis or who did not respond to other treatments for CMV retinitis; the diagnosis should be made after a comprehensive eye exam, including indirect ophthalmoscopy

**Usual Dosage** Treatment with Vitravene™ consists of two phases:

Phase I (induction phase): One injection (6.6 mg) every other week for 2 doses

Phase II (maintenance phase): One injection (6.6 mg) once every 4 weeks

**Dosage Forms** Injection, intravitreal: 6.6 mg

**Foradil® (Can)** *see* formoterol *(Canada only) on this page*

**Forane®** *see* isoflurane *on page 327*

## formoterol *(Canada only)* (for MOT ter ol)

**U.S./Canadian Brand Names** Foradil® (Can)

**Therapeutic Category** Adrenergic Agonist Agent; Beta$_2$-Adrenergic Agonist Agent; Bronchodilator

**Use** Long-term treatment in maintenance of asthma and in prevention of bronchospasm in patients >12 years of age with reversible obstructive airway disease

**Usual Dosage** Inhalation: One capsule (12 mcg) inhaled using the Aerolizer inhaler twice daily, morning and evening

**Dosage Forms** Capsule, for inhalation use, as fumarate: 12 mcg

**Formula Q®** ***(Discontinued)*** *see page 750*

**Formulex® (Can)** *see* dicyclomine *on page 183*

**5-formyl tetrahydrofolate** *see* leucovorin *on page 343*

**Fortabs®** *see* butalbital compound and aspirin *on page 93*

**Fortaz®** *see* ceftazidime *on page 117*

**Fortovase®** *see* saquinavir *on page 537*

**Fosamax®** *see* alendronate *on page 19*

## foscarnet (fos KAR net)

**Synonyms** PFA; phosphonoformic acid

**U.S./Canadian Brand Names** Foscavir®

**Therapeutic Category** Antiviral Agent

**Use** Alternative to ganciclovir for treatment of CMV infections and is possibly the preferred initial agent for the treatment of CMV retinitis except for those patients with decreased renal function; treatment of acyclovir-resistant mucocutaneous herpes simplex virus infections in immunocompromised patients; and acyclovir-resistant herpes zoster infections

**Usual Dosage**

Induction treatment: 60 mg/kg 3 times/day for 14-21 days

Maintenance therapy: 90-120 mg/kg/day

**Dosage Forms** Injection: 24 mg/mL (250 mL, 500 mL)

**Foscavir®** *see* foscarnet *on previous page*

## fosfomycin (fos foe MYE sin)

**U.S./Canadian Brand Names** Monurol™

**Therapeutic Category** Antibiotic, Miscellaneous

**Use** Treatment of uncomplicated urinary tract infections

**Usual Dosage** Adults: Oral: Single dose of 3 g in 4 oz of water

**Dosage Forms** Powder, as tromethamine: 3 g, to be mixed in 4 oz of water

## fosinopril (foe SIN oh pril)

**U.S./Canadian Brand Names** Monopril®

**Therapeutic Category** Angiotensin-Converting Enzyme (ACE) Inhibitor

**Use** Treatment of hypertension, either alone or in combination with other antihypertensive agents

**Usual Dosage** Adults: Oral: 20-40 mg/day

**Dosage Forms** Tablet: 10 mg, 20 mg, 40 mg

## fosinopril and hydrochlorothiazide

(foe SIN oh pril & hye droe klor oh THYE a zide)

**U.S./Canadian Brand Names** Monopril-HCT®

**Therapeutic Category** Angiotensin-Converting Enzyme (ACE) Inhibitor

**Use** Treatment of hypertension

**Usual Dosage** Adults: Oral: Dose is individualized; not for initial therapy

**Dosage Forms** Tablet: Fosinopril 10 mg and hydrochlorothiazide 12.5 mg; fosinopril 20 mg and hydrochlorothiazide 12.5 mg

## fosphenytoin (FOS fen i toyn)

**U.S./Canadian Brand Names** Cerebyx®

**Therapeutic Category** Hydantoin

**Use** Indicated for short-term parenteral administration when other means of phenytoin administration are unavailable, inappropriate or deemed less advantageous; the safety and effectiveness of fosphenytoin in this use has not been systematically evaluated for more than 5 days; may be used for the control of generalized convulsive status epilepticus and prevention and treatment of seizures occurring during neurosurgery

**Usual Dosage The dose, concentration in solutions, and infusion rates for fosphenytoin are expressed as phenytoin sodium equivalents; fosphenytoin should always be prescribed and dispensed in phenytoin sodium equivalents**

Status epilepticus: I.V.: Adults: Loading dose: Phenytoin equivalent 15-20 mg/kg I.V. administered at 100-150 mg/minute

Nonemergent loading and maintenance dosing: I.V. or I.M.: Adults:

Loading dose: Phenytoin equivalent 10-20 mg/kg I.V. or I.M. (max I.V. rate 150 mg/minute)

Initial daily maintenance dose: Phenytoin equivalent 4-6 mg/kg/day I.V. or I.M.

I.M. or I.V. substitution for oral phenytoin therapy: May be substituted for oral phenytoin sodium at the same total daily dose, however, Dilantin® capsules are ~90% bioavailable by the oral route; phenytoin, supplied as fosphenytoin, is 100% bioavailable by both the I.M. and I.V. routes; for this reason, plasma phenytoin concentrations may

(Continued)

## fosphenytoin *(Continued)*

increase when I.M. or I.V. fosphenytoin is substituted for oral phenytoin sodium therapy; in clinical trials I.M. fosphenytoin was administered as a single daily dose utilizing either 1 or 2 injection sites; some patients may require more frequent dosing

**Dosage Forms** Injection, as sodium: 150 mg [equivalent to phenytoin sodium 100 mg]; 750 mg, [equivalent to phenytoin sodium 500 mg]

**Fostex® [OTC]** *see* sulfur and salicylic acid *on page 566*

**Fostex® 10% BPO Gel [OTC]** *see* benzoyl peroxide *on page 74*

**Fostex® 10% Wash [OTC]** *see* benzoyl peroxide *on page 74*

**Fototar® [OTC]** *see* coal tar *on page 149*

**Fragmin®** *see* dalteparin *on page 164*

## framycetin *(Canada only)* (fra mye CEE tin)

**U.S./Canadian Brand Names** Sofra-Tulle® (Can)

**Therapeutic Category** Antibiotic, Topical

**Use** Treatment of infected or potentially infected burns, wounds, ulcers, and graft sites

**Usual Dosage** A single layer to be applied directly to the wound and covered with an appropriate dressing. If exudative, dressings should be changed at least daily. In case of leg ulcers, cut dressing accurately to size of ulcer to decrease the risk of sensitization and to avoid contact with surrounding healthy skin.

**Dosage Forms** Dressing, gauze: 1% (10 cm x 10 cm, 10 cm x 30 cm)

**Fraxiparine™ (Can)** *see* nadroparin *(Canada only) on page 405*

**Freezone® Solution [OTC]** *see* salicylic acid *on page 535*

**Frisium® (Can)** *see* clobazam *(Canada only) on page 143*

**Froben® (Can)** *see* flurbiprofen *on page 259*

**frusemide** *see* furosemide *on next page*

**FS** *see* fibrin sealant kit *on page 248*

**FS Shampoo® Topical *(Discontinued)*** *see page 750*

**5-FU** *see* fluorouracil *on page 256*

**Fucidin® I.V. (Can)** *see* fusidic acid *(Canada only) on next page*

**Fucidin® Oral Suspension (Can)** *see* fusidic acid *(Canada only) on next page*

**Fucidin® Tablet (Can)** *see* fusidic acid *(Canada only) on next page*

**FUDR®** *see* floxuridine *on page 251*

**Ful-Glo® Ophthalmic Strips** *see* fluorescein sodium *on page 254*

**Fulvicin® P/G** *see* griseofulvin *on page 281*

**Fulvicin-U/F®** *see* griseofulvin *on page 281*

**Fumasorb® [OTC]** *see* ferrous fumarate *on page 246*

**Fumerin® [OTC]** *see* ferrous fumarate *on page 246*

**Funduscein® Injection** *see* fluorescein sodium *on page 254*

**Fungi-Gard® [OTC]** *see* tolnaftate *on page 595*

**Fungizone®** *see* amphotericin B (conventional) *on page 37*

**Fungoid® Creme** *see* miconazole *on page 390*

**Fungoid® Solution** *see* clotrimazole *on page 147*

**Fungoid® Tincture** *see* miconazole *on page 390*

**Furacin® Topical** *see* nitrofurazone *on page 422*

**Furadantin®** *see* nitrofurantoin *on page 422*

**Furalan® *(Discontinued)*** *see page 750*

**Furamide®** ***(Discontinued)*** *see page 750*

**Furan®** ***(Discontinued)*** *see page 750*

**Furanite®** ***(Discontinued)*** *see page 750*

## furazolidone (fyoor a ZOE li done)

**U.S./Canadian Brand Names** Furoxone®

**Therapeutic Category** Antiprotozoal

**Use** Treatment of bacterial or protozoal diarrhea and enteritis caused by susceptible organisms: *Giardia lamblia* and *Vibrio cholerae*

**Usual Dosage** Oral:

Children >1 month: 5-8.8 mg/kg/day in 3-4 divided doses for 7-10 days, not to exceed 400 mg/day

Adults: 100 mg 4 times/day for 7-10 days

**Dosage Forms** Liquid: 50 mg/15 mL (60 mL, 473 mL)

**furazosin** *see* prazosin *on page 491*

## furosemide (fyoor OH se mide)

**Synonyms** frusemide

**U.S./Canadian Brand Names** Apo®-Furosemide (Can); Lasix®

**Therapeutic Category** Diuretic, Loop

**Use** Management of edema associated with congestive heart failure and hepatic or renal disease; used alone or in combination with antihypertensives in treatment of hypertension

**Usual Dosage**

Infants and Children:

Oral: 2 mg/kg/dose increased in increments of 1 mg/kg/dose with each succeeding dose until a satisfactory effect is achieved to a maximum of 6 mg/kg/dose no more frequently than 6 hours

I.M., I.V.: 1 mg/kg/dose, increasing by each succeeding dose at 1 mg/kg/dose at intervals of 6-12 hours until a satisfactory response up to 6 mg/kg/dose

Adults:

Oral: Initial: 20-80 mg/dose, increase in increments of 20-40 mg/dose at intervals of 6-8 hours; usual maintenance dose interval is twice daily or every day

I.M., I.V.: 20-40 mg/dose, may be repeated in 1-2 hours as needed and increased by 20 mg/dose with each succeeding dose up to 600 mg/day; usual dosing interval: 6-12 hours

**Dosage Forms**

Injection: 10 mg/mL (2 mL, 4 mL, 5 mL, 6 mL, 8 mL, 10 mL, 12 mL)

Solution, oral: 10 mg/mL (60 mL, 120 mL); 40 mg/5 mL (5 mL, 10 mL, 500 mL)

Tablet: 20 mg, 40 mg, 80 mg

**Furoxone®** *see* furazolidone *on this page*

## fusidic acid *(Canada only)* (fyoo SI dik AS id)

**Synonyms** sodium fusidate

**U.S./Canadian Brand Names** Fucidin® I.V. (Can); Fucidin® Oral Suspension (Can); Fucidin® Tablet (Can)

**Therapeutic Category** Antifungal Agent

**Use** The treatment of the following infections when due to susceptible strains of *S. aureus*, both penicillinase producing and nonpenicillinase producing: skin and soft tissue infections, osteomyelitis. For patients with staphylococcal infections where other antibiotics have failed (ie, patients with staphylococcal septicemia, burns, endocarditis, pneumonia, cystic fibrosis). Appropriate culture and susceptibility studies should be performed. Fucidin® may be administered to those patients in whom a staphylococcal infection is suspected. This antibiotic treatment may subsequently require modification once these results become available.

(Continued)

## fusidic acid *(Canada only)* *(Continued)*

**Usual Dosage** Adults:
I.V.: 500 mg 3 times/day
Oral: 500 mg 3 times/day

**Dosage Forms**
Powder for injection: 500 mg
Suspension, oral (banana flavor): 246 mg/5 mL (50 mL)
Tablet, sodium fusidate: 250 mg (equivalent to 240 mg fusidic acid)

**G-1®** *see* butalbital compound and acetaminophen *on page 93*

## gabapentin (GA ba pen tin)

**U.S./Canadian Brand Names** Neurontin®

**Therapeutic Category** Anticonvulsant

**Use** Adjunct for treatment of drug-refractory partial and secondarily generalized seizures

**Usual Dosage** Adults: Oral: 900-1800 mg/day administered in 3 divided doses; therapy is initiated with a rapid titration, beginning with 300 mg on day 1, 300 mg twice daily on day 2, and 300 mg 3 times/day on day 3

Discontinuing therapy or replacing with an alternative agent should be done gradually over a minimum of 7 days

**Dosage Forms**
Capsule: 100 mg, 300 mg, 400 mg
Tablet: 600 mg, 800 mg

**Gabitril®** *see* tiagabine *on page 589*

## galantamine (ga LAN ta meen)

**U.S./Canadian Brand Names** Reminyl®

**Therapeutic Category** Acetylcholinesterase Inhibitor (Central)

**Use** Treatment of mild to moderate dementia of Alzheimer's disease

**Usual Dosage** **Note:** Take with breakfast and dinner. If therapy is interrupted for ≥3 days, restart at the lowest dose and increase to current dose.

Oral: Adults: Mild to moderate dementia of Alzheimer's: Initial: 4 mg twice a day for 4 weeks
If 8 mg per day tolerated, increase to 8 mg twice daily for ≥4 weeks
If 16 mg per day tolerated, increase to 12 mg twice daily
Range: 16-24 mg/day in 2 divided doses

**Dosage Forms** Tablet, as hydrobromide: 4 mg, 8 mg, 12 mg

## gallium nitrate (GAL ee um NYE trate)

**U.S./Canadian Brand Names** Ganite™

**Therapeutic Category** Antidote

**Use** Treatment of clearly symptomatic cancer-related hypercalcemia that has not responded to adequate hydration

**Usual Dosage** Adults: I.V. infusion: 200 mg/m$^2$ for 5 consecutive days

**Dosage Forms** Injection: 25 mg/mL (20 mL)

**Gamastan®** ***(Discontinued)*** *see page 750*

**Gamimune® N** *see* immune globulin (intravenous) *on page 315*

**gamma benzene hexachloride** *see* lindane *on page 350*

**Gammagard® Injection** ***(Discontinued)*** *see page 750*

**Gammagard® S/D** *see* immune globulin (intravenous) *on page 315*

**gamma globulin** *see* immune globulin (intramuscular) *on page 315*

**gammaphos** *see* amifostine *on page 29*

**Gammar®** ***(Discontinued)*** *see page 750*

**Gammar®-P I.V.** *see* immune globulin (intravenous) *on page 315*

**Gamulin® Rh *(Discontinued)*** *see page 750*

## ganciclovir (gan SYE kloe veer)

**Synonyms** DHPG sodium; GCV sodium; nordeoxyguanosine

**U.S./Canadian Brand Names** Cytovene®; Vitrasert®

**Therapeutic Category** Antiviral Agent

**Use**

Parenteral: Treatment of CMV retinitis in immunocompromised individuals, including patients with acquired immunodeficiency syndrome; prophylaxis of CMV infection in transplant patients

Oral: Alternative to the I.V. formulation for maintenance treatment of CMV retinitis in immunocompromised patients, including patients with AIDS, in whom retinitis is stable following appropriate induction therapy and for whom the risk of more rapid progression is balanced by the benefit associated with avoiding daily I.V. infusions.

**Usual Dosage** Slow I.V. infusion:

Retinitis: Children >3 months and Adults: Induction therapy: 5 mg/kg/dose every 12 hours for 14-21 days followed by maintenance therapy; maintenance therapy: 5 mg/kg/day as a single daily dose for 7 days/week or 6 mg/kg/day for 5 days/week

Other CMV infections: 5 mg/kg/dose every 12 hours for 14-21 days or 2.5 mg/kg/dose every 8 hours; maintenance therapy: 5 mg/kg/day as a single daily dose for 7 days/week or 6 mg/kg/day for 5 days/week

**Dosage Forms**

Capsule: 250 mg, 500 mg

Implant, intravitreal: 4.5 mg released gradually over 5-8 months

Powder for injection, lyophilized: 500 mg (10 mL)

**Ganite™** *see* gallium nitrate *on previous page*

**Gantanol® *(Discontinued)*** *see page 750*

**Gantrisin® Ophthalmic *(Discontinued)*** *see page 750*

**Gantrisin® Pediatric Suspension** *see* sulfisoxazole *on page 566*

**Gantrisin® Tablet *(Discontinued)*** *see page 750*

**Garamycin®** *see* gentamicin *on page 273*

**Garatec (Can)** *see* gentamicin *on page 273*

**Gas-Ban DS® [OTC]** *see* aluminum hydroxide, magnesium hydroxide, and simethicone *on page 27*

**Gas Relief® [OTC]** *see* simethicone *on page 544*

**Gastrocrom®** *see* cromolyn sodium *on page 156*

**Gastrografin®** *see* radiological/contrast media (ionic) *on page 516*

**Gastrosed™** *see* hyoscyamine *on page 309*

**Gas-X® [OTC]** *see* simethicone *on page 544*

## gatifloxacin (ga ti FLOKS a sin)

**U.S./Canadian Brand Names** Tequin®

**Therapeutic Category** Antibiotic, Quinolone

**Use** Treatment of infections due to susceptible strains of the designated microorganisms in the conditions listed: Acute bacterial exacerbation of chronic bronchitis, acute sinusitis, community-acquired pneumonia, uncomplicated urinary tract infections (cystitis), complicated urinary tract infections, pyelonephritis, uncomplicated urethral and cervical gonorrhea, acute, uncomplicated rectal infections in women

**Usual Dosage** I.V. Oral: Adults: 400 mg given once daily, depending on infection, for 1 to 14 days

**Dosage Forms**

Infusion, preservative free, ready-to-use: 200 mg (100 mL); 400 mg (200 mL)

(Continued)

## gatifloxacin *(Continued)*

Injection, preservative free (single use vials): 200 mg (20 mL); 400 mg (40 mL)
Tablet: 200 mg, 400 mg

**Gaviscon®-2 Tablet [OTC]** *see* aluminum hydroxide and magnesium trisilicate *on page 27*

**Gaviscon® Liquid [OTC]** *see* aluminum hydroxide and magnesium carbonate *on page 26*

**Gaviscon® Tablet [OTC]** *see* aluminum hydroxide and magnesium trisilicate *on page 27*

**G-CSF** *see* filgrastim *on page 249*

**GCV sodium** *see* ganciclovir *on previous page*

**Gee Gee® [OTC]** *see* guaifenesin *on page 281*

## gelatin (absorbable) (JEL a tin ab SORB a ble)

**Synonyms** absorbable gelatin sponge
**U.S./Canadian Brand Names** Gelfilm® Ophthalmic; Gelfoam® Topical
**Therapeutic Category** Hemostatic Agent
**Use** Adjunct to provide hemostasis in surgery; also used in oral and dental surgery; in open prostatic surgery
**Usual Dosage** Topical: Hemostasis: Apply packs or sponges dry or saturated with sodium chloride. When applied dry, hold in place with moderate pressure. When applied wet, squeeze to remove air bubbles. Prostatectomy cones are designed for use with the Foley bag catheter. The powder is applied as a paste prepared by adding approximately 4 mL of sterile saline solution to the powder.
**Dosage Forms**
Gelfilm® (sterile)
- Film: 100 mm x 125 mm (1s)
- Ophthalmic: 25 mm x 50 mm (6s)

Gelfoam®
- Cones, prostatectomy:
  - Size 13 cm (13 cm in diameter) (6s)
  - Size 18 cm (18 cm in diameter) (6s)
- Packs:
  - Size 2 cm (40 cm x 2 cm) (1s)
  - Size 6 cm (40 cm x 6 cm) (6s)
- Packs, dental:
  - Size 2 (10 mm x 20 mm x 7 mm) (15s)
  - Size 4 (20 mm x 20 mm x 7 mm) (15s)
- Sponges:
  - Size 12-3 mm (20 mm x 60 mm x 3 mm) (4s)
  - Size 12-7 mm (20 mm x 60 mm x 7 mm) (4s)
  - Size 50 (80 mm x 62.5 mm x 10 mm) (4s)
  - Size 100 (80 mm x 125 mm x 10 mm) (6s)
  - Size 100, compressed (80 mm x 125 mm) (6s)
  - Size 200 (80 mm x 250 mm x 10 mm) (6s)

## gelatin, pectin, and methylcellulose

(JEL a tin, PEK tin, & meth il SEL yoo lose)
**U.S./Canadian Brand Names** Orabase® Plain [OTC]
**Therapeutic Category** Protectant, Topical
**Use** Temporary relief from minor oral irritations
**Usual Dosage** Oral: Press small dabs into place until the involved area is coated with a thin film; do not try to spread onto area; may be used as often as needed
**Dosage Forms** Paste, oral: 5 g, 15 g

**Gelfilm® Ophthalmic** *see* gelatin (absorbable) *on this page*

**Gelfoam® Topical** *see* gelatin (absorbable) *on previous page*

**Gel-Kam®** *see* fluoride *on page 255*

**Gelpirin® [OTC]** *see* acetaminophen, aspirin, and caffeine *on page 6*

**Gel-Tin® [OTC]** *see* fluoride *on page 255*

**Gelucast®** *see* zinc gelatin *on page 639*

**Gelusil® Liquid *(Discontinued)*** *see page 750*

**Gelusil® Tablet (Can)** *see* aluminum hydroxide and magnesium hydroxide *on page 27*

## gemcitabine (jem SIT a been)

**U.S./Canadian Brand Names** Gemzar®

**Therapeutic Category** Antineoplastic Agent

**Use** Treatment of patients with inoperable pancreatic cancer

**Usual Dosage** Adults: I.V.: 1000 mg/$^2$ over 30 minutes once weekly for up to 7 weeks

**Dosage Forms** Powder for injection, as hydrochloride, lyophilized: 20 mg/mL (10 mL, 50 mL)

## gemfibrozil (jem FI broe zil)

**Synonyms** CI-719

**U.S./Canadian Brand Names** Apo®-Gemfibrozil (Can); Gen-Gemfibrozil (Can); Lopid®; Novo-Gemfibrozil (Can); Nu-Gemfibrozil (Can); PMS-Gemfibrozil (Can)

**Therapeutic Category** Antihyperlipidemic Agent, Miscellaneous

**Use** Hypertriglyceridemia in types IV and V hyperlipidemia; increases HDL cholesterol

**Usual Dosage** Oral: 1200 mg/day in 2 divided doses, 30 minutes before breakfast and supper

**Dosage Forms**

Capsule: 300 mg

Tablet, film coated: 600 mg

## gemtuzumab ozogamicin (gem TUZ yu mab oh zog a MY sin)

**U.S./Canadian Brand Names** Mylotarg™

**Therapeutic Category** Antineoplastic Agent

**Use** Treatment of acute myeloid leukemia (CD33 positive) in first relapse in patients who are 60 years of age or older and who are not considered candidates for cytotoxic chemotherapy.

**Usual Dosage** Adults ≥60 years: I.V.: 9 mg/m$^2$, infused over 2 hours. The patient should receive diphenhydramine 50 mg and acetaminophen 650-1000 mg orally 1 hour prior to administration of each dose. Acetaminophen dosage should be repeated as needed every 4 hours for two additional doses. A full treatment course is a total of two doses administered with 14 days between doses. Full hematologic recovery is not necessary for administration of the second dose. There has been only limited experience with repeat courses of gemtuzumab ozogamicin.

**Dosage Forms** Powder for injection: 5 mg

**Gemzar®** *see* gemcitabine *on this page*

**Genabid® *(Discontinued)*** *see page 750*

**Gen-Acebutolol (Can)** *see* acebutolol *on page 3*

**Genac® Tablet [OTC]** *see* triprolidine and pseudoephedrine *on page 609*

**Genagesic® *(Discontinued)*** *see page 750*

**Genahist® Oral** *see* diphenhydramine *on page 191*

**Gen-Alprazolam (Can)** *see* alprazolam *on page 22*

**Gen-Amantadine (Can)** *see* amantadine *on page 28*

**Genamin® Cold Syrup *(Discontinued)*** *see page 750*

**Gen-Minocycline (Can)** *see* minocycline *on page 394*

**Gen-Naproxen EC (Can)** *see* naproxen *on page 409*

**Genoptic®** *see* gentamicin *on this page*

**Genora® 0.5/35** *see* ethinyl estradiol and norethindrone *on page 232*

**Genora® 1/35** *see* ethinyl estradiol and norethindrone *on page 232*

**Genora® 1/50** *see* mestranol and norethindrone *on page 375*

**Genotropin®** *see* human growth hormone *on page 296*

**Gen-Oxybutynin (Can)** *see* oxybutynin *on page 443*

**Gen-Pindolol (Can)** *see* pindolol *on page 472*

**Gen-Piroxicam (Can)** *see* piroxicam *on page 474*

**Genpril® [OTC]** *see* ibuprofen *on page 311*

**Gen-Ranitidine (Can)** *see* ranitidine hydrochloride *on page 519*

**Gen-Selegiline (Can)** *see* selegiline *on page 540*

**Gen-Sotalol (Can)** *see* sotalol *on page 555*

**Gentacidin®** *see* gentamicin *on this page*

**Gent-AK®** *see* gentamicin *on this page*

## gentamicin (jen ta MYE sin)

**U.S./Canadian Brand Names** Alcomicin® (Can); Diogent® (Can); Garamycin®; Garatec (Can); Genoptic®; Gentacidin®; Gent-AK®; Gentrasul®

**Therapeutic Category** Aminoglycoside (Antibiotic); Antibiotic, Ophthalmic; Antibiotic, Topical

**Use** Treatment of susceptible bacterial infections, normally due to gram-negative organisms including *Pseudomonas*, *Proteus*, *Serratia*, and gram-positive *Staphylococcus*; treatment of bone infections, CNS infections, respiratory tract infections, skin and soft tissue infections, as well as abdominal and urinary tract infections, endocarditis, and septicemia; used in combination with ampicillin as empiric therapy for sepsis in newborns; used topically to treat superficial infections of the skin or ophthalmic infections caused by susceptible bacteria

**Usual Dosage** Dosage should be based on an estimate of ideal body weight

Infants and Children >3 months: Intrathecal: 1-2 mg/day

Infants and Children <5 years: 2.5 mg/kg/dose every 8 hours

Children >5 years: 1.5-2.5 mg/kg/dose every 8 hours

Ophthalmic: Solution: 1-2 drops every 2-4 hours, up to 2 drops every hour for severe infections; ointment: 2-3 times/day

Topical: Apply 3-4 times/day

Adults:

I.M., I.V.: 3-5 mg/kg/day in divided doses every 8 hours

Topical: Apply 3-4 times/day

Ophthalmic: Solution: 1-2 drops every 2-4 hours; ointment: 2-3 times/day

**Dosage Forms**

Cream, topical, as sulfate (Garamycin®): 0.1% (15 g)

Infusion, in $D_5W$, as sulfate: 60 mg, 80 mg, 100 mg

Infusion, in NS, as sulfate: 40 mg, 60 mg, 80 mg, 90 mg, 100 mg, 120 mg

Injection, as sulfate: 40 mg/mL (1 mL, 1.5 mL, 2 mL)

Pediatric, as sulfate: 10 mg/mL (2 mL)

Intrathecal, preservative free, as sulfate (Garamycin®): 2 mg/mL (2 mL)

Ointment, as sulfate:

Ophthalmic: 0.3% [3 mg/g] (3.5 g)

Garamycin®, Genoptic® S.O.P., Gentacidin®, Gentak®: 0.3% [3 mg/g] (3.5 g)

Topical, as sulfate (Garamycin®): 0.1% (15 g)

Solution, ophthalmic, as sulfate: 0.3% (5 mL, 15 mL)

Garamycin®, Genoptic®, Gentacidin®, Gentak®: 0.3% (1 mL, 5 mL, 15 mL)

**Gen-Tamoxifen (Can)** *see* tamoxifen *on page 570*

**GenTeal™ [OTC]** *see* hydroxypropyl methylcellulose *on page 307*

**Gen-Temazepam (Can)** *see* temazepam *on page 572*

**Gen-Ticlopidine (Can)** *see* ticlopidine *on page 590*

**Gen-Timolol (Can)** *see* timolol *on page 591*

**Gentlax® [OTC]** *see* senna *on page 541*

**Gentran®** *see* dextran *on page 177*

**Gentrasul®** *see* gentamicin *on previous page*

**Gen-Trazodone (Can)** *see* trazodone *on page 600*

**Gen-Triazolam (Can)** *see* triazolam *on page 603*

**Gen-Valproic (Can)** *see* valproic acid and derivatives *on page 620*

**Gen-Verapamil (Can)** *see* verapamil *on page 625*

**Gen-XENE®** *see* clorazepate *on page 147*

**Gen-Zopiclone (Can)** *see* zopiclone *(Canada only) on page 641*

**Geocillin®** *see* carbenicillin *on page 106*

**Geone®** *see* butalbital compound and acetaminophen *on page 93*

**Geref®** *see* sermorelin acetate *on page 542*

**Geridium®** ***(Discontinued)*** *see page 750*

**German measles vaccine** *see* rubella virus vaccine (live) *on page 533*

**Germinal®** *see* ergoloid mesylates *on page 220*

**Gevrabon® [OTC]** *see* vitamin B complex *on page 630*

**GG** *see* guaifenesin *on page 281*

**GG-Cen®** ***(Discontinued)*** *see page 750*

## glatiramer acetate (gla TIR a mer AS e tate)

**Synonyms** copolymer-1

**U.S./Canadian Brand Names** Copaxone®

**Therapeutic Category** Biological, Miscellaneous

**Use** Reduce the frequency of relapses in relapsing-remitting multiple sclerosis (MS)

**Usual Dosage** Adults: S.C.: 20 mg/day

**Dosage Forms** Injection: 20 mg (2 mL)

**Glaucon®** *see* epinephrine *on page 216*

**Gleevec™** *see* imatinib *on page 313*

**glibenclamide** *see* glyburide *on page 276*

## gliclazide *(Canada only)* (GLYE kla zide)

**U.S./Canadian Brand Names** Diamicron® (Can); Gen-Gliclazide (Can); Novo-Gliclazide (Can)

**Therapeutic Category** Antidiabetic Agent, Oral; Hypoglycemic Agent, Oral; Sulfonylurea Agent

**Use** Control of hyperglycemia in gliclazide-responsive diabetes mellitus of stable, mild, nonketosis prone, maturity onset or adult type which cannot be controlled by proper dietary management and exercise, or when insulin therapy is not appropriate.

**Usual Dosage** Adults: Oral: There is no fixed dosage regimen for the management of diabetes mellitus with gliclazide or any other hypoglycemic agent. Determination of the proper dosage for gliclazide for each patient should be made on the basis of frequent determinations of blood glucose during dose titration and throughout maintenance.

Recommended daily dosage: 80-320 mg; dosage of ≥160 mg should be divided into 2 equal parts for twice daily administration. Gliclazide should be taken preferentially with meals.

Recommended starting dose: 160 mg/day taken as 1 tablet twice daily with meals; total daily dose should not exceed 320 mg

**Dosage Forms** Tablet: 80 mg

## glimepiride (GLYE me pye ride)

**U.S./Canadian Brand Names** Amaryl®

**Therapeutic Category** Antidiabetic Agent, Oral

**Use**

Management of noninsulin-dependent diabetes mellitus (type 2) as an adjunct to diet and exercise to lower blood glucose

In combination with insulin to lower blood glucose in patients whose hyperglycemia cannot be controlled by diet and exercise in conjunction with an oral hypoglycemic agent

**Usual Dosage** Oral (allow several days between dose titrations):

Adults: Initial: 1-2 mg once daily, administered with breakfast or the first main meal; usual maintenance dose: 1-4 mg once daily; after a dose of 2 mg once daily, increase in increments of 2 mg at 1- to 2-week intervals based upon the patient's blood glucose response to a maximum of 8 mg once daily

Elderly: Initial: 1 mg/day

Combination with insulin therapy (fasting glucose level for instituting combination therapy is in the range of >150 mg/dL in plasma or serum depending on the patient): 8 mg once daily with the first main meal

After starting with low-dose insulin, upward adjustments of insulin can be done approximately weekly as guided by frequent measurements of fasting blood glucose. Once stable, combination-therapy patients should monitor their capillary blood glucose on an ongoing basis, preferably daily.

**Dosage Forms** Tablet: 1 mg, 2 mg, 4 mg

## glipizide (GLIP i zide)

**Synonyms** glydiazinamide

**U.S./Canadian Brand Names** Glucotrol®; Glucotrol® XL

**Therapeutic Category** Antidiabetic Agent, Oral

**Use** Management of noninsulin-dependent diabetes mellitus (type 2)

**Usual Dosage** Adults: Oral: 2.5-40 mg/day; doses larger than 15-20 mg/day should be divided and administered twice daily

**Dosage Forms**

Tablet: 5 mg, 10 mg

Tablet, extended release: 2.5 mg, 5 mg, 10 mg

**glivec** *see* imatinib *on page 313*

## glucagon (GLOO ka gon)

**Therapeutic Category** Antihypoglycemic Agent

**Use** Hypoglycemia; diagnostic aid in the radiologic examination of GI tract when a hypotonic state is needed; used with some success as a cardiac stimulant in management of severe cases of beta-adrenergic blocking agent overdosage

**Usual Dosage**

Hypoglycemia or insulin shock therapy: I.M., I.V., S.C.:

Children: 0.025-0.1 mg/kg/dose, not to exceed 1 mg/dose, repeated in 20 minutes as needed

Adults: 0.5-1 mg, may repeat in 20 minutes as needed

Diagnostic aid: Adults: I.M., I.V.: 0.25-2 mg 10 minutes prior to procedure

**Dosage Forms** Powder for injection, lyophilized: 1 mg [1 unit]; 10 mg [10 units]

**glucocerebrosidase** *see* alglucerase *on page 20*

**GlucoNorm® (Can)** *see* repaglinide *on page 521*

**Glucophage®** *see* metformin *on page 377*

**Glucophage® XR** *see* metformin *on page 377*

## glucose (instant) (GLOO kose IN stant)

**U.S./Canadian Brand Names** B-D Glucose® [OTC]; Glutose® [OTC]; Insta-Glucose® [OTC]

**Therapeutic Category** Antihypoglycemic Agent

**Use** Management of hypoglycemia

**Usual Dosage** Oral: 10-20 g

**Dosage Forms**

Gel, oral (Glutose®, Insta-Glucose®): Dextrose 40% (25 g, 30.8 g, 80 g)
Tablet, chewable (B-D Glucose®): 5 g

## glucose polymers (GLOO kose POL i merz)

**U.S./Canadian Brand Names** Moducal® [OTC]; Polycose® [OTC]; Sumacal® [OTC]

**Therapeutic Category** Nutritional Supplement

**Use** Supplies calories for those persons not able to meet the caloric requirement with usual food intake

**Usual Dosage** Adults: Oral: Add to foods or beverages or mix in water

**Dosage Forms**

Liquid (Polycose®): 126 mL
Powder (Moducal®, Polycose®, Sumacal®): 350 g, 368 g, 400 g

**Glucotrol®** *see* glipizide *on previous page*

**Glucotrol® XL** *see* glipizide *on previous page*

**Glucovance™** *see* glyburide and metformin *on next page*

**Glu-K®** *see* potassium gluconate *on page 487*

**Glukor®** ***(Discontinued)*** *see page 750*

## glutamic acid (gloo TAM ik AS id)

**U.S./Canadian Brand Names** Feracid®

**Therapeutic Category** Gastrointestinal Agent, Miscellaneous

**Use** Treatment of hypochlorhydria and achlorhydria

**Usual Dosage** Adults: Oral: 340 mg to 1.02 g 3 times/day before meals or food

**Dosage Forms**

Capsule, as hydrochloride: 340 mg
Powder: 100 g
Tablet: 500 mg

**Glutose® [OTC]** *see* glucose (instant) *on this page*

**Glyate® [OTC]** *see* guaifenesin *on page 281*

## glyburide (GLYE byoor ide)

**Synonyms** glibenclamide

**U.S./Canadian Brand Names** Albert® Glyburide (Can); Apo®-Glyburide (Can); Diaβeta®; Euglucon® (Can); Gen-Glybe (Can); Glynase™ PresTab™; Micronase®; Novo-Glyburide (Can); Nu-Glyburide (Can); PMS-Glyburide (Can)

**Therapeutic Category** Antidiabetic Agent, Oral

**Use** Management of noninsulin-dependent diabetes mellitus (type 2)

**Usual Dosage** Oral:

Diaβeta®, Micronase®:

Adults: Initial: 1.25-5 mg, then increase at weekly intervals to 1.25-20 mg maintenance dose/day divided in 1-2 doses

Elderly: Initial: 1.25-2.5 mg/day, increase by 1.25-2.5 mg/day every 1-3 weeks
Glynase™ PresTab™: Adults: Initial: 0.75-3 mg/day, increase by 1.5 mg/day in weekly intervals, maximum: 12 mg/day

**Dosage Forms**
Tablet (Diaβeta®, Micronase®): 1.25 mg, 2.5 mg, 5 mg
Tablet, micronized (Glynase™ PresTab™): 1.5 mg, 3 mg, 6 mg

## glyburide and metformin (GLYE byoor ide & met FOR min)

**U.S./Canadian Brand Names** Glucovance™

**Therapeutic Category** Antidiabetic Agent, Oral

**Use** Initial therapy for management of type 2 (noninsulin-dependent) diabetes mellitus when hyperglycemia cannot be managed with diet and exercise alone. Second-line therapy for management of type 2 (noninsulin-dependent) diabetes mellitus when hyperglycemia cannot be managed with a sulfonylurea or metformin along with diet and exercise.

**Usual Dosage** Adults: Oral: Dose should be individualized based on effectiveness and tolerance; titrate to minimum effective dose needed to achieve blood glucose control; **do not exceed maximum recommended doses**

Initial therapy: Glucovance™ 1.25 mg/250 mg once daily with a meal; patients with Hb $A_{1c}$ >9% or fasting plasma glucose (FPG) >200 mg/dL may start with Glucovance™ 1.25 mg/250 mg twice daily with meals

Dosage increases may be made every 2 weeks, in increments of Glucovance™ 1.25 mg/250 mg, until a dose of glyburide 10 mg/metformin 2000 mg per day has been reached

**Due to increased risk of hypoglycemia, do not start with Glucovance™ 5 mg/500 mg.**

Second-line therapy: Patients previously treated with a sulfonylurea or metformin alone: Starting dose: Glucovance™ 2.5 mg/500 mg or Glucovance™ 5 mg/500 mg twice daily with the morning and evening meals; doses may be increased in increments no larger than glyburide 5 mg/metformin 500 mg, up to a maximum dose of glyburide 20 mg/ metformin 2000 mg.

When switching patients previously on a sulfonylurea and metformin together, do not exceed the daily dose of glyburide (or glyburide equivalent) or metformin.

**Dosage adjustment in renal impairment:** Risk of lactic acidosis increases with degree of renal impairment; contraindicated in renal disease or renal dysfunction

**Dosage adjustment in hepatic impairment:** Use conservative initial and maintenance doses and avoid use in severe hepatic disease

Elderly: Conservative doses are recommended in the elderly due to potentially decreased renal function; **do not titrate to maximum dose**; should not be used in patients ≥80 years of age unless renal function is verified as normal

**Dosage Forms** Tablet, film-coated:
Glucovance™ 1.25 mg/250 mg: Glyburide 1.25 mg and metformin hydrochloride 250 mg
Glucovance™ 2.5 mg/500 mg: Glyburide 2.5 mg and metformin hydrochloride 500 mg
Glucovance™ 5 mg/500 mg: Glyburide 5 mg and metformin hydrochloride 500 mg

## glycerin (GLIS er in)

**Synonyms** glycerol

**U.S./Canadian Brand Names** Fleet® Babylax® Rectal [OTC]; Ophthalgan® Ophthalmic; Osmoglyn®; Sani-Supp® Suppository [OTC]

**Therapeutic Category** Laxative; Ophthalmic Agent, Miscellaneous

**Use** Constipation; reduction of intraocular pressure; reduction of corneal edema; glycerin has been administered orally to reduce intracranial pressure

**Usual Dosage**
Constipation: Rectal:
Children <6 years: 1 infant suppository 1-2 times/day as needed or 2-5 mL as an enema
Children >6 years and Adults: 1 adult suppository 1-2 times/day as needed or 5-15 mL as an enema
(Continued)

## glycerin *(Continued)*

Children and Adults:

Reduction of intraocular pressure: Oral: 1-1.8 g/kg 1-1½ hours preoperatively; additional doses may be administered at 5-hour intervals

Reduction of corneal edema: Instill 1-2 drops in eye(s) every 3-4 hours

Reduction of intracranial pressure: Oral: 1.5 g/kg/day divided every 4 hours; dose of 1 g/kg/dose every 6 hours has also been used

**Dosage Forms**

Solution:

Ophthalmic, sterile (Ophthalgan®): Glycerin with chlorobutanol 0.55% (7.5 mL)

Oral (lime flavor)(Osmoglyn®): 50% (220 mL)

Rectal (Fleet® Babylax®): 4 mL/applicator (6s)

Suppository, rectal (Sani-Supp®): Glycerin with sodium stearate (infant and adult sizes)

## glycerin, lanolin, and peanut oil (GLIS er in, LAN oh lin, & PEE nut oyl)

**U.S./Canadian Brand Names** Massé® Breast Cream [OTC]

**Therapeutic Category** Topical Skin Product

**Use** Nipple care of pregnant and nursing women

**Usual Dosage** Topical: Apply as often as needed

**Dosage Forms** Cream: 2 oz

**glycerol** *see* glycerin *on previous page*

**glycerol guaiacolate** *see* guaifenesin *on page 281*

**Glycerol-T® *(Discontinued)*** *see page 750*

**glycerol triacetate** *see* triacetin *on page 601*

**glyceryl trinitrate** *see* nitroglycerin *on page 422*

**Glycofed®** *see* guaifenesin and pseudoephedrine *on page 283*

**Glycon (Can)** *see* metformin *on page 377*

## glycopyrrolate (glye koe PYE roe late)

**U.S./Canadian Brand Names** Robinul®; Robinul® Forte

**Therapeutic Category** Anticholinergic Agent

**Use** Adjunct in treatment of peptic ulcer disease; inhibit salivation and excessive secretions of the respiratory tract; reversal of cholinergic agents such as neostigmine and pyridostigmine; control of upper airway secretions

**Usual Dosage**

Children: Control of secretions:

Oral: 40-100 mcg/kg/dose 3-4 times/day

I.M., I.V.: 4-10 mcg/kg/dose every 3-4 hours; maximum: 0.2 mg/dose or 0.8 mg/24 hours

Children:

Intraoperative: I.V.: 4 mcg/kg not to exceed 0.1 mg; repeat at 2- to 3-minute intervals as needed

Preoperative: I.M.:

<2 years: 4.4-8.8 mcg/kg 30-60 minutes before procedure

>2 years: 4.4 mcg/kg 30-60 minutes before procedure

Children and Adults: Reverse neuromuscular blockade: I.V.: 0.2 mg for each 1 mg of neostigmine or 5 mg of pyridostigmine administered

Adults:

Intraoperative: I.V.: 0.1 mg repeated as needed at 2- to 3-minute intervals

Peptic ulcer:

Oral: 1-2 mg 2-3 times/day

I.M., I.V.: 0.1-0.2 mg 3-4 times/day

Preoperative: I.M.: 4.4 mcg/kg 30-60 minutes before procedure

**Dosage Forms**

Injection, as bromide: 0.2 mg/mL (1 mL, 2 mL, 5 mL, 20 mL)

Robinul®: 0.2 mg/mL (1 mL, 2 mL, 5 mL, 20 mL)
Tablet, as bromide:
Robinul®: 1 mg
Robinul® Forte: 2 mg

**Glycotuss® [OTC]** *see* guaifenesin *on page 281*

**Glycotuss-dM® [OTC]** *see* guaifenesin and dextromethorphan *on page 282*

**glydiazinamide** *see* glipizide *on page 275*

**Glynase™ PresTab™** *see* glyburide *on page 276*

**Gly-Oxide® Oral [OTC]** *see* carbamide peroxide *on page 106*

**Glyset™** *see* miglitol *on page 393*

**Glytuss® [OTC]** *see* guaifenesin *on page 281*

**GM-CSF** *see* sargramostim *on page 537*

**G-myticin® *(Discontinued)*** *see page 750*

**GnRH** *see* gonadorelin *on this page*

## gold sodium thiomalate (gold SOW dee um thye oh MAL ate)

**U.S./Canadian Brand Names** Aurolate®

**Therapeutic Category** Gold Compound

**Use** Treatment of progressive rheumatoid arthritis

**Usual Dosage** I.M.:

Children: Initial: Test dose of 10 mg I.M. is recommended, followed by 1 mg/kg I.M. weekly for 20 weeks; not to exceed 50 mg in a single injection; maintenance: 1 mg/kg/dose at 2- to 4-week intervals thereafter for as long as therapy is clinically beneficial and toxicity does not develop. Administration for 2-4 months is usually required before clinical improvement is observed.

Adults: 10 mg first week; 25 mg second week; then 25-50 mg/week until 1 g cumulative dose has been administered. If improvement occurs without adverse reactions, administer 25-50 mg every 2-3 weeks, then every 3-4 weeks.

**Dosage Forms** Injection: 25 mg/mL (1 mL); 50 mg/mL (1 mL, 2 mL, 10 mL)

**GoLYTELY®** *see* polyethylene glycol solution *on page 480*

## gonadorelin (goe nad oh REL in)

**Synonyms** GnRH; gonadotropin-releasing hormone; LHRH; LRH; luteinizing hormone-releasing hormone

**U.S./Canadian Brand Names** Factrel®; Lutrepulse®

**Therapeutic Category** Diagnostic Agent; Gonadotropin

**Use** Evaluation of hypothalamic-pituitary gonadotropic function; used to evaluate abnormal gonadotropin regulation as in precocious puberty and delayed puberty; treatment of primary hypothalamic amenorrhea

**Usual Dosage** Female:

Diagnostic test: Children >12 years and Adults: I.V., S.C. hydrochloride salt: 100 mcg administered in women during early phase of menstrual cycle (day 1-7)

Primary hypothalamic amenorrhea: Adults: Acetate: I.V.: 5 mcg every 90 minutes via Lutrepulse® pump kit at treatment intervals of 21 days (pump will pulsate every 90 minutes for 7 days)

**Dosage Forms**

Injection, as acetate (Lutrepulse®): 0.8 mg, 3.2 mg
Injection, as hydrochloride (Factrel®): 100 mcg, 500 mcg

**gonadotropin-releasing hormone** *see* gonadorelin *on this page*

**Gonak™ [OTC]** *see* hydroxypropyl methylcellulose *on page 307*

**Gonal-F®** *see* follitropin alfa *on page 263*

**Gonic® *(Discontinued)*** *see page 750*

**gonioscopic ophthalmic solution** *see* hydroxypropyl methylcellulose *on page 307*

**Goniosol® [OTC]** *see* hydroxypropyl methylcellulose *on page 307*

**Goody's® Fast Pain Relief® [OTC]** *see* acetaminophen, aspirin, and caffeine *on page 6*

**Goody's® Headache Powders [OTC]** *see* acetaminophen, aspirin, and caffeine *on page 6*

**Gordofilm® Liquid** *see* salicylic acid *on page 535*

**Gormel® Creme [OTC]** *see* urea *on page 617*

## goserelin (GOE se rel in)

**U.S./Canadian Brand Names** Zoladex® Implant

**Therapeutic Category** Gonadotropin Releasing Hormone Analog

**Use** Palliative treatment of advanced prostate cancer and breast cancer

**Usual Dosage** Adults: S.C.:

Breast/prostatic cancer: 3.6 mg as a depot injection every 28 days into upper abdominal wall using sterile technique under the supervision of a physician. At the physician's option, local anesthesia may be used prior to injection. The injection should be repeated every 28 days as long as the patient can tolerate the side effects and there is satisfactory disease regression. While a delay of a few days is permissible, every effort should be made to adhere to the 28-day schedule.

Prostatic cancer: 10.8 mg as a depot injection every 12 weeks into upper abdominal wall using sterile technique under the supervision of a physician. At the physician's option, local anesthesia may be used prior to injection. The injection should be repeated every 12 weeks as long as the patient can tolerate the side effects and there is satisfactory disease regression. While a delay of a few days is permissible, every effort should be made to adhere to the 12-week schedule.

**Dosage Forms** Injection, implant, as acetate: 3.6 mg, 10.8 mg

**GP 47680** *see* oxcarbazepine *on page 441*

## granisetron (gra NI se tron)

**U.S./Canadian Brand Names** Kytril™

**Therapeutic Category** Selective 5-$HT_3$ Receptor Antagonist

**Use** Prophylaxis and treatment of chemotherapy-related emesis

**Usual Dosage**

Oral: 1 tablet (1 mg) twice daily

I.V.:

10-40 mcg/kg for 1-3 doses; doses should be administered as a single IVPB over 5 minutes to 1 hour, administer just prior to chemotherapy (15-60 minutes before)

As intervention therapy for breakthrough nausea and vomiting, during the first 24 hours following chemotherapy, 2 or 3 repeat infusions (same dose) have been administered, separated by at least 10 minutes

**Dosage Forms**

Injection: 1 mg/mL

Tablet: 1 mg (2s), (20s)

**Granulex** *see* trypsin, balsam Peru, and castor oil *on page 612*

**granulocyte colony-stimulating factor** *see* filgrastim *on page 249*

**granulocyte-macrophage colony-stimulating factor** *see* sargramostim *on page 537*

**Gravol® (Can)** *see* dimenhydrinate *on page 188*

**Grifulvin® V** *see* griseofulvin *on next page*

**Grisactin®** *see* griseofulvin *on next page*

**Grisactin® Ultra *(Discontinued)*** *see page 750*

## griseofulvin (gri see oh FUL vin)

**Synonyms** griseofulvin microsize; griseofulvin ultramicrosize

**U.S./Canadian Brand Names** Fulvicin® P/G; Fulvicin-U/F®; Grifulvin® V; Grisactin®; Gris-PEG®

**Therapeutic Category** Antifungal Agent

**Use** Treatment of tinea infections of the skin, hair, and nails caused by susceptible species of *Microsporum*, *Epidermophyton*, or *Trichophyton*

**Usual Dosage** Oral:

Children:

Microsize: 10-15 mg/kg/day in single or divided doses;

Ultramicrosize: >2 years: 5.5-7.3 mg/kg/day in single or divided doses

Adults:

Microsize: 500-1000 mg/day in single or divided doses

Ultramicrosize: 330-375 mg/day in single or divided doses; doses up to 750 mg/day have been used for infections more difficult to eradicate such as tinea unguium

Duration of therapy depends on the site of infection:

Tinea corporis: 2-4 weeks

Tinea capitis: 4-6 weeks or longer

Tinea pedis: 4-8 weeks

Tinea unguium: 3-6 months

**Dosage Forms**

Microsize:

Capsule (Grisactin®): 125 mg, 250 mg

Suspension, oral (Grifulvin® V): 125 mg/5 mL with alcohol 0.2% (120 mL)

Tablet:

Fulvicin-U/F®, Grifulvin® V: 250 mg

Fulvicin-U/F®, Grifulvin® V, Grisactin-500®: 500 mg

Ultramicrosize:

Tablet:

Fulvicin® P/G: 165 mg, 330 mg

Fulvicin® P/G, Grisactin® Ultra, Gris-PEG®: 125 mg, 250 mg

**griseofulvin microsize** *see* griseofulvin *on this page*

**griseofulvin ultramicrosize** *see* griseofulvin *on this page*

**Gris-PEG®** *see* griseofulvin *on this page*

**Guaifed® [OTC]** *see* guaifenesin and pseudoephedrine *on page 283*

**Guaifed-PD®** *see* guaifenesin and pseudoephedrine *on page 283*

## guaifenesin (gwye FEN e sin)

**Synonyms** GG; glycerol guaiacolate

**U.S./Canadian Brand Names** Anti-Tuss® Expectorant [OTC]; Balminil® Expectorant (Can); Benylin-E (Can); Breonesin® [OTC]; Diabetic Tussin® EX [OTC]; Duratuss-G®; Fenesin™; Gee Gee® [OTC]; Genatuss® [OTC]; Glyate® [OTC]; Glycotuss® [OTC]; Glytuss® [OTC]; Guaifenex® LA; GuiaCough® Expectorant [OTC]; Guiatuss® [OTC]; Halotussin® [OTC]; Humibid® L.A.; Humibid® Sprinkle; Hytuss® [OTC]; Hytuss-2X® [OTC]; Koffex Expectorant (Can); Liquibid®; Medi-Tuss® [OTC]; Monafed®; Muco-Fen-LA®; Mytussin® [OTC]; Naldecon® Senior EX [OTC]; Organidin® NR; Pneumomist®; Respa-GF®; Robitussin® [OTC]; Scot-Tussin® [OTC]; Siltussin® [OTC]; Sinumist®-SR Capsulets®; Touro Ex®; Tusibron® [OTC]; Uni-Tussin® [OTC]

**Therapeutic Category** Expectorant

**Use** Temporary control of cough due to minor throat and bronchial irritation

**Usual Dosage** Oral:

Children:

<2 years: 12 mg/kg/day in 6 divided doses

2-5 years: 50-100 mg (2.5-5 mL) every 4 hours, not to exceed 600 mg/day

6-11 years: 100-200 mg (5-10 mL) every 4 hours, not to exceed 1.2 g/day

(Continued)

## guaifenesin *(Continued)*

Children >12 years and Adults: 200-400 mg (10-20 mL) every 4 hours to a maximum of 2.4 g/day (60 mL/day)

**Dosage Forms**

Caplet, sustained release (Touro Ex®): 600 mg
Capsule (Breonesin®, GG-Cen®, Hytuss-2X®): 200 mg
Sustained release (Humibid® Sprinkle): 300 mg
Liquid:
Diabetic Tussin® EX, Organidin® NR, Tusibron®: 100 mg/5 mL (118 mL)
Naldecon® Senior EX: 200 mg/5 mL (118 mL, 480 mL)
Syrup (Anti-Tuss® Expectorant, Genatuss®, Glyate®, GuiaCough® Expectorant, Guiatuss®, Halotussin®, Malotuss®, Medi-Tuss®, Mytussin®, Robitussin®, Scot-Tussin®, Siltussin®, Tusibron®, Uni-Tussin®): 100 mg/5 mL with alcohol 3.5% (30 mL, 120 mL, 240 mL, 473 mL, 946 mL)
Tablet:
Duratuss-G®: 1200 mg
Gee Gee®, Glytuss®, Organidin® NR: 200 mg
Glycotuss®, Hytuss®: 100 mg
Sustained release:
Fenesin™, Guaifenex® LA, Humibid® L.A., Liquibid®, Monafed®, Muco-Fen-LA®, Pneumomist®, Respa-GF®, Sinumist®-SR Capsulets®: 600 mg

## guaifenesin and codeine (gwye FEN e sin & KOE deen)

**U.S./Canadian Brand Names** Brontex® Liquid; Brontex® Tablet; Cheracol®; Guaituss AC®; Guiatussin® With Codeine; Mytussin® AC; Robafen® AC; Robitussin® A-C; Tussi-Organidin® NR

**Therapeutic Category** Antitussive/Expectorant

**Controlled Substance** C-V

**Use** Temporary control of cough due to minor throat and bronchial irritation

**Usual Dosage** Oral:

Children:
2-6 years: 1-1.5 mg/kg codeine/day divided into 4 doses administered every 4-6 hours
6-12 years: 5 mL every 4 hours, not to exceed 30 mL/24 hours
>12 years: 10 mL every 4 hours, up to 60 mL/24 hours
Adults: 10 mL or 1 tablet every 6-8 hours

**Dosage Forms**

Liquid [C-V] (Brontex®): Guaifenesin 75 mg and codeine phosphate 2.5 mg per 5 mL
Syrup [C-V] (Cheracol®, Guaituss AC®, Guiatussin® with Codeine, Mytussin® AC, Robafen® AC, Robitussin® A-C, Tussi-Organidin® NR): Guaifenesin 100 mg and codeine phosphate 10 mg per 5 mL (60 mL, 120 mL, 480 mL)
Tablet [C-III] (Brontex®): Guaifenesin 300 mg and codeine phosphate 10 mg

## guaifenesin and dextromethorphan

(gwye FEN e sin & deks troe meth OR fan)

**U.S./Canadian Brand Names** Balminil DM + Expectorant (Can); Benylin® DM-E (Can); Benylin® Expectorant [OTC]; Cheracol® D [OTC]; Clear Tussin® 30; Contac® Cough Formula Liquid [OTC]; Diabetic Tussin DM® [OTC]; Extra Action Cough Syrup [OTC]; Fenesin™ DM; Genatuss DM® [OTC]; Glycotuss-dM® [OTC]; Guaifenex® DM; GuiaCough® [OTC]; Guiatuss-DM® [OTC]; Halotussin® DM [OTC]; Humibid® DM [OTC]; Iobid DM®; Koffex DM + Expectorant (Can); Kolephrin® GG/DM [OTC]; Monafed® DM; Muco-Fen-DM®; Mytussin® DM [OTC]; Naldecon® Senior DX [OTC]; Phanatuss® Cough Syrup [OTC]; Phenadex® Senior [OTC]; Respa®-DM; Rhinosyn-DMX® [OTC]; Robafen DM® [OTC]; Robitussin®-DM [OTC]; Safe Tussin® 30 [OTC]; Scot-Tussin® Senior Clear [OTC]; Siltussin DM® [OTC]; Synacol® CF [OTC]; Syracol-CF® [OTC]; Tolu-Sed® DM [OTC]; Tusibron-DM® [OTC]; Tuss-DM® [OTC]; Tussi-Organidin® DM NR; Uni-tussin® DM [OTC]; Vicks® 44E [OTC]; Vicks® Pediatric Formula 44E [OTC]

**Therapeutic Category** Antitussive/Expectorant

**Use** Temporary control of cough due to minor throat and bronchial irritation

**Usual Dosage** Oral:

Children:

2-5 years: 2.5 mL every 6-8 hours; maximum: 10 mL/day

6-12 years: 5 mL every 6-8 hours; maximum: 20 mL/24 hours

>12 years: 10 mL every 6-8 hours; maximum: 40 mL/24 hours

Alternatively: 0.1-0.15 mL/kg/dose every 6-8 hours as needed

Adults: 10 mL every 6-8 hours

**Dosage Forms**

Syrup:

Benylin® Expectorant: Guaifenesin 100 mg and dextromethorphan hydrobromide 5 mg per 5 mL (118 mL, 236 mL)

Cheracol® D, Clear Tussin® 30, Genatuss DM®, Mytussin® DM, Robitussin®-DM, Siltussin DM®, Tolu-Sed® DM, Tussi-Organidin® DM NR: Guaifenesin 100 mg and dextromethorphan hydrobromide 10 mg per 5 mL (5 mL, 10 mL, 120 mL, 240 mL, 360 mL, 480 mL, 3780 mL)

Contac® Cough Formula Liquid: Guaifenesin 67 mg and dextromethorphan hydrobromide 10 mg per 5 mL (120 mL)

Extra Action Cough Syrup, GuiaCough®, Guiatuss DM®, Halotussin® DM, Rhinosyn-DMX®, Tusibron-DM®, Uni-tussin® DM: Guaifenesin 100 mg and dextromethorphan hydrobromide 15 mg per 5 mL (120 mL, 240 mL, 480 mL)

Kolephrin® GG/DM: Guaifenesin 150 mg and dextromethorphan hydrobromide 10 mg per 5 mL (120 mL)

Naldecon® Senior DX: Guaifenesin 200 mg and dextromethorphan hydrobromide 15 mg per 5 mL (118 mL, 480 mL)

Phanatuss®: Guaifenesin 85 mg and dextromethorphan hydrobromide 10 mg per 5 mL

Vicks® 44E: Guaifenesin 66.7 mg and dextromethorphan hydrobromide 6.7 mg per 5 mL

Tablet:

Extended release

Guaifenex DM®, Iobid DM®, Fenesin™ DM, Humibid® DM, Monafed® DM, Respa®-DM: Guaifenesin 600 mg and dextromethorphan hydrobromide 30 mg

Glycotuss-dM®: Guaifenesin 100 mg and dextromethorphan hydrobromide 10 mg

Queltuss®: Guaifenesin 100 mg and dextromethorphan hydrobromide 15 mg

Syracol-CF®: Guaifenesin 200 mg and dextromethorphan hydrobromide 15 mg

Tuss-DM®: Guaifenesin 200 mg and dextromethorphan hydrobromide 10 mg

## guaifenesin and phenylephrine (gwye FEN e sin & fen il EF rin)

**U.S./Canadian Brand Names** Deconsal® Sprinkle®; Endal®; Sinupan®

**Therapeutic Category** Cold Preparation

**Use** Symptomatic relief of those respiratory conditions where tenacious mucous plugs and congestion complicate the problem such as sinusitis, pharyngitis, bronchitis, asthma, and as an adjunctive therapy in serous otitis media

**Usual Dosage** Adults: Oral: 1-2 tablets/capsules every 12 hours

**Dosage Forms**

Capsule, sustained release:

Deconsal® Sprinkle®: Guaifenesin 300 mg and phenylephrine hydrochloride 10 mg

Sinupan®: Guaifenesin 200 mg and phenylephrine hydrochloride 40 mg

Tablet, timed release (Endal®): Guaifenesin 300 mg and phenylephrine hydrochloride 20 mg

## guaifenesin and pseudoephedrine (gwye FEN e sin & soo doe e FED rin)

**U.S./Canadian Brand Names** Congess® Jr; Congess® Sr; Congestac®; Deconsal® II; Defen-LA®; Entex® PSE; Eudal®-SR; Fedahist® Expectorant [OTC]; Fedahist® Expectorant Pediatric [OTC]; Glycofed®; Guaifed® [OTC]; Guaifed-PD®; Guaifenex® PSE; GuaiMAX-D®; Guaitab®; Guaivent®; Guai-Vent/PSE®; Guiatuss PE® [OTC]; Halotussin® PE [OTC]; Maxifed®; Maxifed-G®; Nasabid™; Respa-1st®; Respaire®-60 SR; Respaire®-120 SR; Robitussin-PE® [OTC]; Robitussin® Severe Congestion Liqui-Gels® [OTC]; Ru-

(Continued)

## guaifenesin and pseudoephedrine *(Continued)*

Tuss® DE; Rymed®; Sinufed® Timecelles®; Touro LA®; Tuss-LA®; V-Dec-M®; Versacaps®; Zephrex®; Zephrex LA®

**Therapeutic Category** Expectorant/Decongestant

**Use** Enhance the output of respiratory tract fluid and reduce mucosal congestion and edema in the nasal passage

**Usual Dosage** Oral:

Children:

2-6 years: 2.5 mL every 4 hours not to exceed 15 mL/24 hours

6-12 years: 5 mL every 4 hours not to exceed 30 mL/24 hours

Children >12 years and Adults: 10 mL every 4 hours not to exceed 60 mL/24 hours

**Dosage Forms**

Capsule:

Guaivent®: Guaifenesin 250 mg and pseudoephedrine hydrochloride 120 mg

Robitussin® Severe Congestion Liqui-Gels®: Guaifenesin 200 mg and pseudoephedrine hydrochloride 30 mg

Rymed®: Guaifenesin 250 mg and pseudoephedrine hydrochloride 30 mg

Capsule, extended release:

Congess® Jr: Guaifenesin 125 mg and pseudoephedrine hydrochloride 60 mg

Nasabid®: Guaifenesin 250 mg and pseudoephedrine hydrochloride 90 mg

Congess® Sr, Guaifed®, Respaire®-120 SR,: Guaifenesin 250 mg and pseudoephedrine hydrochloride 120 mg

Guaifed-PD®, Sinufed® Timecelles®, Versacaps®: Guaifenesin 300 mg and pseudoephedrine hydrochloride 60 mg

Respaire®-60 SR: Guaifenesin 200 mg and pseudoephedrine hydrochloride 60 mg

Tuss-LA® Capsule: Guaifenesin 500 mg and pseudoephedrine hydrochloride 120 mg

Drops, oral (Fedahist® Expectorant Pediatric): Guaifenesin 40 mg and pseudoephedrine hydrochloride 7.5 mg per mL (30 mL)

Syrup:

Fedahist® Expectorant, Guaifed®: Guaifenesin 200 mg and pseudoephedrine hydrochloride 30 mg per 5 mL (120 mL, 240 mL)

Guiatuss® PE, Halotussin® PE, Robitussin-PE®, Rymed®: Guaifenesin 100 mg and pseudoephedrine hydrochloride 30 mg per 5 mL (120 mL, 240 mL, 480 mL)

Tablet:

Congestac®, Guaitab®, Zephrex®: Guaifenesin 400 mg and pseudoephedrine hydrochloride 60 mg

Glycofed®: Guaifenesin 100 mg and pseudoephedrine hydrochloride 30 mg

Tablet, extended release:

Deconsal® II, Defen-LA®, Respa-1st®: Guaifenesin 600 mg and pseudoephedrine hydrochloride 60 mg

Entex® PSE, Guaifenex® PSE, GuaiMAX-D®, Guai-Vent/PSE®, Ru-Tuss® DE, Sudex®, Zephrex LA®: Guaifenesin 600 mg and pseudoephedrine hydrochloride 120 mg

Eudal®-SR, Histalet® X, Touro LA®: Guaifenesin 400 mg and pseudoephedrine hydrochloride 120 mg

Maxifed®: Guaifenesin 700 mg and pseudoephedrine hydrochloride 80 mg

Maxifed-G®: Guaifenesin 550 mg and pseudoephedrine hydrochloride 60 mg

Tuss-LA® Tablet, V-Dec-M®: Guaifenesin 5 mg and pseudoephedrine hydrochloride 120 mg

## guaifenesin, pseudoephedrine, and codeine

(gwye FEN e sin, soo doe e FED rin, & KOE deen)

**U.S./Canadian Brand Names** Benylin® Codeine (Can); Calmylin with Codeine® (Can); Codafed® Expectorant; Cycofed® Pediatric; Decohistine® Expectorant; Deproist® Expectorant With Codeine; Dihistine® Expectorant; Guiatuss DAC®; Guiatussin® DAC; Halotussin® DAC; Isoclor® Expectorant; Mytussin® DAC; Nucofed®; Nucofed® Pediatric Expectorant; Nucotuss®; Phenhist® Expectorant; Robitussin®-DAC; Ryna-CX®; Tussar® SF Syrup

**Therapeutic Category** Antitussive/Decongestant/Expectorant

**Controlled Substance** C-III; C-V

**Use** Temporarily relieves nasal congestion and controls cough due to minor throat and bronchial irritation; helps loosen phlegm and thin bronchial secretions to make coughs more productive

**Usual Dosage** Oral:

Children 6-12 years: 5 mL every 4 hours, not to exceed 40 mL/24 hours

Children >12 years and Adults: 10 mL every 4 hours, not to exceed 40 mL/24 hours

**Dosage Forms** Liquid:

C-III: Nucofed®, Nucotuss®: Guaifenesin 200 mg, pseudoephedrine hydrochloride 60 mg, and codeine phosphate 20 mg per 5 mL (480 mL)

C-V: Codafed® Expectorant, Decohistine® Expectorant, Deproist® Expectorant with Codeine, Dihistine® Expectorant, Guiatuss DAC®, Guiatussin® DAC, Halotussin® DAC, Isoclor® Expectorant, Mytussin® DAC, Nucofed® Pediatric Expectorant, Phenhist® Expectorant, Robitussin®-DAC, Ryna-CX®, Tussar® SF: Guaifenesin 100 mg, pseudoephedrine hydrochloride 30 mg, and codeine phosphate 10 mg per 5 mL (120 mL, 480 mL, 4000 mL)

## guaifenesin, pseudoephedrine, and dextromethorphan

(gwye FEN e sin, soo doe e FED rin, & deks troe meth OR fan)

**U.S./Canadian Brand Names** Anatuss® DM [OTC]; Benylin® DM-D-E (Can); Calmylin #3 (Can); Dimacol® Caplets [OTC]; Koffex DM + Decongestant (Can); Maxifed® DM; Novahistine DM Decongestant Expectorant (Can); Rhinosyn-X® Liquid [OTC]; Robitussin® Cough & Cold (Can); Ru-Tuss® Expectorant [OTC]; Sudafed® Cold & Cough Liquid Caps [OTC]

**Therapeutic Category** Cold Preparation

**Use** Temporarily relieves nasal congestion and controls cough due to minor throat and bronchial irritation; helps loosen phlegm and thin bronchial secretions to make coughs more productive

**Usual Dosage** Adults: Oral: 2 capsules (caplets) or 10 mL every 4 hours

**Dosage Forms**

Caplets (Dimacol®): Guaifenesin 100 mg, pseudoephedrine hydrochloride 30 mg, and dextromethorphan hydrobromide 10 mg

Capsule (Sudafed® Cold & Cough Liquid Caps): Guaifenesin 100 mg, pseudoephedrine hydrochloride 30 mg, and dextromethorphan hydrobromide 10 mg

Liquid (Anatuss® DM, Rhinosyn-X® Liquid, Ru-Tuss® Expectorant): Guaifenesin 100 mg, pseudoephedrine hydrochloride 30 mg, and dextromethorphan hydrobromide 10 mg per 5 mL

Tablet, sustained release (Maxifed® DM): Guaifenesin 550 mg, pseudoephedrine hydrochloride 60 mg, and dextromethorphan hydrobromide 30 mg

**Guaifenex®** ***(Discontinued)*** *see page 750*

**Guaifenex® DM** *see* guaifenesin and dextromethorphan *on page 282*

**Guaifenex® LA** *see* guaifenesin *on page 281*

**Guaifenex® PPA 75** ***(Discontinued)*** *see page 750*

**Guaifenex® PSE** *see* guaifenesin and pseudoephedrine *on page 283*

**GuaiMAX-D®** *see* guaifenesin and pseudoephedrine *on page 283*

**Guaipax®** ***(Discontinued)*** *see page 750*

**Guaitab®** *see* guaifenesin and pseudoephedrine *on page 283*

**Guaituss AC®** *see* guaifenesin and codeine *on page 282*

**Guaivent®** *see* guaifenesin and pseudoephedrine *on page 283*

**Guai-Vent/PSE®** *see* guaifenesin and pseudoephedrine *on page 283*

## guanabenz (GWAHN a benz)

**U.S./Canadian Brand Names** Wytensin®

**Therapeutic Category** Alpha-Adrenergic Agonist

(Continued)

## guanabenz *(Continued)*

**Use** Management of hypertension

**Usual Dosage** Adults: Oral: Initial: 4 mg twice daily, increase in increments of 4-8 mg/ day every 1-2 weeks to a maximum of 32 mg twice daily

**Dosage Forms** Tablet, as acetate: 4 mg, 8 mg

## guanadrel (GWAHN a drel)

**U.S./Canadian Brand Names** Hylorel®

**Therapeutic Category** Alpha-Adrenergic Agonist

**Use** Step 2 agent in stepped-care treatment of hypertension, usually with a diuretic

**Usual Dosage** Oral: Initial: 10 mg/day (5 mg twice daily); adjust dosage until blood pressure is controlled, usual dosage: 20-75 mg/day, administered twice daily

**Dosage Forms** Tablet, as sulfate: 10 mg

## guanethidine (gwahn ETH i deen)

**U.S./Canadian Brand Names** Apo®-Guanethidine (Can); Ismelin®

**Therapeutic Category** Alpha-Adrenergic Agonist

**Use** Treatment of moderate to severe hypertension

**Usual Dosage** Oral:

Children:

Initial: 0.2 mg/kg/day administered daily

Maximum dose: Up to 3 mg/kg/24 hours

Adults: Initial: 10-12.5 mg/day, then 25-50 mg/day in 3 divided doses

**Dosage Forms** Tablet, as monosulfate: 10 mg, 25 mg

## guanfacine (GWAHN fa seen)

**U.S./Canadian Brand Names** Tenex®

**Therapeutic Category** Alpha-Adrenergic Agonist

**Use** Management of hypertension

**Usual Dosage** Adults: Oral: 1 mg (usually at bedtime), may increase if needed at 3- to 4-week intervals to a maximum of 3 mg/day; 1 mg/day is most common dose

**Dosage Forms** Tablet, as hydrochloride: 1 mg, 2 mg

## guanidine (GWAHN i deen)

**Therapeutic Category** Cholinergic Agent

**Use** Reduction of the symptoms of muscle weakness associated with the myasthenic syndrome of Eaton-Lambert, not for myasthenia gravis

**Usual Dosage** Adults: Oral: Initial: 10-15 mg/kg/day in 3-4 divided doses, gradually increase to 35 mg/kg/day

**Dosage Forms** Tablet, as hydrochloride: 125 mg

**GuiaCough® [OTC]** *see* guaifenesin and dextromethorphan *on page 282*

**GuiaCough® Expectorant [OTC]** *see* guaifenesin *on page 281*

**Guiatex®** ***(Discontinued)*** *see page 750*

**Guiatuss® [OTC]** *see* guaifenesin *on page 281*

**Guiatuss CF®** ***(Discontinued)*** *see page 750*

**Guiatuss DAC®** *see* guaifenesin, pseudoephedrine, and codeine *on page 284*

**Guiatuss-DM® [OTC]** *see* guaifenesin and dextromethorphan *on page 282*

**Guiatussin® DAC** *see* guaifenesin, pseudoephedrine, and codeine *on page 284*

**Guiatussin® With Codeine** *see* guaifenesin and codeine *on page 282*

**Guiatuss PE® [OTC]** *see* guaifenesin and pseudoephedrine *on page 283*

**gum benjamin** *see* benzoin *on page 74*

**GVG** *see* vigabatrin *(Canada only) on page 627*

**G-well® *(Discontinued)*** *see page 750*

**Gynazole•1®** *see* butoconazole *on page 94*

**Gynecort® Topical [OTC]** *see* hydrocortisone (topical) *on page 304*

**GyneCure™ (Can)** *see* tioconazole *on page 592*

**Gyne-Lotrimin® [OTC]** *see* clotrimazole *on page 147*

**Gyne-Lotrimin® 3 [OTC]** *see* clotrimazole *on page 147*

**Gyne-Sulf® *(Discontinued)*** *see page 750*

**Gynodiol™** *see* estradiol *on page 224*

**Gynogen® Injection *(Discontinued)*** *see page 750*

**Gynogen L.A.® Injection** *see* estradiol *on page 224*

**Gynol II® [OTC]** *see* nonoxynol 9 *on page 424*

**$H_2$Oxyl (Can)** *see* benzoyl peroxide *on page 74*

**Habitrol™ Patch** *see* nicotine *on page 419*

## *Haemophilus* B conjugate and hepatitis B vaccine

(hem OF fi lus bee KON joo gate & hep a TYE tis bee vak SEEN)

**U.S./Canadian Brand Names** Comvax®

**Therapeutic Category** Vaccine, Inactivated Virus

**Use** For vaccination against *Haemophilus influenzae* type B and hepatitis B virus in infants 6 weeks to 15 months old of HGsAG-negative mothers

**Usual Dosage** Children: I.M.: 0.5 mL as a single dose should be administered

**Dosage Forms** Injection: *Haemophilus* B conjugate purified capsular polysaccharide 7.5 mcg and Hepatitis B vaccine surface antigen 5 mcg per 0.5 mL (0.5 mL)

## *Haemophilus* B conjugate vaccine

(hem OF fi lus bee KON joo gate vak SEEN)

**Synonyms** HIB polysaccharide conjugate; PRP-D

**U.S./Canadian Brand Names** ActHIB®; HibTITER®; PedvaxHIB®

**Therapeutic Category** Vaccine, Inactivated Bacteria

**Use** Immunization of children 24 months to 6 years of age against diseases caused by *H. influenzae* type B

**Usual Dosage** Children: I.M.: 0.5 mL as a single dose should be administered

**Dosage Forms** Injection:

ActHIB®, HibTITER®: Capsular oligosaccharide 10 mcg and diphtheria $CRM_{197}$ protein ~25 mcg per 0.5 mL (0.5 mL, 2.5 mL, 5 mL)

PedvaxHIB®: Purified capsular polysaccharide 15 mcg and *Neisseria meningitidis* OMPC 250 mcg per dose (0.5 mL)

## halazepam (hal AZ e pam)

**U.S./Canadian Brand Names** Paxipam®

**Therapeutic Category** Benzodiazepine

**Controlled Substance** C-IV

**Use** Management of anxiety disorders; short-term relief of the symptoms of anxiety

**Usual Dosage** Adults: Oral: 20-40 mg 3 or 4 times/day

**Dosage Forms** Tablet: 20 mg, 40 mg

**halazone tablet *(Discontinued)*** *see page 750*

## halcinonide (hal SIN oh nide)

**U.S./Canadian Brand Names** Halog®; Halog®-E

**Therapeutic Category** Corticosteroid, Topical

**Use** Inflammation of corticosteroid-responsive dermatoses

(Continued)

## halcinonide *(Continued)*

**Usual Dosage** Children and Adults: Topical: Apply sparingly 1-3 times/day; occlusive dressing may be used for severe or resistant dermatoses. Therapy should be discontinued when control is achieved. If no improvement is seen, reassessment of diagnosis may be necessary.

**Dosage Forms**
Cream (Halog®): 0.025% (15 g, 60 g, 240 g); 0.1% (15 g, 30 g, 60 g, 240 g)
Cream, emollient base (Halog®-E) : 0.1% (15 g, 30 g, 60 g)
Ointment, topical (Halog®): 0.1% (15 g, 30 g, 60 g, 240 g)
Solution (Halog®): 0.1% (20 mL, 60 mL)

**Halcion®** *see* triazolam *on page 603*

**Haldol®** *see* haloperidol *on this page*

**Haldol® Decanoate** *see* haloperidol *on this page*

**Haldrone® *(Discontinued)*** *see page 750*

**Halenol® [OTC]** *see* acetaminophen *on page 3*

**Halenol® Tablet *(Discontinued)*** *see page 750*

**Haley's M-O® [OTC]** *see* magnesium hydroxide and mineral oil emulsion *on page 362*

**Halfan®** *see* halofantrine *on this page*

**Halfprin® 81® [OTC]** *see* aspirin *on page 55*

## halobetasol (hal oh BAY ta sol)

**U.S./Canadian Brand Names** Ultravate™

**Therapeutic Category** Corticosteroid, Topical

**Use** Relief of inflammatory and pruritic manifestations of corticosteroid-response dermatoses

**Usual Dosage** Children and Adults: Topical: Apply sparingly to skin twice daily; rub in gently and completely. Therapy should be discontinued when control is achieved. If no improvement is seen, reassessment of diagnosis may be necessary.

**Dosage Forms**
Cream, as propionate: 0.05% (15 g, 50 g)
Ointment, topical, as propionate: 0.05% (15 g, 50 g)

## halofantrine (ha loe FAN trin)

**U.S./Canadian Brand Names** Halfan®

**Therapeutic Category** Antimalarial Agent

**Use** Treatment of mild to moderate acute malaria caused by susceptible strains of *Plasmodium falciparum* and *Plasmodium vivax*

**Usual Dosage** Oral:
Children <40 kg: 8 mg/kg every 6 hours for 3 doses
Adults: 500 mg every 6 hours for 3 doses

**Dosage Forms**
Suspension, as hydrochloride: 100 mg/5 mL
Tablet, as hydrochloride: 250 mg

**Halog®** *see* halcinonide *on previous page*

**Halog®-E** *see* halcinonide *on previous page*

## haloperidol (ha loe PER i dole)

**U.S./Canadian Brand Names** Apo®-Haloperidol (Can); Haldol®; Haldol® Decanoate; Novo-Peridol (Can); Peridol (Can); PMS-Haloperidol LA (Can)

**Therapeutic Category** Antipsychotic Agent, Butyrophenone

**Use** Treatment of psychoses, Tourette's disorder, and severe behavioral problems in children

**Usual Dosage**
Children:
<3 years: Not recommended
3-6 years: Dose and indications are not well established
Control of agitation or hyperkinesia in disturbed children: Oral: 0.01-0.03 mg/kg/day once daily
Infantile autism: Oral: Daily doses of 0.5-4 mg have been reported to be helpful in this disorder
6-12 years: Dose not well established
I.M.: 1-3 mg/dose every 4-8 hours, up to a maximum of 0.1 mg/kg/day
Acute psychoses: Oral: Begin with 0.5-1.5 mg/day and increase gradually in increments of 0.5 mg/day, to a maintenance dose of 2-4 mg/day (0.05-0.1 mg/kg/day).
Tourette's syndrome and mental retardation with hyperkinesia: Oral: Begin with 0.5 mg/day and increase by 0.5 mg/day each day until symptoms are controlled or a maximum dose of 15 mg is reached
Children >12 years and Adults:
I.M.:
Acute psychoses: 2-5 mg/dose every 1-8 hours PRN up to a total of 10-30 mg, until control of symptoms is achieved
Mental retardation with hyperkinesia: Begin with 20 mg/day in divided doses, then increase slowly, up to a maximum of 60 mg/day; change to oral administration as soon as symptoms are controlled
Oral:
Acute psychoses: Begin with 1-15 mg/day in divided doses, then gradually increase until symptoms are controlled, up to a maximum of 100 mg/day; after control of symptoms is achieved, reduce dose to the minimal effective dose
Tourette's syndrome: Begin with 6-15 mg/day in divided doses, increase in increments of 2-10 mg/day until symptoms are controlled or adverse reactions become disabling; when symptoms are controlled, reduce to approximately 9 mg/day for maintenance

**Dosage Forms**
Concentrate, oral, as lactate: 2 mg/mL (5 mL, 10 mL, 15 mL, 120 mL, 240 mL)
Injection, as decanoate: 50 mg/mL (1 mL, 5 mL); 100 mg/mL (1 mL, 5 mL)
Injection, as lactate: 5 mg/mL (1 mL, 2 mL, 2.5 mL, 10 mL)
Tablet: 0.5 mg, 1 mg, 2 mg, 5 mg, 10 mg, 20 mg

**Halotestin®** *see* fluoxymesterone *on page 257*

**Halotex®** ***(Discontinued)*** *see page 750*

## halothane (HA loe thane)

**Therapeutic Category** General Anesthetic
**Use** General induction and maintenance of anesthesia (inhalation)
**Usual Dosage** Maintenance concentration varies from 0.5% to 1.5%
**Dosage Forms** Liquid: 125 mL, 250 mL

**Halotussin® [OTC]** *see* guaifenesin *on page 281*

**Halotussin® DAC** *see* guaifenesin, pseudoephedrine, and codeine *on page 284*

**Halotussin® DM [OTC]** *see* guaifenesin and dextromethorphan *on page 282*

**Halotussin® PE [OTC]** *see* guaifenesin and pseudoephedrine *on page 283*

**Haltran® [OTC]** *see* ibuprofen *on page 311*

**hamamelis water** *see* witch hazel *on page 635*

**Harmonyl®** ***(Discontinued)*** *see page 750*

**Havrix®** *see* hepatitis A vaccine *on page 292*

**Hayfebrol® Liquid [OTC]** *see* chlorpheniramine and pseudoephedrine *on page 130*

**H-BIG®** ***(Discontinued)*** *see page 750*

**HBIG** *see* hepatitis B immune globulin *on page 292*

**hBNP** *see* nesiritide *on page 417*

**HCG** *see* chorionic gonadotropin *on page 136*

**HCTZ** *see* hydrochlorothiazide *on page 299*

**HD 85®** *see* radiological/contrast media (ionic) *on page 516*

**HD 200 Plus®** *see* radiological/contrast media (ionic) *on page 516*

**HDCV** *see* rabies virus vaccine *on page 516*

**HDRS** *see* rabies virus vaccine *on page 516*

**Headache Formula PM® [OTC]** *see* acetaminophen and diphenhydramine *on page 5*

**Headache Relief PM® [OTC]** *see* acetaminophen and diphenhydramine *on page 5*

**Headrin® Plus Pain Relief [OTC]** *see* acetaminophen, aspirin, and caffeine *on page 6*

**Head & Shoulders® [OTC]** *see* pyrithione zinc *on page 512*

**Healon® *(Discontinued)*** *see page 750*

**Healon® GV *(Discontinued)*** *see page 750*

**Heartline® [OTC]** *see* aspirin *on page 55*

**Hectorol®** *see* doxercalciferol *on page 203*

**Helidac™** *see* bismuth subsalicylate, metronidazole, and tetracycline *on page 82*

**Helistat®** *see* microfibrillar collagen hemostat *on page 391*

**Helixate®** *see* antihemophilic factor (recombinant) *on page 44*

**Hemabate™** *see* carboprost tromethamine *on page 109*

**HemFe® *(Discontinued)*** *see page 750*

**hemiacidrin** *see* citric acid bladder mixture *on page 140*

## hemin (HEE min)

**U.S./Canadian Brand Names** Panhematin®

**Therapeutic Category** Blood Modifiers

**Use** Treatment of recurrent attacks of acute intermittent porphyria (AIP) only after an appropriate period of alternate therapy has been tried

**Usual Dosage** I.V.: 1-4 mg/kg/day administered over 10-15 minutes for 3-14 days; may be repeated no earlier than every 12 hours; not to exceed 6 mg/kg in any 24-hour period

**Dosage Forms** Powder for injection, preservative free: 313 mg/vial [hematin 7 mg/mL] (43 mL)

**Hemocyte® [OTC]** *see* ferrous fumarate *on page 246*

**Hemofil® M** *see* antihemophilic factor (human) *on page 43*

**Hemonyne®** *see* factor IX complex (human) *on page 238*

**Hemotene®** *see* microfibrillar collagen hemostat *on page 391*

**Hepalean® (Can)** *see* heparin *on this page*

**Hepalean-Lok® (Can)** *see* heparin *on this page*

## heparin (HEP a rin)

**U.S./Canadian Brand Names** Hepalean® (Can); Hepalean-Lok® (Can); Hepflush-10®; Hep-Lock®

**Therapeutic Category** Anticoagulant

**Use** Prophylaxis and treatment of thromboembolic disorders

**Usual Dosage Note:** For full-dose heparin (ie, nonlow-dose), the dose should be titrated according to PTT results. For anticoagulation, an APTT 1.5-2.5 times normal is usually desired. APTT is usually measured prior to heparin therapy, 6-8 hours after initiation of a continuous infusion (following a loading dose), and 6-8 hours after changes in the infusion rate; increase or decrease infusion by 2-4 units/kg/hour dependent on PTT. Continuous I.V. infusion is preferred vs I.V. intermittent injections. For intermittent I.V. injections, PTT is measured 3.5-4 hours after I.V. injection.

Children:
- Intermittent I.V.: Initial: 50-100 units/kg, then 50-100 units/kg every 4 hours
- I.V. infusion: Initial: 50 units/kg, then 15-25 units/kg/hour; increase dose by 2-4 units/kg/hour every 6-8 hours as required

Adults:
- Prophylaxis (low-dose heparin): S.C.: 5000 units every 8-12 hours
- Intermittent I.V.: Initial: 10,000 units, then 50-70 units/kg (5000-10,000 units) every 4-6 hours
- I.V. infusion: Initial: 75-100 units/kg, then 15 units/kg/hour with dose adjusted according to PTT results; usual range: 10-30 units/kg/hour

**Dosage Forms**

Heparin sodium:

Lock flush injection:
- Beef lung source: 10 units/mL (1 mL, 2 mL, 2.5 mL, 3 mL, 5 mL, 10 mL, 30 mL); 100 units/mL (1 mL, 2 mL, 2.5 mL, 3 mL, 5 mL, 10 mL, 30 mL)
- Porcine intestinal mucosa source: 10 units/mL (1 mL, 2 mL, 10 mL, 30 mL); 100 units/mL (1 mL, 2 mL, 10 mL, 30 mL)
- Porcine intestinal mucosa source, preservative free: 10 units/mL (1 mL, 10 mL); 100 units/mL (1 mL)

Multiple-dose vial injection:
- Beef lung source, with preservative: 1000 units/mL (5 mL, 10 mL, 30 mL); 5000 units/mL (10 mL); 10,000 units/mL (4 mL, 5 mL, 10 mL); 20,000 units/mL (2 mL, 5 mL, 10 mL); 40,000 units/mL (5 mL)
- Porcine intestinal mucosa source, with preservative: 1000 units/mL (10 mL, 30 mL); 5000 units/mL (10 mL); 10,000 units/mL (4 mL); 20,000 units/mL (2 mL, 5 mL)

Single-dose vial injection:
- Beef lung source: 1000 units/mL (1 mL); 5000 units/mL (1 mL); 10,000 units/mL (1 mL); 20,000 units/mL (1 mL); 40,000 units/mL (1 mL)
- Porcine intestinal mucosa: 1000 units/mL (1 mL); 5000 units/mL (1 mL); 10,000 units/mL (1 mL); 20,000 units/mL (1 mL); 40,000 units/mL (1 mL)

Unit dose injection:
- Porcine intestinal mucosa source, with preservative: 1000 units/dose (1 mL, 2 mL); 2500 units/dose (1 mL); 5000 units/dose (0.5 mL, 1 mL); 7500 units/dose (1 mL); 10,000 units/dose (1 mL); 15,000 units/dose (1 mL); 20,000 units/dose (1 mL)

Heparin sodium infusion, porcine intestinal mucosa source:
- $D_5W$: 40 units/mL (500 mL); 50 units/mL (250 mL, 500 mL); 100 units/mL (100 mL, 250 mL)
- NaCl 0.45%: 2 units/mL (500 mL, 1000 mL); 50 units/mL (250 mL); 100 units/mL (250 mL)
- NaCl 0.9%: 2 units/mL (500 mL, 1000 mL); 5 units/mL (1000 mL); 50 units/mL (250 mL, 500 mL, 1000 mL)

Heparin calcium:
- Unit dose injection, porcine intestinal mucosa, preservative free: 5000 units/dose (0.2 mL); 12,500 units/dose (0.5 mL); 20,000 units/dose (0.8 mL)

**heparin cofactor I** *see* antithrombin III *on page 45*

## hepatitis A inactivated and hepatitis B (recombinant) vaccine

(hep a TYE tis aye in ak ti VAY ted & hep a TYE tis bee (ree KOM be nant) vak SEEN)

**U.S./Canadian Brand Names** Twinrix®

**Therapeutic Category** Vaccine

**Use** Active immunization against disease caused by hepatitis A virus and hepatitis B virus (all known subtypes) in populations desiring protection against or at high risk of exposure to these viruses.

(Continued)

## hepatitis A inactivated and hepatitis B (recombinant) vaccine *(Continued)*

Populations include travelers to areas of intermediate/high endemicity for **both** HAV and HBV; those at increased risk of HBV infection due to behavioral or occupational factors; patients with chronic liver disease; laboratory workers who handle live HAV and HBV; healthcare workers, police, and other personnel who render first-aid or medical assistance; workers who come in contact with sewage; employees of day care centers and correctional facilities; patients/staff of hemodialysis units; male homosexuals; patients frequently receiving blood products; military personnel; users of injectable illicit drugs; close household contacts of patients with hepatitis A and hepatitis B infection.

**Usual Dosage** I.M.: Adults: Primary immunization: Three doses (1 mL each) given on a 0-, 1-, and 6-month schedule

**Dosage Forms**

Injection [single-dose vial]: Inactivated hepatitis A virus 720 ELISA units and hepatitis B surface antigen 20 mcg per mL (1 mL)

Injection, prefilled syringe [single-dose]: Inactivated hepatitis A virus 720 ELISA units and hepatitis B surface antigen 20 mcg per mL (1 mL)

## hepatitis A vaccine (hep a TYE tis aye vak SEEN)

**U.S./Canadian Brand Names** Havrix®; VAQTA®

**Therapeutic Category** Vaccine, Inactivated Virus

**Use** For populations desiring protection against hepatitis A or for populations at high risk of exposure to hepatitis A virus (travelers to developing countries, household and sexual contacts of persons infected with hepatitis A), child day care employees, illicit drug users, male homosexuals, institutional workers (eg, institutions for the mentally and physically handicapped persons, prisons, etc), and healthcare workers who may be exposed to hepatitis A virus (eg, laboratory employees)

**Usual Dosage** I.M.:

Children: 0.5 mL (360 units) on days 1 and 30, with a booster dose 6-12 months late; completion of the first 2 doses (ie, the primary series) should be accomplished at least 2 weeks before anticipated exposure to hepatitis A

Adults: 1 mL (1440 units), with a booster dose at 6-12 months

**Dosage Forms**

Injection, pediatric (Havrix®): 720 ELISA units/0.5 mL (prefilled syringe, single-dose vials)

Injection, adults (Havrix®): 1440 ELISA units/mL (prefilled syringe, single-dose vials)

Injection, pediatric/adolescents (VAQTA®): 25 units/0.5 mL HAV protein (prefilled syringe, single-dose vials)

Injection, adults (VAQTA®): 50 units/mL HAV protein (prefilled syringe, syringe, single-dose vials)

## hepatitis B immune globulin (hep a TYE tis bee i MYUN GLOB yoo lin)

**Synonyms** HBIG

**U.S./Canadian Brand Names** Bayhep B®; Nabi-HB®

**Therapeutic Category** Immune Globulin

**Use** Provide prophylactic passive immunity to hepatitis B infection to those individuals exposed. Hepatitis B immune globulin is not indicated for treatment of active hepatitis B infections and is ineffective in the treatment of chronic active hepatitis B infection.

**Usual Dosage** I.M.:

Newborns: Hepatitis B: 0.5 mL as soon after birth as possible (within 12 hours)

Adults: Postexposure prophylaxis: 0.06 mL/kg; usual dose: 3-5 mL; repeat at 28-30 days after exposure

**Dosage Forms** Injection: 0.5 mL, 1 mL, 5 mL

## hepatitis B vaccine (hep a TYE tis bee vak SEEN)

**U.S./Canadian Brand Names** Engerix-B®; Recombivax HB®

**Therapeutic Category** Vaccine, Inactivated Virus

**Use** Immunization against infection caused by all known subtypes of hepatitis B virus in individuals considered at high risk of potential exposure to hepatitis B virus or $HB_sAg$-positive materials

**Usual Dosage** I.M.:

Children:

≤11 years: 2.5 mcg doses

11-19 years: 5 mcg doses

Adults >20 years: 10 mcg doses

**Dosage Forms** Injection:

Recombinant DNA (Engerix-B®): Hepatitis B surface antigen 20 mcg/mL (1 mL)

Pediatric, recombinant DNA:

Engerix-B®: Hepatitis B surface antigen 10 mcg/0.5 mL (0.5 mL)

Recombivax HB®: Hepatitis B surface antigen 5 mcg/0.5 mL

Recombinant DNA (Recombivax HB®): Hepatitis B surface antigen 10 mcg/mL (1 mL, 3 mL)

Dialysis formulation, recombinant DNA (Recombivax HB®): Hepatitis B surface antigen 40 mcg/mL (1 mL)

**Hep-B-Gammagee®** ***(Discontinued)*** *see page 750*

**Hepflush-10®** *see* heparin *on page 290*

**Hep-Lock®** *see* heparin *on page 290*

**Heptalac®** *see* lactulose *on page 338*

**Heptovir® (Can)** *see* lamivudine *on page 339*

**Herbogesic (Can)** *see* magnesium salicylate *on page 362*

**Herceptin®** *see* trastuzumab *on page 599*

**Herplex®** ***(Discontinued)*** *see page 750*

**HES** *see* hetastarch *on this page*

**Hespan®** *see* hetastarch *on this page*

## hetastarch (HET a starch)

**Synonyms** HES; hydroxyethyl starch

**U.S./Canadian Brand Names** Hespan®

**Therapeutic Category** Plasma Volume Expander

**Use** Blood volume expander used in treatment of shock or impending shock when blood or blood products are not available; does not have oxygen-carrying capacity and is not a substitute for blood or plasma; an adjunct in leukapheresis to enhance the yield of granulocytes by centrifugal means

**Usual Dosage** I.V.: Up to 1500 mL/day

**Dosage Forms** Infusion, in sodium chloride 0.9%: 6% (500 mL)

**Hetrazan®** ***(Discontinued)*** *see page 750*

**Hexabrix™** *see* radiological/contrast media (ionic) *on page 516*

**hexachlorocyclohexane** *see* lindane *on page 350*

## hexachlorophene (heks a KLOR oh feen)

**U.S./Canadian Brand Names** pHisoHex®

**Therapeutic Category** Antibacterial, Topical

**Use** Surgical scrub and as a bacteriostatic skin cleanser; to control an outbreak of gram-positive staphylococcal infection when other infection control procedures have been unsuccessful

**Usual Dosage** Children and Adults: Topical: Apply 5 mL cleanser and water to area to be cleansed; lather and rinse thoroughly under running water

**Dosage Forms**

Foam (Septisol®): 0.23% with alcohol 56% (180 mL, 600 mL)

Liquid, topical (pHisoHex®): 3% (8 mL, 150 mL, 500 mL, 3840 mL)

**Hexadrol®** *see* dexamethasone (systemic) *on page 174*

**Hexalen®** *see* altretamine *on page 25*

**hexamethylenetetramine** *see* methenamine *on page 379*

**hexamethylmelamine** *see* altretamine *on page 25*

**Hexit® (Can)** *see* lindane *on page 350*

## hexylresorcinol (heks il re ZOR si nole)

**U.S./Canadian Brand Names** Sucrets® Sore Throat [OTC]

**Therapeutic Category** Local Anesthetic

**Use** Minor antiseptic and local anesthetic for sore throat

**Usual Dosage** May be used as needed, allow to dissolve slowly in mouth

**Dosage Forms** Lozenge: 2.4 mg

**Hibiclens® [OTC]** *see* chlorhexidine gluconate *on page 126*

**Hibidil® (Can)** *see* chlorhexidine gluconate *on page 126*

**Hibistat® [OTC]** *see* chlorhexidine gluconate *on page 126*

**HIB polysaccharide conjugate** *see Haemophilus* B conjugate vaccine *on page 287*

**HibTITER®** *see Haemophilus* B conjugate vaccine *on page 287*

**Hi-Cor-1.0® Topical** *see* hydrocortisone (topical) *on page 304*

**Hi-Cor-2.5® Topical** *see* hydrocortisone (topical) *on page 304*

**Hiprex®** *see* methenamine *on page 379*

**hirulog** *see* bivalirudin *on page 83*

**Hismanal®** ***(Discontinued)*** *see page 750*

**Histafed® [OTC]** *see* triprolidine and pseudoephedrine *on page 609*

**Histaject®** ***(Discontinued)*** *see page 750*

**Histalet Forte® Tablet** ***(Discontinued)*** *see page 750*

## histamine (HIS ta meen)

**U.S./Canadian Brand Names** Histatrol®

**Therapeutic Category** Diagnostic Agent

**Use** To test the ability of the gastric mucosa to produce hydrochloric acid

**Usual Dosage** Adults: S.C.: Gastric acid test:

The patient fasts for 12 hours. A plastic duodenal tube is passed into the stomach, the gastric content withdrawn, and its acidity determined. Care should be taken to prevent the patient from swallowing salivary secretions during administration of the test results. The alkalinity of the saliva may interfere with the test results. Histamine phosphate 500 to 750 mcg is then injected.

Gastric content is again removed after 5 minutes and at 15 minute intervals thereafter on 3 occasions

The volume and acidity of each specimen is determined. If no acidity is detected, a maximum histamine stimulation test can be performed using 40 mcg/kg histamine phosphate. Pulse rate and blood pressure should be determined immediately after histamine injection.

**Dosage Forms** Injection, as phosphate: 0.275 mg/mL (5 mL)

**Histatab® Plus Tablet [OTC]** *see* chlorpheniramine and phenylephrine *on page 129*

**Hista-Tabs® [OTC]** *see* triprolidine and pseudoephedrine *on page 609*

**Histatrol®** *see* histamine *on this page*

**Hista-Vadrin® Tablet** ***(Discontinued)*** *see page 750*

**Histerone® Injection** *see* testosterone *on page 576*

**Histinex® D Liquid** *see* hydrocodone and pseudoephedrine *on page 301*

**Histolyn-CYL®** *see* histoplasmin *on this page*

## histoplasmin (his toe PLAZ min)

**Synonyms** histoplasmosis skin test antigen

**U.S./Canadian Brand Names** Histolyn-CYL®

**Therapeutic Category** Diagnostic Agent

**Use** Diagnosing histoplasmosis; to assess cell-mediated immunity

**Usual Dosage** Adults: Intradermally: 0.1 mL of 1:100 dilution 5-10 cm apart into volar surface of forearm; induration of ≥5 mm in diameter indicates a positive reaction

**Dosage Forms** Injection: 1:100 (0.1 mL, 1.3 mL)

**histoplasmosis skin test antigen** *see* histoplasmin *on this page*

**Histor-D® Syrup** *see* chlorpheniramine and phenylephrine *on page 129*

**Histor-D® Timecelles®** *see* chlorpheniramine, phenylephrine, and methscopolamine *on page 131*

## histrelin (his TREL in)

**U.S./Canadian Brand Names** Supprelin™

**Therapeutic Category** Gonadotropin Releasing Hormone Analog

**Use** Central idiopathic precocious puberty; also used to treat estrogen-associated gynecological disorders (ie, endometriosis, intermittent porphyria, possibly premenstrual syndrome, leiomyomata uteri [uterine fibroids])

**Usual Dosage**

Central idiopathic precocious puberty: S.C.: Usual dose is 10 mcg/kg/day administered as a single daily dose at the same time each day

Acute intermittent porphyria in women:

S.C.: 5 mcg/day

Intranasal: 400-800 mcg/day

Endometriosis: S.C.: 100 mcg/day

Leiomyomata uteri: S.C.: 20-50 mcg/day or 4 mcg/kg/day

**Dosage Forms** Injection: 7-day kits of single use: 120 mcg/0.6 mL; 300 mcg/0.6 mL; 600 mcg/0.6 mL

**Histussin D® Liquid** *see* hydrocodone and pseudoephedrine *on page 301*

**Hi-Vegi-Lip®** *see* pancreatin *on page 447*

**Hivid®** *see* zalcitabine *on page 637*

**HMS Liquifilm®** *see* medrysone *on page 369*

**$HN_2$** *see* mechlorethamine *on page 367*

**Hold® DM [OTC]** *see* dextromethorphan *on page 178*

## homatropine (hoe MA troe peen)

**U.S./Canadian Brand Names** Isopto® Homatropine Ophthalmic

**Therapeutic Category** Anticholinergic Agent

**Use** Producing cycloplegia and mydriasis for refraction; treatment of acute inflammatory conditions of the uveal tract

**Usual Dosage** Ophthalmic:

Children:

Mydriasis and cycloplegia for refraction: 1 drop of 2% solution immediately before the procedure; repeat at 10-minute intervals as needed

Uveitis: 1 drop of 2% solution 2-3 times/day

Adults:

Mydriasis and cycloplegia for refraction: 1-2 drops of 2% solution or 1 drop of 5% solution before the procedure; repeat at 5- to 10-minute intervals as needed

Uveitis: 1-2 drops 2-3 times/day up to every 3-4 hours as needed

(Continued)

## homatropine *(Continued)*

**Dosage Forms** Solution, ophthalmic, as hydrobromide:
2% (1 mL, 5 mL); 5% (1 mL, 2 mL, 5 mL)
Isopto® Homatropine 2% (5 mL, 15 mL); 5% (5 mL, 15 mL)

**Honvol® (Can)** *see* diethylstilbestrol *on page 184*

**horse antihuman thymocyte gamma globulin** *see* lymphocyte immune globulin *on page 359*

**H.P. Acthar® Gel** *see* corticotropin *on page 154*

**Humalog®** *see* insulin preparations *on page 319*

**Humalog® Mix 50/50™** *see* insulin preparations *on page 319*

**Humalog® Mix 75/25™** *see* insulin preparations *on page 319*

## human growth hormone (HYU man grothe HOR mone)

**Synonyms** somatrem; somatropin

**U.S./Canadian Brand Names** Genotropin®; Humatrope®; Norditropin®; Nutropin®; Nutropin® AQ; Protropin®; Saizen®; Serostim®

**Therapeutic Category** Growth Hormone

**Use** Long-term treatment of growth failure from lack of adequate endogenous growth hormone secretion

**Usual Dosage** Children: I.M., S.C.:
Somatrem: Up to 0.1 mg (0.26 units)/kg/dose 3 times/week
Somatropin: Up to 0.06 mg (0.16 units)/kg/dose 3 times/week
Therapy should be discontinued when patient has reached satisfactory adult height, when epiphyses have fused, or when the patient ceases to respond

**Dosage Forms** Powder for injection (lyophilized):
Somatrem, Protropin®: 5 mg ~15 units (10 mL); 10 mg ~26 units (10 mL)
Somatropin:
Genotropin®: 1.5 mg ~4.5 units (5 mL); 5.8 mg ~17.4 units (5 mL)
Humatrope®: 5 mg ~15 units
Norditropin®: 4 mg ~12 units; 8 mg ~24 units
Nutropin®: 5 mg ~15 units (10 mL); 10 mg ~30 units (10 mL)
Nutropin® AQ: 10 mg ~30 units (2 mL)
Saizen® (rDNA origin): 5 mg ~15 units
Serostim®: 5 mg ~15 units (5 mL); 6 mg ~18 units (5 mL)

**humanized IgG1 anti-CD52 monoclonal antibody** *see* alemtuzumab *on page 19*

**human thyroid-stimulating hormone** *see* thyrotropin alpha *on page 588*

**Humatin®** *see* paromomycin *on page 452*

**Humatrope®** *see* human growth hormone *on this page*

**Humegon™** *see* menotropins *on page 371*

**Humibid® DM [OTC]** *see* guaifenesin and dextromethorphan *on page 282*

**Humibid® L.A.** *see* guaifenesin *on page 281*

**Humibid® Sprinkle** *see* guaifenesin *on page 281*

**HuMIST® Nasal Mist [OTC]** *see* sodium chloride *on page 549*

**Humorsol® Ophthalmic** *see* demecarium *on page 169*

**Humulin® 50/50** *see* insulin preparations *on page 319*

**Humulin® 70/30** *see* insulin preparations *on page 319*

**Humulin® L** *see* insulin preparations *on page 319*

**Humulin® N** *see* insulin preparations *on page 319*

**Hurricaine®** *see* benzocaine *on page 72*

**Hyalgan®** *see* sodium hyaluronate *on page 550*

**hyaluronic acid** *see* sodium hyaluronate *on page 550*

## hyaluronidase (hye al yoor ON i dase)

**U.S./Canadian Brand Names** Wydase®

**Therapeutic Category** Antidote

**Use** Increase the dispersion and absorption of other drugs; increase rate of absorption of parenteral fluids administered by hypodermoclysis; management of I.V. extravasations

**Usual Dosage**

Infants and Children:

Management of I.V. extravasation: Reconstitute the 150 unit vial of lyophilized powder with 1 mL normal saline; administer 0.1 mL of this solution and dilute with 0.9 mL normal saline to yield 15 units/mL; using a 25- or 26-gauge needle, five 0.2 mL injections are made subcutaneously or intradermally into the extravasation site at the leading edge, changing the needle after each injection

Hypodermoclysis: S.C.: 15 units is added to each 100 mL of I.V. fluid to be administered

Adults: Absorption and dispersion of drugs: 150 units is added to the vehicle containing the drug

**Dosage Forms**

Injection, stabilized solution: 150 units/mL (1 mL, 10 mL)

Powder for injection, lyophilized: 150 units, 1500 units

**Hyate®:C** *see* antihemophilic factor (porcine) *on page 43*

**Hybolin™ Decanoate** *see* nandrolone *on page 408*

**Hybolin™ Improved Injection** *see* nandrolone *on page 408*

**hycamptamine** *see* topotecan *on page 596*

**Hycamtin™** *see* topotecan *on page 596*

**HycoClear Tuss®** *see* hydrocodone and guaifenesin *on page 301*

**Hycodan®** *see* hydrocodone and homatropine *on page 301*

**Hycomine® *(Discontinued)*** *see page 750*

**Hycomine® Compound** *see* hydrocodone, chlorpheniramine, phenylephrine, acetaminophen, and caffeine *on page 302*

**Hycomine® Pediatric *(Discontinued)*** *see page 750*

**Hycort™ (Can)** *see* hydrocortisone (rectal) *on page 302*

**Hycort® Topical** *see* hydrocortisone (topical) *on page 304*

**Hycotuss® Expectorant Liquid** *see* hydrocodone and guaifenesin *on page 301*

**Hydeltra-T.B.A.® *(Discontinued)*** *see page 750*

**Hydergine®** *see* ergoloid mesylates *on page 220*

**Hydergine® LC** *see* ergoloid mesylates *on page 220*

**Hyderm (Can)** *see* hydrocortisone (topical) *on page 304*

## hydralazine (hye DRAL a zeen)

**U.S./Canadian Brand Names** Apo®-Hydralazine (Can); Apresoline®; Novo-Hylazin (Can); Nu-Hydral (Can)

**Therapeutic Category** Vasodilator

**Use** Management of moderate to severe hypertension, congestive heart failure, hypertension secondary to pre-eclampsia/eclampsia, primary pulmonary hypertension

**Usual Dosage**

Children:

Oral: Initial: 0.75-1 mg/kg/day in 2-4 divided doses; increase over 3-4 weeks to maximum of 7.5 mg/kg/day in 2-4 divided doses; maximum daily dose: 200 mg/day

(Continued)

## hydralazine *(Continued)*

I.M., I.V.: 0.1-0.2 mg/kg/dose (not to exceed 20 mg) every 4-6 hours as needed, up to 1.7-3.5 mg/kg/day in 4-6 divided doses

Adults:

Oral: Hypertension:

Initial dose: 10 mg 4 times/day for first 2-4 days; increase to 25 mg 4 times/day for the balance of the first week

Increase by 10-25 mg/dose gradually to 50 mg 4 times/day; 300 mg/day may be required for some patients

Oral: Congestive heart failure:

Initial dose: 10-25 mg 3-4 times/day

Adjustment: Dosage must be adjusted based on individual response

Target dose: 75 mg 4 times/day in combination with isosorbide dinitrate (40 mg 4 times a day)

Range: Typically 200-600 mg daily in 2-4 divided doses. Dosages as high as 3 g/day have been used in some patients for symptomatic and hemodynamic improvement. Hydralazine 75 mg 4 times a day combined with isosorbide dinitrate 40 mg 4 times a day were shown in clinical trials to provide a mortality benefit in the treatment of CHF. Higher doses may be used for symptomatic and hemodynamic improvement following optimization of standard therapy.

I.M., I.V.:

Hypertension: Initial: 10-20 mg/dose every 4-6 hours as needed, may increase to 40 mg/dose; change to oral therapy as soon as possible.

Pre-eclampsia/eclampsia: 5 mg/dose then 5-10 mg every 20-30 minutes as needed.

Hemodialysis: Supplemental dose is not necessary.

Peritoneal dialysis: Supplemental dose is not necessary.

**Dosage Forms**

Injection, as hydrochloride: 20 mg/mL (1 mL)

Tablet, as hydrochloride: 10 mg, 25 mg, 50 mg, 100 mg

## hydralazine and hydrochlorothiazide

(hye DRAL a zeen & hye droe klor oh THYE a zide)

**U.S./Canadian Brand Names** Hydra-Zide®

**Therapeutic Category** Antihypertensive Agent, Combination

**Use** Management of moderate to severe hypertension and treatment of congestive heart failure

**Usual Dosage** Adults: Oral: 1 capsule twice daily

**Dosage Forms** Capsule:

25/25: Hydralazine hydrochloride 25 mg and hydrochlorothiazide 25 mg

50/50: Hydralazine hydrochloride 50 mg and hydrochlorothiazide 50 mg

100/50: Hydralazine hydrochloride 100 mg and hydrochlorothiazide 50 mg

## hydralazine, hydrochlorothiazide, and reserpine

(hye DRAL a zeen, hye droe klor oh THYE a zide, & re SER peen)

**U.S./Canadian Brand Names** Hyserp®; Ser-A-Gen®

**Therapeutic Category** Antihypertensive Agent, Combination

**Use** Hypertensive disorders

**Usual Dosage** Adults: Oral: 1-2 tablets 3 times/day

**Dosage Forms** Tablet: Hydralazine 25 mg, hydrochlorothiazide 15 mg, and reserpine 0.1 mg

**Hydramine® *(Discontinued)*** *see page 750*

**Hydramyn® Syrup [OTC]** *see* diphenhydramine *on page 191*

**Hydrasense® (Can)** *see* sodium chloride *on page 549*

**Hydrate® Injection** *see* dimenhydrinate *on page 188*

**Hydra-Zide®** *see* hydralazine and hydrochlorothiazide *on this page*

**Hydrea®** *see* hydroxyurea *on page 307*

**Hydrobexan® Injection** ***(Discontinued)*** *see page 750*

**Hydrocet®** *see* hydrocodone and acetaminophen *on next page*

## hydrochlorothiazide (hye droe klor oh THYE a zide)

**Synonyms** HCTZ

**U.S./Canadian Brand Names** Apo®-Hydro (Can); Aquazide H®; Esidrix®; Ezide®; Hydrocot®; HydroDIURIL®; Microzide™; Oretic®

**Therapeutic Category** Diuretic, Thiazide

**Use** Management of mild to moderate hypertension; treatment of edema in congestive heart failure and nephrotic syndrome

**Usual Dosage** Oral:

Children (daily dosages should be decreased if used with other antihypertensives):

<6 months: 2-3 mg/kg/day in 2 divided doses

>6 months: 2 mg/kg/day in 2 divided doses

Adults: 25-50 mg/day in 1-2 doses; maximum: 200 mg/day

**Dosage Forms**

Capsule: 12.5 mg

Solution, oral (mint flavor): 50 mg/5 mL (50 mL)

Tablet: 25 mg, 50 mg, 100 mg

## hydrochlorothiazide and spironolactone

(hye droe klor oh THYE a zide & speer on oh LAK tone)

**U.S./Canadian Brand Names** Aldactazide®; Novo-Spirozine (Can)

**Therapeutic Category** Antihypertensive Agent, Combination

**Use** Management of mild to moderate hypertension; treatment of edema in congestive heart failure and nephrotic syndrome

**Usual Dosage** Oral:

Children: 1.66-3.3 mg/kg/day (of spironolactone) in 2-4 divided doses

Adults: 1-8 tablets in 1-2 divided doses

**Dosage Forms** Tablet:

25/25: Hydrochlorothiazide 25 mg and spironolactone 25 mg

50/50: Hydrochlorothiazide 50 mg and spironolactone 50 mg

## hydrochlorothiazide and triamterene

(hye droe klor oh THYE a zide & trye AM ter een)

**Synonyms** triamterene and hydrochlorothiazide

**U.S./Canadian Brand Names** Apo®-Triazide (Can); Dyazide®; Maxzide®; Novo-Triamzide (Can); Nu-Triazide (Can)

**Therapeutic Category** Antihypertensive Agent, Combination

**Use** Management of mild to moderate hypertension; treatment of edema in congestive heart failure and nephrotic syndrome

**Usual Dosage** Adults: Oral:

Triamterene/hydrochlorothiazide 37.5 mg/25 mg: 1-2 tablets/capsules once daily

Triamterene/hydrochlorothiazide 75 mg/50 mg: 1 tablet daily

**Dosage Forms**

Capsule (Dyazide®): Hydrochlorothiazide 25 mg and triamterene 37.5 mg

Tablet:

Maxzide®-25: Hydrochlorothiazide 25 mg and triamterene 37.5 mg

Maxzide®: Hydrochlorothiazide 50 mg and triamterene 75 mg

**Hydrocil® [OTC]** *see* psyllium *on page 509*

**Hydro Cobex®** ***(Discontinued)*** *see page 750*

## hydrocodone and acetaminophen

(hye droe KOE done & a seet a MIN oh fen)

**Synonyms** acetaminophen and hydrocodone

**U.S./Canadian Brand Names** Anexsia®; Anodynos-DHC®; Bancap HC®; Co-Gesic®; Dolacet®; DuoCet™; Duradyne DHC®; Hydrocet®; Hydrogesic®; Hy-Phen®; Lorcet® 10/650; Lorcet®-HD; Lorcet® Plus; Lortab®; Margesic® H; Norcet®; Norco®; Stagesic®; T-Gesic®; Vicodin®; Vicodin® ES; Zydone®

**Therapeutic Category** Analgesic, Narcotic

**Controlled Substance** C-III

**Use** Relief of moderate to severe pain; antitussive (hydrocodone)

**Usual Dosage** Doses should be titrated to appropriate analgesic effect

Adults: Oral: 1-2 tablets or capsules every 4-6 hours

**Dosage Forms**

Capsule:

Bancap HC®, Dolacet®, Hydrocet®, Hydrogesic®, Lorcet®-HD, Margesic® H, Medipain 5®, Norcet®, Stagesic®, T-Gesic®, Zydone®: Hydrocodone bitartrate 5 mg and acetaminophen 500 mg

Elixir (tropical fruit punch flavor) (Lortab®): Hydrocodone bitartrate 2.5 mg and acetaminophen 167 mg per 5 mL with alcohol 7% (480 mL)

Solution, oral (tropical fruit punch flavor) (Lortab®): Hydrocodone bitartrate 2.5 mg and acetaminophen 167 mg per 5 mL with alcohol 7% (480 mL)

Tablet: Hydrocodone bitartrate 5 mg and acetaminophen 400 mg; hydrocodone bitartrate 7.5 mg and acetaminophen 400 mg; hydrocodone bitartrate 10 mg and acetaminophen 400 mg; hydrocodone bitartrate 5 mg and acetaminophen 500 mg; hydrocodone bitartrate 7.5 mg and acetaminophen 750 mg; hydrocodone bitartrate 7.5 mg and acetaminophen 500 mg; hydrocodone bitartrate 7.5 mg and acetaminophen 650 mg; hydrocodone bitartrate 10 mg and acetaminophen 650 mg

Lortab® 2.5/500: Hydrocodone bitartrate 2.5 mg and acetaminophen 500 mg

Anexsia® 5/500, Anodynos-DHC®, Co-Gesic®, DuoCet™, DHC®; Hy-Phen®, Lorcet®, Lortab®® 5/500, Vicodin®: Hydrocodone bitartrate 5 mg and acetaminophen 500 mg

Lortab® 7.5/500: Hydrocodone bitartrate 7.5 mg and acetaminophen 500 mg

Anexsia® 7.5/650, Lorcet® Plus: Hydrocodone bitartrate 7.5 mg and acetaminophen 650 mg

Vicodin® ES: Hydrocodone bitartrate 7.5 mg and acetaminophen 750 mg

Norco®: Hydrocodone bitartrate 10 mg and acetaminophen 325 mg

Lortab® 10/500: Hydrocodone bitartrate 10 mg and acetaminophen 500 mg

Lorcet® 10/650: Hydrocodone bitartrate 10 mg and acetaminophen 650 mg

Vicodin® HP: Hydrocodone bitartrate 10 mg and acetaminophen 660 mg

Zydone®: Hydrocodone bitartrate 5 mg and acetaminophen 400 mg; hydrocodone bitartrate 7.5 mg and acetaminophen 400 mg; hydrocodone bitartrate 10 mg and acetaminophen 400 mg

## hydrocodone and aspirin (hye droe KOE done & AS pir in)

**U.S./Canadian Brand Names** Damason-P®; Lortab® ASA

**Therapeutic Category** Analgesic, Narcotic

**Controlled Substance** C-III

**Use** Relief of moderate to moderately severe pain

**Usual Dosage** Adults: Oral: 1-2 tablets every 4-6 hours as needed for pain

**Dosage Forms** Tablet: Hydrocodone bitartrate 5 mg and aspirin 500 mg

## hydrocodone and chlorpheniramine

(hye droe KOE done & klor fen IR a meen)

**U.S./Canadian Brand Names** Tussionex®

**Therapeutic Category** Antihistamine/Antitussive

**Controlled Substance** C-III

**Use** Symptomatic relief of cough

**Usual Dosage** Oral:
Children 6-12 years: 2.5 mL every 12 hours; do not exceed 5 mL/24 hours
Adults: 5 mL every 12 hours; do not exceed 10 mL/24 hours

**Dosage Forms** Syrup, alcohol free: Hydrocodone polistirex 10 mg and chlorpheniramine polistirex 8 mg per 5 mL (480 mL, 900 mL)

## hydrocodone and guaifenesin (hye droe KOE done & gwye FEN e sin)

**U.S./Canadian Brand Names** Codiclear® DH; HycoClear Tuss®; Hycotuss® Expectorant Liquid; Kwelcof®

**Therapeutic Category** Antitussive/Expectorant

**Controlled Substance** C-III

**Use** Symptomatic relief of nonproductive coughs associated with upper and lower respiratory tract congestion

**Usual Dosage** Oral:
Children:
<2 years: 0.3 mg/kg/day (hydrocodone) in 4 divided doses
2-12 years: 2.5 mL every 4 hours, after meals and at bedtime
>12 years: 5 mL every 4 hours, after meals and at bedtime
Adults: 5 mL every 4 hours, after meals and at bedtime, up to 30 mL/24 hours

**Dosage Forms** Liquid: Hydrocodone bitartrate 5 mg and guaifenesin 100 mg per 5 mL (120 mL, 480 mL)

## hydrocodone and homatropine (hye droe KOE done & hoe MA troe peen)

**U.S./Canadian Brand Names** Hycodan®; Hydromet®; Tussigon®

**Therapeutic Category** Antitussive

**Controlled Substance** C-III

**Use** Symptomatic relief of cough

**Usual Dosage** Oral (based on hydrocodone component):
Children: 0.6 mg/kg/day in 3-4 divided doses; do not administer more frequently than every 4 hours
A single dose should not exceed 10 mg in children >12 years, 5 mg in children 2-12 years, and 1.25 mg in children <2 years of age
Adults: 5-10 mg every 4-6 hours, a single dose should not exceed 15 mg; do not administer more frequently than every 4 hours

**Dosage Forms**
Syrup (Hycodan®, Hydromet®, Hydropane®, Hydrotropine®): Hydrocodone bitartrate 5 mg and homatropine methylbromide 1.5 mg per 5 mL (120 mL, 480 mL, 4000 mL)
Tablet (Hycodan®, Tussigon®): Hydrocodone bitartrate 5 mg and homatropine methylbromide 1.5 mg

## hydrocodone and ibuprofen (hye droe KOE done & eye byoo PROE fen)

**U.S./Canadian Brand Names** Vicoprofen®

**Therapeutic Category** Analgesic, Narcotic

**Controlled Substance** C-III

**Use** Relief of moderate to moderately severe pain (short-term, less than 10 days)

**Usual Dosage** Adults: Oral: 1-2 tablets every 4-6 hours as needed for pain

**Dosage Forms** Tablet: Hydrocodone bitartrate 7.5 mg and ibuprofen 200 mg

## hydrocodone and pseudoephedrine
(hye droe KOE done & soo doe e FED rin)

**U.S./Canadian Brand Names** Detussin® Liquid; Entuss-D® Liquid; Histinex® D Liquid; Histussin D® Liquid; Tyrodone® Liquid

**Therapeutic Category** Cough and Cold Combination

**Use** Symptomatic relief of cough due to colds, etc

**Usual Dosage** Oral: Adults: 5 mL four times/day

(Continued)

## hydrocodone and pseudoephedrine *(Continued)*

**Dosage Forms** Liquid:

Entuss-D®: Hydrocodone bitartrate 5 mg and pseudoephedrine hydrochloride 30 mg per 5 mL

Detussin®, Histussin D®, Tyrodone®: Hydrocodone bitartrate 5 mg and pseudoephedrine hydrochloride 60 mg per 5 mL

## hydrocodone, chlorpheniramine, phenylephrine, acetaminophen, and caffeine

(hye droe KOE done, klor fen IR a meen, fen il EF rin, a seet a MIN oh fen, & KAF een)

**U.S./Canadian Brand Names** Hycomine® Compound

**Therapeutic Category** Antitussive

**Use** Symptomatic relief of cough and symptoms of upper respiratory infections

**Usual Dosage** Adults: Oral: 1 tablet every 4 hours, up to 4 times/day

**Dosage Forms** Tablet: Hydrocodone bitartrate 5 mg, chlorpheniramine maleate 2 mg, phenylephrine hydrochloride 10 mg, acetaminophen 250 mg, and caffeine 30 mg

**Hydrocodone PA® Syrup *(Discontinued)*** *see page 750*

## hydrocodone, phenylephrine, pyrilamine, phenindamine, chlorpheniramine, and ammonium chloride

(hye droe KOE done, fen il EF rin, peer IL a meen, fen IN da meen, klor fen IR a meen, & a MOE nee um KLOR ide)

**U.S./Canadian Brand Names** P-V-Tussin®

**Therapeutic Category** Antihistamine/Decongestant/Antitussive

**Use** Symptomatic relief of cough and nasal congestion

**Usual Dosage** Adults: Oral: 10 mL every 4-6 hours, up to 40 mL/day

**Dosage Forms** Syrup: Hydrocodone bitartrate 2.5 mg, phenylephrine hydrochloride 5 mg, pyrilamine maleate 6 mg, phenindamine tartrate 5 mg, chlorpheniramine maleate 2 mg, and ammonium chloride 50 mg per 5 mL with alcohol 5% (480 mL, 3780 mL)

## hydrocodone, pseudoephedrine, and guaifenesin

(hye droe KOE done, soo doe e FED rin, & gwye FEN e sin)

**U.S./Canadian Brand Names** Cophene XP®; Detussin® Expectorant; SRC® Expectorant; Tussafin® Expectorant

**Therapeutic Category** Antitussive/Decongestant/Expectorant

**Controlled Substance** C-III

**Use** Symptomatic relief of irritating, nonproductive cough associated with respiratory conditions such as bronchitis, bronchial asthma, tracheobronchitis, and the common cold

**Usual Dosage** Adults: Oral: 5 mL every 4-6 hours

**Dosage Forms** Liquid: Hydrocodone bitartrate 5 mg, pseudoephedrine hydrochloride 60 mg, and guaifenesin 200 mg per 5 mL with alcohol 12.5% (480 mL)

## hydrocortisone (rectal) (hye droe KOR ti sone REK tal)

**U.S./Canadian Brand Names** Anusol-HC® Suppository; Colocort™; Cortenema® Rectal; Cortifoam® Rectal; Hycort™ (Can); Proctocort™ Rectal; ProctoCream ® HC Cream

**Therapeutic Category** Adrenal Corticosteroid

**Use** Management of adrenocortical insufficiency; adjunctive treatment of ulcerative colitis

**Usual Dosage** Ulcerative colitis: Adults: Rectal: 10-100 mg 1-2 times/day for 2-3 weeks

**Dosage Forms**

Acetate:

Aerosol, rectal: 10% [90 mg/applicatorful] 20 g

Suppository, rectal: 25 mg
Base:
Cream: 2.5% (30 g)
Rectal: 1% (30 g)
Suspension, rectal: 100 mg/60 mL (7s)

## hydrocortisone (systemic) (hye droe KOR ti sone sis TEM ik)

**Synonyms** compound F

**U.S./Canadian Brand Names** A-hydroCort®; Hydrocortone® Acetate; Solu-Cortef®

**Therapeutic Category** Adrenal Corticosteroid

**Use** Management of adrenocortical insufficiency; relief of inflammation of corticosteroid-responsive dermatoses

**Usual Dosage** Dose should be based on severity of disease and patient response

Acute adrenal insufficiency: I.M., I.V.:
Infants and young Children: Succinate: 1-2 mg/kg/dose bolus, then 25-150 mg/day in divided doses every 6-8 hours
Older Children: Succinate: 1-2 mg/kg bolus then 150-250 mg/day in divided doses every 6-8 hours
Adults: Succinate: 100 mg I.V. bolus, then 300 mg/day in divided doses every 8 hours or as a continuous infusion for 48 hours; once patient is stable change to oral, 50 mg every 8 hours for 6 doses, then taper to 30-50 mg/day in divided doses
Chronic adrenal corticoid insufficiency: Adults: Oral: 20-30 mg/day

Anti-inflammatory or immunosuppressive:
Infants and Children:
Oral: 2.5-10 mg/kg/day **or** 75-300 mg/m$^2$/day every 6-8 hours
I.M., I.V.: Succinate: 1-5 mg/kg/day **or** 30-150 mg/m$^2$/day divided every 12-24 hours
Adolescents and Adults: Oral, I.M., I.V.: Succinate: 15-240 mg every 12 hours
Congenital adrenal hyperplasia: Oral: Initial: 10-20 mg/m$^2$/day in 3 divided doses; a variety of dosing schedules have been used. **Note:** Inconsistencies have occurred with liquid formulations; tablets may provide more reliable levels. Doses must be individualized by monitoring growth, bone age, and hormonal levels. Mineralcorticoid and sodium supplementation may be required based upon electrolyte regulation and plasma renin activity.
Physiologic replacement: Children:
Oral: 0.5-0.75 mg/kg/day **or** 20-25 mg/m$^2$/day every 8 hours
I.M.: Succinate: 0.25-0.35 mg/kg/day **or** 12-15 mg/m$^2$/day once daily
Shock: I.M., I.V.: Succinate:
Children: Initial: 50 mg/kg, then repeated in 4 hours and/or every 24 hours as needed
Adolescents and Adults: 500 mg to 2 g every 2-6 hours
Status asthmaticus: Children and Adults: I.V.: Succinate: 1-2 mg/kg/dose every 6 hours for 24 hours, then maintenance of 0.5-1 mg/kg every 6 hours
Rheumatic diseases:
Adults: Intralesional, intra-articular, soft tissue injection: Acetate:
Large joints: 25 mg (up to 37.5 mg)
Small joints: 10-25 mg
Tendon sheaths: 5-12.5 mg
Soft tissue infiltration: 25-50 mg (up to 75 mg)
Bursae: 25-37.5 mg
Ganglia: 12.5-25 mg
Dermatosis: Children >2 years and Adults: Topical: Apply to affected area 3-4 times/day (Buteprate: Apply once or twice daily)
Ulcerative colitis: Adults: Rectal: 10-100 mg 1-2 times/day for 2-3 weeks

**Dosage Forms**
Injection, suspension: 25 mg/mL (5 mL, 10 mL); 50 mg/mL (5 mL, 10 mL)
Suspension, oral: 10 mg/5 mL (120 mL)
Tablet: 5 mg, 10 mg, 20 mg

## hydrocortisone (topical) (hye droe KOR ti sone TOP i kal)

**U.S./Canadian Brand Names** Acticort® Topical; Aeroseb-HC® Topical; Ala-Cort® Topical; Ala-Scalp® Topical; Anusol® HC-1 Topical [OTC]; Anusol® HC-2.5% Topical [OTC]; Aquacort® (Can); Bactine® Hydrocortisone [OTC]; CaldeCORT® Anti-Itch Topical Spray; CaldeCORT® Topical [OTC]; Cetacort® Topical; Clocort® Maximum Strength [OTC]; CortaGel® Topical [OTC]; Cortaid® Maximum Strength Topical [OTC]; Cortaid® with Aloe Topical [OTC]; Cort-Dome® Topical; Cortef® Feminine Itch Topical; Cortizone®-5 Topical [OTC]; Cortizone®-10 Topical [OTC]; Cortoderm (Can); Delcort® Topical; Dermacort® Topical; Dermarest Dricort® Topical; Dermolate® Topical [OTC]; Dermtex® HC with Aloe Topical [OTC]; Eldecort® Topical; Gynecort® Topical [OTC]; Hi-Cor-1.0® Topical; Hi-Cor-2.5® Topical; Hycort® Topical; Hyderm (Can); Hydrocort® Topical; Hydro-Tex® Topical [OTC]; Hytone® Topical; LactiCare-HC® Topical; Lanacort® Topical [OTC]; Locoid® Topical; Nutracort® Topical; Orabase® HCA Topical; Penecort® Topical; Prevex® HC (Can); Sarna® HC (Can); Scalpicin® Topical; S-T Cort® Topical; Synacort® Topical; Tegrin®-HC Topical [OTC]; Texacort® Topical; U-Cort™ Topical; Westcort® Topical

**Therapeutic Category** Corticosteroid, Topical

**Use** Management of adrenocortical insufficiency; relief of inflammation of corticosteroid-responsive dermatoses; adjunctive treatment of ulcerative colitis

**Usual Dosage** Children >2 years and Adults: Topical: Apply to affected area 3-4 times/day (Buteprate: Apply once or twice daily). Therapy should be discontinued when control is achieved. If no improvement is seen, reassessment of diagnosis may be necessary.

**Dosage Forms**

Aerosol, topical:
Cream: 0.5%, 1%, 2.5%
Gel: 0.5%
Ointment, topical: 0.5%, 1%, 2.5%
Lotion: 0.5%, 1%, 2.5%
Paste: 0.5% (5 g)
Solution, topical; 1%

Butyrate:
- Cream: 0.1%
- Ointment, topical: 0.1%
- Solution, topical: 0.1%

Valerate:
- Cream: 0.2%
- Ointment, topical: 0.2%

**Hydrocortone® Acetate** *see* hydrocortisone (systemic) *on previous page*

**Hydrocort® Topical** *see* hydrocortisone (topical) *on this page*

**Hydrocot®** *see* hydrochlorothiazide *on page 299*

**Hydro-Crysti-12®** ***(Discontinued)*** *see page 750*

**HydroDIURIL®** *see* hydrochlorothiazide *on page 299*

## hydroflumethiazide (hye droe floo meth EYE a zide)

**U.S./Canadian Brand Names** Diucardin®; Saluron®

**Therapeutic Category** Diuretic, Thiazide

**Use** Management of mild to moderate hypertension; treatment of edema in congestive heart failure and nephrotic syndrome

**Usual Dosage** Oral: 1 tablet 1-2 times/day

**Dosage Forms** Tablet: 50 mg

**hydrogenated ergot alkaloids** *see* ergoloid mesylates *on page 220*

**Hydrogesic®** *see* hydrocodone and acetaminophen *on page 300*

**hydromagnesium aluminate** *see* magaldrate *on page 360*

**Hydromet®** *see* hydrocodone and homatropine *on page 301*

**Hydromorph Contin® (Can)** *see* hydromorphone *on this page*

## hydromorphone (hye droe MOR fone)

**Synonyms** dihydromorphinone

**U.S./Canadian Brand Names** Dilaudid® Cough Syrup; Dilaudid-HP® Injection; Dilaudid® Injection; Dilaudid® Oral; Dilaudid® Suppository; Hydromorph Contin® (Can); PMS-Hydromorphone (Can)

**Therapeutic Category** Analgesic, Narcotic

**Controlled Substance** C-II

**Use** Management of moderate to severe pain; antitussive at lower doses

**Usual Dosage** Doses should be titrated to appropriate analgesic effects; when changing routes of administration, note that oral doses are less than half as effective as parenteral doses (may be only $^1/_5$ as effective)

Pain: Older Children and Adults: Oral, I.M., I.V., S.C.: 1-4 mg/dose every 4-6 hours as needed; usual adult dose: 2 mg/dose

Antitussive: Oral:

- Children 6-12 years: 0.5 mg every 3-4 hours as needed
- Children >12 years and Adults: 1 mg every 3-4 hours as needed

**Dosage Forms**

Injection, as hydrochloride:

- Dilaudid®: 1 mg/mL (1 mL); 2 mg/mL (1 mL, 20 mL); 3 mg/mL (1 mL); 4 mg/mL (1 mL)
- Dilaudid-HP®: 10 mg/mL (1 mL, 2 mL, 5 mL)

Liquid, as hydrochloride: 5 mg/5 mL (480 mL)

Powder for injection, as hydrochloride: (Dilaudid-HP®): 250 mg

Solution, oral, as hydrochloride (raspberry flavored): 5 mg/5 mL (120 mL, 250 mL, 500 mL)

Suppository, rectal, as hydrochloride: 3 mg (6s)

Tablet, as hydrochloride: 1 mg, 2 mg, 3 mg, 4 mg, 8 mg

**Hydromox®** ***(Discontinued)*** *see page 750*

**Hydro-Par®** ***(Discontinued)*** *see page 750*

**Hydrophed®** ***(Discontinued)*** *see page 750*

**Hydropres® 25 mg Tablet** ***(Discontinued)*** *see page 750*

**hydroquinol** *see* hydroquinone *on this page*

## hydroquinone (HYE droe kwin one)

**Synonyms** hydroquinol; quinol

**U.S./Canadian Brand Names** Ambi® Skin Tone [OTC]; Eldopaque® [OTC]; Eldopaque Forte®; Eldoquin® [OTC]; Eldoquin® Forte®; Esoterica® Facial [OTC]; Esoterica® Regular [OTC]; Esoterica® Sensitive Skin Formula [OTC]; Esoterica® Sunscreen [OTC]; Lustra®; Lustra-AF®; Melanex®; Neostrata® HQ (Can); Porcelana® [OTC]; Porcelana® Sunscreen [OTC]; Solaquin® [OTC]; Solaquin Forte®; Ultraquin® (Can)

**Therapeutic Category** Topical Skin Product

**Use** Gradual bleaching of hyperpigmented skin conditions

**Usual Dosage** Topical: Apply thin layer and rub in twice daily

**Dosage Forms**

Cream, topical:

- Esoterica® Sensitive Skin Formula: 1.5% [OTC] (85 g)
- Eldopaque®, Eldoquin®, Esoterica® Facial, Esoterica® Regular, Porcelana®: 2% [OTC] (14.2 g, 28.4 g, 60 g, 85 g, 120 g)
- Eldopaque Forte®, Eldoquin® Forte®, Melquin HP®: 4% (14.2 g, 28.4 g)

Cream, topical, with sunblock:

- Esoterica® Sunscreen, Porcelana®, Solaquin®: 2% [OTC] (28.4 g, 120 g)
- Melpaque HP®, Nuquin HP®, Solaquin Forte®: 4% (14.2 g, 28.4 g)

Gel, topical, with sunscreen (Solaquin Forte®): 4% (14.2 g, 28.4 g)

(Continued)

## hydroquinone *(Continued)*

Solution, topical (Melanex®): 3% (30 mL)

**Hydro-Tex® Topical [OTC]** *see* hydrocortisone (topical) *on page 304*

**Hydroxacen® *(Discontinued)*** *see page 750*

## hydroxocobalamin (hye droks oh koe BAL a min)

**Synonyms** vitamin $B_{12a}$

**Therapeutic Category** Vitamin, Water Soluble

**Use** Pernicious anemia, vitamin $B_{12}$ deficiency, increased $B_{12}$ requirements due to pregnancy, thyrotoxicosis, hemorrhage, malignancy, liver or kidney disease

**Usual Dosage**

Children:

Congenital pernicious anemia (if evidence of neurologic involvement): I.M.: 1000 mcg/day for at least 2 weeks; maintenance: 50 mcg/month

Vitamin $B_{12}$ deficiency: I.M., S.C.: 1-5 mg administered in single or S.C. doses of 100 mcg over 2 or more weeks

Adults:

Pernicious anemia: I.M., S.C.: 100 mcg/day for 6-7 days

Vitamin $B_{12}$ deficiency:

Oral: Usually not recommended, maximum absorbed from a single oral dose is 2-3 mcg

I.M., S.C.: 30 mcg/day for 5-10 days, followed by 100-200 mcg/month

**Dosage Forms** Injection: 1000 mcg/mL (10 mL, 30 mL)

## hydroxyamphetamine and tropicamide

(hye droks ee am FET a meen & troe PIK a mide)

**U.S./Canadian Brand Names** Paremyd® Ophthalmic

**Therapeutic Category** Adrenergic Agonist Agent

**Use** Mydriasis with cycloplegia

**Usual Dosage** Adults: Ophthalmic: Instill 1-2 drops into conjunctival sac(s)

**Dosage Forms** Solution, ophthalmic: Hydroxyamphetamine hydrobromide 1% and tropicamide 0.25% (5 mL, 15 mL)

**hydroxycarbamide** *see* hydroxyurea *on next page*

## hydroxychloroquine (hye droks ee KLOR oh kwin)

**U.S./Canadian Brand Names** Plaquenil®

**Therapeutic Category** Aminoquinoline (Antimalarial)

**Use** Suppression or chemoprophylaxis of malaria caused by susceptible *P. vivax*, *P. ovale*, *P. malariae*, and some strains of *P. falciparum* (not active against pre-erythrocytic or exoerythrocytic tissue stages of *Plasmodium*); treatment of systemic lupus erythematosus (SLE) and rheumatoid arthritis

**Usual Dosage** Oral:

Children:

Chemoprophylaxis of malaria: 5 mg/kg (base) once weekly; should not exceed the recommended adult dose; begin 2 weeks before exposure; continue for 8 weeks after leaving endemic area

Acute attack: 10 mg/kg (base) initial dose; followed by 5 mg/kg in 6 hours on day 1; 5 mg/kg in 1 dose on day 2 and on day 3

Juvenile rheumatoid arthritis or SLE: 3-5 mg/kg/day divided 1-2 times/day to a maximum of 400 mg/day; not to exceed 7 mg/kg/day

Adults:

Chemoprophylaxis of malaria: 2 tablets weekly on same day each week; begin 2 weeks before exposure; continue for 6-8 weeks after leaving epidemic area

Acute attack: 4 tablets first dose day 1; 2 tablets in 6 hours day 1; 2 tablets in 1 dose day 2; and 2 tablets in 1 dose on day 3

Rheumatoid arthritis: 2-3 tablets/day to start with food or milk; increase dose until optimum response level is reached; usually after 4-12 weeks dose should be reduced by 1/2 and a maintenance dose of 1-2 tablets/day

Lupus erythematosus: 2 tablets every day or twice daily for several weeks depending on response; 1-2 tablets/day for prolonged maintenance therapy

**Dosage Forms** Tablet, as sulfate: 200 mg [base 155 mg]

**25-hydroxycholecalciferol** *see* calcifediol *on page 95*

**hydroxydaunomycin** *see* doxorubicin *on page 203*

**hydroxyethyl starch** *see* hetastarch *on page 293*

## hydroxyprogesterone caproate

(hye droks ee proe JES te rone KAP roe ate)

**U.S./Canadian Brand Names** Hylutin®; Prodrox®

**Therapeutic Category** Progestin

**Use** Treatment of amenorrhea, abnormal uterine bleeding, submucous fibroids, endometriosis, uterine carcinoma, and testing of estrogen production

**Usual Dosage** Adults: I.M.:

Amenorrhea: 375 mg; if no bleeding, begin cyclic treatment with estradiol valerate

Endometriosis: Start cyclic therapy with estradiol valerate

Uterine carcinoma: 1 g one or more times/day (1-7 g/week) for up to 12 weeks

Test for endogenous estrogen production: 250 mg anytime; bleeding 7-14 days after injection indicate positive test

**Dosage Forms** Injection:

125 mg/mL (10 mL)

Hylutin®, Prodrox®: 250 mg/mL (5 mL)

## hydroxypropyl cellulose (hye droks ee PROE pil SEL yoo lose)

**U.S./Canadian Brand Names** Lacrisert®

**Therapeutic Category** Ophthalmic Agent, Miscellaneous

**Use** Dry eyes

**Usual Dosage** Adults: Ophthalmic: Apply once daily into the inferior cul-de-sac beneath the base of tarsus, not in apposition to the cornea nor beneath the eyelid at the level of the tarsal plate

**Dosage Forms** Insert, ophthalmic: 5 mg

## hydroxypropyl methylcellulose

(hye droks ee PROE pil meth il SEL yoo lose)

**Synonyms** gonioscopic ophthalmic solution

**U.S./Canadian Brand Names** GenTeal™ [OTC]; Gonak™ [OTC]; Goniosol® [OTC]

**Therapeutic Category** Ophthalmic Agent, Miscellaneous

**Use** Ophthalmic surgical aid in cataract extraction and intraocular implantation; gonioscopic examinations

**Usual Dosage** Introduced into anterior chamber of eye with 20-gauge or larger cannula

**Dosage Forms**

Gel, ophthalmic: 0.3% (10 mL)

Solution, ophthalmic: 0.3% (15 mL, 25 mL); 2.5% (15 mL)

## hydroxyurea (hye droks ee yoor EE a)

**Synonyms** hydroxycarbamide

**U.S./Canadian Brand Names** Droxia™; Hydrea®; Mylocel™

**Therapeutic Category** Antineoplastic Agent

**Use** CML in chronic phase; radiosensitizing agent in the treatment of primary brain tumors, head and neck tumors, uterine cervix and nonsmall cell lung cancer, and psoriasis; treatment of hematologic conditions such as essential thrombocythemia, polycythemia vera, hypereosinophilia, and hyperleukocytosis due to acute leukemia. (Continued)

## hydroxyurea *(Continued)*

Has shown activity against renal cell cancer, melanoma, ovarian cancer, head and neck cancer, and prostate cancer.

Sickle cell anemia: Specifically for patients >18 years of age who have had at least three "painful crises" in the previous year - to reduce frequency of these crises and the need for blood transfusions

**Unlabeled use:** Thrombocythemia

**Usual Dosage** Oral (refer to individual protocols): All dosage should be based on ideal or actual body weight, whichever is less:

Children:

No FDA-approved dosage regimens have been established; dosages of 1500-3000 $mg/m^2$ as a single dose in combination with other agents every 4-6 weeks have been used in the treatment of pediatric astrocytoma, medulloblastoma, and primitive neuro-ectodermal tumors

CML: Initial: 10-20 mg/kg/day once daily; adjust dose according to hematologic response

Adults: Dose should always be titrated to patient response and WBC counts; usual oral doses range from 10-30 mg/kg/day or 500-3000 mg/day; if WBC count falls to <2500 cells/$mm^3$, or the platelet count to <100,000/$mm^3$, therapy should be stopped for at least 3 days and resumed when values rise toward normal

Solid tumors:

Intermittent therapy: 80 mg/kg as a single dose every third day

Continuous therapy: 20-30 mg/kg/day given as a single dose/day

Concomitant therapy with irradiation: 80 mg/kg as a single dose every third day starting at least 7 days before initiation of irradiation

Resistant chronic myelocytic leukemia: 20-30 mg/kg/day divided daily

HIV: 1000-1500 mg daily in a single dose or divided doses

Sickle cell anemia (moderate/severe disease): Initial: 15 mg/kg/day, increased by 5 mg/kg every 12 weeks if blood counts are in an acceptable range until the maximum tolerated dose of 35 mg/kg/day is achieved or the dose that does not produce toxic effects

*Acceptable range:*

Neutrophils ≥2500 cells/$mm^3$

Platelets ≥95,000/$mm^3$

Hemoglobin >5.3 g/dL, and

Reticulocytes ≥95,000/$mm^3$ if the hemoglobin concentration is <9 g/dL

*Toxic range:*

Neutrophils <2000 cells/$mm^3$

Platelets <80,000/$mm^3$

Hemoglobin <4.5 g/dL

Reticulocytes <80,000/$mm^3$ if the hemoglobin concentration is <9 g/dL

Monitor for toxicity every 2 weeks; if toxicity occurs, stop treatment until the bone marrow recovers; restart at 2.5 mg/kg/day less than the dose at which toxicity occurs; if no toxicity occurs over the next 12 weeks, then the subsequent dose should be increased by 2.5 mg/kg/day; reduced dosage of hydroxyurea alternating with erythropoietin may decrease myelotoxicity and increase levels of fetal hemoglobin in patients who have not been helped by hydroxyurea alone

**Dosage Forms**

Capsule (Droxia™): 200 mg, 300 mg, 400 mg

Capsule: 500 mg

Tablet (Mylocel™): 1000 mg

**25-hydroxyvitamin $D_3$** *see* calcifediol *on page 95*

## hydroxyzine (hye DROKS i zeen)

**U.S./Canadian Brand Names** Apo®-Hydroxyzine (Can); Atarax®; Hyzine® Injection; Novo-Hydroxyzin (Can); PMS-Hydroxyzine (Can); Restall® Injection; Vistacot® Injection; Vistaril®

**Therapeutic Category** Antiemetic; Antihistamine

**Use** Treatment of anxiety; preoperative sedative; antipruritic; antiemetic

**Usual Dosage**

Children:

Oral: 2 mg/kg/day divided every 6-8 hours

I.M.: 0.5-1 mg/kg/dose every 4-6 hours as needed

Adults:

Antiemetic: I.M.: 25-100 mg/dose every 4-6 hours as needed

Anxiety: Oral: 25-100 mg 4 times/day; maximum dose: 600 mg/day

Preoperative sedation:

Oral: 50-100 mg

I.M.: 25-100 mg

Management of pruritus: Oral: 25 mg 3-4 times/day

**Dosage Forms**

Hydroxyzine hydrochloride:

Injection: 25 mg/mL (1 mL, 2 mL, 10 mL)

Hyzine-50®, Restall®, Vistacot®, Vistaril®: 50 mg/mL (10 mL)

Syrup: 10 mg/5 mL (120 mL, 480 mL, 3840 mL)

Atarax®: 10 mg/5 mL (480 mL)

Tablet: 10 mg, 25 mg, 50 mg, 100 mg

Atarax®: 10 mg, 25 mg, 50 mg, 100 mg

Hydroxyzine pamoate:

Capsule: 25 mg, 50 mg, 100 mg

Vistaril®: 25 mg, 50 mg, 100 mg

Suspension, oral: 25 mg/5 mL (120 mL, 480 mL)

Vistaril®: 25 mg/5 mL (120 mL, 480 mL)

**Hygroton®** ***(Discontinued)*** *see page 750*

**Hylorel®** *see* guanadrel *on page 286*

**Hylutin®** *see* hydroxyprogesterone caproate *on page 307*

**hyoscine** *see* scopolamine *on page 539*

## hyoscyamine (hye oh SYE a meen)

**Synonyms** *l*-hyoscyamine sulfate

**U.S./Canadian Brand Names** Anaspaz®; A-Spas® S/L; Cystospaz®; Cystospaz-M®; Donnamar®; ED-SPAZ®; Gastrosed™; Levbid®; Levsin®; Levsinex®; Levsin/SL®

**Therapeutic Category** Anticholinergic Agent

**Use** GI tract disorders caused by spasm, adjunctive therapy for peptic ulcers

**Usual Dosage**

Children:

<2 years: 1/4 adult dosage

2-10 years: 1/2 adult dosage

Adults:

Oral, S.L.: 0.125-0.25 mg 3-4 times/day before meals or food and at bedtime; 0.375-0.75 mg (timed release) every 12 hours

I.M., I.V., S.C.: 0.25-0.5 mg every 6 hours

**Dosage Forms**

Capsule, as sulfate, timed release (Cystospaz-M®, Levsinex®): 0.375 mg

Elixir, as sulfate (Levsin®): 0.125 mg/5 mL with alcohol 20% (480 mL)

Injection, as sulfate (Levsin®): 0.5 mg/mL (1 mL, 10 mL)

Solution, oral (Gastrosed™, Levsin®): 0.125 mg/mL (15 mL)

Tablet, as sulfate:

Anaspaz®, Gastrosed™, Levsin®, Neoquess®: 0.125 mg

Cystospaz®: 0.15 mg

Extended release (Levbid®): 0.375 mg

Sublingual (Levsin/SL®): 0.125 mg

## hyoscyamine, atropine, scopolamine, and phenobarbital

(hye oh SYE a meen, A troe peen, skoe POL a meen, & fee noe BAR bi tal)

**U.S./Canadian Brand Names** Barbidonna®; Bellatal®; Donnatal®; Hyosophen®; Spasmolin®

**Therapeutic Category** Anticholinergic Agent

**Use** Adjunct in treatment of peptic ulcer disease, irritable bowel, spastic colitis, spastic bladder, and renal colic

**Usual Dosage** Oral:

Children 2-12 years:

Kinesed® dose: 1/2 to 1 tablet 3-4 times/day

Donnatal®: 0.1 mL/kg/dose every 4 hours; maximum dose: 5 mL

Adults: 0.125-0.25 mg (1-2 capsules or tablets) 3-4 times/day; or 0.375-0.75 mg (1 Donnatal® Extentab®) in sustained release form every 12 hours; or 5-10 mL elixir 3-4 times/day or every 8 hours

**Dosage Forms**

Capsule (Donnatal®, Spasmolin®): Hyoscyamine sulfate 0.1037 mg, atropine sulfate 0.0194 mg, scopolamine hydrobromide 0.0065 mg, and phenobarbital 16.2 mg

Elixir (Donnatal®, Hyosophen®, Spasmophen®): Hyoscyamine sulfate 0.1037 mg, atropine sulfate 0.0194 mg, scopolamine hydrobromide 0.0065 mg, and phenobarbital 16.2 mg per 5 mL (120 mL, 480 mL, 4000 mL)

Tablet:

Barbidonna®: Hyoscyamine hydrobromide 0.1286 mg, atropine sulfate 0.025 mg, scopolamine hydrobromide 0.0074 mg, and phenobarbital 16 mg

Barbidonna® No. 2: Hyoscyamine hydrobromide 0.1286 mg, atropine sulfate 0.025 mg, scopolamine hydrobromide 0.0074 mg, and phenobarbital 32 mg

Bellatal®, Donnatal®, Hyosophen®: Hyoscyamine sulfate 0.1037 mg, atropine sulfate 0.0194 mg, scopolamine hydrobromide 0.0065 mg, and phenobarbital 16.2 mg

Long-acting (Donnatal®): Hyoscyamine sulfate 0.3111 mg, atropine sulfate 0.0582 mg, scopolamine hydrobromide 0.0195 mg, and phenobarbital 48.6 mg

Spasmophen®: Hyoscyamine sulfate 0.1037 mg, atropine sulfate 0.0194 mg, scopolamine hydrobromide 0.0065 mg, and phenobarbital 15 mg

## hyoscyamine, atropine, scopolamine, kaolin, and pectin

(hye oh SYE a meen, A troe peen, skoe POL a meen, KAY oh lin, & PEK tin)

**Therapeutic Category** Anticholinergic Agent

**Use** Antidiarrheal; also used in gastritis, enteritis, colitis, and acute gastrointestinal upsets, and nausea which may accompany any of these conditions

**Usual Dosage** Oral:

Children:

10-20 lb: 2.5 mL

20-30 lb: 5 mL

>30 lb: 5-10 mL

Adults:

Diarrhea: 30 mL at once and 15-30 mL with each loose stool

Other conditions: 15 mL every 3 hours as needed

**Dosage Forms** Suspension, oral: Hyoscyamine sulfate 0.1037 mg, atropine sulfate 0.0194 mg, scopolamine hydrobromide 0.0065 mg, kaolin 6 g, and pectin 142.8 mg per 30 mL

## hyoscyamine, atropine, scopolamine, kaolin, pectin, and opium

(hye oh SYE a meen, A troe peen, skoe POL a meen, KAY oh lin, PEK tin, & OH pee um)

**U.S./Canadian Brand Names** Donnapectolin-PG®; Kapectolin PG®

**Therapeutic Category** Anticholinergic Agent

**Controlled Substance** C-V

**Use** Treatment of diarrhea

**Usual Dosage** Oral:

Children 6-12 years: Initial: 10 mL, then 5-10 mL every 3 hours thereafter

Dosage recommendations (body weight/dosage): 10 lb/2.5 mL; 20 lb/5 mL; 30 lb and over/5-10 mL; do not administer more than 4 doses in any 24-hour period

Children >12 years and Adults: Initial: 30 mL (1 fluid oz) followed by 15 mL every 3 hours

**Dosage Forms** Suspension, oral: Hyoscyamine sulfate 0.1037 mg, atropine sulfate 0.0194 mg, scopolamine hydrobromide 0.0065 mg, kaolin 6 g, pectin 142.8 mg, and powdered opium 24 mg per 30 mL with alcohol 5%

**Hyosophen®** *see* hyoscyamine, atropine, scopolamine, and phenobarbital *on previous page*

**Hy-Pam® Oral *(Discontinued)*** *see page 750*

**Hypaque-Cysto®** *see* radiological/contrast media (ionic) *on page 516*

**Hypaque® Meglumine** *see* radiological/contrast media (ionic) *on page 516*

**Hypaque® Sodium** *see* radiological/contrast media (ionic) *on page 516*

**Hyperab® *(Discontinued)*** *see page 750*

**Hyperstat® I.V.** *see* diazoxide *on page 180*

**Hyper-Tet® *(Discontinued)*** *see page 750*

**Hy-Phen®** *see* hydrocodone and acetaminophen *on page 300*

**HypoTears PF Solution [OTC]** *see* artificial tears *on page 53*

**HypoTears Solution [OTC]** *see* artificial tears *on page 53*

**HypRho®-D *(Discontinued)*** *see page 750*

**HypRho®-D Mini-Dose *(Discontinued)*** *see page 750*

**Hyprogest® 250 *(Discontinued)*** *see page 750*

**Hyrexin-50® Injection** *see* diphenhydramine *on page 191*

**Hyserp®** *see* hydralazine, hydrochlorothiazide, and reserpine *on page 298*

**Hytinic® [OTC]** *see* polysaccharide-iron complex *on page 482*

**Hytone® Topical** *see* hydrocortisone (topical) *on page 304*

**Hytrin®** *see* terazosin *on page 574*

**Hytuss® [OTC]** *see* guaifenesin *on page 281*

**Hytuss-2X® [OTC]** *see* guaifenesin *on page 281*

**Hyzaar®** *see* losartan and hydrochlorothiazide *on page 357*

**Hyzine® Injection** *see* hydroxyzine *on page 308*

**ibenzmethyzin** *see* procarbazine *on page 497*

**Iberet-Folic-500®** *see* ferrous sulfate, ascorbic acid, vitamin B-complex, and folic acid *on page 247*

**Iberet®-Liquid [OTC]** *see* ferrous sulfate, ascorbic acid, and vitamin B-complex *on page 247*

**ibidomide** *see* labetalol *on page 336*

**Ibuprin® [OTC]** *see* ibuprofen *on this page*

## ibuprofen (eye byoo PROE fen)

**Synonyms** *p*-isobutylhydratropic acid

**U.S./Canadian Brand Names** Aches-N-Pain® [OTC]; Advil® [OTC]; Apo®-Ibuprofen (Can); Children's Advil® Suspension; Children's Motrin® Suspension [OTC]; Excedrin® IB [OTC]; Genpril® [OTC]; Haltran® [OTC]; Ibuprin® [OTC]; Ibuprohm® [OTC]; Ibu-Tab®; Junior Strength Motrin® [OTC]; Medipren® [OTC]; Menadol® [OTC]; Midol® IB [OTC]; Motrin®; Motrin® IB [OTC]; Novo-Profen® (Can); Nu-Ibuprofen (Can); Nuprin® [OTC]; Pamprin IB® [OTC]; Pedia-Profen™; Saleto-200® [OTC]; Saleto-400®; Trendar® [OTC]; Uni-Pro® [OTC]

(Continued)

## ibuprofen *(Continued)*

**Therapeutic Category** Analgesic, Non-narcotic; Antipyretic; Nonsteroidal Anti-inflammatory Drug (NSAID)

**Use** Inflammatory diseases and rheumatoid disorders including juvenile rheumatoid arthritis (JRA); mild to moderate pain; fever; dysmenorrhea; gout

**Usual Dosage** Oral:

Children:

Antipyretic: 6 months to 12 years: Temperature <102.5°F (39°C): 5 mg/kg/dose; temperature >102.5°F: 10 mg/kg/dose administered every 6-8 hours; maximum daily dose: 40 mg/kg/day

Juvenile rheumatoid arthritis: 30-50 mg/kg/day in 4 divided doses; start at lower end of dosing range and titrate upward; maximum: 2.4 g/day

Analgesic: 4-10 mg/kg/dose every 6-8 hours

Adults:

Inflammatory disease: 400-800 mg/dose 3-4 times/day; maximum dose: 3.2 g/day

Pain/fever/dysmenorrhea: 200-400 mg/dose every 4-6 hours; maximum daily dose: 1.2 g

**Dosage Forms**

Caplet: 100 mg

Drops, oral (berry flavor): 40 mg/mL (15 mL)

Suppository, rectal: 80 mg

Suspension, oral: 100 mg/5 mL [OTC] (60 mL, 120 mL, 480 mL)

Suspension, oral, drops: 40 mg/mL [OTC]

Tablet: 100 mg [OTC], 200 mg [OTC], 300 mg, 400 mg, 600 mg, 800 mg

Tablet, chewable: 50 mg, 100 mg

**Ibuprohm® [OTC]** *see* ibuprofen *on previous page*

**Ibu-Tab®** *see* ibuprofen *on previous page*

## ibutilide (i BYOO ti lide)

**U.S./Canadian Brand Names** Corvert®

**Therapeutic Category** Antiarrhythmic Agent, Class III

**Use** Acute termination of atrial fibrillation or flutter of recent onset; the effectiveness of ibutilide has not been determined in patients with arrhythmias of >90 days in duration

**Usual Dosage** I.V.: Initial:

<60 kg: 0.01 mg/kg over 10 minutes

≥60 kg: 1 mg over 10 minutes

If the arrhythmia does not terminate within 10 minutes after the end of the initial infusion, a second infusion of equal strength may be infused over a 10-minute period

**Dosage Forms** Injection, as fumarate: 0.1 mg/mL (10 mL)

**Icaps® (Can)** *see* vitamin (multiple/oral) *on page 632*

**ICRF-187** *see* dexrazoxane *on page 176*

**Icy Hot Arthritis Therapy®** *see* capsaicin *on page 104*

**I.D.A.®** *see* acetaminophen, isometheptene, and dichloralphenazone *on page 8*

**Idamycin®** *see* idarubicin *on this page*

**Idamycin® PFS** *see* idarubicin *on this page*

**Idarac® (Can)** *see* floctafenine *(Canada only)* *on page 250*

## idarubicin (eye da ROO bi sin)

**Synonyms** 4-demethoxydaunorubicin; 4-dmdr

**U.S./Canadian Brand Names** Idamycin®; Idamycin® PFS

**Therapeutic Category** Antineoplastic Agent

**Use** In combination with other antineoplastic agents for treatment of acute myelogenous leukemia (AML) in adults and acute lymphocytic leukemia (ALL) in children

**Usual Dosage** I.V.:

Children:

Leukemia: 10-12 mg/m$^2$ once daily for 3 days and repeat every 3 weeks

Solid tumors: 5 mg/m$^2$ once daily for 3 days and repeat every 3 weeks

Adults: 12 mg/m$^2$/day for 3 days by slow I.V. injection (10-15 minutes) in combination with Ara-C. The Ara-C may be given as 100 mg/m$^2$/day by continuous infusion for 7 days or 25 mg/m$^2$ bolus followed by Ara-C 200 mg/m$^2$/day for 5 days continuous infusion.

**Dosage Forms** As hydrochloride:

Injection, preservative free (Idamycin® PFS): 1 mg/mL (5 mL, 10 mL, 20 mL)

Powder for injection, lyophilized (Idamycin®): 20 mg

**Ifex®** *see* ifosfamide *on this page*

**IFLrA** *see* interferon alfa-2a *on page 321*

## ifosfamide (eye FOSS fa mide)

**U.S./Canadian Brand Names** Ifex®

**Therapeutic Category** Antineoplastic Agent

**Use** In combination with other antineoplastics in treatment of lung cancer, Hodgkin's and non-Hodgkin's lymphoma, breast cancer, acute and chronic lymphocytic leukemia, ovarian cancer, testicular cancer, and sarcomas

**Usual Dosage** I.V. (refer to individual protocols):

Children: 1800 mg/m$^2$/day for 3-5 days every 21-28 days or 5000 mg/m$^2$ as a single 24-hour infusion or 3 g/m$^2$/day for 2 days

Adults: 700-2000 mg/m$^2$/day for 5 days or 2400 mg/m$^2$/day for 3 days every 21-28 days; 5000 mg/m$^2$ as a single dose over 24 hours

**Dosage Forms** Powder for injection for I.V. infusion, parenteral kit:

Ifosfamide (Ifex®) 1 g and mesna (Mesnex®) 1 g

Ifosfamide (Ifex®) 3 g and mesna (Mesnex®) 1 g

**IG** *see* immune globulin (intramuscular) *on page 315*

**IGIM** *see* immune globulin (intramuscular) *on page 315*

**IGIV** *see* immune globulin (intravenous) *on page 315*

**IL-11** *see* oprelvekin *on page 437*

**Iletin® II Pork (Can)** *see* insulin preparations *on page 319*

**Ilopan-Choline® Oral *(Discontinued)*** *see page 750*

**Ilopan® Injection *(Discontinued)*** *see page 750*

**Ilosone® Pulvules®** *see* erythromycin (systemic) *on page 222*

**Ilozyme®** *see* pancrelipase *on page 448*

## imatinib eye MAT eh nib

**Synonyms** CGP 57148B; glivec; ST1571

**U.S./Canadian Brand Names** Gleevec™

**Therapeutic Category** Antineoplastic Agent

**Use** Treatment of patients with chronic myeloid leukemia (CML) in blast crisis, accelerated phase, or in chronic phase after failure of interferon-alpha therapy

**Usual Dosage** Oral: Adults: Dose should be taken with food and large glass of water:

Chronic myeloid leukemia (CML):

Chronic phase: 400 mg once daily; may be increased to 600 mg daily in the event of disease progression, loss of previously achieved response, or failure to achieve response after at least 3 months of therapy and in the absence of severe adverse reaction

Accelerated phase or blast crisis: 600 mg once daily; may be increased to 800 mg daily (400 mg twice daily) in the event of disease progression, loss of previously achieved response, or failure to achieve response after at least 3 months of therapy and in the absence of severe adverse reaction

(Continued)

## imatinib *(Continued)*

**Dosage Forms** Capsule, as mesylate: 100 mg

**Imdur™** *see* isosorbide mononitrate *on page 329*

**imidazole carboxamide** *see* dacarbazine *on page 163*

## imiglucerase (i mi GLOO ser ace)

**U.S./Canadian Brand Names** Cerezyme®

**Therapeutic Category** Enzyme

**Use** Long-term enzyme replacement therapy for patients with Type 1 Gaucher's disease

**Usual Dosage** I.V.: 2.5 units/kg 3 times/week up to as much as 60 units/kg administered as frequently as once weekly or as infrequently as every 4 weeks; 60 units/kg administered every 2 weeks is the most common dose

**Dosage Forms**

Powder for injection, preservative free (lyophilized):

212 units [equivalent to a withdrawal dose of 200 units]

424 units [equivalent to a withdrawal dose of 400 units]

**imipemide** *see* imipenem and cilastatin *on this page*

## imipenem and cilastatin (i mi PEN em & sye la STAT in)

**Synonyms** imipemide

**U.S./Canadian Brand Names** Primaxin®

**Therapeutic Category** Carbapenem (Antibiotic)

**Use** Treatment of documented multidrug resistant gram-negative infection due to organisms proven or suspected to be susceptible to imipenem/cilastatin; treatment of multiple organism infection in which other agents have an insufficient spectrum of activity or are contraindicated due to toxic potential; therapeutic alternative for treatment of gram negative sepsis in immunocompromised patients

**Usual Dosage** I.V. infusion (dosage recommendation based on imipenem component):

Children: 60-100 mg/kg/day in 4 divided doses

Adults:

Serious infection: 2-4 g/day in 3-4 divided doses

Mild to moderate infection: 1-2 g/day in 3-4 divided doses

**Dosage Forms** Powder for injection:

I.M.:

Imipenem 500 mg and cilastatin 500 mg

Imipenem 750 mg and cilastatin 750 mg

I.V.:

Imipenem 250 mg and cilastatin 250 mg

Imipenem 500 mg and cilastatin 500 mg

## imipramine (im IP ra meen)

**U.S./Canadian Brand Names** Apo®-Imipramine (Can); Tofranil®; Tofranil-PM®

**Therapeutic Category** Antidepressant, Tricyclic (Tertiary Amine)

**Use** Treatment of various forms of depression, often in conjunction with psychotherapy; enuresis in children; analgesic for certain chronic and neuropathic pain

**Usual Dosage**

Children: Oral (safety and efficacy of imipramine therapy for treatment of depression in children $<12$ years have not been established):

Enuresis: $\geq 6$ years: Initial: 10-25 mg at bedtime, if inadequate response still seen after 1 week of therapy, increase by 25 mg/day; dose should not exceed 2.5 mg/kg/day or 50 mg at bedtime if 6-12 years of age or 75 mg at bedtime if $\geq 12$ years of age

Adjunct in the treatment of cancer pain: Initial: 0.2-0.4 mg/kg at bedtime; dose may be increased by 50% every 2-3 days up to 1-3 mg/kg/dose at bedtime

Adolescents: Oral: Initial: 25-50 mg/day; increase gradually; maximum: 100 mg/day in single or divided doses

Adults:
Oral: Initial: 25 mg 3-4 times/day, increase dose gradually, total dose may be administered at bedtime; maximum: 300 mg/day
I.M.: Initial: Up to 100 mg/day in divided doses; change to oral as soon as possible

**Dosage Forms**
Capsule, as pamoate (Tofranil-PM®): 75 mg, 100 mg, 125 mg, 150 mg
Injection, as hydrochloride (Tofranil®): 12.5 mg/mL (2 mL)
Tablet, as hydrochloride (Janimine®, Tofranil®): 10 mg, 25 mg, 50 mg

## imiquimod (i mi KWI mod)

**U.S./Canadian Brand Names** Aldara™
**Therapeutic Category** Immune Response Modifier
**Use** Genital and perianal warts (condyloma acuminata)
**Usual Dosage** Adults: Topical: Apply 3 times/week, prior to bedtime, leave on for 6-10 hours; remove cream by washing area with mild soap and water
**Dosage Forms** Cream: 5% (250 mg single dose packets)

**Imitrex®** *see* sumatriptan succinate *on page 567*

**ImmuCyst® (Can)** *see* BCG vaccine *on page 68*

## immune globulin (intramuscular)

(i MYUN GLOB yoo lin IN tra MUS kyoo ler)

**Synonyms** gamma globulin; IG; IGIM; immune serum globulin; ISG
**Therapeutic Category** Immune Globulin
**Use** Prophylaxis against hepatitis A, measles, varicella, and possibly rubella and immunoglobulin deficiency, idiopathic thrombocytopenia purpura, Kawasaki syndrome, lymphocytic leukemia
**Usual Dosage** I.M.:
Hepatitis A: 0.02 mL/kg
IgG: 1.3 mL/kg then 0.66 mL/kg in 3-4 weeks
Measles: 0.25 mL/kg
Rubella: 0.55 mL/kg
Varicella: 0.6-1.2 mL/kg
**Dosage Forms** Injection: I.M.: 165±15 mg (of protein)/mL (2 mL, 10 mL)

## immune globulin (intravenous) (i MYUN GLOB yoo lin IN tra VEE nus)

**Synonyms** IGIV; IVIG
**U.S./Canadian Brand Names** Gamimune® N; Gammagard® S/D; Gammar®-P I.V.; Polygam® S/D; Sandoglobulin®; Venoglobulin®-I; Venoglobulin®-S
**Therapeutic Category** Immune Globulin
**Use** Immunodeficiency syndrome, idiopathic thrombocytopenic purpura (ITP) and B-cell chronic lymphocytic leukemia (CLL); used in conjunction with appropriate anti-infective therapy to prevent or modify acute bacterial or viral infections in patients with iatrogenically-induced or disease-associated immunodepression; autoimmune neutropenia, bone marrow transplantation patients, Kawasaki disease, Guillain-Barré syndrome, demyelinating polyneuropathies
**Usual Dosage** Children and Adults: I.V. infusion:
Immunodeficiency syndrome: 100-200 mg/kg/dose every month; may increase to 400 mg/kg/dose as needed
Idiopathic thrombocytopenic purpura: 400-1000 mg/kg/dose for 2-5 consecutive days; maintenance dose: 400-1000 mg/kg/dose every 3-6 weeks based on clinical response and platelet count
Kawasaki disease: 400 mg/kg/day for 4 days or 2 g/kg as a single dose
Congenital and acquired antibody deficiency syndrome: 100-400 mg/kg/dose every 3-4 weeks
Bone marrow transplant: 500 mg/kg/week
Severe systemic viral and bacterial infections: Children: 500-1000 mg/kg/week
(Continued)

## immune globulin (intravenous) *(Continued)*

**Dosage Forms**

Injection: Gamimune® N: 5% [50 mg/mL] (10 mL, 50 mL, 100 mL); 10% [100 mg/mL] (50 mL, 100 mL, 200 mL)

Powder for injection, lyophilized:

Gammar-P®-IV: 1 g, 2.5 g, 5 g, 10 g

Sandoglobulin®: 1 g, 3 g, 6 g

Venoglobulin®-I: 2.5 g, 5 g

Detergent treated:

Gammagard® S/D: 2.5 g, 5 g, 10 g

Polygam® S/D: 2.5 g, 5 g, 10 g

Venoglobulin®-S: 2.5 g, 5 g, 10 g

**immune serum globulin** *see* immune globulin (intramuscular) *on previous page*

**Imodium®** *see* loperamide *on page 354*

**Imodium® A-D [OTC]** *see* loperamide *on page 354*

**Imogam® Rabies-HT** *see* rabies immune globulin (human) *on page 515*

**Imogen®** *see* loperamide *on page 354*

**Imotil® [OTC]** *see* loperamide *on page 354*

**Imovane® (Can)** *see* zopiclone *(Canada only) on page 641*

**Imovax® Rabies I.D. Vaccine** *see* rabies virus vaccine *on page 516*

**Imovax® Rabies Vaccine** *see* rabies virus vaccine *on page 516*

**Imperim® [OTC]** *see* loperamide *on page 354*

**Imuran®** *see* azathioprine *on page 61*

## inamrinone (eye NAM ri none)

**Synonyms** amrinone

**Therapeutic Category** Adrenergic Agonist Agent

**Use** Treatment of low cardiac output states (sepsis, congestive heart failure); adjunctive therapy of pulmonary hypertension

To avoid confusion with amiodarone, the generic name "amrinone" changed to "inamrinone" on July, 2000

**Usual Dosage** Dosage is based on clinical response. **Note:** Dose should not exceed 10 mg/kg/24 hours.

Children: 0.75 mg/kg I.V. bolus over 2-3 minutes followed by maintenance infusion 5-10 mcg/kg/minute; I.V. bolus may need to be repeated in 30 minutes

Adults: 0.75 mg/kg I.V. bolus over 2-3 minutes followed by maintenance infusion of 5-10 mcg/kg/minute

**Dosage Forms** Injection, as lactate: 5 mg/mL (20 mL)

**I-Naphline® Ophthalmic** *see* naphazoline *on page 409*

**Inapsine®** *see* droperidol *on page 206*

## indapamide (in DAP a mide)

**U.S./Canadian Brand Names** Apo®-Indapadmide (Can); Lozol®; Novo-Indapamide (Can); PMS-Indapamide (Can)

**Therapeutic Category** Diuretic, Miscellaneous

**Use** Management of mild to moderate hypertension; treatment of edema in congestive heart failure and nephrotic syndrome

**Usual Dosage** Adults: Oral: 2.5-5 mg/day

**Dosage Forms** Tablet: 1.25 mg, 2.5 mg

**Inderal®** *see* propranolol *on page 504*

**Inderal® LA** *see* propranolol *on page 504*

**Inderide®** *see* propranolol and hydrochlorothiazide *on page 505*

## indinavir (in DIN a veer)

**U.S./Canadian Brand Names** Crixivan®

**Therapeutic Category** Antiviral Agent

**Use** Treatment of HIV infection, especially advanced disease; usually administered as part of a three-drug regimen (two nucleosides plus a protease inhibitor) or double therapy (one nucleoside plus a protease inhibitor)

**Usual Dosage** Adults: Oral: 800 mg every 8 hours

**Dosage Forms** Capsule: 100 mg, 200 mg, 333 mg, 400 mg

**Indocid® (Can)** *see* indomethacin *on this page*

**Indocin® I.V. Injection** *see* indomethacin *on this page*

**Indocin® Oral** *see* indomethacin *on this page*

**Indocin® SR Oral** *see* indomethacin *on this page*

## indocyanine green (in doe SYE a neen green)

**Therapeutic Category** Diagnostic Agent

**Use** Determining hepatic function, cardiac output and liver blood flow and for ophthalmic angiography

**Usual Dosage** Dilute dose in sterile water for injection or 0.9% NaCl to final volume of 1 mL if necessary doses may be repeated periodically; total dose should not exceed 2 mg/kg

Infants: 1.25 mg
Children: 2.5 mg
Adults: 5 mg

**Dosage Forms** Injection: 25 mg

**indometacin** *see* indomethacin *on this page*

## indomethacin (in doe METH a sin)

**Synonyms** indometacin

**U.S./Canadian Brand Names** Apo®-Indomethacin (Can); Indocid® (Can); Indocin® I.V. Injection; Indocin® Oral; Indocin® SR Oral; Indotec® (Can); Novo-Methacin (Can); Nu-Indo (Can); Rhodacine® (Can)

**Therapeutic Category** Analgesic, Non-narcotic; Nonsteroidal Anti-inflammatory Drug (NSAID)

**Use** Management of inflammatory diseases and rheumatoid disorders; moderate pain; acute gouty arthritis; I.V. form used as alternative to surgery for closure of patent ductus arteriosus (PDA) in neonates

**Usual Dosage**

Patent ductus arteriosus: Neonates: I.V.: Initial: 0.2 mg/kg; followed with: 2 doses of 0.1 mg/kg at 12- to 24-hour intervals if age <48 hours at time of first dose; 0.2 mg/kg 2 times if 2-7 days old at time of first dose; or 0.25 mg/kg 2 times if over 7 days at time of first dose; discontinue if significant adverse effects occur. Dose should be withheld if patient has anuria or oliguria.

Analgesia:

Children: Oral: Initial: 1-2 mg/kg/day in 2-4 divided doses; maximum: 4 mg/kg/day; not to exceed 150-200 mg/day

Adults: Oral, rectal: 25-50 mg/dose 2-3 times/day; maximum dose: 200 mg/day; extended release capsule should be administered on a 1-2 times/day schedule

**Dosage Forms**

Capsule: 25 mg, 50 mg
Indocin®: 25 mg, 50 mg
Capsule, sustained release (Indocin® SR): 75 mg
Powder for injection, as sodium trihydrate (Indocin® I.V.): 1 mg
Suppository, rectal (Indocin®): 50 mg
(Continued)

**indomethacin** *(Continued)*

Suspension, oral (Indocin®): 25 mg/5 mL (5 mL, 10 mL, 237 mL, 500 mL)

**Indotec® (Can)** *see* indomethacin *on previous page*

**INF-alpha 2** *see* interferon alfa-2b *on page 321*

**Infanrix™** *see* diphtheria, tetanus toxoids, and acellular pertussis vaccine *on page 193*

**Infantaire® [OTC]** *see* acetaminophen *on page 3*

**Infantol® (Can)** *see* vitamin (multiple/oral) *on page 632*

**Infasurf®** *see* calfactant *on page 101*

**INFeD®** *see* iron dextran complex *on page 326*

**Infergen®** *see* interferon alfacon-1 *on page 322*

**Inflamase® Forte Ophthalmic** *see* prednisolone (ophthalmic) *on page 492*

**Inflamase® Mild Ophthalmic** *see* prednisolone (ophthalmic) *on page 492*

## infliximab (in FLIKS e mab)

**U.S./Canadian Brand Names** Remicade®

**Therapeutic Category** Gastrointestinal Agent, Miscellaneous

**Use** Treatment of moderately to severely active Crohn's disease for the reduction of the signs and symptoms in patients who have an inadequate response to conventional therapy or for the treatment of patients with fistulizing Crohn's disease for the reduction in the number of draining enterocutaneous fistula(s)

**Usual Dosage**

Moderately to severely active Crohn's disease: Adults: I.V.: 5 mg/kg as a single infusion over a minimum of 2 hours

Fistulizing Crohn's disease: 5 mg/kg as an infusion over a minimum of 2 hours, dose repeated at 2 and 6 weeks after the initial infusion

**Dosage Forms** Powder for injection: 100 mg

## influenza virus vaccine (in floo EN za VYE rus vak SEEN)

**U.S./Canadian Brand Names** Fluogen®; Fluviral® S/F (Can); Fluzone®

**Therapeutic Category** Vaccine, Inactivated Virus

**Use** Provide active immunity to influenza virus strains contained in the vaccine

**Usual Dosage** Annual vaccination with current vaccine; either whole- or split-virus vaccine may be used

**Dosage Forms** Injection:

Purified surface antigen (Flu-Imune®): 5 mL

Split-virus (Fluogen®, Fluzone®): 0.5 mL, 5 mL

Whole-virus (Fluzone®): 5 mL

**Infufer® (Can)** *see* iron dextran complex *on page 326*

**Infumorph™** *see* morphine sulfate *on page 400*

**INH** *see* isoniazid *on page 327*

**Inhibace® (Can)** *see* cilazapril *(Canada only) on page 137*

**Innerclean® [OTC]** *see* senna *on page 541*

**Innohep®** *see* tinzaparin *on page 591*

**Innovar®** *see* droperidol and fentanyl *on page 206*

**Inocor®** ***(Discontinued)*** *see page 750*

**INOmax®** *see* nitric oxide *on page 421*

## insect sting kit (IN sekt sting kit)

**U.S./Canadian Brand Names** Ana-Kit®

**Therapeutic Category** Antidote

**Use** Anaphylaxis emergency treatment of insect bites or stings by the sensitive patient that may occur within minutes of insect sting or exposure to an allergic substance

**Usual Dosage** Children and Adults:

Epinephrine:

<2 years: 0.05-0.1 mL

2-6 years: 0.15 mL

6-12 years: 0.2 mL

>12 years : 0.3 mL

Chlorpheniramine:

<6 years: 1 tablet

6-12 years: 2 tablets

>12 years: 4 tablets

**Dosage Forms** Kit: Epinephrine hydrochloride 1:1000 (1 mL syringe), chlorpheniramine maleate chewable tablet 2 mg (4), sterile alcohol pads (2), tourniquet

**Insta-Glucose® [OTC]** *see* glucose (instant) *on page 276*

## insulin preparations (IN su lin prep a RAY shuns)

**U.S./Canadian Brand Names** Humalog®; Humalog® Mix 50/50™; Humalog® Mix 75/25™; Humulin® 50/50; Humulin® 70/30; Humulin® L; Humulin® N; Iletin® II Pork (Can); Lantus®; Lente® Iletin® I; Lente® Iletin® II; Lente® Insulin; Lente® L; Novolin® 70/30; Novolin® ge (Can); Novolin® L; Novolin® N; Novolin-Pen® II, -3 (Can); Novolin® R; NovoLog™; NPH Iletin® I; NPH-N; Pork NPH Iletin® II; Pork Regular Iletin® II; Regular (Concentrated) Iletin® II U-500; Regular Iletin® I; Regular Insulin; Regular Purified Pork Insulin; Velosulin® BR Human (Buffered); Velosulin® Human Iletin® (Can)

**Therapeutic Category** Antidiabetic Agent, Parenteral

**Use** Treatment of insulin-dependent diabetes mellitus, also noninsulin-dependent diabetes mellitus unresponsive to treatment with diet and/or oral hypoglycemics; to assure proper utilization of glucose and reduce glucosuria in nondiabetic patients receiving parenteral nutrition whose glucosuria cannot be adequately controlled with infusion rate adjustments or those who require assistance in achieving optimal caloric intakes; hyperkalemia (regular insulin only; use with glucose to shift potassium into cells to lower serum potassium levels)

**Usual Dosage** Dose requires continuous medical supervision; may administer I.V. (regular), I.M., S.C.

Diabetes mellitus: The number and size of daily doses, time of administration, and diet and exercise require continuous medical supervision. In addition, specific formulations may require distinct administration procedures.

Lispro should be given within 15 minutes before or immediately after a meal

Human regular insulin should be given within 30-60 minutes before a meal.

Intermediate-acting insulins may be administered 1-2 times/day.

Long-acting insulins may be administered once daily.

Insulin glargine (Lantus®) should be administered subcutaneously once daily at bedtime. Maintenance doses should be administered subcutaneously and sites should be rotated to prevent lipodystrophy.

Children and Adults: 0.5-1 unit/kg/day in divided doses

Adolescents (growth spurts): 0.8-1.2 units/kg/day in divided doses

Adjust dose to maintain premeal and bedtime blood glucose of 80-140 mg/dL (children <5 years: 100-200 mg/dL)

Insulin glargine (Lantus®):

Type 2 diabetes (patient not already on insulin): 10 units once daily, adjusted according to patient response (range in clinical study 2-100 units/day)

Patients already receiving insulin: In clinical studies, when changing to insulin glargine from once-daily NPH or Ultralente® insulin, the initial dose was not changed; when

(Continued)

## insulin preparations *(Continued)*

changing from twice-daily NPH to once daily insulin glargine, the total daily dose was reduced by 20% and adjusted according to patient response

Hyperkalemia: Administer calcium gluconate and $NaHCO_3$ first then 50% dextrose at 0.5-1 mL/kg and insulin 1 unit for every 4-5 g dextrose given

Diabetic ketoacidosis: Children and Adults: Regular insulin: I.V. loading dose: 0.1 unit/kg, then maintenance continuous infusion: 0.1 unit/kg/hour (range: 0.05-0.2 units/kg/hour depending upon the rate of decrease of serum glucose - too rapid decrease of serum glucose may lead to cerebral edema).

Optimum rate of decrease (serum glucose): 80-100 mg/dL/hour

**Note:** Newly diagnosed patients with IDDM presenting in DKA and patients with blood sugars <800 mg/dL may be relatively "sensitive" to insulin and should receive loading and initial maintenance doses approximately ½ of those indicated above.

### Dosage Forms

**Rapid-Acting:**

Injection, rapid-acting, aspart, human [solution]:
NovoLog™: 100 units/mL (10 mL vial)
NovoLog® PenFill: 100 units/mL (3 mL cartridge)

Injection, rapid-acting, lispro, human (Humalog®): 100 units/mL (1.5 mL cartridge, 3 mL disposable pen, 10 mL vial) [solution]

**Short-Acting:**

Injection, short-acting, regular, human [solution]:
Humlin® R: 100 units/mL (1.5 mL cartridge, 10 mL vial)
Novolin® R: 100 units/mL (10 mL vial)
Novolin R® PenFill: 100 units/mL (1.5 mL cartridge, 3 mL cartridge)
Novolin R®, prefilled: 100 units/mL (1.5 mL prefilled syringe)

Injection, short-acting, regular, human, buffered (Velosulin® BR): 100 units/mL (10 mL vial) [solution]

Injection, short-acting, regular, human, concentrate (Humulin® R U-500): 500 units/mL (20 mL vial) [solution]

Injection, short-acting, regular, purified pork (Regular Iletin® II): 100 units/mL (10 mL vial) [solution]

**Intermediate-Acting:**

Injection, intermediate-acting, lente, human (Humulin® L, Novolin® L): 100 units/mL (10 mL vial) [zinc suspension]

Injection, intermediate-acting, lente, purified pork (Lente® Iletin II): 100 units/mL (10 mL vial) [zinc suspension]

Injection, intermediate-acting, NPH, human [isophane suspension]:
Humulin® N: 100 units/mL (1.5 mL cartridge, 3 mL disposable pen, 10 mL vial)
Novolin® N: 100 units/mL (10 mL vial)
Novolin® N PenFill: 100 units/mL (1.5 mL cartridge, 3 mL cartridge)
Novolin® N, prefilled: 100 units/mL (1.5 mL prefilled syringe)

Injection, intermediate-acting, NPH, purified pork (NPH Iletin® II): 100 units/mL (10 mL vial) [isophane suspension]

**Long-Acting:**

Injection, long-acting, Ultralente®, human (Humulin U Ultralente®): 100 units/mL (10 mL vial) [zinc suspension]

Injection, long-acting, glargine, human (Lantus®): 100 unit/mL (3 mL cartridge, 5 mL vial, 10 mL vial) [solution]

**Combination:**

Injection, combination, intermediate-acting, lispro human suspension 75% and rapid-acting lispro human solution 25% (Humalog® Mix 75/25®): 100 units/mL (3 mL disposable pen, 10 mL vial)

Injection, combination, intermediate-acting, NPH human insulin suspension 50% and short-acting regular human insulin solution 50% (Humulin® 50/50): 100 units/mL (10 mL vial)

Injection, combination, intermediate-acting, NPH human insulin suspension 70% and short-acting regular human insulin solution 30%:

Humulin® 70/30: 100 units/mL (1.5 mL cartridge, 3 ml disposable pen, 10 mL vial)

Novolin® 70/30: 100 units/mL (10 mL vial)

Novolin® 70/30 PenFill: 100 units/mL (1.5 mL cartridge, 3 mL cartridge)

Novolin® 70/30, prefilled: 100 units/mL (1.5 mL prefilled syringe)

**Intal®** *see* cromolyn sodium *on page 156*

**Intal® Inhalation Capsule *(Discontinued)*** *see page 750*

**Integrilin®** *see* eptifibatide *on page 219*

**Intercept™ *(Discontinued)*** *see page 750*

**α-2-interferon** *see* interferon alfa-2b *on this page*

## interferon alfa-2a (in ter FEER on AL fa too aye)

**Synonyms** IFLrA; rIFN-A

**U.S./Canadian Brand Names** Roferon-A®

**Therapeutic Category** Biological Response Modulator; Interferon

**Use** Hairy cell leukemia, AIDS-related Kaposi's sarcoma in patients >18 years of age, multiple unlabeled uses

**Usual Dosage**

Children: S.C.: Pulmonary hemangiomatosis: 1-3 million units/m$^2$/day once daily

Adults >18 years:

Hairy cell leukemia: I.M., S.C.: Induction dose is 3 million units/day for 16-24 weeks; maintenance: 3 million units 3 times/week

AIDS-related Kaposi's sarcoma: I.M., S.C.: Induction dose is 36 million units for 10-12 weeks; maintenance: 36 million units 3 times/week (may begin with dose escalation from 3-9-18 million units each day over 3 consecutive days followed by 36 million units daily for the remainder of the 10-12 weeks of induction)

**Dosage Forms**

Injection: 3 million units/mL (1 mL); 6 million units/mL (3 mL); 9 million units/mL (0.9 mL, 3 mL); 36 million units/mL (1 mL)

Powder for injection: 6 million units/mL when reconstituted

## interferon alfa-2b (in ter FEER on AL fa too bee)

**Synonyms** INF-alpha 2; α-2-interferon; rLFN-α2

**U.S./Canadian Brand Names** Intron® A

**Therapeutic Category** Biological Response Modulator; Interferon

**Use** Induce hairy cell leukemia remission; treatment of AIDS-related Kaposi's sarcoma; condylomata acuminata; chronic hepatitis C

**Usual Dosage** Adults (refer to individual protocols):

Hairy cell leukemia: I.M., S.C.: 2 million units/m$^2$ 3 times/week

AIDS-related Kaposi's sarcoma: I.M., S.C.: 30 million units/m$^2$ 3 times/week or 50 million units/m$^2$ I.V. 5 days/week every other week

Condylomata acuminata: Intralesionally: 1 million units/lesion 3 times/week for 3 weeks; not to exceed 5 million units per treatment (maximum: 5 lesions at one time)

Chronic hepatitis C: I.M., S.C.: 3 million units 3 times/week for approximately a 6-month course

**Dosage Forms**

Injection, albumin free: 3 million units (0.5 mL); 5 million units (0.5 mL); 10 million units (1 mL); 25 million units

Powder for injection, lyophilized: 18 million units, 50 million units

## interferon alfa-2b and ribavirin combination pack

(in ter FEER on AL fa too bee & rye ba VYE rin com bi NAY shun pak)

**U.S./Canadian Brand Names** Rebetron™

**Therapeutic Category** Antiviral Agent; Biological Response Modulator; Interferon

(Continued)

## interferon alfa-2b and ribavirin combination pack *(Continued)*

**Use** The combination therapy is indicated for the treatment of chronic hepatitis C in patients with compensated liver disease who have relapsed following alpha interferon therapy

**Usual Dosage** The recommended dosage of combination therapy is 3 million int. units of Intron® A injected subcutaneously three times per week and 1000-1200 mg of Rebetrol® capsules administered orally in a divided daily (morning and evening) dose for 24 weeks; patients weighing 75 kg (165 pounds) or less should receive 1000 mg of Rebetrol® daily, while patients weighing more than 75 kg should receive 1200 mg of Rebetrol® daily

**Dosage Forms** Combination package:

For patients ≤75 kg:

Each Rebetron™ combination package consists of:

A box containing 6 vials of Intron® A (3 million int. units in 0.5 mL per vial) and 6 syringes and alcohol swabs; two boxes containing 35 Rebetrol® capsules each for a total of 70 capsules (5 capsules per blister card)

One 18 million int. units multidose vial of Intron® A injection (22.8 million int. units per 3.8 mL; 3 million int. units/0.5 mL) and 6 syringes and alcohol swabs; two boxes containing 35 Rebetrol® capsules each for a total of 70 capsules (5 capsules per blister card)

One 18 million int. units Intron® A injection multidose pen (22.5 million int. units per 1.5 mL; 3 million int. units/0.2 mL) and 6 disposable needles and alcohol swabs; two boxes containing 35 Rebetrol® capsules each for a total of 70 capsules (5 capsules per blister card)

For patients >75 kg:

A box containing 6 vials of Intron® A injection (3 million int. units in 0.5 mL per vial) and 6 syringes and alcohol swabs; two boxes containing 42 Rebetrol® capsules each for a total of 84 capsules (6 capsules per blister card)

One 18 million int. units multidose vial of Intron® A injection (22.5 million int. units per 3.8 mL; 3 million int. units/0.5 mL) and 6 syringes and alcohol swabs; two boxes containing 42 Rebetrol® capsules each for a total of 84 capsules (6 capsules per blister card)

One 18 million int. units Intron® A injection multidose pen (22.5 million int. units per 1.5 mL; 3 million int. units/0.2 mL) and 6 disposable needles and alcohol swabs; two boxes containing 42 Rebetrol® capsules each for a total of 84 capsules (6 capsules per blister card)

For Rebetrol® dose reduction:

A box containing 6 vials of Intron® A injection (3 million int. units in 0.5 mL per vial) and 6 syringes and alcohol swabs; one box containing 42 Rebetrol® capsules (6 capsules per blister card)

One 18 million int. units multidose vial of Intron® A injection (22.8 million int. units per 3.8 mL; 3 million int. units/0.5 mL) and 6 syringes and alcohol swabs; one box containing 42 Rebetrol® capsules (6 capsules per blister card)

One 18 million int. units Introl® A injection multidose pen (22.5 million int. units per 1.5 mL; 3 million int. units/0.2 mL) and 6 disposable needles and alcohol swabs; one box containing 42 Rebetrol® capsules (6 capsules per blister card)

## interferon alfacon-1 (in ter FEER on AL fa con one)

**U.S./Canadian Brand Names** Infergen®

**Therapeutic Category** Interferon

**Use** Treatment of chronic hepatitis C virus (HCV) infection in patients ≥18 years of age with compensated liver disease and anti-HCV serum antibodies or HCV RNA.

**Usual Dosage** Adults ≥18 years: S.C.:

Chronic HCV infection: 9 mcg 3 times/week for 24 weeks; allow 48 hours between doses

Patients who have previously tolerated interferon therapy but did not respond or relapsed: 15 mcg 3 times/week for 6 months

Dose reduction for toxicity: Dose should be held in patients who experience a severe adverse reaction, and treatment should be stopped or decreased if the reaction does not become tolerable

Doses were reduced from 9 mcg to 7.5 mcg in the pivotal study

For patients receiving 15 mcg/dose, doses were reduced in 3 mcg increments. Efficacy is decreased with doses <7.5 mcg

**Dosage Forms** Injection (single-dose, preservative-free vials and syringes): 30 mcg/mL (0.3 mL, 0.5 mL)

## interferon alfa-n3 (in ter FEER on AL fa en three)

**U.S./Canadian Brand Names** Alferon® N

**Therapeutic Category** Biological Response Modulator; Interferon

**Use** Intralesional treatment of refractory or recurring genital or venereal warts; useful in patients who do not respond or are not candidates for usual treatments; indications and dosage regimens are specific for a particular brand of interferon

**Usual Dosage** Adults: Inject 250,000 units (0.05 mL) in each wart twice weekly for a maximum of 8 weeks; therapy should not be repeated for at least 3 months after the initial 8-week course of therapy

**Dosage Forms** Injection: 5 million units (1 mL)

## interferon beta-1a (in ter FEER on BAY ta won aye)

**U.S./Canadian Brand Names** Avonex™

**Therapeutic Category** Biological Response Modulator; Interferon

**Use** Treatment of relapsing forms of multiple sclerosis (MS); to slow the accumulation of physical disability and decrease the frequency of clinical exacerbations

**Usual Dosage** Adults >18 years: I.M.: 30 mcg once weekly

**Dosage Forms** Powder for injection, lyophilized: 33 mcg [6.6 million units]

## interferon beta-1b (in ter FEER on BAY ta won bee)

**U.S./Canadian Brand Names** Betaseron®

**Therapeutic Category** Biological Response Modulator; Interferon

**Use** Reduce the frequency of clinical exacerbations in ambulatory patients with relapsing-remitting multiple sclerosis

**Usual Dosage** Adults: S.C.: 0.25 mg every other day

**Dosage Forms** Powder for injection, lyophilized: 0.3 mg [9.6 million units]

## interferon gamma-1b (in ter FEER on GAM ah won bee)

**U.S./Canadian Brand Names** Actimmune®

**Therapeutic Category** Biological Response Modulator; Interferon

**Use** Reduce the frequency and severity of serious infections associated with chronic granulomatous disease

**Usual Dosage** Adults: S.C. (dosing is based on body surface ($m^2$)):

$\leq$0.5: 1.5 mcg/kg/dose

>0.5: 50 mcg/$m^2$ (1.5 million units/$m^2$) 3 times/week

**Dosage Forms** Injection: 100 mcg [3 million units]

**interleukin-2** *see* aldesleukin *on page 18*

**interleukin-11** *see* oprelvekin *on page 437*

**Intralipid®** *see* fat emulsion *on page 241*

**intravenous fat emulsion** *see* fat emulsion *on page 241*

**Intron® A** *see* interferon alfa-2b *on page 321*

**Intropin® *(Discontinued)*** *see page 750*

**Inversine®** *see* mecamylamine *on page 367*

**Invirase®** *see* saquinavir *on page 537*

**Iobid DM®** *see* guaifenesin and dextromethorphan *on page 282*

**Iodex® [OTC]** *see* povidone-iodine *on page 489*

**Iodex-p® [OTC]** *see* povidone-iodine *on page 489*

## iodine (EYE oh dyne)

**Therapeutic Category** Topical Skin Product

**Use** Topically as an antiseptic in the management of minor, superficial skin wounds and has been used to disinfect the skin preoperatively

**Usual Dosage** Topical: Apply as necessary to affected areas of skin

**Dosage Forms**

Solution: 2%

Tincture: 2%

**iodochlorhydroxyquin and hydrocortisone** *see* clioquinol and hydrocortisone *on page 143*

**Iodo-Niacin® Tablet *(Discontinued)*** *see page 750*

**Iodopen®** *see* trace metals *on page 598*

## iodoquinol (eye oh doe KWIN ole)

**Synonyms** diiodohydroxyquin

**U.S./Canadian Brand Names** Diodoquin® (Can); Diquinol®; Yodoxin®

**Therapeutic Category** Amebicide

**Use** Treatment of acute and chronic intestinal amebiasis due to *Entamoeba histolytica*; asymptomatic cyst passers; *Blastocystis hominis* infections; iodoquinol alone is ineffective for amebic hepatitis or hepatic abscess

**Usual Dosage** Oral:

Children: 30-40 mg/kg/day in 3 divided doses for 20 days; not to exceed 1.95 g/day

Adults: 650 mg 3 times/day after meals for 20 days; not to exceed 2 g/day

**Dosage Forms**

Powder: 25 g

Tablet: 210 mg, 650 mg

## iodoquinol and hydrocortisone

(eye oh doe KWIN ole & hye droe KOR ti sone)

**U.S./Canadian Brand Names** Vytone® Topical

**Therapeutic Category** Antifungal/Corticosteroid

**Use** Treatment of eczema; infectious dermatitis; chronic eczematoid otitis externa; mycotic dermatoses

**Usual Dosage** Topical: Apply 3-4 times/day

**Dosage Forms** Cream: Iodoquinol 1% and hydrocortisone 1% (30 g)

**Iofed®** *see* brompheniramine and pseudoephedrine *on page 88*

**Iofed® PD** *see* brompheniramine and pseudoephedrine *on page 88*

**Ionamin®** *see* phentermine *on page 466*

**Iophen® *(Discontinued)*** *see page 750*

**Iophen-C® *(Discontinued)*** *see page 750*

**Iophen-DM® *(Discontinued)*** *see page 750*

**Iophylline® *(Discontinued)*** *see page 750*

**Iopidine®** *see* apraclonidine *on page 50*

**Iotuss® *(Discontinued)*** *see page 750*

**Iotuss-DM® *(Discontinued)*** *see page 750*

## ipecac syrup (IP e kak SIR up)

**Therapeutic Category** Antidote

**Use** Treatment of acute oral drug overdosage and certain poisonings

**Usual Dosage** Oral:
Children:
6-12 months: 5-10 mL followed by 10-20 mL/kg of water; repeat dose one time if vomiting does not occur within 20 minutes
1-12 years: 15 mL followed by 10-20 mL/kg of water; repeat dose one time if vomiting does not occur within 20 minutes
Adults: 30 mL followed by 200-300 mL of water; repeat dose one time if vomiting does not occur within 20 minutes

**Dosage Forms** Syrup: 70 mg/mL (15 mL, 30 mL, 473 mL, 4000 mL)

**I-Pentolate®** *see* cyclopentolate *on page 159*

**I-Phrine® Ophthalmic Solution** *see* phenylephrine *on page 467*

**I-Picamide®** ***(Discontinued)*** *see page 750*

**IPOL™** *see* poliovirus vaccine (inactivated) *on page 480*

## ipratropium (i pra TROE pee um)

**U.S./Canadian Brand Names** Alti-Ipratropium (Can); Apo®-Ipravent (Can); Atrovent®; Gen-Ipratropium (Can); Novo-Ipramide (Can); Nu-Ipratropium (Can); PMS-Ipratropium (Can)

**Therapeutic Category** Anticholinergic Agent

**Use** Bronchodilator used in bronchospasm associated with asthma, COPD, bronchitis, and emphysema; nasal spray used for symptomatic relief of rhinorrhea

**Usual Dosage** Children >12 years and Adults: 2 inhalations 4 times/day up to 12 inhalations/24 hours

**Dosage Forms** Solution, as bromide:
Inhalation: 18 mcg/actuation (14 g)
Nasal spray: 0.03% (30 mL); 0.06% (15 mL)
Nebulizing: 0.02% (2.5 mL)

## ipratropium and albuterol (i pra TROE pee um & al BYOO ter ole)

**U.S./Canadian Brand Names** Combivent®

**Therapeutic Category** Bronchodilator

**Use** Treatment of chronic obstructive pulmonary disease (COPD) in those patients that are currently on a regular bronchodilator who continue to have bronchospasms and require a second bronchodilator

**Usual Dosage** Adults: 2 inhalations 4 times/day, maximum of 12 inhalations/24 hours

**Dosage Forms** Aerosol: Ipratropium bromide 18 mcg and albuterol sulfate 103 mcg per actuation [200 doses] (14.7 g)

**iproveratril** *see* verapamil *on page 625*

**IPV** *see* poliovirus vaccine (inactivated) *on page 480*

## irbesartan (ir be SAR tan)

**U.S./Canadian Brand Names** Avapro®

**Therapeutic Category** Angiotensin II Antagonist

**Use** Treatment of hypertension alone or in combination with other antihypertensives

**Usual Dosage** Adults: Oral: 150 mg once daily with or without food; patients may be titrated to 300 mg once daily

**Dosage Forms** Tablet: 75 mg, 150 mg, 300 mg

## irbesartan and hydrochlorothiazide
(ir be SAR tan & hye droe klor oh THYE a zide)

**U.S./Canadian Brand Names** Avalide®

**Therapeutic Category** Antihypertensive Agent, Combination

**Use** Combination therapy for the management of hypertension

(Continued)

## irbesartan and hydrochlorothiazide *(Continued)*

**Dosage Forms** Tablet: Irbesartan 150 mg and hydrochlorothiazide 12.5 mg; irbesartan 300 mg and hydrochlorothiazide 12.5 mg

**Ircon® [OTC]** *see* ferrous fumarate *on page 246*

## irinotecan (eye rye no TEE kan)

**U.S./Canadian Brand Names** Camptosar®

**Therapeutic Category** Antineoplastic Agent

**Use** Treatment of patients with metastatic carcinoma of the colon or rectum whose disease has progressed following 5-FU based therapy

**Usual Dosage** Adults: I.V.: The recommended starting dose is 125 mg/m$^2$ (I.V. infusion over 90 minutes) once a week for 4 weeks, followed by a 2-week rest period; additional 6-week cycles of treatment may be repeated indefinitely in patients who remain stable or do not develop intolerable toxicities

**Dosage Forms** Injection: 20 mg/mL (5 mL)

## iron dextran complex (EYE ern DEKS tran KOM pleks)

**U.S./Canadian Brand Names** Dexferrum®; Dexiron™ (Can); INFeD®; Infufer® (Can)

**Therapeutic Category** Electrolyte Supplement, Oral

**Use** Treatment of microcytic, hypochromic anemia resulting from iron deficiency when oral iron administration is infeasible or ineffective

**Usual Dosage** I.M., I.V.:

A 0.5 mL test dose (0.25 mL in infants) should be administered prior to starting iron dextran therapy

Iron deficiency anemia: Dose (mL) = 0.0476 x LBW (kg) x (normal hemoglobin - observed hemoglobin) + (1 mL/5 kg of LBW to maximum of 14 mL for iron stores)

$Hb_n$ = desired hemoglobin (g/dL)

$Hb_o$ = measured hemoglobin (g/dL)

Maximum daily dose:

Infants <5 kg: 25 mg iron

Children:

5-10 kg: 50 mg iron

10-50 kg: 100 mg iron

Adults >50 kg: 100 mg iron

**Dosage Forms** Injection: 50 mg/mL (2 mL, 10 mL)

## iron sucrose (EYE ern SOO krose)

**U.S./Canadian Brand Names** Venofer®

**Therapeutic Category** Iron Salt

**Use** Treatment of iron-deficiency anemia in patients undergoing chronic hemodialysis who are receiving supplemental erythropoietin therapy

**Usual Dosage** Doses expressed in mg of **elemental** iron

Iron-deficiency anemia: I.V.: 100 mg (5 mL of iron sucrose injection) administered 1-3 times/week during dialysis, to a total dose of 1000 mg (10 doses); administer no more than 3 times/week; may continue to administer at lowest dose necessary to maintain target hemoglobin, hematocrit, and iron storage parameters

Test dose: Product labeling does not indicate need for a test dose in product-naive patients; test doses were administered in some clinical trials as 50 mg (2.5 mL) in 50 mL 0.9% NaCl administered over 3-10 minutes

**Dosage Forms** Injection: 20 mg of elemental iron/mL (5 mL vial)

**ISD** *see* isosorbide dinitrate *on page 328*

**ISDN** *see* isosorbide dinitrate *on page 328*

**ISG** *see* immune globulin (intramuscular) *on page 315*

**Ismelin®** *see* guanethidine *on page 286*

**ISMN** *see* isosorbide mononitrate *on page 329*

**Ismo®** *see* isosorbide mononitrate *on page 329*

**Ismotic®** ***(Discontinued)*** *see page 750*

**isoamyl nitrite** *see* amyl nitrite *on page 40*

**isobamate** *see* carisoprodol *on page 110*

**Iso-Bid®** ***(Discontinued)*** *see page 750*

**Isocaine® HCl** *see* mepivacaine *on page 373*

**Isocal® [OTC]** *see* nutritional formula, enteral/oral *on page 432*

## isocarboxazid (eye soe kar BOKS a zid)

**U.S./Canadian Brand Names** Marplan®

**Therapeutic Category** Antidepressant, Monoamine Oxidase Inhibitor

**Use** Symptomatic treatment of atypical, nonendogenous or neurotic depression

**Usual Dosage** Adults: Oral: 10 mg 3 times/day; reduce to 10-20 mg/day in divided doses when condition improves

**Dosage Forms** Tablet: 10 mg

**Isoclor® Expectorant** *see* guaifenesin, pseudoephedrine, and codeine *on page 284*

## isoetharine (eye soe ETH a reen)

**Therapeutic Category** Adrenergic Agonist Agent

**Use** Bronchodilator used in asthma and for the reversible bronchospasm occurring with bronchitis and emphysema

**Usual Dosage** Treatments are usually not repeated more often than every 4 hours, except in severe cases, and may be repeated up to 5 times/day if necessary

Nebulizer: Children: 0.1-0.2 mg/kg/dose every 2-6 hours as needed; adult: 0.5 mL diluted in 2-3 mL normal saline or 4 inhalations of undiluted 1% solution

**Dosage Forms** Solution inhalation, hydrochloride: 1% (10 mL, 30 mL)

## isoflurane (eye soe FLURE ane)

**U.S./Canadian Brand Names** Forane®

**Therapeutic Category** General Anesthetic

**Use** General induction and maintenance of anesthesia (inhalation)

**Usual Dosage** 1.5% to 3%

**Dosage Forms** Solution: 100 mL, 125 mL, 250 mL

## isoniazid (eye soe NYE a zid)

**Synonyms** INH; isonicotinic acid hydrazide

**U.S./Canadian Brand Names** Isotamine® (Can); Nydrazid®; PMS-Isoniazid (Can)

**Therapeutic Category** Antitubercular Agent

**Use** Treatment of susceptible mycobacterial infection due to *M. tuberculosis* and prophylactically to those individuals exposed to tuberculosis

**Usual Dosage** Oral, I.M.:

Children: 10-20 mg/kg/day in 1-2 divided doses (maximum: 300 mg total dose)
Prophylaxis: 10 mg/kg/day administered daily (up to 300 mg total dose) for 12 months

Adults: 5 mg/kg/day administered daily (usual dose: 300 mg)
Disseminated disease: 10 mg/kg/day in 1-2 divided doses
Treatment should be continued for 9 months with rifampin or for 6 months with rifampin and pyrazinamide
Prophylaxis: 300 mg/day administered daily for 12 months

American Thoracic Society and CDC currently recommend twice weekly therapy as part of a short-course regimen which follows 1-2 months of daily treatment for uncomplicated pulmonary tuberculosis in compliant patients
Children: 20-40 mg/kg/dose (up to 900 mg) twice weekly

(Continued)

## isoniazid *(Continued)*

Adults: 15 mg/kg/dose (up to 900 mg) twice weekly

**Dosage Forms**

Injection: 100 mg/mL (10 mL)
Syrup (orange flavor): 50 mg/5 mL (473 mL)
Tablet: 100 mg, 300 mg

**isonicotinic acid hydrazide** *see* isoniazid *on previous page*

**isonipecaine** *see* meperidine *on page 372*

## isoproterenol (eye soe proe TER e nole)

**U.S./Canadian Brand Names** Isuprel®

**Therapeutic Category** Adrenergic Agonist Agent

**Use** Asthma or COPD (reversible airway obstruction); ventricular arrhythmias due to A-V nodal block; hemodynamically compromised bradyarrhythmias or atropine-resistant bradyarrhythmias, temporary use in third degree A-V block until pacemaker insertion; low cardiac output or vasoconstrictive shock states

**Usual Dosage** I.V. infusion:

Children: 0.05-2 mcg/kg/minute; rate (mL/hour) = dose (mcg/kg/minute) x weight (kg) x 60 minutes/hour divided by concentration (mcg/mL)
Adults: A-V nodal block: 2-20 mcg/minute

**Dosage Forms** Injection: 0.2 mg/mL (1:5000) (1 mL, 5 mL, 10 mL)

**Isoptin®** *see* verapamil *on page 625*

**Isoptin® SR** *see* verapamil *on page 625*

**Isopto® Atropine** *see* atropine *on page 58*

**Isopto® Carbachol Ophthalmic** *see* carbachol *on page 105*

**Isopto® Carpine Ophthalmic** *see* pilocarpine *on page 471*

**Isopto® Cetapred® Ophthalmic** *see* sulfacetamide and prednisolone *on page 563*

**Isopto® Eserine *(Discontinued)*** *see page 750*

**Isopto® Frin Ophthalmic Solution** *see* phenylephrine *on page 467*

**Isopto® Homatropine Ophthalmic** *see* homatropine *on page 295*

**Isopto® Hyoscine** *see* scopolamine *on page 539*

**Isopto® P-ES *(Discontinued)*** *see page 750*

**Isopto® Plain Solution [OTC]** *see* artificial tears *on page 53*

**Isopto® Tears Solution [OTC]** *see* artificial tears *on page 53*

**Isordil®** *see* isosorbide dinitrate *on this page*

## isosorbide dinitrate (eye soe SOR bide dye NYE trate)

**Synonyms** ISD; ISDN

**U.S./Canadian Brand Names** Apo®-ISDN (Can); Cedocard®-SR (Can); Dilatrate®-SR; Isordil®; Sorbitrate®

**Therapeutic Category** Vasodilator

**Use** Prevention and treatment of angina pectoris; for congestive heart failure; to relieve pain, dysphagia, and spasm in esophageal spasm with GE reflux

**Usual Dosage** Adults:

Oral: 5-30 mg 4 times/day or 40 mg every 6-12 hours in sustained-released dosage form
Chewable: 5-10 mg every 2-3 hours
Sublingual: 2.5-10 mg every 4-6 hours

**Dosage Forms**

Capsule, sustained release: 40 mg

Tablet:
Chewable: 5 mg, 10 mg
Oral: 5 mg, 10 mg, 20 mg, 30 mg
Sublingual: 2.5 mg, 5 mg, 10 mg
Sustained release: 40 mg

## isosorbide mononitrate (eye soe SOR bide mon oh NYE trate)

**Synonyms** ISMN
**U.S./Canadian Brand Names** Imdur™; Ismo®; Monoket®
**Therapeutic Category** Vasodilator
**Use** Long-acting metabolite of the vasodilator isosorbide dinitrate used for the prophylactic treatment of angina pectoris
**Usual Dosage** Adults: Oral:
Regular tablet: 20 mg twice daily separated by 7 hours
Extended-release tablet: 30 mg (1/2 of 60 mg tablet) or 60 mg (administered as a single tablet) once daily; after several days the dosage may be increased to 120 mg (administered as two 60 mg tablets) once daily; the daily dose should be administered in the morning upon arising
**Dosage Forms**
Tablet: 20 mg
Ismo®: 20 mg
Monoket®: 10 mg, 20 mg
Tablet, extended release: 60 mg
Imdur™: 30 mg, 60 mg, 120 mg

**Isotamine® (Can)** *see* isoniazid *on page 327*

## isotretinoin (eye soe TRET i noyn)

**Synonyms** 13-*cis*-retinoic acid
**U.S./Canadian Brand Names** Accutane®; Isotrex® (Can)
**Therapeutic Category** Retinoic Acid Derivative
**Use** Treatment of severe recalcitrant cystic and/or conglobate acne unresponsive to conventional therapy
**Investigational use:** Treatment of children with metastatic neuroblastoma or leukemia that does not respond to conventional therapy
**Usual Dosage** Oral:
Children: Maintenance therapy for neuroblastoma: 100-250 mg/m$^2$/day in 2 divided doses has been used investigationally
Children and Adults: 0.5-2 mg/kg/day in 2 divided doses for 15-20 weeks
**Dosage Forms** Capsule: 10 mg, 20 mg, 40 mg

**Isotrex® (Can)** *see* isotretinoin *on this page*

**Isovex® *(Discontinued)*** *see page 750*

**Isovue®** *see* radiological/contrast media (non-ionic) *on page 518*

## isoxsuprine (eye SOKS syoo preen)

**U.S./Canadian Brand Names** Vasodilan®
**Therapeutic Category** Vasodilator
**Use** Treatment of peripheral vascular diseases, such as arteriosclerosis obliterans and Raynaud's disease
**Usual Dosage** Adults: Oral: 10-20 mg 3-4 times/day
**Dosage Forms** Tablet, as hydrochloride: 10 mg, 20 mg

## isradipine (iz RA di peen)

**U.S./Canadian Brand Names** DynaCirc®
**Therapeutic Category** Calcium Channel Blocker
**Use** Management of hypertension, alone or concurrently with thiazide-type diuretics
(Continued)

## isradipine *(Continued)*

**Usual Dosage** Adults: Oral: Initial: 2.5 mg twice daily, if satisfactory response does not occur after 2-4 weeks the dose may be adjusted in increments of 5 mg/day at 2- to 4-week intervals up to a maximum of 20 mg/day

**Dosage Forms** Capsule: 2.5 mg, 5 mg

**Isuprel®** *see* isoproterenol *on page 328*

**Isuprel® Glossets®** ***(Discontinued)*** *see page 750*

**Itch-X® [OTC]** *see* pramoxine *on page 490*

## itraconazole (i tra KOE na zole)

**U.S./Canadian Brand Names** Sporanox®

**Therapeutic Category** Antifungal Agent

**Use** Treatment of systemic fungal infections in immunocompromised and nonimmunocompromised patients including the treatment of susceptible blastomycosis, histoplasmosis, and aspergillosis in patients who do not respond to or cannot tolerate amphotericin B; it also has activity against *Cryptococcus*, *Coccidioides*, and sporotrichosis species; has also been used for prophylaxis against aspergillosis infection

**Usual Dosage** Oral: Capsule: Absorption is best if taken with food, therefore, it is best to administer itraconazole after meals; Solution: Should be taken on an empty stomach. Absorption of both products is significantly increased when taken with a cola beverage.

Children: Efficacy and safety have not been established; a small number of patients 3-16 years of age have been treated with 100 mg/day for systemic fungal infections with no serious adverse effects reported

Adults:

Oral:

Blastomycosis/histoplasmosis: 200 mg once daily, if no obvious improvement or there is evidence of progressive fungal disease, increase the dose in 100 mg increments to a maximum of 400 mg/day; doses >200 mg/day are given in 2 divided doses; length of therapy varies from 1 day to >6 months depending on the condition and mycological response

Aspergillosis: 200-400 mg/day

Onychomycosis: 200 mg once daily for 12 consecutive weeks

Life-threatening infections: Loading dose: 200 mg 3 times/day (600 mg/day) should be given for the first 3 days of therapy

Oropharyngeal and esophageal candidiasis: Oral solution: 100-200 mg once daily

I.V.: 200 mg twice daily for 4 doses, followed by 200 mg daily

**Dosage Forms**

Capsule: 100 mg

Injection kit: 10 mg/mL - 25 mL ampul, one 50 mL (100 mL capacity) bag 0.9% sodium chloride, one filtered infusion set

Solution, oral: 100 mg/10 mL (150 mL)

**I-Tropine®** *see* atropine *on page 58*

## ivermectin (eye ver MEK tin)

**U.S./Canadian Brand Names** Stromectol®

**Therapeutic Category** Antibiotic, Miscellaneous

**Use** Treatment of the following infections: Strongyloidiasis of the intestinal tract due the nematode parasite *Strongyloides stercoralis*. Onchocerciasis due to the nematode parasite *Onchocerca volvulus*. Note: Ivermectin is ineffective against adult *Onchocerca volvulus* parasites because they reside in subcutaneous nodules which are infrequently palpable. Surgical excision of these nodules may be considered in the management of patients with onchocerciasis.

**Usual Dosage** Oral:

Children >5 years: 150 mcg/kg as a single dose once every 12 months

Adults: 150 mcg/kg as a single dose; may be repeated every 6-12 months

**Dosage Forms** Tablet: 3 mg, 6 mg

**IVIG** *see* immune globulin (intravenous) *on page 315*

**IvyBlock®** *see* bentoquatam *on page 71*

**Janimine®** ***(Discontinued)*** *see page 750*

## Japanese encephalitis virus vaccine (inactivated)

(jap a NEESE en sef a LYE tis VYE rus vak SEEN in ak ti VAY ted)

**U.S./Canadian Brand Names** JE-VAX®

**Therapeutic Category** Vaccine, Inactivated Virus

**Use** Active immunization against Japanese encephalitis for persons spending a month or longer in endemic areas, especially if travel will include rural areas

**Usual Dosage** S.C. (administered on days 0, 7, and 30):

Children 1-3 years: 3 doses of 0.5 mL; booster doses of 0.5 mL may administer 2 years after primary immunization series

Children >3 years and Adults: 3 doses of 1 mL; booster doses of 1 mL may be administered 2 years after primary immunization series

**Dosage Forms** Powder for injection, lyophilized: 1 mL, 10 mL

**Jenamicin®** ***(Discontinued)*** *see page 750*

**Jenest-28™** *see* ethinyl estradiol and norethindrone *on page 232*

**JE-VAX®** *see* Japanese encephalitis virus vaccine (inactivated) *on this page*

**Junior Strength Motrin® [OTC]** *see* ibuprofen *on page 311*

**Just Tears® Solution [OTC]** *see* artificial tears *on page 53*

**K+ 10®** *see* potassium chloride *on page 485*

**K-99®** *see* potassium gluconate *on page 487*

**Kabikinase®** *see* streptokinase *on page 558*

**Kadian™ Oral** *see* morphine sulfate *on page 400*

**Kalcinate®** ***(Discontinued)*** *see page 750*

**Kaletra™** *see* lopinavir and ritonavir *on page 355*

## kanamycin (kan a MYE sin)

**U.S./Canadian Brand Names** Kantrex®

**Therapeutic Category** Aminoglycoside (Antibiotic)

**Use**

Oral: Preoperative bowel preparation in the prophylaxis of infections and adjunctive treatment of hepatic coma (oral kanamycin is not indicated in the treatment of systemic infections)

Parenteral: Initial therapy of severe infections where the strain is thought to be susceptible in patients allergic to other antibiotics, or in mixed staphylococcal or gram-negative infections

**Usual Dosage**

Children: Infections: I.M., I.V.: 15 mg/kg/day in divided doses every 8-12 hours

Adults:

Infections: I.M., I.V.: 15 mg/kg/day in divided doses every 8-12 hours

Preoperative intestinal antisepsis: Oral: 1 g every 4-6 hours for 36-72 hours

**Dosage Forms**

Capsule, as sulfate: 500 mg

Injection, as sulfate:

Pediatric: 75 mg (2 mL)

Adults: 500 mg (2 mL); 1 g (3 mL)

**Kantrex®** *see* kanamycin *on this page*

**Kaochlor®** *see* potassium chloride *on page 485*

**Kaochlor-Eff® *(Discontinued)*** *see page 750*

**Kaochlor® SF** *see* potassium chloride *on page 485*

**Kaodene® [OTC]** *see* kaolin and pectin *on this page*

**Kaodene A-D® [OTC]** *see* loperamide *on page 354*

## kaolin and pectin (KAY oh lin & PEK tin)

**U.S./Canadian Brand Names** Kaodene® [OTC]; Kao-Spen® [OTC]; Kapectolin® [OTC]

**Therapeutic Category** Antidiarrheal

**Use** Treatment of uncomplicated diarrhea

**Usual Dosage** Oral:

Children:

<6 years: Do not use

6-12 years: 30-60 mL after each loose stool

Adults: 60-120 mL after each loose stool

**Dosage Forms** Suspension, oral: Kaolin 975 mg and pectin 22 mg per 5 mL

## kaolin and pectin with opium (KAY oh lin & PEK tin with OH pee um)

**U.S./Canadian Brand Names** Donnagel®-PG Suspension® (Can)

**Therapeutic Category** Antidiarrheal

**Controlled Substance** C-V

**Use** Symptomatic relief of diarrhea

**Usual Dosage** Oral:

Children:

3-6 years: 7.5 mL with each loose bowel movement, not to exceed 30 mL in 12 hours

6-12 years: 5-10 mL with each loose bowel movement, not to exceed 40 mL in 12 hours

Children >12 years and Adults: 15-30 mL with each loose bowel movement, not to exceed 120 mL in 12 hours

**Dosage Forms** Suspension, oral: Kaolin 5.5 g, pectin 162 mg, and opium 15 mg per 30 mL [3.7 mL paregoric] (240 mL)

**Kaon®** *see* potassium gluconate *on page 487*

**Kaon-Cl®** *see* potassium chloride *on page 485*

**Kaon-Cl-10®** *see* potassium chloride *on page 485*

**Kao-Paverin® [OTC]** *see* loperamide *on page 354*

**Kaopectate® Advanced Formula [OTC]** *see* attapulgite *on page 60*

**Kaopectate® Children's Tablet *(Discontinued)*** *see page 750*

**Kaopectate® II *(Discontinued)*** *see page 750*

**Kaopectate® Maximum Strength Caplets** *see* attapulgite *on page 60*

**Kao-Spen® [OTC]** *see* kaolin and pectin *on this page*

**Kapectolin® [OTC]** *see* kaolin and pectin *on this page*

**Kapectolin PG®** *see* hyoscyamine, atropine, scopolamine, kaolin, pectin, and opium *on page 310*

**Karidium®** *see* fluoride *on page 255*

**Karigel®** *see* fluoride *on page 255*

**Karigel®-N** *see* fluoride *on page 255*

**Kasof® [OTC]** *see* docusate *on page 197*

**Kato® Powder *(Discontinued)*** *see page 750*

**Kaybovite-1000®** *see* cyanocobalamin *on page 158*

**Kay Ciel®** *see* potassium chloride *on page 485*

**Kayexalate®** *see* sodium polystyrene sulfonate *on page 553*

**K+ Care®** *see* potassium chloride *on page 485*

**K+ Care® Effervescent** *see* potassium bicarbonate *on page 484*

**KCl** *see* potassium chloride *on page 485*

**K-Dur® 10** *see* potassium chloride *on page 485*

**K-Dur® 20** *see* potassium chloride *on page 485*

**Keflex®** *see* cephalexin *on page 120*

**Keflin® *(Discontinued)*** *see page 750*

**Keftab®** *see* cephalexin *on page 120*

**Kefurox® Injection** *see* cefuroxime *on page 118*

**Kefzol®** *see* cefazolin *on page 114*

**K-Electrolyte® Effervescent** *see* potassium bicarbonate *on page 484*

**Kemadrin®** *see* procyclidine *on page 498*

**Kemsol® (Can)** *see* dimethyl sulfoxide *on page 189*

**Kenacort® Oral** *see* triamcinolone (systemic) *on page 602*

**Kenaject® Injection** *see* triamcinolone (systemic) *on page 602*

**Kenalog® Injection** *see* triamcinolone (systemic) *on page 602*

**Kenalog® in Orabase®** *see* triamcinolone (topical) *on page 602*

**Kenalog® Topical** *see* triamcinolone (topical) *on page 602*

**Kenonel® Topical** *see* triamcinolone (topical) *on page 602*

**Keppra®** *see* levetiracetam *on page 344*

**Keralyt® Gel** *see* salicylic acid and propylene glycol *on page 535*

**Kerlone® Oral** *see* betaxolol *on page 78*

**Kestrin® Injection *(Discontinued)*** *see page 750*

**Kestrone®** *see* estrone *on page 228*

**Ketalar®** *see* ketamine *on this page*

## ketamine (KEET a meen)

**U.S./Canadian Brand Names** Ketalar®

**Therapeutic Category** General Anesthetic

**Controlled Substance** C-III

**Use** Anesthesia, short surgical procedures, dressing changes

**Usual Dosage**

Children:

I.M.: 3-7 mg/kg

I.V.: Range: 0.5-2 mg/kg, use smaller doses (0.5-1 mg/kg) for sedation for minor procedures; usual induction dosage: 1-2 mg/kg

Adults:

I.M.: 3-8 mg/kg

I.V.: Range: 1-4.5 mg/kg; usual induction dosage: 1-2 mg/kg

Children and Adults: Maintenance: Supplemental doses of $^1/_3$ to $^1/_2$ of initial dose

**Dosage Forms** Injection, as hydrochloride: 10 mg/mL (20 mL, 25 mL, 50 mL); 50 mg/mL (10 mL); 100 mg/mL (5 mL)

## ketoconazole (kee toe KOE na zole)

**U.S./Canadian Brand Names** Apo®-Ketoconazole (Can); Nizoral®; Nizoral® A-D Shampoo [OTC]; Novo-Ketoconazol (Can)

**Therapeutic Category** Antifungal Agent

**Use** Treatment of susceptible fungal infections, including candidiasis, oral thrush, blastomycosis, histoplasmosis, coccidioidomycosis, paracoccidioidomycosis, chronic mucocutaneous candidiasis, as well as certain recalcitrant cutaneous dermatophytoses; used

(Continued)

## ketoconazole *(Continued)*

topically for treatment of tinea corporis, tinea cruris, tinea versicolor, and cutaneous candidiasis; shampoo is used for dandruff

**Usual Dosage**

Children: Oral: 5-10 mg/kg/day divided every 12-24 hours until lesions clear

Adults:

Oral: 200-400 mg/day as a single daily dose

Topical: Rub gently into the affected area once daily to twice daily for two weeks

**Dosage Forms**

Cream: 2% (15 g, 30 g, 60 g)

Shampoo: 1% (207 mL); 2% (120 mL)

Tablet: 200 mg

## ketoprofen (kee toe PROE fen)

**U.S./Canadian Brand Names** Actron® [OTC]; Apo®-Keto (Can); Apo®-Keto-E (Can); Novo-Keto (Can); Novo-Keto-EC (Can); Nu-Ketoprofen (Can); Nu-Ketoprofen-E (Can); Orafen (Can); Orudis®; Orudis® KT [OTC]; Oruvail®; Rhodis™ (Can); Rhodis-EC™ (Can); Rhovail® (Can)

**Therapeutic Category** Analgesic, Non-narcotic; Nonsteroidal Anti-inflammatory Drug (NSAID)

**Use** Acute or long-term treatment of rheumatoid arthritis and osteoarthritis; primary dysmenorrhea; mild to moderate pain

**Usual Dosage** Oral:

Children 3 months to 14 years: Fever: 0.5-1 mg/kg

Children >12 years and Adults:

Rheumatoid arthritis or osteoarthritis: 50-75 mg 3-4 times/day up to a maximum of 300 mg/day

Mild to moderate pain: 25-50 mg every 6-8 hours up to a maximum of 300 mg/day

**Dosage Forms**

Capsule (Orudis®): 25 mg, 50 mg, 75 mg

Capsule, extended release

Actron®: 200 mg

Oruvail®: 100 mg, 150 mg

Tablet (Orudis® KT): 12.5 mg

## ketorolac tromethamine (KEE toe role ak troe METH a meen)

**U.S./Canadian Brand Names** Acular® Ophthalmic; Apo®-Ketorolac (Can); Novo-Ketorolac (Can); Toradol®

**Therapeutic Category** Analgesic, Non-narcotic; Nonsteroidal Anti-inflammatory Drug (NSAID)

**Use**

Oral, I.M., I.V.,: Short-term (≤5 days) management of moderate to severe pain, including postoperative pain, visceral pain associated with cancer, pain associated with trauma, acute renal colic

Ophthalmic: Ocular itch associated with seasonal allergic conjunctivitis

**Usual Dosage** Adults (pain relief usually begins within 10 minutes with parenteral forms):

Oral: 10 mg every 4-6 hours as needed for a maximum of 40 mg/day; on day of transition from I.M. to oral: maximum oral dose: 40 mg (or 120 mg combined oral and I.M.); maximum 5 days administration

I.M.: Initial: 30-60 mg, then 15-30 mg every 6 hours as needed for up to 5 days maximum; maximum dose in the first 24 hours: 150 mg with 120 mg/24 hours for up to 5 days total

I.V.: Initial: 30 mg, then 15-30 mg every 6 hours as needed for up to 5 days **maximum**; maximum daily dose: 120 mg for up to 5 days total

Ophthalmic: Instill 1 drop in eye(s) 4 times/day

**Dosage Forms**
Injection: 15 mg/mL (1 mL); 30 mg/mL (1 mL, 2 mL)
Solution, ophthalmic: 0.5% (5 mL)
Tablet: 10 mg

## ketotifen (kee toe TYE fen)

**U.S./Canadian Brand Names** Apo®-Ketotifen (Can); Novo-Ketotifen (Can); Zaditen® (Can); Zaditor™
**Therapeutic Category** Antihistamine, $H_1$ Blocker, Ophthalmic
**Use** Temporary prevention of eye itching due to allergic conjunctivitis
**Usual Dosage** Adults: Ophthalmic: Instill 1 drop in the affected eye(s) every 8-12 hours
**Dosage Forms** Solution, ophthalmic: 0.025% (5 mL)

**Key-Pred® Injection** *see* prednisolone (systemic) *on page 493*
**Key-Pred-SP® Injection** *see* prednisolone (systemic) *on page 493*
**K-Gen® Effervescent** *see* potassium bicarbonate *on page 484*
**K-Glucon®** *see* potassium gluconate *on page 487*
**KI** *see* potassium iodide *on page 487*
**K-Ide®** *see* potassium bicarbonate and potassium citrate, effervescent *on page 485*
**Kidrolase (Can)** *see* asparaginase *on page 55*
**Kinevac®** *see* sincalide *on page 545*
**Kionex™** *see* sodium polystyrene sulfonate *on page 553*
**Klaron®** *see* sulfacetamide *on page 562*
**Klean-Prep® (Can)** *see* polyethylene glycol solution *on page 480*
**K-Lease®** *see* potassium chloride *on page 485*
**Klerist-D® Tablet [OTC]** *see* chlorpheniramine and pseudoephedrine *on page 130*
**Klonopin™** *see* clonazepam *on page 145*
**K-Lor™** *see* potassium chloride *on page 485*
**Klor-Con®** *see* potassium chloride *on page 485*
**Klor-Con® 8** *see* potassium chloride *on page 485*
**Klor-Con® 10** *see* potassium chloride *on page 485*
**Klor-Con®/25** *see* potassium chloride *on page 485*
**Klor-Con®/EF** *see* potassium bicarbonate and potassium citrate, effervescent *on page 485*
**Klorvess® Effervescent** *see* potassium bicarbonate and potassium chloride, effervescent *on page 485*
**Klotrix®** *see* potassium chloride *on page 485*
**K-Lyte®** *see* potassium bicarbonate and potassium citrate, effervescent *on page 485*
**K/Lyte/CL®** *see* potassium bicarbonate and potassium chloride, effervescent *on page 485*
**K-Lyte® Effervescent** *see* potassium bicarbonate *on page 484*
**K-Norm®** *see* potassium chloride *on page 485*
**Koāte®-DVI** *see* antihemophilic factor (human) *on page 43*
**Koāte®-HP** *see* antihemophilic factor (human) *on page 43*
**Koāte®-HS Injection *(Discontinued)*** *see page 750*
**Koāte®-HT Injection *(Discontinued)*** *see page 750*
**Koffex DM-D (Can)** *see* pseudoephedrine and dextromethorphan *on page 508*

**Koffex DM + Decongestant (Can)** *see* guaifenesin, pseudoephedrine, and dextromethorphan *on page 285*

**Koffex DM + Expectorant (Can)** *see* guaifenesin and dextromethorphan *on page 282*

**Koffex Expectorant (Can)** *see* guaifenesin *on page 281*

**Kogenate®** *see* antihemophilic factor (recombinant) *on page 44*

**Kogenate® FS** *see* antihemophilic factor (recombinant) *on page 44*

**Kolephrin® [OTC]** *see* acetaminophen, chlorpheniramine, and pseudoephedrine *on page 6*

**Kolephrin® GG/DM [OTC]** *see* guaifenesin and dextromethorphan *on page 282*

**Kolyum® Powder *(Discontinued)*** *see page 750*

**Konakion® Injection *(Discontinued)*** *see page 750*

**Kondon's Nasal® *(Discontinued)*** *see page 750*

**Konsyl® [OTC]** *see* psyllium *on page 509*

**Konsyl-D® [OTC]** *see* psyllium *on page 509*

**Konȳne® 80** *see* factor IX complex (human) *on page 238*

**Konyne-HT® Injection *(Discontinued)*** *see page 750*

**Koromex® [OTC]** *see* nonoxynol 9 *on page 424*

**K-Pek II® [OTC]** *see* loperamide *on page 354*

**K-Phos® Neutral** *see* potassium phosphate and sodium phosphate *on page 488*

**K-Phos® Original** *see* potassium acid phosphate *on page 484*

**Kristalose™** *see* lactulose *on page 338*

**K-Tab®** *see* potassium chloride *on page 485*

**Kutrase®** *see* pancrelipase *on page 448*

**Ku-Zyme®** *see* pancrelipase *on page 448*

**Ku-Zyme® HP** *see* pancrelipase *on page 448*

**K-Vescent®** *see* potassium bicarbonate and potassium citrate, effervescent *on page 485*

**Kwelcof®** *see* hydrocodone and guaifenesin *on page 301*

**Kwell® *(Discontinued)*** *see page 750*

**Kwellada-P™ (Can)** *see* permethrin *on page 462*

**Kytril™** *see* granisetron *on page 280*

***L*-3-hydroxytyrosine** *see* levodopa *on page 345*

**LA-12® *(Discontinued)*** *see page 750*

## labetalol (la BET a lole)

**Synonyms** ibidomide

**U.S./Canadian Brand Names** Normodyne®; Trandate®

**Therapeutic Category** Alpha-/Beta- Adrenergic Blocker

**Use** Treatment of mild to severe hypertension; I.V. for hypertensive emergencies

**Usual Dosage**

Children: Limited information regarding labetalol use in pediatric patients is currently available in literature. Some centers recommend initial oral doses of 4 mg/kg/day in 2 divided doses. Reported oral doses have started at 3 mg/kg/day and 20 mg/kg/day and have increased up to 40 mg/kg/day.

I.V., intermittent bolus doses of 0.3-1 mg/kg/dose have been reported

For treatment of pediatric hypertensive emergencies, initial continuous infusions of 0.4-1 mg/kg/hour with a maximum of 3 mg/kg/hour have been used.

Due to limited documentation of its use, labetalol should be initiated cautiously in pediatric patients with careful dosage adjustment and blood pressure monitoring

Adults:

Oral: Initial: 100 mg twice daily, may increase as needed every 2-3 days by 100 mg until desired response is obtained; usual dose: 200-400 mg twice daily; not to exceed 2.4 g/day

I.V.: 20 mg or 1-2 mg/kg whichever is lower, IVP over 2 minutes, may administer 40-80 mg at 10-minute intervals, up to 300 mg total dose

I.V. infusion: Initial: 2 mg/minute; titrate to response

**Dosage Forms**

Injection, as hydrochloride: 5 mg/mL (20 mL, 40 mL, 60 mL)

Tablet, as hydrochloride: 100 mg, 200 mg, 300 mg

**Lac-Hydrin®** *see* lactic acid with ammonium hydroxide *on this page*

**Lacril® Ophthalmic Solution [OTC]** *see* artificial tears *on page 53*

**Lacrinorm (Can)** *see* carbopol 940 *(Canada only) on page 109*

**Lacrisert®** *see* hydroxypropyl cellulose *on page 307*

**LactAid® [OTC]** *see* lactase *on this page*

## lactase (LAK tase)

**U.S./Canadian Brand Names** Dairyaid® (Can); Dairy Ease® [OTC]; LactAid® [OTC]; Lactrase® [OTC]

**Therapeutic Category** Nutritional Supplement

**Use** Help digest lactose in milk for patients with lactose intolerance

**Usual Dosage** Oral:

Capsule: 1-2 capsules administered with milk or meal; pretreat milk with 1-2 capsules per quart of milk

Liquid: 5-15 drops per quart of milk

Tablet: 1-3 tablets with meals

**Dosage Forms**

Caplet: 3000 FCC lactase units

Capsule: 250 mg

Liquid: 1250 neutral lactase units/5 drops

Tablet, chewable: 3300 FCC lactase units

## lactic acid and sodium-PCA (LAK tik AS id & SOW dee um-pee see aye)

**Synonyms** sodium-pca and lactic acid

**U.S./Canadian Brand Names** LactiCare® [OTC]

**Therapeutic Category** Topical Skin Product

**Use** Lubricate and moisturize the skin counteracting dryness and itching

**Usual Dosage** Topical: Apply as needed

**Dosage Forms** Lotion, topical: Lactic acid 5% and sodium-PCA 2.5% (240 mL)

## lactic acid with ammonium hydroxide

(LAK tik AS id with a MOE nee um hye DROKS ide)

**Synonyms** ammonium lactate

**U.S./Canadian Brand Names** Lac-Hydrin®

**Therapeutic Category** Topical Skin Product

**Use** Treatment of moderate to severe xerosis and ichthyosis vulgaris

**Usual Dosage** Topical: Shake well; apply to affected areas, use twice daily, rub in well

**Dosage Forms** Lotion: Lactic acid 12% with ammonium hydroxide (150 mL)

**LactiCare® [OTC]** *see* lactic acid and sodium-PCA *on this page*

**LactiCare-HC® Topical** *see* hydrocortisone (topical) *on page 304*

**Lactinex® [OTC]** *see* Lactobacillus *on next page*

## Lactobacillus (lak toe ba SIL us)

**Synonyms** *Lactobacillus acidophilus*; *Lactobacillus acidophilus* and *Lactobacillus bulgaricus*

**U.S./Canadian Brand Names** Bacid® [OTC]; Fermalac (Can); Lactinex® [OTC]; More-Dophilus® [OTC]

**Therapeutic Category** Gastrointestinal Agent, Miscellaneous

**Use** Uncomplicated diarrhea particularly that caused by antibiotic therapy; re-establish normal physiologic and bacterial flora of the intestinal tract

**Usual Dosage** Children >3 years and Adults: Oral:

Capsules: 2 capsules 2-4 times/day

Granules: 1 packet added to or taken with cereal, food, milk, fruit juice, or water, 3-4 times/day

Powder: ¼-1 teaspoonful 1-3 times/daily with liquid

Tablet, chewable: 4 tablets 3-4 times/day; may follow each dose with a small amount of milk, fruit juice, or water

**Dosage Forms**

Capsule:

Bacid®: *Lactobacillus acidophilus* cultured strain ≥500 million viable (50s, 100s)

Pro-Bionate®: *Lactobacillus acidophilus* strain NAS 2 billion units/g

Granules (Lactinex®): *Lactobacillus acidophilus* and *Lactobacillus bulgaricus* mixed culture (1 g/packet-12s)

Powder:

MoreDophilus®: Acidophilus-carrot derivative 4 billion units/g

Pro-Bionate®: *Lactobacillus acidophilus* strain NAS 2 billion units/g

Tablet, chewable (Lactinex®): *Lactobacillus acidophilus* and *Lactobacillus bulgaricus* mixed culture (50s)

***Lactobacillus acidophilus*** *see* Lactobacillus *on this page*

***Lactobacillus acidophilus* and *Lactobacillus bulgaricus*** *see* Lactobacillus *on this page*

**lactoflavin** *see* riboflavin *on page 525*

**Lactrase® [OTC]** *see* lactase *on previous page*

## lactulose (LAK tyoo lose)

**U.S./Canadian Brand Names** Acilac (Can); Cephulac®; Cholac®; Chronulac®; Constilac®; Constulose®; Duphalac®; Enulose®; Evalose®; Heptalac®; Kristalose™; Lactulose PSE®; Laxilose (Can); PMS-Lactulose (Can)

**Therapeutic Category** Ammonium Detoxicant; Laxative

**Use** Adjunct in the prevention and treatment of portal-systemic encephalopathy (PSE); treatment of chronic constipation

**Usual Dosage** Oral:

Infants: 2.5-10 mL/day divided 3-4 times/day

Children: 40-90 mL/day divided 3-4 times/day

Adults:

Acute episodes of portal systemic encephalopathy: 30-45 mL at 1- to 2-hour intervals until laxative effect observed

Chronic therapy: 30-45 mL/dose 3-4 times/day; titrate dose to produce 2-3 soft stools per day

Rectal: 300 mL diluted with 700 mL of water or normal saline, and administered via a rectal balloon catheter and retained for 30-60 minutes; may administer every 4-6 hours

**Dosage Forms**

Powder for reconstitution: 10 g, 20 g,

Syrup: 10 g/15 mL (15 mL, 30 mL, 237 mL, 473 mL, 946 mL, 1890 mL)

**Lactulose PSE®** *see* lactulose *on this page*

**L-AmB** *see* amphotericin B liposomal *on page 38*

**Lamictal®** *see* lamotrigine *on this page*

**Lamictal® CD** *see* lamotrigine *on this page*

**Lamisil® Cream** *see* terbinafine (topical) *on page 574*

**Lamisil® Oral** *see* terbinafine (oral) *on page 574*

## lamivudine (la MI vyoo deen)

**Synonyms** 3TC

**U.S./Canadian Brand Names** Epivir®; Epivir®-HBV™; Heptovir® (Can); 3TC® (Can)

**Therapeutic Category** Antiviral Agent

**Use**

Epivir®: In combination with zidovudine for treatment of HIV infection when therapy is warranted based on clinical and/or immunological evidence of disease progression

Epivir®-HBV™: Treatment of chronic hepatitis B associated with evidence of hepatitis B viral replication and active liver inflammation

**Usual Dosage** Oral:

Hepatitis B virus (HBV): 100 mg once daily

HIV:

Adolescents 12-16 years and Adults: 150 mg twice daily with zidovudine

Adults <50 kg: 2 mg/kg twice daily with zidovudine

**Dosage Forms**

Solution, oral:

Epivir®: 10 mg/mL (240 mL)

Epivir®-HBV™: 5 mg/mL (240 mL)

Tablet:

Epivir®: 150 mg

Epivir®-HBV™: 100 mg

## lamotrigine (la MOE tri jeen)

**Synonyms** LTG

**U.S./Canadian Brand Names** Lamictal®; Lamictal® CD

**Therapeutic Category** Anticonvulsant

**Use** Adjunctive treatment of partial seizures, with or without secondary generalized seizures; investigations for absence, generalized tonic-clonic, atypical absence, myoclonic seizures, and Lennox-Gastaut syndrome are in progress

**Usual Dosage** Oral:

Children: 2-12 years: **Note:** Only whole tablets should be used for dosing, rounded down to the nearest whole tablet

With concomitant antiepileptic drug (AED) regimen with valproic acid (VPA) therapy: 0.15 mg/kg/day in 1-2 divided doses for 2 weeks, then 0.3 mg/kg/day in 1-2 divided doses for 2 weeks; thereafter, titrate by additional 0.3 mg/kg/day every 1-2 weeks; usual maintenance dose: 1-5 mg/kg/day (maximum: 200 mg/day)

With concomitant enzyme-inducing AED regimen without VPA: 0.6 mg/kg/day for 2 weeks, then 1.2 mg/kg/day for 2 weeks; thereafter, titrate by additional 1.2 mg/kg/day every 1-2 weeks; usual maintenance dose: 5-15 mg/kg/day (maximum: 400 mg/day)

Adults: Initial dose: 50 mg/day for 2 weeks, then 100 mg in 2 doses for 2 weeks; thereafter, daily dose can be increased by 100 mg every 1-2 weeks to 300-500 mg/day given in 2 divided doses

With concomitant VPA therapy and other AEDs: 25 mg every other day for 2 weeks; 25 mg/day for 2 weeks; thereafter, dose may be increased by 25-50 mg/day every 1-2 weeks to 150 mg/day given in 2 divided doses

**Dosage Forms**

Tablet: 25 mg, 100 mg, 150 mg, 200 mg

Tablet, dispersible, chewable: 2 mg, 5 mg, 25 mg

**Lamprene®** *see* clofazimine *on page 144*

**Lamprene® 100 mg *(Discontinued)*** *see page 750*

**Lanacane® [OTC]** *see* benzocaine *on page 72*

**Lanacort® Topical [OTC]** *see* hydrocortisone (topical) *on page 304*

**Lanaphilic® Topical [OTC]** *see* urea *on page 617*

**Laniazid® Tablet *(Discontinued)*** *see page 750*

**Laniroif®** *see* butalbital compound and aspirin *on page 93*

## lanolin, cetyl alcohol, glycerin, and petrolatum

(LAN oh lin, SEE til AL koe hol, GLIS er in, & pe troe LAY tum)

**U.S./Canadian Brand Names** Lubriderm® [OTC]

**Therapeutic Category** Topical Skin Product

**Use** Treatment of dry skin

**Usual Dosage** Topical: Apply to skin as necessary

**Dosage Forms** Lotion: 480 mL

**Lanorinal® *(Discontinued)*** *see page 750*

**Lanoxicaps®** *see* digoxin *on page 185*

**Lanoxin®** *see* digoxin *on page 185*

## lansoprazole (lan SOE pra zole)

**U.S./Canadian Brand Names** Prevacid®

**Therapeutic Category** Gastric Acid Secretion Inhibitor

**Use** Short-term treatment of active duodenal ulcers; maintenance treatment of healed duodenal ulcers; as part of a multidrug regimen for *H. pylori* eradication to reduce the risk of duodenal ulcer recurrence; short-term treatment of active benign gastric ulcer; treatment of NSAID-associated gastric ulcer; to reduce the risk of NSAID-associated gastric ulcer in patients with a history of gastric ulcer who require an NSAID; short-term treatment of symptomatic GERD; short-term treatment for all grades of erosive esophagitis; to maintain healing of erosive esophagitis; long-term treatment of pathological hypersecretory conditions, including Zollinger-Ellison syndrome

**Usual Dosage**

Duodenal or gastric ulcer:

Treatment: 15 mg once daily for 4 weeks

Maintenance (healed): 15 mg once daily

Erosive esophagitis:

Treatment: 30 mg once daily for up to 8 weeks; may give for additional 8 weeks for patients who do not heal with the first 8 weeks; if recurrence or erosive esophagitis, consider an additional 8-week course

Maintenance (healing): 15 mg once daily

Hypersecretory conditions: 30-180 mg once daily, titrated to reduce acid secretion to <10 mEq/hour (5 mEq/hour in patients with prior gastric surgery)

**Dosage Forms** Capsule, delayed release: 15 mg, 30 mg

## lansoprazole, amoxicillin, and clarithromycin

(lan SOE pra zole, a moks i SIL in, & kla RITH roe mye sin)

**U.S./Canadian Brand Names** Prevpac™

**Therapeutic Category** Antibiotic, Macrolide Combination; Antibiotic, Penicillin; Gastrointestinal Agent, Miscellaneous

**Use** Eradication of *H. pylori* to reduce the risk of recurrent duodenal ulcer

**Dosage Forms** The package contains:

Amoxicillin: 500 mg capsules

Clarithromycin: 500 mg tablets

Lansoprazole: 30 mg capsules

**Lantus®** *see* insulin preparations *on page 319*

**Lanvis® (Can)** *see* thioguanine *on page 585*

**Largactil® (Can)** *see* chlorpromazine *on page 132*

**Largon®** ***(Discontinued)*** *see page 750*

**Lariam®** *see* mefloquine *on page 369*

**Larodopa®** *see* levodopa *on page 345*

**Lasan™ HP-1 Topical** ***(Discontinued)*** *see page 750*

**Lasan™ Topical** ***(Discontinued)*** *see page 750*

**Lasix®** *see* furosemide *on page 267*

**Lassar's zinc paste** *see* zinc oxide *on page 639*

## latanoprost (la TAN oh prost)

**U.S./Canadian Brand Names** Xalatan®

**Therapeutic Category** Prostaglandin

**Use** Prostaglandin analog to reduce intraocular pressure that occurs in patients with glaucoma who cannot tolerate or have not responded to any other available treatments

**Usual Dosage** Ophthalmic:

Children: Not recommended

Adults: 1 drop in affected eye(s) once daily in the evening

**Dosage Forms** Solution, ophthalmic: 0.005% (2.5 mL, 3 mL, 25 mL)

***Latrodectus mactans*** **antivenin** *see* antivenin (*Latrodectus mactans*) *on page 46*

**Lavacol® [OTC]** *see* alcohol (ethyl) *on page 18*

**lavage solution** *see* polyethylene glycol solution *on page 480*

**Laxagel® [OTC]** *see* senna *on page 541*

**Laxilose (Can)** *see* lactulose *on page 338*

***l*-bunolol** *see* levobunolol *on page 344*

***l*-carnitine** *see* levocarnitine *on page 345*

**LCD** *see* coal tar *on page 149*

**LCR** *see* vincristine *on page 628*

***l*-deprenyl** *see* selegiline *on page 540*

***l*-dopa** *see* levodopa *on page 345*

**Lectopam® (Can)** *see* bromazepam *(Canada only) on page 86*

**Ledercillin VK®** ***(Discontinued)*** *see page 750*

**Lederplex® [OTC]** *see* vitamin B complex *on page 630*

## leflunomide (le FLU no mide)

**U.S./Canadian Brand Names** Arava™

**Therapeutic Category** Anti-inflammatory Agent

**Use** Treatment of active rheumatoid arthritis to reduce signs and symptoms and to retard structural damage as evidenced by X-ray erosions and joint space narrowing

**Usual Dosage** Oral:

Adults: Initial: 100 mg/day for 3 days, followed by 20 mg/day; dosage may be decreased to 10 mg/day in patients who have difficulty tolerating the 20 mg dose. Due to the long half-life of the active metabolite, plasma levels may require a prolonged period to decline after dosage reduction.

Guidelines for dosage adjustment or discontinuation based on the severity and persistence of ALT elevation have been developed. For ALT elevations >2 times the upper limit of normal, dosage reduction to 10 mg/day may allow continued administration. Cholestyramine 8 g 3 times/day for 1-3 days may be administered to decrease plasma levels. If elevations >2 times but less than or equal to 3 times the upper limit of normal persist, liver biopsy is recommended. If elevations >3 times the upper limit of normal

(Continued)

## leflunomide *(Continued)*

persist despite cholestyramine administration and dosage reduction, leflunomide should be discontinued and drug elimination should be enhanced with additional cholestyramine as indicated.

Elderly: Although hepatic function may decline with age, no specific dosage adjustment is recommended; patients should be monitored closely for adverse effects which may require dosage adjustment

**Dosage Forms** Tablet: 10 mg, 20 mg, 100 mg

**Legatrin® PM Advanced Formula [OTC]** *see* acetaminophen and diphenhydramine *on page 5*

**Leg Cramp Relief PM® [OTC]** *see* acetaminophen and diphenhydramine *on page 5*

**Lenoltec No 1, 2, 3, 4 (Can)** *see* acetaminophen and codeine *on page 4*

**Lente® Iletin® I** *see* insulin preparations *on page 319*

**Lente® Iletin® II** *see* insulin preparations *on page 319*

**Lente® Insulin** *see* insulin preparations *on page 319*

**Lente® L** *see* insulin preparations *on page 319*

## lepirudin (leh puh ROO din)

**U.S./Canadian Brand Names** Refludan®

**Therapeutic Category** Anticoagulant

**Use** Indicated for anticoagulation in patient with heparin-induced thrombocytopenia (HIT) and associated thromboembolic disease in order to prevent further thromboembolic complications

**Usual Dosage** Maximum dose: Do not exceed 0.21 mg/kg/hour unless an evaluation of coagulation abnormalities limiting response has been completed; dosing is weight-based, however patients weighing >110 kg should not receive doses greater than the recommended dose for a patient weighing 110 kg (44 mg bolus and initial maximal infusion rate of 16.5 mg/hour)

Use in patients with heparin-induced thrombocytopenia: Bolus dose: 0.4 mg/kg IVP (over 15-20 seconds), followed by continuous infusion at 0.15 mg/kg/hour; bolus and infusion must be reduced in renal insufficiency

Concomitant use with thrombolytic therapy: Bolus dose: 0.2 mg/kg IVP (over 15-20 seconds), followed by continuous infusion at 0.1 mg/kg/hour

Dosing adjustments during infusions: Monitor first APTT 4 hours after the start of the infusion; subsequent determinations of APTT should be obtained at least once daily during treatment; more frequent monitoring is recommended in renally impaired patients; any APTT out of range should be confirmed prior to adjusting dose, unless a clinical need for immediate reaction exists; if the APTT is below target range, increase infusion by 20%; if the APTT is in excess of the target range, decrease infusion rate by 50%; a repeat APTT should be obtained 4 hours after any dosing change

**Dosage Forms** Injection: 50 mg

**Lescol®** *see* fluvastatin *on page 262*

**Lescol® XL** *see* fluvastatin *on page 262*

## letrozole (LET roe zole)

**U.S./Canadian Brand Names** Femara®

**Therapeutic Category** Antineoplastic Agent

**Use** Treatment of advanced breast cancer in postmenopausal women with disease progression following tamoxifen therapy. Patients with ER-negative disease and patients who did not respond to tamoxifen therapy rarely responded to anastrozole.

**Usual Dosage** Adults: Oral: 2.5 mg once/day, without regard to meals

**Dosage Forms** Tablet: 2.5 mg

## leucovorin (loo koe VOR in)

**Synonyms** citrovorum factor; folinic acid; 5-formyl tetrahydrofolate

**U.S./Canadian Brand Names** Wellcovorin®

**Therapeutic Category** Folic Acid Derivative

**Use** Antidote for folic acid antagonists; treatment of folate deficient megaloblastic anemias of infancy, sprue, pregnancy; nutritional deficiency when oral folate therapy is not possible

**Usual Dosage** Children and Adults:

Adjunctive therapy with antimicrobial agents (pyrimethamine): Oral: 2-15 mg/day for 3 days or until blood counts are normal or 5 mg every 3 days; doses of 6 mg/day are needed for patients with platelet counts <100,000/mm$^3$

Folate-deficient megaloblastic anemia: I.M.: 1 mg/day

Megaloblastic anemia secondary to congenital deficiency of dihydrofolate reductase: I.M.: 3-6 mg/day

Rescue dose: I.V.: 10 mg/m$^2$ to start, then 10 mg/m$^2$ every 6 hours orally for 72 hours; if serum creatinine 24 hours after methotrexate is elevated 50% or more **or** the serum MTX concentration is >5 x 10$^{-6}$M, increase dose to 100 mg/m$^2$/dose every 3 hours until serum methotrexate level is less than 1 x 10$^{-8}$M

**Dosage Forms**

Injection, as calcium: 3 mg/mL (1 mL)

Powder for injection, as calcium: 25 mg, 50 mg, 100 mg, 350 mg

Powder for oral solution, as calcium: 1 mg/mL (60 mL)

Tablet, as calcium: 5 mg, 10 mg, 15 mg, 25 mg

**Leukeran®** *see* chlorambucil *on page 124*

**Leukine™** *see* sargramostim *on page 537*

## leuprolide acetate (loo PROE lide AS e tate)

**U.S./Canadian Brand Names** Lupron®; Lupron Depot®; Lupron Depot-3® Month; Lupron Depot-4® Month; Lupron Depot-Ped®

**Therapeutic Category** Antineoplastic Agent; Luteinizing Hormone-Releasing Hormone Analog

**Use** Treatment of precocious puberty; palliative treatment of advanced prostate carcinoma

**Usual Dosage**

Children: S.C.: Precocious puberty: 20-45 mcg/kg/day

Adults:

Advanced prostatic carcinoma:

S.C.: 1 mg/day **or**

I.M. (suspension): 7.5 mg/dose administered monthly

Endometriosis: ≥18 years: I.M.: 3.75 mg/month for 6 months

**Dosage Forms**

Injection: 5 mg/mL (2.8 mL)

Powder for injection (depot):

Depot®: 3.75 mg, 7.5 mg

Depot-3® Month: 11.25 mg, 22.5 mg

Depot-4® Month: 30 mg

Depot-Ped™: 7.5 mg, 11.25 mg, 15 mg

**leurocristine** *see* vincristine *on page 628*

**Leustatin™** *see* cladribine *on page 140*

## levalbuterol (leve al BYOO ter ole)

**Synonyms** R-albuterol

**U.S./Canadian Brand Names** Xopenex™

**Therapeutic Category** Adrenergic Agonist Agent; Beta$_2$-Adrenergic Agonist Agent; Bronchodilator

(Continued)

## levalbuterol *(Continued)*

**Use** Treatment or prevention of bronchospasm in adults and adolescents ≥12 years of age with reversible obstructive airway disease

**Usual Dosage**

Children: Safety and efficacy in patients <12 years of age not established

Children >12 years and Adults: Inhalation: 0.63 mg 3 times/day at intervals of 6-8 hours, via nebulization. Dosage may be increased to 1.25 mg 3 times/day with close monitoring for adverse effects. Most patients gain optimal benefit from regular use

Elderly: Only a small number of patients have been studied. Although greater sensitivity of some elderly patients cannot be ruled out, no overall differences in safety or effectiveness were observed. An initial dose of 0.63 mg should be used in all patients >65 years of age.

**Dosage Forms** Solution, inhalation: 0.63 mg/3 mL, 1.25 mg/3 mL

## levamisole (lee VAM i sole)

**U.S./Canadian Brand Names** Ergamisol®; Novo-Levamisole (Can)

**Therapeutic Category** Immune Modulator

**Use** Adjuvant treatment with fluorouracil in Dukes stage C colon cancer

**Usual Dosage** Oral: Initial: 50 mg every 8 hours for 3 days, then 50 mg every 8 hours for 3 days every 2 weeks (fluorouracil is always administered concomitantly)

**Dosage Forms** Tablet, as base: 50 mg

**Levaquin™** *see* levofloxacin *on page 346*

**Levatol®** *see* penbutolol *on page 454*

**Levbid®** *see* hyoscyamine *on page 309*

## levetiracetam (lev e tir AS e tam)

**U.S./Canadian Brand Names** Keppra®

**Therapeutic Category** Anticonvulsant, Miscellaneous

**Use** Indicated as adjunctive therapy in the treatment of partial onset seizures in adults with epilepsy

**Usual Dosage** Adults: Initial: 500 mg twice daily; additional dosing increments may be given (1000 mg/day additional every 2 weeks) to a maximum recommended daily dose of 3000 mg

**Dosage Forms** Tablet: 250 mg, 500 mg, 750 mg

**Levlen®** *see* ethinyl estradiol and levonorgestrel *on page 232*

**Levlite™** *see* ethinyl estradiol and levonorgestrel *on page 232*

## levobetaxolol (lee voe be TAX oh lol)

**U.S./Canadian Brand Names** Betaxon®

**Therapeutic Category** Beta-Adrenergic Blocker

**Use** Lowers intraocular pressure in patients with chronic open-angle glaucoma or ocular hypertension

**Usual Dosage** Adults: Ophthalmic: Instill 1 drop in affected eye(s) twice daily

**Dosage Forms** Solution, ophthalmic: 0.5% (5 mL, 10 mL, 15 mL)

## levobunolol (lee voe BYOO noe lole)

**Synonyms** *l*-bunolol

**U.S./Canadian Brand Names** Betagan® Liquifilm® Ophthalmic; Novo-Levobunolol (Can); Ophtho-Bunolol® (Can); PMS-Levobunolol (Can)

**Therapeutic Category** Beta-Adrenergic Blocker

**Use** To lower intraocular pressure in chronic open-angle glaucoma or ocular hypertension

**Usual Dosage** Adults: Ophthalmic: 1-2 drops of 0.5% solution in eye(s) once daily or 1-2 drops of 0.25% solution twice daily

**Dosage Forms** Solution, ophthalmic, as hydrochloride: 0.25% (5 mL, 10 mL, 15 mL); 0.5% (2 mL, 5 mL, 10 mL, 15 mL)

## levobupivacaine (LEE voe byoo PIV a kane)

**U.S./Canadian Brand Names** Chirocaine®

**Therapeutic Category** Local Anesthetic; Local Anesthetic, Injectable

**Use** Production of local or regional anesthesia for surgery and obstetrics, and for postoperative pain management

**Usual Dosage** Adults: **Note:** Rapid injection of a large volume of local anesthetic solution should be avoided. Fractional (incremental) doses are recommended.

**Maximum dosage:** Epidural doses up to 375 mg have been administered incrementally to patients during a surgical procedure

Intraoperative block and postoperative pain: 695 mg in 24 hours

Postoperative epidural infusion over 24 hours: 570 mg

Single-fractionated injection for brachial plexus block: 300 mg

**Dosage Forms** Injection: 2.5 mg/mL (10 mL, 30 mL); 5 mg/mL (10 mL, 30 mL); 7.5 mg/mL (10 mL, 30 mL)

## levocabastine (LEE voe kab as teen)

**U.S./Canadian Brand Names** Livostin®

**Therapeutic Category** Antihistamine

**Use** Temporary relief of the signs and symptoms of seasonal allergic conjunctivitis

**Usual Dosage** Adults: Ophthalmic: Instill 1 drop in affected eye 4 times/day for up to 2 weeks

**Dosage Forms** Suspension, ophthalmic, as hydrochloride: 0.05% (5 mL, 10 mL)

## levocarnitine (lee voe KAR ni teen)

**Synonyms** *l*-carnitine

**U.S./Canadian Brand Names** Carnitor® Injection; Carnitor® Oral; VitaCarn® Oral

**Therapeutic Category** Dietary Supplement

**Use** Treatment of primary or secondary carnitine deficiency

**Usual Dosage** Oral:

Children: 50-100 mg/kg/day divided 2-3 times/day, maximum: 3 g/day; dosage must be individualized based upon patient response; higher dosages have been used

Adults: 1-3 g/day for 50 kg subject; start at 1 g/day, increase slowly assessing tolerance and response

**Dosage Forms**

Capsule: 250 mg

Injection: 1 g/5 mL (5 mL)

Liquid (cherry flavor): 100 mg/mL (10 mL)

Tablet: 330 mg

## levodopa (lee voe DOE pa)

**Synonyms** *L*-3-hydroxytyrosine; *l*-dopa

**U.S./Canadian Brand Names** Larodopa®

**Therapeutic Category** Diagnostic Agent; Dopaminergic Agent (Anti-Parkinson's)

**Use** Diagnostic agent for growth hormone deficiency

**Usual Dosage** Children: Oral (administered as a single dose to evaluate growth hormone deficiency): 0.5 g/m$^2$

**or**

<30 lbs: 125 mg

30-70 lbs: 250 mg

>70 lbs: 500 mg

**Dosage Forms** Tablet: 100 mg, 250 mg, 500 mg

## levodopa and benserazide *(Canada only)*

(lee voe DOE pa & ben SER a zide)

**U.S./Canadian Brand Names** Prolopa® (Can)

**Therapeutic Category** Anti-Parkinson's Agent

**Use** Treatment of Parkinson's syndrome with exception of drug-induced parkinsonism

**Usual Dosage** Adult: Oral: The optimal dose for most patients is usually 4-8 capsules of 100-25 daily (400-800 mg levodopa) divided into 4-6 doses

**Dosage Forms** Capsule:

50-12.5: Levodopa 50 and benserazide 12.5 mg
100-25: Levodopa 100 mg and benserazide 25 mg
200-50: Levodopa 200 mg and benserazide 50 mg

**levodopa and carbidopa** *see* carbidopa and levodopa *on page 107*

**Levo-Dromoran®** *see* levorphanol *on next page*

## levofloxacin (lee voe FLOKS a sin)

**U.S./Canadian Brand Names** Levaquin™; Quixin™ Ophthalmic

**Therapeutic Category** Antibiotic, Ophthalmic; Antibiotic, Quinolone

**Use**

Systemic:

Acute bacterial exacerbation of chronic bronchitis and community-acquired pneumonia due to *S. aureus*, *S. pneumoniae* (including penicillin-resistant strains), *H. influenzae*, *H. parainfluenzae*, or *M. catarrhalis*, *C. pneumoniae*, *L. pneumophila*, or *M. pneumoniae*

Acute maxillary sinusitis due to *S. pneumoniae*, *H. influenzae*, or *M. catarrhalis*

Acute pyelonephritis caused by *E. coli*

Skin or skin structure infections:

Complicated, due to methcillin-susceptible *S. aureus*, *Enterococcus fecalis*, *S. pyogenes*, or *Proteus mirabilis*

Uncomplicated, due to *S. aureus* or *S. pyogenes*

Urinary tract infections:

Complicated, due to gram-negative bacteria (*E. coli*, *Enterobacter cloacae*, *Klebsiella pneumoniae*, *Proteus mirabilis*, *Enterococcus fecalis*, or *Pseudomonas aeruginosa*)

Uncomplicated, due to *E. coli*, *K. pneumoniae*, or *S. saprophyticus*

Ophthalmic: Bacterial conjunctivitis due to *S. aureus* (methicillin-susceptible strains), *S. epidermidis* (methicillin-susceptible strains), *S. pneumoniae*, *Streptococcus* (groups C/F), *Streptococcus* (group G), Viridans group streptococci, *Corynebacterium* spp, *H. influenzae*, *Acinetobacter lwoffii*, or *Serratia marcescens*

**Usual Dosage**

Adults: Oral, I.V. (infuse I.V. solution over 60 minutes):

Acute bacterial exacerbation of chronic bronchitis: 500 mg every 24 hours for at least 7 days

Community-acquired pneumonia: 500 mg every 24 hours for 7-14 days

Acute maxillary sinusitis: 500 mg every 24 hours for 10-14 days

Uncomplicated skin infections: 500 mg every 24 hours for 7-10 days

Complicated skin infections: 750 mg every 24 hours for 7-14 days

Uncomplicated urinary tract infections: 250 mg once daily for 3 days

Complicated urinary tract infections, including acute pyelonephritis: 250 mg every 24 hours for 10 days

Children ≥1 year and Adults: Ophthalmic:

Treatment day 1 and day 2: Instill 1-2 drops into affected eye(s) every 2 hours while awake, up to 8 times/day

Treatment day 3 through day 7: Instill 1-2 drops into affected eye(s) every 4 hours while awake, up to 4 times/day

**Dosage Forms**

Infusion, in $D_5W$: 5 mg/mL (50 mL, 100 mL)
Injection: 25 mg/mL (20 mL)
Solution, ophthalmic: 0.5% (2.5 mL, 5 mL)

Tablet: 250 mg, 500 mg, 750 mg

**levomepromazine** *see* methotrimeprazine *(Canada only)* *on page 381*

## levomethadyl acetate hydrochloride

(lee voe METH a dil AS e tate hye droe KLOR ide)

**U.S./Canadian Brand Names** ORLAAM®

**Therapeutic Category** Analgesic, Narcotic

**Controlled Substance** C-II

**Use** Management of opiate dependence

**Usual Dosage** Adults: Oral: 20-40 mg 3 times/week; range: 10 mg to as high as 140 mg 3 times/week

**Dosage Forms** Solution, oral: 10 mg/mL (474 mL)

## levonorgestrel (LEE voe nor jes trel)

**U.S./Canadian Brand Names** Mirena®; Norplant® Implant; Plan B™

**Therapeutic Category** Contraceptive, Implant (Progestin); Contraceptive, Progestin Only

**Use** Prevention of pregnancy

**Usual Dosage** Adults:

**Long-term prevention of pregnancy:**

Subdermal capsules: Total administration doses (implanted): 216 mg in 6 capsules which should be implanted during the first 7 days of onset of menses subdermally in the upper arm; each Norplant® silastic capsule releases 80 mcg of levonorgestrel/day for 6-18 months, following which a rate of release of 25-30 mcg/day is maintained for ≤5 years; capsules should be removed by end of 5th year

Intrauterine system: To be inserted into uterine cavity; should be inserted within 7 days of onset of menstruation or immediately after first trimester abortion; releases 20 mcg levonorgestrel/day over 5 years. May be removed and replaced with a new unit at anytime during menstrual cycle; do not leave any one system in place for >5 years

**Emergency contraception:** Oral tablet: One 0.75 mg tablet as soon as possible within 72 hours of unprotected sexual intercourse; a second 0.75 mg tablet should be taken 12 hours after the first dose; may be used at any time during menstrual cycle

**Dosage Forms**

Capsule, subdermal implantation (Norplant®): 36 mg (6s)

Intrauterine device (Mirena®): 52 mg

Tablet (Plan B™): 0.75 mg

**Levophed®** *see* norepinephrine *on page 425*

**Levora®** *see* ethinyl estradiol and levonorgestrel *on page 232*

## levorphanol (lee VOR fa nole)

**U.S./Canadian Brand Names** Levo-Dromoran®

**Therapeutic Category** Analgesic, Narcotic

**Controlled Substance** C-II

**Use** Relief of moderate to severe pain; also used parenterally for preoperative sedation and an adjunct to nitrous oxide/oxygen anesthesia

**Usual Dosage** Adults: Oral, S.C.: 2 mg, up to 3 mg if necessary

**Dosage Forms**

Injection, as tartrate: 2 mg/mL (1 mL, 10 mL)

Tablet, as tartrate: 2 mg

**Levo-T™** *see* levothyroxine *on next page*

**Levotabs®** *see* levothyroxine *on next page*

**Levothroid®** *see* levothyroxine *on next page*

## levothyroxine (lee voe thye ROKS een)

**Synonyms** *l*-thyroxine; $t_4$ thyroxine

**U.S./Canadian Brand Names** Eltroxin® (Can); Levo-T™; Levotabs®; Levothroid®; Levoxyl®; Synthroid®; Thyrox®; Unithroid®

**Therapeutic Category** Thyroid Product

**Use** Replacement or supplemental therapy in hypothyroidism; management of nontoxic goiter, chronic lymphocytic thyroiditis, as an adjunct to thyrotoxicosis

**Usual Dosage**

Children:

Oral:

0-6 months: 8-10 mcg/kg/day

6-12 months: 6-8 mcg/kg/day

1-5 years: 5-6 mcg/kg/day

6-12 years: 4-5 mcg/kg/day

>12 years: 2-3 mcg/kg/day

I.M., I.V.: 75% of the oral dose

Adults:

Oral: 12.5-50 mcg/day to start, then increase by 25-50 mcg/day at intervals of 2-4 weeks; average adult dose: 100-200 mcg/day

I.M., I.V.: 50% of the oral dose

Myxedema coma or stupor: I.V.: 200-500 mcg one time, then 100-300 mcg the next day if necessary

**Dosage Forms**

Powder for injection, as sodium, lyophilized: 200 mcg/vial (6 mL, 10 mL); 500 mcg/vial (6 mL, 10 mL)

Tablet, as sodium: 25 mcg, 50 mcg, 75 mcg, 88 mcg, 100 mcg, 112 mcg, 125 mcg, 137 mcg, 150 mcg, 175 mcg, 200 mcg, 300 mcg

**Levoxyl®** *see* levothyroxine *on this page*

**Levsin®** *see* hyoscyamine *on page 309*

**Levsinex®** *see* hyoscyamine *on page 309*

**Levsin/SL®** *see* hyoscyamine *on page 309*

**Levulan® Kerastick™** *see* aminolevulinic acid *on page 31*

**Lexxel™** *see* enalapril and felodipine *on page 213*

**LHRH** *see* gonadorelin *on page 279*

***l*-hyoscyamine sulfate** *see* hyoscyamine *on page 309*

**Librax®** *see* clidinium and chlordiazepoxide *on page 142*

**Libritabs® (all products) *(Discontinued)*** *see page 750*

**Librium®** *see* chlordiazepoxide *on page 125*

**Lice-Enz® Shampoo [OTC]** *see* pyrethrins *on page 510*

**Lida-Mantle HC® Topical** *see* lidocaine and hydrocortisone *on page 350*

**Lidemol® (Can)** *see* fluocinonide *on page 254*

**Lidex®** *see* fluocinonide *on page 254*

**Lidex-E®** *see* fluocinonide *on page 254*

## lidocaine (LYE doe kane)

**Synonyms** lignocaine

**U.S./Canadian Brand Names** Anestacon® Topical Solution; Dilocaine® Injection; Duo-Trach® Injection; Lidodan™ (Can); LidoPen® I.M. Injection Auto-Injector; Nervocaine® Injection; Xylocaine® HCl I.V. Injection for Cardiac Arrhythmias; Xylocaine® Oral; Xylocaine® Topical Ointment; Xylocaine® Topical Solution; Xylocaine® Topical Spray; Xylocard® (Can)

**Therapeutic Category** Analgesic, Topical; Antiarrhythmic Agent, Class I-B; Local Anesthetic

**Use** Drug of choice for ventricular ectopy, ventricular tachycardia (VT), ventricular fibrillation (VF); for pulseless VT or VF preferably administer **after** defibrillation and epinephrine; control of premature ventricular contractions, wide-complex PSVT; local anesthetic

**Usual Dosage**

Topical: Apply to affected area as needed; maximum: 3 mg/kg/dose; do not repeat within 2 hours

Injectable local anesthetic: Varies with procedure, degree of anesthesia needed, vascularity of tissue, duration of anesthesia required, and physical condition of patient; maximum: 4.5 mg/kg/dose; do not repeat within 2 hours

Children: Endotracheal, I.O., I.V.: Loading dose: 1 mg/kg; may repeat in 10-15 minutes to a maximum total dose of 5 mg/kg; after loading dose, start I.V. continuous infusion 20-50 mcg/kg/minute. Use 20 mcg/kg/minute in patients with shock, hepatic disease, mild congestive heart failure (CHF); moderate to severe CHF may require $^1/_2$ loading dose and lower infusion rates to avoid toxicity. Endotracheal doses should be diluted to 1-2 mL with normal saline prior to endotracheal administration and may need 2-3 times the I.V. dose.

Adults: Antiarrhythmic:

Endotracheal: Total dose: 5 mg/kg; follow with 0.5 mg/kg in 10 minutes if effective

I.M.: 300 mg may be repeated in 1-1$^1/_2$ hours

I.V.: Loading dose: 1 mg/kg/dose, then 50-100 mg bolus over 2-3 minutes; may repeat in 5-10 minutes up to 200-300 mg in a 1-hour period; continuous infusion of 20-50 mcg/kg/minute or 1-4 mg/minute; decrease the dose in patients with CHF, shock, or hepatic disease

**Dosage Forms**

Cream, as hydrochloride: 2% (56 g)

Injection, as hydrochloride: 0.5% [5 mg/mL] (50 mL); 1% [10 mg/mL] (2 mL, 5 mL, 10 mL, 20 mL, 30 mL, 50 mL); 1.5% [15 mg/mL] (20 mL); 2% [20 mg/mL] (2 mL, 5 mL, 10 mL, 20 mL, 30 mL, 50 mL); 4% [40 mg/mL] (5 mL); 10% [100 mg/mL] (10 mL); 20% [200 mg/mL] (10 mL, 20 mL)

Injection, as hydrochloride:

I.M. use: 10% [100 mg/mL] (3 mL, 5 mL)

Direct I.V.: 1% [10 mg/mL] (5 mL, 10 mL); 20 mg/mL (5 mL)

I.V. admixture, preservative free: 4% [40 mg/mL] (25 mL, 30 mL); 10% [100 mg/mL] (10 mL); 20% [200 mg/mL] (5 mL, 10 mL)

I.V. infusion, in $D_5W$: 0.2% [2 mg/mL] (500 mL); 0.4% [4 mg/mL] (250 mL, 500 mL, 1000 mL); 0.8% [8 mg/mL] (250 mL, 500 mL)

Gel, as hydrochloride, topical: 2% (30 mL); 2.5% (15 mL)

Kit: 4 g

Liquid, as hydrochloride, topical: 2.5% (7.5 mL)

Liquid, as hydrochloride, viscous: 2% (20 mL, 100 mL)

Ointment, as hydrochloride, topical: 2.5% [OTC], 5% (35 g)

Solution, as hydrochloride, topical: 2% (15 mL, 240 mL); 4% (50 mL)

## lidocaine and epinephrine (LYE doe kane & ep i NEF rin)

**U.S./Canadian Brand Names** Xylocaine® With Epinephrine

**Therapeutic Category** Local Anesthetic

**Use** Local infiltration anesthesia

**Usual Dosage** Children (dosage varies with the anesthetic procedure): Use lidocaine concentrations of 0.5% or 1% (or even more dilute) to decrease possibility of toxicity; lidocaine dose should not exceed 4.5 mg/kg/dose; do not repeat within 2 hours

**Dosage Forms** Injection with epinephrine:

Epinephrine 1:200,000: Lidocaine hydrochloride 0.5% [5 mg/mL] (50 mL); 1% [10 mg/mL] (30 mL); 1.5% [15 mg/mL] (5 mL, 10 mL, 30 mL); 2% [20 mg/mL] (20 mL)

Epinephrine 1:100,000: Lidocaine hydrochloride 1% [10 mg/mL] (20 mL, 50 mL); 2% [20 mg/mL] (1.8 mL, 20 mL, 30 mL, 50 mL)

Epinephrine 1:50,000: Lidocaine hydrochloride 2% [20 mg/mL] (1.8 mL)

## lidocaine and hydrocortisone (LYE doe kane & hye droe KOR ti sone)

**U.S./Canadian Brand Names** Lida-Mantle HC® Topical

**Therapeutic Category** Anesthetic/Corticosteroid

**Use** Topical anti-inflammatory and anesthetic for skin disorders

**Usual Dosage** Topical: Apply 2-4 times/day

**Dosage Forms** Cream: Lidocaine 3% and hydrocortisone 0.5% (15 g, 30 g)

## lidocaine and prilocaine (LYE doe kane & PRIL oh kane)

**U.S./Canadian Brand Names** EMLA®

**Therapeutic Category** Analgesic, Topical

**Use** Topical anesthetic for use on normal intact skin to provide local analgesia for minor procedures such as I.V. cannulation or venipuncture; has also been used for painful procedures such as lumbar puncture and skin graft harvesting

**Usual Dosage** Children and Adults: Topical: Apply a thick layer of cream to intact skin and cover with an occlusive dressing; for minor procedures, apply 2.5 g/site for at least 60 minutes; for painful procedures, apply 2 g/10 $cm^2$ of skin and leave on for at least 2 hours

**Dosage Forms**

Cream: Lidocaine 2.5% and prilocaine 2.5% [2 Tegaderm® dressings] (5 g, 30 g)

Patch: Single-dose, in the form of an occlusive dressing contains: a laminate backing, an absorbent cellulose disc, and an adhesive tape ring; the disc contains 1 g of the EMLA® emulsion, the active contact surface area being approximately 10 $cm^2$; surface area of the entire patch is approximately 40 $cm^2$

**Lidodan™ (Can)** *see* lidocaine *on page 348*

**LidoPen® I.M. Injection Auto-Injector** *see* lidocaine *on page 348*

**lignocaine** *see* lidocaine *on page 348*

**Limbitrol® DS 10-25** *see* amitriptyline and chlordiazepoxide *on page 33*

**Lin-Amox (Can)** *see* amoxicillin *on page 35*

**Lincocin®** *see* lincomycin *on this page*

## lincomycin (lin koe MYE sin)

**U.S./Canadian Brand Names** Bactramycin®; Lincocin®; Lincorex® Injection

**Therapeutic Category** Macrolide (Antibiotic)

**Use** Treatment of susceptible bacterial infections, mainly those caused by streptococci and staphylococci

**Usual Dosage**

Children >1 month:

- I.M.: 10 mg/kg every 12-24 hours
- I.V.: 10-20 mg/kg/day in divided doses 2-3 times/day

Adults:

- I.M.: 600 mg every 12-24 hours
- I.V.: 600-1 g every 8-12 hours up to 8 g/day

**Dosage Forms** Injection, as hydrochloride: 300 mg/mL (2 mL, 10 mL)

**Lincorex® Injection** *see* lincomycin *on this page*

## lindane (LIN dane)

**Synonyms** benzene hexachloride; gamma benzene hexachloride; hexachlorocyclohexane

**U.S./Canadian Brand Names** Hexit® (Can); PMS-Lindane (Can)

**Therapeutic Category** Scabicides/Pediculicides

**Use** Treatment of scabies (*Sarcoptes scabiei*), *Pediculus capitis* (head lice), and *Pediculus pubis* (crab lice)

**Usual Dosage** Children and Adults: Topical:

Scabies: Apply a thin layer of lotion and massage it on skin from the neck to the toes. For adults, bathe and remove the drug after 8-12 hours; for children, wash off 6 hours after application.

Pediculosis: 15-30 mL of shampoo is applied and lathered for 4-5 minutes; rinse hair thoroughly and comb with a fine tooth comb to remove nits; repeat treatment in 7 days if lice or nits are still present

**Dosage Forms**

Lotion: 1% (60 mL, 473 mL, 4000 mL)

Shampoo: 1% (60 mL, 473 mL, 4000 mL)

## linezolid (li NE zoh lid)

**U.S./Canadian Brand Names** Zyvox™

**Therapeutic Category** Antibiotic, Oxozolidinone

**Use** Treatment of vancomycin-resistant *Enterococcus faecium* (VRE) infections, nosocomial pneumonia caused by *Staphylococcus aureus* including MRSA or *Streptococcus pneumoniae* (penicillin-susceptible strains only), complicated and uncomplicated skin and skin structure infections, and community-acquired pneumonia caused by susceptible gram-positive organisms.

**Usual Dosage** Adult:

Oral, I.V.:

VRE infections: 600 mg every 12 hours for 14-28 days

Nosocomial pneumonia, complicated skin and skin structure infections, community-acquired pneumonia including concurrent bacteremia: 600 mg every 12 hours for 10-14 days

Oral: Uncomplicated skin and skin structure infections: 400 mg every 12 hours for 10-14 days

**Dosage Forms**

Infusion: 2 mg/mL (100 mL, 200 mL, 300 mL)

Suspension, oral (orange-flavored): 20 mg/mL (150 mL)

Tablet: 400 mg, 600 mg

**Lin-Megestrol (Can)** *see* megestrol acetate *on page 370*

**Lin-Pravastatin (Can)** *see* pravastatin *on page 491*

**Lioresal®** *see* baclofen *on page 66*

**Liotec (Can)** *see* baclofen *on page 66*

## liothyronine (lye oh THYE roe neen)

**Synonyms** *l*-triiodothyronine; $t_3$ thyronine

**U.S./Canadian Brand Names** Cytomel® Oral; Triostat™ Injection

**Therapeutic Category** Thyroid Product

**Use** Replacement or supplemental therapy in hypothyroidism, management of nontoxic goiter, chronic lymphocytic thyroiditis, as an adjunct in thyrotoxicosis and as a diagnostic aid; levothyroxine is recommended for chronic therapy; (if rapid correction of thyroid is needed, $T_3$ is preferred, but use cautiously and with lower recommended doses)

**Usual Dosage**

Mild hypothyroidism: 25 mcg/day; daily dosage may then be increased by 12.5 or 25 mcg/day every 1 or 2 weeks; maintenance: 25-75 mcg/day

Myxedema: 5mcg/day; may be increased by 5-10 mcg/day every 1-2 weeks; when 25 mcg is reached, dosage may often be increased by 12.5 or 25 mcg every 1 or 2 weeks; maintenance: 50-100 mcg/day

Cretinism: 5 mcg/day with a 5 mcg increment every 3-4 days until the desired response is achieved

Simple (nontoxic) goiter: 5 mcg/day; may be increased every week or two by 5 or 10 mcg; when 25 mcg/day is reached, dosage may be increased every week or two by 12.5 or 25 mcg; maintenance: 75 mcg/day

(Continued)

## liothyronine *(Continued)*

$T_3$ suppression test: $I^{131}$ thyroid uptake is in the borderline-high range, administer 75-100 mcg/day for 7 days then repeat $I^{131}$ thyroid uptake test

Children and Elderly: Start therapy with 5 mcg/day; increase only by 5 mcg increments at the recommended intervals

**Dosage Forms**

Injection, as sodium: 10 mcg/mL (1 mL)

Tablet, as sodium: 5 mcg, 25 mcg, 50 mcg

## liotrix (LYE oh triks)

**Synonyms** $t_3/t_4$ liotrix

**U.S./Canadian Brand Names** Thyrolar®

**Therapeutic Category** Thyroid Product

**Use** Replacement or supplemental therapy in hypothyroidism

**Usual Dosage** Congenital hypothyroidism: Oral:

Children (dose/day):

0-6 months: 8-10 mcg/kg

6-12 months: 6-8 mcg/kg

1-5 years: 5-6 mcg/kg

6-12 years: 4-5 mcg/kg

>12 years: 2-3 mcg/kg

Adults: 30 mg/day, increasing by 15 mg/day at 2- to 3-week intervals to a maximum of 180 mg/day

**Dosage Forms** Tablet: 15 mg, 30 mg, 60 mg, 120 mg, 180 mg [thyroid equivalent]

**lipancreatin** *see* pancrelipase *on page 448*

**lipase, protease, and amylase** *see* pancrelipase *on page 448*

**Lipitor®** *see* atorvastatin *on page 57*

**Liposyn®** *see* fat emulsion *on page 241*

**Lipovite® [OTC]** *see* vitamin B complex *on page 630*

**Lipram®** *see* pancrelipase *on page 448*

**Liquaemin®** ***(Discontinued)*** *see page 750*

**Liquibid®** *see* guaifenesin *on page 281*

**Liqui-Char® [OTC]** *see* charcoal *on page 123*

**liquid antidote** *see* charcoal *on page 123*

**Liquid Barosperse®** *see* radiological/contrast media (ionic) *on page 516*

**Liquid Pred®** ***(Discontinued)*** *see page 750*

**Liqui-E®** *see* tocophersolan *on page 594*

**Liquifilm® Forte Solution [OTC]** *see* artificial tears *on page 53*

**Liquifilm® Tears Solution [OTC]** *see* artificial tears *on page 53*

**Liquipake®** *see* radiological/contrast media (ionic) *on page 516*

## lisinopril (lyse IN oh pril)

**U.S./Canadian Brand Names** Apo®-Lisinopril (Can); Prinivil®; Zestril®

**Therapeutic Category** Angiotensin-Converting Enzyme (ACE) Inhibitor

**Use** Treatment of hypertension, either alone or in combination with other antihypertensive agents

**Usual Dosage** Adults: Oral: 10-40 mg/day in a single dose

**Dosage Forms** Tablet: 2.5 mg, 5 mg, 10 mg, 20 mg, 30 mg, 40 mg

## lisinopril and hydrochlorothiazide

(lyse IN oh pril & hye droe klor oh THYE a zide)

**U.S./Canadian Brand Names** Prinzide®; Zestoretic®

**Therapeutic Category** Antihypertensive Agent, Combination

**Use** Treatment of hypertension

**Usual Dosage** Adults: Oral: Dosage is individualized; see each component for appropriate dosing suggestions

**Dosage Forms** Tablet:

Lisinopril 10 mg and hydrochlorothiazide 12.5 mg
[12.5]-Lisinopril 20 mg and hydrochlorothiazide 12.5 mg
[25]-Lisinopril 20 mg and hydrochlorothiazide 25 mg

**Listerex® Scrub *(Discontinued)*** *see page 750*

**Listermint® with Fluoride [OTC]** *see* fluoride *on page 255*

**Lithane® *(Discontinued)*** *see page 750*

## lithium (LITH ee um)

**U.S./Canadian Brand Names** Carbolith™ (Can); Duralith® (Can); Eskalith®; Eskalith CR®; Lithobid®; PMS-Lithium Carbonate (Can); PMS-Lithium Citrate (Can)

**Therapeutic Category** Antimanic Agent

**Use** Management of acute manic episodes, bipolar disorders, and depression

**Usual Dosage** Oral: Monitor serum concentrations and clinical response (efficacy and toxicity) to determine proper dose

Children: 15-60 mg/kg/day in 3-4 divided doses; dose not to exceed usual adult dosage
Adults: 300 mg 3-4 times/day; usual maximum maintenance dose: 2.4 g/day

**Dosage Forms**

Lithium carbonate:
- Capsule: 150 mg, 300 mg, 600 mg
- Tablet: 300 mg
- Tablet, controlled release: 450 mg (Eskalith CR®)
- Tablet, slow release: 300 mg (Lithobid®)

Lithium citrate:
- Syrup: 300 mg/5 mL (5 mL, 10 mL, 480 mL)

**Lithobid®** *see* lithium *on this page*

**Lithonate® *(Discontinued)*** *see page 750*

**Lithostat®** *see* acetohydroxamic acid *on page 9*

**Lithotabs® *(Discontinued)*** *see page 750*

**Livostin®** *see* levocabastine *on page 345*

**LKV-Drops® [OTC]** *see* vitamin (multiple/pediatric) *on page 632*

## l-lysine (el LYE seen)

**U.S./Canadian Brand Names** Enisyl® [OTC]; Lycolan® Elixir [OTC]

**Therapeutic Category** Dietary Supplement

**Use** Improves utilization of vegetable proteins

**Usual Dosage** Adults: Oral: 334-1500 mg/day

**Dosage Forms** l-lysine hydrochloride:

- Capsule: 500 mg
- Elixir: 100 mg/15 mL with glycine 1800 mg/15 mL and alcohol 12%
- Tablet: 312 mg, 334 mg, 500 mg, 1000 mg

**LMD®** *see* dextran *on page 177*

**LoCHOLEST®** *see* cholestyramine resin *on page 134*

**LoCHOLEST® Light** *see* cholestyramine resin *on page 134*

**Locoid® Topical** *see* hydrocortisone (topical) *on page 304*

**Lodine®** *see* etodolac *on page 236*

**Lodine® XL** *see* etodolac *on page 236*

**Lodosyn®** *see* carbidopa *on page 107*

## lodoxamide tromethamine (loe DOKS a mide troe METH a meen)

**U.S./Canadian Brand Names** Alomide® Ophthalmic

**Therapeutic Category** Mast Cell Stabilizer

**Use** Symptomatic treatment of vernal keratoconjunctivitis, vernal conjunctivitis, and vernal keratitis

**Usual Dosage** Children >2 years and Adults: Ophthalmic: Instill 1-2 drops in eye(s) 4 times/day for up to 3 months

**Dosage Forms** Solution, ophthalmic: 0.1% (10 mL)

**Loestrin®** *see* ethinyl estradiol and norethindrone *on page 232*

**Logen®** ***(Discontinued)*** *see page 750*

**Lomanate®** ***(Discontinued)*** *see page 750*

## lomefloxacin (loe me FLOKS a sin)

**U.S./Canadian Brand Names** Maxaquin®

**Therapeutic Category** Quinolone

**Use** Quinolone antibiotic for skin and skin structure, lower respiratory and urinary tract infections, and sexually transmitted diseases

**Usual Dosage** Adults: Oral: 400 mg once daily for 10-14 days

**Dosage Forms** Tablet, as hydrochloride: 400 mg

**Lomine (Can)** *see* dicyclomine *on page 183*

**Lomocot®** *see* diphenoxylate and atropine *on page 192*

**Lomotil®** *see* diphenoxylate and atropine *on page 192*

## lomustine (loe MUS teen)

**Synonyms** CCNU

**U.S./Canadian Brand Names** CeeNU®

**Therapeutic Category** Antineoplastic Agent

**Use** Treatment of brain tumors, Hodgkin's and non-Hodgkin's lymphomas, melanoma, renal carcinoma, lung cancer, colon cancer

**Usual Dosage** Oral (refer to individual protocol):

Children: 75-150 mg/m$^2$ as a single dose every 6 weeks. Subsequent doses are readjusted after initial treatment according to platelet and leukocyte counts

Adults: 100-130 mg/m$^2$ as a single dose every 6 weeks; readjust after initial treatment according to platelet and leukocyte counts

**Dosage Forms**

Capsule: 10 mg, 40 mg, 100 mg

Dose Pack: 10 mg (2s); 100 mg (2s); 40 mg (2s)

**Loniten® Oral** *see* minoxidil *on page 394*

**Lonox®** *see* diphenoxylate and atropine *on page 192*

**Lo/Ovral®** *see* ethinyl estradiol and norgestrel *on page 233*

**Loperacap (Can)** *see* loperamide *on this page*

## loperamide (loe PER a mide)

**U.S./Canadian Brand Names** Apo®-Loperamide (Can); Diamode® [OTC]; Diarr-Eze (Can); Diarrid® [OTC]; Imodium®; Imodium® A-D [OTC]; Imogen®; Imotil® [OTC]; Imperim® [OTC]; Kaodene A-D® [OTC]; Kao-Paverin® [OTC]; K-Pek II® [OTC]; Loperacap (Can); Novo-Loperamide (Can); PMS-Loperamide (Can); Rho®-Loperamide (Can); Riva-Loperamide (Can)

**Therapeutic Category** Antidiarrheal

**Use** Treatment of acute diarrhea and chronic diarrhea associated with inflammatory bowel disease; chronic functional diarrhea (idiopathic), chronic diarrhea caused by bowel resection or organic lesions; to decrease the volume of ileostomy discharge

**Usual Dosage** Oral:

Children:

Acute diarrhea: 0.4-0.8 mg/kg/day divided every 6-12 hours, maximum: 2 mg/dose

Chronic diarrhea: 0.08-0.24 mg/kg/day divided 2-3 times/day, maximum: 2 mg/dose

Adults: Initial: 4 mg (2 capsules), followed by 2 mg after each loose stool, up to 16 mg/day (8 capsules)

**Dosage Forms**

Caplet, as hydrochloride: 2 mg

Capsule, as hydrochloride: 2 mg

Liquid, oral, as hydrochloride: 1 mg/5 mL (60 mL, 90 mL, 120 mL)

Tablet, as hydrochloride: 2 mg

**Lopid®** *see* gemfibrozil *on page 271*

**lopinavir** *see* lopinavir and ritonavir *on this page*

## lopinavir and ritonavir (loe PIN a veer & rye TON a veer)

**Synonyms** lopinavir

**U.S./Canadian Brand Names** Kaletra™

**Therapeutic Category** Antiretroviral Agent, Non-nucleoside Reverse Transcriptase Inhibitor (NNRTI)

**Use** For use in combination with other antiretroviral agents in the treatment of HIV infection

**Usual Dosage** Oral (take with food):

Children 6 months to 12 years: Dosage based on weight, presented based on mg of lopinavir (maximum dose: 400 mg lopinavir/100 mg ritonavir)

7-<15 kg: 12 mg/kg twice daily

15-40 kg: 10 mg/kg twice daily

>40 kg: Refer to adult dosing

Children >12 years and Adults: 400 mg lopinavir/100 mg ritonavir twice daily

**Dosage adjustment when taken with efavirenz or nevirapine:**

Children 6 months to 12 years:

7-<15 kg: 13 mg/kg twice daily

15-50 kg: 11 mg/kg twice daily

>50 kg: Refer to adult dosing

Children >12 years and Adults: 533 mg lopinavir/133 mg ritonavir twice daily

**Dosage Forms**

Capsule: Lopinavir 133.3 mg and ritonavir 33.3 mg

Solution, oral: Lopinavir 80 mg and ritonavir 20 mg per mL

**lopremone** *see* protirelin *on page 506*

**Lopressor®** *see* metoprolol *on page 388*

**Loprox®** *see* ciclopirox *on page 136*

**Lorabid™** *see* loracarbef *on this page*

## loracarbef (lor a KAR bef)

**U.S./Canadian Brand Names** Lorabid™

**Therapeutic Category** Antibiotic, Carbacephem

**Use** Treatment of mild to moderate community-acquired infections of the respiratory tract, skin and skin structure, and urinary tract that are caused by susceptible *S. pneumoniae*, *H. influenzae*, *B. catarrhalis*, *S. aureus*, and *E. coli*

**Usual Dosage** Oral:

Acute otitis media: Children: 15 mg/kg twice a day for 10 days

Urinary tract infections: Women: 200 mg once a day for 7 days

(Continued)

## loracarbef *(Continued)*

**Dosage Forms**
Capsule: 200 mg, 400 mg
Suspension, oral: 100 mg/5 mL (50 mL, 100 mL); 200 mg/5 mL (50 mL, 100 mL)

## loratadine (lor AT a deen)

**U.S./Canadian Brand Names** Claritin®; Claritin® RediTab®
**Therapeutic Category** Antihistamine
**Use** Relief of nasal and non-nasal symptoms of seasonal allergic rhinitis; treatment of chronic idiopathic urticaria
**Usual Dosage**
Children 2-5 years: Seasonal allergic rhinitis, chronic idiopathic urticaria: Oral: 5 mg once daily
Children ≥6 years and Adults: Seasonal allergic rhinitis, chronic idiopathic urticaria: Oral: 10 mg once daily
**Dosage Forms**
Syrup: 1 mg/mL (480 mL)
Tablet: 10 mg
Tablet, rapid-disintegrating (RediTabs®): 10 mg

## loratadine and pseudoephedrine (lor AT a deen & soo doe e FED rin)

**U.S./Canadian Brand Names** Chlor-Tripolon® N.D. (Can); Claritin-D®; Claritin-D® 24-Hour; Claritin® Extra (Can)
**Therapeutic Category** Antihistamine/Decongestant Combination
**Use** Temporary relief of symptoms of seasonal and perennial allergic rhinitis, and vasomotor rhinitis, including nasal obstruction
**Usual Dosage** Adults: Oral: 1 tablet every 12 hours
**Dosage Forms**
Tablet: Loratadine 5 mg and pseudoephedrine sulfate 120 mg
Tablet, extended release: Loratadine 10 mg and pseudoephedrine sulfate 240 mg

## lorazepam (lor A ze pam)

**U.S./Canadian Brand Names** Apo®-Lorazepam (Can); Ativan®; Novo-Lorazem (Can); Novo-Lorazepam (Can); Nu-Loraz (Can); Riva-Lorazepam (Can)
**Therapeutic Category** Benzodiazepine
**Controlled Substance** C-IV
**Use** Management of anxiety; status epilepticus; preoperative sedation and amnesia
**Usual Dosage**
Anxiety and sedation:
Infants and Children: Oral, I.V.: Usual: 0.05 mg/kg/dose (range: 0.02-0.09 mg/kg) every 4-8 hours
Adults: Oral: 1-10 mg/day in 2-3 divided doses; usual dose: 2-6 mg/day in divided doses
Insomnia: Adults: Oral: 2-4 mg at bedtime

Preoperative: Adults:
I.M.: 0.05 mg/kg administered 2 hours before surgery; maximum: 4 mg/dose
I.V.: 0.044 mg/kg 15-20 minutes before surgery; usual maximum: 2 mg/dose
Operative amnesia: Adults: I.V.: up to 0.05 mg/kg; maximum: 4 mg/dose
Status epilepticus: I.V.:
Infants and Children: 0.1 mg/kg slow I.V. over 2-5 minutes, do not exceed 4 mg/single dose; may repeat second dose of 0.05 mg/kg slow I.V. in 10-15 minutes if needed
Adolescents: 0.07 mg/kg slow I.V. over 2-5 minutes; maximum: 4 mg/dose; may repeat in 10-15 minutes
Adults: 4 mg/dose administered slowly over 2-5 minutes; may repeat in 10-15 minutes; usual maximum dose: 8 mg
**Dosage Forms**
Injection: 2 mg/mL (1 mL, 10 mL); 4 mg/mL (1 mL, 10 mL)

Solution, oral concentrated, alcohol and dye free: 2 mg/mL (30 mL)
Tablet: 0.5 mg, 1 mg, 2 mg

**Lorcet® *(Discontinued)*** *see page 750*

**Lorcet® 10/650** *see* hydrocodone and acetaminophen *on page 300*

**Lorcet®-HD** *see* hydrocodone and acetaminophen *on page 300*

**Lorcet® Plus** *see* hydrocodone and acetaminophen *on page 300*

**Lorelco® *(Discontinued)*** *see page 750*

**Loroxide® [OTC]** *see* benzoyl peroxide *on page 74*

**Lorsin® [OTC]** *see* acetaminophen, chlorpheniramine, and pseudoephedrine *on page 6*

**Lortab®** *see* hydrocodone and acetaminophen *on page 300*

**Lortab® ASA** *see* hydrocodone and aspirin *on page 300*

## losartan (loe SAR tan)

**Synonyms** DuP 753; MK594

**U.S./Canadian Brand Names** Cozaar®

**Therapeutic Category** Angiotensin II Antagonist

**Use** Treatment of hypertension alone or in combination with other antihypertensives; in considering the use of monotherapy with Cozaar®, it should be noted that in controlled trials Cozaar® had an effect on blood pressure that was notably less in black patients than in nonblacks, a finding similar to the small effect of ACE inhibitors in blacks

**Usual Dosage** Adults: Oral: Initial: 50 mg once daily, with 25 mg used in patients with possible depletion of intravascular volume (eg, patients treated with diuretics) and patients with a history of hepatic impairment; can be administered once or twice daily with total daily doses ranging from 25-100 mg; if the antihypertensive effect measured at trough using once daily dosing is inadequate, a twice daily regimen at the same total daily dose or an increase in dose may give a more satisfactory response; if blood pressure is not controlled by Cozaar® alone, a low dose of a diuretic may be added; hydrochlorothiazide has been shown to have an additive effect

**Dosage Forms** Tablet, film coated, as potassium: 25 mg, 50 mg

## losartan and hydrochlorothiazide

(loe SAR tan & hye droe klor oh THYE a zide)

**U.S./Canadian Brand Names** Hyzaar®

**Therapeutic Category** Antihypertensive Agent, Combination

**Use** Treatment of hypertension

**Usual Dosage** Adults: Oral: 1 tablet daily

**Dosage Forms** Tablet: Losartan potassium 50 mg and hydrochlorothiazide 12.5 mg; losartan potassium 100 mg and hydrochlorothiazide 25 mg

**Losopan®** *see* magaldrate and simethicone *on page 360*

**Lotemax™** *see* loteprednol *on this page*

**Lotensin®** *see* benazepril *on page 70*

**Lotensin® HCT** *see* benazepril and hydrochlorothiazide *on page 70*

## loteprednol (loe te PRED nol)

**U.S./Canadian Brand Names** Alrex™; Lotemax™

**Therapeutic Category** Corticosteroid, Ophthalmic

**Use** Temporary relief of signs and symptoms of seasonal allergic conjunctivitis

**Usual Dosage** Adults: Ophthalmic: Instill 1 drop in eye(s) 4 times/day

**Dosage Forms** Suspension, ophthalmic, as etabonate:

0.2% (Alrex™): 5 mL, 10 mL
0.5% (Lotemax™): 2.5 mL, 5 mL, 10 mL, 15 mL

**Lotrel®** *see* amlodipine and benazepril *on page 34*

**Lotriderm® (Can)** *see* betamethasone and clotrimazole *on page 77*

**Lotrimin®** *see* clotrimazole *on page 147*

**Lotrimin® AF Cream [OTC]** *see* clotrimazole *on page 147*

**Lotrimin® AF Lotion [OTC]** *see* clotrimazole *on page 147*

**Lotrimin® AF Powder [OTC]** *see* miconazole *on page 390*

**Lotrimin® AF Solution [OTC]** *see* clotrimazole *on page 147*

**Lotrimin® AF Spray Liquid [OTC]** *see* miconazole *on page 390*

**Lotrimin® AF Spray Powder [OTC]** *see* miconazole *on page 390*

**Lotrisone®** *see* betamethasone and clotrimazole *on page 77*

**Lotronex®** ***(Discontinued)*** *see page 750*

## lovastatin (LOE va sta tin)

**Synonyms** mevinolin; monacolin k

**U.S./Canadian Brand Names** Apo®-Lovastatin (Can); Mevacor®

**Therapeutic Category** HMG-CoA Reductase Inhibitor

**Use** Adjunct to dietary therapy to decrease elevated serum total and LDL cholesterol concentrations in primary hypercholesterolemia

**Usual Dosage** Adults: Oral: Initial: 20 mg with evening meal, then adjust at 4-week intervals; maximum dose: 80 mg/day

**Dosage Forms** Tablet: 10 mg, 20 mg, 40 mg

**Lovenox®** *see* enoxaparin *on page 215*

**Loxapac® (Can)** *see* loxapine *on this page*

## loxapine (LOKS a peen)

**Synonyms** oxilapine

**U.S./Canadian Brand Names** Apo®-Loxapine (Can); Loxapac® (Can); Loxitane®; Nu-Loxapine (Can); PMS-Loxapine (Can)

**Therapeutic Category** Antipsychotic Agent, Dibenzoxazepine

**Use** Management of psychotic disorders

**Usual Dosage** Adults:

Oral: 10 mg twice daily, increase dose until psychotic symptoms are controlled; usual dose range: 60-100 mg/day in divided doses 2-4 times/day; dosages >250 mg/day are not recommended

I.M.: 12.5-50 mg every 4-6 hours or longer as needed and change to oral therapy as soon as possible

**Dosage Forms**

Loxapine hydrochloride:

Concentrate, oral: 25 mg/mL (120 mL dropper bottle)

Injection: 50 mg/mL (1 mL)

Loxapine succinate:

Capsule: 5 mg, 10 mg, 25 mg, 50 mg

**Loxitane®** *see* loxapine *on this page*

**Lozi-Tab®** *see* fluoride *on page 255*

**Lozol®** *see* indapamide *on page 316*

**l-PAM** *see* melphalan *on page 370*

**LRH** *see* gonadorelin *on page 279*

**l-sarcolysin** *see* melphalan *on page 370*

**LTG** *see* lamotrigine *on page 339*

***l*-thyroxine** *see* levothyroxine *on page 348*

**l-triiodothyronine** *see* liothyronine *on page 351*

**Lubriderm® [OTC]** *see* lanolin, cetyl alcohol, glycerin, and petrolatum *on page 340*

**LubriTears® Solution [OTC]** *see* artificial tears *on page 53*

**Ludiomil®** *see* maprotiline *on page 365*

**Lufyllin®** *see* dyphylline *on page 208*

**Lugol's solution** *see* potassium iodide *on page 487*

**Lumigan™** *see* bimatoprost *on page 80*

**Luminal®** *see* phenobarbital *on page 464*

**Lumitene™** *see* beta-carotene *on page 76*

**Lunelle™** *see* estradiol cypionate and medroxyprogesterone acetate *on page 226*

**Lupron®** *see* leuprolide acetate *on page 343*

**Lupron Depot®** *see* leuprolide acetate *on page 343*

**Lupron Depot-3® Month** *see* leuprolide acetate *on page 343*

**Lupron Depot-4® Month** *see* leuprolide acetate *on page 343*

**Lupron Depot-Ped®** *see* leuprolide acetate *on page 343*

**Luride®** *see* fluoride *on page 255*

**Luride®-SF** *see* fluoride *on page 255*

**Lustra®** *see* hydroquinone *on page 305*

**Lustra-AF®** *see* hydroquinone *on page 305*

**luteinizing hormone-releasing hormone** *see* gonadorelin *on page 279*

**Lutrepulse®** *see* gonadorelin *on page 279*

**Luvox®** *see* fluvoxamine *on page 262*

**LY170053** *see* olanzapine *on page 434*

**Lycolan® Elixir [OTC]** *see* l-lysine *on page 353*

**Lyderm (Can)** *see* fluocinonide *on page 254*

**Lydonide (Can)** *see* fluocinonide *on page 254*

## Lyme disease vaccine (LIME dee seas vak SEEN)

**U.S./Canadian Brand Names** LYMErix™

**Therapeutic Category** Vaccine

**Use** Active immunization against Lyme disease in individuals between 15-70 years of age

**Usual Dosage** Adults: I.M.: Vaccination with three doses of 30 mcg (0.5 mL), administered at 0, 1 and 12 months, is recommended for optimal protection

**Dosage Forms** Injection:

Vial: 30 mcg/0.5 mL

Prefilled syringe (Tip-Lok™): 30 mcg/0.5 mL

**LYMErix™** *see* Lyme disease vaccine *on this page*

**Lymphazurin®** *see* radiological/contrast media (ionic) *on page 516*

## lymphocyte immune globulin (LIM foe site i MYUN GLOB yoo lin)

**Synonyms** antithymocyte globulin (equine); ATG; horse antihuman thymocyte gamma globulin

**U.S./Canadian Brand Names** Atgam®

**Therapeutic Category** Immunosuppressant Agent

**Use** Prevention and treatment of acute allograft rejection; treatment of moderate to severe aplastic anemia in patients not considered suitable candidates for bone marrow transplantation; prevention of graft-vs-host disease following bone marrow transplantation

(Continued)

## lymphocyte immune globulin *(Continued)*

**Usual Dosage** An intradermal skin test is recommended prior to administration of the initial dose of ATG. Use 0.1 mL of a 1:1000 dilution of ATG in normal saline

Aplastic anemia protocol: I.V.: 10-20 mg/kg/day for 8-14 days, then administer every other day for 7 more doses

Rejection prevention: Children and Adults: I.V.: 15 mg/kg/day for 14 days, then administer every other day for 7 more doses; initial dose should be administered within 24 hours before or after transplantation

Rejection treatment: Children and Adults: I.V. 10-15 mg/kg/day for 14 days, then administer every other day for 7 more doses

**Dosage Forms** Injection: 50 mg/mL (5 mL)

**Lyphocin® Injection** *see* vancomycin *on page 621*

**Lysodren®** *see* mitotane *on page 396*

**Maalox® [OTC]** *see* aluminum hydroxide and magnesium hydroxide *on page 27*

**Maalox Anti-Gas® [OTC]** *see* simethicone *on page 544*

**Maalox® Plus [OTC]** *see* aluminum hydroxide, magnesium hydroxide, and simethicone *on page 27*

**Maalox® Therapeutic Concentrate [OTC]** *see* aluminum hydroxide and magnesium hydroxide *on page 27*

**Macrobid®** *see* nitrofurantoin *on page 422*

**Macrodantin®** *see* nitrofurantoin *on page 422*

**Macrodex®** *see* dextran *on page 177*

## mafenide (MA fe nide)

**Synonyms** succinate mafenide acetate

**U.S./Canadian Brand Names** Sulfamylon® Topical

**Therapeutic Category** Antibacterial, Topical

**Use** Adjunct in the treatment of second and third degree burns to prevent septicemia caused by susceptible organisms such as *Pseudomonas aeruginosa*

**Usual Dosage** Children and Adults: Topical: Apply once or twice daily with a sterile gloved hand; apply to a thickness of approximately 16 mm; the burned area should be covered with cream at all times

**Dosage Forms** Cream, topical, as acetate: 85 mg/g (56.7 g, 113.4 g, 411 g)

## magaldrate (MAG al drate)

**Synonyms** hydromagnesium aluminate

**U.S./Canadian Brand Names** Riopan® [OTC]

**Therapeutic Category** Antacid

**Use** Symptomatic relief of hyperacidity associated with peptic ulcer, gastritis, peptic esophagitis and hiatal hernia

**Usual Dosage** Adults: Oral: 540-1080 mg between meals and at bedtime

**Dosage Forms** Suspension, oral: 540 mg/5 mL (360 mL)

## magaldrate and simethicone (MAG al drate & sye METH i kone)

**U.S./Canadian Brand Names** Losopan®; Ri-Mag®; Riopan Plus® [OTC]

**Therapeutic Category** Antacid; Antiflatulent

**Use** Relief of hyperacidity associated with peptic ulcer, gastritis, peptic esophagitis and hiatal hernia which are accompanied by symptoms of gas

**Usual Dosage** Adults: Oral: 5-10 mL between meals and at bedtime

**Dosage Forms** Suspension, oral: Magaldrate 540 mg and simethicone 40 mg per 5 mL (360 mL)

**Magalox Plus® [OTC]** *see* aluminum hydroxide, magnesium hydroxide, and simethicone *on page 27*

**Magan®** *see* magnesium salicylate *on next page*

**Mag Delay®** *see* magnesium chloride *on this page*

**Magnacal® [OTC]** *see* nutritional formula, enteral/oral *on page 432*

**magnesia magma** *see* magnesium hydroxide *on this page*

## magnesium chloride (mag NEE zhum KLOR ide)

**U.S./Canadian Brand Names** Chloromag®; Mag Delay®; Mag-SR®; Slow-Mag® [OTC]

**Therapeutic Category** Electrolyte Supplement, Oral

**Use** Correct or prevent hypomagnesemia

**Usual Dosage** I.V. in TPN:

Children: 2-10 mEq/day; the usual recommended pediatric maintenance intake of magnesium ranges from 0.2-0.6 mEq/kg/day. The dose of magnesium may also be based on the caloric intake; on that basis, 3-10 mEq/day of magnesium are needed; maximum maintenance dose: 8-16 mEq/day

Adults: 8-24 mEq/day

**Dosage Forms**

Injection: 200 mg/mL [1.97 mEq/mL] (50 mL)

Tablet: Elemental magnesium 64 mg

Tablet, extended release: 535 mg

## magnesium citrate (mag NEE zhum SIT rate)

**Synonyms** citrate of magnesia

**U.S./Canadian Brand Names** Citro-Mag (Can)

**Therapeutic Category** Laxative

**Use** Evacuation of bowel prior to certain surgical and diagnostic procedures

**Usual Dosage** Cathartic: Oral:

Children:

<6 years: 2-4 mL/kg administered as a single daily dose or in divided doses

6-12 years: $^1/_3$ to $^1/_2$ bottle

Children ≥12 years and Adults: $^1/_2$ to 1 full bottle

**Dosage Forms** Solution, oral: 300 mL

## magnesium gluconate (mag NEE zhum GLOO koe nate)

**U.S./Canadian Brand Names** Magonate® [OTC]

**Therapeutic Category** Electrolyte Supplement, Oral

**Use** Dietary supplement for treatment of magnesium deficiencies

**Usual Dosage** The recommended dietary allowance (RDA) of magnesium is 4.5 mg/kg which is a total daily allowance of 350-400 mg for adult men and 280-300 mg for adult women. During pregnancy the RDA is 300 mg and during lactation the RDA is 355 mg. Average daily intakes of dietary magnesium have declined in recent years due to processing of food. The latest estimate of the average American dietary intake was 349 mg/day.

Dietary supplement: Oral:

Children: 3-6 mg/kg/day in divided doses 3-4 times/day; maximum: 400 mg/day

Adults: 27-54 mg 2-3 times/day or 100 mg 4 times/day

**Dosage Forms** Tablet: 500 mg [elemental magnesium 27 mg]

## magnesium hydroxide (mag NEE zhum hye DROKS ide)

**Synonyms** magnesia magma; milk of magnesia; MOM

**U.S./Canadian Brand Names** Phillips'® Milk of Magnesia [OTC]

**Therapeutic Category** Antacid; Electrolyte Supplement, Oral; Laxative

**Use** Short-term treatment of occasional constipation and symptoms of hyperacidity

(Continued)

## magnesium hydroxide *(Continued)*

**Usual Dosage** Oral:

Laxative:

<2 years: 0.5 mL/kg/dose
2-5 years: 5-15 mL/day or in divided doses
6-12 years: 15-30 mL/day or in divided doses
≥12 years: 30-60 mL/day or in divided doses

Antacid:

Children: 2.5-5 mL as needed
Adults: 5-15 mL as needed

**Dosage Forms**

Liquid: 390 mg/5 mL (10 mL, 15 mL, 20 mL, 30 mL, 100 mL, 120 mL, 180 mL, 360 mL, 720 mL)
Liquid, concentrate: 10 mL equivalent to 30 mL milk of magnesia USP (3 times as potent as regular strength product)
Suspension, oral: 2.5 g/30 mL (10 mL, 15 mL, 30 mL)
Tablet: 300 mg, 600 mg

## magnesium hydroxide and mineral oil emulsion

(mag NEE zhum hye DROKS ide & MIN er al oyl e MUL shun)

**Synonyms** mom/mineral oil emulsion

**U.S./Canadian Brand Names** Haley's M-O® [OTC]

**Therapeutic Category** Laxative

**Use** Short-term treatment of occasional constipation

**Usual Dosage** Adults: Oral: 5-45 mL at bedtime

**Dosage Forms** Suspension, oral: Equivalent to magnesium hydroxide 24 mL/mineral oil emulsion 6 mL (30 mL unit dose)

## magnesium oxide (mag NEE zhum OKS ide)

**U.S./Canadian Brand Names** Mag-Ox® 400 [OTC]; Maox® [OTC]; Uro-Mag® [OTC]

**Therapeutic Category** Antacid; Electrolyte Supplement, Oral; Laxative

**Use** Treatment of magnesium deficiencies, short-term treatment of occasional constipation, and symptoms of hyperacidity

**Usual Dosage** Oral:

Antacid: 250 mg to 1.5 g with water or milk 4 times/day after meals and at bedtime
Laxative: 2-4 g at bedtime with full glass of water

**Dosage Forms**

Capsule: 140 mg
Tablet: 400 mg, 420 mg, 500 mg

## magnesium salicylate (mag NEE zhum sa LIS i late)

**U.S./Canadian Brand Names** Back-Ese M (Can); Doan's Backache Pills (Can); Doan's®, Original [OTC]; Extra Strength Doan's® [OTC]; Herbogesic (Can); Magan®; Magsal®; Mobidin®

**Therapeutic Category** Nonsteroidal Anti-inflammatory Drug (NSAID)

**Use** Mild to moderate pain, fever, various inflammatory conditions

**Usual Dosage** Adults: Oral: 650 mg 4 times/day or 1090 mg 3 times/day; may increase to 3.6-4.8 mg/day in 3-4 divided doses

**Dosage Forms**

Caplet:

Doan's®, Original: 325 mg
Extra Strength Doan's®: 500 mg

Tablet:

Magan®: 545 mg
Magsal®: 600 mg
Mobidin®: 600 mg

## magnesium sulfate (mag NEE zhum SUL fate)

**Synonyms** epsom salts

**Therapeutic Category** Anticonvulsant; Electrolyte Supplement, Oral; Laxative

**Use** Treatment and prevention of hypomagnesemia; hypertension; encephalopathy and seizures associated with acute nephritis in children; also used as a cathartic

**Usual Dosage** Dose represented as $MgSO_4$ unless stated otherwise

Hypomagnesemia:

Children:

I.M., I.V.: 25-50 mg/kg/dose (0.2-0.4 mEq/kg/dose) every 4-6 hours for 3-4 doses, maximum single dose: 2000 mg (16 mEq), may repeat if hypomagnesemia persists (higher dosage up to 100 mg/kg/dose $MgSO_4$ I.V. has been used)

Oral: 100-200 mg/kg/dose 4 times/day

Maintenance: I.V.: 30-60 mg/kg/day (0.25-0.5 mEq/kg/day)

Adults: I.M., I.V.: 1 g every 6 hours for 4 doses or 250 mg/kg over a 4-hour period; for severe hypomagnesemia: 8-12 g $MgSO_4$/day in divided doses has been used; Oral: 3 g every 6 hours for 4 doses as needed

Management of seizures and hypertension: Children: I.M., I.V.: 20-100 mg/kg/dose every 4-6 hours as needed; in severe cases doses as high as 200 mg/kg/dose have been used

Cathartic: Oral:

Children: 0.25 g/kg/dose

Adults: 10-30 g

**Dosage Forms**

Granules: ~40 mEq magnesium/5 g (240 g)

Injection: 100 mg/mL (20 mL); 125 mg/mL (8 mL); 200 mg/mL (50 mL); 250 mg/mL (150 mL); 500 mg/mL (2 mL, 5 mL, 10 mL, 30 mL, 50 mL)

Solution, oral: 50% [500 mg/mL] (30 mL)

**Magnevist®** *see* radiological/contrast media (ionic) *on page 516*

**Magonate® [OTC]** *see* magnesium gluconate *on page 361*

**Mag-Ox® 400 [OTC]** *see* magnesium oxide *on previous page*

**Magsal®** *see* magnesium salicylate *on previous page*

**Mag-SR®** *see* magnesium chloride *on page 361*

**Majeptil® (Can)** *see* thioproperazine *(Canada only)* *on page 586*

**Major-Gesic® [OTC]** *see* acetaminophen and phenyltoloxamine *on page 5*

**Malarone™** *see* atovaquone and proguanil *on page 58*

**Malatal®** ***(Discontinued)*** *see page 750*

## malathion (mal a THYE on)

**U.S./Canadian Brand Names** Ovide™ Topical

**Therapeutic Category** Scabicides/Pediculicides

**Use** Treatment of head lice and their ova

**Usual Dosage** Topical: Sprinkle Ovide™ lotion on dry hair and rub gently until the scalp is thoroughly moistened; pay special attention to the back of the head and neck. Allow to dry naturally, use no heat and leave uncovered. After 8-12 hours, the hair should be washed with a nonmedicated shampoo; rinse and use a fine-toothed comb to remove dead lice and eggs. If required, repeat with second application in 7-9 days. Further treatment is generally not necessary. Other family members should be evaluated to determine if infested and if so, receive treatment.

**Dosage Forms** Lotion: 0.5% (59 mL)

**Mallamint® [OTC]** *see* calcium carbonate *on page 97*

**Mallisol®** ***(Discontinued)*** *see page 750*

**Malotuss® Syrup** ***(Discontinued)*** *see page 750*

**Maltlevol® (Can)** *see* vitamin (multiple/oral) *on page 632*

## malt soup extract (malt soop EKS trakt)

**U.S./Canadian Brand Names** Maltsupex® [OTC]

**Therapeutic Category** Laxative

**Use** Short-term treatment of constipation

**Usual Dosage** Oral:

Infants >1 month:

Breast fed: 1-2 teaspoonfuls in 2-4 oz of water or fruit juice 1-2 times/day

Bottle fed: $^1/_2$ to 2 tablespoonfuls/day in formula for 3-4 days, then 1-2 teaspoonfuls/day

Children 2-11 years: 1-2 tablespoonfuls 1-2 times/day

Adults ≥12 years: 2 tablespoonfuls twice daily for 3-4 days, then 1-2 tablespoonfuls every evening

**Dosage Forms**

Liquid: Nondiastatic barley malt extract 16 g/15 mL

Powder: Nondiastatic barley malt extract 16 g/heaping tablespoonful

Tablet: Nondiastatic barley malt extract 750 mg

**Maltsupex® [OTC]** *see* malt soup extract *on this page*

**Mandelamine®** *see* methenamine *on page 379*

**Mandol®** *see* cefamandole *on page 114*

**mandrake** *see* podophyllum resin *on page 479*

**Manerix® (Can)** *see* moclobemide *(Canada only) on page 397*

**manganese injection** *see* trace metals *on page 598*

## mannitol (MAN i tole)

**Synonyms** *d*-mannitol

**U.S./Canadian Brand Names** Osmitrol® Injection; Resectisol® Irrigation Solution

**Therapeutic Category** Diuretic, Osmotic

**Use** Reduction of increased intracranial pressure (ICP) associated with cerebral edema; promotion of diuresis in the prevention and/or treatment of oliguria or anuria due to acute renal failure; reduction of increased intraocular pressure; promotion of urinary excretion of toxic substances

**Usual Dosage**

Children:

Test dose (to assess adequate renal function): 200 mg/kg over 3-5 minutes to produce a urine flow of at least 1 mL/kg/hour for 1-3 hours

Initial: 0.5-1 g/kg

Maintenance: 0.25-0.5 g/kg/hour administered every 4-6 hours

Adults:

Test dose: 12.5 g (200 mg/kg) over 3-5 minutes to produce a urine flow of at least 30-50 mL of urine per hour over the next 2-3 hours

Initial: 0.5-1 g/kg

Maintenance: 0.25-0.5 g/kg every 4-6 hours

**Dosage Forms**

Injection: 5% [50 mg/mL] (1000 mL); 10% [100 mg/mL] (500 mL, 1000 mL); 15% [150 mg/mL] (150 mL, 500 mL); 20% [200 mg/mL] (150 mL, 250 mL, 500 mL); 25% [250 mg/mL] (50 mL)

Solution, urogenital: 0.54% [5.4 mg/mL] (2000 mL)

**Mantadil® Cream *(Discontinued)*** *see page 750*

**Mantoux** *see* tuberculin tests *on page 612*

**Maolate® *(Discontinued)*** *see page 750*

**Maox® [OTC]** *see* magnesium oxide *on page 362*

**Mapap® [OTC]** *see* acetaminophen *on page 3*

**Mapap® Children's [OTC]** *see* acetaminophen *on page 3*

**Mapap® Extra Strength [OTC]** *see* acetaminophen *on page 3*

**Mapap® Infants' [OTC]** *see* acetaminophen *on page 3*

**Mapap® Multi-Symptom Cold [OTC]** *see* acetaminophen, dextromethorphan, and pseudoephedrine *on page 7*

**Mapap-PM® [OTC]** *see* acetaminophen and diphenhydramine *on page 5*

**Mapap Sinus® Maximum Strength [OTC]** *see* acetaminophen and pseudoephedrine *on page 6*

## maprotiline (ma PROE ti leen)

**U.S./Canadian Brand Names** Ludiomil®; Novo-Maprotiline (Can)

**Therapeutic Category** Antidepressant, Tetracyclic

**Use** Treatment of depression and anxiety associated with depression

**Usual Dosage** Oral:

Children 6-14 years: 10 mg/day, increase to a maximum daily dose of 75 mg

Adults: 75 mg/day to start, increase by 25 mg every 2 weeks up to 150-225 mg/day; administered in 3 divided doses or in a single daily dose

**Dosage Forms** Tablet, as hydrochloride: 25 mg, 50 mg, 75 mg

**Marax® *(Discontinued)*** *see page 750*

**Marcaine®** *see* bupivacaine *on page 90*

**Marcillin®** *see* ampicillin *on page 39*

**Mardol® [OTC]** *see* acetaminophen *on page 3*

**Marezine® Injection *(Discontinued)*** *see page 750*

**Marezine® Oral [OTC]** *see* cyclizine *on page 158*

**Margesic®** *see* butalbital compound and acetaminophen *on page 93*

**Margesic® H** *see* hydrocodone and acetaminophen *on page 300*

**Marinol®** *see* dronabinol *on page 205*

**Marmine® Injection** *see* dimenhydrinate *on page 188*

**Marmine® Oral [OTC]** *see* dimenhydrinate *on page 188*

**Marplan®** *see* isocarboxazid *on page 327*

**Marthritic® *(Discontinued)*** *see page 750*

**Marvelon® (Can)** *see* ethinyl estradiol and desogestrel *on page 230*

**Massé® Breast Cream [OTC]** *see* glycerin, lanolin, and peanut oil *on page 278*

**Massengill® Medicated Douche w/Cepticin [OTC]** *see* povidone-iodine *on page 489*

**Materna®** *see* vitamin (multiple/prenatal) *on page 632*

**Matulane®** *see* procarbazine *on page 497*

**Mavik®** *see* trandolapril *on page 598*

**Maxair™ Inhalation Aerosol** *see* pirbuterol *on page 473*

**Maxalt®** *see* rizatriptan *on page 530*

**Maxalt-MLT™** *see* rizatriptan *on page 530*

**Maxaquin®** *see* lomefloxacin *on page 354*

**Max-Caro® *(Discontinued)*** *see page 750*

**Maxidex®** *see* dexamethasone (ophthalmic) *on page 174*

**Maxifed®** *see* guaifenesin and pseudoephedrine *on page 283*

**Maxifed® DM** *see* guaifenesin, pseudoephedrine, and dextromethorphan *on page 285*

**Maxifed-G®** *see* guaifenesin and pseudoephedrine *on page 283*

**Maxiflor®** *see* diflorasone *on page 185*

**Maximum Strength Anbesol® [OTC]** *see* benzocaine *on page 72*

**Maximum Strength Desenex® Antifungal Cream [OTC]** *see* miconazole *on page 390*

**Maximum Strength Dex-A-Diet®** ***(Discontinued)*** *see page 750*

**Maximum Strength Dexatrim®** ***(Discontinued)*** *see page 750*

**Maximum Strength Nytol® [OTC]** *see* diphenhydramine *on page 191*

**Maximum Strength Orajel® [OTC]** *see* benzocaine *on page 72*

**Maxipime®** *see* cefepime *on page 114*

**Maxitrol®** *see* neomycin, polymyxin B, and dexamethasone *on page 414*

**Maxivate® Topical** *see* betamethasone (topical) *on page 78*

**Maxolon®** ***(Discontinued)*** *see page 750*

**Maxzide®** *see* hydrochlorothiazide and triamterene *on page 299*

**may apple** *see* podophyllum resin *on page 479*

**Mazanor®** ***(Discontinued)*** *see page 750*

**MCH** *see* microfibrillar collagen hemostat *on page 391*

## m-cresyl acetate (em-KREE sil AS e tate)

**U.S./Canadian Brand Names** Cresylate®

**Therapeutic Category** Otic Agent, Anti-infective

**Use** Provides an acid medium; for external otitis infections caused by susceptible bacteria or fungus

**Usual Dosage** Otic: Instill 2-4 drops as required

**Dosage Forms** Solution: 25% with isopropanol 25%, chlorobutanol 1%, benzyl alcohol 1%, and castor oil 5% in propylene glycol (15 mL dropper bottle)

**MCT Oil® [OTC]** *see* medium chain triglycerides *on page 368*

**MD-Gastroview®** *see* radiological/contrast media (ionic) *on page 516*

**MDL-71754** *see* vigabatrin *(Canada only) on page 627*

## measles and rubella vaccines, combined

(MEE zels & roo BEL a vak SEENS, kom BINED)

**U.S./Canadian Brand Names** MoRu-Viraten Berna™ (Can); M-R-VAX® II

**Therapeutic Category** Vaccine, Live Virus

**Use** Simultaneous immunization against measles and rubella

**Usual Dosage** S.C.: Inject into outer aspect of upper arm

**Dosage Forms** Injection: 1000 $TCID_{50}$ each of live attenuated measles virus vaccine and live rubella virus vaccine

## measles, mumps, and rubella vaccines, combined

(MEE zels, mumpz, & roo BEL a vak SEENS, kom BINED)

**Synonyms** MMR

**U.S./Canadian Brand Names** M-M-R® II; Priorix™ (Can)

**Therapeutic Category** Vaccine, Live Virus

**Use** Measles, mumps, and rubella prophylaxis

**Usual Dosage** S.C.: Inject in outer aspect of the upper arm to children ≥15 months of age; each dose contains 1000 $TCID_{50}$ (tissue culture infectious doses) of live attenuated measle virus vaccine, 5000 $TCID_{50}$ of live mumps virus vaccine and 1000 $TCID_{50}$ of live rubella virus vaccine

**Dosage Forms** Injection: 1000 $TCID_{50}$ each of measles virus vaccine and rubella virus vaccine, 5000 $TCID_{50}$ mumps virus vaccine

## measles virus vaccine (live) (MEE zels VYE rus vak SEEN live)

**Synonyms** more attenuated enders strain; rubeola vaccine

**U.S./Canadian Brand Names** Attenuvax®

**Therapeutic Category** Vaccine, Live Virus

**Use** Immunization against measles (rubeola) in persons ≥15 months of age

**Usual Dosage** Children >15 months and Adults: S.C.: 0.5 mL in outer aspect of the upper arm

**Dosage Forms** Injection: 1000 $TCID_{50}$ per dose

**Mebaral®** *see* mephobarbital *on page 372*

## mebendazole (me BEN da zole)

**U.S./Canadian Brand Names** Vermox®

**Therapeutic Category** Anthelmintic

**Use** Treatment of enterobiasis (pinworm infection), trichuriasis (whipworm infections), ascariasis (roundworm infection), and hookworm infections caused by *Necator americanus* or *Ancylostoma duodenale*; drug of choice in the treatment of capillariasis

**Usual Dosage** Children and Adults: Oral:

Pinworms: Single chewable tablet; may need to repeat after 2 weeks

Whipworms, roundworms, hookworms: 1 tablet twice daily, morning and evening on 3 consecutive days; if patient is not cured within 3-4 weeks, a second course of treatment may be administered

**Dosage Forms** Tablet, chewable: 100 mg

## mecamylamine (mek a MIL a meen)

**U.S./Canadian Brand Names** Inversine®

**Therapeutic Category** Ganglionic Blocking Agent

**Use** Treatment of moderately severe to severe hypertension and in uncomplicated malignant hypertension

**Usual Dosage** Adults: Oral: 2.5 mg twice daily after meals for 2 days; increased by increments of 2.5 mg at intervals of ≥2 days until desired blood pressure response is achieved

**Dosage Forms** Tablet, as hydrochloride: 2.5 mg

## mechlorethamine (me klor ETH a meen)

**Synonyms** $HN_2$; mustine; nitrogen mustard

**U.S./Canadian Brand Names** Mustargen® Hydrochloride

**Therapeutic Category** Antineoplastic Agent

**Use** Combination therapy of Hodgkin's disease, brain tumors, non-Hodgkin's lymphoma, and malignant lymphomas; palliative treatment of bronchogenic, breast, and ovarian carcinoma; sclerosing agent in intracavitary therapy of pleural, pericardial, and other malignant effusions

**Usual Dosage** Refer to individual protocols

Children: MOPP: I.V.: 6 $mg/m^2$ on days 1 and 8 of a 28-day cycle

Adults:

I.V.: 0.4 mg/kg or 12-16 $mg/m^2$ for one dose or divided into 0.1 mg/kg/day for 4 days

Intracavitary: 10-20 mg or 0.2-0.4 mg/kg

**Dosage Forms** Powder for injection, as hydrochloride: 10 mg

**Meclan® Topical *(Discontinued)*** *see page 750*

## meclizine (MEK li zeen)

**U.S./Canadian Brand Names** Antivert®; Antrizine®; Bonamine™ (Can); Bonine® [OTC]; Dizmiss® [OTC]; Dramamine® II [OTC]; Meni-D®; Nico-Vert® [OTC]; Ru-Vert-M®; Vergon® [OTC]

**Therapeutic Category** Antihistamine

**Use** Prevention and treatment of motion sickness; management of vertigo

(Continued)

## meclizine *(Continued)*

**Usual Dosage** Children >12 years and Adults: Oral:

Motion sickness: 25-50 mg 1 hour before travel, repeat dose every 24 hours if needed

Vertigo: 25-100 mg/day in divided doses

**Dosage Forms**

Capsule, as hydrochloride: 15 mg, 25 mg, 30 mg

Tablet, as hydrochloride: 12.5 mg, 25 mg, 50 mg

Tablet, as hydrochloride:

Chewable: 25 mg

Film coated: 25 mg

## meclofenamate (me kloe fen AM ate)

**Therapeutic Category** Analgesic, Non-narcotic; Nonsteroidal Anti-inflammatory Drug (NSAID)

**Use** Treatment of inflammatory disorders

**Usual Dosage** Adults: Oral: 200-300 mg 3-4 times/day

**Dosage Forms** Capsule, as sodium: 50 mg, 100 mg

**Meclomen® *(Discontinued)*** *see page 750*

**Meda-Cap® [OTC]** *see* acetaminophen *on page 3*

**medicinal carbon** *see* charcoal *on page 123*

**Medigesic®** *see* butalbital compound and acetaminophen *on page 93*

**Medihaler-Epi® *(Discontinued)*** *see page 750*

**Medihaler Ergotamine® *(Discontinued)*** *see page 750*

**Medihaler-Iso® *(Discontinued)*** *see page 750*

**Medi-Lice® [OTC]** *see* permethrin *on page 462*

**Medi-Phedrine® Severe Cold Formula [OTC]** *see* acetaminophen, dextromethorphan, and pseudoephedrine *on page 7*

**Mediplast® Plaster [OTC]** *see* salicylic acid *on page 535*

**Medipren® [OTC]** *see* ibuprofen *on page 311*

**Medi-Quick® Topical Ointment [OTC]** *see* bacitracin, neomycin, and polymyxin B *on page 65*

**Medi-Tuss® [OTC]** *see* guaifenesin *on page 281*

## medium chain triglycerides (mee DEE um chane trye GLIS er ides)

**Synonyms** triglycerides, medium chain

**U.S./Canadian Brand Names** MCT Oil® [OTC]

**Therapeutic Category** Nutritional Supplement

**Use** Dietary supplement for those who cannot digest long chain fats; malabsorption associated with disorders such as pancreatic insufficiency, bile salt deficiency, and bacterial overgrowth of the small bowel; induce ketosis as a prevention for seizures (akinetic, clonic, and petit mal)

**Usual Dosage** Oral: 15 mL 3-4 times/day

**Dosage Forms** Oil: 14 g/15 mL (960 mL)

**Medralone® Injection** *see* methylprednisolone *on page 385*

**Medrapred® *(Discontinued)*** *see page 750*

**Medrol® Acetate Topical *(Discontinued)*** *see page 750*

**Medrol® Oral** *see* methylprednisolone *on page 385*

## medroxyprogesterone acetate (me DROKS ee proe JES te rone AS e tate)

**Synonyms** acetoxymethylprogesterone; methylacetoxyprogesterone

**U.S./Canadian Brand Names** Alti-MPA (Can); Depo-Provera® Injection; Gen-Medroxy (Can); Novo-Medrone (Can); Provera® Oral

**Therapeutic Category** Contraceptive, Progestin Only; Progestin

**Use** Secondary amenorrhea or abnormal uterine bleeding due to hormonal imbalance

**Usual Dosage**

Adolescents and Adults: Oral:

Amenorrhea: 5-10 mg/day for 5-10 days or 2.5 mg/day

Abnormal uterine bleeding: 5-10 mg for 5-10 days starting on day 16 or 21 of cycle

Accompanying cyclic estrogen therapy, postmenopausal: 2.5-10 mg the last 10-13 days of estrogen dosing each month

Adults:

Contraception: Deep I.M.: 150 mg every 3 months or 450 mg every 6 months

Endometrial or renal carcinoma: I.M.: 400-1000 mg/week

**Dosage Forms**

Injection, suspension: 100 mg/mL (5 mL); 150 mg/mL (1 mL); 400 mg/mL (1 mL, 2.5 mL, 10 mL)

Tablet: 2.5 mg, 5 mg, 10 mg

## medrysone (ME dri sone)

**U.S./Canadian Brand Names** HMS Liquifilm®

**Therapeutic Category** Adrenal Corticosteroid

**Use** Treatment of allergic conjunctivitis, vernal conjunctivitis, episcleritis, ophthalmic epinephrine sensitivity reaction

**Usual Dosage** Children and Adults: Ophthalmic: 1 drop in conjunctival sac 2-4 times/day up to every 4 hours; may use every 1-2 hours during first 1-2 days

**Dosage Forms** Solution, ophthalmic: 1% (5 mL, 10 mL)

## mefenamic acid (me fe NAM ik AS id)

**U.S./Canadian Brand Names** Apo®-Mefenamic (Can); Nu-Mefenamic (Can); PMS-Mefenamic Acid (Can); Ponstan® (Can); Ponstel®

**Therapeutic Category** Analgesic, Non-narcotic; Nonsteroidal Anti-inflammatory Drug (NSAID)

**Use** Short-term relief of mild to moderate pain including primary dysmenorrhea

**Usual Dosage** Children >14 years and Adults: Oral: 500 mg to start then 250 mg every 4 hours as needed; maximum therapy: 1 week

**Dosage Forms** Capsule: 250 mg

## mefloquine (ME floe kwin)

**U.S./Canadian Brand Names** Lariam®

**Therapeutic Category** Antimalarial Agent

**Use** Treatment of acute malarial infections and prevention of malaria

**Usual Dosage** Adults: Oral:

Mild to moderate malaria infection: 5 tablets (1250 mg) as a single dose with at least 8 oz of water

Malaria prophylaxis: 1 tablet (250 mg) weekly starting 1 week before travel, continuing weekly during travel and for 4 weeks after leaving endemic area

**Dosage Forms** Tablet, as hydrochloride: 250 mg

**Mefoxin®** *see* cefoxitin *on page 116*

**Mega B® [OTC]** *see* vitamin B complex *on page 630*

**Megace®** *see* megestrol acetate *on next page*

**Megaton™ [OTC]** *see* vitamin B complex *on page 630*

## megestrol acetate (me JES trole AS e tate)

**U.S./Canadian Brand Names** Apo®-Megestrol (Can); Lin-Megestrol (Can); Megace®; Nu-Megestrol (Can)

**Therapeutic Category** Antineoplastic Agent; Progestin

**Use** Palliative treatment of breast and endometrial carcinomas, appetite stimulation and promotion of weight gain in cachexia

**Usual Dosage** Adults: Oral:

Breast carcinoma: 40 mg 4 times/day

Endometrial: 40-320 mg/day in divided doses

**Dosage Forms**

Suspension, oral: 40 mg/mL with alcohol 0.06% (240 mL)

Tablet: 20 mg, 40 mg

**Melanex®** *see* hydroquinone *on page 305*

**Melfiat®** *see* phendimetrazine *on page 463*

**Melfiat® Tablet *(Discontinued)*** *see page 750*

**Mellaril®** *see* thioridazine *on page 586*

**Mellaril-S® *(Discontinued)*** *see page 750*

## meloxicam (mel OX ee cam)

**U.S./Canadian Brand Names** Mobic®

**Therapeutic Category** Nonsteroidal Anti-inflammatory Drug (NSAID)

**Use** Relief of signs and symptoms of osteoarthritis

**Usual Dosage** Adult: Oral: Initial: 7.5 mg once daily; some patients may receive additional benefit from an increased dose of 15 mg once daily

**Dosage Forms** Tablet: 7.5 mg, 15 mg

## melphalan (MEL fa lan)

**Synonyms** l-PAM; l-sarcolysin; phenylalanine mustard

**U.S./Canadian Brand Names** Alkeran®

**Therapeutic Category** Antineoplastic Agent

**Use** Palliative treatment of multiple myeloma and nonresectable epithelial ovarian carcinoma; neuroblastoma, rhabdomyosarcoma, breast cancer, sarcoma; I.V. formulation: Use in patients in whom oral therapy is not appropriate

**Usual Dosage** Refer to individual protocols

Children: I.V. (investigational, distributed under the auspices of the NCI for authorized studies):

Pediatric rhabdomyosarcoma: 10-35 mg/m$^2$ bolus every 21-28 days

Chemoradiotherapy supported by marrow infusions for neuroblastoma: 70-140 mg/m$^2$ on day 7 and 6 before BMT

Adults: Oral:

Multiple myeloma: 6 mg/day or 10 mg/day for 7-10 days, or 0.15 mg/kg/day for 7 days

Ovarian carcinoma: 0.2 mg/kg/day for 5 days, repeat in 4-5 weeks

**Dosage Forms**

Powder for injection: 50 mg

Tablet: 2 mg

**Menadol® [OTC]** *see* ibuprofen *on page 311*

**Menest®** *see* estrogens (esterified) *on page 228*

**Meni-D®** *see* meclizine *on page 367*

## meningococcal polysaccharide vaccine (groups A, C, Y, and W-135)

(me NIN joe kok al pol i SAK a ride vak SEEN groops aye, see, why, & dubl yoo won thur tee fyve)

**U.S./Canadian Brand Names** Menomune®-A/C/Y/W-135

**Therapeutic Category** Vaccine, Live Bacteria

**Use** Immunization against infection caused by *Neisseria meningitidis* groups A,C,Y, and W-135 in persons ≥2 years

**Usual Dosage** S.C.: 0.5 mL; do not inject intradermally or I.V.

**Dosage Forms** Injection: 10 dose, 50 dose

**Menomune®-A/C/Y/W-135** *see* meningococcal polysaccharide vaccine (groups A, C, Y, and W-135) *on this page*

## menotropins (men oh TROE pins)

**U.S./Canadian Brand Names** Humegon™; Pergonal®; Repronex®

**Therapeutic Category** Gonadotropin

**Use** Sequentially with hCG to induce ovulation and pregnancy in the infertile woman with functional anovulation or in patients who have previously received pituitary suppression; used with hCG in men to stimulate spermatogenesis in those with primary hypogonadotropic hypogonadism

**Usual Dosage** Adults: I.M.:

Male: Following pretreatment with hCG, 1 ampul 3 times/week and hCG 2000 units twice weekly until sperm is detected in the ejaculate (4-6 months) then may be increased to 2 ampuls of menotropins (150 units FSH/150 units LH) 3 times/week

Female: 1 ampul/day (75 units of FSH and LH) for 9-12 days followed by 10,000 units hCG 1 day after the last dose; repeated at least twice at same level before increasing dosage to 2 ampuls (150 units FSH/150 units LH)

Repronex®: I.M., S.C.:

Infertile patients with oligo-anovulation: Initial: 150 int. units daily for the first 5 days of treatment. Adjustments should not be made more frequently than once every 2 days and should not exceed 75-150 int. units per adjustment. Maximum daily dose should not exceed 450 int. units and dosing beyond 12 days is not recommended. If patient's response to Repronex® is appropriate, hCG 5000-10,000 units should be given one day following the last dose of Repronex®.

Assisted reproductive technologies: Initial (in patients who have received GnRH agonist or antagonist pituitary suppression): 225 int. units; adjustments in dose should not be made more frequently than once every 2 days and should not exceed more than 75-50 int. units per adjustment. The maximum daily doses of Repronex® given should not exceed 450 int. units and dosing beyond 12 days is not recommended. Once adequate follicular development is evident, hCG (5000-10,000 units) should be administered to induce final follicular maturation in preparation for oocyte retrieval.

**Dosage Forms** Injection: Follicle stimulating hormone activity 75 units and luteinizing hormone activity 75 units per 2 mL ampul

**Mentax®** *see* butenafine *on page 93*

## mepenzolate (me PEN zoe late)

**U.S./Canadian Brand Names** Cantil®

**Therapeutic Category** Anticholinergic Agent

**Use** Management of peptic ulcer disease; inhibit salivation and excessive secretions in respiratory tract preoperatively

**Usual Dosage** Adults: Oral: 25-50 mg 4 times/day with meals and at bedtime

**Dosage Forms** Tablet, as bromide: 25 mg

**Mepergan®** *see* meperidine and promethazine *on next page*

## meperidine (me PER i deen)

**Synonyms** isonipecaine; pethidine
**U.S./Canadian Brand Names** Demerol®
**Therapeutic Category** Analgesic, Narcotic
**Controlled Substance** C-II
**Use** Management of moderate to severe pain; adjunct to anesthesia and preoperative sedation
**Usual Dosage** Doses should be titrated to appropriate analgesic effect; when changing route of administration, note that oral doses are about half as effective as parenteral dose

Oral, I.M., I.V., S.C.:
Children: 1-1.5 mg/kg/dose every 3-4 hours as needed; 1-2 mg/kg as a single dose preoperative medication may be used; maximum 100 mg/dose
Adults: 50-150 mg/dose every 3-4 hours as needed

**Dosage Forms**
Injection, as hydrochloride:
Multiple dose vials: 50 mg/mL (30 mL); 100 mg/mL (20 mL)
Single dose: 10 mg/mL (5 mL, 10 mL, 30 mL); 25 mg/dose (0.5 mL, 1 mL); 50 mg/dose (1 mL); 75 mg/dose (1 mL, 1.5 mL); 100 mg/dose (1 mL)
Syrup, as hydrochloride: 50 mg/5 mL (500 mL)
Tablet, as hydrochloride: 50 mg, 100 mg

## meperidine and promethazine (me PER i deen & proe METH a zeen)

**U.S./Canadian Brand Names** Mepergan®
**Therapeutic Category** Analgesic, Narcotic
**Controlled Substance** C-II
**Use** Management of moderate to severe pain
**Usual Dosage** Adults:
Oral: 1 capsule every 4-6 hours
I.M.: 1-2 mL every 3-4 hours

**Dosage Forms**
Capsule: Meperidine hydrochloride 50 mg and promethazine hydrochloride 25 mg
Injection: Meperidine hydrochloride 25 mg and promethazine hydrochloride 25 per mL (2 mL, 10 mL)

## mephentermine (me FEN ter meen)

**U.S./Canadian Brand Names** Wyamine® Sulfate
**Therapeutic Category** Adrenergic Agonist Agent
**Use** Treatment of hypotension secondary to ganglionic blockade or spinal anesthesia; may be used as an emergency measure to maintain blood pressure until whole blood replacement becomes available
**Usual Dosage**
Hypotension: I.M., I.V.:
Children: 0.4 mg/kg
Adults: 0.5 mg/kg
Hypotensive emergency: I.V. infusion: 20-60 mg
**Dosage Forms** Injection, as sulfate: 15 mg/mL (2 mL)

## mephobarbital (me foe BAR bi tal)

**Synonyms** methylphenobarbital
**U.S./Canadian Brand Names** Mebaral®
**Therapeutic Category** Barbiturate
**Controlled Substance** C-IV
**Use** Treatment of generalized tonic-clonic and simple partial seizures
**Usual Dosage** Epilepsy: Oral:
Children: 4-10 mg/kg/day in 2-4 divided doses
Adults: 200-600 mg/day in 2-4 divided doses

**Dosage Forms** Tablet: 32 mg, 50 mg, 100 mg

**Mephyton® Oral** *see* phytonadione *on page 470*

## mepivacaine (me PIV a kane)

**U.S./Canadian Brand Names** Carbocaine®; Isocaine® HCl; Polocaine®

**Therapeutic Category** Local Anesthetic

**Use** Local anesthesia by nerve block; infiltration in dental procedures

**Usual Dosage**

Injectable local anesthetic: Varies with procedure, degree of anesthesia needed, vascularity of tissue, duration of anesthesia required, and physical condition of patient

Topical: Apply to affected area as needed

**Dosage Forms** Injection, as hydrochloride: 1% [10 mg/mL] (30 mL, 50 mL); 1.5% [15 mg/mL] (30 mL); 2% [20 mg/mL] (20 mL, 50 mL); 3% [30 mg/mL] (1.8 mL)

## meprobamate (me proe BA mate)

**U.S./Canadian Brand Names** Apo®-Meprobamate (Can); Equanil®; Miltown®

**Therapeutic Category** Antianxiety Agent, Miscellaneous

**Controlled Substance** C-IV

**Use** Management of anxiety disorders

**Usual Dosage** Oral:

Children 6-12 years: 100-200 mg 2-3 times/day

Sustained release: 200 mg twice daily

Adults: 400 mg 3-4 times/day, up to 2400 mg/day

Sustained release: 400-800 mg twice daily

**Dosage Forms**

Capsule, sustained release: 200 mg, 400 mg

Tablet: 200 mg, 400 mg, 600 mg

**Mepron™** *see* atovaquone *on page 57*

**Meprospan®** ***(Discontinued)*** *see page 750*

## mequinol and tretinoin (ME kwi nol & TRET i noyn)

**U.S./Canadian Brand Names** Solagé™ Topical Solution

**Therapeutic Category** Retinoic Acid Derivative; Vitamin A Derivative; Vitamin, Topical

**Use** Treatment of solar lentigines; the efficacy of using Solagé™ daily for >24 weeks has not been established. The local cutaneous safety of Solagé™ in non-Caucasians has not been adequately established.

**Usual Dosage** Adults: Topical: Apply twice daily to solar lentigines using the applicator tip while avoiding application to the surrounding skin. Separate application by at least 8 hours or as directed by physician.

**Dosage Forms** Liquid, topical: Mequinol 2% and tretinoin 0.01% (30 mL)

## merbromin (mer BROE min)

**U.S./Canadian Brand Names** Mercurochrome®

**Therapeutic Category** Topical Skin Product

**Use** Topical antiseptic

**Usual Dosage** Topical: Apply freely, until injury has healed

**Dosage Forms** Solution, topical: 2%

## mercaptopurine (mer kap toe PYOOR een)

**Synonyms** 6-mercaptopurine; 6-MP

**U.S./Canadian Brand Names** Purinethol®

**Therapeutic Category** Antineoplastic Agent

**Use** Treatment of acute leukemias (ALL, CML)

(Continued)

## mercaptopurine *(Continued)*

**Usual Dosage** Oral (refer to individual protocols):

Induction: 2.5 mg/kg/day for several weeks or more; if, after 4 weeks there is no improvement and no myelosuppression, increase dosage up to 5 mg/kg/day

Maintenance: 1.5-2.5 mg/kg/day

**Dosage Forms** Tablet: 50 mg

**6-mercaptopurine** *see* mercaptopurine *on previous page*

**mercapturic acid** *see* acetylcysteine *on page 10*

## mercuric oxide (mer KYOOR ik OKS ide)

**Synonyms** yellow mercuric oxide

**U.S./Canadian Brand Names** Ocu-Merox®

**Therapeutic Category** Antibiotic, Ophthalmic

**Use** Treatment of irritation and minor infections of the eyelids

**Usual Dosage** Ophthalmic: Apply small amount to inner surface of lower eyelid once or twice daily

**Dosage Forms** Ointment, ophthalmic: 1%, 2% [OTC]

**Mercurochrome®** *see* merbromin *on previous page*

**Meridia™** *see* sibutramine *on page 543*

## meropenem (mer oh PEN em)

**U.S./Canadian Brand Names** Merrem® I.V.

**Therapeutic Category** Carbapenem (Antibiotic)

**Use** Meropenem is indicated as single agent therapy for the treatment of intra-abdominal infections including complicated appendicitis and peritonitis in adults and bacterial meningitis in pediatric patients >3 months of age caused by *S. pneumoniae*, *H. influenzae*, and *N. meningitidis* (penicillin-resistant pneumococci have not been studied in clinical trials); it is better tolerated than imipenem and highly effective against a broad range of bacteria

**Usual Dosage**

Children:

Intra-abdominal infections: 20 mg/kg every 8 hours (maximum dose: 1 g every 8 hours)

Meningitis: 40 mg/kg every 8 hours (maximum dose: 2 g every 8 hours)

Adults: 1 g every 8 hours

**Dosage Forms**

Infusion: 500 mg (100 mL); 1 g (100 mL)

Infusion, ADD-Vantage®: 500 mg (15 mL); 1 g (15 mL)

Injection: 25 mg/mL (20 mL); 33.3 mg/mL (30 mL)

**Merrem® I.V.** *see* meropenem *on this page*

**Mersol® [OTC]** *see* thimerosal *on page 585*

**Merthiolate® [OTC]** *see* thimerosal *on page 585*

**Meruvax® II** *see* rubella virus vaccine (live) *on page 533*

## mesalamine (me SAL a meen)

**Synonyms** 5-aminosalicylic acid; 5-ASA; fisalamine; mesalazine

**U.S./Canadian Brand Names** Asacol® Oral; Canasa® Rectal; Mesasal® (Can); Novo-5 ASA (Can); Pentasa® Oral; Quintasa® (Can); Rowasa® Rectal; Salofalk® (Can)

**Therapeutic Category** 5-Aminosalicylic Acid Derivative

**Use** Treatment of ulcerative colitis, proctosigmoiditis, and proctitis

**Usual Dosage** Adults (usual course of therapy is 3-6 weeks): Oral: 800 mg 3 times/day

Retention enema: 60 mL (4 g) at bedtime, retained overnight, approximately 8 hours

Rectal suppository: Insert 1 suppository in rectum twice daily

**Dosage Forms**
Capsule, controlled release (Pentasa®): 250 mg
Suppository, rectal (Canasa®, Rowasa®): 500 mg
Suspension, rectal (Rowasa®): 4 g/60 mL (7s)
Tablet, enteric coated (Asacol®): 400 mg

**mesalazine** *see* mesalamine *on previous page*

**Mesantoin® *(Discontinued)*** *see page 750*

**Mesasal® (Can)** *see* mesalamine *on previous page*

**M-Eslon® (Can)** *see* morphine sulfate *on page 400*

## mesna (MES na)

**Synonyms** sodium 2-mercaptoethane sulfonate
**U.S./Canadian Brand Names** Mesnex™; Uromitexan™ (Can)
**Therapeutic Category** Antidote
**Use** Detoxifying agent used as a protectant against hemorrhagic cystitis induced by ifosfamide and cyclophosphamide
**Usual Dosage** Children and Adults (refer to individual protocols):
Ifosfamide: I.V.: 20% W/W of ifosfamide dose at time of administration and 4 and 8 hours after each dose of ifosfamide
Cyclophosphamide: I.V.: 20% W/W of cyclophosphamide dose prior to administration and 3, 6, 9, 12 hours after cyclophosphamide dose (total daily dose: 120% to 180% of cyclophosphamide dose)
Oral dose: 40% W/W of the antineoplastic agent dose in 3 doses at 4-hour intervals
**Dosage Forms** Injection: 100 mg/mL (2 mL, 4 mL, 10 mL)

**Mesnex™** *see* mesna *on this page*

## mesoridazine (mez oh RID a zeen)

**U.S./Canadian Brand Names** Serentil®
**Therapeutic Category** Phenothiazine Derivative
**Use** Symptomatic management of psychotic disorders, including schizophrenia, behavioral problems, alcoholism as well as reducing anxiety and tension occurring in neurosis
**Usual Dosage** Initial: 25 mg for most patients; may repeat dose in 30-60 minutes, if necessary; usual optimum dosage range: 25-200 mg/day. Concentrate may be diluted just prior to administration with distilled water, acidified tap water, orange or grape juice; do not prepare and store bulk dilutions.
**Dosage Forms**
Injection, as besylate: 25 mg/mL (1 mL)
Liquid, oral, as besylate: 25 mg/mL (118 mL)
Tablet, as besylate: 10 mg, 25 mg, 50 mg, 100 mg

**Mestinon® Injection** *see* pyridostigmine *on page 511*

**Mestinon® Oral** *see* pyridostigmine *on page 511*

## mestranol and norethindrone (MES tra nole & nor eth IN drone)

**U.S./Canadian Brand Names** Genora® 1/50; Nelova® 1/50M; Norinyl® 1+50; Ortho-Novum® 1/50
**Therapeutic Category** Contraceptive, Oral
**Use** Prevention of pregnancy; treatment of hypermenorrhea, endometriosis, female hypogonadism
**Usual Dosage** See ethinyl estradiol and desogestrel
**Dosage Forms** Tablet: Mestranol 0.05 mg and norethindrone 1 mg (21s and 28s)

**metacortandralone** *see* prednisolone (systemic) *on page 493*

**Metadate® CD** *see* methylphenidate *on page 384*

**Metadate™ ER** *see* methylphenidate *on page 384*

**Metadol™ (Can)** *see* methadone *on page 378*

**Metahydrin® *(Discontinued)*** *see page 750*

**Metamucil® [OTC]** *see* psyllium *on page 509*

**Metamucil® Instant Mix [OTC]** *see* psyllium *on page 509*

**Metaprel® Aerosol *(Discontinued)*** *see page 750*

**Metaprel® Inhalation Solution *(Discontinued)*** *see page 750*

**Metaprel® Syrup *(Discontinued)*** *see page 750*

**Metaprel® Tablet *(Discontinued)*** *see page 750*

## metaproterenol (met a proe TER e nol)

**Synonyms** orciprenaline

**U.S./Canadian Brand Names** Alupent®

**Therapeutic Category** Adrenergic Agonist Agent

**Use** Bronchodilator in reversible airway obstruction due to asthma or COPD

**Usual Dosage**

Oral:

Children:

<2 years: 0.4 mg/kg/dose administered 3-4 times/day; in infants, the dose can be administered every 8-12 hours

2-6 years: 1-2.6 mg/kg/day divided every 6-8 hours

6-9 years: 10 mg/dose administered 3-4 times/day

Children >9 years and Adults: 20 mg/dose administered 3-4 times/day

Inhalation: Children >12 years and Adults: 2-3 inhalations every 3-4 hours, up to 12 inhalations in 24 hours

Nebulizer:

Infants: 6 mg/dose administered over 5 minutes

Children <12 years: 0.01-0.02 mL/kg of 5% solution; diluted in 2-3 mL normal saline every 4-6 hours (may be administered more frequently according to need), maximum dose: 15 mg/dose every 4-6 hours

Adolescents and Adults: 5-20 breaths of full strength 5% metaproterenol **or** 0.2-0.3 mL of 5% metaproterenol in 2.5-3 mL normal saline nebulized every 4-6 hours (can be administered more frequently according to need)

**Dosage Forms**

Aerosol, oral, as sulfate: 0.65 mg/dose (5 mL, 10 mL)

Solution for inhalation, as sulfate, preservative free: 0.4% [4 mg/mL] (2.5 mL); 0.6% [6 mg/mL] (2.5 mL); 5% [50 mg/mL] (10 mL, 30 mL)

Syrup, as sulfate: 10 mg/5 mL (480 mL)

Tablet, as sulfate: 10 mg, 20 mg

## metaraminol (met a RAM i nole)

**U.S./Canadian Brand Names** Aramine®

**Therapeutic Category** Adrenergic Agonist Agent

**Use** Acute hypotensive crisis in the treatment of shock

**Usual Dosage** Adults:

Prevention of hypotension: I.M., S.C.: 2-10 mg

Adjunctive treatment of hypotension: I.V.: 15-100 mg in 250-500 mL NS or 5% dextrose in water

Severe shock: I.V.: 0.5-5 mg direct I.V. injection then use I.M. dose

**Dosage Forms** Injection, as bitartrate: 10 mg/mL (10 mL)

**Metasep® [OTC]** *see* parachlorometaxylenol *on page 450*

**Metastron®** *see* strontium-89 *on page 560*

## metaxalone (me TAKS a lone)

**U.S./Canadian Brand Names** Skelaxin®

**Therapeutic Category** Skeletal Muscle Relaxant

**Use** Relief of discomfort associated with acute, painful musculoskeletal conditions

**Usual Dosage** Children >12 years and Adults: Oral: 800 mg 3-4 times/day

**Dosage Forms** Tablet: 400 mg

**Meted® Shampoo (Can)** *see* sulfur and salicylic acid *on page 566*

## metformin (met FOR min)

**U.S./Canadian Brand Names** Apo®-Metformin (Can); Gen-Metformin (Can); Glucophage®; Glucophage® XR; Glycon (Can); Novo-Metformin (Can); Nu-Metformin (Can); Rho®-Metformin (Can)

**Therapeutic Category** Antidiabetic Agent, Oral

**Use** Management of noninsulin-dependent diabetes mellitus (type 2) as monotherapy when hyperglycemia cannot be managed on diet alone. May be used concomitantly with a sulfonylurea when diet and metformin or sulfonylurea alone do not result in adequate glycemic control.

**Usual Dosage** Oral (allow 1-2 weeks between dose titrations):

Adults:

500 mg tablets: Initial: 500 mg twice daily (administered with the morning and evening meals). Dosage increases should be made in increments of one tablet every week, administered in divided doses, up to a maximum of 2,500 mg/day. Doses of up to 2000 mg/day may be administered twice daily. If a dose of 2,500 mg/day is required, it may be better tolerated 3 times/day (with meals).

850 mg tablets: Initial: 850 mg once daily (administered with the morning meal). Dosage increases should be made in increments of one tablet every OTHER week, administered in divided doses, up to a maximum of 2550 mg/day. The usual maintenance dose is 850 mg twice daily (with the morning and evening meals). Some patients may be administered 850 mg 3 times/day (with meals).

Elderly patients: The initial and maintenance dosing should be conservative, due to the potential for decreased renal function. Generally, elderly patients should not be titrated to the maximum dose of metformin.

**Transfer from other antidiabetic agents:** No transition period is generally necessary except when transferring from chlorpropamide. When transferring from chlorpropamide, care should be exercised during the first 2 weeks because of the prolonged retention of chlorpropamide in the body, leading to overlapping drug effects and possible hypoglycemia.

**Concomitant metformin and oral sulfonylurea therapy:** If patients have not responded to 4 weeks of the maximum dose of metformin monotherapy, consideration to a gradually addition of an oral sulfonylurea while continuing metformin at the maximum dose, even if prior primary or secondary failure to a sulfonylurea has occurred.

**Dosage Forms**

Tablet, as hydrochloride: 500 mg, 850 mg, 1000 mg

Tablet, extended release, as hydrochloride: 500 mg

## methacholine (meth a KOLE leen)

**U.S./Canadian Brand Names** Provocholine®

**Therapeutic Category** Diagnostic Agent

**Use** Diagnosis of bronchial airway hyperactivity in subjects who do not have clinically apparent asthma

**Usual Dosage** The table is a suggested schedule for administration of methacholine challenge. Calculate cumulative units by multiplying number of breaths by concentration given. Total cumulative units is the sum of cumulative units for each concentration given.

**Dosage Forms** Powder for reconstitution, inhalation, as chloride: 100 mg/5 mL

| Vial | Serial Concentration (mg/mL) | No. of Breaths | Cumulative Units per Concentration | Total Cumulative Units |
|---|---|---|---|---|
| E | 0.025 | 5 | 0.125 | 0.125 |
| D | 0.25 | 5 | 1.25 | 1.375 |
| C | 2.5 | 5 | 12.5 | 13.88 |
| B | 10 | 5 | 50 | 63.88 |
| A | 25 | 5 | 125 | 188.88 |

## methadone (METH a done)

**U.S./Canadian Brand Names** Dolophine®; Metadol™ (Can); Methadose® (Can)

**Therapeutic Category** Analgesic, Narcotic

**Controlled Substance** C-II

**Use** Management of severe pain, used in narcotic detoxification maintenance programs and for the treatment of iatrogenic narcotic dependency

**Usual Dosage** Doses should be titrated to appropriate effects:

Children: Analgesia:

Oral, I.M., S.C.: 0.7 mg/kg/24 hours divided every 4-6 hours as needed or 0.1-0.2 mg/kg every 4-12 hours as needed; maximum: 10 mg/dose

I.V.: Initial: 0.1 mg/kg every 4 hours for 2-3 doses, then every 6-12 hours as needed; maximum: 10 mg/dose

Adults:

Analgesia: Oral, I.M., S.C.: 2.5-10 mg every 3-8 hours as needed, up to 5-20 mg every 6-8 hours

Detoxification: Oral: 15-40 mg/day

Maintenance of opiate dependence: Oral: 20-120 mg/day

**Dosage Forms**

Injection, as hydrochloride: 10 mg/mL (1 mL, 10 mL, 20 mL)

Solution, as hydrochloride:

Oral: 5 mg/5 mL (5 mL, 500 mL); 10 mg/5 mL (500 mL)

Oral, concentrate: 10 mg/mL (30 mL, 960 mL)

Tablet, as hydrochloride: 5 mg, 10 mg

Tablet, dispersible, as hydrochloride: 40 mg

**Methadose® (Can)** *see* methadone *on this page*

**methaminodiazepoxide** *see* chlordiazepoxide *on page 125*

## methamphetamine (meth am FET a meen)

**Synonyms** desoxyephedrine

**U.S./Canadian Brand Names** Desoxyn®

**Therapeutic Category** Amphetamine

**Controlled Substance** C-II

**Use** Narcolepsy; exogenous obesity; abnormal behavioral syndrome in children (minimal brain dysfunction)

**Usual Dosage** Oral:

Attention deficit disorder: Children >6 years: 2.5-5 mg 1-2 times/day, may increase by 5 mg increments weekly until optimum response is achieved, usually 20-25 mg/day

Exogenous obesity: Children >12 years and Adults: 5 mg, 30 minutes before each meal, 10-15 mg in morning; treatment duration should not exceed a few weeks

**Dosage Forms** Tablet, as hydrochloride: 5 mg

## methazolamide (meth a ZOE la mide)

**U.S./Canadian Brand Names** Neptazane®

**Therapeutic Category** Carbonic Anhydrase Inhibitor

**Use** Adjunctive treatment of open-angle or secondary glaucoma; short-term therapy of narrow-angle glaucoma when delay of surgery is desired

**Usual Dosage** Adults: Oral: 50-100 mg 2-3 times/day

**Dosage Forms** Tablet: 25 mg, 50 mg

## methenamine (meth EN a meen)

**Synonyms** hexamethylenetetramine

**U.S./Canadian Brand Names** Dehydral® (Can); Hiprex®; Mandelamine®; Urasal® (Can); Urex®

**Therapeutic Category** Antibiotic, Miscellaneous

**Use** Prophylaxis or suppression of recurrent urinary tract infections

**Usual Dosage** Oral:

Children:

Hippurate: 6-12 years: 25-50 mg/kg/day divided every 12 hours

Mandelate: 50-75 mg/kg/day divided every 6 hours

Adults:

Hippurate: 1 g twice daily

Mandelate: 1 g 4 times/day after meals and at bedtime

**Dosage Forms**

Methenamine hippurate:

Tablet, (Hiprex®, Urex®): 1 g (Hiprex® contains tartrazine dye)

Methenamine mandelate:

Suspension, oral: 500 mg/5 mL (480 mL)

Tablet, enteric coated: 500 mg, 1 g

## methenamine, phenyl salicylate, atropine, hyoscyamine, benzoic acid, and methylene blue

(meth EN a meen, fen nil sa LIS i late, A troe peen, hye oh SYE a meen, ben ZOE ik AS id, & METH i leen bloo)

**U.S./Canadian Brand Names** Atrosept®; Dolsed®; UAA®; Uridon Modified®; Urised®; Uritin®

**Therapeutic Category** Antibiotic, Urinary Anti-infective; Urinary Tract Product

**Usual Dosage** Adults: Oral: Two tablets four/daily

**Dosage Forms** Tablet: Methenamine 40.8 mg, phenyl salicylate 18.1 mg, atropine sulfate 0.03 mg, hyoscyamine sulfate 0.03 mg, benzoic acid 4.5 mg, and methylene blue 5.4 mg

**Methergine®** *see* methylergonovine *on page 384*

## methimazole (meth IM a zole)

**Synonyms** thiamazole

**U.S./Canadian Brand Names** Tapazole®

**Therapeutic Category** Antithyroid Agent

**Use** Palliative treatment of hyperthyroidism, to return the hyperthyroid patient to a normal metabolic state prior to thyroidectomy, and to control thyrotoxic crisis that may accompany thyroidectomy

**Usual Dosage** Oral:

Children: Initial: 0.4 mg/kg/day in 3 divided doses; maintenance: 0.2 mg/kg/day in 3 divided doses

Adults: Initial: 10 mg every 8 hours; maintenance dose ranges from 5-30 mg/day

**Dosage Forms** Tablet: 5 mg, 10 mg

## methionine (me THYE oh neen)

**U.S./Canadian Brand Names** Pedameth®

**Therapeutic Category** Dietary Supplement

**Use** Treatment of diaper rash and control of odor, dermatitis and ulceration caused by ammoniacal urine

(Continued)

## methionine *(Continued)*

**Usual Dosage** Oral:

Children: Control of diaper rash: 75 mg in formula or other liquid 3-4 times/day for 3-5 days

Adults:

Control of odor in incontinent adults: 200-400 mg 3-4 times/day

Dietary supplement: 500 mg/day

**Dosage Forms**

Capsule: 500 mg

Liquid: 75 mg/5 mL (473 mL)

Tablet: 500 mg

## methocarbamol (meth oh KAR ba mole)

**U.S./Canadian Brand Names** Robaxin®

**Therapeutic Category** Skeletal Muscle Relaxant

**Use** Treatment of muscle spasm associated with acute painful musculoskeletal conditions; supportive therapy in tetanus

**Usual Dosage**

Children: Recommended **only** for use in tetanus I.V.: 15 mg/kg/dose or 500 $mg/m^2$/dose, may repeat every 6 hours if needed; maximum dose: 1.8 $g/m^2$/day for 3 days only

Adults: Muscle spasm:

Oral: 1.5 g 4 times/day for 2-3 days, then decrease to 4-4.5 g/day in 3-6 divided doses

I.M., I.V.: 1 g every 8 hours if oral not possible

**Dosage Forms**

Injection: 100 mg/mL in polyethylene glycol 50% (10 mL)

Tablet: 500 mg, 750 mg

## methocarbamol and aspirin (meth oh KAR ba mole & AS pir in)

**U.S./Canadian Brand Names** Aspirin® Backache (Can); Methoxisal (Can); Robaxisal®

**Therapeutic Category** Skeletal Muscle Relaxant

**Use** Adjunct to rest, physical therapy, and other measures for the relief of discomfort associated with acute, painful musculoskeletal disorders

**Usual Dosage** Children >12 years and Adults: Oral: 2 tablets 4 times/day

**Dosage Forms** Tablet: Methocarbamol 400 mg and aspirin 325 mg

## methohexital (meth oh HEKS i tal)

**U.S./Canadian Brand Names** Brevital® Sodium; Brietal Sodium® (Can)

**Therapeutic Category** Barbiturate

**Controlled Substance** C-IV

**Use** Induction and maintenance of general anesthesia for short procedures

**Usual Dosage** Doses must be titrated to effect

Children:

I.M.: Preop: 5-10 mg/kg/dose

I.V.: Induction: 1-2 mg/kg/dose

Rectal: Preop/induction: 20-35 mg/kg/dose; usual: 25 mg/kg/dose; administer as 10% aqueous solution

Adults: I.V.: Induction: 50-120 mg to start; 20-40 mg every 4-7 minutes

**Dosage Forms** Injection, as sodium: 500 mg, 2.5 g, 5 g

## methotrexate (meth oh TREKS ate)

**Synonyms** amethopterin; MTX

**U.S./Canadian Brand Names** Rheumatrex®

**Therapeutic Category** Antineoplastic Agent

**Use** Treatment of trophoblastic neoplasms, leukemias, osteosarcoma, non-Hodgkin's lymphoma; psoriasis, rheumatoid arthritis

**Usual Dosage** Refer to individual protocols

Children:

High-dose MTX for acute lymphocytic leukemia: I.V.: Loading dose of 200 mg/m$^2$ and a 24-hour infusion of 1200 mg/m$^2$/day

Induction of remission in acute lymphoblastic leukemias: Oral, I.M., I.V.: 3.3 mg/m$^2$/day for 4-6 weeks

Leukemia: Remission maintenance: Oral, I.M.: 20-30 mg/m$^2$ 2 times/week

Juvenile rheumatoid arthritis: Oral: 5-15 mg/m$^2$/week as a single dose or as 3 divided doses administered 12 hours apart

Osteosarcoma:

I.T.: 10-15 mg/m$^2$ (maximum dose: 15 mg) by protocol

I.V.: <12 years: 12 g/m$^2$ (12-18 g); >12 years: 8 g/m$^2$ (maximum dose: 18 g)

Non-Hodgkin's lymphoma: I.V.: 200-300 mg/m$^2$

Adults:

Trophoblastic neoplasms: Oral, I.M.: 15-30 mg/day for 5 days, repeat in 7 days for 3-5 courses

Rheumatoid arthritis: Oral: 7.5 mg once weekly or 2.5 mg every 12 hours for 3 doses/ week; not to exceed 20 mg/week

**Dosage Forms**

Injection, as sodium, with preservatives: 25 mg/mL (2 mL, 4 mL, 8 mL, 10 mL)

Injection, as sodium, preservative free: 2.5 mg/mL (2 mL); 25 mg/mL (2 mL, 4 mL, 8 mL, 10 mL)

Powder for injection, lyophilized, preservative free: 20 mg, 50 mg, 1 g

Tablet, as sodium: 2.5 mg

Tablet, as sodium, dose pack: 2.5 mg (4 cards with 2, 3, 4, 5, or 6 tablets each)

## methotrimeprazine *(Canada only)* (meth oh trye MEP ra zeen)

**Synonyms** levomepromazine

**U.S./Canadian Brand Names** Apo®-Methoprazine (Can); Novo-Meprazine (Can); Nozinan® (Can)

**Therapeutic Category** Neuroleptic Agent

**Use** Acute and chronic schizophrenias, senile psychoses, manic-depressive syndromes. Conditions associated with anxiety and tension: autonomic disturbances, personality disturbances, emotional troubles secondary to such physical conditions as resistant pruritus. Methotrimeprazine is also employed: As an analgesic: In pain due to cancer, zona, trigeminal neuralgia and neurocostal neuralgia and in phantom limb pains and muscular discomforts.

**Usual Dosage** Adults: I.M.:

Sedation analgesia: 10-20 mg every 4-6 hours as needed

Preoperative medication: 2-20 mg, 45 minutes to 3 hours before surgery

Postoperative analgesia: 2.5-7.5 mg every 4-6 hours is suggested as necessary since residual effects of anesthetic may be present

Pre- and postoperative hypotension: I.M.: 5-10 mg

**Dosage Forms** Injection, as hydrochloride: 20 mg/mL (10 mL)

**Methoxisal (Can)** *see* methocarbamol and aspirin *on previous page*

## methoxsalen (meth OKS a len)

**Synonyms** methoxypsoralen

**U.S./Canadian Brand Names** Oxsoralen® Topical; Oxsoralen-Ultra®; Ultramop™ (Can); Uvadex® Injection

**Therapeutic Category** Psoralen

**Use** Symptomatic control of severe, recalcitrant, disabling psoriasis in conjunction with long wave ultraviolet radiation; induce repigmentation in vitiligo topical repigmenting agent in conjunction with controlled doses of ultraviolet A (UVA) or sunlight

**Usual Dosage**

Psoriasis: Adults: Oral: 10-70 mg 1½-2 hours before exposure to UVA light, 2-3 times at least 48 hours apart; dosage is based upon patient's body weight and skin type

<30 kg: 10 mg

(Continued)

## methoxsalen *(Continued)*

30-50 kg: 20 mg
51-65 kg: 30 mg
66-80 kg: 40 mg
81-90 kg: 50 mg
91-115 kg: 60 mg
>115 kg: 70 mg

Vitiligo: Children >12 years and Adults:

Oral: 20 mg 2-4 hours before exposure to UVA light or sunlight; limit exposure to 15-40 minutes based on skin basic color and exposure

Topical: Apply lotion 1-2 hours before exposure to UVA light, no more than once weekly

**Dosage Forms**

Capsule: 10 mg
Injection: 20 mcg/mL (10 mL)
Lotion: 1% (30 mL)

## methoxycinnamate and oxybenzone

(meth OKS ee SIN a mate & oks i BEN zone)

**U.S./Canadian Brand Names** PreSun® 29 [OTC]; Ti-Screen® [OTC]

**Therapeutic Category** Sunscreen

**Use** Reduce the chance of premature aging of the skin and skin cancer from overexposure to the sun

**Usual Dosage** Adults: Topical: Apply liberally to all exposed areas at least 30 minutes prior to sun exposure

**Dosage Forms** Lotion:

SPF 15: 120 mL
SPF 29: 120 mL

## methoxyflurane (meth oks ee FLOO rane)

**U.S./Canadian Brand Names** Penthrane®

**Therapeutic Category** General Anesthetic

**Use** Adjunct to provide anesthesia procedures <4 hours in duration

**Usual Dosage** 0.3% to 0.8% for analgesia and anesthesia, with 0.1% to 2% for maintenance when used with nitrous oxide

**Dosage Forms** Liquid: 15 mL

**methoxypsoralen** *see* methoxsalen *on previous page*

## methscopolamine (meth skoe POL a meen)

**U.S./Canadian Brand Names** Pamine®

**Therapeutic Category** Anticholinergic Agent

**Use** Adjunctive therapy in the treatment of peptic ulcer

**Usual Dosage** Adults: Oral: 2.5 mg 30 minutes before meals or food and 2.5-5 mg at bedtime

**Dosage Forms** Tablet, as bromide: 2.5 mg

## methsuximide (meth SUKS i mide)

**U.S./Canadian Brand Names** Celontin®

**Therapeutic Category** Anticonvulsant

**Use** Control of absence (petit mal) seizures; useful adjunct in refractory, partial complex (psychomotor) seizures

**Usual Dosage** Oral:

Children: Initial: 10-15 mg/kg/day in 3-4 divided doses; increase weekly up to maximum of 30 mg/kg/day

Adults: 300 mg/day for the first week; may increase by 300 mg/day at weekly intervals up to 1.2 g in 2-4 divided doses/day

**Dosage Forms** Capsule: 150 mg, 300 mg

## methyclothiazide (meth i kloe THYE a zide)

**U.S./Canadian Brand Names** Aquatensen®; Enduron®

**Therapeutic Category** Diuretic, Thiazide

**Use** Management of mild to moderate hypertension; treatment of edema in congestive heart failure and nephrotic syndrome

**Usual Dosage** Adults: Oral:

Edema: 2.5-10 mg/day

Hypertension: 2.5-5 mg/day

**Dosage Forms** Tablet: 2.5 mg, 5 mg

## methyclothiazide and deserpidine

(meth i kloe THYE a zide & de SER pi deen)

**U.S./Canadian Brand Names** Enduronyl®; Enduronyl® Forte

**Therapeutic Category** Antihypertensive Agent, Combination

**Use** Management of mild to moderately severe hypertension

**Usual Dosage** Oral: Individualized, normally 1-4 tablets/day

**Dosage Forms** Tablet: Methyclothiazide 5 mg and deserpidine 0.25 mg; methyclothiazide 5 mg and deserpidine 0.5 mg

**methylacetoxyprogesterone** *see* medroxyprogesterone acetate *on page 369*

## methylbenzethonium chloride (meth il ben ze THOE nee um KLOR ide)

**U.S./Canadian Brand Names** Diaparene® [OTC]; Puri-Clens™ [OTC]; Sween Cream® [OTC]

**Therapeutic Category** Topical Skin Product

**Use** Treatment of diaper rash and ammonia dermatitis

**Usual Dosage** Topical: Apply to area as needed

**Dosage Forms**

Cream: 0.1% (30 g, 60 g, 120 g)

Ointment, topical: 0.1% (30 g, 60 g, 120 g)

Powder: 0.055% (120 g, 270 g, 420 g)

## methylcellulose (meth il SEL yoo lose)

**U.S./Canadian Brand Names** Citrucel® [OTC]

**Therapeutic Category** Laxative

**Use** Adjunct in treatment of constipation

**Usual Dosage** Oral:

Children: 5-10 mL 1-2 times/day

Adults: 5-20 mL 3 times/day

**Dosage Forms** Powder: 105 mg/g

## methyldopa (meth il DOE pa)

**U.S./Canadian Brand Names** Aldomet®; Apo®-Methyldopa (Can); Novo-Medopa® (Can); Nu-Medopa (Can)

**Therapeutic Category** Alpha-Adrenergic Blocking Agent

**Use** Management of moderate to severe hypertension

**Usual Dosage**

Children:

Oral: Initial: 10 mg/kg/day in 2-4 divided doses; increase every 2 days as needed to maximum dose of 65 mg/kg/day; do not exceed 3 g/day

I.V.: 5-10 mg/kg/dose every 6-8 hours

Adults:

Oral: Initial: 250 mg 2-3 times/day; increase every 2 days as needed; usual dose 1-1.5 g/day in 2-4 divided doses; maximum dose: 3 g/day

I.V.: 250-1000 mg every 6-8 hours

(Continued)

## methyldopa *(Continued)*

**Dosage Forms**

Injection, as methyldopate hydrochloride: 50 mg/mL (5 mL, 10 mL)
Suspension, oral: 250 mg/5 mL (5 mL, 473 mL)
Tablet: 125 mg, 250 mg, 500 mg

## methyldopa and hydrochlorothiazide

(meth il DOE pa & hye droe klor oh THYE a zide)

**U.S./Canadian Brand Names** Aldoril®; Apo®-Methazide (Can)

**Therapeutic Category** Antihypertensive Agent, Combination

**Use** Management of moderate to severe hypertension

**Usual Dosage** Oral: 1 tablet 2-3 times/day for first 48 hours, then decrease or increase at intervals of not less than 2 days until an adequate response is achieved

**Dosage Forms** Tablet:

15: Methyldopa 250 mg and hydrochlorothiazide 15 mg
25: Methyldopa 250 mg and hydrochlorothiazide 25 mg
D30: Methyldopa 500 mg and hydrochlorothiazide 30 mg

## methylene blue (METH i leen bloo)

**U.S./Canadian Brand Names** Urolene Blue®

**Therapeutic Category** Antidote

**Use** Antidote for cyanide poisoning and drug-induced methemoglobinemia, indicator dye, bacteriostatic genitourinary antiseptic

**Usual Dosage**

Children:

NADH-methemoglobin reductase deficiency: Oral: 1.5-5 mg/kg/day (maximum: 300 mg/day) administered with 5-8 mg/kg/day of ascorbic acid
Methemoglobinemia: I.V.: 1-2 mg/kg over several minutes

Adults:

Genitourinary antiseptic: Oral: 55-130 mg 3 times/day (maximum: 390 mg/day)
Methemoglobinemia: I.V.: 1-2 mg/kg over several minutes; may be repeated in 1 hour if necessary

**Dosage Forms**

Injection: 10 mg/mL (1 mL, 10 mL)
Tablet: 65 mg

## methylergonovine (meth il er goe NOE veen)

**U.S./Canadian Brand Names** Methergine®

**Therapeutic Category** Ergot Alkaloid and Derivative

**Use** Prevention and treatment of postpartum and postabortion hemorrhage caused by uterine atony or subinvolution

**Usual Dosage** Adults:

Oral: 0.2-0.4 mg every 6-12 hours for 2-7 days
I.M., I.V.: 0.2 mg every 2-4 hours for 5 doses then change to oral dosage

**Dosage Forms**

Injection, as maleate: 0.2 mg/mL (1 mL)
Tablet, as maleate: 0.2 mg

**Methylin™** *see* methylphenidate *on this page*

**Methylin™ ER** *see* methylphenidate *on this page*

**methylmorphine** *see* codeine *on page 150*

## methylphenidate (meth il FEN i date)

**U.S./Canadian Brand Names** Concerta™; Metadate® CD; Metadate™ ER; Methylin™; Methylin™ ER; PMS-Methylphenidate (Can); Riphenidate® (Can); Ritalin®; Ritalin-SR®

**Therapeutic Category** Central Nervous System Stimulant, Nonamphetamine

**Controlled Substance** C-II

**Use** Attention-deficit/hyperactivity disorder (ADHD); narcolepsy

**Usual Dosage** Oral (discontinue periodically to re-evaluate or if no improvement occurs within 1 month):

Children ≥6 years: ADHD: Initial: 0.3 mg/kg/dose or 2.5-5 mg/dose given before breakfast and lunch; increase by 0.1 mg/kg/dose or by 5-10 mg/day at weekly intervals; usual dose: 0.5-1 mg/kg/day; maximum dose: 2 mg/kg/day or 90 mg/day

Extended release products:

Metadate™ ER, Methylin™ ER, Ritalin® SR: Duration of action is 8 hours. May be given in place of regular tablets, once the daily dose is titrated using the regular tablets and the titrated 8-hour dosage corresponds to sustained release tablet size.

Metadate® CD: Initial: 20 mg once daily; may be adjusted in 20 mg increments at weekly intervals; maximum: 60 mg/day

Concerta™: Duration of action is 12 hours:

Children not currently taking methylphenidate:

Initial: 18 mg once daily in the morning

Adjustment: May increase to 54 mg/day; dose may be adjusted at weekly intervals

Children currently taking methylphenidate: **Note:** Dosing based on current regimen and clinical judgment; suggested dosing listed below:

Patients taking methylphenidate 5 mg 2-3 times/day or 20 mg/day sustained release formulation: Initial dose: 18 mg once every morning (maximum: 54 mg/day)

Patients taking methylphenidate 10 mg 2-3 times/day or 40 mg/day sustained release formulation: Initial dose: 36 mg once every morning (maximum: 54 mg/day)

Patients taking methylphenidate 15 mg 2-3 times/day or 60 mg/day sustained release formulation: Initial dose: 54 mg once every morning (maximum: 54 mg/day)

Adults:

Narcolepsy: 10 mg 2-3 times/day, up to 60 mg/day

Depression (unlabeled use): Initial: 2.5 mg every morning before 9 AM; dosage may be increased by 2.5-5 mg every 2-3 days as tolerated to a maximum of 20 mg/day; may be divided (ie, 7 AM and 12 noon), but should not be given after noon; do not use sustained release product

**Dosage Forms**

Capsule, extended release, as hydrochloride (Metadate® CD): 20 mg

Tablet, as hydrochloride: 5 mg, 10 mg, 20 mg

Methylin™, Ritalin®: 5 mg, 10 mg, 20 mg

Tablet, extended release, as hydrochloride (Metadate™ ER): 10 mg, 20 mg

Tablet, osmotic controlled release, as hydrochloride (Concerta™): 18 mg, 36 mg, 54 mg

Tablet, sustained release, as hydrochloride: 20 mg

Methylin™ ER: 10 mg, 20 mg

Ritalin-SR®: 20 mg

**methylphenobarbital** *see* mephobarbital *on page 372*

**methylphenyl isoxazolyl penicillin** *see* oxacillin *on page 440*

**methylphytyl napthoquinone** *see* phytonadione *on page 470*

## methylprednisolone (meth il pred NIS oh lone)

**Synonyms** 6-α-methylprednisolone

**U.S./Canadian Brand Names** Adlone® Injection; A-methaPred® Injection; depMedalone® Injection; Depoject® Injection; Depo-Medrol® Injection; Depopred® Injection; D-Med® Injection; Duralone® Injection; Medralone® Injection; Medrol® Oral; M-Prednisol® Injection; Solu-Medrol® Injection

**Therapeutic Category** Adrenal Corticosteroid

**Use** Anti-inflammatory or immunosuppressant agent in the treatment of a variety of diseases including those of hematologic, allergic, inflammatory, neoplastic, and autoimmune origin

**Usual Dosage** Methylprednisolone sodium succinate is highly soluble and has a rapid effect by I.M. and I.V. routes. Methylprednisolone acetate has a low solubility and has a sustained I.M. effect.

(Continued)

## methylprednisolone *(Continued)*

Children:

Anti-inflammatory or immunosuppressive: Oral, I.M., I.V. (sodium succinate): 0.16-0.8 mg/kg/day or 5-25 mg/m$^2$/day in divided doses every 6-12 hours

Status asthmaticus: I.V. (sodium succinate): Loading dose: 2 mg/kg/dose, then 0.5-1 mg/kg/dose every 6 hours for up to 5 days

Lupus nephritis: I.V. (sodium succinate): 30 mg/kg every other day for 6 doses

Adults:

Anti-inflammatory or immunosuppressive: Oral: 4-48 mg/day to start, followed by gradual reduction in dosage to the lowest possible level consistent with maintaining an adequate clinical response

I.M. (sodium succinate): 10-80 mg/day once daily

I.M. (acetate): 40-120 mg every 1-2 weeks

I.V. (sodium succinate): 10-40 mg over a period of several minutes and repeated I.V. or I.M. at intervals depending on clinical response; when high dosages are needed, administer 30 mg/kg over a period of 10-20 minutes and may be repeated every 4-6 hours for 48 hours

Status asthmaticus: I.V. (sodium succinate): Loading dose: 2 mg/kg/dose, then 0.5-1 mg/kg/dose every hours for up to 5 days

Lupus nephritis:

I.V. (sodium succinate): 1 g/day for 3 days

Intra-articular (acetate):

Large joints: 20-80 mg

Small joints: 4-10 mg

Intralesional (acetate): 20-60 mg

**Dosage Forms**

Injection:

As acetate: 20 mg/mL (5 mL, 10 mL); 40 mg/mL (1 mL, 5 mL, 10 mL); 80 mg/mL (1 mL, 5 mL)

As sodium succinate: 40 mg (1 mL, 3 mL); 125 mg (2 mL, 5 mL); 500 mg (1 mL, 4 mL, 8 mL, 20 mL); 1000 mg (1 mL, 8 mL, 50 mL); 2000 mg (30.6 mL)

Tablet: 2 mg, 4 mg, 8 mg, 16 mg, 24 mg, 32 mg

Dose pack: 4 mg (21s)

**6-α-methylprednisolone** *see* methylprednisolone *on previous page*

**4-methylpyrazole** *see* fomepizole *on page 264*

## methyltestosterone (meth il tes TOS te rone)

**U.S./Canadian Brand Names** Android®; Testred®; Virilon®

**Therapeutic Category** Androgen

**Use**

Male: Hypogonadism; delayed puberty; impotence and climacteric symptoms

Female: Palliative treatment of metastatic breast cancer; postpartum breast pain and/or engorgement

**Usual Dosage** Adults:

Male:

Oral: 10-40 mg/day

Buccal: 5-20 mg/day

Female:

Breast pain/engorgement:

Oral: 80 mg/day for 3-5 days

Buccal: 40 mg/day for 3-5 days

Breast cancer:

Oral: 200 mg/day

Buccal: 100 mg/day

**Dosage Forms**

Capsule: 10 mg

Tablet: 10 mg, 25 mg

## methysergide (meth i SER jide)

**U.S./Canadian Brand Names** Sansert®

**Therapeutic Category** Ergot Alkaloid and Derivative

**Use** Prophylaxis of vascular headache

**Usual Dosage** Oral: 4-8 mg/day with meals; if no improvement is noted after 3 weeks, drug is unlikely to be beneficial; must not be administered continuously for longer than 6 months, and a drug-free interval of 3-4 weeks must follow each 6-month course; dosage should be tapered over the 2- to 3-week period before drug discontinuation to avoid rebound headaches

**Dosage Forms** Tablet, as maleate: 2 mg

**Meticorten®** *see* prednisone *on page 493*

**Metimyd® Ophthalmic** *see* sulfacetamide and prednisolone *on page 563*

## metipranolol (met i PRAN oh lol)

**U.S./Canadian Brand Names** OptiPranolol® Ophthalmic

**Therapeutic Category** Beta-Adrenergic Blocker

**Use** Agent for lowering intraocular pressure

**Usual Dosage** Adults: Ophthalmic: 1 drop in the affected eye(s) twice daily

**Dosage Forms** Solution, ophthalmic, as hydrochloride: 0.3% (5 mL, 10 mL)

**Metizol® Tablet *(Discontinued)*** *see page 750*

## metoclopramide (met oh kloe PRA mide)

**U.S./Canadian Brand Names** Apo®-Metoclop (Can); Nu-Metoclopramide (Can); Reglan®

**Therapeutic Category** Gastrointestinal Agent, Prokinetic

**Use** Gastroesophageal reflux; prevention of nausea associated with chemotherapy; facilitates intubation of the small intestine and symptomatic treatment of diabetic gastric stasis

**Usual Dosage**

Children:

Gastroesophageal reflux: Oral: 0.1 mg/kg/dose up to 4 times/day; efficacy of continuing metoclopramide beyond 12 weeks in reflux has not been determined; total daily dose should not exceed 0.5 mg/kg/day

Gastrointestinal hypomotility: Oral, I.M., I.V.: 0.1 mg/kg/dose up to 4 times/day, not to exceed 0.5 mg/kg/day

Antiemetic: I.V.: 1-2 mg/kg 30 minutes before chemotherapy and every 2-4 hours

Facilitate intubation: I.V.: <6 years: 0.1 mg/kg; 6-14 years: 2.5-5 mg

Adults:

Stasis/reflux: Oral: 10-15 mg/dose up to 4 times/day 30 minutes before meals or food and at bedtime; efficacy of continuing metoclopramide beyond 12 weeks in reflux has not been determined

Gastrointestinal hypomotility: Oral, I.M., I.V.: 10 mg 30 minutes before each meal and at bedtime

Antiemetic: I.V.: 1-2 mg/kg 30 minutes before chemotherapy and every 2-4 hours

Facilitate intubation: I.V.: 10 mg

**Dosage Forms**

Injection, as hydrochloride: 5 mg/mL (2 mL, 10 mL, 30 mL, 50 mL, 100 mL)

Solution, as hydrochloride, oral, concentrated: 10 mg/mL (10 mL, 30 mL)

Syrup, as hydrochloride, sugar free: 5 mg/5 mL (10 mL, 480 mL)

Tablet, as hydrochloride: 5 mg, 10 mg

## metolazone (me TOLE a zone)

**U.S./Canadian Brand Names** Mykrox®; Zaroxolyn®

**Therapeutic Category** Diuretic, Miscellaneous

(Continued)

## metolazone (Continued)

**Use** Management of mild to moderate hypertension; treatment of edema in congestive heart failure, nephrotic syndrome, and impaired renal function

**Usual Dosage** Oral:

Children: 0.2-0.4 mg/kg/day divided every 12-24 hours

Adults:

Edema: 5-20 mg/dose every 24 hours

Hypertension: 2.5-5 mg/dose every 24 hours

**Dosage Forms** Tablet:

Mykrox® (rapidly acting): 0.5 mg

Zaroxolyn® (slow acting): 2.5 mg, 5 mg, 10 mg

**Metopirone®** *see* metyrapone *on next page*

## metoprolol (me toe PROE lole)

**U.S./Canadian Brand Names** Apo®-Metoprolol (Can); Betaloc® (Can); Gen-Metoprolol (Can); Lopressor®; Novo-Metoprol (Can); Novo-Metoprolol (Can); Nu-Metop (Can); PMS-Metoprolol (Can); Toprol XL®

**Therapeutic Category** Beta-Adrenergic Blocker

**Use** Treatment of hypertension and angina pectoris; prevention of myocardial infarction; selective inhibitor of $beta_1$-adrenergic receptors

**Usual Dosage** Safety and efficacy in children have not been established.

Children: Oral: 1-5 mg/kg/24 hours divided twice daily; allow 3 days between dose adjustments

Adults:

Oral: 100-450 mg/day in 2-3 divided doses, begin with 50 mg twice daily and increase doses at weekly intervals to desired effect

I.V.: 5 mg every 2 minutes for 3 doses in early treatment of myocardial infarction; thereafter administer 50 mg orally every 6 hours 15 minutes after last I.V. dose and continue for 48 hours; then administer a maintenance dose of 100 mg twice daily

**Dosage Forms**

Metoprolol succinate:

Tablet, sustained release: 50 mg, 100 mg, 200 mg

Metoprolol tartrate:

Injection: 1 mg/mL (5 mL)

Tablet: 50 mg, 100 mg

**Metra® *(Discontinued)*** *see page 750*

**Metreton® Ophthalmic** *see* prednisolone (ophthalmic) *on page 492*

**Metrocream (Can)** *see* metronidazole *on this page*

**Metrodin®** *see* urofollitropin *on page 618*

**MetroGel® Topical** *see* metronidazole *on this page*

**MetroGel®-Vaginal** *see* metronidazole *on this page*

**Metro I.V.® Injection** *see* metronidazole *on this page*

## metronidazole (me troe NI da zole)

**U.S./Canadian Brand Names** Apo®-Metronidazole (Can); Flagyl® Oral; Metrocream (Can); MetroGel® Topical; MetroGel®-Vaginal; Metro I.V.® Injection; Neo-Metric (Can); NidaGel™ (Can); Noritate™; Novo-Nidazol (Can); Protostat® Oral

**Therapeutic Category** Amebicide; Antibiotic, Topical; Antibiotic, Miscellaneous; Antiprotozoal

**Use** Treatment of susceptible anaerobic bacterial and protozoal infections in the following conditions: amebiasis (liver abscess, dysentery), giardiasis, symptomatic and asymptomatic trichomoniasis; skin and skin structure infections, CNS infections, intra-abdominal infections, and systemic anaerobic bacterial infections; topically for the treatment of acne rosacea; treatment of antibiotic-associated pseudomembranous colitis (AAPC) caused by *C. difficile*; bacterial vaginosis

**Usual Dosage**

Infants and Children:

Amebiasis: Oral: 35-50 mg/kg/day in divided doses every 8 hours

Other parasitic infections: Oral: 15-30 mg/kg/day in divided doses every 8 hours

Anaerobic infections: Oral, I.V.: 30 mg/kg/day in divided doses every 6 hours

*Clostridium difficile* (antibiotic-associated colitis): Oral: 20 mg/kg/day divided every 6 hours

Maximum dose: 2 g/day

Adults:

Amebiasis: Oral: 500-750 mg every 8 hours

Other parasitic infections: Oral: 250 mg every 8 hours or 2 g as a single dose

Anaerobic infections: Oral, I.V.: 30 mg/kg/day in divided doses every 6 hours; not to exceed 4 g/day

AAPC: Oral: 250-500 mg 3-4 times/day for 10-14 days

Topical: Apply a thin film twice daily to affected areas

Vaginal: One applicatorful in vagina each morning and evening or given once daily at bedtime

**Dosage Forms**

Capsule: 375 mg

Cream: 0.75% (45 g); 1% (30 g)

Gel, topical: 0.75% [7.5 mg/mL] (30 g)

Gel, vaginal: 0.75% (5 g applicator delivering 37.5 mg in 70 g tube)

Injection, ready to use: 5 mg/mL (100 mL)

Lotion: 0.75%

Powder for injection, as hydrochloride: 500 mg

Tablet: 250 mg, 500 mg

Tablet, extended release: 750 mg

**Metubine® Iodide *(Discontinued)*** *see page 750*

## metyrapone (me TEER a pone)

**U.S./Canadian Brand Names** Metopirone®

**Therapeutic Category** Diagnostic Agent

**Use** Diagnostic test for hypothalamic-pituitary ACTH function

**Usual Dosage** Oral:

Children: 15 mg/kg every 4 hours for 6 doses; minimum dose: 250 mg

Adults: 750 mg every 4 hours for 6 doses

**Dosage Forms** Capsule, as tartrate: 250 mg

## metyrosine (me TYE roe seen)

**Synonyms** AMPT; OGMT

**U.S./Canadian Brand Names** Demser®

**Therapeutic Category** Tyrosine Hydroxylase Inhibitor

**Use** Short-term management of pheochromocytoma before surgery, long-term management when surgery is contraindicated or when malignant

**Usual Dosage** Children >12 years and Adults: Oral: Initial: 250 mg 4 times/day, increased by 250-500 mg/day up to 4 g/day; maintenance: 2-3 g/day in 4 divided doses; for preoperative preparation, administer optimum effective dosage for 5-7 days

**Dosage Forms** Capsule: 250 mg

**Mevacor®** *see* lovastatin *on page 358*

**mevinolin** *see* lovastatin *on page 358*

## mexiletine (MEKS i le teen)

**U.S./Canadian Brand Names** Mexitil®; Novo-Mexiletine (Can)

**Therapeutic Category** Antiarrhythmic Agent, Class I-B

(Continued)

## mexiletine *(Continued)*

**Use** Management of serious ventricular arrhythmias; suppression of PVCs

**Unlabeled use:** Diabetic neuropathy

**Usual Dosage** Oral:

Children: Range: 1.4-5 mg/kg/dose (mean: 3.3 mg/kg/dose) administered every 8 hours; start with lower initial dose and increase according to effects and serum concentrations

Adults: Initial: 200 mg every 8 hours (may load with 400 mg if necessary); adjust dose every 2-3 days; usual dose: 200-300 mg every 8 hours; maximum dose: 1.2 g/day (some patients respond to every 12-hour dosing)

**Dosage Forms** Capsule: 150 mg, 200 mg, 250 mg

**Mexitil®** *see* mexiletine *on previous page*

**Mezlin®** *see* mezlocillin *on this page*

## mezlocillin (mez loe SIL in)

**U.S./Canadian Brand Names** Mezlin®

**Therapeutic Category** Penicillin

**Use** Treatment of infections caused by susceptible gram-negative aerobic bacilli (*Klebsiella, Proteus, Escherichia coli, Enterobacter, Pseudomonas aeruginosa, Serratia*) involving the skin and skin structure, bone and joint, respiratory tract, urinary tract, gastrointestinal tract, as well as septicemia

**Usual Dosage** I.M., I.V.:

Children: 200-300 mg/kg/day divided every 4-6 hours; maximum: 24 g/day

Adults:

Uncomplicated urinary tract infection: 1.5-2 g every 6 hours

Serious infections: 3-4 g every 4-6 hours

**Dosage Forms** Powder for injection, as sodium: 2 g

**Miacalcin®** *see* calcitonin *on page 96*

**Micanol® Cream** *see* anthralin *on page 42*

**Micardis®** *see* telmisartan *on page 572*

**Micardis® HCT** *see* telmisartan and hydrochlorothiazide *on page 572*

**Micatin® Topical [OTC]** *see* miconazole *on this page*

## miconazole (mi KON a zole)

**U.S./Canadian Brand Names** Absorbine® Antifungal Foot Powder [OTC]; Breezee® Mist Antifungal [OTC]; Femizol-M® [OTC]; Fungoid® Creme; Fungoid® Tincture; Lotrimin® AF Powder [OTC]; Lotrimin® AF Spray Liquid [OTC]; Lotrimin® AF Spray Powder [OTC]; Maximum Strength Desenex® Antifungal Cream [OTC]; Micatin® Topical [OTC]; Mitrazol® [OTC]; Monazole-7® (Can); Monistat-Derm™ Topical; Monistat i.v.™ Injection; Monistat™ Vaginal; M-Zole® 7 Dual Pack [OTC]; Prescription Strength Desenex® [OTC]; Zeasorb-AF® Powder [OTC]

**Therapeutic Category** Antifungal Agent

**Use**

I.V.: Treatment of severe systemic fungal infections and fungal meningitis due to susceptible *Cryptococcus* neoformans, *Candida albicans, Candida tropicalis, Candida parapsilosis, Coccidioides immitis*, and *Histoplasma capsulatum* that are refractory to standard treatment

Topical: Treatment of vulvovaginal candidiasis; topical treatment of superficial fungal infections

**Usual Dosage**

Children:

I.V.: 20-40 mg/kg/day divided every 8 hours

Topical: Apply twice daily for 2-4 weeks

Vaginal: Insert contents of one applicator of vaginal cream or 100 mg suppository at bedtime for 7 days, or 200 mg suppository at bedtime for 3 days

Adults:

I.T.: 20 mg every 3-7 days

I.V.: Candidiasis: 600-1800 mg/day divided every 8 hours

Topical: Apply twice daily for 2-4 weeks

Vaginal: Insert contents of one applicator of vaginal cream or 100 mg suppository at bedtime for 7 days, or 200 mg suppository at bedtime for 3 days

Coccidioidomycosis: 1800-3600 mg/day divided every 8 hours

Cryptococcosis: 1200-2400 mg/day divided every 8 hours

Paracoccidioidomycosis: 200-1200 mg/day divided every 8 hours

**Dosage Forms**

Cream:

Topical, as nitrate: 2% (15 g, 30 g, 56.7 g, 85 g)

Vaginal, as nitrate: 2% (45 g is equivalent to 7 doses)

Dual pack: Vaginal suppositories and external vulvar cream 2%

Injection: 1% [10 mg/mL] (20 mL)

Lotion, as nitrate: 2% (30 mL, 60 mL)

Powder, topical: 2% (45 g, 90 g, 113 g)

Spray, topical: 2% (105 mL)

Suppository, vaginal, as nitrate: 100 mg (7s); 200 mg (3s)

Tincture: 2% with alcohol (7.39 mL, 29.57 mL)

**MICRhoGAM™** *see* $Rh_0$(D) immune globulin (intramuscular) *on page 523*

## microfibrillar collagen hemostat

(mye kro FI bri lar KOL la jen HEE moe stat)

**Synonyms** MCH

**U.S./Canadian Brand Names** Avitene®; Helistat®; Hemotene®

**Therapeutic Category** Hemostatic Agent

**Use** Adjunct to hemostasis when control of bleeding by ligature is ineffective or impractical

**Usual Dosage** Apply dry directly to source of bleeding

**Dosage Forms**

Fibrous: 1 g, 5 g

Nonwoven web: 70 mm x 70 mm x 1 mm; 70 mm x 35 mm x 1 mm

Sponge: 1" x 2" (10s); 3" x 4" (10s); 9" x 10" (5s)

**Micro-K® 10** *see* potassium chloride *on page 485*

**Micro-K® 10 Extencaps®** *see* potassium chloride *on page 485*

**Micro-K® LS** *see* potassium chloride *on page 485*

**Microlipid™ [OTC]** *see* nutritional formula, enteral/oral *on page 432*

**Micronase®** *see* glyburide *on page 276*

**microNefrin® [OTC]** *see* epinephrine *on page 216*

**Micronor®** *see* norethindrone *on page 425*

**Microzide™** *see* hydrochlorothiazide *on page 299*

**Midamor®** *see* amiloride *on page 30*

## midazolam (MID aye zoe lam)

**U.S./Canadian Brand Names** Versed®

**Therapeutic Category** Benzodiazepine

**Controlled Substance** C-IV

**Use** Preoperative sedation; conscious sedation prior to diagnostic or radiographic procedures

(Continued)

## midazolam *(Continued)*

**Usual Dosage**

Preoperative sedation: Children:

Oral:

<5 years: 0.5 mg/kg;

>5 years: 0.4-0.5 mg/kg; doses as high as 0.5-0.75 mg/kg have provided effective preanesthetic sedation

I.M.: 0.07-0.08 mg/kg 30 minutes to 1 hour before surgery; range: 0.05-0.1 mg/kg

I.V.: 0.035 mg/kg/dose, repeat over several minutes as required to achieve the desired sedative effect up to a total dose of 0.1-0.2 mg/kg or 5 mg total

Conscious sedation during mechanical ventilation:

Neonates: I.V. continuous infusion: 0.15-1 mcg/kg/minute

Children:

I.V.: 0.1-0.2 mg/kg; follow loading dose with a 1-2 mcg/kg/minute continuous infusion; titrate to the desired effect; range: 0.4-6 mcg/kg/minute

I.V. intermittent infusion: 0.05-0.2 mg/kg every 1-2 hours as needed

Conscious sedation for procedures:

Children:

Oral: 0.2-0.4 mg/kg; dose as high as 1 mg/kg have been used in younger (6 months to <6 years of age) and less cooperative patients; (maximum: 20 mg) 30-45 minutes before the procedure

Intranasal: 0.2-0.4 mg/kg (use undiluted 5 mg/mL injectable drug for intranasal administration)

I.V.: 0.05-0.1 mg/kg 3 minutes before procedure

Adolescents >12 years:

Sedation for procedure: I.V.: 0.5 mg every 3-4 minutes until effect achieved

Preoperative sedation: I.M.: 0.07-0.08 mg/kg 30-60 minutes before surgery; usual dose: 5 mg

Conscious sedation: I.V.: Initial: 0.5-2 mg; slowly titrate to effect by repeating doses every 2-3 minutes; usual total dose: 2.5-5 mg

Adults, healthy <60 years: Some patients respond to doses as low as 1 mg; no more than 2.5 mg should be administered over a period of 2 minutes. Additional doses of midazolam may be administered after a 2-minute waiting period and evaluation of sedation after each dose increment. A total dose >5 mg is generally not needed. If narcotics or other CNS depressants are administered concomitantly, the midazolam dose should be reduced by 30%.

**Dosage Forms** Injection, as hydrochloride: 1 mg/mL (2 mL, 5 mL, 10 mL); 5 mg/mL (1 mL, 2 mL, 5 mL, 10 mL)

## midodrine (MI doe dreen)

**U.S./Canadian Brand Names** Amatine® (Can); ProAmatine

**Therapeutic Category** Alpha-Adrenergic Agonist

**Use** Treatment of symptomatic orthostatic hypotension in patients whose lives are considerably impaired despite standard clinical care.

**Usual Dosage** Adults: Oral: 10 mg 3 times/day (every 3-4 hours); dosing should take place during daytime hours when the patient needs to be upright, pursuing activities of daily living; a suggested dosing schedule is as follows:

Dose 1: Shortly before or upon rising in the morning

Dose 2: At midday

Dose 3: In the late afternoon (not later than 6 PM)

**Dosage Forms** Tablet, as hydrochloride: 2.5 mg, 5 mg

**Midol® IB [OTC]** *see* ibuprofen *on page 311*

**Midol® PM [OTC]** *see* acetaminophen and diphenhydramine *on page 5*

**Midrin®** *see* acetaminophen, isometheptene, and dichloralphenazone *on page 8*

**Mifeprex™** *see* mifepristone *on this page*

## mifepristone (mi fe PRIS tone)

**Synonyms** RU-486; RU-38486

**U.S./Canadian Brand Names** Mifeprex™

**Therapeutic Category** Abortifacient; Antineoplastic Agent; Antiprogestin

**Use** Medical termination of intrauterine pregnancy, through day 49 of pregnancy. Patients may need treatment with misoprostol and possibly surgery to complete therapy

**Unlabeled use:** Treatment of unresectable meningioma; has been studied in the treatment of breast cancer, ovarian cancer, and adrenal cortical carcinoma

**Usual Dosage** Oral:

Adults: Termination of pregnancy: Treatment consists of three office visits by the patient; the patient must read medication guide and sign patient agreement prior to treatment:

Day 1: 600 mg (three 200 mg tablets) taken as a single dose under physician supervision

Day 3: Patient must return to the healthcare provider 2 days following administration of mifepristone; if termination of pregnancy cannot be confirmed using ultrasound or clinical examination: 400 mcg (two 200 mcg tablets) of misoprostol; patient may need treatment for cramps or gastrointestinal symptoms at this time

Day 14: Patient must return to the healthcare provider ~14 days after administration of mifepristone; confirm complete termination of pregnancy by ultrasound or clinical exam. Surgical termination is recommended to manage treatment failures.

**Dosage Forms** Tablet: 200 mcg

**Miflex® Tablet *(Discontinued)*** *see page 750*

## miglitol (MIG li tol)

**U.S./Canadian Brand Names** Glyset™

**Therapeutic Category** Antidiabetic Agent, Oral

**Use** As an adjunct to diet to lower blood glucose in patients with noninsulin-dependent diabetes mellitus (NIDDM)

**Usual Dosage** Adults: Oral: 25 mg 3 times/day with the first bite of food at each meal; dose may be increased to 50 mg 3 times/day after 4-8 weeks; maximum recommended dose: 100 mg 3 times/day

**Dosage Forms** Tablet: 25 mg, 50 mg, 100 mg

**Migquin®** *see* acetaminophen, isometheptene, and dichloralphenazone *on page 8*

**Migraine®** *see* acetaminophen, isometheptene, and dichloralphenazone *on page 8*

**Migranal® Nasal Spray** *see* dihydroergotamine *on page 186*

**Migrapap®** *see* acetaminophen, isometheptene, and dichloralphenazone *on page 8*

**Migratine®** *see* acetaminophen, isometheptene, and dichloralphenazone *on page 8*

**Migrazone®** *see* acetaminophen, isometheptene, and dichloralphenazone *on page 8*

**MIH** *see* procarbazine *on page 497*

**Miles Nervine® Caplets [OTC]** *see* diphenhydramine *on page 191*

**Milkinol® *(Discontinued)*** *see page 750*

**milk of magnesia** *see* magnesium hydroxide *on page 361*

**Milontin® *(Discontinued)*** *see page 750*

**Milophene® *(Discontinued)*** *see page 750*

**Milprem® *(Discontinued)*** *see page 750*

## milrinone (MIL ri none)

**U.S./Canadian Brand Names** Primacor®

**Therapeutic Category** Cardiovascular Agent, Other

**Use** Short-term I.V. therapy of congestive heart failure

**Usual Dosage** Adults: I.V.: Loading dose: 50 mcg/kg administered over 10 minutes, then 0.375-0.75 mcg/kg/min as a continuous infusion for a total daily dose of 0.59-1.13 mg/kg

**Dosage Forms**

Infusion, as lactate, in $D_5W$: 200 mcg/mL (100 mL, 200 mL)
Injection, as lactate: 1 mg/mL (5 mL, 10 mL, 20 mL)

**Miltown®** *see* meprobamate *on page 373*

**Minestrin™ (Can)** *see* ethinyl estradiol and norethindrone *on page 232*

**Minidyne® [OTC]** *see* povidone-iodine *on page 489*

**Mini-Gamulin® Rh *(Discontinued)*** *see page 750*

**Minipress®** *see* prazosin *on page 491*

**Minitran™ Patch** *see* nitroglycerin *on page 422*

**Minizide®** *see* prazosin and polythiazide *on page 491*

**Minocin®** *see* minocycline *on this page*

**Minocin® IV Injection** *see* minocycline *on this page*

**Minocin® Tablet *(Discontinued)*** *see page 750*

## minocycline (mi noe SYE kleen)

**U.S./Canadian Brand Names** Alti-Minocycline (Can); Apo®-Minocycline (Can); Dynacin® Oral; Gen-Minocycline (Can); Minocin®; Minocin® IV Injection; Rhoxal-minocycline (Can); Vectrin®

**Therapeutic Category** Tetracycline Derivative

**Use** Treatment of susceptible bacterial infections of both gram-negative and gram-positive organisms; acne

**Usual Dosage**

Children 8-12 years: 4 mg/kg stat, then 4 mg/kg/day (maximum: 200 mg/day) in divided doses every 12 hours
Adults:
Infection: Oral, I.V.: 200 mg stat, 100 mg every 12 hours
Acne: Oral: 50 mg 1-3 times/day

**Dosage Forms**

Capsule, as hydrochloride: 50 mg, 100 mg
Capsule, as hydrochloride (Dynacin®): 50 mg, 75 mg, 100 mg
Capsule, as hydrochloride (Vectrin®): 50 mg, 100 mg
Capsule, pellet-filled, as hydrochloride (Minocin®): 50 mg, 100 mg
Injection, as hydrochloride (Minocin® IV): 100 mg
Suspension, oral, as hydrochloride (Minocin®)50 mg/5 mL (60 mL)

**Min-Ovral® (Can)** *see* ethinyl estradiol and levonorgestrel *on page 232*

**Minox (Can)** *see* minoxidil *on this page*

## minoxidil (mi NOKS i dil)

**U.S./Canadian Brand Names** Apo®-Gain (Can); Loniten® Oral; Minox (Can); Rogaine® Topical

**Therapeutic Category** Topical Skin Product; Vasodilator

**Use** Management of severe hypertension; topically for management of alopecia or male pattern alopecia

**Usual Dosage**

Children <12 years: Hypertension: Oral: Initial: 0.1-0.2 mg/kg once daily; maximum: 5 mg/day; increase gradually every 3 days; usual dosage: 0.25-1 mg/kg/day in 1-2 divided doses; maximum: 50 mg/day

Adults:

Hypertension: Oral: Initial: 5 mg once daily, increase gradually every 3 days; usual dose: 10-40 mg/day in 1-2 divided doses; maximum: 100 mg/day

Alopecia: Topical: Apply twice daily

**Dosage Forms**

Solution, topical: 2% = 20 mg/metered dose (60 mL); 5% = 50 mg/metered dose (60 mL)

Tablet: 2.5 mg, 10 mg

**Mintezol®** *see* thiabendazole *on page 584*

**Minute-Gel®** *see* fluoride *on page 255*

**Miocarpine® (Can)** *see* pilocarpine *on page 471*

**Miochol® *(Discontinued)*** *see page 750*

**Miochol-E®** *see* acetylcholine *on page 9*

**Mio-Rel®** *see* orphenadrine *on page 438*

**Miostat® Intraocular** *see* carbachol *on page 105*

**MiraLax™** *see* polyethylene glycol solution *on page 480*

**Mirapex®** *see* pramipexole *on page 490*

**Mircette®** *see* ethinyl estradiol and desogestrel *on page 230*

**Mirena®** *see* levonorgestrel *on page 347*

## mirtazapine (mir TAZ a peen)

**U.S./Canadian Brand Names** Remeron®; Remeron® SolTab™

**Therapeutic Category** Antidepressant, Alpha-2 Antagonist

**Use** Treatment of depression, works through noradrenergic and serotonergic pharmacologic action

**Usual Dosage** Adults: Oral: Initial: 15 mg/day, then 15-45 mg/day

**Dosage Forms**

Tablet: 15 mg, 30 mg, 45 mg

Tablet, orally disintegrating, orange flavor: 15 mg [phenylalanine 2.6 mg/tablet]; 30 mg [phenylalanine 5.2 mg/tablet]; 45 mg [phenylalanine 7.8 mg/tablet]

## misoprostol (mye soe PROST ole)

**U.S./Canadian Brand Names** Cytotec®

**Therapeutic Category** Prostaglandin

**Use** Prevention of NSAID-induced gastric ulcers

**Usual Dosage** Oral: 200 mcg 4 times/day with food

**Dosage Forms** Tablet: 100 mcg, 200 mcg

**Mithracin®** *see* plicamycin *on page 475*

**mithramycin** *see* plicamycin *on page 475*

## mitomycin (mye toe MYE sin)

**Synonyms** mitomycin-c; MTC

**U.S./Canadian Brand Names** Mutamycin®

**Therapeutic Category** Antineoplastic Agent

**Use** Therapy of disseminated adenocarcinoma of stomach, colon, or pancreas in combination with other approved chemotherapeutic agents; bladder cancer, breast cancer

(Continued)

## mitomycin *(Continued)*

**Usual Dosage** Children and Adults (refer to individual protocols): I.V.: 10-20 mg/m²/dose every 6-8 weeks, or 2 mg/m²/day for 5 days, stop for 2 days then repeat; subsequent doses should be adjusted to platelet and leukocyte response

**Dosage Forms** Powder for injection: 5 mg, 20 mg, 40 mg

**mitomycin-c** *see* mitomycin *on previous page*

## mitotane (MYE toe tane)

**Synonyms** o,p′-DDD

**U.S./Canadian Brand Names** Lysodren®

**Therapeutic Category** Antineoplastic Agent

**Use** Treatment of inoperable adrenal cortical carcinoma

**Usual Dosage** Adults: Oral: 8-10 g/day in 3-4 divided doses; dose is changed based on side effects with aim of administering as high a dose as tolerated

**Dosage Forms** Tablet: 500 mg

## mitoxantrone (mye toe ZAN trone)

**Synonyms** DHAD

**U.S./Canadian Brand Names** Novantrone®

**Therapeutic Category** Antineoplastic Agent

**Use** FDA approved for remission-induction therapy of acute nonlymphocytic leukemia (ANLL); mitoxantrone is also active against other various leukemias, lymphoma, and breast cancer, and moderately active against pediatric sarcoma

**Usual Dosage** I.V. (refer to individual protocols):

Leukemias:

Children ≤2 years: 0.4 mg/kg/day once daily for 3-5 days

Children >2 years and Adults: 8-12 mg/m²/day once daily for 5 days or 12 mg/m²/day once daily for 3 days

Solid tumors:

Children: 18-20 mg/m² every 3-4 weeks

Adults: 12-14 mg/m² every 3-4 weeks

**Dosage Forms** Injection, as base: 2 mg/mL (10 mL, 12.5 mL, 15 mL)

**Mitran® Oral *(Discontinued)*** *see page 750*

**Mitrazol® [OTC]** *see* miconazole *on page 390*

**Mitrolan® Chewable Tablet [OTC]** *see* calcium polycarbophil *on page 101*

**Mivacron®** *see* mivacurium *on this page*

## mivacurium (mye va KYOO ree um)

**U.S./Canadian Brand Names** Mivacron®

**Therapeutic Category** Skeletal Muscle Relaxant

**Use** Short-acting nondepolarizing neuromuscular blocking agent; an adjunct to general anesthesia; facilitates endotracheal intubation; provides skeletal muscle relaxation during surgery or mechanical ventilation

**Usual Dosage** I.V.:

Children 2-12 years: 0.2 mg/kg over 5-15 seconds; continuous infusion: 14 mcg/kg

Adults: Initial: 0.15 mg/kg administered over 5-15 seconds

**Dosage Forms** Injection, as chloride: 2 mg/mL (5 mL, 10 mL, 20 mL, 50 mL)

**MK594** *see* losartan *on page 357*

**MMR** *see* measles, mumps, and rubella vaccines, combined *on page 366*

**M-M-R® II** *see* measles, mumps, and rubella vaccines, combined *on page 366*

**Moban®** *see* molindone *on page 398*

**Mobic®** *see* meloxicam *on page 370*

**Mobidin®** *see* magnesium salicylate *on page 362*

## moclobemide *(Canada only)* (moe KLOE be mide)

**Synonyms** Ro 11-1163

**U.S./Canadian Brand Names** Alti-Moclobemide (Can); Apo®-Moclobemide (Can); Manerix® (Can); Novo-Moclobemide (Can); Nu-Moclobemide (Can)

**Therapeutic Category** Antidepressant, Monoamine Oxidase Inhibitor

**Use** Depression; smoking cessation

**Usual Dosage** Oral:

Depression: Initial: 100 mg 3 times/day immediately following a meal; maximum dose/day: 600 mg; reduce dosage by 30% to 50% in patients with hepatic disease

Smoking cessation: 400 mg/day for 2 months, then, 200 mg/day for 1 month

**Dosage Forms** Tablet: 100 mg, 150 mg, 300 mg

**Moctanin®** *see* monoctanoin *on page 399*

## modafinil (moe DAF i nil)

**U.S./Canadian Brand Names** Alertec® (Can); Provigil®

**Therapeutic Category** Central Nervous System Stimulant, Nonamphetamine

**Controlled Substance** C-IV

**Use** Indicated to improve wakefulness in patients with excessive daytime sleepiness associated with narcolepsy

**Usual Dosage** Adults: Oral: Initial: 200 mg as a single daily dose

**Dosage Forms** Tablet: 100 mg, 200 mg

**Modane® Bulk [OTC]** *see* psyllium *on page 509*

**Modane® Soft [OTC]** *see* docusate *on page 197*

**Modecate® (Can)** *see* fluphenazine *on page 258*

**Modicon™** *see* ethinyl estradiol and norethindrone *on page 232*

**modified Dakin's solution** *see* sodium hypochlorite solution *on page 550*

**Moducal® [OTC]** *see* glucose polymers *on page 276*

**Modulon® (Can)** *see* trimebutine *(Canada only) on page 606*

**Moduret® (Can)** *see* amiloride and hydrochlorothiazide *on page 30*

**Moduretic®** *see* amiloride and hydrochlorothiazide *on page 30*

## moexipril (mo EKS i pril)

**U.S./Canadian Brand Names** Univasc®

**Therapeutic Category** Angiotensin-Converting Enzyme (ACE) Inhibitor

**Use** Treatment of hypertension, alone or in combination with thiazide diuretics

**Usual Dosage** Oral:

Patients not receiving diuretics: Initial: 7.5 mg 1 hour prior to meals once daily; if antihypertensive effect diminishes toward end of dosing interval, increase or divide dose; maintenance dose of 7.5-30 mg/day in 1 or 2 divided doses

Patients receiving diuretics: Discontinue diuretic 2-3 days before starting moexipril to avoid symptomatic hypotension; if blood pressure is not controlled, resume diuretic therapy; if diuretic cannot be held, initiate moexipril at 3.75 mg/day

**Dosage Forms** Tablet, as hydrochloride: 7.5 mg, 15 mg

## moexipril and hydrochlorothiazide

(mo EKS i pril & hye droe klor oh THYE a zide)

**U.S./Canadian Brand Names** Uniretic™

**Therapeutic Category** Angiotensin-Converting Enzyme (ACE) Inhibitor; Diuretic, Thiazide

**Use** Treatment of hypertension

(Continued)

**moexipril and hydrochlorothiazide** *(Continued)*

**Usual Dosage** Adults: Oral: 7.5-30 mg of moexipril, taken either in a single or divided dose one hour before meals

**Dosage Forms** Tablet: Moexipril hydrochloride 7.5 mg and hydrochlorothiazide 12.5 mg; moexipril hydrochloride 15 mg and hydrochlorothiazide 25 mg

**Moi-Stir® Solution [OTC]** *see* saliva substitute *on page 536*

**Moi-Stir® Swabsticks [OTC]** *see* saliva substitute *on page 536*

**Moisturel® Lotion *(Discontinued)*** *see page 750*

**Moisture® Ophthalmic Drops [OTC]** *see* artificial tears *on page 53*

## molindone (moe LIN done)

**U.S./Canadian Brand Names** Moban®

**Therapeutic Category** Antipsychotic Agent, Dihydroindoline

**Use** Management of psychotic disorder

**Usual Dosage** Oral: 50-75 mg/day; up to 225 mg/day

**Dosage Forms**

Concentrate, oral, as hydrochloride: 20 mg/mL (120 mL)

Tablet, as hydrochloride: 5 mg, 10 mg, 25 mg, 50 mg, 100 mg

**Mol-Iron® [OTC]** *see* ferrous sulfate *on page 247*

**Mollifene® Ear Wax Removing Formula [OTC]** *see* carbamide peroxide *on page 106*

**molybdenum injection** *see* trace metals *on page 598*

**Molypen®** *see* trace metals *on page 598*

**MOM** *see* magnesium hydroxide *on page 361*

## mometasone furoate (moe MET a sone FYOOR oh ate)

**U.S./Canadian Brand Names** Elocom® (Can); Elocon®; Nasonex®

**Therapeutic Category** Corticosteroid, Intranasal; Corticosteroid, Topical

**Use** Topical forms for the relief of the inflammatory and pruritic manifestations of corticosteroid-responsive dermatoses (medium potency topical corticosteroid); nasal spray used for the prophylaxis and treatment of nasal symptoms of seasonal allergic rhinitis and the treatment of nasal symptoms of perennial allergic rhinitis in adults and children 12 years of age and older

**Usual Dosage** Adults:

Nasally: 200 mcg (two sprays per nostril) once daily

Topical: Apply sparingly to area once daily, do not use occlusive dressings

**Dosage Forms**

Cream: 0.1% (15 g, 45 g)

Lotion: 0.1% (30 mL, 60 mL)

Ointment, topical: 0.1% (15 g, 45 g)

Spray, nasal, as monohydrate: 50 mcg/spray (17 g)

**mom/mineral oil emulsion** *see* magnesium hydroxide and mineral oil emulsion *on page 362*

**monacolin k** *see* lovastatin *on page 358*

**Monafed®** *see* guaifenesin *on page 281*

**Monafed® DM** *see* guaifenesin and dextromethorphan *on page 282*

**Monarc-M®** *see* antihemophilic factor (human) *on page 43*

**Monazole-7® (Can)** *see* miconazole *on page 390*

***Monilia* skin test** *see Candida albicans (Monilia) on page 103*

**Monistat® 1 [OTC]** *see* tioconazole *on page 592*

**Monistat-Derm™ Topical** *see* miconazole *on page 390*

**Monistat i.v.™ Injection** *see* miconazole *on page 390*

**Monistat™ Vaginal** *see* miconazole *on page 390*

**Monitan® (Can)** *see* acebutolol *on page 3*

## monobenzone (mon oh BEN zone)

**U.S./Canadian Brand Names** Benoquin®

**Therapeutic Category** Topical Skin Product

**Use** Final depigmentation in extensive vitiligo

**Usual Dosage** Adults: Topical: Apply 2-3 times/day

**Dosage Forms** Cream: 20% (35.4 g)

**Monocete® Topical Liquid *(Discontinued)*** *see page 750*

**Monocid®** *see* cefonicid *on page 115*

**monoclonal antibody** *see* muromonab-CD3 *on page 403*

**monoclonal antibody purified** *see* factor IX (purified/human) *on page 239*

**Monocor® (Can)** *see* bisoprolol *on page 82*

## monoctanoin (mon OK ta noyn)

**Synonyms** monooctanoin

**U.S./Canadian Brand Names** Moctanin®

**Therapeutic Category** Gallstone Dissolution Agent

**Use** Solubilize cholesterol gallstones that are retained in the biliary tract after cholecystectomy

**Usual Dosage** Administer via T-tube into common bile duct at rate of 3-5 mL/hour at pressure of 10 mL water for 7-21 days

**Dosage Forms** Solution: 120 mL

**Monodox®** *see* doxycycline *on page 204*

**Mono-Gesic®** *see* salsalate *on page 536*

**Monoket®** *see* isosorbide mononitrate *on page 329*

**Mononine®** *see* factor IX (purified/human) *on page 239*

**monooctanoin** *see* monoctanoin *on this page*

**Monopril®** *see* fosinopril *on page 265*

**Monopril-HCT®** *see* fosinopril and hydrochlorothiazide *on page 265*

## montelukast (mon te LOO kast)

**U.S./Canadian Brand Names** Singulair®

**Therapeutic Category** Leukotriene Receptor Antagonist

**Use** Prophylaxis and chronic treatment of asthma in adults and children ≥6 years

**Usual Dosage** Oral:

Children 6-14 years: 5 mg once daily

Children >14 years and Adults: 10 mg once daily

**Dosage Forms**

Tablet, as sodium: 10 mg

Tablet, chewable (cherry), as sodium: 4 mg, 5 mg

**Monurol™** *see* fosfomycin *on page 265*

**more attenuated enders strain** *see* measles virus vaccine (live) *on page 367*

**More-Dophilus® [OTC]** *see* Lactobacillus *on page 338*

## moricizine (mor EYE siz een)

**U.S./Canadian Brand Names** Ethmozine®

**Therapeutic Category** Antiarrhythmic Agent, Class I

(Continued)

## moricizine *(Continued)*

**Use** Treatment of ventricular tachycardia and life-threatening ventricular arrhythmias; a Class I antiarrhythmic agent

**Usual Dosage** Adults: Oral: 200-300 mg every 8 hours, adjust dosage at 150 mg/day at 3-day intervals

**Dosage Forms** Tablet, as hydrochloride: 200 mg, 250 mg, 300 mg

## morphine sulfate (MOR feen SUL fate)

**Synonyms** MS

**U.S./Canadian Brand Names** Duramorph® Injection; Infumorph™; Kadian™ Oral; M-Eslon® (Can); MS Contin® Oral; MSIR® Oral; Oramorph SR™ Oral; RMS® Rectal; Roxanol™ Oral; Roxanol SR™ Oral; Roxanol-T™; Statex® (Can)

**Therapeutic Category** Analgesic, Narcotic

**Controlled Substance** C-II

**Use** Relief of moderate to severe acute and chronic pain; pain of myocardial infarction; relieves dyspnea of acute left ventricular failure and pulmonary edema; preanesthetic medication

**Usual Dosage** Doses should be titrated to appropriate effect; when changing routes of administration in chronically treated patients, please note that oral doses are approximately $^1/_6$ as effective as parenteral dose

Infants and Children:

- Oral: Tablet and solution (prompt-release): 0.2-0.5 mg/kg/dose every 4-6 hours as needed; tablet (controlled-release): 0.3-0.6 mg/kg/dose every 12 hours
- I.M., I.V., S.C.: 0.1-0.2 mg/kg/dose every 2-4 hours as needed; usual maximum: 15 mg/dose; may initiate at 0.05 mg/kg/dose
- I.V., S.C. continuous infusion: Sickle cell or cancer pain: 0.025-2 mg/kg/hour; postoperative pain: 0.01-0.04 mg/kg/hour
- Sedation/analgesia for procedures: I.V.: 0.05-0.1 mg/kg 5 minutes before the procedure

Adolescents >12 years: Sedation/analgesia for procedures: I.V.: 3-4 mg and repeat in 5 minutes if necessary

Adults:

- Oral: Prompt-release: 10-30 mg every 4 hours as needed; controlled release: 15-30 mg every 8-12 hours
- I.M., I.V., S.C.: 2.5-20 mg/dose every 2-6 hours as needed; usual: 10 mg/dose every 4 hours as needed
- I.V., S.C. continuous infusion: 0.8-10 mg/hour; may increase depending on pain relief/adverse effects; usual range up to 80 mg/hour
- Epidural: Initial: 5 mg in lumbar region; if inadequate pain relief within 1 hour, administer 1-2 mg, maximum dose: 10 mg/24 hours
- Intrathecal ($^1/_{10}$ of epidural dose): 0.2-1 mg/dose; repeat doses **not** recommended

**Dosage Forms**

Capsule (MSIR®): 15 mg, 30 mg

Capsule, sustained release (Kadian™): 20 mg, 30 mg, 50 mg, 60 mg, 100 mg

Infusion: 0.2 mg/mL in $D_5W$ (250 mL, 500 mL); 1 mg/mL in $D_5W$ (100 mL, 250 mL, 500 mL)

Injection: 0.5 mg/mL (30 mL); 1 mg/mL (10 mL, 30 mL, 50 mL, 60 mL); 2 mg/mL (1 mL, 60 mL); 4 mg/mL (1 mL); 5 mg/mL (1 mL, 30 mL, 50 mL); 8 mg/mL (1 mL); 10 mg/mL (1 mL, 10 mL, 20 mL); 15 mg/mL (1 mL, 20 mL); 25 mg/mL (4 mL, 10 mL, 20 mL, 40 mL, 50 mL); 50 mg/mL (10 mL, 20 mL, 40 mL, 50 mL)

- Astramorph™ PF [preservative free]: 0.5 mg/mL (2 mL, 10 mL); 1 mg/mL (2 mL, 10 mL)
- Infumorph™: 10 mg/mL (20 mL); 25 mg/mL (20 mL)
- Duramorph® [preservative free]: 0.5 mg/mL (2 mL, 10 mL); 1 mg/mL (2 mL, 10 mL)

Injection, I.V. infusion preparation: 25 mg/mL (4 mL, 10 mL, 20 mL)

Injection, I.V. via PCA pump: 1 mg/mL (10 mL, 30 mL, 60 mL); 5 mg/mL (30 mL)

Solution, oral: 10 mg/5 mL (5 mL, 100 mL, 500 mL); 20 mg/5 mL (5 mL, 100 mL, 120 mL, 500 mL)

MSIR®: 10 mg/5 mL (5 mL, 120 mL); 20 mg/5 mL (5 mL, 120 mL); 20 mg/mL (30 mL, 120 mL)
Roxanol™: 20 mg/mL (30 mL, 120 mL)
Roxanol™ T: 20 mg/mL (30 mL, 120 mL) [flavored] [tinted]
Roxanol 100™: 100 mg/5 mL (240 mL) [with calibrated spoon]
Suppository, rectal: 5 mg, 10 mg, 20 mg, 30 mg
MS/S®, RMS®, Roxanol™: 5 mg, 10 mg, 20 mg, 30 mg
Tablet: 15 mg, 30 mg
MSIR®: 15 mg, 30 mg
Tablet, controlled release: MS Contin®: 15 mg, 30 mg, 60 mg, 100 mg, 200 mg
Tablet, extended release: 15 mg, 30 mg, 60 mg
Tablet, sustained release (Oramorph SR™): 15 mg, 30 mg, 60 mg, 100 mg

## morrhuate sodium (MOR yoo ate SOW dee um)

**U.S./Canadian Brand Names** Scleromate™

**Therapeutic Category** Sclerosing Agent

**Use** Treatment of small, uncomplicated varicose veins of the lower extremities

**Usual Dosage** I.V.:

Children 1-18 years: Esophageal hemorrhage: 2, 3, or 4 mL of 5% solution repeated every 3-4 days until bleeding is controlled, then every 6 weeks until varices obliterated

Adults: 50-250 mg, repeat at 5- to 7-day intervals (50-100 mg for small veins, 150-250 mg for large veins)

**Dosage Forms** Injection: 50 mg/mL (30 mL)

**MoRu-Viraten Berna™ (Can)** *see* measles and rubella vaccines, combined *on page 366*

**Motilium® (Can)** *see* domperidone *(Canada only) on page 200*

**Motofen®** *see* difenoxin and atropine *on page 184*

**Motrin®** *see* ibuprofen *on page 311*

**Motrin® IB [OTC]** *see* ibuprofen *on page 311*

**Motrin® IB Sinus [OTC]** *see* pseudoephedrine and ibuprofen *on page 508*

**Mouthkote® Solution [OTC]** *see* saliva substitute *on page 536*

**Moxam® Injection *(Discontinued)*** *see page 750*

## moxifloxacin (mox i FLOX a sin)

**U.S./Canadian Brand Names** Avelox™

**Therapeutic Category** Antibiotic, Quinolone

**Use** Treatment of mild to moderate community-acquired pneumonia, acute bacterial exacerbation of chronic bronchitis, acute bacterial sinusitis, uncomplicated skin infections

**Usual Dosage** Adults: Oral:

Community-acquired pneumonia or acute bacterial sinusitis: 400 mg every 24 hours for 10 days

Chronic bronchitis, acute bacterial exacerbation: 400 mg every 24 hours for 5 days

Uncomplicated skin infections: 400 mg every 24 hours for 7 days

**Dosage Forms** Tablet: 400 mg

**4-MP** *see* fomepizole *on page 264*

**6-MP** *see* mercaptopurine *on page 373*

**M-Prednisol® Injection** *see* methylprednisolone *on page 385*

**M-R-VAX® II** *see* measles and rubella vaccines, combined *on page 366*

**MS** *see* morphine sulfate *on previous page*

**MS Contin® Oral** *see* morphine sulfate *on previous page*

**MSIR® Oral** *see* morphine sulfate *on previous page*

**MSTA** *see* mumps skin test antigen *on this page*

**MSTA® Mumps** *see* mumps skin test antigen *on this page*

**MTC** *see* mitomycin *on page 395*

**M.T.E.-4®** *see* trace metals *on page 598*

**M.T.E.-5®** *see* trace metals *on page 598*

**M.T.E.-6®** *see* trace metals *on page 598*

**MTX** *see* methotrexate *on page 380*

**Muco-Fen-DM®** *see* guaifenesin and dextromethorphan *on page 282*

**Muco-Fen-LA®** *see* guaifenesin *on page 281*

**Mucomyst®** *see* acetylcysteine *on page 10*

**Mucoplex® [OTC]** *see* vitamin B complex *on page 630*

**MulTE-PAK-4®** *see* trace metals *on page 598*

**MulTE-PAK-5®** *see* trace metals *on page 598*

**Multitest CMI®** *see* skin test antigens, multiple *on page 546*

**multivitamins/fluoride** *see* vitamin (multiple/pediatric) *on page 632*

**Multi Vit® Drops [OTC]** *see* vitamin (multiple/pediatric) *on page 632*

## mumps skin test antigen (mumpz skin test AN ti jen)

**Synonyms** MSTA

**U.S./Canadian Brand Names** MSTA® Mumps

**Therapeutic Category** Diagnostic Agent

**Use** Assess the status of cell-mediated immunity

**Usual Dosage** Children and Adults: 0.1 mL intradermally into flexor surface of the forearm; examine reaction site in 24-48 hours; a positive reaction is ≥1.5 mm diameter induration

**Dosage Forms** Injection: 1 mL (10 tests)

**Mumpsvax®** *see* mumps virus vaccine, live, attenuated *on this page*

## mumps virus vaccine, live, attenuated

(mumpz VYE rus vak SEEN, live, a ten YOO ate ed)

**U.S./Canadian Brand Names** Mumpsvax®

**Therapeutic Category** Vaccine, Live Virus

**Use** Immunization against mumps in children ≥12 months and adults

**Usual Dosage** S.C.: 1 vial (5000 units) in outer aspect of the upper arm

**Dosage Forms** Injection: Single dose

## mupirocin (myoo PEER oh sin)

**Synonyms** pseudomonic acid A

**U.S./Canadian Brand Names** Bactroban®; Bactroban® Nasal

**Therapeutic Category** Antibiotic, Topical

**Use** Topical treatment of impetigo caused by *Staphylococcus aureus* and *Streptococcus pyogenes*; also effective for the topical treatment of folliculitis, furunculosis, minor wounds, burns, and ulcers caused by susceptible organisms; used as a prophylactic agent applied to intravenous catheter exit sites; used for eradication of *S. aureus* from nasal and perineal carriage sites

**Usual Dosage**

Children and Adults: Topical: Apply small amount to affected area 2-5 times/day for 5-14 days

Children ≥12 years and Adults: Intranasal: ~½ of a single-use tube (0.5 g) to each nostril twice daily for 5 days

**Dosage Forms**

Cream: 2% (15 g, 30 g)

Ointment, as calcium:
Intranasal: 2% (1 g single use tube)
Topical: 2% (15 g, 30 g)

**Murine® Ear Drops [OTC]** *see* carbamide peroxide *on page 106*

**Murine® Plus Ophthalmic [OTC]** *see* tetrahydrozoline *on page 580*

**Murine® Solution [OTC]** *see* artificial tears *on page 53*

**Muro 128® Ophthalmic [OTC]** *see* sodium chloride *on page 549*

**Murocel® Ophthalmic Solution [OTC]** *see* artificial tears *on page 53*

**Murocoll-2® Ophthalmic** *see* phenylephrine and scopolamine *on page 468*

## muromonab-CD3 (myoo roe MOE nab see dee three)

**Synonyms** monoclonal antibody; OKT3

**U.S./Canadian Brand Names** Orthoclone® OKT3

**Therapeutic Category** Immunosuppressant Agent

**Use** Treatment of acute allograft rejection in renal transplant patients; effective in reversing acute hepatic, cardiac, and bone marrow transplant rejection episodes resistant to conventional treatment

**Usual Dosage** I.V. (refer to individual protocols):
Children <30 kg: 2.5 mg/day once daily for 10-14 days
Adults: 5 mg/day once daily for 10-14 days
Children and Adults: Methylprednisolone sodium succinate 1 mg/kg I.V. administered prior to first muromonab-CD3 administration and I.V. hydrocortisone sodium succinate 50-100 mg administered 30 minutes after administration are strongly recommended to decrease the incidence of reactions to the first dose; patient temperature should not exceed 37.8°C (100°F) at time of administration

**Dosage Forms** Injection: 1 mg/mL (5 mL)

**Muroptic-5® [OTC]** *see* sodium chloride *on page 549*

**Muse® Pellet** *see* alprostadil *on page 23*

**Mus-Lax® *(Discontinued)*** *see page 750*

**Mustargen® Hydrochloride** *see* mechlorethamine *on page 367*

**mustine** *see* mechlorethamine *on page 367*

**Mutamycin®** *see* mitomycin *on page 395*

**M.V.C.® 9 + 3** *see* vitamin (multiple/injectable) *on page 632*

**M.V.I.®-12** *see* vitamin (multiple/injectable) *on page 632*

**M.V.I.® Concentrate** *see* vitamin (multiple/injectable) *on page 632*

**M.V.I.® Pediatric** *see* vitamin (multiple/injectable) *on page 632*

**Myambutol®** *see* ethambutol *on page 229*

**Mycelex®** *see* clotrimazole *on page 147*

**Mycelex®-7** *see* clotrimazole *on page 147*

**Mycelex®-G** *see* clotrimazole *on page 147*

**Mycifradin® Sulfate** *see* neomycin *on page 413*

**Mycil® (Can)** *see* chlorphenesin *(Canada only) on page 129*

**Mycinettes® [OTC]** *see* benzocaine *on page 72*

**Mycitracin® Topical [OTC]** *see* bacitracin, neomycin, and polymyxin B *on page 65*

**Mycobutin®** *see* rifabutin *on page 526*

**Mycogen II Topical** *see* nystatin and triamcinolone *on page 433*

**Mycolog®-II Topical** *see* nystatin and triamcinolone *on page 433*

**Myco-Nail® [OTC]** *see* triacetin *on page 601*

**Myconel® Topical *(Discontinued)*** *see page 750*

## mycophenolate (mye koe FEN oh late)

**U.S./Canadian Brand Names** CellCept®

**Therapeutic Category** Immunosuppressant Agent

**Use** Prophylaxis of organ rejection concomitantly with cyclosporine and corticosteroids in patients receiving allogenic renal, cardiac, or hepatic transplants. Intravenous formulation is an alternative dosage form to oral capsules, suspension, and tablets.

**Unlabeled uses:** Treatment of rejection in liver transplant patients unable to tolerate tacrolimus or cyclosporine due to neurotoxicity; mild rejection in heart transplant patients; treatment of moderate-severe psoriasis

**Usual Dosage** Adults: I.V./Oral: 1 g twice daily (2 g daily dose), administered within 72 hours of transplantation, when administered in combination with corticosteroids and cyclosporine

**Dosage Forms**

Capsule, as mofetil: 250 mg
Powder for injection, as hydrochloride: 500 mg
Suspension, oral, as mofetil: 200 mg/mL (175 mL)
Tablet, as mofetil: 500 mg

**Mycostatin®** *see* nystatin *on page 432*

**Myco-Triacet® II** *see* nystatin and triamcinolone *on page 433*

**Mydfrin® Ophthalmic Solution** *see* phenylephrine *on page 467*

**Mydral®** *see* tropicamide *on page 611*

**Mydriacyl®** *see* tropicamide *on page 611*

**Myferon® 150 [OTC]** *see* polysaccharide-iron complex *on page 482*

**Mykrox®** *see* metolazone *on page 387*

**Mylanta® [OTC]** *see* aluminum hydroxide, magnesium hydroxide, and simethicone *on page 27*

**Mylanta AR®** *see* famotidine *on page 240*

**Mylanta Gas® [OTC]** *see* simethicone *on page 544*

**Mylanta® Gelcaps® [OTC]** *see* Calcium Carbonate and Magnesium Hydroxide *on page 98*

**Mylanta®-II [OTC]** *see* aluminum hydroxide, magnesium hydroxide, and simethicone *on page 27*

**Mylanta® Tablets [OTC]** *see* Calcium Carbonate and Magnesium Hydroxide *on page 98*

**Mylanta® Ultra Tablet [OTC]** *see* Calcium Carbonate and Magnesium Hydroxide *on page 98*

**Mylaxen® Injection *(Discontinued)*** *see page 750*

**Myleran®** *see* busulfan *on page 92*

**Mylicon® [OTC]** *see* simethicone *on page 544*

**Mylocel™** *see* hydroxyurea *on page 307*

**Mylotarg™** *see* gemtuzumab ozogamicin *on page 271*

**Myminic® Expectorant *(Discontinued)*** *see page 750*

**Myobloc®** *see* botulinum toxin type B *on page 84*

**Myochrysine® *(Discontinued)*** *see page 750*

**Myoflex® [OTC]** *see* triethanolamine salicylate *on page 605*

**Myotonachol™ *(Discontinued)*** *see page 750*

**Myphetane DC® *(Discontinued)*** *see page 750*

**Mysoline®** *see* primidone *on page 495*

**Mytelase® Caplets®** *see* ambenonium *on page 28*

**Mytrex® F Topical** *see* nystatin and triamcinolone *on page 433*

**Mytussin® [OTC]** *see* guaifenesin *on page 281*

**Mytussin® AC** *see* guaifenesin and codeine *on page 282*

**Mytussin® DAC** *see* guaifenesin, pseudoephedrine, and codeine *on page 284*

**Mytussin® DM [OTC]** *see* guaifenesin and dextromethorphan *on page 282*

**M-Zole® 7 Dual Pack [OTC]** *see* miconazole *on page 390*

**Nabi-HB®** *see* hepatitis B immune globulin *on page 292*

## nabumetone (na BYOO me tone)

**U.S./Canadian Brand Names** Apo®-Nabumetone (Can); Relafen®

**Therapeutic Category** Analgesic, Non-narcotic; Nonsteroidal Anti-inflammatory Drug (NSAID)

**Use** Management of osteoarthritis and rheumatoid arthritis

**Usual Dosage** Adults: Oral: 1000 mg/day; an additional 500-1000 mg may be needed in some patients to obtain more symptomatic relief; may be administered once or twice daily

**Dosage Forms** Tablet: 500 mg, 750 mg

**NAC** *see* acetylcysteine *on page 10*

***N*-acetylcysteine** *see* acetylcysteine *on page 10*

***N*-acetyl-L-cysteine** *see* acetylcysteine *on page 10*

**n-acetyl-p-aminophenol** *see* acetaminophen *on page 3*

**NaCl** *see* sodium chloride *on page 549*

## nadolol (nay DOE lole)

**U.S./Canadian Brand Names** Alti-Nadolol (Can); Apo®-Nadol (Can); Corgard®; Novo-Nadolol (Can)

**Therapeutic Category** Beta-Adrenergic Blocker

**Use** Treatment of hypertension and angina pectoris; prevention of myocardial infarction; prophylaxis of migraine headaches

**Usual Dosage** Adults: Oral: Initial: 40 mg once daily; increase gradually; usual dosage: 40-80 mg/day; may need up to 240-320 mg/day; doses as high as 640 mg/day have been used

**Dosage Forms** Tablet: 20 mg, 40 mg, 80 mg, 120 mg, 160 mg

**Nadopen-V® (Can)** *see* penicillin V potassium *on page 457*

## nadroparin *(Canada only)* (nad roe PA rin)

**U.S./Canadian Brand Names** Fraxiparine™ (Can)

**Therapeutic Category** Anticoagulant

**Use** Prevention of clotting during hemodialysis; Prophylaxis of thromboembolic disorders (particularly deep vein thrombosis and pulmonary embolism) in general surgery and in orthopedic surgery; treatment of deep vein thrombosis

**Usual Dosage** Adult: S.C.:

Thromboembolism prophylaxis: 0.3 mL daily S.C for 7 days.

Orthopedic surgery: 0.2-0.4 mL daily for 3 days then 0.3-0.6 mL daily; doses should be adjusted for bodyweight.

Thromboembolism treatment: 0.4-0.9 mL twice daily for 10 days. Doses should be adjusted for bodyweight.

Hemodialysis: 0.3-0.6 mL into the arterial line at start of 4 hour session. Dose should be adjusted for bodyweight.

(Continued)

## nadroparin *(Canada only)* *(Continued)*

Child: Hemodialysis: 60-120 int. units/kg at the start of 4 hour session. Duration of therapy should be determined by the clinical need. Dosage should be individualized.

**Dosage Forms** Injection, as calcium: in prefilled syringes or graduated syringes: 9500 int. units anti-Xa/mL (0.2mL, 0.3 mL, 0.4 mL, 0.6 mL, 0.8 mL, 1 mL)

## nafarelin (NAF a re lin)

**U.S./Canadian Brand Names** Synarel®

**Therapeutic Category** Hormone, Posterior Pituitary

**Use** Treatment of endometriosis, including pain and reduction of lesions; treatment of central precocious puberty (gonadotropin-dependent precocious puberty) in children of both sexes

**Usual Dosage** Adults: 1 spray in one nostril each morning and evening for 6 months

**Dosage Forms** Solution, nasal, as acetate: 2 mg/mL (10 mL)

**Nafazair® Ophthalmic** *see* naphazoline *on page 409*

**Nafcil™ *(Discontinued)*** *see page 750*

## nafcillin (naf SIL in)

**Synonyms** ethoxynaphthamido penicillin sodium

**Therapeutic Category** Penicillin

**Use** Treatment of bacterial infections such as osteomyelitis, septicemia, endocarditis, and CNS infections due to susceptible penicillinase-producing strains of *Staphylococcus*

**Usual Dosage**

Children:

I.M.: 25 mg/kg twice daily

I.V.:

Mild to moderate infections: 50-100 mg/kg/day in divided doses every 6 hours

Severe infections: 100-200 mg/kg/day in divided doses every 4-6 hours

Maximum dose: 12 g/day

Adults:

I.M.: 500 mg every 4-6 hours

I.V.: 500-2000 mg every 4-6 hours

**Dosage Forms** Powder for injection, as sodium: 1 g, 2 g, 10 g

## naftifine (NAF ti feen)

**U.S./Canadian Brand Names** Naftin®

**Therapeutic Category** Antifungal Agent

**Use** Topical treatment of tinea cruris and tinea corporis

**Usual Dosage** Adults: Topical: Apply twice daily

**Dosage Forms**

Cream, as hydrochloride: 1% (15 g, 30 g, 60 g)

Gel, topical, as hydrochloride: 1% (20 g, 40 g, 60 g)

**Naftin®** *see* naftifine *on this page*

**$NaHCO_3$** *see* sodium bicarbonate *on page 548*

## nalbuphine (NAL byoo feen)

**U.S./Canadian Brand Names** Nubain®

**Therapeutic Category** Analgesic, Narcotic

**Use** Relief of moderate to severe pain

**Usual Dosage** I.M., I.V., S.C.: 10 mg/70 kg every 3-6 hours

**Dosage Forms** Injection, as hydrochloride: 1.5 mg/mL (30 mL); 10 mg/mL (1 mL, 10 mL); 20 mg/mL (1 mL, 10 mL)

**Nalcrom® (Can)** *see* cromolyn sodium *on page 156*

**Naldecon®** ***(Discontinued)*** *see page 750*

**Naldecon® DX Adult Liquid** ***(Discontinued)*** *see page 750*

**Naldecon-EX® Children's Syrup** ***(Discontinued)*** *see page 750*

**Naldecon® Senior DX [OTC]** *see* guaifenesin and dextromethorphan *on page 282*

**Naldecon® Senior EX [OTC]** *see* guaifenesin *on page 281*

**Naldelate®** ***(Discontinued)*** *see page 750*

**Nalfon®** *see* fenoprofen *on page 243*

**Nalgest®** ***(Discontinued)*** *see page 750*

## nalidixic acid (nal i DIKS ik AS id)

**Synonyms** nalidixinic acid

**U.S./Canadian Brand Names** NegGram®

**Therapeutic Category** Quinolone

**Use** Lower urinary tract infections due to susceptible gram-negative organisms including *E. coli*, *Enterobacter*, *Klebsiella*, and *Proteus* (inactive against *Pseudomonas*)

**Usual Dosage** Oral:

Children: 55 mg/kg/day divided every 6 hours; suppressive therapy is 33 mg/kg/day divided every 6 hours

Adults: 1 g 4 times/day for 2 weeks; then suppressive therapy of 500 mg 4 times/day

**Dosage Forms**

Suspension, oral (raspberry flavor): 250 mg/5 mL (473 mL)

Tablet: 250 mg, 500 mg, 1 g

**nalidixinic acid** *see* nalidixic acid *on this page*

***n*-allylnoroxymorphone** *see* naloxone *on this page*

## nalmefene (NAL me feen)

**U.S./Canadian Brand Names** Revex®

**Therapeutic Category** Antidote

**Use** Complete or partial of opioid drug effects; management of known or suspected opioid overdose

**Usual Dosage** Titrate to reverse the undesired effects of opioids; once adequate reversal has been established, additional administration is not required and may actually be harmful due to unwanted reversal of analgesia or precipitated withdrawal; the recommended initial dose for nonopioid dependent patient is 0.5 mg/70 kg, a second dose of 1 mg/70 kg 2-5 minutes later may be administered, after a total dose of 1.5 mg/70 kg has been administered with no clinical response, additional nalmefene is not likely to have an effect

**Dosage Forms** Injection, as hydrochloride: 100 mcg/mL [blue label] (1 mL); 1000 mcg/mL [green label] (2 mL)

## naloxone (nal OKS one)

**Synonyms** *n*-allylnoroxymorphone

**U.S./Canadian Brand Names** Narcan®

**Therapeutic Category** Antidote

**Use** Reverses CNS and respiratory depression in suspected narcotic overdose; neonatal opiate depression; coma of unknown etiology

**Investigational use:** Shock, phencyclidine, and alcohol ingestion

**Usual Dosage** I.M., I.V. (preferred), intratracheal, S.C. (administer undiluted injection):

Infants and Children:

Postanesthesia narcotic reversal: 0.01 mg/kg; may repeat every 2-3 minutes as needed based on response

(Continued)

## naloxone *(Continued)*

Opiate intoxication:

Birth (including premature infants) to 5 years or <20 kg: 0.1 mg/kg; repeat every 2-3 minutes if needed; may need to repeat doses every 20-60 minutes

>5 years or ≥20 kg: 2 mg/dose; if no response, repeat every 2-3 minutes; may need to repeat doses every 20-60 minutes

Children and Adults: Continuous infusion: I.V.: If continuous infusion is required, calculate dosage/hour based on effective intermittent dose used and duration of adequate response seen, titrate dose 0.04-0.16 mg/kg/hour for 2-5 days in children, adult dose typically 0.25-6.25 mg/hour (short-term infusions as high as 2.4 mg/kg/hour have been tolerated in adults during treatment for septic shock); alternatively, continuous infusion utilizes 2/3 of the initial naloxone bolus on an hourly basis; add 10 times this dose to each liter of $D_5W$ and infuse at a rate of 100 mL/hour; 1/2 of the initial bolus dose should be readministered 15 minutes after initiation of the continuous infusion to prevent a drop in naloxone levels; increase infusion rate as needed to assure adequate ventilation

Adults: 0.4-2 mg every 2-3 minutes as needed; may need to repeat doses every 20-60 minutes; if no response is observed for a total of 10 mg, re-evaluate patient for possibility of a drug or disease process unresponsive to naloxone. **Note:** Use 0.1-0.2 mg increments in patients who are opioid dependent and in postoperative patients to avoid large cardiovascular changes

**Dosage Forms**

Injection, as hydrochloride: 0.4 mg/mL (1 mL, 2 mL, 10 mL); 1 mg/mL (2 mL, 10 mL)

Injection, neonatal, as hydrochloride: 0.02 mg/mL (2 mL)

**Nalspan® *(Discontinued)*** *see page 750*

## naltrexone (nal TREKS one)

**U.S./Canadian Brand Names** Depade®; ReVia®

**Therapeutic Category** Antidote

**Use** Adjunct to the maintenance of an opioid-free state in detoxified individual

**Usual Dosage** Do not administer until patient is opioid-free for 7-10 days as required by urine analysis

Adults: Oral: 25 mg; if no withdrawal signs within 1 hour administer another 25 mg; maintenance regimen is flexible, variable and individualized (50 mg/day to 100-150 mg 3 times/week)

**Dosage Forms** Tablet, as hydrochloride: 50 mg

**Nandrobolic® Injection *(Discontinued)*** *see page 750*

## nandrolone (NAN droe lone)

**U.S./Canadian Brand Names** Deca-Durabolin®; Hybolin™ Decanoate; Hybolin™ Improved Injection

**Therapeutic Category** Androgen

**Controlled Substance** C-III

**Use** Control of metastatic breast cancer; management of anemia of renal insufficiency

**Usual Dosage**

Children 2-13 years: 25-50 mg every 3-4 weeks

Adults:

Male: 100-200 mg/week

Female: 50-100 mg/week

**Dosage Forms**

Nandrolone phenpropionate: Injection in oil: 25 mg/mL (5 mL); 50 mg/mL (2 mL)

Nandrolone decanoate:

Injection in oil: 50 mg/mL (1 mL, 2 mL); 100 mg/mL (1 mL, 2 mL); 200 mg/mL (1 mL)

Injection, repository: 50 mg/mL (2 mL); 100 mg/mL (2 mL); 200 mg/mL (2 mL)

## naphazoline (naf AZ oh leen)

**U.S./Canadian Brand Names** AK-Con® Ophthalmic; Albalon® Liquifilm® Ophthalmic; Allerest® Eye Drops [OTC]; Clear Eyes® [OTC]; Comfort® Ophthalmic [OTC]; Degest® 2 Ophthalmic [OTC]; Estivin® II Ophthalmic [OTC]; I-Naphline® Ophthalmic; Nafazair® Ophthalmic; Naphcon Forte® Ophthalmic; Naphcon® Ophthalmic [OTC]; Opcon® Ophthalmic; Privine® Nasal [OTC]; VasoClear® Ophthalmic [OTC]; Vasocon Regular® Ophthalmic

**Therapeutic Category** Adrenergic Agonist Agent

**Use** Topical ocular vasoconstrictor (to soothe, refresh, moisturize, and relieve redness due to minor eye irritation); temporarily relieves nasal congestion associated with rhinitis, sinusitis, hay fever, or the common cold

**Usual Dosage**

Nasal:

Children:

<6 years: Not recommended (especially infants) due to CNS depression

6-12 years: 1 spray of 0.05% into each nostril, repeat in 3 hours if necessary

Children >12 years and Adults: 0.05%, instill 2 drops or sprays every 3-6 hours if needed; therapy should not exceed 3-5 days or more frequently than every 3 hours

Ophthalmic:

Children <6 years: Not recommended for use due to CNS depression (especially in infants)

Children >6 years and Adults: Instill 1-2 drops into conjunctival sac of affected eye(s) every 3-4 hours; therapy generally should not exceed 3-4 days

**Dosage Forms** Solution, as hydrochloride:

Nasal:

Drops: 0.05% (20 mL)

Spray: 0.05% (15 mL)

Ophthalmic: 0.012% (7.5 mL, 30 mL); 0.02% (15 mL); 0.03% (15 mL); 0.1% (15 mL)

## naphazoline and antazoline (naf AZ oh leen & an TAZ oh leen)

**U.S./Canadian Brand Names** Albalon-A® Ophthalmic; Antazoline-V® Ophthalmic; Vasocon-A® [OTC] Ophthalmic

**Therapeutic Category** Antihistamine/Decongestant Combination

**Use** Topical ocular congestion, irritation, and itching

**Usual Dosage** Ophthalmic: 1-2 drops every 3-4 hours

**Dosage Forms** Solution: Naphazoline hydrochloride 0.05% and antazoline phosphate 0.5% (15 mL)

## naphazoline and pheniramine (naf AZ oh leen & fen NIR a meen)

**U.S./Canadian Brand Names** Naphcon-A® Ophthalmic [OTC]

**Therapeutic Category** Antihistamine/Decongestant Combination

**Use** Topical ocular vasoconstrictor

**Usual Dosage** Ophthalmic: 1-2 drops every 3-4 hours

**Dosage Forms** Solution, ophthalmic: Naphazoline hydrochloride 0.025% and pheniramine 0.3% (15 mL)

**Naphcon-A® Ophthalmic [OTC]** *see* naphazoline and pheniramine *on this page*

**Naphcon Forte® Ophthalmic** *see* naphazoline *on this page*

**Naphcon® Ophthalmic [OTC]** *see* naphazoline *on this page*

**Naprelan®** *see* naproxen *on this page*

**Naprosyn®** *see* naproxen *on this page*

## naproxen (na PROKS en)

**U.S./Canadian Brand Names** Aleve® [OTC]; Anaprox®; Apo®-Napro-Na (Can); Apo®-Naproxen (Can); Gen-Naproxen EC (Can); Naprelan®; Naprosyn®; Naxen® (Can);

(Continued)

## naproxen *(Continued)*

Novo-Naprox (Can); Nu-Naprox (Can); Riva-Naproxen (Can); Synflex® (Can); Synflex® DS (Can)

**Therapeutic Category** Analgesic, Non-narcotic; Antipyretic; Nonsteroidal Anti-inflammatory Drug (NSAID)

**Use** Management of inflammatory disease and rheumatoid disorders (including juvenile rheumatoid arthritis); acute gout; mild to moderate pain; dysmenorrhea; fever

**Usual Dosage** Oral (as naproxen):

Children >2 years:

Antipyretic or analgesic: 5-7 mg/kg/dose every 8-12 hours

Juvenile rheumatoid arthritis: 10 mg/kg/day, up to a maximum of 1000 mg/day divided twice daily

Adults:

Rheumatoid arthritis, osteoarthritis, and ankylosing spondylitis: 500-1000 mg/day in 2 divided doses

Mild to moderate pain or dysmenorrhea: Initial: 500 mg, then 250 mg every 6-8 hours; maximum: 1250 mg/day

**Dosage Forms**

Suspension, oral: 125 mg/5 mL (15 mL, 30 mL, 480 mL)

Tablet:

Aleve®: 200 mg

Naprosyn®: 250 mg, 375 mg, 500 mg

Tablet, controlled release (Naprelan®): 375 mg, 500 mg

Naproxen sodium:

Tablet, as sodium: 220 mg (200 mg base)

Anaprox®: 220 mg (200 mg base); 275 mg (250 mg base); 550 mg (500 mg base)

**Naqua®** *see* trichlormethiazide *on page 604*

## naratriptan (NAR a trip tan)

**U.S./Canadian Brand Names** Amerge®

**Therapeutic Category** Antimigraine Agent; Serotonin Agonist

**Use** Acute treatment of migraine with or without aura

**Usual Dosage** Oral: Adults: 1 mg or 2.5 mg (maximum dose: 5 mg); if no response, dose may be repeated in 4 hours

**Dosage Forms** Tablet, as hydrochloride: 1 mg, 2.5 mg

**Narcan®** *see* naloxone *on page 407*

**Nardil®** *see* phenelzine *on page 464*

**Naropin™** *see* ropivacaine *on page 532*

**Nasabid™** *see* guaifenesin and pseudoephedrine *on page 283*

**Nasacort®** *see* triamcinolone (inhalation, nasal) *on page 601*

**Nasacort® AQ** *see* triamcinolone (inhalation, nasal) *on page 601*

**Nasahist B®** *see* brompheniramine *on page 87*

**NaSal™ [OTC]** *see* sodium chloride *on page 549*

**Nasalcrom® [OTC]** *see* cromolyn sodium *on page 156*

**Nasalide® Nasal Aerosol** *see* flunisolide *on page 253*

**Nasal Moist® [OTC]** *see* sodium chloride *on page 549*

**Nasarel® Nasal Spray** *see* flunisolide *on page 253*

**Nasonex®** *see* mometasone furoate *on page 398*

**Natabec® [OTC]** *see* vitamin (multiple/prenatal) *on page 632*

**Natabec® FA [OTC]** *see* vitamin (multiple/prenatal) *on page 632*

**Natabec® Rx** *see* vitamin (multiple/prenatal) *on page 632*

**Natacyn®** *see* natamycin *on this page*

**Natalins® [OTC]** *see* vitamin (multiple/prenatal) *on page 632*

**Natalins® Rx** *see* vitamin (multiple/prenatal) *on page 632*

## natamycin (na ta MYE sin)

**Synonyms** pimaricin

**U.S./Canadian Brand Names** Natacyn®

**Therapeutic Category** Antifungal Agent

**Use** Treatment of blepharitis, conjunctivitis, and keratitis caused by susceptible fungi (*Aspergillus, Candida, Cephalosporium, Curvularia, Fusarium, Penicillium, Microsporum, Epidermophyton, Blastomyces dermatitidis, Coccidioides immitis, Cryptococcus neoformans, Histoplasma capsulatum, Sporothrix schenckii, Trichomonas vaginalis*)

**Usual Dosage** Adults: Ophthalmic: 1 drop in conjunctival sac every 1-2 hours, after 3-4 days dose may be reduced to one drop 6-8 times/day; usual course of therapy: 2-3 weeks

**Dosage Forms** Suspension, ophthalmic: 5% (15 mL)

## nateglinide (na TEG li nide)

**U.S./Canadian Brand Names** Starlix®

**Therapeutic Category** Antidiabetic Agent, Oral

**Use** Management of type 2 diabetes mellitus (noninsulin dependent, NIDDM) as monotherapy when hyperglycemia cannot be managed by diet and exercise alone; in combination with metformin to lower blood glucose in patients whose hyperglycemia cannot be controlled by exercise, diet, and metformin alone.

**Usual Dosage**

Children: Safety and efficacy have not been established

Adults: Management of type 2 diabetes mellitus: Oral: Initial and maintenance dose: 120 mg 3 times/day, 1-30 minutes before meals; may be given alone or in combination with metformin; patients close to Hb $A_{1c}$ goal may be started at 60 mg 3 times/day

**Dosage Forms** Tablet: 60 mg, 120 mg

**Natrecor®** *see* nesiritide *on page 417*

**natriuretic peptide** *see* nesiritide *on page 417*

**Natulan® (Can)** *see* procarbazine *on page 497*

**natural lung surfactant** *see* beractant *on page 76*

**Nature's Tears® Solution [OTC]** *see* artificial tears *on page 53*

**Naturetin®** *see* bendroflumethiazide *on page 71*

**Naus-A-Way® [OTC]** *see* phosphorated carbohydrate solution *on page 469*

**Nausetrol® [OTC]** *see* phosphorated carbohydrate solution *on page 469*

**Navane® Capsule** *see* thiothixene *on page 587*

**Navane® Concentrate & Injection *(Discontinued)*** *see page 750*

**Navelbine®** *see* vinorelbine *on page 628*

**Naxen® (Can)** *see* naproxen *on page 409*

**N-B-P® Ointment *(Discontinued)*** *see page 750*

**ND-Stat®** *see* brompheniramine *on page 87*

**Nebcin® Injection** *see* tobramycin *on page 593*

**NebuPent™ Inhalation** *see* pentamidine *on page 458*

## nedocromil (inhalation) (ne doe KROE mil in hil LA shun)

**U.S./Canadian Brand Names** Tilade® Inhalation Aerosol

**Therapeutic Category** Mast Cell Stabilizer

**Use** Maintenance therapy in patients with mild to moderate bronchial asthma

(Continued)

## nedocromil (inhalation) *(Continued)*

**Usual Dosage** Adults: Inhalation: 2 inhalations 4 times/day
**Dosage Forms** Aerosol, as sodium: 1.75 mg/activation (16.2 g)

## nedocromil (ophthalmic) (ne doe KROE mil op THAL mik)

**U.S./Canadian Brand Names** Alocril™
**Therapeutic Category** Mast Cell Stabilizer
**Use** Treatment of itching associated with allergic conjunctivitis
**Usual Dosage** Adults: Ophthalmic: 1-2 drops in eye(s) twice daily
**Dosage Forms** Solution, ophthalmic, as sodium: 2% (5 mL)

## nefazodone (nef AY zoe done)

**U.S./Canadian Brand Names** Serzone®
**Therapeutic Category** Antidepressant, Miscellaneous
**Use** Treatment of depression
**Usual Dosage** Adults: Oral: Initial: 200 mg/day administered in two divided doses with a range of 300-600 mg/day in two divided doses thereafter
**Dosage Forms** Tablet, as hydrochloride: 50 mg, 100 mg, 150 mg, 200 mg, 250 mg

**NegGram®** *see* nalidixic acid *on page 407*

## nelfinavir (nel FIN a veer)

**U.S./Canadian Brand Names** Viracept®
**Therapeutic Category** Antiviral Agent
**Use** As monotherapy or preferably in combination with nucleoside analogs in the treatment of HIV infection, in adults and children, when antiretroviral therapy is warranted
**Usual Dosage** Oral:
Children 2-13 years: 20-30 mg/kg 3 times/day with a meal or light snack; if tablets are unable to be taken, use oral powder in small amount of water, milk, formula, or dietary supplements; do not use acidic food/juice or store for >6 hours
Adults: 750 mg 3 times/day with meals
**Dosage Forms**
Powder, oral: 50 mg/g (contains 11.2 mg phenylalanine)
Tablet: 250 mg

**Nelova™ 0.5/35E** *see* ethinyl estradiol and norethindrone *on page 232*
**Nelova® 1/50M** *see* mestranol and norethindrone *on page 375*
**Nelova™ 10/11** *see* ethinyl estradiol and norethindrone *on page 232*
**Nemasol® (Can)** *see* aminosalicylate sodium *on page 32*
**Nembutal®** *see* pentobarbital *on page 459*
**Neoasma®** *see* theophylline and guaifenesin *on page 583*
**Neo-Calglucon® [OTC]** *see* calcium glubionate *on page 99*
**Neo-Castaderm *(Discontinued)*** *see page 750*
**Neo-Cortef® Ophthalmic *(Discontinued)*** *see page 750*
**Neo-Cortef® Topical *(Discontinued)*** *see page 750*
**NeoDecadron® Ophthalmic** *see* neomycin and dexamethasone *on next page*
**NeoDecadron® Topical *(Discontinued)*** *see page 750*
**Neo-Dexameth® Ophthalmic** *see* neomycin and dexamethasone *on next page*
**Neo-Durabolic *(Discontinued)*** *see page 750*
**Neofed® [OTC]** *see* pseudoephedrine *on page 507*
**Neo-fradin®** *see* neomycin *on next page*
**Neoloid® [OTC]** *see* castor oil *on page 112*

**Neo-Medrol® Acetate Topical *(Discontinued)*** *see page 750*

**Neo-Metric (Can)** *see* metronidazole *on page 388*

**Neomixin® Topical** *see* bacitracin, neomycin, and polymyxin B *on page 65*

## neomycin (nee oh MYE sin)

**U.S./Canadian Brand Names** Mycifradin® Sulfate; Neo-fradin®; Neo-Tabs®

**Therapeutic Category** Aminoglycoside (Antibiotic); Antibiotic, Topical

**Use** Administered orally to prepare GI tract for surgery; treat minor skin infections; treat diarrhea caused by *E. coli*; adjunct in the treatment of hepatic encephalopathy

**Usual Dosage**

Children: Oral:

Preoperative intestinal antisepsis: 90 mg/kg/day divided every 4 hours for 2 days; or 25 mg/kg at 1 PM, 2 PM, and 11 PM on the day preceding surgery as an adjunct to mechanical cleansing of the intestine and in combination with erythromycin base

Hepatic coma: 50-100 mg/kg/day in divided doses every 6-8 hours or 2.5-7 g/m$^2$/day divided every 4-6 hours for 5-6 days not to exceed 12 g/day

Children and Adults: Topical: Apply ointment 1-4 times/day; topical solutions containing 0.1% to 1% neomycin have been used for irrigation

Adults: Oral:

Preoperative intestinal antisepsis: 1 g each hour for 4 doses then 1 g every 4 hours for 5 doses; or 1 g at 1 PM, 2 PM, and 11 PM on day preceding surgery as an adjunct to mechanical cleansing of the bowel and oral erythromycin; or 6 g/day divided every 4 hours for 2-3 days

Hepatic coma: 500-2000 mg every 6-8 hours or 4-12 g/day divided every 4-6 hours for 5-6 days

Chronic hepatic insufficiency: Oral: 4 g/day for an indefinite period

**Dosage Forms**

Cream, as sulfate: 0.5% (15 g)

Injection, as sulfate: 500 mg

Ointment, topical, as sulfate: 0.5% (15 g, 30 g, 120 g)

Solution, oral, as sulfate: 125 mg/5 mL (480 mL)

Tablet, as sulfate: 500 mg [base 300 mg]

## neomycin and dexamethasone (nee oh MYE sin & deks a METH a sone)

**U.S./Canadian Brand Names** NeoDecadron® Ophthalmic; Neo-Dexameth® Ophthalmic

**Therapeutic Category** Antibiotic/Corticosteroid, Ophthalmic; Antibiotic/Corticosteroid, Topical

**Use** Treatment of steroid responsive inflammatory conditions of the palpebral and bulbar conjunctiva, lid, cornea, and anterior segment of the globe

**Usual Dosage**

Ophthalmic: Instill 1-2 drops in eye(s) every 3-4 hours

Topical: Apply thin coat 3-4 times/day until favorable response is observed, then reduce dose to one application/day. Therapy should be discontinued when control is achieved. If no improvement is seen, reassessment of diagnosis may be necessary.

**Dosage Forms** Solution, ophthalmic: Neomycin sulfate 0.35% [3.5 mg/mL] and dexamethasone 0.1% [1 mg/mL] (5 mL)

## neomycin and hydrocortisone (nee oh MYE sin & hye droe KOR ti sone)

**Therapeutic Category** Antibiotic/Corticosteroid, Ophthalmic; Antibiotic/Corticosteroid, Topical

**Use** Treatment of susceptible topical bacterial infections with associated inflammation

**Usual Dosage** Topical: Apply to area in a thin film 2-4 times/day. Therapy should be discontinued when control is achieved. If no improvement is seen, reassessment of diagnosis may be necessary.

**Dosage Forms** Ointment, topical: Neomycin sulfate 0.5% and hydrocortisone 1% (20 g)

## neomycin and polymyxin B (nee oh MYE sin & pol i MIKS in bee)

**U.S./Canadian Brand Names** Neosporin® Cream [OTC]; Neosporin® G.U. Irrigant

**Therapeutic Category** Antibiotic, Topical; Genitourinary Irrigant

**Use** Short-term use as a continuous irrigant or rinse in the urinary bladder to prevent bacteriuria and gram-negative rod septicemia associated with the use of indwelling catheters; to help prevent infection in minor cuts, scrapes, and burns

**Usual Dosage** Children and Adults:

Topical: Apply cream 2-4 times/day

Bladder irrigation: Continuous irrigant or rinse in the urinary bladder for up to 10 days where 1 mL is added to 1 L of normal saline with administration rate adjusted to patient's urine output; usually no more than 1 L of irrigant is used per day

**Dosage Forms**

Cream: Neomycin sulfate 3.5 mg and polymyxin B sulfate 10,000 units per g (0.94 g, 15 g)

Solution, irrigant: Neomycin sulfate 40 mg and polymyxin B sulfate 200,000 units per mL (1 mL, 20 mL)

## neomycin, colistin, hydrocortisone, and thonzonium

(nee oh MYE sin, koe LIS tin, hye droe KOR ti sone, & thon ZOE nee um)

**U.S./Canadian Brand Names** Cortisporin®-TC® Otic Suspension

**Therapeutic Category** Antibiotic/Corticosteroid, Otic

**Use** Treatment of superficial and susceptible bacterial infections of the external auditory canal; for treatment of susceptible bacterial infections of mastoidectomy and fenestration cavities

**Usual Dosage**

Children: 4 drops in affected ear 3-4 times/day

Adults: 5 drops in affected ear 3-4 times/day

**Dosage Forms** Suspension, otic: Neomycin sulfate 3.3 mg, colistin sulfate 3 mg, hydrocortisone acetate 1%, and thonzonium bromide 0.5 mg per mL (10 mL)

## neomycin, polymyxin B, and dexamethasone

(nee oh MYE sin, pol i MIKS in bee, & deks a METH a sone)

**U.S./Canadian Brand Names** AK-Trol®; Dexacidin®; Dexasporin®; Dioptrol® (Can); Maxitrol®

**Therapeutic Category** Antibiotic/Corticosteroid, Ophthalmic

**Use** Steroid-responsive inflammatory ocular conditions in which a corticosteroid is indicated and where bacterial infection or a risk of bacterial infection exists

**Usual Dosage** Children and Adults: Ophthalmic:

Ointment: Place a small amount (~½") in the affected eye 3-4 times/day or apply at bedtime as an adjunct with drops

Solution: Instill 1-2 drops into affected eye(s) every 4-6 hours; in severe disease, drops may be used hourly and tapered to discontinuation

**Dosage Forms**

Ointment, ophthalmic: Neomycin sulfate 3.5 mg, polymyxin B sulfate 10,000 units, and dexamethasone 0.1% per g (3.5 g)

Suspension, ophthalmic: Neomycin sulfate 3.5 mg, polymyxin B sulfate 10,000 units, and dexamethasone 0.1% per mL (5 mL)

## neomycin, polymyxin B, and gramicidin

(nee oh MYE sin, pol i MIKS in bee, & gram i SYE din)

**U.S./Canadian Brand Names** AK-Spore® Ophthalmic Solution; Neosporin® Ophthalmic Solution; Optimyxin® Plus® (Can)

**Therapeutic Category** Antibiotic, Ophthalmic

**Use** Treatment of superficial ocular infection, infection prophylaxis in minor skin abrasions

**Usual Dosage** Ophthalmic: Drops: 1-2 drops 4-6 times/day or more frequently as required for severe infections

**Dosage Forms** Solution, ophthalmic: Neomycin sulfate 1.75 mg, polymyxin B sulfate 10,000 units, and gramicidin 0.025 mg per mL (2 mL, 10 mL)

## neomycin, polymyxin B, and hydrocortisone

(nee oh MYE sin, pol i MIKS in bee, & hye droe KOR ti sone)

**U.S./Canadian Brand Names** AK-Spore® H.C. Ophthalmic Suspension; AK-Spore® H.C. Otic; AntibiOtic® Otic; Cortatrigen® Otic; Cortimyxin® (Can); Cortisporin® Ophthalmic Suspension; Cortisporin® Otic; Cortisporin® Topical Cream; Octicair® Otic; Otic-Care® Otic; Otocort® Otic; Otosporin® Otic; Pediotic® Otic; UAD Otic®

**Therapeutic Category** Antibiotic/Corticosteroid, Ophthalmic; Antibiotic/Corticosteroid, Otic; Antibiotic/Corticosteroid, Topical

**Use** Steroid-responsive inflammatory condition for which a corticosteroid is indicated and where bacterial infection or a risk of bacterial infection exists

**Usual Dosage** Duration of use should be limited to 10 days unless otherwise directed by the physician

Ophthalmic: Adults and Children:
- Ointment: Apply to the affected eye every 3-4 hours
- Suspension: 1 drop every 3-4 hours

Otic: Solution/suspension:
- Children: 3 drops into affected ear 3-4 times/day
- Adults: 4 drops into affected ear 3-4 times/day

**Dosage Forms**

Cream, topical: Neomycin sulfate 5 mg, polymyxin B sulfate 10,000 units, and hydrocortisone 10 mg per mL (7.5 g)

Solution, otic: Neomycin sulfate 5 mg, polymyxin B sulfate 10,000 units, and hydrocortisone 10 mg per mL (10 mL)

Suspension:
- Ophthalmic: Neomycin sulfate 5 mg, polymyxin B sulfate 10,000 units, and hydrocortisone 10 mg per mL (7.5 mL)
- Otic: Neomycin sulfate 5 mg, polymyxin B sulfate 10,000 units, and hydrocortisone 10 mg per mL (10 mL)

## neomycin, polymyxin B, and prednisolone

(nee oh MYE sin, pol i MIKS in bee, & pred NIS oh lone)

**U.S./Canadian Brand Names** Poly-Pred® Ophthalmic Suspension

**Therapeutic Category** Antibiotic/Corticosteroid, Ophthalmic

**Use** Steroid-responsive inflammatory ocular condition in which bacterial infection or a risk of bacterial ocular infection exists

**Usual Dosage** Children and Adults: Ophthalmic: Instill 1-2 drops every 3-4 hours; acute infections may require every 30-minute instillation initially with frequency of administration reduced as the infection is brought under control. To treat the lids: Instill 1-2 drops every 3-4 hours, close the eye and rub the excess on the lids and lid margins.

**Dosage Forms** Suspension, ophthalmic: Neomycin sulfate 0.35%, polymyxin B sulfate 10,000 units, and prednisolone acetate 0.5% per mL (5 mL, 10 mL)

**neonatal trace metals** *see* trace metals *on page 598*

**Neoquess® Injection *(Discontinued)*** *see page 750*

**Neoquess® Tablet *(Discontinued)*** *see page 750*

**Neoral®** *see* cyclosporine *on page 160*

**Neosar®** *see* cyclophosphamide *on page 159*

**Neosporin® Cream [OTC]** *see* neomycin and polymyxin B *on previous page*

**Neosporin® G.U. Irrigant** *see* neomycin and polymyxin B *on previous page*

**Neosporin® Ophthalmic Ointment** *see* bacitracin, neomycin, and polymyxin B *on page 65*

**Neosporin® Ophthalmic Solution** *see* neomycin, polymyxin B, and gramicidin *on previous page*

**Neosporin® Topical Ointment [OTC]** *see* bacitracin, neomycin, and polymyxin B *on page 65*

## neostigmine (nee oh STIG meen)

**U.S./Canadian Brand Names** Prostigmin®

**Therapeutic Category** Cholinergic Agent

**Use** Treatment of myasthenia gravis; prevention and treatment of postoperative bladder distention and urinary retention; reversal of the effects of nondepolarizing neuromuscular blocking agents after surgery

**Usual Dosage**

Myasthenia gravis: Diagnosis: I.M.:
- Children: 0.04 mg/kg as a single dose
- Adults: 0.02 mg/kg as a single dose

Myasthenia gravis: Treatment:
- Children:
  - Oral: 2 mg/kg/day divided every 3-4 hours
  - I.M., I.V., S.C.: 0.01-0.04 mg/kg every 2-4 hours
- Adults:
  - Oral: 15 mg/dose every 3-4 hours
  - I.M., I.V., S.C.: 0.5-2.5 mg every 1-3 hours

Reversal of nondepolarizing neuromuscular blockade after surgery in conjunction with atropine or glycopyrrolate: I.V.:
- Infants: 0.025-0.1 mg/kg/dose
- Children: 0.025-0.08 mg/kg/dose
- Adults: 0.5-2.5 mg; total dose not to exceed 5 mg

Bladder atony: Adults: I.M., S.C.:
- Prevention: 0.25 mg every 4-6 hours for 2-3 days
- Treatment: 0.5-1 mg every 3 hours for 5 doses after bladder has emptied

**Dosage Forms**

Injection, as methylsulfate: 0.5 mg/mL (1 mL, 10 mL); 1 mg/mL (10 mL)

Tablet, as bromide: 15 mg

**Neostrata® HQ (Can)** *see* hydroquinone *on page 305*

**Neo-Synalar® Topical *(Discontinued)*** *see page 750*

**Neo-Synephrine® 12 Hour Nasal Solution [OTC]** *see* oxymetazoline *on page 444*

**Neo-Synephrine® Nasal Solution [OTC]** *see* phenylephrine *on page 467*

**Neo-Synephrine® Ophthalmic Solution** *see* phenylephrine *on page 467*

**Neo-Tabs®** *see* neomycin *on page 413*

**Neotopic (Can)** *see* bacitracin, neomycin, and polymyxin B *on page 65*

**Neotrace-4®** *see* trace metals *on page 598*

**Neotricin HC® Ophthalmic Ointment** *see* bacitracin, neomycin, polymyxin B, and hydrocortisone *on page 65*

**NeoVadrin® [OTC]** *see* vitamin (multiple/oral) *on page 632*

**NeoVadrin® B Complex [OTC]** *see* vitamin B complex *on page 630*

**Nephro-Calci® [OTC]** *see* calcium carbonate *on page 97*

**Nephrocaps®** *see* vitamin B complex with vitamin C and folic acid *on page 631*

**Nephro-Fer™ [OTC]** *see* ferrous fumarate *on page 246*

**Nephrox Suspension [OTC]** *see* aluminum hydroxide *on page 26*

**Neptazane®** *see* methazolamide *on page 378*

**Nervocaine® Injection** *see* lidocaine *on page 348*

**Nesacaine®** *see* chloroprocaine *on page 127*

**Nesacaine®-MPF** *see* chloroprocaine *on page 127*

## nesiritide (ni SIR i tide)

**Synonyms** B-type natriuretic peptide (Human); hBNP; natriuretic peptide

**U.S./Canadian Brand Names** Natrecor®

**Therapeutic Category** Vasodilator

**Use** Treatment of acutely decompensated congestive heart failure (CHF) in patients with dyspnea at rest or with minimal activity

**Dosage Forms** Powder for injection: 1.5 mg

**Nestrex® *(Discontinued)*** *see page 750*

**Netromycin® *(Discontinued)*** *see page 750*

**Neucalm-50® Injection *(Discontinued)*** *see page 750*

**Neuleptil® (Can)** *see* pericyazine *(Canada only) on page 461*

**Neumega®** *see* oprelvekin *on page 437*

**Neupogen®** *see* filgrastim *on page 249*

**Neuramate® *(Discontinued)*** *see page 750*

**Neurontin®** *see* gabapentin *on page 268*

**Neut®** *see* sodium bicarbonate *on page 548*

**Neutra-Phos®** *see* potassium phosphate and sodium phosphate *on page 488*

**Neutra-Phos® Capsule *(Discontinued)*** *see page 750*

**Neutra-Phos®-K** *see* potassium phosphate *on page 488*

**Neutrexin®** *see* trimetrexate glucuronate *on page 608*

**Neutrogena® Acne Mask [OTC]** *see* benzoyl peroxide *on page 74*

**Neutrogena® On-The-Spot [OTC]** *see* benzoyl peroxide *on page 74*

**Neutrogena® T/Derm** *see* coal tar *on page 149*

## nevirapine (ne VYE ra peen)

**U.S./Canadian Brand Names** Viramune®

**Therapeutic Category** Antiviral Agent

**Use** In combination therapy with nucleoside antiretroviral agents in HIV-1 infected adults previously treated for whom current therapy is deemed inadequate

**Usual Dosage** Adults: Oral: 200 mg once daily for 2 weeks followed by 200 mg twice daily

**Dosage Forms**

Suspension, oral: 50 mg/5 mL (240 mL)

Tablet: 200 mg

**New Decongestant® *(Discontinued)*** *see page 750*

**Nexium™** *see* esomeprazole *on page 224*

**N.G.A.® Topical** *see* nystatin and triamcinolone *on page 433*

**Niac® *(Discontinued)*** *see page 750*

**Niacels™ *(Discontinued)*** *see page 750*

## niacin (NYE a sin)

**Synonyms** nicotinic acid; vitamin $B_3$

**U.S./Canadian Brand Names** Niaspan®; Nicobid® [OTC]; Nicolar® [OTC]; Nicotinex [OTC]; Slo-Niacin® [OTC]

**Therapeutic Category** Vitamin, Water Soluble

**Use** Adjunctive treatment of hyperlipidemias; peripheral vascular disease and circulatory disorders; treatment of pellagra; dietary supplement

**Usual Dosage**

Children: Pellagra: Oral, I.M., I.V.: 50-100 mg/dose 3 times/day

(Continued)

## niacin *(Continued)*

Oral: Recommended daily allowances:
0-1 year: 6-8 mg/day
2-6 years: 9-11 mg/day
7-10 years: 16 mg/day
>10 years: 15-18 mg/day
Adults: Oral:
Hyperlipidemia: 1.5-6 g/day in 3 divided doses with or after meals
Pellagra: 50 mg 3-10 times/day, maximum: 500 mg/day
Niacin deficiency: 10-20 mg/day, maximum: 100 mg/day

**Dosage Forms**
Capsule, timed release: 125 mg, 250 mg, 300 mg, 400 mg, 500 mg
Elixir: 50 mg/5 mL (473 mL, 4000 mL)
Injection: 100 mg/mL (30 mL)
Tablet: 25 mg, 50 mg, 100 mg, 250 mg, 500 mg
Extended release: 500 mg, 750 mg, 1000 mg
Timed release: 150 mg, 250 mg, 500 mg, 750 mg

## niacinamide (nye a SIN a mide)

**Synonyms** nicotinamide
**Therapeutic Category** Vitamin, Water Soluble
**Use** Prophylaxis and treatment of pellagra
**Usual Dosage** Oral:
Children: Pellagra: 100-300 mg/day
Adults: 50 mg 3-10 times/day
Pellagra: 300-500 mg/day
Hyperlipidemias: 1-2 g 3 times/day
**Dosage Forms** Tablet: 50 mg, 100 mg, 125 mg, 250 mg, 500 mg

**Niaspan®** *see* niacin *on previous page*

## nicardipine (nye KAR de peen)

**U.S./Canadian Brand Names** Cardene®; Cardene® SR
**Therapeutic Category** Calcium Channel Blocker
**Use** Chronic stable angina; management of essential hypertension
**Usual Dosage** Adults:
Oral: 40 mg 3 times/day (allow 3 days between dose increases)
Oral, sustained release: Initial: 30 mg twice daily, titrate up to 60 mg twice daily
I.V.: (Dilute to 0.1 mg/mL) Initial: 5 mg/hour increased by 2.5 mg/hour every 15 minutes to a maximum of 15 mg/hour
Oral to I.V. dose:
20 mg every 8 hours = I.V. 0.5 mg/hour
30 mg every 8 hours = I.V. 1.2 mg/hour
40 mg every 8 hours = I.V. 2.2 mg/hour

**Dosage Forms**
Capsule, as hydrochloride: 20 mg, 30 mg
Capsule, as hydrochloride, sustained release: 30 mg, 45 mg, 60 mg
Injection, as hydrochloride: 2.5 mg/mL (10 mL)

**N'ice®** *see* ascorbic acid *on page 54*

**Niclocide®** ***(Discontinued)*** *see page 750*

**Nicobid® [OTC]** *see* niacin *on previous page*

**NicoDerm® Patch** *see* nicotine *on next page*

**Nicolar® [OTC]** *see* niacin *on previous page*

**Nicorette® DS Gum** *see* nicotine *on next page*

**Nicorette® Gum** *see* nicotine *on next page*

**Nicorette® Plus (Can)** *see* nicotine *on this page*

**nicotinamide** *see* niacinamide *on previous page*

## nicotine (nik oh TEEN)

**U.S./Canadian Brand Names** Habitrol™ Patch; NicoDerm® Patch; Nicorette® DS Gum; Nicorette® Gum; Nicorette® Plus (Can); Nicotrol® Inhaler; Nicotrol® NS Nasal Spray; Nicotrol® Patch [OTC]; ProStep® Patch

**Therapeutic Category** Smoking Deterrent

**Use** Treatment aid to giving up smoking while participating in a behavioral modification program, under medical supervision

**Usual Dosage**

Gum: Chew 1 piece of gum when urge to smoke, up to 30 pieces/day; most patients require 10-12 pieces of gum/day

Inhaler: Usually 6 to 16 cartridges per day; best effect was achieved by frequent continuous puffing (20 minutes); recommended duration of treatment is 3 months, after which patients may be weaned from the inhaler by gradual reduction of the daily dose over 6-12 weeks

Transdermal patch (patients should be advised to completely stop smoking upon initiation of therapy): Apply new patch every 24 hours to nonhairy, clean, dry skin on the upper body or upper outer arm; each patch should be applied to a different site

Initial starting dose: 21 mg/day for 4-8 weeks for most patients

First weaning dose: 14 mg/day for 2-4 weeks

Second weaning dose: 7 mg/day for 2-4 weeks

Initial starting dose for patients <100 pounds, smoke <10 cigarettes/day, have a history of cardiovascular disease: 14 mg/day for 4-8 weeks followed by 7 mg/day for 2-4 weeks

In patients who are receiving >600 mg/day of cimetidine: Decrease to the next lower patch size

Benefits of use of nicotine transdermal patches beyond 3 months have not been demonstrated

Spray: 1-2 sprays/hour; do not exceed more than 5 doses (10 sprays) per hour; each dose (2 sprays) contains 1 mg of nicotine. **Warning:** A dose of 40 mg can cause fatalities

**Dosage Forms**

Inhaler, oral (cartridge): 10 mg [delivering 4 mg] (42s); each unit consists of one mouthpiece, 7 storage trays each containing 6 cartridges and one storage case

Patch, transdermal:

Habitrol™: 21 mg/day; 14 mg/day; 7 mg/day (30 systems/box)

NicoDerm®: 21 mg/day; 14 mg/day; 7 mg/day (14 systems/box)

Nicotrol® [OTC]: 15 mg/day (gradually released over 16 hours)

ProStep®: 22 mg/day; 11 mg/day (7 systems/box)

Pieces, chewing gum, as polacrilex: 2 mg/square [OTC] (96 pieces/box); 4 mg/square (96 pieces/box)

Spray, nasal: 0.5 mg/actuation [10 mg/mL - 200 actuations] (10 mL)

**Nicotinex [OTC]** *see* niacin *on page 417*

**nicotinic acid** *see* niacin *on page 417*

**Nicotrol® Inhaler** *see* nicotine *on this page*

**Nicotrol® NS Nasal Spray** *see* nicotine *on this page*

**Nicotrol® Patch [OTC]** *see* nicotine *on this page*

## nicoumalone *(Canada only)* (nye KYOO ma lone)

**U.S./Canadian Brand Names** Sintrom® (Can)

**Therapeutic Category** Anticoagulant

(Continued)

## nicoumalone *(Canada only)* *(Continued)*

**Use** Prophylaxis and treatment of venous thrombosis and its extension, the treatment of atrial fibrillation with embolization, the prophylaxis and treatment of pulmonary embolism, and as an adjunct in the treatment of coronary occlusion and transient cerebral ischemic attacks

**Usual Dosage** Adults: Oral:

First day: 8-12 mg

Second day: 4-8 mg; if the thromboplastin time is initially abnormal, treatment must be commenced with great caution

Maintenance therapy and coagulation tests: In view of the marked individual differences encountered, the maintenance dose should be established and adjusted by reference to the results of periodically performed laboratory tests to determine the patient's blood coagulation time.

**Dosage Forms** Tablet: 1 mg, 4 mg

**Nico-Vert® [OTC]** *see* meclizine *on page 367*

**NidaGel™ (Can)** *see* metronidazole *on page 388*

**Nidryl®** ***(Discontinued)*** *see page 750*

## nifedipine (nye FED i peen)

**U.S./Canadian Brand Names** Adalat® CC; Adalat PA® (Can); Apo®-Nifed (Can); Novo-Nifedin (Can); Nu-Nifed (Can); Nu-Nifedin (Can); Procardia®; Procardia XL®

**Therapeutic Category** Calcium Channel Blocker

**Use** Angina, hypertrophic cardiomyopathy, hypertension

**Usual Dosage** Oral:

Children:

Hypertensive emergencies: 0.25-0.5 mg/kg/dose

Hypertrophic cardiomyopathy: 0.6-0.9 mg/kg/24 hours in 3-4 divided doses

Adults: Initial: 10 mg 3 times/day as capsules or 30-60 mg once daily as sustained release tablet; maintenance: 10-30 mg 3-4 times/day (capsules); maximum: 180 mg/24 hours (capsules) or 120 mg/day (sustained release)

**Dosage Forms**

Capsule, liquid-filled: 10 mg, 20 mg

Capsule, liquid-filled (Procardia®): 10 mg, 20 mg

Tablet, extended release (Adalat® CC): 30 mg, 60 mg, 90 mg

Tablet, sustained release (Procardia XL®): 30 mg, 60 mg, 90 mg

**Niferex® [OTC]** *see* polysaccharide-iron complex *on page 482*

**Niferex Forte®** ***(Discontinued)*** *see page 750*

**Niferex®-PN** *see* vitamin (multiple/oral) *on page 632*

**Night-Time Cramp Relief® [OTC]** *see* acetaminophen and diphenhydramine *on page 5*

**Night-Time Pain Reliever/Sleep [OTC]** *see* acetaminophen and diphenhydramine *on page 5*

**Nilandron™** *see* nilutamide *on this page*

**Niloric®** ***(Discontinued)*** *see page 750*

**Nilstat®** *see* nystatin *on page 432*

## nilutamide (ni LU ta mide)

**U.S./Canadian Brand Names** Anandron® (Can); Nilandron™

**Therapeutic Category** Antineoplastic Agent

**Use** With orchiectomy (surgical castration) for the treatment of metastatic prostate cancer

**Usual Dosage** Adults: Oral: 300 mg (6-50 mg tablets) once daily for 30 days, then 150 mg (3-50 mg tablets) once daily; starting on the same day or day after surgical castration

**Dosage Forms** Tablet: 50 mg

**Nimbex®** *see* cisatracurium *on page 139*

## nimodipine (nye MOE di peen)

**U.S./Canadian Brand Names** Nimotop®

**Therapeutic Category** Calcium Channel Blocker

**Use** Improvement of neurological deficits due to spasm following subarachnoid hemorrhage from ruptured congenital intracranial aneurysms who are in good neurological condition postictus

**Usual Dosage** Adults: Oral: 60 mg every 4 hours for 21 days, start therapy within 96 hours after subarachnoid hemorrhage

**Dosage Forms** Capsule, liquid-filled: 30 mg

**Nimotop®** *see* nimodipine *on this page*

**Nipent™** *see* pentostatin *on page 460*

**Nipride® Injection *(Discontinued)*** *see page 750*

**Nisaval® *(Discontinued)*** *see page 750*

## nisoldipine (NYE sole di peen)

**U.S./Canadian Brand Names** Sular®

**Therapeutic Category** Calcium Channel Blocker

**Use** Management of hypertension, may be used alone or in combination with other antihypertensive agents

**Usual Dosage** Adults: Oral: Initial: 20 mg once daily, then increase by 10 mg per week (or longer intervals) to attain adequate control of blood pressure; doses >60 mg once daily are not recommended

**Dosage Forms** Tablet, extended release: 10 mg, 20 mg, 30 mg, 40 mg

**nitalapram** *see* citalopram *on page 140*

**Nitoman® (Can)** *see* tetrabenazine *(Canada only)* *on page 578*

## nitric oxide (NYE trik OKS ide)

**U.S./Canadian Brand Names** INOmax®

**Therapeutic Category** Vasodilator, Pulmonary

**Use** Treatment of term and near-term (>34 weeks) neonates with hypoxic respiratory failure associated with pulmonary hypertension; used concurrently with ventilatory support and other agents

**Usual Dosage** Neonates (up to 14 days old): 20 ppm. Treatment should be maintained up to 14 days or until the underlying oxygen desaturation has resolved and the neonate is ready to be weaned from therapy. In the CINRGI trial, patients whose oxygenation improved had their dose reduced to 5 ppm at the end of 4 hours of treatment. Doses above 20 ppm should not be used because of the risk of methemoglobinemia and elevated $NO_2$.

**Dosage Forms** Aluminum cylinders: 353 L, 1963 L

**Nitro-Bid® I.V. Injection** *see* nitroglycerin *on next page*

**Nitro-Bid® Ointment** *see* nitroglycerin *on next page*

**Nitro-Bid® Oral *(Discontinued)*** *see page 750*

**Nitrocine® Oral *(Discontinued)*** *see page 750*

**Nitrodisc® Patch *(Discontinued)*** *see page 750*

**Nitro-Dur® Patch** *see* nitroglycerin *on next page*

**nitrofural** *see* nitrofurazone *on next page*

## nitrofurantoin (nye troe fyoor AN toyn)

**U.S./Canadian Brand Names** Apo®-Nitrofurantoin (Can); Furadantin®; Macrobid®; Macrodantin®; Novo-Furantoin (Can)

**Therapeutic Category** Antibiotic, Miscellaneous

**Use** Prevention and treatment of urinary tract infections caused by susceptible gram-negative and some gram-positive organisms including *E. coli*, *Klebsiella*, *Enterobacter*, *Enterococa*, and *S. aureus*; *Pseudomonas*, *Serratia*, and most species of *Proteus* are generally resistant to nitrofurantoin

**Usual Dosage** Oral:

Children >1 month: 5-7 mg/kg/day divided every 6 hours; maximum: 400 mg/day

Chronic therapy: 1-2 mg/kg/day in divided doses every 12-24 hours; maximum dose: 400 mg/day

Adults: 50-100 mg/dose every 6 hours (not to exceed 400 mg/24 hours)

Prophylaxis: 50-100 mg/dose at bedtime

**Dosage Forms**

Capsule: 50 mg, 100 mg

Capsule:

Macrocrystal: 25 mg, 50 mg, 100 mg

Macrocrystal/monohydrate: 100 mg

Suspension, oral: 25 mg/5 mL (470 mL)

## nitrofurazone (nye troe FYOOR a zone)

**Synonyms** nitrofural

**U.S./Canadian Brand Names** Furacin® Topical

**Therapeutic Category** Antibacterial, Topical

**Use** Antibacterial agent used in second- and third-degree burns and skin grafting

**Usual Dosage** Children and Adults: Topical: Apply once daily or every few days to lesion or place on gauze

**Dosage Forms**

Cream: 0.2% (28 g)

Ointment, soluble dressing: 0.2% (28 g, 56 g, 454 g, 480 g)

Solution, topical: 0.2% (480 mL)

**Nitrogard® Buccal** *see* nitroglycerin *on this page*

**nitrogen mustard** *see* mechlorethamine *on page 367*

## nitroglycerin (nye troe GLI ser in)

**Synonyms** glyceryl trinitrate; nitroglycerol; NTG

**U.S./Canadian Brand Names** Deponit® Patch; Minitran™ Patch; Nitro-Bid® I.V. Injection; Nitro-Bid® Ointment; Nitro-Dur® Patch; Nitrogard® Buccal; Nitroglyn® Oral; Nitrolingual® Translingual Spray; Nitrol® Ointment; Nitrong® Oral Tablet; Nitrostat® Sublingual; NitroTab®; Transdermal-NTG® Patch; Transderm-Nitro® Patch; Tridil® Injection

**Therapeutic Category** Vasodilator

**Use** Angina pectoris; I.V. for congestive heart failure (especially when associated with acute myocardial infarction); pulmonary hypertension; hypertensive emergencies occurring perioperatively (especially during cardiovascular surgery)

**Usual Dosage Note:** Hemodynamic and antianginal tolerance often develops within 24-48 hours of continuous nitrate administration

Children: Pulmonary hypertension: Continuous infusion: Start 0.25-0.5 mcg/kg/minute and titrate by 1 mcg/kg/minute at 20- to 60-minute intervals to desired effect; usual dose: 1-3 mcg/kg/minute; maximum: 5 mcg/kg/minute

Adults:

Oral: 2.5-9 mg 2-4 times/day (up to 26 mg 4 times/day)

I.V.: 5 mcg/minute, increase by 5 mcg/minute every 3-5 minutes to 20 mcg/minute; if no response at 20 mcg/minute increase by 10 mcg/minute every 3-5 minutes, up to 200 mcg/minute

Sublingual: 0.2-0.6 mg every 5 minutes for maximum of 3 doses in 15 minutes; may also use prophylactically 5-10 minutes prior to activities which may provoke an attack

Ointment: 1" to 2" every 8 hours up to 4" to 5" every 4 hours

Patch, transdermal: 0.2-0.4 mg/hour initially and titrate to doses of 0.4-0.8 mg/hour; tolerance is minimized by using a patch on period of 12-14 hours and patch off period of 10-12 hours

Translingual: 1-2 sprays into mouth under tongue every 3-5 minutes for maximum of 3 doses in 15 minutes, may also be used 5-10 minutes prior to activities which may provoke an attack prophylactically

Buccal: Initial: 1 mg every 3-5 hours while awake (3 times/day); titrate dosage upward if angina occurs with tablet in place

May need to use nitrate-free interval (10-12 hours/day) to avoid tolerance development; tolerance may possibly be reversed with acetylcysteine; gradually decrease dose in patients receiving NTG for prolonged period to avoid withdrawal reaction

**Dosage Forms**

Capsule, sustained release: 2.5 mg, 6.5 mg, 9 mg

Injection: 0.5 mg/mL (10 mL); 0.8 mg/mL (10 mL); 5 mg/mL (1 mL, 5 mL, 10 mL, 20 mL); 10 mg/mL (5 mL, 10 mL)

Ointment, topical (Nitrol®): 2% [20 mg/g] (30 g, 60 g)

Patch, transdermal, topical: Systems designed to deliver 2.5, 5, 7.5, 10, or 15 mg NTG over 24 hours

Spray, translingual: 0.4 mg/metered spray (13.8 g)

Tablet:

Buccal, controlled release: 1 mg, 2 mg, 3 mg

Sublingual (Nitrostat®, NitroTab®): 0.3 mg, 0.4 mg, 0.6 mg

Sustained release: 2.6 mg, 6.5 mg, 9 mg

**nitroglycerol** *see* nitroglycerin *on previous page*

**Nitroglyn® Oral** *see* nitroglycerin *on previous page*

**Nitrolingual® Translingual Spray** *see* nitroglycerin *on previous page*

**Nitrol® Ointment** *see* nitroglycerin *on previous page*

**Nitrong® Oral Tablet** *see* nitroglycerin *on previous page*

**Nitropress®** *see* nitroprusside *on this page*

## nitroprusside (nye troe PRUS ide)

**Synonyms** sodium nitroferricyanide

**U.S./Canadian Brand Names** Nitropress®

**Therapeutic Category** Vasodilator

**Use** Management of hypertensive crises; congestive heart failure; used for controlled hypotension during anesthesia

**Usual Dosage** I.V.:

Children: Continuous infusion:

Initial: 1 mcg/kg/minute by continuous I.V. infusion; increase in increments of 1 mcg/kg/minute at intervals of 20-60 minutes; titrating to the desired response

Usual dose: 3 mcg/kg/minute; rarely need >4 mcg/kg/minute

Maximum: 10 mcg/kg/minute. Dilute 15 mg x weight (kg) to 250 mL $D_5W$, then dose in mcg/kg/minute = infusion rate in mL/hour

Adults: Begin at 5 mcg/kg/minute; increase in increments of 5 mcg/kg/minute (up to 20 mcg/kg/minute), then in increments of 10-20 mcg/kg/minute; titrating to the desired hemodynamic effect or the appearance of headache or nausea. When >500 mcg/kg is administered by prolonged infusion of faster than 2 mcg/kg/minute, cyanide is generated faster than an unaided patient can handle.

**Dosage Forms** Injection, as sodium: 10 mg/mL (5 mL); 25 mg/mL (2 mL)

**Nitrostat® 0.15 mg Tablet *(Discontinued)*** *see page 750*

**Nitrostat® Sublingual** *see* nitroglycerin *on previous page*

**NitroTab®** *see* nitroglycerin *on page 422*

**nitrous oxide** (NYE trus OKS ide)

**Therapeutic Category** Anesthetic, Gas

**Use** Produces sedation and analgesia; principal adjunct to inhalation and intravenous general anesthesia

**Usual Dosage** Children and Adults: For sedation and analgesia: Concentrations of 25% to 50% nitrous oxide with oxygen. For general anesthesia, concentrations of 40% to 70% via mask or endotracheal tube. Minimal alveolar concentration or (MAC) $ED_{50}$ is 105%, therefore delivery in a hyperbaric chamber is necessary to use as a complete anesthetic; when administered at 70%, reduces the MAC of other anesthetics by half.

**Dosage Forms** Cylinder

**Nix™ Creme Rinse** *see* permethrin *on page 462*

**nizatidine** (ni ZA ti deen)

**U.S./Canadian Brand Names** Apo®-Nizatidine (Can); Axid®; Axid® AR [OTC]; Novo-Nizatidine (Can)

**Therapeutic Category** Histamine $H_2$ Antagonist

**Use** Treatment and maintenance of duodenal ulcer; treatment of gastroesophageal reflux disease (GERD)

**Usual Dosage** Adults: Active duodenal ulcer: Oral:

Treatment: 300 mg at bedtime or 150 mg twice daily

Maintenance: 150 mg/day

**Dosage Forms**

Capsule: 150 mg, 300 mg

Tablet: 75 mg

**Nizoral®** *see* ketoconazole *on page 333*

**Nizoral® A-D Shampoo [OTC]** *see* ketoconazole *on page 333*

**n-methylhydrazine** *see* procarbazine *on page 497*

**Noctec®** ***(Discontinued)*** *see page 750*

**Nolahist® [OTC]** *see* phenindamine *on page 464*

**Nolamine®** ***(Discontinued)*** *see page 750*

**Nolex® LA** ***(Discontinued)*** *see page 750*

**Noludar®** ***(Discontinued)*** *see page 750*

**Nolvadex®** *see* tamoxifen *on page 570*

**nonoxynol 9** (non OKS i nole nine)

**U.S./Canadian Brand Names** Advantage 24™ (Can); Because® [OTC]; Delfen® [OTC]; Emko® [OTC]; Encare® [OTC]; Gynol II® [OTC]; Koromex® [OTC]; Ramses® [OTC]; Semicid® [OTC]; Shur-Seal® [OTC]

**Therapeutic Category** Spermicide

**Use** Spermatocide in contraception

**Usual Dosage** Insert into vagina at least 15 minutes before intercourse

**Dosage Forms** Vaginal:

Cream: 2% (103.5 g)

Foam: 12.5% (60 g)

Jelly: 2% (81 g, 126 g)

**No Pain-HP®** ***(Discontinued)*** *see page 750*

**noradrenaline acid tartrate** *see* norepinephrine *on next page*

**Norcet®** *see* hydrocodone and acetaminophen *on page 300*

**Norco®** *see* hydrocodone and acetaminophen *on page 300*

**Norcuron®** *see* vecuronium *on page 624*

**nordeoxyguanosine** *see* ganciclovir *on page 269*

**Nordette®** *see* ethinyl estradiol and levonorgestrel *on page 232*

**Norditropin®** *see* human growth hormone *on page 296*

**Nordryl® Injection** *see* diphenhydramine *on page 191*

**Nordryl® Oral** *see* diphenhydramine *on page 191*

## norepinephrine (nor ep i NEF rin)

**Synonyms** noradrenaline acid tartrate

**U.S./Canadian Brand Names** Levophed®

**Therapeutic Category** Adrenergic Agonist Agent

**Use** Treatment of shock which persists after adequate fluid volume replacement; severe hypotension; cardiogenic shock

**Usual Dosage Note:** Dose stated in terms of norepinephrine base. I.V.:

Children: Initial: 0.05-0.1 mcg/kg/minute, titrate to desired effect; rate (mL/hour) = dose (mcg/kg/minute) x weight (kg) x 60 minutes/hour divided by concentration (mcg/mL)

Adults: 8-12 mcg/minute as an infusion; initiate at 4 mcg/minute and titrate to desired response

**Dosage Forms** Injection, as bitartrate: 1 mg/mL (4 mL)

**Norethin™ 1/35E** *see* ethinyl estradiol and norethindrone *on page 232*

## norethindrone (nor eth IN drone)

**Synonyms** norethisterone

**U.S./Canadian Brand Names** Aygestin®; Micronor®; NOR-QD®

**Therapeutic Category** Contraceptive, Progestin Only; Progestin

**Use** Treatment of amenorrhea; abnormal uterine bleeding; endometriosis

**Usual Dosage** Adolescents and Adults: Oral:

Amenorrhea and abnormal uterine bleeding: 2.5-10 mg on days 5-25 of menstrual cycle

Endometriosis: 5 mg/day for 14 days; increase at increments of 2.5 mg/day every 2 weeks up to 15 mg/day

**Dosage Forms**

Tablet: 0.35 mg, 5 mg

Tablet, as acetate: 5 mg

**norethisterone** *see* norethindrone *on this page*

**Norflex™** *see* orphenadrine *on page 438*

## norfloxacin (nor FLOKS a sin)

**U.S./Canadian Brand Names** Apo®-Norflox (Can); Chibroxin™ Ophthalmic; Noroxin® Oral; Novo-Norfloxacin (Can); Riva-Norfloxacin (Can)

**Therapeutic Category** Quinolone

**Use** Complicated and uncomplicated urinary tract infections caused by susceptible gram-negative and gram-positive bacteria

**Usual Dosage**

Children >1 year and Adults: Ophthalmic: Instill 1-2 drops in affected eye(s) 4 times/day for up to 7 days

Adults: Oral: 400 mg twice daily for 7-21 days depending on infection

**Dosage Forms**

Solution, ophthalmic: 0.3% [3 mg/mL] (5 mL)

Tablet: 400 mg

**Norgesic™** *see* orphenadrine, aspirin, and caffeine *on page 439*

**Norgesic™ Forte** *see* orphenadrine, aspirin, and caffeine *on page 439*

## norgestrel (nor JES trel)

**U.S./Canadian Brand Names** Ovrette®

**Therapeutic Category** Contraceptive, Progestin Only

**Use** Prevention of pregnancy; treatment of hypermenorrhea, endometriosis, female hypogonadism

**Usual Dosage** Oral: Administer daily, starting the first day of menstruation, administer one tablet at the same time each day, every day of the year. If one dose is missed, administer as soon as remembered, then next tablet at regular time; if two doses are missed, administer one tablet and discard the other, then administer daily at usual time; if three doses are missed, use an additional form of birth control until menses or pregnancy is ruled out

**Dosage Forms** Tablet: 0.075 mg

**Norinyl® 1+35** *see* ethinyl estradiol and norethindrone *on page 232*

**Norinyl® 1+50** *see* mestranol and norethindrone *on page 375*

**Noritate™** *see* metronidazole *on page 388*

**Norlutate®** ***(Discontinued)*** *see page 750*

**Norlutin®** ***(Discontinued)*** *see page 750*

**normal saline** *see* sodium chloride *on page 549*

**Normiflo®** ***(Discontinued)*** *see page 750*

**Normodyne®** *see* labetalol *on page 336*

**Noroxin® Oral** *see* norfloxacin *on previous page*

**Norpace®** *see* disopyramide *on page 195*

**Norpace® CR** *see* disopyramide *on page 195*

**Norplant® Implant** *see* levonorgestrel *on page 347*

**Norpramin®** *see* desipramine *on page 172*

**NOR-QD®** *see* norethindrone *on previous page*

**North American coral snake antivenin** *see* antivenin (*Micrurus fulvius*) *on page 46*

**North and South American antisnake-bite serum** *see* antivenin (*Crotalidae*) polyvalent *on page 45*

## nortriptyline (nor TRIP ti leen)

**U.S./Canadian Brand Names** Apo®-Nortriptyline (Can); Aventyl® Hydrochloride; Pamelor®

**Therapeutic Category** Antidepressant, Tricyclic (Secondary Amine)

**Use** Treatment of various forms of depression, often in conjunction with psychotherapy; nocturnal enuresis

**Usual Dosage** Oral:
Adults: 25 mg 3-4 times/day up to 150 mg/day
Adolescents and Elderly: 30-50 mg/day in divided doses

**Dosage Forms**
Capsule, as hydrochloride: 10 mg, 25 mg, 50 mg, 75 mg
Solution, as hydrochloride: 10 mg/5 mL (473 mL)

**Norvasc®** *see* amlodipine *on page 34*

**Norvir®** *see* ritonavir *on page 529*

**Norzine®** ***(Discontinued)*** *see page 750*

**Nōstrilla® [OTC]** *see* oxymetazoline *on page 444*

**Nostril® Nasal Solution [OTC]** *see* phenylephrine *on page 467*

**Novacet® Topical** *see* sulfur and sulfacetamide *on page 566*

**Novafed®** ***(Discontinued)*** *see page 750*

**Novagesic® [OTC]** *see* acetaminophen and phenyltoloxamine *on page 5*

**Novahistex® DM** *see* pseudoephedrine and dextromethorphan *on page 508*

**Novahistine® DH** *see* chlorpheniramine, pseudoephedrine, and codeine *on page 132*

**Novahistine® DM** *see* pseudoephedrine and dextromethorphan *on page 508*

**Novahistine DM Decongestant Expectorant (Can)** *see* guaifenesin, pseudoephedrine, and dextromethorphan *on page 285*

**Novahistine DMX® Liquid *(Discontinued)*** *see page 750*

**Novahistine® Elixir *(Discontinued)*** *see page 750*

**Novahistine® Expectorant *(Discontinued)*** *see page 750*

**Novamilor (Can)** *see* amiloride and hydrochlorothiazide *on page 30*

**Novamoxin® (Can)** *see* amoxicillin *on page 35*

**Novantrone®** *see* mitoxantrone *on page 396*

**Novarel™** *see* chorionic gonadotropin *on page 136*

**Novo-5 ASA (Can)** *see* mesalamine *on page 374*

**Novo-Acebutolol (Can)** *see* acebutolol *on page 3*

**Novo-Alprazol (Can)** *see* alprazolam *on page 22*

**Novo-Amiodarone (Can)** *see* amiodarone *on page 32*

**Novo-AZT (Can)** *see* zidovudine *on page 638*

**Novo-Baclofen (Can)** *see* baclofen *on page 66*

**Novo-Benzydamine (Can)** *see* benzydamine *(Canada only) on page 75*

**Novo-Bromazepam (Can)** *see* bromazepam *(Canada only) on page 86*

**Novocain®** *see* procaine *on page 497*

**Novo-Captopril (Can)** *see* captopril *on page 104*

**Novo-Carbamaz (Can)** *see* carbamazepine *on page 105*

**Novo-Cefaclor (Can)** *see* cefaclor *on page 113*

**Novo-Cefadroxil (Can)** *see* cefadroxil *on page 113*

**Novo-Cholamine (Can)** *see* cholestyramine resin *on page 134*

**Novo-Cimetine (Can)** *see* cimetidine *on page 137*

**Novo-Clobazam (Can)** *see* clobazam *(Canada only) on page 143*

**Novo-Clobetasol (Can)** *see* clobetasol *on page 143*

**Novo-Clonazepam (Can)** *see* clonazepam *on page 145*

**Novo-Clonidine (Can)** *see* clonidine *on page 146*

**Novo-Clopamine (Can)** *see* clomipramine *on page 145*

**Novo-Clopate (Can)** *see* clorazepate *on page 147*

**Novo-Cloxin (Can)** *see* cloxacillin *on page 148*

**Novo-Cycloprine (Can)** *see* cyclobenzaprine *on page 159*

**Novo-Cyproterone (Can)** *see* cyproterone *(Canada only) on page 161*

**Novo-Desipramine (Can)** *see* desipramine *on page 172*

**Novo-Difenac-K (Can)** *see* diclofenac *on page 181*

**Novo-Difenac®-SR (Can)** *see* diclofenac *on page 181*

**Novo-Diflunisal (Can)** *see* diflunisal *on page 185*

**Novo-Diltazem (Can)** *see* diltiazem *on page 187*

**Novo-Dipiradol (Can)** *see* dipyridamole *on page 194*

**Novo-Divalproex® (Can)** *see* valproic acid and derivatives *on page 620*

**Novo-Domperidone (Can)** *see* domperidone *(Canada only) on page 200*

**Novo-Doxepin (Can)** *see* doxepin *on page 202*

**Novo-Doxylin (Can)** *see* doxycycline *on page 204*

**Novo-Famotidine (Can)** *see* famotidine *on page 240*

**Novo-Fluoxetine (Can)** *see* fluoxetine *on page 256*

**Novo-Flurprofen (Can)** *see* flurbiprofen *on page 259*

**Novo-Flutamide (Can)** *see* flutamide *on page 259*

**Novo-Fluvoxamine (Can)** *see* fluvoxamine *on page 262*

**Novo-Furantoin (Can)** *see* nitrofurantoin *on page 422*

**Novo-Gemfibrozil (Can)** *see* gemfibrozil *on page 271*

**Novo-Gliclazide (Can)** *see* gliclazide *(Canada only) on page 274*

**Novo-Glyburide (Can)** *see* glyburide *on page 276*

**Novo-Hydroxyzin (Can)** *see* hydroxyzine *on page 308*

**Novo-Hylazin (Can)** *see* hydralazine *on page 297*

**Novo-Indapamide (Can)** *see* indapamide *on page 316*

**Novo-Ipramide (Can)** *see* ipratropium *on page 325*

**Novo-Keto (Can)** *see* ketoprofen *on page 334*

**Novo-Ketoconazol (Can)** *see* ketoconazole *on page 333*

**Novo-Keto-EC (Can)** *see* ketoprofen *on page 334*

**Novo-Ketorolac (Can)** *see* ketorolac tromethamine *on page 334*

**Novo-Ketotifen (Can)** *see* ketotifen *on page 335*

**Novo-Levamisole (Can)** *see* levamisole *on page 344*

**Novo-Levobunolol (Can)** *see* levobunolol *on page 344*

**Novo-Lexin® (Can)** *see* cephalexin *on page 120*

**Novolin® 70/30** *see* insulin preparations *on page 319*

**Novolin® ge (Can)** *see* insulin preparations *on page 319*

**Novolin® L** *see* insulin preparations *on page 319*

**Novolin® N** *see* insulin preparations *on page 319*

**Novolin-Pen® II, -3 (Can)** *see* insulin preparations *on page 319*

**Novolin® R** *see* insulin preparations *on page 319*

**NovoLog™** *see* insulin preparations *on page 319*

**Novo-Loperamide (Can)** *see* loperamide *on page 354*

**Novo-Lorazem (Can)** *see* lorazepam *on page 356*

**Novo-Lorazepam (Can)** *see* lorazepam *on page 356*

**Novo-Maprotiline (Can)** *see* maprotiline *on page 365*

**Novo-Medopa® (Can)** *see* methyldopa *on page 383*

**Novo-Medrone (Can)** *see* medroxyprogesterone acetate *on page 369*

**Novo-Meprazine (Can)** *see* methotrimeprazine *(Canada only) on page 381*

**Novo-Metformin (Can)** *see* metformin *on page 377*

**Novo-Methacin (Can)** *see* indomethacin *on page 317*

**Novo-Metoprol (Can)** *see* metoprolol *on page 388*

**Novo-Metoprolol (Can)** *see* metoprolol *on page 388*

**Novo-Mexiletine (Can)** *see* mexiletine *on page 389*

**Novo-Moclobemide (Can)** *see* moclobemide *(Canada only) on page 397*

**Nu-Ketoprofen (Can)** *see* ketoprofen *on page 334*
**Nu-Ketoprofen-E (Can)** *see* ketoprofen *on page 334*
**Nu-Levocarb (Can)** *see* carbidopa and levodopa *on page 107*
**Nullo® [OTC]** *see* chlorophyll *on page 127*
**Nu-Loraz (Can)** *see* lorazepam *on page 356*
**Nu-Loxapine (Can)** *see* loxapine *on page 358*
**NuLytely®** *see* polyethylene glycol solution *on page 480*
**Nu-Medopa (Can)** *see* methyldopa *on page 383*
**Nu-Mefenamic (Can)** *see* mefenamic acid *on page 369*
**Nu-Megestrol (Can)** *see* megestrol acetate *on page 370*
**Nu-Metformin (Can)** *see* metformin *on page 377*
**Nu-Metoclopramide (Can)** *see* metoclopramide *on page 387*
**Nu-Metop (Can)** *see* metoprolol *on page 388*
**Nu-Moclobemide (Can)** *see* moclobemide *(Canada only) on page 397*
**Numorphan®** *see* oxymorphone *on page 445*
**Numzitdent® [OTC]** *see* benzocaine *on page 72*
**Numzit Teething® [OTC]** *see* benzocaine *on page 72*
**Nu-Naprox (Can)** *see* naproxen *on page 409*
**Nu-Nifed (Can)** *see* nifedipine *on page 420*
**Nu-Nifedin (Can)** *see* nifedipine *on page 420*
**Nu-Oxybutyn (Can)** *see* oxybutynin *on page 443*
**Nu-Pentoxifylline-SR (Can)** *see* pentoxifylline *on page 460*
**Nu-Pen-VK (Can)** *see* penicillin V potassium *on page 457*
**Nupercainal® [OTC]** *see* dibucaine *on page 181*
**Nu-Pindol (Can)** *see* pindolol *on page 472*
**Nu-Pirox (Can)** *see* piroxicam *on page 474*
**Nu-Prazo (Can)** *see* prazosin *on page 491*
**Nuprin® [OTC]** *see* ibuprofen *on page 311*
**Nu-Prochlor (Can)** *see* prochlorperazine *on page 497*
**Nu-Propranolol (Can)** *see* propranolol *on page 504*
**Nu-Ranit (Can)** *see* ranitidine hydrochloride *on page 519*
**Nuromax®** *see* doxacurium *on page 201*
**Nursoy®** ***(Discontinued)*** *see page 750*
**Nu-Selegiline (Can)** *see* selegiline *on page 540*
**Nu-Sotalol (Can)** *see* sotalol *on page 555*
**Nu-Sucralfate (Can)** *see* sucralfate *on page 561*
**Nu-Sulfinpyrazone (Can)** *see* sulfinpyrazone *on page 566*
**Nu-Sulindac (Can)** *see* sulindac *on page 567*
**Nu-Tears® II Solution [OTC]** *see* artificial tears *on page 53*
**Nu-Tears® Solution [OTC]** *see* artificial tears *on page 53*
**Nu-Temazepam (Can)** *see* temazepam *on page 572*
**Nu-Terazosin (Can)** *see* terazosin *on page 574*
**Nu-Tetra (Can)** *see* tetracycline *on page 579*
**Nu-Tiaprofenic (Can)** *see* tiaprofenic acid *(Canada only) on page 589*

**Nu-Ticlopidine (Can)** *see* ticlopidine *on page 590*

**Nu-Timolol (Can)** *see* timolol *on page 591*

**Nutracort® Topical** *see* hydrocortisone (topical) *on page 304*

**Nutraplus® Topical [OTC]** *see* urea *on page 617*

**Nu-Trazodone (Can)** *see* trazodone *on page 600*

**Nu-Triazide (Can)** *see* hydrochlorothiazide and triamterene *on page 299*

**Nutrilipid®** *see* fat emulsion *on page 241*

**Nu-Trimipramine (Can)** *see* trimipramine *on page 608*

## nutritional formula, enteral/oral

(noo TRISH un al FOR myoo la, EN ter al/OR al)

**Synonyms** dietary supplements

**U.S./Canadian Brand Names** Carnation Instant Breakfast® [OTC]; Citrotein® [OTC]; Criticare HN® [OTC]; Ensure® [OTC]; Ensure Plus® [OTC]; Isocal® [OTC]; Magnacal® [OTC]; Microlipid™ [OTC]; Osmolite® HN [OTC]; Pedialyte® [OTC]; Portagen® [OTC]; Pregestimil® [OTC]; Propac™ [OTC]; Soyalac® [OTC]; Vital HN® [OTC]; Vitaneed™ [OTC]; Vivonex® [OTC]; Vivonex® T.E.N. [OTC]

**Therapeutic Category** Nutritional Supplement

**Dosage Forms**

Liquid: Calcium and sodium caseinate, maltodextrin, sucrose, partially hydrogenated soy oil, soy lecithin

Powder: Amino acids, predigested carbohydrates, safflower oil

**Nutropin®** *see* human growth hormone *on page 296*

**Nutropin® AQ** *see* human growth hormone *on page 296*

**Nu-Valproic (Can)** *see* valproic acid and derivatives *on page 620*

**Nu-Verap (Can)** *see* verapamil *on page 625*

**Nu-Zopiclone (Can)** *see* zopiclone *(Canada only) on page 641*

**Nyaderm (Can)** *see* nystatin *on this page*

**Nydrazid®** *see* isoniazid *on page 327*

## nystatin (nye STAT in)

**U.S./Canadian Brand Names** Bio-Statin®; Candistatin® (Can); Mycostatin®; Nilstat®; Nyaderm (Can); Nystat-Rx®; Nystex®; Pedi-Dri® Topical Powder; PMS-Nystatin (Can)

**Therapeutic Category** Antifungal Agent

**Use** Treatment of susceptible cutaneous, mucocutaneous, oral cavity and vaginal fungal infections normally caused by the *Candida* species

**Usual Dosage**

Oral candidiasis:

Infants: 200,000 units 4 times/day or 100,000 units to each side of mouth 4 times/day

Children and Adults: 400,000-600,000 units 4 times/day; troche: 200,000-400,000 units 4-5 times/day

Cutaneous candidal infections: Children and Adults: Topical: Apply 3-4 times/day

Intestinal infections: Adults: Oral: 500,000-1,000,000 units every 8 hours

Vaginal infections: Adults: Vaginal tablets: Insert 1-2 tablets/day at bedtime for 2 weeks

**Dosage Forms**

Capsule: 500,000 units, 1 million units

Cream: 100,000 units/g (15 g, 30 g)

Ointment, topical: 100,000 units/g (15 g, 30 g)

Powder, for preparation of oral suspension: 50 million units, 1 billion units, 2 billion units, 5 billion units

Powder, topical: 100,000 units/g (15 g, 56.7 g)

Suspension, oral: 100,000 units/mL (5 mL, 60 mL, 480 mL)

Tablet:
Oral: 500,000 units
Vaginal: 100,000 units (15 and 30/box with applicator)
Troche: 200,000 units

## nystatin and triamcinolone (nye STAT in & trye am SIN oh lone)

**U.S./Canadian Brand Names** Mycogen II Topical; Mycolog®-II Topical; Myco-Triacet® II; Mytrex® F Topical; N.G.A.® Topical; Quenalog®

**Therapeutic Category** Antifungal/Corticosteroid

**Use** Treatment of cutaneous candidiasis

**Usual Dosage** Topical: Apply twice daily

**Dosage Forms**
Cream: Nystatin 100,000 units and triamcinolone acetonide 0.1% (15 g, 30 g, 45 g, 60 g, 240 g)
Ointment, topical: Nystatin 100,000 units and triamcinolone acetonide 0.1% (15 g, 30 g, 60 g, 120 g)

**Nystat-Rx®** *see* nystatin *on previous page*

**Nystex®** *see* nystatin *on previous page*

**Nytol® Oral [OTC]** *see* diphenhydramine *on page 191*

**Obezine®** *see* phendimetrazine *on page 463*

**Occlusal®-HP Liquid** *see* salicylic acid *on page 535*

**Ocean Nasal Mist [OTC]** *see* sodium chloride *on page 549*

**OCL®** *see* polyethylene glycol solution *on page 480*

**Octamide®** ***(Discontinued)*** *see page 750*

**Octicair® Otic** *see* neomycin, polymyxin B, and hydrocortisone *on page 415*

**Octocaine®** ***(Discontinued)*** *see page 750*

## octreotide (ok TREE oh tide)

**U.S./Canadian Brand Names** Sandostatin®; Sandostatin LAR®

**Therapeutic Category** Somatostatin Analog

**Use** Control of symptoms in patients with metastatic carcinoid and vasoactive intestinal peptide-secreting tumors (VIPomas); acromegaly, insulinomas, Zollinger-Ellison syndrome, pancreatic tumors, gastrinoma, postgastrectomy dumping syndrome, bleeding esophageal varices, small bowel fistulas, AIDS-associated secretory diarrhea, chemotherapy-induced diarrhea, GVHD-induced diarrhea, control of bleeding of esophageal varices; depot suspension is indicated for long term maintenance therapy in acromegalic patients for whom medical treatment is appropriate and who have been shown to respond to and can tolerate the injection

**Usual Dosage** Adults: S.C.: Initial: 50 mcg 1-2 times/day and titrate dose based on patient tolerance and response

Carcinoid: 100-600 mcg/day in 2-4 divided doses
VIPomas: 200-300 mcg/day in 2-4 divided doses
Diarrhea: Initial: I.V.: 50-100 mcg every 8 hours; increase by 100 mcg/dose at 48-hour intervals; maximum dose: 500 mcg every 8 hours

**Dosage Forms**
Injection: 0.05 mg/mL (1 mL); 0.1 mg/mL (1 mL); 0.2 mg/mL (5 mL); 0.5 mg/mL (1 mL); 1 mg/mL (5 mL)
Injection, suspension, depot: 10 mg (5 mL); 20 mg (5 mL); 30 mg (5 mL)

**Ocu-Caine®** *see* proparacaine *on page 502*

**Ocu-Carpine® Ophthalmic** *see* pilocarpine *on page 471*

**Ocu-Chlor®** *see* chloramphenicol *on page 125*

**OcuClear® Ophthalmic [OTC]** *see* oxymetazoline *on page 444*

**OcuCoat® Ophthalmic Solution [OTC]** *see* artificial tears *on page 53*

**OcuCoat® PF Ophthalmic Solution [OTC]** *see* artificial tears *on page 53*

**Ocufen® Ophthalmic** *see* flurbiprofen *on page 259*

**Ocuflox™ Ophthalmic** *see* ofloxacin *on this page*

**Ocu-Merox®** *see* mercuric oxide *on page 374*

**Ocupress® Ophthalmic** *see* carteolol *on page 111*

**Ocusert Pilo-20® Ophthalmic** *see* pilocarpine *on page 471*

**Ocusert Pilo-40® Ophthalmic** *see* pilocarpine *on page 471*

**Ocu-Sul®** *see* sulfacetamide *on page 562*

**Ocutricin® Topical Ointment** *see* bacitracin, neomycin, and polymyxin B *on page 65*

**Ocu-Tropic®** *see* tropicamide *on page 611*

**Ocuvite™ (Can)** *see* vitamin (multiple/oral) *on page 632*

**Oestrilin (Can)** *see* estrone *on page 228*

## ofloxacin (oh FLOKS a sin)

**U.S./Canadian Brand Names** Apo®-Oflox (Can); Floxin®; Ocuflox™ Ophthalmic

**Therapeutic Category** Antibiotic, Ophthalmic; Antibiotic, Otic; Quinolone

**Use** Quinolone antibiotic for skin and skin structure, lower respiratory and urinary tract infections, and sexually transmitted diseases; bacterial conjunctivitis caused by susceptible organisms; otitis externa in adults and pediatric ≥1 year of age caused by susceptible organisms; otitis media in patients ≥12 years of age with perforated tympanic membranes caused by susceptible organisms; acute otitis media in pediatric patients ≥1 year of age with tympanostomy tubes caused by susceptible organisms

**Usual Dosage**

Children >1 year and Adults: Ophthalmic: Instill 1-2 drops in affected eye(s) every 2-4 hours for the first 2 days, then use 4 times/day for an additional 5 days

Children >1 year to 12 years: Otic: Instill 5 drops in affected ear(s) twice daily for 10 days

Children ≥12 years: Otic: Instill 10 drops in affected ear(s) twice daily for 10 days

Adults: Oral, I.V.: 200-400 mg every 12 hours for 7-10 days for most infections or for 6 weeks for prostatitis

**Dosage Forms**

Injection: 200 mg (50 mL); 400 mg (10 mL, 20 mL, 100 mL)

Solution:

Ophthalmic: 0.3% (5 mL)

Otic: 0.3% (5 mL)

Tablet: 200 mg, 300 mg, 400 mg

**Ogen® Oral** *see* estropipate *on page 228*

**Ogen® Vaginal** *see* estropipate *on page 228*

**OGMT** *see* metyrosine *on page 389*

**Ohmni-Gesic® [OTC]** *see* acetaminophen and phenyltoloxamine *on page 5*

**OKT3** *see* muromonab-CD3 *on page 403*

## olanzapine (oh LAN za peen)

**Synonyms** LY170053

**U.S./Canadian Brand Names** Zyprexa®; Zyprexa® Zydis®

**Therapeutic Category** Antipsychotic Agent

**Use** Treatment of the manifestations of psychotic disorders; short-term treatment of acute mania episodes associated with bipolar I disorder

**Usual Dosage**
Schizophrenia: Usual starting dose: 5-10 mg once daily; increase to 10 mg once daily within 5-7 days, thereafter adjust by 5 mg/day at 1-week intervals, up to a maximum of 20 mg/day; doses of 30-50 mg/day have been used
Bipolar mania: Usual starting dose: 10-15 mg once daily; increase by 5 mg/day at intervals of not less than 24 hours; maximum dose: 20 mg/day

**Dosage Forms**
Tablet: 2.5 mg, 5 mg, 7.5 mg, 10 mg, 15 mg, 20 mg
Tablet, orally-disintegrating: 5 mg, 10 mg, 15 mg, 20 mg

**old tuberculin** *see* tuberculin tests *on page 612*

**oleovitamin A** *see* vitamin A *on page 629*

**oleum ricini** *see* castor oil *on page 112*

## olopatadine (oh LOP ah tah deen)

**U.S./Canadian Brand Names** Patanol®
**Therapeutic Category** Antihistamine
**Use** Allergic conjunctivitis
**Usual Dosage** Adults: Ophthalmic: 1 drop in affected eye(s) every 6-8 hours (twice daily)
**Dosage Forms** Solution, ophthalmic: 0.1% (5 mL)

## olsalazine (ole SAL a zeen)

**U.S./Canadian Brand Names** Dipentum®
**Therapeutic Category** 5-Aminosalicylic Acid Derivative
**Use** Maintenance of remission of ulcerative colitis in patients intolerant to sulfasalazine
**Usual Dosage** Adults: Oral: 1 g daily in 2 divided doses
**Dosage Forms** Capsule, as sodium: 250 mg

**Olux™** *see* clobetasol *on page 143*

## omeprazole (oh ME pray zol)

**U.S./Canadian Brand Names** Prilosec™
**Therapeutic Category** Gastric Acid Secretion Inhibitor
**Use** Short-term (4-8 weeks) treatment of erosive esophagitis (grade 2 or above), diagnosed by endoscopy; maintain healing of erosive esophagitis; short-term treatment of symptomatic gastroesophageal reflux disease (GERD) poorly responsive to customary medical treatment; short-term treatment of active duodenal ulcer; long-term treatment of pathological hypersecretory conditions
**Usual Dosage** Adults: Oral:
Duodenal ulcer: 20 mg/day for 4-8 weeks
GERD or erosive esophagitis: 20 mg/day for 4-8 weeks
Maintenance of healing erosive esophagitis: 20 mg/day
Pathological hypersecretory conditions: 60 mg once daily initially; doses up to 120 mg 3 times/day have been administered; administer daily doses >80 mg in divided doses; patients with Zollinger-Ellison syndrome have been treated continuously for over 5 years
**Dosage Forms** Capsule, delayed release: 10 mg, 20 mg, 40 mg

**Omnicef®** *see* cefdinir *on page 114*

**OmniHIB™** ***(Discontinued)*** *see page 750*

**Omnipaque®** *see* radiological/contrast media (non-ionic) *on page 518*

**Omnipen®** ***(Discontinued)*** *see page 750*

**Omnipen®-N** ***(Discontinued)*** *see page 750*

**Oncaspar®** *see* pegaspargase *on page 453*

**Oncet®** ***(Discontinued)*** *see page 750*

**OncoTICE™ (Can)** *see* BCG vaccine *on page 68*

**Oncovin®** *see* vincristine *on page 628*

## ondansetron (on DAN se tron)

**U.S./Canadian Brand Names** Zofran®; Zofran® ODT

**Therapeutic Category** Selective 5-$HT_3$ Receptor Antagonist

**Use** Prevention of nausea and vomiting associated with initial and repeat courses of emetogenic cancer chemotherapy and prevention of postoperative nausea and vomiting; prevent postoperative nausea/vomiting (I.M.)

**Usual Dosage**

Oral:

Children 4-11 years: 4 mg 30 minutes before chemotherapy; repeat 4 and 8 hours after initial dose

Children >11 years and Adults: 8 mg 30 minutes before chemotherapy; repeat 4 and 8 hours after initial dose or every 8 hours for a maximum of 48 hours

I.V.: Administer either three 0.15 mg/kg doses or a single 32 mg dose; with the 3-dose regimen, the initial dose is given 30 minutes prior to chemotherapy with subsequent doses administered 4 and 8 hours after the first dose. With the single-dose regimen 32 mg is infused over 15 minutes beginning 30 minutes before the start of emetogenic chemotherapy. Dosage should be calculated based on weight:

Children: Pediatric dosing should follow the manufacturer's guidelines for 0.15 mg/kg/dose administered 30 minutes prior to chemotherapy, 4 and 8 hours after the first dose. While not as yet FDA-approved, literature supports the day's total dose administered as a single dose 30 minutes prior to chemotherapy.

Adults:

>80 kg: 12 mg IVPB

45-80 kg: 8 mg IVPB

<45 kg: 0.15 mg/kg/dose IVPB

**Dosage Forms**

Injection, as hydrochloride: 2 mg/mL (2 mL, 20 mL); 32 mg (single-dose vials)

Solution, as hydrochloride: 4 mg/5 mL (50 mL)

Tablet, as hydrochloride: 4 mg, 8 mg, 24 mg

Tablet, as hydrochloride, orally disintegrating: 4 mg, 8 mg

**Ontak®** *see* denileukin diftitox *on page 170*

**Onxel®** *see* paclitaxel *on page 446*

**Ony-Clear® [OTC]** *see* benzalkonium chloride *on page 72*

**OP-CCK** *see* sincalide *on page 545*

**Opcon® Ophthalmic** *see* naphazoline *on page 409*

**o,p′-DDD** *see* mitotane *on page 396*

**Operand® [OTC]** *see* povidone-iodine *on page 489*

**Ophthaine® *(Discontinued)*** *see page 750*

**Ophthalgan® Ophthalmic** *see* glycerin *on page 277*

**Ophthetic®** *see* proparacaine *on page 502*

**Ophtho-Bunolol® (Can)** *see* levobunolol *on page 344*

**Ophthochlor® Ophthalmic *(Discontinued)*** *see page 750*

**Ophthocort® *(Discontinued)*** *see page 750*

**Ophtho-Pipivefrin™ (Can)** *see* dipivefrin *on page 194*

**Ophtho-Tate® (Can)** *see* prednisolone (ophthalmic) *on page 492*

## opium tincture (OH pee um TINGK chur)

**Synonyms** deodorized opium tincture; DTO

**Therapeutic Category** Analgesic, Narcotic

**Controlled Substance** C-II

**Use** Treatment of diarrhea or relief of pain; **a 25-fold dilution with water** (final concentration 0.4 mg/mL morphine) can be used to treat neonatal abstinence syndrome (opiate withdrawal)

**Usual Dosage** Oral:

Children:

Diarrhea: 0.005-0.01 mL/kg/dose every 3-4 hours

Analgesia: 0.01-0.02 mL/kg/dose every 3-4 hours

Adults: 0.6 mL 4 times/day

**Dosage Forms** Liquid: 10% [0.6 mL equivalent to morphine 6 mg] with alcohol 19%

## oprelvekin (oh PREL ve kin)

**Synonyms** IL-11; interleukin-11; recombinant human interleukin-11; recombinant interleukin-11; rhIL-11; rIL-11

**U.S./Canadian Brand Names** Neumega®

**Therapeutic Category** Platelet Growth Factor

**Use** Prevention and treatment of severe thrombocytopenia following myelosuppressive chemotherapy

**Usual Dosage** Refer to individual protocols

Children: 75-100 mcg/kg/day for 10-21 days (until platelet count >50,000/mm$^3$)

Adults: 50 mcg/kg/day for 10-21 days (until platelet count >50,000/mm$^3$)

**Dosage Forms** Powder for injection, lyophilized: 5 mg

**Opticrom®** *see* cromolyn sodium *on page 156*

**Optigene® Ophthalmic [OTC]** *see* tetrahydrozoline *on page 580*

**Optimine®** *see* azatadine *on page 61*

**Optimoist® Solution [OTC]** *see* saliva substitute *on page 536*

**Optimyxin® Plus® (Can)** *see* neomycin, polymyxin B, and gramicidin *on page 414*

**OptiPranolol® Ophthalmic** *see* metipranolol *on page 387*

**Optiray®** *see* radiological/contrast media (non-ionic) *on page 518*

**Optivar™ Ophthalmic Solution** *see* azelastine *on page 62*

**OPV** *see* poliovirus vaccine, live, trivalent, oral *on page 480*

**Orabase®-B [OTC]** *see* benzocaine *on page 72*

**Orabase® HCA Topical** *see* hydrocortisone (topical) *on page 304*

**Orabase®-O [OTC]** *see* benzocaine *on page 72*

**Orabase® Plain [OTC]** *see* gelatin, pectin, and methylcellulose *on page 270*

**Orabase® With Benzocaine [OTC]** *see* benzocaine, gelatin, pectin, and sodium carboxymethylcellulose *on page 73*

**Oradex-C®** ***(Discontinued)*** *see page 750*

**Orafen (Can)** *see* ketoprofen *on page 334*

**Oragrafin® Calcium** *see* radiological/contrast media (ionic) *on page 516*

**Oragrafin® Sodium** *see* radiological/contrast media (ionic) *on page 516*

**Orajel® Brace-Aid Oral Anesthetic [OTC]** *see* benzocaine *on page 72*

**Orajel® Maximum Strength [OTC]** *see* benzocaine *on page 72*

**Orajel® Mouth-Aid [OTC]** *see* benzocaine *on page 72*

**Orajel® Perioseptic® [OTC]** *see* carbamide peroxide *on page 106*

**Oramorph SR™ Oral** *see* morphine sulfate *on page 400*

**Oranyl Plus® [OTC]** *see* acetaminophen and pseudoephedrine *on page 6*

**Orap™** *see* pimozide *on page 471*

**Oraphen PD® [OTC]** *see* acetaminophen *on page 3*

**Orasept® [OTC]** *see* benzocaine *on page 72*

**Orasol® [OTC]** *see* benzocaine *on page 72*

**Orasone® *(Discontinued)*** *see page 750*

**Oratect® *(Discontinued)*** *see page 750*

**Orazinc® Oral [OTC]** *see* zinc sulfate *on page 639*

**orciprenaline** *see* metaproterenol *on page 376*

**Ordrine AT® Extended Release Capsule *(Discontinued)*** *see page 750*

**Oretic®** *see* hydrochlorothiazide *on page 299*

**Oreticyl® *(Discontinued)*** *see page 750*

**Oreton® Methyl *(Discontinued)*** *see page 750*

**Orexin® [OTC]** *see* vitamin B complex *on page 630*

**Organidin® *(Discontinued)*** *see page 750*

**Organidin® NR** *see* guaifenesin *on page 281*

**Orgaran®** *see* danaparoid *on page 165*

**ORG NC 45** *see* vecuronium *on page 624*

**Orifer® F (Can)** *see* vitamin (multiple/oral) *on page 632*

**Orimune®** *see* poliovirus vaccine, live, trivalent, oral *on page 480*

**Orinase® Diagnostic Injection** *see* tolbutamide *on page 594*

**Orinase® Oral *(Discontinued)*** *see page 750*

**ORLAAM®** *see* levomethadyl acetate hydrochloride *on page 347*

## orlistat (OR li stat)

**U.S./Canadian Brand Names** Xenical®

**Therapeutic Category** Lipase Inhibitor

**Use** Management of obesity, including weight loss and weight management when used in conjunction with a reduced-calorie diet; reduce the risk of weight regain after prior weight loss; indicated for obese patients with an initial body mass index (BMI) ≥30 kg/m$^2$ or ≥27 kg/m$^2$ in the presence of other risk factors

**Usual Dosage** Adults: Oral: 120 mg 3 times/day with each main meal containing fat (during or up to 1 hour after the meal); omit dose if meal is occasionally missed or contains no fat

**Dosage Forms** Capsule: 120 mg

**Ormazine® *(Discontinued)*** *see page 750*

**Ornade® Spansule® *(Discontinued)*** *see page 750*

**Ornex® [OTC]** *see* acetaminophen and pseudoephedrine *on page 6*

**Ornex® Maximum Strength [OTC]** *see* acetaminophen and pseudoephedrine *on page 6*

**Ornidyl® Injection** *see* eflornithine *on page 211*

**Oro-Clense (Can)** *see* chlorhexidine gluconate *on page 126*

## orphenadrine (or FEN a dreen)

**U.S./Canadian Brand Names** Antiflex®; Mio-Rel®; Norflex™; Orphenate®

**Therapeutic Category** Skeletal Muscle Relaxant

**Use** Treatment of muscle spasm associated with acute painful musculoskeletal conditions; supportive therapy in tetanus

**Usual Dosage** Adults:

Oral: 100 mg twice daily

I.M., I.V.: 60 mg every 12 hours

**Dosage Forms**
Injection, as citrate: 30 mg/mL (2 mL, 10 mL)
Tablet, as citrate, sustained release: 100 mg

## orphenadrine, aspirin, and caffeine

(or FEN a dreen, AS pir in, & KAF een)

**U.S./Canadian Brand Names** Norgesic™; Norgesic™ Forte; Orphengesic®

**Therapeutic Category** Analgesic, Non-narcotic; Skeletal Muscle Relaxant

**Use** Relief of discomfort associated with skeletal muscular conditions

**Usual Dosage** Oral: 1-2 tablets 3-4 times/day

**Dosage Forms**
Tablet: Orphenadrine citrate 25 mg, aspirin 385 mg, and caffeine 30 mg
Tablet (Norgesic® Forte): Orphenadrine citrate 50 mg, aspirin 770 mg, and caffeine 60 mg

**Orphenate®** *see* orphenadrine *on previous page*

**Orphengesic®** *see* orphenadrine, aspirin, and caffeine *on this page*

**Ortho® 0.5/35 (Can)** *see* ethinyl estradiol and norethindrone *on page 232*

**Ortho-Cept®** *see* ethinyl estradiol and desogestrel *on page 230*

**Orthoclone® OKT3** *see* muromonab-CD3 *on page 403*

**Ortho-Cyclen®** *see* ethinyl estradiol and norgestimate *on page 233*

**Ortho®-Dienestrol Vaginal** *see* dienestrol *on page 184*

**Ortho-Est® Oral** *see* estropipate *on page 228*

**Ortho-Novum® 1/35** *see* ethinyl estradiol and norethindrone *on page 232*

**Ortho-Novum® 1/50** *see* mestranol and norethindrone *on page 375*

**Ortho-Novum® 7/7/7** *see* ethinyl estradiol and norethindrone *on page 232*

**Ortho-Novum® 10/11** *see* ethinyl estradiol and norethindrone *on page 232*

**Ortho-Prefest®** *see* ethinyl estradiol and norgestimate *on page 233*

**Ortho Tri-Cyclen®** *see* ethinyl estradiol and norgestimate *on page 233*

**Or-Tyl® Injection** *see* dicyclomine *on page 183*

**Orudis®** *see* ketoprofen *on page 334*

**Orudis® KT [OTC]** *see* ketoprofen *on page 334*

**Oruvail®** *see* ketoprofen *on page 334*

**Os-Cal® 500 [OTC]** *see* calcium carbonate *on page 97*

## oseltamivir (o sel TAM e veer)

**U.S./Canadian Brand Names** Tamiflu™

**Therapeutic Category** Antiviral Agent

**Controlled Substance** [FS100]influenza

**Use** Treatment of uncomplicated acute illness due to influenza (A or B) infection in adults and children >1 year of age who have been symptomatic for no more than 2 days; prophylaxis against influenza (A or B) infection in adults and adolescents ≥13 years of age

**Usual Dosage** Oral:
Treatment: Initiate treatment within 2 days of onset of symptoms; duration of treatment: 5 days:
Children: 1-12 years:
≤15 kg: 30 mg twice daily
>15 kg - ≤23 kg: 45 mg twice daily
>23 kg - ≤40 kg: 60 mg twice daily
>40 kg: 75 mg twice daily
Adolescents and Adults: 75 mg twice daily
(Continued)

## oseltamivir *(Continued)*

Prophylaxis: Adolescents and Adults: 75 mg once daily for at least 7 days; treatment should begin within 2 days of contact with an infected individual. During community outbreaks, dosing is 75 mg once daily. May be used for up to 6 weeks; duration of protection lasts for length of dosing period

**Dosage Forms**

Capsule, as phosphate: 75 mg (blister package 10)
Powder for oral suspension (tutti-frutti flavor): 12 mg/mL (100 mL)

**Osmitrol® Injection** *see* mannitol *on page 364*

**Osmoglyn®** *see* glycerin *on page 277*

**Osmolite® HN [OTC]** *see* nutritional formula, enteral/oral *on page 432*

**Ostac® (Can)** *see* clodronate disodium *(Canada only) on page 144*

**Osteocalcin® *(Discontinued)*** *see page 750*

**Ostoforte® (Can)** *see* ergocalciferol *on page 220*

**Otic-Care® Otic** *see* neomycin, polymyxin B, and hydrocortisone *on page 415*

**Otic Domeboro®** *see* aluminum acetate and acetic acid *on page 25*

**Oticort® HC Otic** *see* acetic acid, propylene glycol diacetate, and hydrocortisone *on page 9*

**Otic Tridesilon® *(Discontinued)*** *see page 750*

**Otobiotic® Otic** *see* polymyxin B and hydrocortisone *on page 482*

**Otocort® Otic** *see* neomycin, polymyxin B, and hydrocortisone *on page 415*

**Otosporin® Otic** *see* neomycin, polymyxin B, and hydrocortisone *on page 415*

**Otrivin® Nasal [OTC]** *see* xylometazoline *on page 636*

**Ovcon® 35** *see* ethinyl estradiol and norethindrone *on page 232*

**Ovcon® 50** *see* ethinyl estradiol and norethindrone *on page 232*

**Ovide™ Topical** *see* malathion *on page 363*

**Ovidrel®** *see* chorionic gonadotropin (recombinant) *on page 136*

**Ovol® (Can)** *see* simethicone *on page 544*

**Ovral®** *see* ethinyl estradiol and norgestrel *on page 233*

**Ovrette®** *see* norgestrel *on page 426*

**O-V Staticin® *(Discontinued)*** *see page 750*

## oxacillin (oks a SIL in)

**Synonyms** methylphenyl isoxazolyl penicillin

**Therapeutic Category** Penicillin

**Use** Treatment of bacterial infections such as osteomyelitis, septicemia, endocarditis, and CNS infections due to susceptible penicillinase-producing strains of *Staphylococcus*

**Usual Dosage**

Infants and Children:
I.M., I.V.: 150-200 mg/kg/day in divided doses every 6 hours; maximum dose: 12 g/day
Oral: 50-100 mg/kg/day divided every 6 hours

Adults:
Oral: 500-1000 mg every 4-6 hours for at least 5 days
I.M., I.V.: 250 mg to 2 g/dose every 4-6 hours

**Dosage Forms**

Capsule, as sodium: 250 mg, 500 mg
Powder:
For injection, as sodium: 500 mg, 1 g, 2 g, 10 g
For oral solution, as sodium: 250 mg/5 mL (100 mL)

**Oxandrin®** *see* oxandrolone *on this page*

## oxandrolone (oks AN droe lone)

**U.S./Canadian Brand Names** Oxandrin®

**Therapeutic Category** Androgen

**Controlled Substance** C-III

**Use** Treatment of catabolic or tissue-depleting processes

**Usual Dosage** Adults: Oral: 2.5 mg 2-4 times/day

**Dosage Forms** Tablet: 2.5 mg

## oxaprozin (oks a PROE zin)

**U.S./Canadian Brand Names** Daypro™

**Therapeutic Category** Analgesic, Non-narcotic; Nonsteroidal Anti-inflammatory Drug (NSAID)

**Use** Acute and long-term use in the management of signs and symptoms of osteoarthritis and rheumatoid arthritis

**Usual Dosage** Adults: Oral (individualize the dosage to the lowest effective dose to minimize adverse effects):

Osteoarthritis: 600-1200 mg once daily

Rheumatoid arthritis: 1200 mg once daily

Maximum dose: 1800 mg/day or 26 mg/kg (whichever is lower) in divided doses

**Dosage Forms** Tablet: 600 mg

## oxazepam (oks A ze pam)

**U.S./Canadian Brand Names** Apo®-Oxazepam (Can); Serax®

**Therapeutic Category** Anticonvulsant; Benzodiazepine

**Controlled Substance** C-IV

**Use** Treatment of anxiety and management of alcohol withdrawal; may also be used as an anticonvulsant in management of simple partial seizures

**Usual Dosage** Oral:

Children: 1 mg/kg/day has been administered

Adults:

Anxiety: 10-30 mg 3-4 times/day

Alcohol withdrawal: 15-30 mg 3-4 times/day

Hypnotic: 15-30 mg

**Dosage Forms**

Capsule: 10 mg, 15 mg, 30 mg

Tablet: 15 mg

## oxcarbazepine (ox car BAZ e peen)

**Synonyms** GP 47680

**U.S./Canadian Brand Names** Trileptal®

**Therapeutic Category** Anticonvulsant, Miscellaneous

**Use** Monotherapy or adjunctive therapy in the treatment of partial seizures in adults with epilepsy and as adjunctive therapy in the treatment of partial seizures in children ages 4-16 with epilepsy

**Unlabeled use:** Antimanic

**Usual Dosage**

Children:

Adjunctive therapy: 8-10 mg/kg/day, not to exceed 600 mg/day, given in two divided daily doses. Maintenance dose should be achieved over 2 weeks, and is dependent upon patient weight, according to the following:

20-29 kg: 900 mg/day in 2 divided doses

29.1-39 kg: 1200 mg/day in 2 divided doses

>39 kg: 1800 mg/day in 2 divided doses

(Continued)

## oxcarbazepine *(Continued)*

Adults:

Adjunctive therapy: Initial: 300 mg twice daily; dose may be increased by as much as 600 mg/day at weekly intervals; recommended daily dose: 1200 mg/day in 2 divided doses

Conversion to monotherapy: Oxcarbazepine 600 mg/day in twice daily divided doses while simultaneously initiating the reduction of the dose of the concomitant antiepileptic drug. The concomitant dosage should be withdrawn over 3-6 weeks, while the maximum dose of oxcarbazepine should be reached in about 2-4 weeks. Recommended daily dose: 2400 mg/day.

Initiation of monotherapy: Oxcarbazepine should be initiated at a dose of 600 mg/day in twice daily divided doses; doses may be titrated upward by 300 mg/day every third day to a final dose of 1200 mg/day given in 2 daily divided doses

**Dosage Forms** Tablet: 150 mg, 300 mg, 600 mg

## oxiconazole (oks i KON a zole)

**U.S./Canadian Brand Names** Oxistat® Topical

**Therapeutic Category** Antifungal Agent

**Use** Treatment of tinea pedis, tinea cruris, and tinea corporis

**Usual Dosage** Topical: Apply once daily to affected areas for 2 weeks to 1 month

**Dosage Forms**

Cream, as nitrate: 1% (15 g, 30 g, 60 g)

Lotion, as nitrate: 1% (30 mL)

**oxilapine** *see* loxapine *on page 358*

**Oxistat® Topical** *see* oxiconazole *on this page*

**oxpentifylline** *see* pentoxifylline *on page 460*

## oxprenolol *(Canada only)* (ox PREN oh lole)

**U.S./Canadian Brand Names** Slow-Trasicor® (Can); Trasicor® (Can)

**Therapeutic Category** Beta-Adrenergic Blocker

**Use** Treatment of mild to moderate hypertension

**Usual Dosage** Adults: Oral: Start with 20 mg three times/day, titrated upward to a maximum dose of 480 mg/day

**Dosage Forms** Tablet: 40 mg, 80 mg

**Oxsoralen® Oral *(Discontinued)*** *see page 750*

**Oxsoralen® Topical** *see* methoxsalen *on page 381*

**Oxsoralen-Ultra®** *see* methoxsalen *on page 381*

## oxtriphylline (oks TRYE fi lin)

**Synonyms** choline theophyllinate

**U.S./Canadian Brand Names** Apo®-Oxtriphylline (Can); Choledyl SA®

**Therapeutic Category** Theophylline Derivative

**Use** Bronchodilator in symptomatic treatment of asthma and reversible bronchospasm

**Usual Dosage** Oral:

Children:

1-9 years: 6.2 mg/kg/dose every 6 hours

9-16 years: 4.7 mg/kg/dose every 6 hours

Adults: 4.7 mg/kg every 8 hours; sustained release: administer every 12 hours

**Dosage Forms**

Elixir: 100 mg/5 mL (5 mL, 10 mL, 473 mL)

Syrup: 50 mg/5 mL (473 mL)

Tablet: 100 mg, 200 mg

Sustained release: 400 mg, 600 mg

**Oxy-10® Balance Spot Treatment [OTC]** *see* benzoyl peroxide *on page 74*

**Oxybutyn (Can)** *see* oxybutynin *on this page*

## oxybutynin (oks i BYOO ti nin)

**U.S./Canadian Brand Names** Albert® Oxybutynin (Can); Apo®-Oxybutynin (Can); Ditropan®; Ditropan® XL; Gen-Oxybutynin (Can); Novo-Oxybutynin (Can); Nu-Oxybutyn (Can); Oxybutyn (Can); PMS-Oxybutynin (Can)

**Therapeutic Category** Antispasmodic Agent, Urinary

**Use** Relief of bladder spasms associated with voiding in patients with uninhibited and reflex neurogenic bladder

**Usual Dosage** Oral:

Children:

1-5 years: 0.2 mg/kg/dose 2-4 times/day

>5 years: 5 mg twice daily, up to 5 mg 3 times/day

Adults: 5 mg 2-3 times/day up to 5 mg 4 times/day maximum

**Dosage Forms**

Syrup, as chloride: 5 mg/5 mL (473 mL)

Tablet, as chloride: 5 mg

Tablet, extended release, as chloride: 5 mg, 10 mg, 15 mg

**Oxycel®** *see* cellulose, oxidized *on page 119*

## oxychlorosene (oks i KLOR oh seen)

**U.S./Canadian Brand Names** Clorpactin® WCS-90

**Therapeutic Category** Antibiotic, Topical

**Use** Treating localized infections

**Usual Dosage** Topical (0.1% to 0.5% solutions): Apply by irrigation, instillation, spray, soaks, or wet compresses

**Dosage Forms** Powder for solution, as sodium: 2 g, 5 g

**Oxycocet® (Can)** *see* oxycodone and acetaminophen *on next page*

**Oxycodan® (Can)** *see* oxycodone and aspirin *on next page*

## oxycodone (oks i KOE done)

**Synonyms** dihydrohydroxycodeinone

**U.S./Canadian Brand Names** Endocodone®; OxyContin®; OxyIR™; Percolone®; Roxicodone™; Supeudol® (Can)

**Therapeutic Category** Analgesic, Narcotic

**Controlled Substance** C-II

**Use** Management of moderate to severe pain, normally used in combination with non-narcotic analgesics

**Usual Dosage** Oral:

Children:

6-12 years: 1.25 mg every 6 hours as needed

>12 years: 2.5 mg every 6 hours as needed

Adults: 5 mg every 6 hours as needed

**Dosage Forms**

Capsule, as hydrochloride, immediate release (OxyIR™): 5 mg

Liquid, oral, as hydrochloride: 5 mg/5 mL (500 mL)

Solution, oral concentrate, as hydrochloride: 20 mg/mL (30 mL)

Tablet, as hydrochloride: 5 mg

Percolone®: 5 mg

Roxicodone™: 5 mg, 15 mg, 30 mg

Tablet, controlled release, as hydrochloride (OxyContin®): 10 mg, 20 mg, 40 mg, 80 mg, 160 mg

## oxycodone and acetaminophen (oks i KOE done & a seet a MIN oh fen)

**U.S./Canadian Brand Names** Endocet®; Oxycocet® (Can); Percocet® 2.5/325; Percocet® 5/325; Percocet® 7.5/500; Percocet® 10/650; Percocet®-Demi (Can); Roxicet® 5/500; Roxilox™; Tylox®

**Therapeutic Category** Analgesic, Narcotic

**Controlled Substance** C-II

**Use** Management of moderate to severe pain

**Usual Dosage** Oral (doses should be titrated to appropriate analgesic effects):

Children: Oxycodone: 0.05-0.15 mg/kg/dose to 5 mg/dose (maximum) every 4-6 hours as needed

Adults: 1-2 tablets every 4-6 hours as needed for pain

Maximum daily dose of acetaminophen: 4 g/day

**Dosage Forms**

Caplet: Oxycodone hydrochloride 5 mg and acetaminophen 500 mg

Capsule: Oxycodone hydrochloride 5 mg and acetaminophen 500 mg

Solution, oral: Oxycodone hydrochloride 5 mg and acetaminophen 325 mg per 5 mL (5 mL, 500 mL)

Tablet: Oxycodone hydrochloride 2.5 mg and acetaminophen 325 mg; oxycodone hydrochloride 5 mg and acetaminophen 325 mg; oxycodone hydrochloride 7.5 mg and acetaminophen 500 mg; oxycodone hydrochloride 10 mg and acetaminophen 650 mg

## oxycodone and aspirin (oks i KOE done & AS pir in)

**U.S./Canadian Brand Names** Endodan®; Oxycodan® (Can); Percodan®; Percodan®-Demi

**Therapeutic Category** Analgesic, Narcotic

**Controlled Substance** C-II

**Use** Relief of moderate to moderately severe pain

**Usual Dosage** Oral (based on oxycodone combined salts):

Children: 0.05-0.15 mg/kg/dose every 4-6 hours as needed; maximum: 5 mg/dose (1 tablet Percodan® or 2 tablets Percodan®-Demi/dose) **or**

Alternatively:

6-12 years: Percodan®-Demi: $^1/_4$ tablet every 6 hours as needed for pain

>12 years: $^1/_2$ tablet every 6 hours as needed for pain

Adults: Percodan®: 1 tablet every 6 hours as needed for pain or Percodan®-Demi: 1-2 tablets every 6 hours as needed for pain

**Dosage Forms** Tablet:

Percodan®, Endodan®: Oxycodone hydrochloride 4.5 mg, oxycodone terephthalate 0.38 mg, and aspirin 325 mg

Percodan®-Demi: Oxycodone hydrochloride 2.25 mg, oxycodone terephthalate 0.19 mg, and aspirin 325 mg

**OxyContin®** *see* oxycodone *on previous page*

**OxyIR™** *see* oxycodone *on previous page*

## oxymetazoline (oks i met AZ oh leen)

**U.S./Canadian Brand Names** Afrin® Children's Nose Drops [OTC]; Afrin® Nasal Solution [OTC]; Allerest® 12 Hour Nasal Solution [OTC]; Chlorphed®-LA Nasal Solution [OTC]; Dristan® Long Lasting Nasal Solution [OTC]; Duramist Plus® [OTC]; Duration® Nasal Solution [OTC]; Neo-Synephrine® 12 Hour Nasal Solution [OTC]; Nōstrilla® [OTC]; NTZ® Long Acting Nasal Solution [OTC]; OcuClear® Ophthalmic [OTC]; Sinarest® 12 Hour Nasal Solution; Sinex® Long-Acting [OTC]; Twice-A-Day® Nasal Solution [OTC]; Visine® L.R. Ophthalmic [OTC]; 4-Way® Long Acting Nasal Solution [OTC]

**Therapeutic Category** Adrenergic Agonist Agent

**Use** Symptomatic relief of nasal mucosal congestion associated with acute or chronic rhinitis, the common cold, sinusitis, hay fever, or other allergies

**Usual Dosage**

Intranasal:

Children 2-5 years: 0.025% solution: Instill 2-3 drops in each nostril twice daily

Children ≥6 years and Adults: 0.05% solution: Instill 2-3 drops or 2-3 sprays into each nostril twice daily

Ophthalmic: Adults: Instill 1-2 drops into affected eye(s) every 6 hours

**Dosage Forms**

Nasal solution, as hydrochloride:

Drops:

Afrin® Children's Nose Drops: 0.025% (20 mL)

Afrin®, NTZ® Long Acting Nasal Solution: 0.05% (15 mL, 20 mL)

Spray: Afrin® Sinus, Allerest® 12 Hours, Chlorphed®-LA, Dristan® Long Lasting, Duration®, 4-Way® Long Acting, Genasal®, Nasal Relief®, Neo-Synephrine® 12 Hour, Nōstrilla®, NTZ® Long Acting Nasal Solution, Sinex® Long-Acting, Twice-A-Day®: 0.05% (15 mL, 30 mL)

Ophthalmic solution, as hydrochloride (OcuClear®, Visine® L.R.): 0.025% (15 mL, 30 mL)

## oxymetholone (oks i METH oh lone)

**U.S./Canadian Brand Names** Anadrol®

**Therapeutic Category** Anabolic Steroid

**Controlled Substance** C-III

**Use** Anemias caused by the administration of myelotoxic drugs

**Usual Dosage** Erythropoietic effects: 1-5 mg/kg/day as a single dose; maximum: 100 mg/day

**Dosage Forms** Tablet: 50 mg

## oxymorphone (oks i MOR fone)

**U.S./Canadian Brand Names** Numorphan®

**Therapeutic Category** Analgesic, Narcotic

**Controlled Substance** C-II

**Use** Management of moderate to severe pain and preoperatively as a sedative and a supplement to anesthesia

**Usual Dosage** Adults:

I.M., S.C.: Initial: 0.5 mg, then 1-1.5 mg every 4-6 hours as needed

I.V.: Initial: 0.5 mg

Rectal: 5 mg every 4-6 hours

**Dosage Forms**

Injection, as hydrochloride: 1 mg/mL (1 mL); 1.5 mg/mL (10 mL)

Suppository, rectal, as hydrochloride: 5 mg

**oxyphenbutazone *(Discontinued)*** *see page 750*

## oxytetracycline (oks i tet ra SYE kleen)

**U.S./Canadian Brand Names** Terramycin® I.M. Injection

**Therapeutic Category** Tetracycline Derivative

**Use** Treatment of susceptible bacterial infections; both gram-positive and gram-negative, as well as *Rickettsia* and *Mycoplasma* organisms

**Usual Dosage** I.M.:

Children >8 years: 15-25 mg/kg/day (maximum: 250 mg/dose) in divided doses every 8-12 hours

Adults: 250-500 mg every 24 hours or 300 mg/day divided every 8-12 hours

**Dosage Forms** Injection, as hydrochloride, with lidocaine 2%: 5% [50 mg/mL] (2 mL, 10 mL); 12.5% [125 mg/mL] (2 mL)

## oxytetracycline and polymyxin B

(oks i tet ra SYE kleen & pol i MIKS in bee)

**U.S./Canadian Brand Names** Terak® Ophthalmic Ointment; Terramycin® Ophthalmic Ointment; Terramycin® w/Polymyxin B Ophthalmic Ointment

**Therapeutic Category** Antibiotic, Ophthalmic

**Use** Treatment of superficial ocular infections involving the conjunctiva and/or cornea

**Usual Dosage** Ophthalmic: Apply 1/2" of ointment onto the lower lid of affected eye 2-4 times/day

**Dosage Forms**

Ointment, ophthalmic/otic: Oxytetracycline hydrochloride 5 mg and polymyxin B 10,000 units per g (3.5 g)

Tablet, vaginal: Oxytetracycline hydrochloride 100 mg and polymyxin B 100,000 units (10s)

## oxytocin (oks i TOE sin)

**Synonyms** PIT

**U.S./Canadian Brand Names** Pitocin®

**Therapeutic Category** Oxytocic Agent

**Use** Induce labor at term; control postpartum bleeding

**Usual Dosage** Adults:

Induction of labor: I.V.: 0.001-0.002 unit/minute; increase by 0.001-0.002 units every 15-30 minutes until contraction pattern has been established

Postpartum bleeding: I.V.: 0.001-0.002 unit/minute as needed

**Dosage Forms** Injection: 10 units/mL (1 mL, 10 mL, 25 mL)

**Oyst-Cal 500 [OTC]** *see* calcium carbonate *on page 97*

**Oystercal® 500** *see* calcium carbonate *on page 97*

**P-071** *see* cetirizine *on page 121*

**Pacerone®** *see* amiodarone *on page 32*

**PACIS™ (Can)** *see* BCG vaccine *on page 68*

## paclitaxel (PAK li taks el)

**U.S./Canadian Brand Names** Onxel®; Taxol®

**Therapeutic Category** Antineoplastic Agent

**Use** Treatment of metastatic carcinoma of the ovary after failure of first-line or subsequent chemotherapy; treatment for AIDS-related Kaposi's sarcoma

**Usual Dosage** Adults: I.V.: 135 mg/m$^2$ over 24 hours every 3 weeks

**Dosage Forms** Injection: 6 mg/mL (5 mL, 16.7 mL, 25 mL, 50 mL)

**Pain Enz®** *see* capsaicin *on page 104*

**Pain-Eze® [OTC]** *see* acetaminophen *on page 3*

**Pain-Gesic® [OTC]** *see* acetaminophen and phenyltoloxamine *on page 5*

**Pain-Off® [OTC]** *see* acetaminophen, aspirin, and caffeine *on page 6*

**Palafer® (Can)** *see* ferrous fumarate *on page 246*

## palivizumab (pah li VIZ u mab)

**U.S./Canadian Brand Names** Synagis®

**Therapeutic Category** Monoclonal Antibody

**Use** Prevention of serious lower respiratory tract disease caused by respiratory syncytial virus (RSV) in pediatric patients at high risk of RSV disease; safety and efficacy were established in infants with bronchopulmonary dysplasia (BPD) and infants with a history of prematurity ≤35 weeks gestational age

**Usual Dosage** Children: I.M.: 15 mg/kg of body weight, monthly throughout RSV season (First dose administered prior to commencement of RSV season)

**Dosage Forms** Injection, lyophilized: 50 mg, 100 mg

**Palmitate-A® 5000 [OTC]** *see* vitamin A *on page 629*

**PALS® [OTC]** *see* chlorophyll *on page 127*

**2-PAM** *see* pralidoxime *on page 489*

**Pamelor®** *see* nortriptyline *on page 426*

## pamidronate (pa mi DROE nate)

**U.S./Canadian Brand Names** Aredia™

**Therapeutic Category** Bisphosphonate Derivative

**Use** Symptomatic treatment of Paget's disease; hypercalcemia associated with malignancy

**Usual Dosage** Drug must be diluted properly before administration and infused slowly (at least over 2 hours)

Adults: I.V.:

Moderate cancer-related hypercalcemia (12-13 mg/dL): 60-90 mg administered as a slow infusion over 2-24 hours

Severe cancer-related hypercalcemia (>13.5 mg/dL): 90 mg as a slow infusion over 2-24 hours

A period of 7 days should elapse before the use of second course; repeat infusions every 2-3 weeks have been suggested, however, could be administered every 2-3 months according to the degree and of severity of hypercalcemia and/or the type of malignancy

Paget's disease: 60 mg as a single 2- to 24-hour infusion

**Dosage Forms** Powder for injection, lyophilized, as disodium: 30 mg, 90 mg

**Pamine®** *see* methscopolamine *on page 382*

**Pamix® [OTC]** *see* pyrantel pamoate *on page 509*

**Pamprin IB® [OTC]** *see* ibuprofen *on page 311*

**Panasal® 5/500 *(Discontinued)*** *see page 750*

**Pan-B antibodies** *see* rituximab *on page 529*

**Pancrease®** *see* pancrelipase *on next page*

**Pancrease® MT 4** *see* pancrelipase *on next page*

**Pancrease® MT 10** *see* pancrelipase *on next page*

**Pancrease® MT 16** *see* pancrelipase *on next page*

**Pancrease® MT 20** *see* pancrelipase *on next page*

## pancreatin (PAN kree a tin)

**U.S./Canadian Brand Names** Creon®; Digepepsin®; Donnazyme®; Hi-Vegi-Lip®

**Therapeutic Category** Enzyme

**Use** Replacement therapy in symptomatic treatment of malabsorption syndrome caused by pancreatic insufficiency

**Usual Dosage** Enteric coated microspheres: The following dosage recommendations are only an approximation for initial dosages. The actual dosage will depend on the digestive requirements of the individual patient.

Oral:

Children:

<1 year: 2000 units of lipase with meals/feedings

1-6 years: 4000-8000 units of lipase with meals and 4000 units with snacks

7-12 years: 4000-12,000 units of lipase with meals and snacks

Adults: 4000-16,000 units of lipase with meals and with snacks

**Dosage Forms**

Capsule, enteric coated microspheres (Creon®): Lipase 8000 units, amylase 30,000 units, protease 13,000 units and pancreatin 300 mg

Tablet:

Digepepsin®: Pancreatin 300 mg, pepsin 250 mg, and bile salts 150 mg

(Continued)

## pancreatin *(Continued)*

Donnazyme®: Lipase 1000 units, amylase 12,500 units, protease 12,500 units and pancreatin 500 mg

Hi-Vegi-Lip®: Lipase 4800 units, amylase 60,000 units, protease 60,000 units and pancreatin 2400 mg

**Pancrecarb MS-4®** *see* pancrelipase *on this page*

**Pancrecarb MS-8®** *see* pancrelipase *on this page*

## pancrelipase (pan kre LI pase)

**Synonyms** lipancreatin; lipase, protease, and amylase

**U.S./Canadian Brand Names** Cotazym®; Cotazym-S®; Creon® 5; Creon® 10; Creon® 20; Ilozyme®; Kutrase®; Ku-Zyme®; Ku-Zyme® HP; Lipram®; Pancrease®; Pancrease® MT 4; Pancrease® MT 10; Pancrease® MT 16; Pancrease® MT 20; Pancrecarb MS-4®; Pancrecarb MS-8®; Protilase®; Ultrase®; Ultrase® MT12; Ultrase® MT18; Ultrase® MT20; Viokase®; Zymase®

**Therapeutic Category** Enzyme

**Use** Replacement therapy in symptomatic treatment of malabsorption syndrome caused by pancreatic insufficiency

**Usual Dosage** Oral:

Powder: Actual dose depends on the digestive requirements of the patient

Children <1 year: Start with 1/8 teaspoonful with feedings

Enteric coated microspheres and microtablets: The following dosage recommendations are only an approximation for initial dosages. The actual dosage will depend on the digestive requirements of the individual patient.

Children:

<1 year: 2000 units of lipase with meals/feedings

1-6 years: 4000-8000 units of lipase with meals and 4000 units with snacks

7-12 years: 4000-12,000 units of lipase with meals and snacks

Adults: 4000-16,000 units of lipase with meals and with snacks

**Dosage Forms**

Capsule:

Cotazym®: Lipase 8000 units, protease 30,000 units, amylase 30,000 units

Kutrase®: Lipase 2400 units, protease 30,000 units, amylase 30,000 units

Ku-Zyme®: Lipase 1200 units, protease 15,000 units, amylase 15,000 units

Ku-Zyme® HP: Lipase 8000 units, protease 30,000 units, amylase 30,000 units

Lipram-PN16®: Lipase 16,000 units, protease 48,000 units, amylase 48, 000 units

Lipram-CR20®: Lipase 20,000 units, protease 75,000 units, amylase 66,400 units

Lipram-UL12®: Lipase 12,000 units, protease 39,000 units, amylase 39,000 units

Lipram-PN10®: Lipase 10,000 units, protease 30,000 units, amylase 30,000 units

Lipram-UL18®: Lipase 18,000 units, protease 58,500 units, amylase 58,500 units

Lipram-UL20®: Lipase 20,000 units, protease 65,000 units, amylase 65,000 units

Ultrase®: Lipase 4500 units, protease 25,000 units, amylase 20,000 units

Ultrase® MT12: Lipase 12,000 units, protease 39,000 units, amylase 39,000 units

Ultrase® MT18: Lipase 18,000 units, protease 58,500 units, amylase 58,500 units

Ultrase® MT20: Lipase 20,000 units, protease 65,000 units, amylase 65,000 units

Enteric coated microspheres (Pancrease®): Lipase 4000 units, protease 25,000 units, amylase 20,000 units

Enteric coated microtablets:

Pancrease® MT 4: Lipase 4500 units, protease 12,000 units, amylase 12,000 units

Pancrease® MT 10: Lipase 10,000 units, protease 30,000 units, amylase 30,000 units

Pancrease® MT 16: Lipase 16,000 units, protease 48,000 units, amylase 48,000 units

Pancrease® MT 20: Lipase 20,000 units, protease 44,000 units, amylase 56,000 units

Pancrecarb MS-4®: Lipase 4000 units, protease 25,000 units, amylase 25,000 units

Pancrecarb MS-8®: Lipase 8000 units, protease 45,000 units, amylase 40,000 units

Enteric coated spheres:

Cotazym-S®: Lipase 5000 units, protease 20,000 units, amylase 20,000 units

Pancrelipase, Protilase®: Lipase 4000 units, protease 25,000 units, amylase 20,000 units

Zymase®: Lipase 12,000 units, protease 24,000 units, amylase 24,000 units

Delayed release:

Creon® 5: Lipase 5000 units, protease 18,750 units, amylase 16,600 units

Creon® 10: Lipase 10,000 units, protease 37,500 units, amylase 33,200 units

Creon® 20: Lipase 20,000 units, protease 75,000 units, amylase 66,400 units

Powder (Viokase®): Lipase 16,800 units, protease 70,000 units, amylase 70,000 units per 0.7 g

Tablet:

Ilozyme®: Lipase 11,000 units, protease 30,000 units, amylase 30,000 units

Viokase®: Lipase 8000 units, protease 30,000 units, amylase 30,000 units

## pancuronium (pan kyoo ROE nee um)

**Therapeutic Category** Skeletal Muscle Relaxant

**Use** Produces skeletal muscle relaxation during surgery after induction of general anesthesia, increases pulmonary compliance during assisted mechanical respiration, facilitates endotracheal intubation

**Usual Dosage** Infants >1 month, Children, and Adults: I.V.: 0.04-0.1 mg/kg; maintenance dose: 0.02-0.1 mg/kg/dose every 30-60 minutes as needed

**Dosage Forms** Injection, as bromide: 1 mg/mL (10 mL); 2 mg/mL (2 mL, 5 mL)

**Panectyl® (Can)** *see* trimeprazine *(Canada only)* *on page 607*

**Panhematin®** *see* hemin *on page 290*

**PanOxyl®-AQ 2.5** *see* benzoyl peroxide *on page 74*

**PanOxyl®-AQ 5** *see* benzoyl peroxide *on page 74*

**PanOxyl®-AQ 10** *see* benzoyl peroxide *on page 74*

**PanOxyl® Bar 5 [OTC]** *see* benzoyl peroxide *on page 74*

**PanOxyl® Bar 10 [OTC]** *see* benzoyl peroxide *on page 74*

**Panretin™** *see* alitretinoin *on page 20*

**Panscol® Lotion [OTC]** *see* salicylic acid *on page 535*

**Panscol® Ointment [OTC]** *see* salicylic acid *on page 535*

**Panthoderm® Cream [OTC]** *see* dexpanthenol *on page 176*

**Panto™ I.V. (Can)** *see* pantoprazole *on this page*

**Pantoloc™ (Can)** *see* pantoprazole *on this page*

**Pantopon® *(Discontinued)*** *see page 750*

## pantoprazole (pan TOE pra zole)

**U.S./Canadian Brand Names** Panto™ I.V. (Can); Pantoloc™ (Can); Protonix®

**Therapeutic Category** Proton Pump Inhibitor

**Use** Short-term treatment of erosive esophagitis associated with GERD

**Usual Dosage** Adults:

I.V. (Canada only): 1 vial (pantoprazole 40 mg/day, administered either by slow I.V. injection or by I.V. infusion over 15 minutes). Patients should be switched to pantoprazole tablet when feasible. In switching, the same dose mg per mg should be administered. Divided doses of up to 240 mg pantoprazole I.V. were administered and were well tolerated.

Oral: 40 mg every day for up to 8 weeks; an additional 8 weeks may be used in patients who have not healed after an 8-week course

**Dosage Forms**

Injection, lyophilized: 40 mg

Tablet, enteric coated: 40 mg

## pantothenic acid (pan toe THEN ik AS id)

**Synonyms** calcium pantothenate; vitamin $B_5$

**Therapeutic Category** Vitamin, Water Soluble

**Use** Pantothenic acid deficiency

**Usual Dosage** Adults: Oral: Recommended daily dose: 4-7 mg/day

**Dosage Forms** Tablet: 25 mg, 50 mg, 100 mg, 218 mg, 250 mg, 500 mg, 545 mg, 1000 mg

**pantothenyl alcohol** *see* dexpanthenol *on page 176*

**Panwarfarin® *(Discontinued)*** *see page 750*

**Papacon®** *see* papaverine *on this page*

## papain and urea (pa PAY in & yoor EE a)

**U.S./Canadian Brand Names** Accuzyme™

**Therapeutic Category** Enzyme, Topical Debridement; Topical Skin Product

**Use** Enzymatic debriding ointment for treatment of chronic and acute wounds

**Usual Dosage** Cleanse wound with cleanser or saline (not hydrogen peroxide); apply directly to the wound, cover with appropriate dressing, secure into place and reapply 1-2 times/day. Irrigate wound at each dressing.

**Dosage Forms** Ointment, topical: Papain 1.1 x $10^4$ int. units and urea 10% in hydrophilic ointment (30 g)

## papaverine (pa PAV er een)

**U.S./Canadian Brand Names** Papacon®; Para-Time S.R.®; Pavacot®

**Therapeutic Category** Vasodilator

**Use** Relief of peripheral and cerebral ischemia associated with arterial spasm

**Investigational use:** Prophylaxis of migraine headache

**Usual Dosage** Adults: Oral, sustained release: 150-300 mg every 12 hours; in difficult cases: 150 mg every 8 hours

**Dosage Forms**

Capsule, sustained release, as hydrochloride: 150 mg

Injection: 30 mg/mL (2 mL, 10 mL)

**Paplex® *(Discontinued)*** *see page 750*

**parabromdylamine** *see* brompheniramine *on page 87*

**paracetaldehyde** *see* paraldehyde *on next page*

**paracetamol** *see* acetaminophen *on page 3*

## parachlorometaxylenol (PAIR a klor oh met a ZYE le nol)

**Synonyms** PCMX

**U.S./Canadian Brand Names** Metasep® [OTC]

**Therapeutic Category** Antiseborrheic Agent, Topical

**Use** Aid in relief of dandruff and associated conditions

**Usual Dosage** Massage to a foamy lather, allow to remain on hair for 5 minutes, rinse thoroughly and repeat

**Dosage Forms** Shampoo: 2% with isopropyl alcohol 9%

**Paradione® *(Discontinued)*** *see page 750*

**Paraflex® *(Discontinued)*** *see page 750*

**Parafon Forte™ DSC** *see* chlorzoxazone *on page 134*

**Para-Hist AT® *(Discontinued)*** *see page 750*

**Paral®** *see* paraldehyde *on next page*

**paraldehyde** (par AL de hyde)

**Synonyms** paracetaldehyde

**U.S./Canadian Brand Names** Paral®

**Therapeutic Category** Anticonvulsant

**Controlled Substance** C-IV

**Use** Treatment of status epilepticus and tetanus-induced seizures; has been used as a sedative/hypnotic and in the treatment of alcohol withdrawal symptoms

**Usual Dosage** Dilute in milk or iced fruit juice to mask taste and odor

Oral, rectal:

Children: 0.15-0.3 mL/kg

Adults:

Hypnotic: 10-30 mL

Sedative: 5-10 mL

Rectal: Mix paraldehyde 2:1 with oil (cottonseed or olive)

**Dosage Forms** Liquid, oral or rectal: 1 g/mL (30 mL)

**Paraplatin®** *see* carboplatin *on page 109*

**Parathar™** *see* teriparatide *on page 575*

**Para-Time S.R.®** *see* papaverine *on previous page*

**Parcaine®** *see* proparacaine *on page 502*

**Par Decon®** ***(Discontinued)*** *see page 750*

**Paredrine®** ***(Discontinued)*** *see page 750*

**paregoric** (par e GOR ik)

**Synonyms** camphorated tincture of opium

**Therapeutic Category** Analgesic, Narcotic

**Controlled Substance** C-III

**Use** Treatment of diarrhea or relief of pain; neonatal abstinence syndrome (neonatal opiate withdrawal)

**Usual Dosage** Oral:

Neonatal opiate withdrawal: 3-6 drops every 3-6 hours as needed, or initially 0.2 mL every 3 hours; increase dosage by approximately 0.05 mL every 3 hours until withdrawal symptoms are controlled; it is rare to exceed 0.7 mL/dose. Stabilize withdrawal symptoms for 3-5 days, then gradually decrease dosage over a 2- to 4-week period.

Children: 0.25-0.5 mL/kg 1-4 times/day

Adults: 5-10 mL 1-4 times/day

**Dosage Forms** Liquid: 2 mg morphine equivalent/5 mL [equivalent to 20 mg opium powder] (5 mL, 60 mL, 473 mL, 4000 mL)

**Paremyd® Ophthalmic** *see* hydroxyamphetamine and tropicamide *on page 306*

**Parepectolin®** ***(Discontinued)*** *see page 750*

**Pargen Fortified®** ***(Discontinued)*** *see page 750*

**Par Glycerol®** ***(Discontinued)*** *see page 750*

**paricalcitol** (par eh CAL ci tol)

**U.S./Canadian Brand Names** Zemplar™

**Therapeutic Category** Vitamin D Analog

**Use** Prevention and treatment of secondary hyperparathyroidism associated with chronic renal failure

**Usual Dosage** Adults: I.V.: 0.04-0.1 mcg/kg (2.8-7 mcg) given as a bolus dose no more frequently than every other day at any time during dialysis; doses as high as 0.24 mcg/kg (16.8 mcg) have been administered safely

**Dosage Forms** Injection: 5 mcg/mL (1 mL, 2 mL)

**pariprazole** *see* rabeprazole *on page 515*

**Parlodel®** *see* bromocriptine *on page 86*

**Parnate®** *see* tranylcypromine *on page 599*

## paromomycin (par oh moe MYE sin)

**U.S./Canadian Brand Names** Humatin®

**Therapeutic Category** Amebicide

**Use** Treatment of acute and chronic intestinal amebiasis due to susceptible *Entamoeba histolytica* (not effective in the treatment of extraintestinal amebiasis); tapeworm infestations; adjunctive management of hepatic coma; treatment of cryptosporidial diarrhea

**Usual Dosage** Oral:

Intestinal amebiasis: Children and Adults: 25-35 mg/kg/day in 3 divided doses for 5-10 days

Tapeworm (fish, dog, bovine, porcine):

Children: 11 mg/kg every 15 minutes for 4 doses

Adults: 1 g every 15 minutes for 4 doses

Hepatic coma: Adults: 4 g/day in 2-4 divided doses for 5-6 days

Dwarf tapeworm: Children and Adults: 45 mg/kg/dose every day for 5-7 days

**Dosage Forms** Capsule, as sulfate: 250 mg

## paroxetine (pa ROKS e teen)

**U.S./Canadian Brand Names** Paxil™

**Therapeutic Category** Antidepressant, Selective Serotonin Reuptake Inhibitor

**Use** Treatment of depression, obsessive compulsive disorder (OCD) and panic disorder (PD)

**Usual Dosage** Adults: Oral: 20 mg once daily, preferably in the morning

**Dosage Forms**

Suspension, oral: 10 mg/5 mL (250 mL)

Tablet: 10 mg, 20 mg, 30 mg, 40 mg

**Parsidol®** ***(Discontinued)*** *see page 750*

**Parsitan® (Can)** *see* ethopropazine *(Canada only) on page 234*

**Partuss® LA** ***(Discontinued)*** *see page 750*

**Parvolex® (Can)** *see* acetylcysteine *on page 10*

**PAS** *see* aminosalicylate sodium *on page 32*

**Patanol®** *see* olopatadine *on page 435*

**Pathilon®** ***(Discontinued)*** *see page 750*

**Pathocil®** ***(Discontinued)*** *see page 750*

**Pavabid® (all products)** ***(Discontinued)*** *see page 750*

**Pavacot®** *see* papaverine *on page 450*

**Pavasule®** ***(Discontinued)*** *see page 750*

**Pavatine®** ***(Discontinued)*** *see page 750*

**Pavatym®** ***(Discontinued)*** *see page 750*

**Pavesed®** ***(Discontinued)*** *see page 750*

**Pavulon®** ***(Discontinued)*** *see page 750*

**Paxene®** ***(Discontinued)*** *see page 750*

**Paxil™** *see* paroxetine *on this page*

**Paxipam®** *see* halazepam *on page 287*

**PBZ® (all products)** ***(Discontinued)*** *see page 750*

**PCE®** *see* erythromycin (systemic) *on page 222*

**PCMX** *see* parachlorometaxylenol *on page 450*

**PCV7** *see* pneumococcal conjugate vaccine (7-valent) *on page 477*

**Pedameth®** *see* methionine *on page 379*

**PediaCare® Oral** *see* pseudoephedrine *on page 507*

**Pediacof®** *see* chlorpheniramine, phenylephrine, and codeine *on page 131*

**Pediaflor®** *see* fluoride *on page 255*

**Pedialyte® [OTC]** *see* nutritional formula, enteral/oral *on page 432*

**PediaPatch Transdermal Patch [OTC]** *see* salicylic acid *on page 535*

**Pediapred® Oral** *see* prednisolone (systemic) *on page 493*

**Pedia-Profen™** *see* ibuprofen *on page 311*

**Pediatric Triban®** ***(Discontinued)*** *see page 750*

**Pediatrix (Can)** *see* acetaminophen *on page 3*

**Pediazole®** *see* erythromycin and sulfisoxazole *on page 221*

**Pedi-Boro® [OTC]** *see* aluminum sulfate and calcium acetate *on page 28*

**Pedi-Dri® Topical Powder** *see* nystatin *on page 432*

**Pediotic® Otic** *see* neomycin, polymyxin B, and hydrocortisone *on page 415*

**Pedituss®** *see* chlorpheniramine, phenylephrine, and codeine *on page 131*

**PedTE-PAK-4®** *see* trace metals *on page 598*

**Pedtrace-4®** *see* trace metals *on page 598*

**PedvaxHIB®** *see* *Haemophilus* B conjugate vaccine *on page 287*

## pegademase (bovine) (peg A de mase BOE vine)

**U.S./Canadian Brand Names** Adagen™

**Therapeutic Category** Enzyme

**Use** Enzyme replacement therapy for adenosine deaminase (ADA) deficiency in patients with severe combined immunodeficiency disease (SCID) who can not benefit from bone marrow transplant

**Usual Dosage** Children: I.M.: Dose administered every 7 days, 10 units/kg the first dose, 15 units/kg the second dose, and 20 units/kg the third; maintenance dose: 20 units/kg/week is recommended depending on patient's ADA level

**Dosage Forms** Injection: 250 units/mL (1.5 mL)

**Peganone®** *see* ethotoin *on page 235*

## pegaspargase (peg AS par jase)

**Synonyms** PEG-L-asparaginase

**U.S./Canadian Brand Names** Oncaspar®

**Therapeutic Category** Antineoplastic Agent

**Use** Induction treatment of acute lymphoblastic leukemia in combination with other chemotherapeutic agents in patients who have developed hypersensitivity to native forms of asparaginase derived from *E. coli* and/or *Erwinia chrysanthem*, treatment of lymphoma

**Usual Dosage** **Refer to individual protocols**; I.M. administration may decrease the risk of anaphylaxis; dose must be individualized based upon clinical response and tolerance of the patient

I.M., I.V.: 2000 units/m$^2$ every 14 days

**Dosage Forms** Injection, preservative free: 750 units/mL

**PEG-ES** *see* polyethylene glycol solution *on page 480*

## peginterferon alfa-2b (peg in ter FEER on AL fa-too bee)

**U.S./Canadian Brand Names** PEG-Intron™

**Therapeutic Category** Interferon

(Continued)

## peginterferon alfa-2b *(Continued)*

**Use** Treatment of chronic hepatitis C in adult patients who have never received interferon alpha and have compensated liver disease

**Usual Dosage**

Children: Safety and efficacy has not been established

Adults: Chronic hepatitis C: S.C.: Initial:

37-45 kg: 40 mcg
46-56 kg: 50 mcg
57-72 kg: 64 mcg
73-88 kg: 80 mcg
89-106 kg: 96 mcg
107-136 kg: 120 mcg
137-160 kg: 150 mcg

**Note:** Administer dose once weekly for 1 year; after 24 weeks of treatment, if serum HCV RNA is not below the limit of detection of the assay, consider discontinuation

**Dosage Forms** Powder for injection: 100 mcg/mL, 160 mcg/mL, 240 mcg/mL, 300 mcg/mL

**PEG-Intron™** *see* peginterferon alfa-2b *on previous page*

**PEG-L-asparaginase** *see* pegaspargase *on previous page*

**Peglyte® (Can)** *see* polyethylene glycol solution *on page 480*

**PemADD®** *see* pemoline *on this page*

**PemADD CT®** *see* pemoline *on this page*

## pemirolast (pe MIR oh last)

**U.S./Canadian Brand Names** Alamast™

**Therapeutic Category** Mast Cell Stabilizer; Ophthalmic Agent, Miscellaneous

**Use** Prevention of itchy eyes due to allergic conjunctivitis.

**Dosage Forms** Solution, ophthalmic: 0.1% (10 mL)

## pemoline (PEM oh leen)

**Synonyms** phenylisohydantoin; PIO

**U.S./Canadian Brand Names** Cylert®; PemADD®; PemADD CT®

**Therapeutic Category** Central Nervous System Stimulant, Nonamphetamine

**Controlled Substance** C-IV

**Use** Treatment of attention-deficit/hyperactivity disorder (ADHD); narcolepsy

**Usual Dosage** Oral:

Children <6 years: Not recommended

Children ≥6 years and Adults: Initial: 37.5 mg administered once daily in the morning, increase by 18.75 mg/day at weekly intervals; effective dose range: 56.25-75 mg/day; maximum: 112.5 mg/day; dosage range: 0.5-3 mg/kg/24 hours

**Dosage Forms**

Tablet: 18.75 mg, 37.5 mg, 75 mg

Tablet, chewable: 37.5 mg

## penbutolol (pen BYOO toe lole)

**U.S./Canadian Brand Names** Levatol®

**Therapeutic Category** Beta-Adrenergic Blocker

**Use** Treatment of mild to moderate arterial hypertension

**Usual Dosage** Adults: Oral: Initial: 20 mg once daily, full effect of a 20 or 40 mg dose is seen by the end of a 2-week period, doses of 40-80 mg have been tolerated but have shown little additional antihypertensive effects

**Dosage Forms** Tablet, as sulfate: 20 mg

## penciclovir (pen SYE kloe veer)

**U.S./Canadian Brand Names** Denavir™

**Therapeutic Category** Antiviral Agent

**Use** Antiviral cream for the treatment of recurrent herpes labialis (cold sores) in adults

**Usual Dosage** Apply cream at the first sign or symptom of cold sore (eg, tingling, swelling); apply every 2 hours during waking hours for 4 days

**Dosage Forms** Cream: 1% [10 mg/g] (1.5 g)

**Penecort® Topical** *see* hydrocortisone (topical) *on page 304*

**Penetrex™** *see* enoxacin *on page 214*

## penicillamine (pen i SIL a meen)

**Synonyms** d-3-mercaptovaline; β,β-dimethylcysteine; d-penicillamine

**U.S./Canadian Brand Names** Cuprimine®; Depen®

**Therapeutic Category** Chelating Agent

**Use** Treatment of Wilson's disease, cystinuria, adjunct in the treatment of severe rheumatoid arthritis; lead poisoning, primary biliary cirrhosis

**Usual Dosage** Oral:

Rheumatoid arthritis:

Children: Initial: 3 mg/kg/day (≤250 mg/day) for 3 months, then 6 mg/kg/day (≤500 mg/day) in divided doses twice daily for 3 months to a maximum of 10 mg/kg/day in 3-4 divided doses

Adults: 125-250 mg/day, may increase dose at 1- to 3-month intervals up to 1-1.5 g/day

Wilson's disease (doses titrated to maintain urinary copper excretion >1 mg/day):

Infants <6 months: 250 mg/dose once daily

Children <12 years: 250 mg/dose 2-3 times/day

Adults: 250 mg 4 times/day

Cystinuria:

Children: 30 mg/kg/day in 4 divided doses

Adults: 1-4 g/day in divided doses every 6 hours

Lead poisoning (continue until blood lead level is <60 mcg/dL):

Children: 25-40 mg/kg/day in 3 divided doses

Adults: 250 mg/dose every 8-12 hours

Primary biliary cirrhosis: 250 mg/day to start, increase by 250 mg every 2 weeks up to a maintenance dose of 1 g/day, usually administered 250 mg 4 times/day

Arsenic poisoning: Children: 100 mg/kg/day in divided doses every 6 hours for 5 days; maximum: 1 g/day

**Dosage Forms**

Capsule: 125 mg, 250 mg

Tablet: 250 mg

## penicillin G benzathine (pen i SIL in jee BENZ a theen)

**Synonyms** benzathine benzylpenicillin; benzathine penicillin G; benzylpenicillin benzathine

**U.S./Canadian Brand Names** Bicillin® L-A; Permapen®

**Therapeutic Category** Penicillin

**Use** Active against most gram-positive organisms and some spirochetes; used only for the treatment of mild to moderately severe infections (ie, *Streptococcus* pharyngitis) caused by organisms susceptible to low concentrations of penicillin G, or for prophylaxis of infections caused by these organisms such as rheumatic fever prophylaxis

**Usual Dosage** I.M.: Administer undiluted injection, very slowly released from site of injection, providing uniform levels over 2-4 weeks; higher doses result in more sustained rather than higher levels. Use a penicillin G benzathine-penicillin G procaine combination to achieve early peak levels in acute infections

Infants and Children:

Group A streptococcal upper respiratory infection: 25,000 units/kg as a single dose; maximum: 1.2 million units

(Continued)

## penicillin G benzathine *(Continued)*

Prophylaxis of recurrent rheumatic fever: 25,000 units/kg every 3-4 weeks; maximum: 1.2 million units/dose

Early syphilis: 50,000 units/kg as a single injection; maximum: 2.4 million units

Syphilis of more than 1-year duration: 50,000 units/kg every week for 3 doses; maximum: 2.4 million units/dose

Adults:

Group A streptococcal upper respiratory infection: 1.2 million units as a single dose

Prophylaxis of recurrent rheumatic fever: 1.2 million units every 3-4 weeks or 600,000 units twice monthly; a single dose of 600,000 to 1,2000,000 units is effective in the prevention of rheumatic fever secondary to streptococcal pharyngitis

Early syphilis: 2.4 million units as a single dose

Syphilis of more than 1-year duration: 2.4 million units once weekly for 3 doses

**Dosage Forms** Injection: 300,000 units/mL (10 mL); 600,000 units/mL (1 mL, 2 mL, 4 mL)

## penicillin G benzathine and procaine combined

(pen i SIL in jee BENZ a theen & PROE kane KOM bined)

**U.S./Canadian Brand Names** Bicillin® C-R; Bicillin® C-R 900/300

**Therapeutic Category** Penicillin

**Use** Active against most gram-positive organisms, mostly streptococcal and pneumococcal

**Usual Dosage** I.M.:

Children:

<30 lb: 600,000 units in a single dose

30-60 lb: 900,000 units to 1.2 million units in a single dose

Children >60 lb and Adults: 2.4 million units in a single dose

**Dosage Forms**

Injection:

300,000 units [150,000 units each of penicillin G benzathine and penicillin G procaine] (10 mL)

600,000 units [300,000 units each penicillin G benzathine and penicillin G procaine] (1 mL)

1,200,000 units [600,000 units each penicillin G benzathine and penicillin G procaine] (2 mL)

2,400,000 units [1,200,000 units each penicillin G benzathine and penicillin G procaine] (4 mL)

Injection: Penicillin G benzathine 900,000 units and penicillin G procaine 300,000 units per dose (2 mL)

## penicillin G (parenteral/aqueous)

(pen i SIL in jee pa REN ter al/AYE kwee us)

**Synonyms** benzylpenicillin; crystalline penicillin

**U.S./Canadian Brand Names** Pfizerpen®

**Therapeutic Category** Penicillin

**Use** Active against most gram-positive organisms except *Staphylococcus aureus*; some gram-negative such as *Neisseria gonorrhoeae* and some anaerobes and spirochetes; although ceftriaxone is now the drug of choice for Lyme disease and gonorrhea

**Usual Dosage** I.M., I.V.:

Infants and Children (sodium salt is preferred in children): 100,000-250,000 units/kg/day in divided doses every 4 hours; maximum: 4.8 million units/24 hours

Severe infections: Up to 400,000 units/kg/day in divided doses every 4 hours; maximum dose: 24 million units/day

Adults: 2-24 million units/day in divided doses every 4 hours

**Dosage Forms** Injection:

Penicillin G potassium:

Frozen premixed: 1 million units, 2 million units, 3 million units

Powder: 1 million units, 5 million units, 10 million units, 20 million units
Penicillin G sodium: 5 million units

## penicillin G procaine (pen i SIL in jee PROE kane)

**Synonyms** APPG; aqueous procaine penicillin G; procaine benzylpenicillin; procaine penicillin G

**U.S./Canadian Brand Names** Ayercillin® (Can); Crysticillin® A.S.; Wycillin®

**Therapeutic Category** Penicillin

**Use** Moderately severe infections due to *Neisseria gonorrhoeae*, *Treponema pallidum*, and other penicillin G-sensitive microorganisms that are susceptible to low but prolonged serum penicillin concentrations

**Usual Dosage** I.M.:

Newborns: 50,000 units/kg/day administered every day (avoid using in this age group since sterile abscesses and procaine toxicity occur more frequently with neonates than older patients)

Children: 25,000-50,000 units/kg/day in divided doses 1-2 times/day; not to exceed 4.8 million units/24 hours

Gonorrhea: 100,000 units/kg one time (in 2 injection sites) along with probenecid 25 mg/kg (maximum: 1 g) orally 30 minutes prior to procaine penicillin

Adults: 0.6-4.8 million units/day in divided doses 1-2 times/day

Uncomplicated gonorrhea: 1 g probenecid orally, then 4.8 million units procaine penicillin divided into 2 injection sites 30 minutes later. When used in conjunction with an aminoglycoside for the treatment of endocarditis caused by susceptible *S. viridans*: 1.2 million units every 6 hours for 2-4 weeks

**Dosage Forms** Injection, suspension: 300,000 units/mL (10 mL); 500,000 units/mL (1.2 mL); 600,000 units/mL (1 mL, 2 mL, 4 mL)

## penicillin V potassium (pen i SIL in vee poe TASS ee um)

**Synonyms** pen VK; phenoxymethyl penicillin

**U.S./Canadian Brand Names** Apo®-Pen VK (Can); Nadopen-V® (Can); Novo-Pen-VK® (Can); Nu-Pen-VK (Can); Truxcillin VK®; Veetids®

**Therapeutic Category** Penicillin

**Use** Treatment of mild to moderately severe susceptible bacterial infections involving the upper respiratory tract, skin, and urinary tract; prophylaxis of pneumococcal infections and rheumatic fever

**Usual Dosage** Oral:

Systemic infections:

Children <12 years: 25-50 mg/kg/day in divided doses every 6-8 hours; maximum dose: 3 g/day

Children >12 years and Adults: 125-500 mg every 6-8 hours

Prophylaxis of pneumococcal infections:

Children <5 years: 125 mg twice daily

Children ≥5 years: 250 mg twice daily

Prophylaxis of recurrent rheumatic fever:

Children <5 years: 125 mg

Children ≥5 years and Adults: 250 mg twice daily

**Dosage Forms**

Powder for oral solution: 125 mg/5 mL (100 mL, 200 mL); 250 mg/5 mL (100 mL, 150 mL, 200 mL)

Tablet: 250 mg, 500 mg

**penicilloyl-polylysine** *see* benzylpenicilloyl-polylysine *on page 75*

**Penlac™** *see* ciclopirox *on page 136*

**Penta/3B® Plus (Can)** *see* vitamin (multiple/oral) *on page 632*

**Pentacarinat® Injection** *see* pentamidine *on next page*

**Pentam-300® Injection** *see* pentamidine *on next page*

## pentamidine (pen TAM i deen)

**U.S./Canadian Brand Names** NebuPent™ Inhalation; Pentacarinat® Injection; Pentam-300® Injection; Pneumopent (Can)

**Therapeutic Category** Antiprotozoal

**Use** Treatment and prevention of pneumonia caused by *Pneumocystis carinii* in patients who cannot tolerate co-trimoxazole or who fail to respond to this drug; treatment of African trypanosomiasis; treatment of visceral leishmaniasis caused by *L. donovani*

**Usual Dosage**

Children:

Treatment: I.M., I.V. (I.V. preferred): 4 mg/kg/day once daily for 14-21 days

Prevention:

I.M., I.V.: 4 mg/kg monthly or biweekly

Inhalation (aerosolized pentamidine in children ≥5 years): 300 mg/dose administered every 3 weeks or monthly via Respirgard® II inhaler (8 mg/kg dose has also been used in children <5 years)

Treatment of trypanosomiasis: I.V.: 4 mg/kg/day once daily for 10 days

Adults:

Treatment: I.M., I.V. (I.V. preferred): 4 mg/kg/day once daily for 14 days

Prevention: Inhalation: 300 mg every 4 weeks via Respirgard® II nebulizer

**Dosage Forms**

Inhalation, as isethionate: 300 mg

Powder for injection, as isethionate, lyophilized: 300 mg

**Pentamycetin® (Can)** *see* chloramphenicol *on page 125*

**Pentasa® Oral** *see* mesalamine *on page 374*

**Pentaspan®** *see* pentastarch *on this page*

## pentastarch (PEN ta starch)

**U.S./Canadian Brand Names** Pentaspan®

**Therapeutic Category** Blood Modifiers

**Use** Adjunct in leukapheresis to improve the harvesting and increase the yield of leukocytes by centrifugal means

**Usual Dosage** 250-700 mL to which citrate anticoagulant has been added is administered by adding to the input line of the centrifugation apparatus at a ratio of 1:8-1:13 to venous whole blood

**Dosage Forms** Injection, in NS: 10% (500 mL)

## pentazocine (pen TAZ oh seen)

**U.S./Canadian Brand Names** Talwin®; Talwin® NX

**Therapeutic Category** Analgesic, Narcotic

**Controlled Substance** C-IV

**Use** Relief of moderate to severe pain; a sedative prior to surgery; supplement to surgical anesthesia

**Usual Dosage**

Children: I.M., S.C.:

5-8 years: 15 mg

8-14 years: 30 mg

Children >12 years and Adults: Oral: 50 mg every 3-4 hours; may increase to 100 mg/dose if needed, but should not exceed 600 mg/day

Adults:

I.M., S.C.: 30-60 mg every 3-4 hours, not to exceed total daily dose of 360 mg

I.V.: 30 mg every 3-4 hours

**Dosage Forms**

Injection, as lactate: 30 mg/mL (1 mL, 1.5 mL, 2 mL, 10 mL)

Tablet: Pentazocine hydrochloride 50 mg and naloxone hydrochloride 0.5 mg

## pentazocine compound (pen TAZ oh seen KOM pownd)

**U.S./Canadian Brand Names** Talacen®; Talwin® Compound

**Therapeutic Category** Analgesic, Narcotic

**Use** Relief of moderate to severe pain; has also been used as a sedative prior to surgery and as a supplement to surgical anesthesia

**Usual Dosage** Adults: Oral: 2 tablets 3-4 times/day

**Dosage Forms** Tablet:

Talacen®: Pentazocine hydrochloride 25 mg and acetaminophen 650 mg
Talwin® Compound: Pentazocine hydrochloride 12.5 mg and aspirin 325 mg

**Penthrane®** *see* methoxyflurane *on page 382*

**Pentids® (all products)** ***(Discontinued)*** *see page 750*

## pentobarbital (pen toe BAR bi tal)

**U.S./Canadian Brand Names** Nembutal®

**Therapeutic Category** Barbiturate

**Controlled Substance** C-II

**Use** Short-term treatment of insomnia; preoperative sedation; high-dose barbiturate coma for treatment of increased intracranial pressure or status epilepticus unresponsive to other therapy

**Usual Dosage**

Children:
- Sedative: Oral: 2-6 mg/kg/day divided in 3 doses; maximum: 100 mg/day
- Hypnotic: I.M.: 2-6 mg/kg; maximum: 100 mg/dose
- Rectal:
  - 2 months to 1 year (10-20 lb): 30 mg
  - 1-4 years (20-40 lb): 30-60 mg
  - 5-12 years (40-80 lb): 60 mg
  - 12-14 years (80-110 lb): 60-120 mg **or**
  - <4 years: 3-6 mg/kg/dose
  - >4 years: 1.5-3 mg/kg/dose
- Preoperative/preprocedure sedation: ≥6 months:
  - Oral, I.M., rectal: 2-6 mg/kg; maximum: 100 mg/dose
  - I.V.: 1-3 mg/kg to a maximum of 100 mg until asleep
- Children 5-12 years: Conscious sedation prior to a procedure: I.V.: 2 mg/kg 5-10 minutes before procedures, may repeat one time

Adolescents: Conscious sedation: Oral, I.V.: 100 mg prior to a procedure

Children and Adults: Barbiturate coma in head injury patients: I.V.:
- Loading dose: 5-10 mg/kg administered slowly over 1-2 hours; monitor blood pressure and respiratory rate
- Maintenance infusion: Initial: 1 mg/kg/hour; may increase to 2-3 mg/kg/hour; maintain burst suppression on EEG

Adults:
- Hypnotic:
  - Oral: 100-200 mg at bedtime or 20 mg 3-4 times/day for daytime sedation
  - I.M.: 150-200 mg
  - I.V.: Initial: 100 mg, may repeat every 1-3 minutes up to 200-500 mg total dose
- Rectal: 120-200 mg at bedtime
- Preoperative sedation: I.M.: 150-200 mg

**Dosage Forms**

Capsule, as sodium (C-II): 50 mg, 100 mg
Injection, as sodium (C-II): 50 mg/mL (20 mL, 50 mL)
Suppository, rectal (C-III): 60 mg, 200 mg

## pentosan polysulfate sodium (PEN toe san pol i SUL fate SOW dee um)

**Synonyms** PPS

**U.S./Canadian Brand Names** Elmiron®

(Continued)

## pentosan polysulfate sodium *(Continued)*

**Therapeutic Category** Analgesic, Urinary

**Use** Bladder pain relief or discomfort associated with interstitial cystitis

**Usual Dosage** Adults: Oral: 100 mg capsule 3 times/day; administer with water at least 1 hour before meals or 2 hours after meals

**Dosage Forms** Capsule: 100 mg

## pentostatin (PEN toe stat in)

**Synonyms** DCF; 2′-deoxycoformycin

**U.S./Canadian Brand Names** Nipent™

**Therapeutic Category** Antineoplastic Agent

**Use** Treatment of adult patients with alpha-interferon-refractory hairy cell leukemia; significant antitumor activity in various lymphoid neoplasms has been demonstrated; pentostatin also is known as 2′-deoxycoformycin; it is a purine analogue capable of inhibiting adenosine deaminase

**Usual Dosage** Refractory hairy cell leukemia: Adults: I.V.: 4 mg/m$^2$ every other week

**Dosage Forms** Powder for injection: 10 mg/vial

**Pentothal® Sodium** *see* thiopental *on page 585*

## pentoxifylline (pen toks I fi leen)

**Synonyms** oxpentifylline

**U.S./Canadian Brand Names** Albert® Pentoxifylline (Can); Apo®-Pentoxifylline SR (Can); Nu-Pentoxifylline-SR (Can); Trental®

**Therapeutic Category** Blood Viscosity Reducer Agent

**Use** Symptomatic management of peripheral vascular disease, mainly intermittent claudication

**Investigational use:** AIDS patients with increased tumor necrosis factor, cerebrovascular accidents, cerebrovascular diseases, new onset type I diabetes mellitus, diabetic atherosclerosis, diabetic neuropathy, gangrene, cutaneous polyarteritis nodosa, hemodialysis shunt thrombosis, cerebral malaria, septic shock, sepsis in premature neonates, sickle cell syndromes, vasculitis, Kawasaki disease, Raynaud's syndrome, cystic fibrosis, and persistent pulmonary hypertension of the newborn (case report)

**Usual Dosage** Adults: Oral: 400 mg 3 times/day with meals; may reduce to 400 mg twice daily if GI or CNS side effects occur

**Dosage Forms** Tablet, controlled release: 400 mg

**Pentrax® [OTC]** *see* coal tar *on page 149*

**Pen.Vee® K *(Discontinued)*** *see page 750*

**pen VK** *see* penicillin V potassium *on page 457*

**Pepcid®** *see* famotidine *on page 240*

**Pepcid® AC Acid Controller [OTC]** *see* famotidine *on page 240*

**Pepcid® Complete [OTC]** *see* famotidine, calcium carbonate, and magnesium hydroxide *on page 240*

**Pepcid RPD®** *see* famotidine *on page 240*

**Peptavlon® *(Discontinued)*** *see page 750*

**Pepto-Bismol® [OTC]** *see* bismuth subsalicylate *on page 81*

**Pepto® Diarrhea Control *(Discontinued)*** *see page 750*

**Perchloracap®** *see* radiological/contrast media (ionic) *on page 516*

**Percocet® 2.5/325** *see* oxycodone and acetaminophen *on page 444*

**Percocet® 5/325** *see* oxycodone and acetaminophen *on page 444*

**Percocet® 7.5/500** *see* oxycodone and acetaminophen *on page 444*

**Percocet® 10/650** *see* oxycodone and acetaminophen *on page 444*

**Percocet®-Demi (Can)** *see* oxycodone and acetaminophen *on page 444*

**Percodan®** *see* oxycodone and aspirin *on page 444*

**Percodan®-Demi** *see* oxycodone and aspirin *on page 444*

**Percogesic® [OTC]** *see* acetaminophen and phenyltoloxamine *on page 5*

**Percolone®** *see* oxycodone *on page 443*

**Perdiem® Plain [OTC]** *see* psyllium *on page 509*

## pergolide (PER go lide)

**U.S./Canadian Brand Names** Permax®

**Therapeutic Category** Anti-Parkinson's Agent; Dopaminergic Agent (Anti-Parkinson's); Ergot Alkaloid and Derivative

**Use** Adjunctive treatment to levodopa/carbidopa in the management of Parkinson's Disease

**Usual Dosage** Adults: Oral: Initial: 0.05 mg/day for 2 days, then increase dosage by 0.1 or 0.15 mg/day every 3 days over next 12 days, increase dose by 0.25 mg/day every 3 days until optimal therapeutic dose is achieved

**Dosage Forms** Tablet, as mesylate: 0.05 mg, 0.25 mg, 1 mg

**Pergonal®** *see* menotropins *on page 371*

**Periactin®** *see* cyproheptadine *on page 161*

**Peri-Colace® [OTC]** *see* docusate and casanthranol *on page 198*

## pericyazine *(Canada only)* (per ee CYE ah zeen)

**U.S./Canadian Brand Names** Neuleptil® (Can)

**Therapeutic Category** Phenothiazine Derivative

**Use** As adjunctive medication in some psychotic patients, for the control of residual prevailing hostility, impulsiveness and aggressiveness

**Usual Dosage** Oral:

Children and adolescents (5 years of age and over): 2.5-10 mg in the morning and 5-30 mg in the evening. These dosages approximate a daily dosage range of 1-3 mg/year of age.

Adults: 5-20 mg in the morning and 10-40 mg in the evening. For maintenance therapy, the dosage should be reduced to the minimum effective dose. Lower doses of 2.5-15 mg in the morning, and 5-30 mg in the evening have been suggested. For elderly patients the initial total daily dosage should be in the order of 5 mg and increased gradually as tolerated, until an adequate response is obtained. A daily dosage of more than 30 mg will rarely be needed. Children and adolescents (5 years of age and over): 2.5-10 mg in the morning and 5-30 mg in the evening. These dosages approximate a daily dosage range of 1-3 mg/year of age.

**Dosage Forms**

Capsule: 5 mg, 10 mg, 20 mg

Drops, oral: 10 mg/mL (100 mL)

**Peridex®** *see* chlorhexidine gluconate *on page 126*

**Peridol (Can)** *see* haloperidol *on page 288*

## perindopril erbumine (per IN doe pril er BYOO meen)

**U.S./Canadian Brand Names** Aceon®; Coversyl® (Can)

**Therapeutic Category** Miscellaneous Product

**Use** Treatment of hypertension

**Usual Dosage** Adults: Oral: 4 mg once daily; usual range: 4-8 mg/day; maximum: 16 mg/day

**Dosage Forms** Tablet: 2 mg, 4 mg, 8 mg

**Periochip®** *see* chlorhexidine gluconate *on page 126*

**PerioGard®** *see* chlorhexidine gluconate *on page 126*

**Peritrate® *(Discontinued)*** *see page 750*

**Peritrate® SA *(Discontinued)*** *see page 750*

**Permapen®** *see* penicillin G benzathine *on page 455*

**Permax®** *see* pergolide *on previous page*

## permethrin (per METH rin)

**U.S./Canadian Brand Names** A-200™ Lice [OTC]; Acticin® Cream; Elimite™ Cream; Kwellada-P™ (Can); Medi-Lice® [OTC]; Nix™ Creme Rinse; R&C® Lice

**Therapeutic Category** Scabicides/Pediculicides

**Use** Single application treatment of infestation with *Pediculus humanus capitis* (head louse) and its nits, or *Sarcoptes scabiei* (scabies)

**Usual Dosage**

Head lice: Children >2 months and Adults: Topical: After hair has been washed with shampoo, rinsed with water and towel-dried, apply a sufficient volume to saturate the hair and scalp. Leave on hair for 10 minutes before rinsing off with water; remove remaining nits.

Scabies: Apply cream from head to toe; leave on for 8-14 hours before washing off with water

**Dosage Forms**

Cream: 5% (60 g)
Creme rinse: 1% (60 mL with comb)
Lotion: 1% (60 mL)
Spray: 0.4% (150 mL); 0.5% (142 g)

**Permitil® Oral** *see* fluphenazine *on page 258*

**Pernox® [OTC]** *see* sulfur and salicylic acid *on page 566*

## perphenazine (per FEN a zeen)

**U.S./Canadian Brand Names** Apo®-Perphenazine (Can); Trilafon®

**Therapeutic Category** Phenothiazine Derivative

**Use** Symptomatic management of psychotic disorders, as well as severe nausea and vomiting

**Usual Dosage**

Children:
- Psychoses: Oral:
  - 1-6 years: 4-6 mg/day in divided doses
  - 6-12 years: 6 mg/day in divided doses
  - >12 years: 4-16 mg 2-4 times/day
  - I.M.: 5 mg every 6 hours
- Nausea/vomiting: I.M.: 5 mg every 6 hours

Adults:
- Psychoses:
  - Oral: 4-16 mg 2-4 times/day not to exceed 64 mg/day
  - I.M.: 5 mg every 6 hours up to 15 mg/day in ambulatory patients and 30 mg/day in hospitalized patients
- Nausea/vomiting:
  - Oral: 8-16 mg/day in divided doses up to 24 mg/day
  - I.M.: 5-10 mg every 6 hours as necessary up to 15 mg/day in ambulatory patients and 30 mg/day in hospitalized patients
  - I.V. (severe): 1 mg at 1- to 2-minute intervals up to a total of 5 mg

**Dosage Forms**

Injection: 5 mg/mL (1 mL)
Tablet: 2 mg, 4 mg, 8 mg, 16 mg

**Persantine®** *see* dipyridamole *on page 194*

**Pertussin® CS [OTC]** *see* dextromethorphan *on page 178*

**Pertussin® ES [OTC]** *see* dextromethorphan *on page 178*

**pethidine** *see* meperidine *on page 372*

**PFA** *see* foscarnet *on page 264*

**Pfizerpen®** *see* penicillin G (parenteral/aqueous) *on page 456*

**Pfizerpen-AS®** ***(Discontinued)*** *see page 750*

**PGE$_1$** *see* alprostadil *on page 23*

**PGE$_2$** *see* dinoprostone *on page 189*

**PGF$_{2\alpha}$** *see* dinoprost tromethamine *on page 190*

**Phanatuss® Cough Syrup [OTC]** *see* guaifenesin and dextromethorphan *on page 282*

**Pharmacist's Capsaicin®** *see* capsaicin *on page 104*

**Pharmaflur®** *see* fluoride *on page 255*

**Pharmorubicin® (Can)** *see* epirubicin *on page 217*

**Phazyme® [OTC]** *see* simethicone *on page 544*

**Phenadex® Senior [OTC]** *see* guaifenesin and dextromethorphan *on page 282*

**Phenahist-TR®** ***(Discontinued)*** *see page 750*

**Phenameth® DM** *see* promethazine and dextromethorphan *on page 501*

**Phenapap® [OTC]** *see* acetaminophen and pseudoephedrine *on page 6*

**Phenaphen®** ***(Discontinued)*** *see page 750*

**Phenaphen®/Codeine #4** ***(Discontinued)*** *see page 750*

**Phenaphen® With Codeine #3** *see* acetaminophen and codeine *on page 4*

**Phenaseptic®** ***(Discontinued)*** *see page 750*

**Phenazine® Injection** *see* promethazine *on page 500*

**Phenazo™ (Can)** *see* phenazopyridine *on this page*

## phenazopyridine (fen az oh PEER i deen)

**Synonyms** phenylazo diamino pyridine hydrochloride

**U.S./Canadian Brand Names** Azo-Dine® [OTC]; Azo-Gesic® [OTC]; Azo-Standard®; Baridium®; Phenazo™ (Can); Prodium™ [OTC]; Pyridiate®; Pyridium®; Uristat® [OTC]; Urodol® [OTC]; Urofemme® [OTC]; Urogesic®

**Therapeutic Category** Analgesic, Urinary

**Use** Symptomatic relief of urinary burning, itching, frequency and urgency in association with urinary tract infection, or following urologic procedures

**Usual Dosage** Oral:

Children 6-12 years: 12 mg/kg/day in 3 divided doses administered after meals for 2 days

Adults: 100-200 mg 3-4 times/day for 2 days

**Dosage Forms** Tablet, as hydrochloride: 95 mg, 97.2 mg, 100 mg, 200 mg

**Phencen-50®** ***(Discontinued)*** *see page 750*

**Phenclor® S.H.A.** ***(Discontinued)*** *see page 750*

**Phendiet®** *see* phendimetrazine *on this page*

**Phendiet-105®** *see* phendimetrazine *on this page*

## phendimetrazine (fen dye ME tra zeen)

**U.S./Canadian Brand Names** Bontril PDM®; Bontril® Slow-Release; Melfiat®; Obezine®; Phendiet®; Phendiet-105®; Prelu-2®

**Therapeutic Category** Anorexiant

**Controlled Substance** C-III

(Continued)

## phendimetrazine *(Continued)*

**Use** Appetite suppressant during the first few weeks of dieting to help establish new eating habits; its effectiveness lasts only for short periods 3-12 weeks

**Usual Dosage** Adults: Oral:

Regular capsule or tablet: 35 mg 2-3 times/day one hour before meals

Sustained release: 105 mg once daily in the morning before breakfast

**Dosage Forms**

Capsule, as tartrate: 35 mg

Capsule, sustained release, as tartrate (Bontril® Slow Release, Melfiat®, Phendiet®-105, Prelu-2®): 105 mg

Tablet, as tartrate (Bontril PDM®, Obenzine®, Phendiet®): 35 mg

**Phendry® Oral [OTC]** *see* diphenhydramine *on page 191*

## phenelzine (FEN el zeen)

**U.S./Canadian Brand Names** Nardil®

**Therapeutic Category** Antidepressant, Monoamine Oxidase Inhibitor

**Use** Symptomatic treatment of atypical, nonendogenous or neurotic depression

**Usual Dosage** Adults: Oral: 15 mg 3 times/day; may increase to 60-90 mg/day during early phase of treatment, then reduce to dose for maintenance therapy slowly after maximum benefit is obtained; takes 2-4 weeks for a significant response to occur

**Dosage Forms** Tablet, as sulfate: 15 mg

**Phenerbel-S®** ***(Discontinued)*** *see page 750*

**Phenergan® Injection** *see* promethazine *on page 500*

**Phenergan® Oral** *see* promethazine *on page 500*

**Phenergan® Rectal** *see* promethazine *on page 500*

**Phenergan® VC Syrup** *see* promethazine and phenylephrine *on page 501*

**Phenergan® VC With Codeine** *see* promethazine, phenylephrine, and codeine *on page 501*

**Phenergan® With Codeine** *see* promethazine and codeine *on page 500*

**Phenergan® With Dextromethorphan** *see* promethazine and dextromethorphan *on page 501*

**Phenetron®** ***(Discontinued)*** *see page 750*

**Phenhist® Expectorant** *see* guaifenesin, pseudoephedrine, and codeine *on page 284*

## phenindamine (fen IN dah meen)

**U.S./Canadian Brand Names** Nolahist® [OTC]

**Therapeutic Category** Antihistamine

**Use** Treatment of perennial and seasonal allergic rhinitis and chronic urticaria

**Usual Dosage** Oral:

Children <6 years: As directed by physician

Children 6 to <12 years: 12.5 mg every 4-6 hours, up to 75 mg/24 hours

Adults: 25 mg every 4-6 hours, up to 150 mg/24 hours

**Dosage Forms** Tablet, as tartrate: 25 mg

## phenobarbital (fee noe BAR bi tal)

**Synonyms** phenobarbitone; phenylethylmalonylurea

**U.S./Canadian Brand Names** Luminal®

**Therapeutic Category** Anticonvulsant; Barbiturate

**Controlled Substance** C-IV

**Use** Management of generalized tonic-clonic (grand mal) and partial seizures; neonatal seizures; febrile seizures in children; sedation; may also be used for prevention and treatment of neonatal hyperbilirubinemia and lowering of bilirubin in chronic cholestasis

**Usual Dosage**

Children:

Sedation: Oral: 2 mg/kg 3 times/day

Hypnotic: I.M., I.V., S.C.: 3-5 mg/kg at bedtime

Hyperbilirubinemia: <12 years: Oral: 3-8 mg/kg/day in 2-3 divided doses; doses up to 12 mg/kg/day have been used

Preoperative sedation: Oral, I.M., I.V.: 1-3 mg/kg 1-1.5 hours before procedure

Adults:

Sedation: Oral, I.M.: 30-120 mg/day in 2-3 divided doses

Hypnotic: Oral, I.M., I.V., S.C.: 100-320 mg at bedtime

Hyperbilirubinemia: Oral: 90-180 mg/day in 2-3 divided doses

Preoperative sedation: I.M.: 100-200 mg 1-1½ hours before procedure

Anticonvulsant: Status epilepticus: **Loading dose:** I.V.:

Infants, Children, and Adults: 15-18 mg/kg in a single or divided dose; usual maximum loading dose: 20 mg/kg; in select patients may administer additional 5 mg/kg/dose every 15-30 minutes until seizure is controlled or a total dose of 30 mg/kg is reached

Anticonvulsant: Maintenance dose: Oral, I.V.:

Infants: 5-6 mg/kg/day in 1-2 divided doses

Children:

1-5 years: 6-8 mg/kg/day in 1-2 divided doses

5-12 years: 4-6 mg/kg/day in 1-2 divided doses

Children >12 years and Adults: 1-3 mg/kg/day in divided doses

**Dosage Forms**

Capsule: 16 mg

Elixir: 15 mg/5 mL (5 mL, 10 mL, 20 mL); 20 mg/5 mL (3.75 mL, 5 mL, 7.5 mL, 120 mL, 473 mL, 946 mL, 4000 mL)

Injection, as sodium: 30 mg/mL (1 mL); 60 mg/mL (1 mL); 65 mg/mL (1 mL); 130 mg/mL (1 mL)

Powder for injection: 120 mg

Tablet: 8 mg, 15 mg, 16 mg, 30 mg, 32 mg, 60 mg, 65 mg, 100 mg

**phenobarbitone** *see* phenobarbital *on previous page*

## phenol (FEE nol)

**Synonyms** carbolic acid

**U.S./Canadian Brand Names** Baker's P&S Topical [OTC]; Cēpastat® [OTC]; Chloraseptic® Oral [OTC]; Ulcerease® [OTC]

**Therapeutic Category** Pharmaceutical Aid

**Use** Relief of sore throat pain, mouth, gum, and throat irritations

**Usual Dosage** Oral: Allow to dissolve slowly in mouth; may be repeated every 2 hours as needed

**Dosage Forms**

Liquid:

Oral, sugar free (Ulcerease®): 6% with glycerin (180 mL)

Topical (Baker's P&S): 1% with sodium chloride, liquid paraffin oil and water (120 mL, 240 mL)

Lozenge:

Cēpastat®: 1.45% with menthol and eucalyptus oil

Cēpastat® Cherry: 0.72% with menthol and eucalyptus oil

Chloraseptic®: 32.5 mg total phenol, sugar, corn syrup

Mouthwash (Chloraseptic®): 1.4% with thymol, sodium borate, menthol, and glycerin (180 mL)

Solution (Liquified Phenol): 88% [880 mg/mL]

Aqueous: 6% [60 mg/mL]

**phenolsulfonphthalein** ***(Discontinued)*** *see page 750*

**Phenoxine®** ***(Discontinued)*** *see page 750*

**phenoxybenzamine** (fen oks ee BEN za meen)

**U.S./Canadian Brand Names** Dibenzyline®

**Therapeutic Category** Alpha-Adrenergic Blocking Agent

**Use** Symptomatic management of hypertension and sweating in patients with pheochromocytoma

**Usual Dosage** Oral:

Children: Initial: 0.2 mg/kg (maximum: 10 mg) once daily, increase by 0.2 mg/kg increments; usual maintenance dose: 0.4-1.2 mg/kg/day every 6-8 hours, maximum single dose: 10 mg

Adults: 10-40 mg every 8-12 hours

**Dosage Forms** Capsule, as hydrochloride: 10 mg

**phenoxymethyl penicillin** *see* penicillin V potassium *on page 457*

**Phentercot®** *see* phentermine *on this page*

**phentermine** (FEN ter meen)

**U.S./Canadian Brand Names** Adipex-P®; Ionamin®; Phentercot®; Phentride®; Pro-Fast Hs®; Pro-Fast SA®; Pro-Fast SR®

**Therapeutic Category** Anorexiant

**Controlled Substance** C-IV

**Use** Short-term adjunct in exogenous obesity

**Usual Dosage** Oral:

Children 3-15 years: 5-15 mg/day for 4 weeks

Adults: 8 mg 3 times/day 30 minutes before meals or food or 15-37.5 mg/day before breakfast or 10-14 hours before retiring

**Dosage Forms**

Capsule, as hydrochloride: 15 mg, 18.75 mg, 30 mg, 37.5 mg

Capsule, resin complex, as hydrochloride: 15 mg, 30 mg

Tablet, as hydrochloride: 8 mg, 37.5 mg

**phentolamine** (fen TOLE a meen)

**U.S./Canadian Brand Names** Rogitine® (Can)

**Therapeutic Category** Alpha-Adrenergic Blocking Agent; Diagnostic Agent

**Use** Diagnosis of pheochromocytoma; treatment of hypertension associated with pheochromocytoma or other causes of excess sympathomimetic amines; local treatment of dermal necrosis after extravasation of drugs with alpha-adrenergic effects (dobutamine, dopamine, epinephrine, metaraminol, norepinephrine, phenylephrine)

**Usual Dosage**

Treatment of extravasation: Infiltrate area S.C. with small amount of solution made by diluting 5-10 mg in 10 mL 0.9% NaCl within 12 hours of extravasation; for children, use 0.1-0.2 mg/kg up to a maximum of 10 mg

Children: I.M., I.V.:

Diagnosis of pheochromocytoma: 0.05-0.1 mg/kg/dose, maximum single dose: 5 mg

Hypertension: 0.05-0.1 mg/kg/dose administered 1-2 hours before procedure; repeat as needed until hypertension is controlled; maximum single dose: 5 mg

Adults: I.M., I.V.:

Diagnosis of pheochromocytoma: 5 mg

Hypertension: 5 mg administered 1-2 hours before procedure

**Dosage Forms** Injection, as mesylate: 5 mg/mL (1 mL)

**Phentride®** *see* phentermine *on this page*

**Phenurone®** ***(Discontinued)*** *see page 750*

**phenylalanine mustard** *see* melphalan *on page 370*

**phenylazo diamino pyridine hydrochloride** *see* phenazopyridine *on page 463*

**Phenyldrine®** ***(Discontinued)*** *see page 750*

## phenylephrine (fen il EF rin)

**U.S./Canadian Brand Names** AK-Dilate® Ophthalmic Solution; AK-Nefrin® Ophthalmic Solution; Alconefrin® Nasal Solution [OTC]; Dionephrine® (Can); Doktors® Nasal Solution [OTC]; I-Phrine® Ophthalmic Solution; Isopto® Frin Ophthalmic Solution; Mydfrin® Ophthalmic Solution; Neo-Synephrine® Nasal Solution [OTC]; Neo-Synephrine® Ophthalmic Solution; Nostril® Nasal Solution [OTC]; Prefrin™ Ophthalmic Solution; Relief® Ophthalmic Solution; Rhinall® Nasal Solution [OTC]; Sinarest® Nasal Solution [OTC]; St. Joseph® Measured Dose Nasal Solution [OTC]; Vicks® Sinex® Nasal Solution [OTC]

**Therapeutic Category** Adrenergic Agonist Agent

**Use** Treatment of hypotension and vascular failure in shock; supraventricular tachycardia; as a vasoconstrictor in regional analgesia; symptomatic relief of nasal and nasopharyngeal mucosal congestion; as a mydriatic in ophthalmic procedures and treatment of wide-angle glaucoma

**Usual Dosage**

Ophthalmic procedures:

Infants <1 year: Instill 1 drop of 2.5% 15-30 minutes before procedures

Children and Adults: Instill 1 drop of 2.5% or 10% solution, may repeat in 10-60 minutes as needed

Nasal decongestant:

Children:

2-6 years: Instill 1 drop every 2-4 hours of 0.125% solution as needed

6-12 years: Instill 1-2 sprays or instill 1-2 drops every 4 hours of 0.25% solution as needed

Children >12 years and Adults: Instill 1-2 sprays or instill 1-2 drops every 4 hours of 0.25% to 0.5% solution as needed; 1% solution may be used in adult in cases of extreme nasal congestion; do not use nasal solutions more than 3 days

Hypotension/shock:

Children:

I.M., S.C.: 0.1 mg/kg/dose every 1-2 hours as needed (maximum: 5 mg)

I.V. bolus: 5-20 mcg/kg/dose every 10-15 minutes as needed

I.V. infusion: 0.1-0.5 mcg/kg/minute; the concentration and rate of infusion can be calculated using the following formulas: Dilute 0.6 mg x weight (kg) to 100 mL; then the dose in mcg/kg/minute = 0.1 x the infusion rate in mL/hour

Adults:

I.M., S.C.: 2-5 mg/dose every 1-2 hours as needed (initial dose should not exceed 5 mg)

I.V. bolus: 0.1-0.5 mg/dose every 10-15 minutes as needed (initial dose should not exceed 0.5 mg)

I.V. infusion: 10 mg in 250 mL $D_5W$ or NS (1:25,000 dilution) (40 mcg/mL); start at 100-180 mcg/minute (2-5 mL/minute; 50-90 drops/minute) initially. When blood pressure is stabilized, maintenance rate: 40-60 mcg/minute (20-30 drops/minute)

Paroxysmal supraventricular tachycardia: I.V.:

Children: 5-10 mcg/kg/dose over 20-30 seconds

Adults: 0.25-0.5 mg/dose over 20-30 seconds

**Dosage Forms**

Injection, as hydrochloride (Neo-Synephrine®): 1% [10 mg/mL] (1 mL)

Solution, intranasal, as hydrochloride [drops]:

Alconefrin®, Neo-Synephrine®: 0.5% (15 mL, 30 mL)

Alconefrin® 12: 0.16% (30 mL)

Alconefrin® 25, Neo-Synephrine®, Children's Nostril®, Rhinall®: 0.25% (15 mL, 30 mL, 40 mL)

Neo-Synephrine®: 0.125% (15 mL)

Solution, intranasal, as hydrochloride [spray]:

Alconefrin® 25, Neo-Synephrine®, Rhinall®: 0.25% (15 mL, 30 mL, 40 mL)

Neo-Synephrine®: 1% (15 mL)

Neo-Synephrine®, Nostril®, Sinex®: 0.5% (15 mL, 30 mL)

(Continued)

## phenylephrine *(Continued)*

Solution, ophthalmic, as hydrochloride:

AK-Dilate®, Mydfrin®, Neo-Synephrine®, Phenoptic®: 2.5% (2 mL, 3 mL, 5 mL, 15 mL)

AK-Dilate®, Neo-Synephrine®, Neo-Synephrine® Viscous: 10% (1 mL, 2 mL, 5 mL, 15 mL)

AK-Nefrin®, Prefrin™ Liquifilm®, Relief®: 0.12% (0.3 mL, 15 mL, 20 mL)

## phenylephrine and scopolamine (fen il EF rin & skoe POL a meen)

**U.S./Canadian Brand Names** Murocoll-2® Ophthalmic

**Therapeutic Category** Anticholinergic/Adrenergic Agonist

**Use** Mydriasis, cycloplegia and to break posterior synechiae in iritis

**Usual Dosage** Ophthalmic: Instill 1-2 drops into eye(s); repeat in 5 minutes

**Dosage Forms** Solution, ophthalmic: Phenylephrine hydrochloride 10% and scopolamine hydrobromide 0.3% (7.5 mL)

## phenylephrine and zinc sulfate (fen il EF rin & zingk SUL fate)

**U.S./Canadian Brand Names** Zincfrin® Ophthalmic [OTC]

**Therapeutic Category** Adrenergic Agonist Agent

**Use** Soothe, moisturize, and remove redness due to minor eye irritation

**Usual Dosage** Ophthalmic: Instill 1-2 drops in eye(s) 2-4 times/day as needed

**Dosage Forms** Solution, ophthalmic: Phenylephrine hydrochloride 0.12% and zinc sulfate 0.25% (15 mL)

**phenylethylmalonylurea** *see* phenobarbital *on page 464*

**Phenylfenesin® L.A. *(Discontinued)*** *see page 750*

**Phenylgesic® [OTC]** *see* acetaminophen and phenyltoloxamine *on page 5*

**phenylisohydantoin** *see* pemoline *on page 454*

## phenytoin (FEN i toyn)

**Synonyms** diphenylhydantoin; DPH

**U.S./Canadian Brand Names** Dilantin®; Tremytoine® (Can)

**Therapeutic Category** Antiarrhythmic Agent, Class I-B; Hydantoin

**Use** Management of generalized tonic-clonic (grand mal), simple partial and complex partial seizures; prevention of seizures following head trauma/neurosurgery; ventricular arrhythmias, including those associated with digitalis intoxication, prolonged QT interval and surgical repair of congenital heart diseases in children; epidermolysis bullosa

**Usual Dosage**

Status epilepticus: I.V.:

Infants and Children: Loading dose: 15-18 mg/kg in a single or divided dose; maintenance, anticonvulsant: Initial: 5 mg/kg/day in 2 divided doses, usual doses:

6 months to 3 years: 8-10 mg/kg/day

4-6 years: 7.5-9 mg/kg/day

7-9 years: 7-8 mg/kg/day

10-16 years: 6-7 mg/kg/day, some patients may require every 8 hours dosing

Adults: Loading dose: 15-18 mg/kg in a single or divided dose; maintenance, anticonvulsant: usual: 300 mg/day or 5-6 mg/kg/day in 3 divided doses or 1-2 divided doses using extended release

Anticonvulsant: Children and Adults: Oral: Loading dose: 15-20 mg/kg; based on phenytoin serum concentrations and recent dosing history; administer oral loading dose in 3 divided doses administered every 2-4 hours to decrease GI adverse effects and to ensure complete oral absorption; maintenance dose: same as I.V.

Arrhythmias:

Children and Adults: Loading dose: I.V.: 1.25 mg/kg IVP every 5 minutes may repeat up to total loading dose: 15 mg/kg

Children: Maintenance dose: Oral, I.V.: 5-10 mg/kg/day in 2 divided doses

Adults: Maintenance dose: Oral: 250 mg 4 times/day for 1 day, 250 mg twice daily for 2 days, then maintenance at 300-400 mg/day in divided doses 1-4 times/day

**Dosage Forms**

Capsule, as sodium:

Extended: 30 mg, 100 mg

Prompt: 30 mg, 100 mg

Injection, as sodium: 50 mg/mL (2 mL, 5 mL)

Suspension, oral: 30 mg/5 mL (5 mL, 240 mL); 125 mg/5 mL (5 mL, 240 mL)

Tablet, chewable: 50 mg

**Pherazine® VC w/ Codeine** *see* promethazine, phenylephrine, and codeine *on page 501*

**Pherazine® w/DM** *see* promethazine and dextromethorphan *on page 501*

**Pherazine® With Codeine** *see* promethazine and codeine *on page 500*

**Phicon® [OTC]** *see* pramoxine *on page 490*

**Phillips'® Milk of Magnesia [OTC]** *see* magnesium hydroxide *on page 361*

**pHisoHex®** *see* hexachlorophene *on page 293*

**Phos-Ex® 62.5** ***(Discontinued)*** *see page 750*

**Phos-Ex® 125** ***(Discontinued)*** *see page 750*

**Phos-Ex® 167** ***(Discontinued)*** *see page 750*

**Phos-Ex® 250** ***(Discontinued)*** *see page 750*

**Phos-Flur®** *see* fluoride *on page 255*

**PhosLo®** *see* calcium acetate *on page 97*

**pHos-pHaid®** ***(Discontinued)*** *see page 750*

**Phosphaljel®** ***(Discontinued)*** *see page 750*

**Phospholine Iodide® Ophthalmic** *see* echothiophate iodide *on page 209*

**phosphonoformic acid** *see* foscarnet *on page 264*

## phosphorated carbohydrate solution

(FOS for ate ed kar boe HYE drate soe LOO shun)

**U.S./Canadian Brand Names** Emecheck® [OTC]; Emetrol® [OTC]; Naus-A-Way® [OTC]; Nausetrol® [OTC]

**Therapeutic Category** Antiemetic

**Use** Relief of nausea associated with upset stomach that occurs with intestinal flu, pregnancy, food indiscretions, and emotional upsets

**Usual Dosage** Oral:

Morning sickness: 15-30 mL on arising; repeat every 3 hours or when nausea threatens

Motion sickness and vomiting due to drug therapy: 5 mL doses for young children; 15 mL doses for older children and adults

Regurgitation in infants: 5 or 10 mL, 10-15 minutes before each feeding; in refractory cases: 10-15 mL, 30 minutes before each feeding

Vomiting due to psychogenic factors:

Children: 5-10 mL; repeat dose every 15 minutes until distress subsides; do not take for more than 1 hour

Adults: 15-30 mL; repeat dose every 15 minutes until distress subsides; do not take for more than 1 hour

**Dosage Forms** Liquid, oral: Fructose, dextrose, and orthophosphoric acid (120 mL, 480 mL, 4000 mL)

**Photofrin®** *see* porfimer *on page 483*

**Phrenilin®** *see* butalbital compound and acetaminophen *on page 93*

**Phrenilin Forte®** *see* butalbital compound and acetaminophen *on page 93*

***p*-hydroxyampicillin** *see* amoxicillin *on page 35*

**phylloquinone** *see* phytonadione *on this page*

## physostigmine (fye zoe STIG meen)

**Therapeutic Category** Cholinesterase Inhibitor

**Use** Reverse toxic CNS and cardiac effects caused by anticholinergics and tricyclic antidepressants; ophthalmic solution is used to treat open-angle glaucoma

**Usual Dosage**

Children: Reserve for life-threatening situations only: I.V.: 0.01-0.03 mg/kg/dose; may repeat after 15-20 minutes to a maximum total dose of 2 mg

Adults:

I.M., I.V., S.C.: 0.5-2 mg to start, repeat every 20 minutes until response occurs or adverse effect occurs

I.M., I.V. to reverse the anticholinergic effects of atropine or scopolamine administered as preanesthetic medications: Administer twice the dose, on a weight basis of the anticholinergic drug

Ophthalmic: 1-2 drops of 0.25% or 0.5% solution every 4-8 hours (up to 4 times/day); the ointment can be instilled at night

**Dosage Forms**

Injection, as salicylate: 1 mg/mL (2 mL)

Ointment, ophthalmic, as sulfate: 0.25% (3.5 g, 3.75 g)

**phytomenadione** *see* phytonadione *on this page*

## phytonadione (fye toe na DYE one)

**Synonyms** methylphytyl napthoquinone; phylloquinone; phytomenadione; vitamin $K_1$

**U.S./Canadian Brand Names** AquaMEPHYTON® Injection; Mephyton® Oral

**Therapeutic Category** Vitamin, Fat Soluble

**Use** Prevention and treatment of hypoprothrombinemia caused by vitamin K deficiency or anticoagulant-induced hypoprothrombinemia; hemorrhagic disease of the newborn

**Usual Dosage** I.V. route should be restricted for emergency use only

Hemorrhagic disease of the newborn:

Prophylaxis: I.M., S.C.: 0.5-1 mg within 1 hour of birth

Treatment: I.M., S.C.: 1-2 mg/dose/day

Oral anticoagulant overdose:

Infants: I.M., I.V., S.C.: 1-2 mg/dose every 4-8 hours

Children and Adults: Oral, I.M., I.V., S.C.: 2.5-10 mg/dose; rarely up to 25-50 mg has been used; may repeat in 6-8 hours if administered by I.M., I.V., S.C. route; may repeat 12-48 hours after oral route

Vitamin K deficiency: Due to drugs, malabsorption or decreased synthesis of vitamin K

Infants and Children:

Oral: 2.5-5 mg/24 hours

I.M., I.V.: 1-2 mg/dose as a single dose

Adults:

Oral: 5-25 mg/24 hours

I.M., I.V.: 10 mg

Minimum daily requirement: Not well established

Infants: 1-5 mcg/kg/day

Adults: 0.03 mcg/kg/day

**Dosage Forms**

Injection:

Aqueous colloidal: 2 mg/mL (0.5 mL); 10 mg/mL (1 mL, 2.5 mL, 5 mL)

Aqueous (I.M. only): 2 mg/mL (0.5 mL); 10 mg/mL (1 mL)

Tablet: 5 mg

**Pilagan® Ophthalmic *(Discontinued)*** *see page 750*

**Pilocar® Ophthalmic** *see* pilocarpine *on next page*

## pilocarpine (pye loe KAR peen)

**U.S./Canadian Brand Names** Diocarpine (Can); Isopto® Carpine Ophthalmic; Miocarpine® (Can); Ocu-Carpine® Ophthalmic; Ocusert Pilo-20® Ophthalmic; Ocusert Pilo-40® Ophthalmic; Pilocar® Ophthalmic; Pilopine HS® Ophthalmic; Piloptic® Ophthalmic; Salagen® Oral

**Therapeutic Category** Cholinergic Agent

**Use**

Ophthalmic: Management of chronic simple glaucoma, chronic and acute angle-closure glaucoma; counter effects of cycloplegics

Oral: Symptomatic treatment of xerostomia caused by salivary gland hypofunction resulting from radiotherapy for cancer of the head and neck

**Usual Dosage** Adults:

Oral: 5 mg 3 times/day, titration up to 10 mg 3 times/day may be considered for patients who have not responded adequately

Ophthalmic:

Nitrate solution: Shake well before using; instill 1-2 drops 2-4 times/day

Hydrochloride solution:

Instill 1-2 drops up to 6 times/day; adjust the concentration and frequency as required to control elevated intraocular pressure

To counteract the mydriatic effects of sympathomimetic agents: Instill 1 drop of a 1% solution in the affected eye

Gel: Instill 0.5" ribbon into lower conjunctival sac once daily at bedtime

Ocular systems: Systems are labeled in terms of mean rate of release of pilocarpine over 7 days; begin with 20 mcg/hour at night and adjust based on response

**Dosage Forms**

Ocular therapeutic system (Ocusert® Pilo): Releases 20 or 40 mcg/hour for 1 week (8s)

Tablet: 5 mg

Pilocarpine hydrochloride:

Gel, ophthalmic (Pilopine HS®): 4% (3.5 g)

Solution, ophthalmic: 0.25% (15 mL); 0.5% (15 mL, 30 mL); 1% (1 mL, 2 mL, 15 mL, 30 mL); 2% (1 mL, 2 mL, 15 mL, 30 mL); 3% (15 mL, 30 mL); 4% (1 mL, 2 mL, 15 mL, 30 mL); 5% (15 mL); 6% (15 mL, 30 mL); 8% (2 mL); 10% (15 mL)

Pilocarpine nitrate: Solution, ophthalmic (Pilagan®): 1% (15 mL); 2% (15 mL); 4% (15 mL)

## pilocarpine and epinephrine (pye loe KAR peen & ep i NEF rin)

**U.S./Canadian Brand Names** E-Pilo-x® Ophthalmic; $P_xE_x$® Ophthalmic

**Therapeutic Category** Cholinergic Agent

**Use** Treatment of glaucoma; counter effect of cycloplegics

**Usual Dosage** Ophthalmic: Instill 1-2 drops up to 6 times/day

**Dosage Forms** Solution, ophthalmic: Epinephrine bitartrate 1% and pilocarpine hydrochloride 1%, 2%, 3%, 4%, 6% (15 mL)

**Pilopine HS® Ophthalmic** *see* pilocarpine *on this page*

**Piloptic® Ophthalmic** *see* pilocarpine *on this page*

**Pilostat® Ophthalmic *(Discontinued)*** *see page 750*

**Pima®** *see* potassium iodide *on page 487*

**pimaricin** *see* natamycin *on page 411*

## pimozide (PI moe zide)

**U.S./Canadian Brand Names** Orap™

**Therapeutic Category** Neuroleptic Agent

**Use** Suppression of severe motor and phonic tics in patients with Tourette's disorder

**Usual Dosage** Children >12 years and Adults: Oral: Initial: 1-2 mg/day, then increase dosage as needed every other day; range: 7-16 mg/day, maximum dose: 20 mg/day or 0.3 mg/kg/day should not be exceeded

(Continued)

## pimozide *(Continued)*

**Dosage Forms** Tablet: 1 mg, 2 mg

## pinaverium *(Canada only)* (pin ah VEER ee um)

**U.S./Canadian Brand Names** Dicetel® (Can)

**Therapeutic Category** Calcium Antagonist; Gastrointestinal Agent, Miscellaneous

**Use** For the treatment and relief of symptoms associated with irritable bowel syndrome (IBS): abdominal pain, bowel disturbances and intestinal discomfort; treatment of symptoms related to functional disorders of the biliary tract

**Usual Dosage** Adults: Oral: Three 50 mg tablets (1 tablet 3 times a day). In exceptional cases, the dosage may be increased up to 6 tablets a day (2 tablets 3 times/day). It is recommended that the tablet be taken with a glass of water during meals or snacks. The tablet should not be swallowed when in the lying position or just before bedtime.

**Dosage Forms** Tablet, as bromide: 50 mg

## pindolol (PIN doe lole)

**U.S./Canadian Brand Names** Apo®-Pindol (Can); Gen-Pindolol (Can); Novo-Pindol (Can); Nu-Pindol (Can); PMS-Pindolol (Can); Visken®

**Therapeutic Category** Beta-Adrenergic Blocker

**Use** Management of hypertension

**Usual Dosage** Oral: 5 mg twice daily

**Dosage Forms** Tablet: 5 mg, 10 mg

**pink bismuth** *see* bismuth subsalicylate *on page 81*

**Pin-Rid® *(Discontinued)*** *see page 750*

**Pin-X® [OTC]** *see* pyrantel pamoate *on page 509*

**PIO** *see* pemoline *on page 454*

## pioglitazone (pye oh GLI ta zone)

**U.S./Canadian Brand Names** Actos™

**Therapeutic Category** Antidiabetic Agent, Oral; Thiazolidinedione Derivative

**Use**

Type 2 diabetes, monotherapy: Adjunct to diet and exercise, to improve glycemic control

Type 2 diabetes, combination therapy with sulfonylurea, metformin, or insulin: When diet, exercise, and a single agent alone does not result in adequate glycemic control

**Usual Dosage** Adults: Oral:

Monotherapy: Initial: 15-30 mg once daily; if response is inadequate, the dosage may be increased in increments up to 45 mg once daily; maximum recommended dose: 45 mg once daily

Combination therapy:

With sulfonylureas: Initial: 15-30 mg once daily; dose of sulfonylurea should be reduced if the patient reports hypoglycemia

With metformin: Initial: 15-30 mg once daily; it is unlikely that the dose of metformin will need to be reduced due to hypoglycemia

With insulin: Initial: 15-30 mg once daily; dose of insulin should be reduced by 10% to 25% if the patient reports hypoglycemia or if the plasma glucose falls to below 100 mg/dL. Doses greater than 30 mg/day have not been evaluated in combination regimens.

A 1-week washout period is recommended in patients with normal liver enzymes who are changed from troglitazone to pioglitazone therapy.

**Dosage Forms** Tablet: 15 mg, 30 mg, 45 mg

## pipecuronium (pi pe kur OH nee um)

**U.S./Canadian Brand Names** Arduan®

**Therapeutic Category** Skeletal Muscle Relaxant

**Use** Adjunct to general anesthesia, to provide skeletal muscle relaxation during surgery and to provide skeletal muscle relaxation for endotracheal intubation; recommended only for procedures anticipated to last 90 minutes or longer

**Usual Dosage** I.V.:

Children:

3 months to 1 year: Adult dosage

1-14 years: May be less sensitive to effects

Adults: Dose is individualized based on ideal body weight, ranges are 85-100 mcg/kg initially to a maintenance dose of 5-25 mcg/kg

**Dosage Forms** Injection, as bromide: 10 mg (10 mL)

## piperacillin (pi PER a sil in)

**U.S./Canadian Brand Names** Pipracil®

**Therapeutic Category** Penicillin

**Use** Treatment of serious infections caused by susceptible strains of gram-positive, gram-negative, and anaerobic bacilli; mixed aerobic-anaerobic bacterial infections or empiric antibiotic therapy in granulocytopenic patients. Its primary use is in the treatment of serious carbenicillin-resistant or ticarcillin-resistant *Pseudomonas aeruginosa* infections susceptible to piperacillin.

**Usual Dosage**

Infants and Children: I.M., I.V.: 200-300 mg/kg/day in divided doses every 4-6 hours; maximum dose: 24 g/day

Higher doses have been used in cystic fibrosis: 350-500 mg/kg/day in divided doses every 4 hours

Adults:

I.M.: 2-3 g/dose every 6-12 hours I.M.; maximum 24 g/24 hours

I.V.: 3-4 g/dose every 4-6 hours; maximum 24 g/24 hours

**Dosage Forms** Powder for injection, as sodium: 2 g, 3 g, 4 g

## piperacillin and tazobactam sodium

(pi PER a sil in & ta zoe BAK tam SOW dee um)

**U.S./Canadian Brand Names** Tazocin® (Can); Zosyn™

**Therapeutic Category** Penicillin

**Use** Treatment of infections caused by piperacillin-resistant, beta-lactamase-producing strains that are piperacillin/tazobactam susceptible involving the lower respiratory tract, urinary tract, skin and skin structures, gynecologic, intra-abdominal, and septicemia. Tazobactam expands activity of piperacillin to include beta-lactamase-producing strains of *S. aureus*, *H. influenzae*, *B. fragilis*, *Klebsiella*, *E. coli*, and *Acinetobacter*.

**Usual Dosage** Adults: I.V.: 3.375 g (3 g piperacillin/0.375 g tazobactam) every 6 hours

**Dosage Forms** Injection: Piperacillin sodium 2 g and tazobactam sodium 0.25 g; piperacillin sodium 3 g and tazobactam sodium 0.375 g; piperacillin sodium 4 g and tazobactam sodium 0.5 g (vials at an 8:1 ratio of piperacillin sodium to tazobactam sodium)

**piperazine estrone sulfate** *see* estropipate *on page 228*

**Pipracil®** *see* piperacillin *on this page*

## pirbuterol (peer BYOO ter ole)

**U.S./Canadian Brand Names** Maxair™ Inhalation Aerosol

**Therapeutic Category** Adrenergic Agonist Agent

**Use** Prevention and treatment of reversible bronchospasm including asthma

**Usual Dosage** Children >12 years and Adults: 2 inhalations every 4-6 hours for prevention; 2 inhalations at an interval of at least 1-3 minutes, followed by a third inhalation in treatment of bronchospasm, not to exceed 12 inhalations/day

**Dosage Forms**

Aerosol, oral, as acetate: 0.2 mg per actuation (25.6 g (300 inhalations))

Autohaler™: 0.2 mg per actuation (2.8 g (80 inhalations); 14 g (400 inhalations))

## piroxicam (peer OKS i kam)

**U.S./Canadian Brand Names** Alti-Piroxicam (Can); Apo®-Piroxicam (Can); Feldene®; Fexicam (Can); Gen-Piroxicam (Can); Novo-Pirocam (Can); Novo-Piroxicam (Can); Nu-Pirox (Can)

**Therapeutic Category** Analgesic, Non-narcotic; Nonsteroidal Anti-inflammatory Drug (NSAID)

**Use** Management of inflammatory disorders; symptomatic treatment of acute and chronic rheumatoid arthritis, osteoarthritis, and ankylosing spondylitis; also used to treat sunburn; dysmenorrhea

**Usual Dosage** Oral:

Children: 0.2-0.3 mg/kg/day once daily; maximum dose: 15 mg/day

Adults: 10-20 mg/day once daily; although associated with increases in GI adverse effects, doses >20 mg/day have been used (ie, 30-40 mg/day)

Therapeutic efficacy of the drug should not be assessed for at least 2 weeks after initiation of therapy or adjustment of dosage

**Dosage Forms** Capsule: 10 mg, 20 mg

## piroxicam and cyclodextrin *(Canada only)*

(peer OKS i kam & sye kloe DEKS trin)

**Therapeutic Category** Analgesic, Non-narcotic; Nonsteroidal Anti-inflammatory Drug (NSAID)

**Use** For the short-term relief of mild to moderately severe acute pain. Complexation with cyclodextrin allows faster absorption of piroxicam

**Dosage Forms** Tablet: Piroxicam-cyclodextrin 191.2 mg, equivalent to piroxicam 20 mg and cyclodextrin 171.2 mg

***p*-isobutylhydratropic acid** *see* ibuprofen *on page 311*

**PIT** *see* oxytocin *on page 446*

**Pitocin®** *see* oxytocin *on page 446*

**Pitressin®** *see* vasopressin *on page 623*

**Pitrex (Can)** *see* tolnaftate *on page 595*

**pit vipers antivenin** *see* antivenin (*Crotalidae*) polyvalent *on page 45*

## pivampicillin *(Canada only)* (piv am pi SIL in)

**U.S./Canadian Brand Names** Pondocillin® (Can)

**Therapeutic Category** Antibiotic, Penicillin

**Use** For the treatment of respiratory tract infections (including acute bronchitis, acute exacerbations of chronic bronchitis and pneumonia); ear, nose and throat infections; gynecological infections; urinary tract infections (including acute uncomplicated gonococcal urethritis) when caused by nonpenicillinase-producing susceptible strains of the following organisms: gram-positive organisms, ie, streptococci, pneumococci and staphylococci; gram-negative organisms, ie, *H. influenzae*, *N. gonorrhoeae*, *E. coli*, *P. mirabilis*.

**Usual Dosage** Oral

Suspension:

Infants 3 to 12 months: 40-60 mg/kg body weight daily divided into 2 equal doses

Children:

1 to 3 years: 5 mL (175 mg) twice daily

4 to 6 years: 7.5 mL (262.5 mg) twice daily

7 to 10 years: 10 mL (350 mg) twice daily

In children 10 years of age or less the dosage range is 25 to 35 mg/kg/day and should not exceed the recommended adult dose of 500 mg twice daily

Children over 10 years and adults: 15 mL (525 mg) twice daily. For severe infections: Dosage may be doubled.

Tablet: Adults and children over 10 years: 500 mg twice daily; double in severe infections

In gonococcal urethritis: 1.5 g as a single dose with 1 g probenecid concurrently

**Dosage Forms**

Suspension, oral: 35 mg/5 mL (100 mL, 150 mL, 200 mL)

Tablet: 500 mg (equivalent to ampicillin 377 mg)

**pix carbonis** *see* coal tar *on page 149*

## pizotifen *(Canada only)* (pi ZOE ti fen)

**U.S./Canadian Brand Names** Sandomigran® (Can); Sandomigran DS® (Can)

**Therapeutic Category** Antimigraine Agent

**Use** Migraine prophylaxis; also used for cyclical vomiting

**Usual Dosage**

Migraine prophylaxis:

Children: Up to 1.5 mg/day in divided doses

Adult: Initial: 0.5 mg; usual adult daily dose: ~1.5 mg; maximum daily dose: 4.5 mg

Cyclical vomiting: Children: 1.5 mg nightly

**Dosage Forms** Tablet, as maleate: 0.5 mg, 1 mg

**Placidyl®** *see* ethchlorvynol *on page 230*

## plague vaccine (plaig vak SEEN)

**Therapeutic Category** Vaccine, Inactivated Bacteria

**Use** Vaccination of persons at high risk exposure to plaque

**Usual Dosage** Three I.M. doses: First dose 1 mL, second dose (0.2 mL) 1 month later, third dose (0.2 mL) 5 months after the second dose; booster doses (0.2 mL) at 1- to 2-year intervals if exposure continues

**Dosage Forms** Injection: 2 mL, 20 mL

**Plan B™** *see* levonorgestrel *on page 347*

**plantago seed** *see* psyllium *on page 509*

**plantain seed** *see* psyllium *on page 509*

**Plaquenil®** *see* hydroxychloroquine *on page 306*

**Plasbumin®** *see* albumin *on page 16*

**Plasmanate®** *see* plasma protein fraction *on this page*

## plasma protein fraction (PLAS mah PROE teen FRAK shun)

**U.S./Canadian Brand Names** Plasmanate®

**Therapeutic Category** Blood Product Derivative

**Use** Plasma volume expansion and maintenance of cardiac output in the treatment of certain types of shock or impending shock

**Usual Dosage** I.V.: 250-1500 mL/day

**Dosage Forms** Injection: 5% (50 mL, 250 mL, 500 mL)

**Plasmatein®** ***(Discontinued)*** *see page 750*

**Platinol®** *see* cisplatin *on page 139*

**Platinol®-AQ** *see* cisplatin *on page 139*

**Plavix®** *see* clopidogrel *on page 146*

**Plendil®** *see* felodipine *on page 242*

**Pletal®** *see* cilostazol *on page 137*

## plicamycin (plye kay MYE sin)

**Synonyms** mithramycin

**U.S./Canadian Brand Names** Mithracin®

**Therapeutic Category** Antidote; Antineoplastic Agent

(Continued)

## plicamycin *(Continued)*

**Use** Malignant testicular tumors; treatment of hypercalcemia and hypercalciuria of malignancy not responsive to conventional treatment; chronic myelogenous leukemia in blast phase; Paget's disease

**Usual Dosage** Refer to individual protocols. Adults: I.V. (dose based on ideal body weight):

Testicular cancer: 25-50 mcg/kg/day or every other day for 5-10 days

Blastic chronic granulocytic leukemia: 25 mcg/kg over 2-4 hours every other day for 3 weeks

Paget's disease: 15 mcg/kg/day once daily for 10 days

Hypercalcemia:

25 mcg/kg single dose which may be repeated in 48 hours if no response occurs

**or** 25 mcg/kg/day for 3-4 days

**or** 25-50 mcg/kg/dose every other day for 3-8 doses

**Dosage Forms** Powder for injection: 2.5 mg

**PMS-Baclofen (Can)** *see* baclofen *on page 66*

**PMS-Benzydamine (Can)** *see* benzydamine *(Canada only) on page 75*

**PMS-Bezafibrate (Can)** *see* bezafibrate *(Canada only) on page 79*

**PMS-Bromocriptine (Can)** *see* bromocriptine *on page 86*

**PMS-Captopril (Can)** *see* captopril *on page 104*

**PMS-Carbamazepine (Can)** *see* carbamazepine *on page 105*

**PMS-Cefaclor (Can)** *see* cefaclor *on page 113*

**PMS-Cephalexin (Can)** *see* cephalexin *on page 120*

**PMS-Chloral Hydrate (Can)** *see* chloral hydrate *on page 124*

**PMS-Cholestyramine (Can)** *see* cholestyramine resin *on page 134*

**PMS-Cimetidine (Can)** *see* cimetidine *on page 137*

**PMS-Clonazepam (Can)** *see* clonazepam *on page 145*

**PMS-Conjugated Estrogens (Can)** *see* estrogens (conjugated/equine) *on page 227*

**PMS-Desipramine (Can)** *see* desipramine *on page 172*

**PMS-Dexamethasone (Can)** *see* dexamethasone (systemic) *on page 174*

**PMS-Diclofenac (Can)** *see* diclofenac *on page 181*

**PMS-Diphenhydramine (Can)** *see* diphenhydramine *on page 191*

**PMS-Dipivefrin (Can)** *see* dipivefrin *on page 194*

**PMS-Domperidone (Can)** *see* domperidone *(Canada only) on page 200*

**PMS-Erythromycin (Can)** *see* erythromycin (systemic) *on page 222*

**PMS-Fluoxetine (Can)** *see* fluoxetine *on page 256*

**PMS-Fluphenazine Decanoate (Can)** *see* fluphenazine *on page 258*

**PMS-Flutamide (Can)** *see* flutamide *on page 259*

**PMS-Fluvoxamine (Can)** *see* fluvoxamine *on page 262*

**PMS-Gemfibrozil (Can)** *see* gemfibrozil *on page 271*

**PMS-Glyburide (Can)** *see* glyburide *on page 276*

**PMS-Haloperidol LA (Can)** *see* haloperidol *on page 288*

**PMS-Hydromorphone (Can)** *see* hydromorphone *on page 305*

**PMS-Hydroxyzine (Can)** *see* hydroxyzine *on page 308*

**PMS-Indapamide (Can)** *see* indapamide *on page 316*

**PMS-Ipratropium (Can)** *see* ipratropium *on page 325*

**PMS-Isoniazid (Can)** *see* isoniazid *on page 327*

**PMS-Lactulose (Can)** *see* lactulose *on page 338*

**PMS-Levobunolol (Can)** *see* levobunolol *on page 344*

**PMS-Lindane (Can)** *see* lindane *on page 350*

**PMS-Lithium Carbonate (Can)** *see* lithium *on page 353*

**PMS-Lithium Citrate (Can)** *see* lithium *on page 353*

**PMS-Loperamide (Can)** *see* loperamide *on page 354*

**PMS-Loxapine (Can)** *see* loxapine *on page 358*

**PMS-Mefenamic Acid (Can)** *see* mefenamic acid *on page 369*

**PMS-Methylphenidate (Can)** *see* methylphenidate *on page 384*

**PMS-Metoprolol (Can)** *see* metoprolol *on page 388*

**PMS-Nystatin (Can)** *see* nystatin *on page 432*

**PMS-Oxybutynin (Can)** *see* oxybutynin *on page 443*

**PMS-Pindolol (Can)** *see* pindolol *on page 472*

**PMS-Sodium Polystyrene Sulfonate (Can)** *see* sodium polystyrene sulfonate *on page 553*

**PMS-Sotalol (Can)** *see* sotalol *on page 555*

**PMS-Sucralfate (Can)** *see* sucralfate *on page 561*

**PMS-Tamoxifen (Can)** *see* tamoxifen *on page 570*

**PMS-Temazepam (Can)** *see* temazepam *on page 572*

**PMS-Tiaprofenic (Can)** *see* tiaprofenic acid *(Canada only) on page 589*

**PMS-Timolol (Can)** *see* timolol *on page 591*

**PMS-Tobramycin (Can)** *see* tobramycin *on page 593*

**PMS-Trazodone (Can)** *see* trazodone *on page 600*

**PMS-Valproic Acid (Can)** *see* valproic acid and derivatives *on page 620*

**pneumococcal 7-valent conjugate vaccine** *see* pneumococcal conjugate vaccine (7-valent) *on this page*

## pneumococcal conjugate vaccine (7-valent)

(noo moe KOK al KON ju gate vak SEEN seven-vay lent)

**Synonyms** diphtheria $CRM_{197}$ protein; PCV7; pneumococcal 7-valent conjugate vaccine

**U.S./Canadian Brand Names** Prevnar™

**Therapeutic Category** Vaccine

**Use** Immunization of infants and toddlers against *Streptococcus pneumoniae* infection caused by serotypes included in the vaccine

American Academy of Pediatrics policy statement: Recommended for all children ≤23 months of age; it is administered concurrently with other recommended vaccines at 2-, 4-, 6-, and 12-15 months. The number of doses required depends upon the age of initiation. All children 24-59 months of age who are at high risk should receive the vaccine (see Usual Dosage).

**High Risk (attack rate of invasive pneumococcal disease >150/100,000 cases per year)**: Sickle cell disease, congenital or acquired asplenia, or splenic dysfunction, HIV infection

**Presumed High Risk (attack rate not calculated)**:

Congenital immune deficiency; Some B- (humoral) or T-lymphocyte deficiencies, complement deficiencies (particularly C1, C2, C3, and C4 deficiencies), or phagocytic disorders (excluding chronic granulomatous disease)

Chronic cardiac disease (particularly cyanotic congenital heart disease and cardiac failure)

(Continued)

## pneumococcal conjugate vaccine (7-valent) *(Continued)*

Chronic pulmonary disease (including asthma treated with high-dose oral corticosteroid therapy)

Cerebrospinal fluid leaks

Chronic renal insufficiency (including nephrotic syndrome)

Diseases associated with immunosuppressive therapy or radiation therapy (including malignant neoplasms, leukemias, lymphomas, and Hodgkin's disease) and solid organ transplant (guidelines for use of pneumococcal vaccines for children who have undergone bone marrow transplants are currently under revision)

Diabetes mellitus

**Moderate Risk (attack rate of invasive pneumococcal disease >20/100,000 per year)**:

All children 24-35 months of age

Children 36-59 months of age attending "out of home" care

Children 36-59 months of age who are Native American (American Indian or Alaska Native) or are of African American descent

**Usual Dosage** Dosing as recommended in the policy statement of the American Academy of Pediatrics: I.M. (0.5 mL each dose):

Previously unvaccinated Infants and Children:

2-6 months: Primary series: Three doses (0.5 mL each dose) at 6- to 8-week intervals; booster dose: 0.5 mL at 12-15 months of age (booster dose given at least 6-8 weeks after the final dose of primary series)

7-11 months: Primary series: Two doses (0.5 mL each dose) at 6- to 8-week intervals; booster dose: 0.5 mL at 12-15 months of age (booster dose given at least 6-8 weeks after the final dose of primary series)

12-23 months: Primary series: Two doses (0.5 mL each dose) at 6- to 8-week intervals

≥24 months: 0.5 mL as a single dose

Dosing recommendations for "High-Risk" Children (see Use):

≤23 months:

Previous doses: None

Recommendation: See dosing for "Previously Unvaccinated Infants and Children"

24-59 months:

Previous doses: Four doses PCV7

Recommendations: One dose 23PS vaccine at 24 months, at least 6-8 weeks after last dose of PCV7; one dose 23PS vaccine 3-5 years after the first dose of 23PS

Previous doses: 1-3 doses PCV7

Recommendations: One dose PCV7; one dose 23PS vaccine, at least 6-8 weeks after last dose of PCV7; one dose 23PS vaccine 3-5 years after the first dose of 23PS

Previous doses: One dose 23PS

Recommendations: Two doses PCV7 6-8 weeks apart, beginning at least 6-8 weeks after the last dose of 23PS; one dose 23PS vaccine 3-5 years after the first dose of 23PS

Previous dose: None

Recommendations: Two doses PCV7 6-8 weeks apart; one dose 23PS vaccine, at least 6-8 weeks after last dose of PCV7; one dose 23PS vaccine 3-5 years after the first dose of 23PS

**Dosage Forms** Injection; 2 mcg of each saccharide for each of six serotypes and 4 mcg of a seventh serotype; also 20 mcg of CRM197 carrier protein and 0.125 mg of aluminum phosphate adjuvant per 0.5 mL per dose

## pneumococcal polysaccharide vaccine

*see* pneumococcal vaccine *on this page*

## pneumococcal vaccine (noo moe KOK al vak SEEN)

**Synonyms** pneumococcal polysaccharide vaccine

**U.S./Canadian Brand Names** Pneumovax® 23; Pnu-Imune® 23

**Therapeutic Category** Vaccine, Inactivated Bacteria

**Use** Immunity to pneumococcal lobar pneumonia and bacteremia in individuals ≥2 years of age who are at high risk of morbidity and mortality from pneumococcal infection

**Usual Dosage** Children >2 years and Adults: I.M., S.C.: 0.5 mL

Revaccination should be considered if ≥6 years since initial vaccination; revaccination is recommended in patients who received 14-valent pneumococcal vaccine and are at highest risk (asplenic) for fatal infection, or at ≥6 years in patients with nephrotic syndrome, renal failure, or transplant recipients, or 3-5 years in children with nephrotic syndrome, asplenia, or sickle cell disease

**Dosage Forms** Injection: 25 mcg each of 23 polysaccharide isolates/0.5 mL dose (0.5 mL, 1 mL, 5 mL)

**Pneumomist®** *see* guaifenesin *on page 281*

**Pneumopent (Can)** *see* pentamidine *on page 458*

**Pneumovax® 23** *see* pneumococcal vaccine *on previous page*

**Pnu-Imune® 23** *see* pneumococcal vaccine *on previous page*

**Podactin® [OTC]** *see* tolnaftate *on page 595*

**Pod-Ben-25®** *see* podophyllum resin *on this page*

**Podocon-25™** *see* podophyllum resin *on this page*

**Podofilm® (Can)** *see* podophyllum resin *on this page*

## podofilox (po do FIL oks)

**U.S./Canadian Brand Names** Condyline™ (Can); Condylox®; Wartec® (Can)

**Therapeutic Category** Keratolytic Agent

**Use** Treatment of external genital warts

**Usual Dosage** Adults: Topical: Apply twice daily (morning and evening) for 3 consecutive days, then withhold use for 4 consecutive days; cycle may be repeated up to 4 times until there is no visible wart tissue

**Dosage Forms**

Gel, topical: 0.5% (3.5 mL)

Solution, topical: 0.5% (3.5 mL)

**Podofin®** *see* podophyllum resin *on this page*

## podophyllum resin (po DOF fil um REZ in)

**Synonyms** mandrake; may apple

**U.S./Canadian Brand Names** Pod-Ben-25®; Podocon-25™; Podofilm® (Can); Podofin®

**Therapeutic Category** Keratolytic Agent

**Use** Topical treatment of benign growths including external genital and perianal warts (condylomata acuminata), papillomas, fibroids

**Usual Dosage** Topical:

Children and Adults: 10% to 25% solution in compound benzoin tincture; apply drug to dry surface, use 1 drop at a time allowing drying between drops until area is covered; total volume should be limited to <0.5 mL per treatment session

Condylomata acuminatum: 25% solution is applied daily; use a 10% solution when applied to or near mucous membranes

Verrucae: 25% solution is applied 3-5 times/day directly to the wart

**Dosage Forms** Liquid, topical: 25% in benzoin tincture (5 mL, 7.5 mL, 30 mL)

**Point-Two®** *see* fluoride *on page 255*

**Poladex®** ***(Discontinued)*** *see page 750*

**Polaramine®** *see* dexchlorpheniramine *on page 175*

**Polargen®** ***(Discontinued)*** *see page 750*

**poliomyelitis vaccine** *see* poliovirus vaccine (inactivated) *on next page*

**Poliovax® Injection** ***(Discontinued)*** *see page 750*

## poliovirus vaccine (inactivated)

(POE lee oh VYE rus vak SEEN in ak ti VAY ted)

**Synonyms** IPV; poliomyelitis vaccine; Salk vaccine

**U.S./Canadian Brand Names** IPOL™

**Therapeutic Category** Vaccine, Live Virus and Inactivated Virus

**Use** Active immunization for the prevention of poliomyelitis

**Usual Dosage**

S.C.: 3 doses of 0.5 mL; the first 2 doses should be administered at an interval of 8 weeks; the third dose should be administered at least 6 and preferably 12 months after the second dose

Booster dose: All children who have received the 3 dose primary series in infancy and early childhood should receive a booster dose of 0.5 mL before entering school. However, if the third dose of the primary series is administered on or after the fourth birthday, a fourth (booster) dose is not required at school entry.

**Dosage Forms** Injection, Suspension: Three types of poliovirus (Types 1, 2, and 3) grown in monkey kidney cell cultures (0.5 mL)

## poliovirus vaccine, live, trivalent, oral

(POE lee oh VYE rus vak SEEN, live, try VAY lent, OR al)

**Synonyms** OPV; Sabin vaccine; TOPV

**U.S./Canadian Brand Names** Orimune®

**Therapeutic Category** Vaccine, Live Virus

**Use** Poliovirus immunization

**Usual Dosage** Oral:

Infants: 0.5 mL dose at age 2 months, 4 months, and 18 months; optional dose may be administered at 6 months in areas where poliomyelitis is endemic

Older Children, Adolescents and Adults: Two 0.5 mL doses 8 weeks apart; third dose of 0.5 mL 6-12 months after second dose; a reinforcing dose of 0.5 mL should be administered before entry to school, in children who received the third primary dose before their fourth birthday

**Dosage Forms** Solution, oral: Mixture of type 1, 2, and 3 viruses in monkey kidney tissue (0.5 mL)

**Polocaine®** *see* mepivacaine *on page 373*

**Polycillin-N® Injection *(Discontinued)*** *see page 750*

**Polycillin® Oral *(Discontinued)*** *see page 750*

**Polycillin-PRB® *(Discontinued)*** *see page 750*

**Polycitra®** *see* sodium citrate and potassium citrate mixture *on page 550*

**Polycitra®-K** *see* potassium citrate and citric acid *on page 486*

**Polycose® [OTC]** *see* glucose polymers *on page 276*

**Polydine® [OTC]** *see* povidone-iodine *on page 489*

## polyethylene glycol solution (pol i ETH i leen GLY kol soe LOO shun)

**Synonyms** lavage solution; PEG-ES

**U.S./Canadian Brand Names** Colyte®; GoLYTELY®; Klean-Prep® (Can); MiraLax™; NuLytely®; OCL®; Peglyte® (Can)

**Therapeutic Category** Laxative

**Use** For bowel cleansing prior to GI examination

**Usual Dosage** The recommended dose for adults is 4 L of solution prior to gastrointestinal examination, as ingestion of this dose produces a satisfactory preparation in >95% of patients. The solution is usually administered orally, but may be administered via nasogastric tube to patients who are unwilling or unable to drink the solution.

Children: Oral: 25-40 mL/kg/hour for 4-10 hours

Adults:

Oral: At a rate of 240 mL (8 oz) every 10 minutes, until 4 liters are consumed or the rectal effluent is clear; rapid drinking of each portion is preferred to drinking small amounts continuously

Nasogastric tube: At the rate of 20-30 mL/minute (1.2-1.8 L/hour); the first bowel movement should occur approximately one hour after the start of administration

**Dosage Forms**

Oral solution (OCL®): PEG 3350 6 g, sodium sulfate decahydrate 1.29 g, sodium bicarbonate 168 mg, potassium chloride 75 mg, and polysorbate 80 30 mg per 100 mL (1500 mL)

Powder for oral solution

Colyte®:

Regular & Pineapple flavor [to make 1 gallon]: PEG 3350 227.1 g, sodium sulfate 21.5 g, sodium bicarbonate 6.36 g, sodium chloride 5.53 g, and potassium chloride 2.82 g

Citrus berry, lemon lime, cherry, pineapple [to make 4000 mL]: PEG 3350 240 g, sodium sulfate 22.72 g, sodium bicarbonate 6.72 g, sodium chloride 5.84 g, and potassium chloride 2.98 g

GoLYTELY®:

Disposable jugs [to make 4000 mL]: PEG 3350 236 g, sodium sulfate 22.74 g, sodium bicarbonate 6.74 g, sodium chloride 5.86 g, and potassium chloride 2.97 g

Packets [to make 4000 mL]: PEG 3350 227.1 g, sodium sulfate 21.5 g, sodium bicarbonate 6.36 g, sodium chloride 5.53 g, and potassium chloride 2.82 g

MiraLax™ [does not contain electrolytes]: PEG 3350 255 g (to make 14 oz); PEG 3350 527 g (to make 26 oz)

NuLytely® (cherry and lemon-lime) [to make 4000 mL]: PEG 3350 420 g, sodium bicarbonate 5.72 g, sodium chloride 11.2 g, and potassium chloride 1.48 g

**Polyflex® Tablet *(Discontinued)*** *see page 750*

**Polygam® Injection *(Discontinued)*** *see page 750*

**Polygam® S/D** *see* immune globulin (intravenous) *on page 315*

**Poly-Histine CS® *(Discontinued)*** *see page 750*

**Poly-Histine-D® Capsule *(Discontinued)*** *see page 750*

**Polyminic® Sore Throat Formula [OTC]** *see* acetaminophen, dextromethorphan, and pseudoephedrine *on page 7*

**Polymox® *(Discontinued)*** *see page 750*

## polymyxin B (pol i MIKS in bee)

**Therapeutic Category** Antibiotic, Irrigation; Antibiotic, Miscellaneous

**Use** Parenteral use of polymyxin B has mainly been replaced by less toxic antibiotics; it is reserved for life-threatening infections caused by organisms resistant to the preferred drugs (eg, pseudomonal meningitis - intrathecal administration)

**Usual Dosage**

Otic: 1-2 drops, 3-4 times/day; should be used sparingly to avoid accumulation of excess debris

Infants <2 years:

I.M.: Up to 40,000 units/kg/day divided every 6 hours (not routinely recommended due to pain at injection sites)

I.V.: Up to 40,000 units/kg/day by continuous I.V. infusion

Intrathecal: 20,000 units/day for 3-4 days, then 25,000 units every other day for at least 2 weeks after CSF cultures are negative and CSF (glucose) has returned to within normal limits

Children ≥2 years and Adults:

I.M.: 25,000-30,000 units/kg/day divided every 4-6 hours (not routinely recommended due to pain at injection sites)

I.V.: 15,000-25,000 units/kg/day divided every 12 hours or by continuous infusion

Intrathecal: 50,000 units/day for 3-4 days, then every other day for at least 2 weeks after CSF cultures are negative and CSF (glucose) has returned to within normal limits

(Continued)

## polymyxin B *(Continued)*

Total daily dose should not exceed 2,000,000 units/day

Bladder irrigation: Continuous irrigant or rinse in the urinary bladder for up to 10 days using 20 mg (equal to 200,000 units) added to 1 L of normal saline; usually no more than 1 L of irrigant is used per day unless urine flow rate is high; administration rate is adjusted to patient's urine output

Topical irrigation or topical solution: 500,000 units/L of normal saline; topical irrigation should not exceed 2 million units/day in adults

Gut sterilization: Oral: 15,000-25,000 units/kg/day in divided doses every 6 hours

*Clostridium difficile* enteritis: Oral: 25,000 units every 6 hours for 10 days

Ophthalmic: A concentration of 0.1% to 0.25% is administered as 1-3 drops every hour, then increasing the interval as response indicates to 1-2 drops 4-6 times/day

**Dosing adjustment/interval in renal impairment:**

$Cl_{cr}$ 20-50 mL/minute: Administer 75% to 100% of normal dose every 12 hours

$Cl_{cr}$ 5-20 mL/minute: Administer 50% of normal dose every 12 hours

$Cl_{cr}$ <5 mL/minute: Administer 15% of normal dose every 12 hours

**Dosage Forms** Injection: 500,000 units (20 mL)

## polymyxin B and hydrocortisone

(pol i MIKS in bee & hye droe KOR ti sone)

**U.S./Canadian Brand Names** Otobiotic® Otic

**Therapeutic Category** Antibiotic/Corticosteroid, Otic

**Use** Treatment of superficial bacterial infections of external ear canal

**Usual Dosage** Otic: Instill 4 drops 3-4 times/day

**Dosage Forms** Solution, otic: Polymyxin B sulfate 10,000 units and hydrocortisone 0.5% [5 mg/mL] per mL (10 mL, 15 mL)

**Poly-Pred® Ophthalmic Suspension** *see* neomycin, polymyxin B, and prednisolone *on page 415*

## polysaccharide-iron complex (pol i SAK a ride-EYE ern KOM pleks)

**U.S./Canadian Brand Names** Ferrex® 150 [OTC]; Fe-Tinic® 150 [OTC]; Hytinic® [OTC]; Myferon® 150 [OTC]; Niferex® [OTC]; Nu-Iron® [OTC]

**Therapeutic Category** Electrolyte Supplement, Oral

**Use** Prevention and treatment of iron deficiency anemias

**Usual Dosage** Oral:

Children: 3 mg/kg 3 times/day

Adults: 200 mg 3-4 times/day

**Dosage Forms**

Capsule: Elemental iron 150 mg

Elixir: Elemental iron 100 mg/5 mL (240 mL)

Tablet: Elemental iron 50 mg

**Polysporin® Ophthalmic** *see* bacitracin and polymyxin B *on page 64*

**Polysporin® Topical** *see* bacitracin and polymyxin B *on page 64*

**Polytar® [OTC]** *see* coal tar *on page 149*

## polythiazide (pol i THYE a zide)

**U.S./Canadian Brand Names** Renese®

**Therapeutic Category** Diuretic, Thiazide

**Use** Adjunctive therapy in treatment of edema and hypertension

**Usual Dosage** Adults: Oral: 1-4 mg/day

**Dosage Forms** Tablet: 1 mg, 2 mg, 4 mg

**Polytrim® Ophthalmic** *see* trimethoprim and polymyxin B *on page 607*

**Poly-Vi-Flor®** *see* vitamin (multiple/pediatric) *on page 632*

**polyvinyl alcohol** *see* artificial tears *on page 53*

**Poly-Vi-Sol® [OTC]** *see* vitamin (multiple/pediatric) *on page 632*

**Pondimin®** ***(Discontinued)*** *see page 750*

**Pondocillin® (Can)** *see* pivampicillin *(Canada only)* *on page 474*

**Ponstan® (Can)** *see* mefenamic acid *on page 369*

**Ponstel®** *see* mefenamic acid *on page 369*

**Pontocaine®** *see* tetracaine *on page 578*

**Pontocaine® With Dextrose** *see* tetracaine and dextrose *on page 579*

## poractant alfa (por AKT ant AL fa)

**U.S./Canadian Brand Names** Curosurf®

**Therapeutic Category** Lung Surfactant

**Use** Treatment of respiratory distress syndrome (RDS) in premature infants

**Usual Dosage** Intratracheal use **only**: Premature infant with RDS: Initial dose is 2.5 mL/kg of birth weight. Up to 2 subsequent doses of 1.25 mL/kg birth weight can be administered at 12-hour intervals if needed in infants who continue to require mechanical ventilation and supplemental oxygen.

**Dosage Forms** Suspension, inhalation: 80 mg/mL (1.5 mL, 3 mL)

**Porcelana® [OTC]** *see* hydroquinone *on page 305*

**Porcelana® Sunscreen [OTC]** *see* hydroquinone *on page 305*

## porfimer (POR fi mer)

**U.S./Canadian Brand Names** Photofrin®

**Therapeutic Category** Antineoplastic Agent

**Use** Esophageal cancer: Photodynamic therapy (PDT) with porfimer for palliation of patients with completely obstructing esophageal cancer, or of patients with partially obstructing esophageal cancer who cannot be satisfactorily treated with Nd:YAG laser therapy; early-stage lung cancer (endobronchial microinvasive nonsmall cell)

**Usual Dosage** I.V. (refer to individual protocols):

Children: Safety and efficacy have not been established

Adults: I.V.: 2 mg/kg over 3-5 minutes

Photodynamic therapy is a two-stage process requiring administration of both drug and light. The first stage of PDT is the I.V. injection of porfimer. Illumination with laser light 40-50 hours following the injection with porfimer constitutes the second stage of therapy. A second laser light application may be administered 90-120 hours after injection, preceded by gentle debridement of residual tumor.

Patients may receive a second course of PDT a minimum of 30 days after the initial therapy; up to three courses of PDT (each separated by a minimum of 30 days) can be given. Before each course of treatment, evaluate patients for the presence of a tracheoesophageal or bronchoesophageal fistula.

**Dosage Forms** Powder for injection, as sodium: 75 mg

**Pork NPH Iletin® II** *see* insulin preparations *on page 319*

**Pork Regular Iletin® II** *see* insulin preparations *on page 319*

**Portagen® [OTC]** *see* nutritional formula, enteral/oral *on page 432*

**Posicor®** ***(Discontinued)*** *see page 750*

**Posture® [OTC]** *see* calcium phosphate (dibasic) *on page 100*

**Potasalan®** *see* potassium chloride *on page 485*

## potassium acetate (poe TASS ee um AS e tate)

**Therapeutic Category** Electrolyte Supplement, Oral

**Use** Potassium deficiency, treatment of hypokalemia, correction of metabolic acidosis through conversion of acetate to bicarbonate

(Continued)

## potassium acetate *(Continued)*

**Usual Dosage** I.V. infusion:

Children: Not to exceed 3 mEq/kg/day

Adults: Up to 150 mEq/day administered at a rate up to 20 mEq/hour; maximum concentration: 40 mEq/L

**Dosage Forms** Injection: 2 mEq/mL (20 mL, 50 mL, 100 mL); 4 mEq/mL (50 mL)

## potassium acetate, potassium bicarbonate, and potassium citrate

(poe TASS ee um AS e tate, poe TASS ee um bye KAR bun ate, & poe TASS ee um SIT rate)

**U.S./Canadian Brand Names** Tri-K®

**Therapeutic Category** Electrolyte Supplement, Oral

**Use** Treatment or prevention of hypokalemia

**Usual Dosage** Oral:

Children: 1-4 mEq/kg/24 hours in divided doses as required to maintain normal serum potassium

Adults:

Prevention: 16-24 mEq/day in 2-4 divided doses

Treatment: 40-100 mEq/day in 2-4 divided doses

**Dosage Forms** Solution, oral: 45 mEq/15 mL from potassium acetate 1500 mg, potassium bicarbonate 1500 mg, and potassium citrate 1500 mg per 15 mL

## potassium acid phosphate (poe TASS ee um AS id FOS fate)

**U.S./Canadian Brand Names** K-Phos® Original

**Therapeutic Category** Urinary Acidifying Agent

**Use** Acidify the urine and lower urinary calcium concentration; reduces odor and rash caused by ammoniacal urine

**Usual Dosage** Adults: Oral: 1000 mg dissolved in 6-8 oz of water 4 times/day with meals and at bedtime

**Dosage Forms** Tablet, sodium free: 500 mg [potassium 3.67 mEq]

## potassium bicarbonate (poe TASS ee um bye KAR bun ate)

**U.S./Canadian Brand Names** K+ Care® Effervescent; K-Electrolyte® Effervescent; K-Gen® Effervescent; K-Lyte® Effervescent

**Therapeutic Category** Electrolyte Supplement, Oral

**Use** Potassium deficiency, hypokalemia

**Usual Dosage** Oral:

Normal daily requirements:

Children: 2-3 mEq/kg/day

Adults: 40-80 mEq/day

Prevention during diuretic therapy:

Children: 1-2 mEq/kg/day in 1-2 divided doses

Adults: 20-40 mEq/day in 1-2 divided doses

Treatment of hypokalemia: Children: 1-2 mEq/kg initially, then as needed based on frequently obtained lab values. If deficits are severe or ongoing losses are great, I.V. route should be considered.

Treatment of hypokalemia: Adults:

Potassium >2.5 mEq/L: 60-80 mEq/day plus additional amounts if needed

Potassium <2.5 mEq/L: Up to 40-60 mEq initial dose, followed by further doses based on lab values; deficits at a plasma level of 2 mEq/L may be as high as 400-800 mEq of potassium

**Dosage Forms**

Tablet for oral solution, effervescent: 6.5 mEq, 25 mEq

K+ Care® Effervescent; K-Electrolyte® Effervescent; K-Gen® Effervescent; K-Ide®; Klor-Con®/EF; K-Lyte® Effervescent: 25 mEq

## potassium bicarbonate and potassium chloride, effervescent

(poe TASS ee um bye KAR bun ate & poe TASS ee um KLOR ide, ef er VES ent)

**U.S./Canadian Brand Names** Klorvess® Effervescent; K/Lyte/CL®

**Therapeutic Category** Electrolyte Supplement, Oral

**Use** Treatment or prevention of hypokalemia

**Usual Dosage** Oral:

Children: 1-4 mEq/kg/24 hours in divided doses as required to maintain normal serum potassium

Adults:

Prevention: 16-24 mEq/day in 2-4 divided doses

Treatment: 40-100 mEq/day in 2-4 divided doses

**Dosage Forms**

Granules for oral solution, effervescent (Klorvess®): 20 mEq per packet

Tablet for oral solution, effervescent

Klorvess®: 20 mEq per packet

K/Lyte/Cl®: 25 mEq, 50 mEq per packet

## potassium bicarbonate and potassium citrate, effervescent

(poe TASS ee um bye KAR bun ate & poe TASS ee um SIT rate, ef er VES ent)

**U.S./Canadian Brand Names** Effer-K™; K-Ide®; Klor-Con®/EF; K-Lyte®; K-Vescent®

**Therapeutic Category** Electrolyte Supplement, Oral

**Use** Treatment or prevention of hypokalemia

**Usual Dosage** Oral:

Children: 1-4 mEq/kg/24 hours as required to maintain normal serum potassium

Adults:

Prevention: 16-24 mEq/day in 2-4 divided doses

Treatment: 40-100 mEq/day in 2-4 divided doses

**Dosage Forms**

Capsule, extended release: 8 mEq, 10 mEq

Powder for oral solution: 15 mEq/packet; 20 mEq/packet; 25 mEq/packet

Tablet, effervescent: 25 mEq, 50 mEq

## potassium chloride (poe TASS ee um KLOR ide)

**Synonyms** KCl

**U.S./Canadian Brand Names** Apo®-K (Can); Cena-K®; Gen-K®; K+ 10®; Kaochlor®; Kaochlor® SF; Kaon-Cl®; Kaon-Cl-10®; Kay Ciel®; K+ Care®; K-Dur® 10; K-Dur® 20; K-Lease®; K-Lor™; Klor-Con®; Klor-Con® 8; Klor-Con® 10; Klor-Con®/25; Klotrix®; K-Norm®; K-Tab®; Micro-K® 10; Micro-K® 10 Extencaps®; Micro-K® LS; Potasalan®; Roychlor® (Can); Rum-K®; Slow-K®; Ten-K®

**Therapeutic Category** Electrolyte Supplement, Oral

**Use** Potassium deficiency, treatment or prevention of hypokalemia

**Usual Dosage** I.V. doses should be incorporated into the patient's maintenance I.V. fluids, intermittent I.V. potassium administration should be reserved for severe depletion situations in patients undergoing EKG monitoring.

Normal daily requirement: Oral, I.V.:

Newborns: 2-6 mEq/kg/day

Children: 2-3 mEq/kg/day

Adults: 40-80 mEq/day

Prevention during diuretic therapy: Oral:

Children: 1-2 mEq/kg/day in 1-2 divided doses

Adults: 20-40 mEq/day in 1-2 divided doses

Treatment: Oral, I.V.:

Children: 2-3 mEq/kg/day

Adults: 40-100 mEq/day

I.V. intermittent infusion:

Children: Dose should not exceed 0.5 mEq/kg/hour, not to exceed 20 mEq/hour

Adults: 10-20 mEq/hour, not to exceed 40 mEq/hour and 150 mEq/day

(Continued)

## potassium chloride *(Continued)*

**Dosage Forms**

Capsule, controlled release (microcapsulated): 600 mg [8 mEq]; 750 mg [10 mEq]
Micro-K® Extencaps®: 600 mg [8 mEq]
K-Lease®, K-Norm®, Micro-K® 10: 750 mg [10 mEq]
Crystals for oral suspension, extended release (Micro-K® LS®): 20 mEq per packet
Infusion, concentrate: 0.1 mEq/mL, 0.2 mEq/mL, 0.3 mEq/mL, 0.4 mEq/mL
Injection, concentrate: 1.5 mEq/mL, 2 mEq/mL, 3 mEq/mL
Liquid: 10% [20 mEq/15 mL] (480 mL, 4000 mL); 20% [40 mEq/15 mL] (480 mL, 4000 mL)
Cena-K®, Kaochlor®, Kaochlor® SF, Kay Ciel®, Potasalan®: 10% [20 mEq/15 mL] (480 mL, 4000 mL)
Rum-K®: 15% [30 mEq/15 mL] (480 mL, 4000 mL)
Cena-K®, Kaon-Cl® 20%: 20% [40 mEq/15 mL]
Powder: 20 mEq per packet (30s, 100s)
K+ Care®, K-Lor™: 15 mEq per packet (30s, 100s)
Gen-K®, Kay Ciel®, K+ Care®, K-Lor™, Klor-Con®: 20 mEq per packet (30s, 100s)
K+ Care®, Klor-Con®/25: 25 mEq per packet (30s, 100s)
Tablet, controlled release (microencapsulated)
K-Dur® 10, Ten-K®: 750 mg [10 mEq]
K-Dur® 20: 1500 mg [20 mEq]
Tablet, controlled release (wax matrix): 600 mg [8 mEq]; 750 mg [10 mEq]
Kaon-Cl®: 500 mg [6.7 mEq]
Klor-Con® 8, Slow-K®: 600 mg [8 mEq]
K+ 10®, Kaon-Cl-10®, Klor-Con® 10, Klotrix®, K-Tab®: 750 mg [10 mEq]

## potassium chloride and potassium gluconate

(poe TASS ee um KLOR ide & poe TASS ee um GLOO coe nate)

**Therapeutic Category** Electrolyte Supplement, Oral

**Use** Treatment or prevention of hypokalemia

**Usual Dosage** Oral:

Children: 1-4 mEq/kg/24 hours in divided doses as required to maintain normal serum potassium
Adults:
Prevention: 16-24 mEq/day in 2-4 divided doses
Treatment: 40-100 mEq/day in 2-4 divided doses

**Dosage Forms** Solution, oral: Potassium 20 mEq/15 mL

## potassium citrate (poe TASS ee um SIT rate)

**U.S./Canadian Brand Names** Urocit®-K

**Therapeutic Category** Alkalinizing Agent

**Use** Prevention of uric acid nephrolithiasis; prevention of calcium renal stones in patients with hypocitraturia; urinary alkalinizer when sodium citrate is contraindicated

**Usual Dosage** Adults: Oral: 10-20 mEq 3 times/day with meals, up to 100 mEq/day

**Dosage Forms** Tablet: 540 mg [5 mEq], 1080 mg [10 mEq]

## potassium citrate and citric acid

(poe TASS ee um SIT rate & SI trik AS id)

**U.S./Canadian Brand Names** Polycitra®-K

**Therapeutic Category** Alkalinizing Agent

**Use** Treatment of metabolic acidosis; alkalinizing agent in conditions where long-term maintenance of an alkaline urine is desirable

**Usual Dosage** Oral:

Mild to moderate hypocitraturia: 10 mEq 3 times/day with meals
Severe hypocitraturia: Initial: 20 mEq 3 times/day or 15 mEq 4 times/day with meals or within 30 minutes after meals; do not exceed 100 mEq/day

**Dosage Forms**
Crystals for reconstitution: Potassium citrate 3300 mg and citric acid 1002 mg per packet
Solution, oral: Potassium citrate 1100 mg and citric acid 334 mg per 5 mL

## potassium citrate and potassium gluconate
(poe TASS ee um SIT rate & poe TASS ee um GLOO coe nate)
**U.S./Canadian Brand Names** Twin-K®
**Therapeutic Category** Electrolyte Supplement, Oral
**Use** Treatment or prevention of hypokalemia
**Usual Dosage** Oral:
Children: 1-4 mEq/kg/24 hours in divided doses as required to maintain normal serum potassium
Adults:
Prevention: 16-24 mEq/day in 2-4 divided doses
Treatment: 40-100 mEq/day in 2-4 divided doses
**Dosage Forms** Solution, oral: 20 mEq/5 mL from potassium citrate 170 mg and potassium gluconate 170 mg per 5 mL

## potassium gluconate (poe TASS ee um GLOO coe nate)
**U.S./Canadian Brand Names** Glu-K®; K-99®; Kaon®; K-Glucon®
**Therapeutic Category** Electrolyte Supplement, Oral
**Use** Treatment or prevention of hypokalemia
**Usual Dosage** Oral:
Normal daily requirement:
Children: 2-3 mEq/kg/day
Adults: 40-80 mEq/day
Prevention during diuretic therapy:
Children: 1-2 mEq/kg/day in 1-2 divided doses
Adults: 20-40 mEq/day in 1-2 divided doses
Treatment of hypokalemia:
Children: 2-3 mEq/kg/day in 2-4 divided doses
Adults: 40-100 mEq/day in 2-4 divided doses
**Dosage Forms**
Elixir: 20 mEq/15 mL
K-G®, Kaon®, Kaylixir®: 20 mEq/15 mL
Tablet:
Glu-K®: 2 mEq
Kaon®: 5 mEq

## potassium iodide (poe TASS ee um EYE oh dide)
**Synonyms** KI; Lugol's solution; strong iodine solution
**U.S./Canadian Brand Names** Pima®; SSKI®
**Therapeutic Category** Antithyroid Agent; Expectorant
**Use** Facilitate bronchial drainage and cough; to reduce thyroid vascularity prior to thyroidectomy and management of thyrotoxic crisis; block thyroidal uptake of radioactive isotopes of iodine in a radiation emergency
**Usual Dosage** Oral:
Adults RDA: 130 mcg
Expectorant:
Children: 60-250 mg every 6-8 hours; maximum single dose: 500 mg
Adults: 300-1000 mg 2-3 times/day, may increase to 1-1.5 g 3 times/day
Preoperative thyroidectomy: Children and Adults: 50-250 mg 3 times/day (2-6 drops strong iodine solution); administer for 10 days before surgery
Thyrotoxic crisis:
Infants <1 year: ½ adult dosage
Children and Adults: 300 mg = 6 drops SSKI® every 8 hours
Graves' disease in neonates: 1 drop of Lugol's solution every 8 hours
(Continued)

## potassium iodide *(Continued)*

Sporotrichosis:
Initial:
Preschool: 50 mg/dose 3 times/day
Children: 250 mg/dose 3 times/day
Adults: 500 mg/dose 3 times/day
Oral increase 50 mg/dose daily
Maximum dose:
Preschool: 500 mg/dose 3 times/day
Children and Adults: 1-2 g/dose 3 times/day
Continue treatment for 4-6 weeks after lesions have completely healed

**Dosage Forms**
Solution, oral:
SSKI®: 1 g/mL (30 mL, 240 mL, 473 mL)
Lugol's solution, strong iodine: 100 mg/mL with iodine 50 mg/mL (120 mL)
Syrup: 325 mg/5 mL
Tablet: 130 mg

## potassium phosphate (poe TASS ee um FOS fate)

**U.S./Canadian Brand Names** Neutra-Phos®-K
**Therapeutic Category** Electrolyte Supplement, Oral
**Use** Treatment and prevention of hypophosphatemia
**Usual Dosage** I.V. doses should be incorporated into the patient's maintenance I.V. fluids; intermittent I.V. infusion should be reserved for severe depletion situations and requires continuous cardiac monitoring. It is difficult to determine total body phosphorus deficit, the following dosages are empiric guidelines: **Note:** Doses listed as mmol of **phosphate**:

Replacement intermittent infusion: I.V.:
Children:
Low dose: 0.08 mmol/kg over 6 hours; use if recent losses and uncomplicated
Intermediate dose: 0.16-0.24 mmol/kg over 4-6 hours; use if serum phosphorus level 0.5-1 mg/dL
High dose: 0.36 mmol/kg over 6 hours; use if serum phosphorus <0.5 mg/dL
Adults: Varying dosages: 0.15-0.3 mmol/kg/dose over 12 hours; may repeat as needed to achieve desired serum level **or**
15 mmol/dose over 2 hours; use if serum phosphorus <2 mg/dL **or**
Low dose: 0.16 mmol/kg over 4-6 hours; use if serum phosphorus level 2.3-3 mg/dL
Intermediate dose: 0.32 mmol/kg over 4-6 hours; use if serum phosphorus level 1.6-2.2 mg/dL
High dose: 0.64 mmol/kg over 8-12 hours; use if serum phosphorus <1.5 mg/dL
Maintenance:
Children: 0.5-1.5 mmol/kg/24 hours I.V. or 2-3 mmol/kg/24 hours orally in divided doses
Adults: 50-70 mmol/24 hours I.V. or 50-150 mmol/24 hours orally in divided doses

**Dosage Forms**
Capsule: Neutra-Phos®-K: Phosphorus 250 mg [8 mmol] and potassium 556 mg [14.25 mEq] per capsule
Injection: Potassium phosphate monobasic anhydrous 224 mg and potassium phosphate dibasic anhydrous 236 mg per mL; [phosphorus 3 mmol and potassium 4.4 mEq per mL] (15 mL)
Powder: Neutra-Phos®-K: Phosphorus 250 mg [8 mmol] and potassium 556 mg [14.25 mEq] per packet

## potassium phosphate and sodium phosphate

(poe TASS ee um FOS fate & SOW dee um FOS fate)
**U.S./Canadian Brand Names** K-Phos® Neutral; Neutra-Phos®; Uro-KP-Neutral®
**Therapeutic Category** Electrolyte Supplement, Oral

**Use** Treatment of conditions associated with excessive renal phosphate loss or inadequate GI absorption of phosphate

**Usual Dosage** All dosage forms to be mixed in 6-8 oz of water prior to administration

Children: 2-3 mmol phosphate/kg/24 hours administered 4 times/day

Adults: 100-150 mmol phosphate/24 hours in divided doses after meals and at bedtime; 1-8 tablets or capsules/day, administered 4 times/day

**Dosage Forms**

Powder, concentrate: Phosphate 8 mmol, sodium 7.125 mEq, and potassium 7.125 mEq per 75 mL when reconstituted

Tablet: Phosphate 8 mmol, sodium 13 mEq, and potassium 1.1 mEq (114 mg of phosphorus)

## povidone-iodine (POE vi done-EYE oh dyne)

**U.S./Canadian Brand Names** ACU-dyne® [OTC]; Betadine® [OTC]; Betadine® 5% Sterile Ophthalmic Prep Solution; Betagan® [OTC]; Iodex® [OTC]; Iodex-p® [OTC]; Massengill® Medicated Douche w/Cepticin [OTC]; Minidyne® [OTC]; Operand® [OTC]; Polydine® [OTC]; Proviodine® (Can); Summer's Eve® Medicated Douche [OTC]; Yeast-Gard® Medicated Douche

**Therapeutic Category** Antibacterial, Topical

**Use** External antiseptic with broad microbicidal spectrum against bacteria, fungi, viruses, protozoa, and yeasts

**Usual Dosage** Apply as needed for treatment and prevention of susceptible microbial infections

**Dosage Forms**

Aerosol: 5% (90 mL)

Cleanser, topical: 7.5% (30 mL, 120 mL)

Concentrate:

Whirlpool: 10% (3840 mL)

Perineal wash: 10% (240 mL)

Douche: 10% [0.3% when reconstituted]

Foam, topical: 10% (250 g)

Gel, vaginal: 10% (3 oz)

Mouthwash: 0.5% (180 mL)

Ointment, topical: 10% (0.9 g foil packet, 0.94 g, 28 g, 480 g)

Pads, antiseptic gauze: 10% (3" x 9", 5" x 9")

Scrub, surgical: 7.5% (480 mL, 946 mL)

Shampoo: 7.5% (120 mL)

Solution:

Ophthalmic, sterile prep: 5% (50 mL)

Swab aid: 10% (100s)

Swabsticks, 4": 10%

Topical: 10% (240 mL, 480 mL, 946 mL)

Suppository, vaginal: 10%

**PPD** *see* tuberculin tests *on page 612*

**PPL** *see* benzylpenicilloyl-polylysine *on page 75*

**PPS** *see* pentosan polysulfate sodium *on page 459*

## pralidoxime (pra li DOKS eem)

**Synonyms** 2-PAM; 2-pyridine aldoxime methochloride

**U.S./Canadian Brand Names** Protopam® Injection

**Therapeutic Category** Antidote

**Use** Reverse muscle paralysis associated with toxic exposure to organophosphate anticholinesterase pesticides and chemicals; control of overdosage by anticholinesterase drugs used to treat myasthenia gravis

**Usual Dosage** Poisoning: I.V.:

Children: 20-50 mg/kg/dose; repeat in 1-2 hours if muscle weakness has not been relieved, then at 10- to 12-hour intervals if cholinergic signs recur

(Continued)

## pralidoxime *(Continued)*

Adults: 1-2 g; repeat in 1-2 hours if muscle weakness has not been relieved, then at 10- to 12-hour intervals if cholinergic signs recur

**Dosage Forms**

Injection: 20 mL vial containing 1 g each pralidoxime chloride with one 20 mL ampul diluent, disposable syringe, needle, and alcohol swab

Pralidoxime chloride:

Injection: 300 mg/mL (2 mL)

**PrameGel® [OTC]** *see* pramoxine *on this page*

**Pramet® FA** *see* vitamin (multiple/prenatal) *on page 632*

**Pramilet® FA** *see* vitamin (multiple/prenatal) *on page 632*

## pramipexole (pra mi PEX ole)

**U.S./Canadian Brand Names** Mirapex®

**Therapeutic Category** Dopaminergic Agent (Anti-Parkinson's)

**Use** Treatment of the signs and symptoms of idiopathic Parkinson's Disease

**Usual Dosage** Adults: Oral: Initial: 0.375 mg/day given in 3 divided doses, increase gradually by 0.125 mg/dose every 5-7 days; range: 1.5-4.5 mg/day

**Dosage Forms** Tablet: 0.125 mg, 0.25 mg, 0.5 mg, 1 mg, 1.5 mg

**Pramosone®** *see* pramoxine and hydrocortisone *on this page*

**Pramox® HC (Can)** *see* pramoxine and hydrocortisone *on this page*

## pramoxine (pra MOKS een)

**U.S./Canadian Brand Names** Anusol® Ointment [OTC]; Caladryl® Lotion; Fleet® Pain Relief [OTC]; Itch-X® [OTC]; Phicon® [OTC]; PrameGel® [OTC]; Prax® [OTC]; ProctoFoam® NS [OTC]; Tronolane® [OTC]

**Therapeutic Category** Local Anesthetic

**Use** Temporary relief of pain and itching associated with anogenital pruritus or irritation; dermatosis, minor burns or hemorrhoids

**Usual Dosage** Apply as directed, usually every 3-4 hours

**Dosage Forms**

Aerosol foam, as hydrochloride (ProctoFoam® NS): 1% (15 g)

Cream, as hydrochloride:

Prax®: 1% (30 g, 113.4 g, 454 g)

Tronolane®: 1% (30 g, 60 g)

Tronothane® HCl: 1% (28.4 g)

Gel, topical, as hydrochloride:

Itch-X®: 1% (35.4 g)

PrameGel®: 1% (118 g)

Lotion, as hydrochloride:

Caladryl® Clear: 1% (180 mL)

Prax®: 1% (15 mL, 120 mL, 240 mL)

Ointment, as hydrochloride (Anusol®): 1% (30 g)

Pads, as hydrochloride (Fleet® Pain Relief): 1% (100s)

Spray, as hydrochloride (Itch-X®): 1% (60 mL)

## pramoxine and hydrocortisone (pra MOKS een & hye droe KOR ti sone)

**U.S./Canadian Brand Names** Enzone®; Pramosone®; Pramox® HC (Can); ProctoFoam®-HC; Zone-A Forte®

**Therapeutic Category** Anesthetic/Corticosteroid

**Use** Treatment of severe anorectal or perianal inflammation

**Usual Dosage** Apply to affected areas 3-4 times/day

**Dosage Forms**

Cream, topical: Pramoxine hydrochloride 1% and hydrocortisone acetate 0.5% (30 g); pramoxine hydrochloride 1% and hydrocortisone acetate 1%

Foam, rectal: Pramoxine hydrochloride 1% and hydrocortisone acetate 1% (10 g)
Lotion, topical: Pramoxine hydrochloride 1% and hydrocortisone 0.25%; pramoxine hydrochloride 1% and hydrocortisone 2.5%; pramoxine hydrochloride 2.5% and hydrocortisone 1% (37.5 mL, 120 mL, 240 mL)

**Prandase® (Can)** *see* acarbose *on page 3*

**Prandin™** *see* repaglinide *on page 521*

**Pravachol®** *see* pravastatin *on this page*

## pravastatin (PRA va stat in)

**U.S./Canadian Brand Names** Lin-Pravastatin (Can); Pravachol®
**Therapeutic Category** HMG-CoA Reductase Inhibitor
**Use** Adjunct to diet for the reduction of elevated total and LDL-cholesterol levels in patients with hypercholesterolemia (Type IIa and IIb)
**Usual Dosage** Adults: Oral: 10-20 mg once daily at bedtime
**Dosage Forms** Tablet, as sodium: 10 mg, 20 mg, 40 mg

**Prax® [OTC]** *see* pramoxine *on previous page*

## praziquantel (pray zi KWON tel)

**U.S./Canadian Brand Names** Biltricide®
**Therapeutic Category** Anthelmintic
**Use** All stages of schistosomiasis caused by all *Schistosoma* species pathogenic to humans; clonorchiasis and opisthorchiasis
**Usual Dosage** Children >4 years and Adults: Oral:
Schistosomiasis: 20 mg/kg/dose 2-3 times/day for 1 day at 4- to 6-hour intervals
Flukes: 25 mg/kg/dose every 8 hours for 1-2 days
Cysticercosis: 50 mg/kg/day divided every 8 hours for 14 days
Tapeworms: 10-20 mg/kg as a single dose (25 mg/kg for *Hymenolepis nana*)
Clonorchiasis/opisthorchiasis: 3 doses of 25 mg/kg as a 1-day treatment
**Dosage Forms** Tablet, tri-scored: 600 mg

## prazosin (PRA zoe sin)

**Synonyms** furazosin
**U.S./Canadian Brand Names** Alti-Prazosin (Can); Apo®-Prazo (Can); Minipress®; Novo-Prazin (Can); Nu-Prazo (Can)
**Therapeutic Category** Alpha-Adrenergic Blocking Agent
**Use** Hypertension, severe congestive heart failure (in conjunction with diuretics and cardiac glycosides)
**Unlabeled use:** Symptoms of benign prostatic hyperplasia
**Usual Dosage** Oral:
Children: Initial: 5 mcg/kg/dose (to assess hypotensive effects); usual dosing interval every 6 hours; increase dosage gradually up to maintenance of 25-150 mcg/kg/day divided every 6 hours
Adults: Initial: 1 mg/dose 2-3 times/day; usual maintenance dose: 3-15 mg/day in divided doses 2-4 times/day; maximum daily dose: 20 mg
**Dosage Forms** Capsule, as hydrochloride: 1 mg, 2 mg, 5 mg

## prazosin and polythiazide (PRA zoe sin & pol i THYE a zide)

**U.S./Canadian Brand Names** Minizide®
**Therapeutic Category** Antihypertensive Agent, Combination
**Use** Management of mild to moderate hypertension
**Usual Dosage** Adults: Oral: 1 capsule 2-3 times/day
**Dosage Forms** Capsule:
1: Prazosin 1 mg and polythiazide 0.5 mg
2: Prazosin 2 mg and polythiazide 0.5 mg
5: Prazosin 5 mg and polythiazide 0.5 mg

**Precedex™** *see* dexmedetomidine *on page 176*

**Precose®** *see* acarbose *on page 3*

**Predair®** ***(Discontinued)*** *see page 750*

**Predaject-50®** ***(Discontinued)*** *see page 750*

**Predalone®** ***(Discontinued)*** *see page 750*

**Predcor®** ***(Discontinued)*** *see page 750*

**Predcor-TBA®** ***(Discontinued)*** *see page 750*

**Pred Forte® Ophthalmic** *see* prednisolone (ophthalmic) *on this page*

**Pred-G® Ophthalmic** *see* prednisolone and gentamicin *on this page*

**Predicort-50®** ***(Discontinued)*** *see page 750*

**Pred Mild® Ophthalmic** *see* prednisolone (ophthalmic) *on this page*

## prednicarbate (PRED ni kar bate)

**U.S./Canadian Brand Names** Dermatop®

**Therapeutic Category** Corticosteroid, Topical

**Use** Relief of the inflammatory and pruritic manifestations of corticosteroid-responsive dermatoses

**Usual Dosage** Adults: Topical: Apply a thin film to affected area twice daily. Therapy should be discontinued when control is achieved. If no improvement is seen, reassessment of diagnosis may be necessary.

**Dosage Forms**

Cream: 0.1% (15 g, 60 g)

Ointment, topical: 0.1% (15 g, 60 g)

**Prednicen-M®** ***(Discontinued)*** *see page 750*

**Prednicot®** *see* prednisone *on next page*

## prednisolone and gentamicin (pred NIS oh lone & jen ta MYE sin)

**U.S./Canadian Brand Names** Pred-G® Ophthalmic

**Therapeutic Category** Antibiotic/Corticosteroid, Ophthalmic

**Use** Treatment of steroid responsive inflammatory conditions and superficial ocular infections due to strains of microorganisms susceptible to gentamicin such as *Staphylococcus*, *E. coli*, *H. influenzae*, *Klebsiella*, *Neisseria*, *Pseudomonas*, *Proteus*, and *Serratia* species

**Usual Dosage** Children and Adults: Ophthalmic: 1 drop 2-4 times/day; during the initial 24-48 hours, the dosing frequency may be increased if necessary

**Dosage Forms**

Ointment, ophthalmic: Prednisolone acetate 0.6% and gentamicin sulfate 0.3% (3.5 g)

Suspension, ophthalmic: Prednisolone acetate 1% and gentamicin sulfate 0.3% (2 mL, 5 mL, 10 mL)

## prednisolone (ophthalmic) (pred NIS oh lone op THAL mik)

**U.S./Canadian Brand Names** AK-Pred® Ophthalmic; Econopred® Ophthalmic; Econopred® Plus Ophthalmic; Inflamase® Forte Ophthalmic; Inflamase® Mild Ophthalmic; Metreton® Ophthalmic; Ophtho-Tate® (Can); Pred Forte® Ophthalmic; Pred Mild® Ophthalmic

**Therapeutic Category** Adrenal Corticosteroid

**Use** Treatment of palpebral and bulbar conjunctivitis; corneal injury from chemical, radiation, thermal burns, or foreign body penetration

**Usual Dosage** Adults: Ophthalmic: 1-2 drops into conjunctival sac every hour during day, every 2 hours at night until favorable response is obtained, then use 1 drop every 4 hours

**Dosage Forms**

Solution, ophthalmic, as sodium phosphate: 0.125% (5 mL, 10 mL, 15 mL); 1% (5 mL, 10 mL, 15 mL)

Suspension, ophthalmic, as acetate: 0.12% (5 mL, 10 mL); 0.125% (5 mL, 10 mL, 15 mL); 1% (1 mL, 5 mL, 10 mL, 15 mL)

## prednisolone (systemic) (pred NIS oh lone sis TEM ik)

**Synonyms** deltahydrocortisone; metacortandralone

**U.S./Canadian Brand Names** Delta-Cortef® Oral; Key-Pred® Injection; Key-Pred-SP® Injection; Pediapred® Oral; Prednisol® TBA Injection; Prelone® Oral

**Therapeutic Category** Adrenal Corticosteroid

**Use** Treatment of endocrine disorders, rheumatic disorders, collagen diseases, dermatologic diseases, allergic states, ophthalmic diseases, respiratory diseases, hematologic disorders, neoplastic diseases, edematous states, and gastrointestinal diseases

**Usual Dosage** Dose depends upon condition being treated and response of patient; dosage for infants and children should be based on severity of the disease and response of the patient rather than on strict adherence to dosage indicated by age, weight, or body surface area. Consider alternate day therapy for long-term therapy. Discontinuation of long-term therapy requires gradual withdrawal by tapering the dose.

Children:

Acute asthma:

Oral: 1-2 mg/kg/day in divided doses 1-2 times/day for 3-5 days

I.V.: 2-4 mg/kg/day divided 3-4 times/day

Anti-inflammatory or immunosuppressive dose: Oral, I.V.: 0.1-2 mg/kg/day in divided doses 1-4 times/day

Nephrotic syndrome: Oral: Initial: 2 mg/kg/day (maximum: 80 mg/day) in divided doses 3-4 times/day until urine is protein free for 5 days (maximum: 28 days); if proteinuria persists, use 4 mg/kg/dose every other day for an additional 28 days (maximum: 120 mg/day); maintenance: 2 mg/kg/dose every other day for 28 days (maximum: 80 mg/dose); then taper over 4-6 weeks

Adults:

Oral, I.V.: 5-60 mg/day

**Dosage Forms**

Injection, as acetate (for I.M., intralesional, intra-articular, or soft tissue administration only): 25 mg/mL (10 mL, 30 mL); 50 mg/mL (30 mL)

Injection, as sodium phosphate (for I.M., I.V., intra-articular, intralesional, or soft tissue administration): 20 mg/mL (2 mL, 5 mL, 10 mL)

Injection, as tebutate (for intra-articular, intralesional, soft tissue administration only): 20 mg/mL (1 mL, 5 mL, 10 mL)

Liquid, oral, as sodium phosphate: 5 mg/5 mL (120 mL)

Syrup: 15 mg/5 mL (240 mL)

Tablet: 5 mg

**Prednisol® TBA Injection** *see* prednisolone (systemic) *on this page*

## prednisone (PRED ni sone)

**Synonyms** deltacortisone; deltadehydrocortisone

**U.S./Canadian Brand Names** Apo®-Prednisone (Can); Deltasone®; Meticorten®; Prednicot®; Strerapred®; Winpred™ (Can)

**Therapeutic Category** Adrenal Corticosteroid

**Use** Management of adrenocortical insufficiency; used for its anti-inflammatory or immunosuppressant effects

**Usual Dosage** Dose depends upon condition being treated and response of patient; dosage for infants and children should be based on severity of the disease and response of the patient rather than on strict adherence to dosage indicated by age, weight, or body surface area. Consider alternate day therapy for long-term therapy. Discontinuation of long-term therapy requires gradual withdrawal by tapering the dose.

(Continued)

## prednisone *(Continued)*

Children: Oral: 0.05-2 mg/kg/day (anti-inflammatory or immunosuppressive dose) divided 1-4 times/day

Acute asthma: Oral: 1-2 mg/kg/day in divided doses 1-2 times/day for 3-5 days

Nephrotic syndrome: Oral: Initial: 2 mg/kg/day (maximum: of 80 mg/day) in divided doses 3-4 times/day until urine is protein free for 5 days (maximum: 28 days); if proteinuria persists, use 4 mg/kg/dose every other day (maximum: 120 mg/day) for an additional 28 days; maintenance: 2 mg/kg/dose every other day for 28 days (maximum: 80 mg/day); then taper over 4-6 weeks

Children and Adults: Physiologic replacement: 4-5 mg/m$^2$/day

Adults: Oral: 5-60 mg/day in divided doses 1-4 times/day

### Dosage Forms

Solution:

Concentrate: 5 mg/mL (5 mL, 30 mL)

Oral: 5 mg/5 mL (10 mL, 20 mL, 500 mL)

Syrup: 5 mg/5 mL (120 mL, 240 mL)

Tablet: 1 mg, 2.5 mg, 5 mg, 10 mg, 20 mg, 50 mg

**Prefrin™ Ophthalmic Solution** *see* phenylephrine *on page 467*

**Pregestimil® [OTC]** *see* nutritional formula, enteral/oral *on page 432*

**pregnenedione** *see* progesterone *on page 498*

**Pregnyl®** *see* chorionic gonadotropin *on page 136*

**Prelone® Oral** *see* prednisolone (systemic) *on previous page*

**Prelu-2®** *see* phendimetrazine *on page 463*

**Preludin® *(Discontinued)*** *see page 750*

**Premarin®** *see* estrogens (conjugated/equine) *on page 227*

**Premarin® With Methyltestosterone** *see* estrogens and methyltestosterone *on page 227*

**Premphase®** *see* estrogens and medroxyprogesterone *on page 227*

**Prempro™** *see* estrogens and medroxyprogesterone *on page 227*

**prenatal vitamins** *see* vitamin (multiple/prenatal) *on page 632*

**Prenavite® [OTC]** *see* vitamin (multiple/prenatal) *on page 632*

**Prenavite® Forte (Can)** *see* vitamin (multiple/oral) *on page 632*

**Preparation H® Cleansing Pads (Can)** *see* witch hazel *on page 635*

**Prepcat®** *see* radiological/contrast media (ionic) *on page 516*

**Pre-Pen®** *see* benzylpenicilloyl-polylysine *on page 75*

**Prepidil® Vaginal Gel** *see* dinoprostone *on page 189*

**Prescription Strength Desenex® [OTC]** *see* miconazole *on page 390*

**Pressyn® (Can)** *see* vasopressin *on page 623*

**PreSun® 29 [OTC]** *see* methoxycinnamate and oxybenzone *on page 382*

**Pretz® [OTC]** *see* sodium chloride *on page 549*

**Pretz-D® [OTC]** *see* ephedrine *on page 215*

**Prevacid®** *see* lansoprazole *on page 340*

**Prevalite®** *see* cholestyramine resin *on page 134*

**Preven™** *see* ethinyl estradiol and levonorgestrel *on page 232*

**Prevex® HC (Can)** *see* hydrocortisone (topical) *on page 304*

**PreviDent®** *see* fluoride *on page 255*

**Prevnar™** *see* pneumococcal conjugate vaccine (7-valent) *on page 477*

**Prevpac™** *see* lansoprazole, amoxicillin, and clarithromycin *on page 340*

**Priftin®** *see* rifapentine *on page 527*

## prilocaine (PRIL oh kane)

**U.S./Canadian Brand Names** Citanest® Forte; Citanest® Plain

**Therapeutic Category** Local Anesthetic

**Use** In dentistry for infiltration anesthesia and for nerve block anesthesia

**Usual Dosage** Dose varies with procedure, desired depth, and duration of anesthesia, desired muscle relaxation, vascularity of tissues, physical condition, and age of patient

**Dosage Forms** Injection:

Citanest® Plain: 4% (1.8 mL)

Citanest® Forte: 4% with epinephrine bitartrate 1:200,000 (1.8 mL)

**Prilosec™** *see* omeprazole *on page 435*

**primaclone** *see* primidone *on this page*

**Primacor®** *see* milrinone *on page 394*

## primaquine (PRIM a kween)

**Synonyms** prymaccone

**Therapeutic Category** Aminoquinoline (Antimalarial)

**Use** In conjunction with a blood schizonticidal agent to provide radical cure of *P. vivax* or *P. ovale* malaria after a clinical attack has been confirmed by blood smear or serologic titer; prevention of relapse of *P. ovale* or *P. vivax* malaria; malaria postexposure prophylaxis

**Usual Dosage** Oral:

Children: 0.3 mg base/kg/day once daily for 14 days not to exceed 15 mg/day or 0.9 mg base/kg once weekly for 8 weeks not to exceed 45 mg base/week

Adults: 15 mg/day (base) once daily for 14 days or 45 mg base once weekly for 8 weeks

**Dosage Forms** Tablet, as phosphate: 26.3 mg [15 mg base]

**Primatene® Mist [OTC]** *see* epinephrine *on page 216*

**Primaxin®** *see* imipenem and cilastatin *on page 314*

## primidone (PRI mi done)

**Synonyms** desoxyphenobarbital; primaclone

**U.S./Canadian Brand Names** Apo®-Primidone (Can); Mysoline®

**Therapeutic Category** Anticonvulsant; Barbiturate

**Use** Management of generalized tonic-clonic (grand mal), complex partial and simple partial (focal) seizures

**Usual Dosage** Oral:

Children <8 years: Initial: 50-125 mg/day given at bedtime; increase by 50-125 mg/day increments every 3-7 days; usual dose: 10-25 mg/kg/day in divided doses 3-4 times/day

Children >8 years and Adults: Initial: 125-250 mg/day at bedtime; increase by 125-250 mg/day every 3-7 days; usual dose: 750-1500 mg/day in divided doses 3-4 times/day with maximum dosage of 2 g/day

**Dosage Forms**

Suspension, oral: 250 mg/5 mL (240 mL)

Tablet: 50 mg, 250 mg

**Primsol®** *see* trimethoprim *on page 607*

**Principen®** *see* ampicillin *on page 39*

**Prinivil®** *see* lisinopril *on page 352*

**Prinzide®** *see* lisinopril and hydrochlorothiazide *on page 353*

**Priorix™ (Can)** *see* measles, mumps, and rubella vaccines, combined *on page 366*

**Priscoline®** *see* tolazoline *on page 594*

**pristinamycin** *see* quinupristin and dalfopristin *on page 515*

**Privine® Nasal [OTC]** *see* naphazoline *on page 409*

**ProAmatine** *see* midodrine *on page 392*

**Proampacin®** ***(Discontinued)*** *see page 750*

**Pro-Banthine®** ***(Discontinued)*** *see page 750*

**Pro-Banthine® (Can)** *see* propantheline *on page 502*

## probenecid (proe BEN e sid)

**U.S./Canadian Brand Names** Benuryl™ (Can)

**Therapeutic Category** Uricosuric Agent

**Use** Prevention of gouty arthritis; hyperuricemia; prolong serum levels of penicillin/cephalosporin

**Usual Dosage** Oral:

Children:

<2 years: Not recommended

2-14 years: Prolong penicillin serum levels: 25 mg/kg starting dose, then 40 mg/kg/day administered 4 times/day

Gonorrhea: <45 kg: 25 mg/kg x 1 (maximum: 1 g/dose) 30 minutes before penicillin, ampicillin or amoxicillin

Adults:

Hyperuricemia with gout: 250 mg twice daily for one week; increase to 500 mg 2 times/day; may increase by 500 mg/month, if needed, to maximum of 2-3 g/day (dosages may be decreased by 500 mg every 6 months if serum urate concentrations are controlled)

Prolong penicillin serum levels: 500 mg 4 times/day

Gonorrhea: 1 g 30 minutes before penicillin, ampicillin or amoxicillin

**Dosage Forms** Tablet: 500 mg

## procainamide (proe kane A mide)

**Synonyms** procaine amide hydrochloride

**U.S./Canadian Brand Names** Apo®-Procainamide (Can); Procanbid®; Procan™ SR (Can); Pronestyl®; Pronestyl-SR®

**Therapeutic Category** Antiarrhythmic Agent, Class I-A

**Use** Ventricular tachycardia, premature ventricular contractions, paroxysmal atrial tachycardia, and atrial fibrillation; to prevent recurrence of ventricular tachycardia, paroxysmal supraventricular tachycardia, atrial fibrillation or flutter

**Usual Dosage** Must be titrated to patient's response

Children:

Oral: 15-50 mg/kg/24 hours divided every 3-6 hours; maximum 4 g/24 hours

I.M.: 20-30 mg/kg/24 hours divided every 4-6 hours in divided doses; maximum 4 g/24 hours

I.V.: Load: 3-6 mg/kg/dose over 5 minutes not to exceed 100 mg/dose; may repeat every 5-10 minutes to maximum of 15 mg/kg/load; maintenance as continuous I.V. infusion: 20-80 mcg/kg/minute; maximum: 2 g/24 hours

Adults:

Oral: 250-500 mg/dose every 3-6 hours or 500 mg to 1 g every 6 hours sustained release; usual dose: 50 mg/kg/24 hours or 2-4 g/24 hours

I.V.: Load: 50-100 mg/dose, repeated every 5-10 minutes until patient controlled; or load with 15-18 mg/kg, maximum loading dose: 1-1.5 g; maintenance: 2-6 mg/minute continuous I.V. infusion, usual maintenance: 3-4 mg/minute

**Dosage Forms**

Capsule, as hydrochloride: 250 mg, 375 mg, 500 mg

Injection, as hydrochloride: 100 mg/mL (10 mL); 500 mg/mL (2 mL)

Tablet, as hydrochloride: 250 mg, 375 mg, 500 mg

Tablet, as hydrochloride, sustained release: 250 mg, 500 mg, 750 mg, 1000 mg

Tablet, as hydrochloride, sustained release (Procanbid®): 500 mg, 1000 mg

**procaine** (PROE kane)

**U.S./Canadian Brand Names** Novocain®

**Therapeutic Category** Local Anesthetic

**Use** Produce spinal anesthesia and epidural and peripheral nerve block by injection and infiltration methods

**Usual Dosage** Dose varies with procedure, desired depth and duration of anesthesia, desired muscle relaxation, vascularity of tissues, physical condition, and age of patient

**Dosage Forms** Injection, as hydrochloride: 1% [10 mg/mL] (2 mL, 6 mL, 30 mL, 100 mL); 2% [20 mg/mL] (30 mL, 100 mL); 10% (2 mL)

**procaine amide hydrochloride** *see* procainamide *on previous page*

**procaine benzylpenicillin** *see* penicillin G procaine *on page 457*

**procaine penicillin G** *see* penicillin G procaine *on page 457*

**Pro-Cal-Sof® [OTC]** *see* docusate *on page 197*

**Procanbid®** *see* procainamide *on previous page*

**Procan SR® *(Discontinued)*** *see page 750*

**Procan™ SR (Can)** *see* procainamide *on previous page*

**procarbazine** (proe KAR ba zeen)

**Synonyms** ibenzmethyzin; MIH; n-methylhydrazine

**U.S./Canadian Brand Names** Matulane®; Natulan® (Can)

**Therapeutic Category** Antineoplastic Agent

**Use** Treatment of Hodgkin's disease, non-Hodgkin's lymphoma, brain tumor, bronchogenic carcinoma

**Usual Dosage** Refer to individual protocols. Oral:

Children: 50-100 mg/m$^2$/day in a single dose; doses as high as 100-200 mg/m$^2$/day once daily have been used for neuroblastoma and medulloblastoma

Adults: Initial: 2-4 mg/kg/day in single or divided doses for 7 days then increase dose to 4-6 mg/kg/day until response is obtained or leukocyte count decreased <4000/mm$^3$ or the platelet count decreased <100,000/mm$^3$; maintenance: 1-2 mg/kg/day

**Dosage Forms** Capsule, as hydrochloride: 50 mg

**Procardia®** *see* nifedipine *on page 420*

**Procardia XL®** *see* nifedipine *on page 420*

**procetofene** *see* fenofibrate *on page 243*

**prochlorperazine** (proe klor PER a zeen)

**U.S./Canadian Brand Names** Compazine®; Nu-Prochlor (Can); Stemetil® (Can)

**Therapeutic Category** Phenothiazine Derivative

**Use** Management of nausea and vomiting; acute and chronic psychoses

**Usual Dosage**

Children: Oral, rectal:

>10 kg: 0.4 mg/kg/24 hours in 3-4 divided doses; **or**

9-14 kg: 2.5 mg every 12-24 hours as needed; maximum: 7.5 mg/day

14-18 kg: 2.5 mg every 8-12 hours as needed; maximum: 10 mg/day

18-39 kg: 2.5 mg every 8 hours or 5 mg every 12 hours as needed; maximum: 15 mg/day

I.M.: 0.1-0.15 mg/kg/dose; usual: 0.13 mg/kg/dose; change to oral as soon as possible

I.V.: Not recommended

Adults:

Oral: 5-10 mg 3-4 times/day; usual maximum: 40 mg/day; doses up to 150 mg/day may be required in some patients

I.M.: 5-10 mg every 3-4 hours; usual maximum: 40 mg/day; doses up to 10-20 mg every 4-6 hours may be required in some patients

(Continued)

## prochlorperazine *(Continued)*

I.V.: 2.5-10 mg; maximum 10 mg/dose or 40 mg/day; may repeat dose every 3-4 hours as needed

Rectal: 25 mg twice daily

**Dosage Forms**

Suppository, rectal: 2.5 mg, 5 mg, 25 mg (12/box)

Prochlorperazine edisylate:

Injection: 5 mg/mL (2 mL, 10 mL)

Syrup: 5 mg/5 mL (120 mL)

Prochlorperazine maleate:

Capsule, sustained action: 10 mg, 15 mg, 30 mg

Tablet: 5 mg, 10 mg, 25 mg

**Procrit®** *see* epoetin alfa *on page 218*

**Proctocort™ Rectal** *see* hydrocortisone (rectal) *on page 302*

**ProctoCream ® HC Cream** *see* hydrocortisone (rectal) *on page 302*

**proctofene** *see* fenofibrate *on page 243*

**ProctoFoam®-HC** *see* pramoxine and hydrocortisone *on page 490*

**ProctoFoam® NS [OTC]** *see* pramoxine *on page 490*

**Procyclid™ (Can)** *see* procyclidine *on this page*

## procyclidine (proe SYE kli deen)

**U.S./Canadian Brand Names** Kemadrin®; Procyclid™ (Can)

**Therapeutic Category** Anticholinergic Agent; Anti-Parkinson's Agent

**Use** Relief of symptoms of Parkinsonian syndrome and drug-induced extrapyramidal symptoms

**Usual Dosage** Adults: Oral: 2-2.5 mg 3 times/day after meals; if tolerated, gradually increase dose to 4-5 mg 3 times/day

**Dosage Forms** Tablet, as hydrochloride: 5 mg

**Procytox® (Can)** *see* cyclophosphamide *on page 159*

**Prodium™ [OTC]** *see* phenazopyridine *on page 463*

**Prodrox®** *see* hydroxyprogesterone caproate *on page 307*

**Profasi® HP** *see* chorionic gonadotropin *on page 136*

**Pro-Fast Hs®** *see* phentermine *on page 466*

**Pro-Fast SA®** *see* phentermine *on page 466*

**Pro-Fast SR®** *see* phentermine *on page 466*

**Profenal® *(Discontinued)*** *see page 750*

**Profen II® *(Discontinued)*** *see page 750*

**Profen II DM® *(Discontinued)*** *see page 750*

**Profen LA® *(Discontinued)*** *see page 750*

**Profilate-HP® *(Discontinued)*** *see page 750*

**Profilnine® SD** *see* factor IX complex (human) *on page 238*

**Proflavanol C™** *see* ascorbic acid *on page 54*

**Progestaject® Injection *(Discontinued)*** *see page 750*

**Progestasert®** *see* progesterone *on this page*

## progesterone (proe JES ter one)

**Synonyms** pregnenedione; progestin

**U.S./Canadian Brand Names** Crinone®; Progestasert®; Prometrium®

**Therapeutic Category** Progestin

**Use** Intrauterine contraception in women who have had at least 1 child, are in a stable, mutually monogamous relationship, and have no history of pelvic inflammatory disease; amenorrhea; functional uterine bleeding; replacement therapy

Oral: Prevention of endometrial hyperplasia in nonhysterectomized postmenopausal women who are receiving conjugated estrogen tablets; secondary amenorrhea

Intravaginal gel: Part of assisted reproductive technology for infertile women with progesterone deficiency; secondary amenorrhea (8% gel is used in those who fail to respond to 4%)

**Usual Dosage** Adults:

Amenorrhea: I.M.: 5-10 mg/day for 6-8 consecutive days

Functional uterine bleeding: I.M.: 5-10 mg/day for 6 doses

Contraception: Female: Intrauterine device: Insert a single system into the uterine cavity; contraceptive effectiveness is retained for 1 year and system must be replaced 1 year after insertion

Replacement therapy: Gel: Administer 90 mg once daily in women who require progesterone supplementation

Oral:

Prevention of endometrial hyperplasia (in postmenopausal women with a uterus who are receiving daily conjugated estrogen tablets): 200 mg as a single daily dose every evening for 12 days sequentially per 28 day cycle.

Amenorrhea: 400 mg every evening for 10 days.

Intravaginal gel:

Partial or complete ovarian failure (assisted reproductive technology): 90 mg (8% gel) intravaginally once daily; if pregnancy is achieved, may continue up to 10-12 weeks

Secondary amenorrhea: 45 mg (4% gel) intravaginally every other day for up to 6 doses; women who fail to respond may be increased to 90 mg (8% gel) every other day for up to 6 doses

**Dosage Forms**

Capsule: 100 mg

Gel: 4% (45 mg), 8% (90 mg)

Injection, in oil: 50 mg/mL (10 mL)

Intrauterine system, reservoir: 38 mg in silicone fluid

**progestin** *see* progesterone *on previous page*

**Proglycem® Oral** *see* diazoxide *on page 180*

**ProHIBiT® *(Discontinued)*** *see page 750*

**Prokine™ Injection *(Discontinued)*** *see page 750*

**Prolamine® *(Discontinued)*** *see page 750*

**Prolastin®** *see* alpha$_1$-proteinase inhibitor *on page 22*

**Proleukin®** *see* aldesleukin *on page 18*

**Prolixin Decanoate® Injection** *see* fluphenazine *on page 258*

**Prolixin Enanthate® Injection** *see* fluphenazine *on page 258*

**Prolixin® Injection** *see* fluphenazine *on page 258*

**Prolixin® Oral** *see* fluphenazine *on page 258*

**Proloid® *(Discontinued)*** *see page 750*

**Prolopa® (Can)** *see* levodopa and benserazide *(Canada only)* *on page 346*

**Proloprim®** *see* trimethoprim *on page 607*

**Promatussin® DM (Can)** *see* promethazine and dextromethorphan *on page 501*

## promazine (PROE ma zeen)

**Therapeutic Category** Phenothiazine Derivative

**Use** Treatment of psychoses

**Usual Dosage** I.M.:

Children >12 years: Antipsychotic: 10-25 mg every 4-6 hours

(Continued)

## promazine *(Continued)*

Adults:

Psychosis: 10-200 mg every 4-6 hours not to exceed 1000 mg/day

Antiemetic: 25-50 mg every 4-6 hours as needed

**Dosage Forms** Injection, as hydrochloride: 25 mg/mL (10 mL); 50 mg/mL (1 mL, 2 mL, 10 mL)

**Prometa® *(Discontinued)*** *see page 750*

**Prometh® *(Discontinued)*** *see page 750*

## promethazine (proe METH a zeen)

**U.S./Canadian Brand Names** Phenazine® Injection; Phenergan® Injection; Phenergan® Oral; Phenergan® Rectal; Prorex® Injection

**Therapeutic Category** Antiemetic; Phenothiazine Derivative

**Use** Symptomatic treatment of various allergic conditions and motion sickness; sedative and an antiemetic

**Usual Dosage**

Children:

Antihistamine: Oral: 0.1 mg/kg/dose every 6 hours during the day and 0.5 mg/kg/dose at bedtime as needed

Antiemetic: Oral, I.M., I.V., rectal: 0.25-1 mg/kg 4-6 times/day as needed

Motion sickness: Oral: 0.5 mg/kg 30 minutes to 1 hour before departure, then every 12 hours as needed

Sedation: Oral, I.M., I.V., rectal: 0.5-1 mg/kg/dose every 6 hours as needed

Adults:

Antihistamine:

Oral: 25 mg at bedtime or 12.5 mg 3 times/day

I.M., I.V., rectal: 25 mg, may repeat in 2 hours

Antiemetic: Oral, I.M., I.V., rectal: 12.5-25 mg every 4 hours as needed

Motion sickness: Oral: 25 mg 30 minutes to 1 hour before departure, then every 12 hours as needed

Sedation: Oral, I.M., I.V., rectal: 25-50 mg/dose

**Dosage Forms**

Injection, as hydrochloride: 25 mg/mL (1 mL, 10 mL); 50 mg/mL (1 mL, 10 mL)

Suppository, rectal, as hydrochloride: 12.5 mg, 25 mg, 50 mg

Syrup, as hydrochloride: 6.25 mg/5 mL (5 mL, 120 mL, 240 mL, 480 mL, 4000 mL); 25 mg/5 mL (120 mL, 480 mL, 4000 mL)

Tablet, as hydrochloride: 12.5 mg, 25 mg, 50 mg

## promethazine and codeine (proe METH a zeen & KOE deen)

**U.S./Canadian Brand Names** Phenergan® With Codeine; Pherazine® With Codeine; Prothazine-DC®

**Therapeutic Category** Antihistamine/Antitussive

**Controlled Substance** C-V

**Use** Temporary relief of coughs and upper respiratory symptoms associated with allergy or the common cold

**Usual Dosage** Oral (in terms of codeine):

Children: 1-1.5 mg/kg/day every 4 hours as needed; maximum: 30 mg/day **or**

2-6 years: 1.25-2.5 mL every 4-6 hours or 2.5-5 mg/dose every 4-6 hours as needed; maximum: 30 mg codeine/day

6-12 years: 2.5-5 mL every 4-6 hours as needed or 5-10 mg/dose every 4-6 hours as needed; maximum: 60 mg codeine/day

Adults: 10-20 mg/dose every 4-6 hours as needed; maximum: 120 mg codeine/day; or 5-10 mL every 4-6 hours as needed

**Dosage Forms** Syrup: Promethazine hydrochloride 6.25 mg and codeine phosphate 10 mg per 5 mL (120 mL, 180 mL, 473 mL)

## promethazine and dextromethorphan
(proe METH a zeen & deks troe meth OR fan)

**U.S./Canadian Brand Names** Phenameth® DM; Phenergan® With Dextromethorphan; Pherazine® w/DM; Promatussin® DM (Can)

**Therapeutic Category** Antihistamine/Antitussive

**Use** Temporary relief of coughs and upper respiratory symptoms associated with allergy or the common cold

**Usual Dosage** Oral:

Children:

2-6 years: 1.25-2.5 mL every 4-6 hours up to 10 mL in 24 hours

6-12 years: 2.5-5 mL every 4-6 hours up to 20 mL in 24 hours

Adults: 5 mL every 4-6 hours up to 30 mL in 24 hours

**Dosage Forms** Syrup: Promethazine hydrochloride 6.25 mg and dextromethorphan hydrobromide 15 mg per 5 mL with alcohol 7% (120 mL, 480 mL, 4000 mL)

## promethazine and phenylephrine (proe METH a zeen & fen il EF rin)

**U.S./Canadian Brand Names** Phenergan® VC Syrup; Promethazine VC Plain Syrup; Promethazine VC Syrup; Prometh® VC Plain Liquid

**Therapeutic Category** Antihistamine/Decongestant Combination

**Use** Temporary relief of upper respiratory symptoms associated with allergy or the common cold

**Usual Dosage** Oral:

Children:

2-6 years: 1.25 mL every 4-6 hours, not to exceed 7.5 mL in 24 hours

6-12 years: 2.5 mL every 4-6 hours, not to exceed 15 mL in 24 hours

Children >12 years and Adults: 5 mL every 4-6 hours, not to exceed 30 mL in 24 hours

**Dosage Forms** Liquid: Promethazine hydrochloride 6.25 mg and phenylephrine hydrochloride 5 mg per 5 mL (120 mL, 240 mL, 473 mL)

## promethazine, phenylephrine, and codeine
(proe METH a zeen, fen il EF rin, & KOE deen)

**U.S./Canadian Brand Names** Phenergan® VC With Codeine; Pherazine® VC w/ Codeine; Promethist® With Codeine; Prometh® VC With Codeine

**Therapeutic Category** Antihistamine/Decongestant/Antitussive

**Controlled Substance** C-V

**Use** Temporary relief of coughs and upper respiratory symptoms including nasal congestion

**Usual Dosage** Oral:

Children (expressed in terms of codeine dosage): 1-1.5 mg/kg/day every 4 hours, maximum: 30 mg/day **or**

<2 years: Not recommended

2 to 6 years:

Weight 25 lb: 1.25-2.5 mL every 4-6 hours, not to exceed 6 mL/24 hours

Weight 30 lb: 1.25-2.5 mL every 4-6 hours, not to exceed 7 mL/24 hours

Weight 35 lb: 1.25-2.5 mL every 4-6 hours, not to exceed 8 mL/24 hours

Weight 40 lb: 1.25-2.5 mL every 4-6 hours, not to exceed 9 mL/24 hours

6 to <12 years: 2.5-5 mL every 4-6 hours, not to exceed 15 mL/24 hours

Adults: 5 mL every 4-6 hours, not to exceed 30 mL/24 hours

**Dosage Forms** Liquid: Promethazine hydrochloride 6.25 mg, phenylephrine hydrochloride 5 mg, and codeine phosphate 10 mg per 5 mL with alcohol 7% (120 mL, 240 mL, 480 mL, 4000 mL)

**Promethazine VC Plain Syrup** *see* promethazine and phenylephrine *on this page*

**Promethazine VC Syrup** *see* promethazine and phenylephrine *on this page*

**Promethist® With Codeine** *see* promethazine, phenylephrine, and codeine *on this page*

**Prometh® VC Plain Liquid** *see* promethazine and phenylephrine *on previous page*

**Prometh® VC With Codeine** *see* promethazine, phenylephrine, and codeine *on previous page*

**Prometrium®** *see* progesterone *on page 498*

**Promit®** *see* dextran 1 *on page 177*

**Pronap-100®** *see* propoxyphene and acetaminophen *on page 504*

**Pronestyl®** *see* procainamide *on page 496*

**Pronestyl-SR®** *see* procainamide *on page 496*

**Pronto® Shampoo [OTC]** *see* pyrethrins *on page 510*

**Propac™ [OTC]** *see* nutritional formula, enteral/oral *on page 432*

**Propacet® *(Discontinued)*** *see page 750*

**Propaderm® (Can)** *see* beclomethasone *on page 68*

## propafenone (proe pa FEEN one)

**U.S./Canadian Brand Names** Rythmol®

**Therapeutic Category** Antiarrhythmic Agent, Class I-C

**Use** Life-threatening ventricular arrhythmias; an oral sodium channel blocker similar to encainide and flecainide; in clinical trials was used effectively to treat atrial flutter, atrial fibrillation and other arrhythmias, but are not labeled indications; can worsen or even cause new ventricular arrhythmias (proarrhythmic effect)

**Usual Dosage** Adults: Oral: 150 mg every 8 hours, up to 300 mg every 8 hours

**Dosage Forms** Tablet, as hydrochloride: 150 mg, 225 mg, 300 mg

**Propagest® *(Discontinued)*** *see page 750*

**Propanthel™ (Can)** *see* propantheline *on this page*

## propantheline (proe PAN the leen)

**U.S./Canadian Brand Names** Pro-Banthine® (Can); Propanthel™ (Can)

**Therapeutic Category** Anticholinergic Agent

**Use** Adjunctive treatment of peptic ulcer, irritable bowel syndrome, pancreatitis, ureteral and urinary bladder spasm; to reduce duodenal motility during diagnostic radiologic procedures

**Usual Dosage** Oral:

Antisecretory:

Children: 1-2 mg/kg/day in 3-4 divided doses

Elderly patients: 7.5 mg 3 times/day before meals and at bedtime

Antispasmodic:

Children: 2-3 mg/kg/day in divided doses every 4-6 hours and at bedtime

Adults: 15 mg 3 times/day before meals or food and 30 mg at bedtime

**Dosage Forms** Tablet, as bromide: 15 mg

## proparacaine (proe PAR a kane)

**Synonyms** proxymetacaine

**U.S./Canadian Brand Names** AK-Taine®; Alcaine®; Diocaine® (Can); Ocu-Caine®; Ophthetic®; Parcaine®

**Therapeutic Category** Local Anesthetic

**Use** Local anesthesia for tonometry, gonioscopy; suture removal from cornea; removal of corneal foreign body; cataract extraction, glaucoma surgery; short operative procedure involving the cornea and conjunctiva

**Usual Dosage** Children and Adults:

Ophthalmic surgery: Instill 1 drop of 0.5% solution in eye every 5-10 minutes for 5-7 doses

Tonometry, gonioscopy, suture removal: Instill 1-2 drops 0.5% solution in eye just prior to procedure

**Dosage Forms** Ophthalmic, solution, as hydrochloride: 0.5% (15 mL)

## proparacaine and fluorescein (proe PAR a kane & FLURE e seen)

**U.S./Canadian Brand Names** Fluoracaine® Ophthalmic

**Therapeutic Category** Diagnostic Agent; Local Anesthetic

**Use** Anesthesia for tonometry, gonioscopy; suture removal from cornea; removal of corneal foreign body; cataract extraction, glaucoma surgery

**Usual Dosage**

Tonometry, gonioscopy, suture removal: Adults: Instill 1-2 drops 0.5% solution in eye just prior to procedure

Ophthalmic surgery: Children and Adults: Instill 1 drop of 0.5% solution in eye every 5-10 minutes for 5-7 doses

**Dosage Forms** Solution: Proparacaine hydrochloride 0.5% and fluorescein sodium 0.25% (2 mL, 5 mL)

**Propine®** *see* dipivefrin *on page 194*

**Proplex® SX-T Injection *(Discontinued)*** *see page 750*

**Proplex® T** *see* factor IX complex (human) *on page 238*

## propofol (PROE po fole)

**U.S./Canadian Brand Names** Diprivan®

**Therapeutic Category** General Anesthetic

**Use** Induction or maintenance of anesthesia; sedation

**Usual Dosage** Dosage must be individualized and titrated to the desired clinical effect; however, as a general guideline:

No pediatric dose has been established

Induction: I.V.:

Adults ≤55 years, and/or ASA I or II patients: 2-2.5 mg/kg of body weight (approximately 40 mg every 10 seconds until onset of induction)

Elderly, debilitated, hypovolemic, and/or ASA III or IV patients: 1-1.5 mg/kg of body weight (approximately 20 mg every 10 seconds until onset of induction)

Maintenance: I.V. infusion:

Adults ≤55 years, and/or ASA I or II patients: 0.1-0.2 mg/kg of body weight/minute (6-12 mg/kg of body weight/hour)

Elderly, debilitated, hypovolemic, and/or ASA III or IV patients: 0.05-0.1 mg/kg of body weight/minute (3-6 mg/kg of body weight/hour)

I.V. intermittent: 25-50 mg increments, as needed

**Dosage Forms** Injection: 10 mg/mL (20 mL, 50 mL, 100 mL)

**Propoxacet-N®** *see* propoxyphene and acetaminophen *on next page*

## propoxyphene (proe POKS i feen)

**Synonyms** dextropropoxyphene

**U.S./Canadian Brand Names** Darvon®; Darvon-N®; 624® Tablets (Can)

**Therapeutic Category** Analgesic, Narcotic

**Controlled Substance** C-IV

**Use** Management of mild to moderate pain

**Usual Dosage** Adults: Oral:

Hydrochloride: 65 mg every 3-4 hours as needed for pain; maximum: 390 mg/day

Napsylate: 100 mg every 4 hours as needed for pain; maximum: 600 mg/day

**Dosage Forms**

Capsule, as hydrochloride: 65 mg

Tablet, as napsylate: 100 mg

## propoxyphene and acetaminophen

(proe POKS i feen & a seet a MIN oh fen)

**U.S./Canadian Brand Names** Darvocet-N®; Darvocet-N® 100; Pronap-100®; Propoxacet-N®; Wygesic®

**Therapeutic Category** Analgesic, Narcotic

**Controlled Substance** C-IV

**Use** Management of mild to moderate pain

**Usual Dosage** Adults: Oral:

Darvocet-N®: 1-2 tablets every 4 hours as needed; maximum: 600 mg propoxyphene napsylate/day

Darvocet-N® 100: 1 tablet every 4 hours as needed; maximum: 600 mg propoxyphene napsylate/day

**Dosage Forms** Tablet:

Darvocet-N®: Propoxyphene napsylate 50 mg and acetaminophen 325 mg

Darvocet-N® 100: Propoxyphene napsylate 100 mg and acetaminophen 650 mg

Wygesic®: Propoxyphene hydrochloride 65 mg and acetaminophen 650 mg

## propoxyphene and aspirin (proe POKS i feen & AS pir in)

**U.S./Canadian Brand Names** Darvon® Compound-65 Pulvules®

**Therapeutic Category** Analgesic, Narcotic

**Controlled Substance** C-IV

**Use** Management of mild to moderate pain

**Usual Dosage** Oral: 1-2 capsules every 4 hours as needed

**Dosage Forms**

Capsule: Propoxyphene hydrochloride 65 mg and aspirin 389 mg with caffeine 32.4 mg

Tablet (Darvon-N® with A.S.A.): Propoxyphene napsylate 100 mg and aspirin 325 mg

## propranolol (proe PRAN oh lole)

**U.S./Canadian Brand Names** Apo®-Propranolol (Can); Inderal®; Inderal® LA; Nu-Propranolol (Can)

**Therapeutic Category** Antiarrhythmic Agent, Class II; Beta-Adrenergic Blocker

**Use** Management of hypertension, angina pectoris, pheochromocytoma, essential tremor, tetralogy of Fallot cyanotic spells, and arrhythmias (such as atrial fibrillation and flutter, A-V nodal re-entrant tachycardias, and catecholamine-induced arrhythmias); prevention of myocardial infarction, migraine headache; symptomatic treatment of hypertrophic subaortic stenosis; short-term adjunctive therapy of thyrotoxicosis

**Usual Dosage**

Tachyarrhythmias:

Oral:

Children: Initial: 0.5-1 mg/kg/day in divided doses every 6-8 hours; titrate dosage upward every 3-7 days; usual dose: 2-4 mg/kg/day; higher doses may be needed; do not exceed 16 mg/kg/day or 60 mg/day

Adults: 10-80 mg/dose every 6-8 hours

I.V.:

Children: 0.01-0.1 mg/kg slow IVP over 10 minutes; maximum dose: 1 mg

Adults: 1 mg/dose slow IVP; repeat every 5 minutes up to a total of 5 mg

Hypertension: Oral:

Children: Initial: 0.5-1 mg/kg/day in divided doses every 6-12 hours; increase gradually every 3-7 days; maximum: 2 mg/kg/24 hours

Adults: Initial: 40 mg twice daily or 60-80 mg once daily as sustained release capsules; increase dosage every 3-7 days; usual dose: ≤320 mg divided in 2-3 doses/day or once daily as sustained release; maximum daily dose: 640 mg

Migraine headache prophylaxis: Oral:

Children: 0.6-1.5 mg/kg/day **or**

≤35 kg: 10-20 mg 3 times/day

>35 kg: 20-40 mg 3 times/day

Adults: Initial: 80 mg/day divided every 6-8 hours; increase by 20-40 mg/dose every 3-4 weeks to a maximum of 160-240 mg/day administered in divided doses every 6-8 hours; if satisfactory response not achieved within 6 weeks of starting therapy, drug should be withdrawn gradually over several weeks

Tetralogy spells: Children: Oral: 1-2 mg/kg/day every 6 hours as needed, may increase by 1 mg/kg/day to a maximum of 5 mg/kg/day, or if refractory may increase slowly to a maximum of 10-15 mg/kg/day

Thyrotoxicosis:

Adolescents and Adults: Oral: 10-40 mg/dose every 6 hours

Adults: I.V.: 1-3 mg/dose slow IVP as a single dose

Adults: Oral:

Angina: 80-320 mg/day in doses divided 2-4 times/day or 80-160 mg of sustained release once daily

Pheochromocytoma: 30-60 mg/day in divided doses

Myocardial infarction prophylaxis: 180-240 mg/day in 3-4divided doses

Hypertrophic subaortic stenosis: 20-40 mg 3-4 times/day

Essential tremor: 40 mg twice daily initially; maintenance doses: usually 120-320 mg/day

**Dosage Forms**

Capsule, as hydrochloride, sustained action: 60 mg, 80 mg, 120 mg, 160 mg

Injection, as hydrochloride: 1 mg/mL (1 mL)

Solution, oral, as hydrochloride (strawberry-mint flavor): 4 mg/mL (5 mL, 500 mL); 8 mg/mL (5 mL, 500 mL)

Solution, oral, concentrate, as hydrochloride: 80 mg/mL (30 mL)

Tablet, as hydrochloride: 10 mg, 20 mg, 40 mg, 60 mg, 80 mg, 90 mg

## propranolol and hydrochlorothiazide

(proe PRAN oh lole & hye droe klor oh THYE a zide)

**U.S./Canadian Brand Names** Inderide®

**Therapeutic Category** Antihypertensive Agent, Combination

**Use** Management of hypertension

**Usual Dosage** Dose is individualized

**Dosage Forms**

Capsule, long-acting (Inderide® LA):

80/50 Propranolol hydrochloride 80 mg and hydrochlorothiazide 50 mg

120/50 Propranolol hydrochloride 120 mg and hydrochlorothiazide 50 mg

160/50 Propranolol hydrochloride 160 mg and hydrochlorothiazide 50 mg

Tablet (Inderide®):

40/25 Propranolol hydrochloride 40 mg and hydrochlorothiazide 25 mg

80/25 Propranolol hydrochloride 80 mg and hydrochlorothiazide 25 mg

**Propulsid®** *see* cisapride *on page 139*

## propylhexedrine (proe pil HEKS e dreen)

**U.S./Canadian Brand Names** Benzedrex® [OTC]

**Therapeutic Category** Adrenergic Agonist Agent

**Use** Topical nasal decongestant

**Usual Dosage** Inhale through each nostril while blocking the other

**Dosage Forms** Inhaler: 250 mg

**2-propylpentanoic acid** *see* valproic acid and derivatives *on page 620*

## propylthiouracil (proe pil thye oh YOOR a sil)

**Synonyms** PTU

**U.S./Canadian Brand Names** Propyl-Thyracil® (Can)

**Therapeutic Category** Antithyroid Agent

(Continued)

## propylthiouracil *(Continued)*

**Use** Palliative treatment of hyperthyroidism, adjunct to ameliorate hyperthyroidism in preparation for surgical treatment or radioactive iodine therapy, management of thyrotoxic crisis

**Usual Dosage** Oral:

Children: Initial: 5-7 mg/kg/day in divided doses every 8 hours or
6-10 years: 50-150 mg/day
>10 years: 150-300 mg/day
Maintenance: 1/3 to 2/3 of the initial dose in divided doses every 8-12 hours

Adults: Initial: 300-450 mg/day in divided doses every 8 hours; maintenance: 100-150 mg/day in divided doses every 8-12 hours

**Dosage Forms** Tablet: 50 mg

**Propyl-Thyracil® (Can)** *see* propylthiouracil *on previous page*

**2-propylvaleric acid** *see* valproic acid and derivatives *on page 620*

**Prorex® Injection** *see* promethazine *on page 500*

**Proscar®** *see* finasteride *on page 249*

**Pro-Sof® *(Discontinued)*** *see page 750*

**Pro-Sof® Plus [OTC]** *see* docusate and casanthranol *on page 198*

**ProSom™** *see* estazolam *on page 224*

**prostaglandin $E_1$** *see* alprostadil *on page 23*

**prostaglandin $E_2$** *see* dinoprostone *on page 189*

**prostaglandin $F_2$ alpha** *see* dinoprost tromethamine *on page 190*

**Prostaphlin® *(Discontinued)*** *see page 750*

**ProStep® Patch** *see* nicotine *on page 419*

**Prostigmin®** *see* neostigmine *on page 416*

**Prostin $E_2$® Vaginal Suppository** *see* dinoprostone *on page 189*

**Prostin $F_2$ Alpha®** *see* dinoprost tromethamine *on page 190*

**Prostin VR Pediatric® Injection** *see* alprostadil *on page 23*

## protamine sulfate (PROE ta meen SUL fate)

**Therapeutic Category** Antidote

**Use** Treatment of heparin overdosage; neutralize heparin during surgery or dialysis procedures

**Usual Dosage** Children and Adults: I.V.: 1 mg of protamine neutralizes 90 USP units of heparin (lung) and 115 USP units of heparin (intestinal); heparin neutralization occurs within 5 minutes following I.V. injection; administer 1 mg for each 100 units of heparin administered in preceding 3-4 hours up to a maximum dose of 50 mg

**Dosage Forms** Injection: 10 mg/mL (5 mL, 25 mL)

**Protenate® *(Discontinued)*** *see page 750*

**Prothazine-DC®** *see* promethazine and codeine *on page 500*

**Protilase®** *see* pancrelipase *on page 448*

## protirelin (proe TYE re lin)

**Synonyms** lopremone

**U.S./Canadian Brand Names** Thyrel® TRH

**Therapeutic Category** Diagnostic Agent

**Use** Adjunct in the diagnostic assessment of thyroid function, and an adjunct to other diagnostic procedures in assessment of patients with pituitary or hypothalamic dysfunction; also causes release of prolactin from the pituitary and is used to detect defective control of prolactin secretion.

**Usual Dosage** I.V.:
Children: 7 mcg/kg to a maximum dose of 500 mcg
Adults: 500 mcg (range: 200-500 mcg)
**Dosage Forms** Injection: 500 mcg/mL (1 mL)

**Protonix®** *see* pantoprazole *on page 449*

**Protopam® Injection** *see* pralidoxime *on page 489*

**Protopam® Tablet *(Discontinued)*** *see page 750*

**Protopic® Topical: Prograf®** *see* tacrolimus *on page 569*

**Protostat® Oral** *see* metronidazole *on page 388*

## protriptyline (proe TRIP ti leen)

**U.S./Canadian Brand Names** Triptil® (Can); Vivactil®
**Therapeutic Category** Antidepressant, Tricyclic (Secondary Amine)
**Use** Treatment of various forms of depression, often in conjunction with psychotherapy
**Usual Dosage** Oral:
Adolescents: 15-20 mg/day
Adults: 15-60 mg in 3-4 divided doses
Elderly: 15-20 mg/day
**Dosage Forms** Tablet, as hydrochloride: 5 mg, 10 mg

**Protropin®** *see* human growth hormone *on page 296*

**Protylol (Can)** *see* dicyclomine *on page 183*

**Provatene® *(Discontinued)*** *see page 750*

**Proventil®** *see* albuterol *on page 16*

**Proventil® HFA** *see* albuterol *on page 16*

**Proventil® Repetabs®** *see* albuterol *on page 16*

**Provera® Oral** *see* medroxyprogesterone acetate *on page 369*

**Provigil®** *see* modafinil *on page 397*

**Proviodine® (Can)** *see* povidone-iodine *on page 489*

**Provisc®** *see* sodium hyaluronate *on page 550*

**Provocholine®** *see* methacholine *on page 377*

**Proxigel® Oral [OTC]** *see* carbamide peroxide *on page 106*

**proxymetacaine** *see* proparacaine *on page 502*

**Prozac®** *see* fluoxetine *on page 256*

**Prozac® Weekly™** *see* fluoxetine *on page 256*

**PRP-D** *see Haemophilus* B conjugate vaccine *on page 287*

**prymaccone** *see* primaquine *on page 495*

**Pseudo-Car® DM** *see* carbinoxamine, pseudoephedrine, and dextromethorphan *on page 108*

**Pseudocot-T® [OTC]** *see* triprolidine and pseudoephedrine *on page 609*

## pseudoephedrine (soo doe e FED rin)

**Synonyms** *d*-isoephedrine
**U.S./Canadian Brand Names** Actifed® Allergy Tablet (Day) [OTC]; Afrinol® [OTC]; Balminil® Decongestant (Can); Cenafed® [OTC]; Children's Silfedrine® [OTC]; Decofed® Syrup [OTC]; Drixoral® Non-Drowsy [OTC]; Efidac/24® [OTC]; Eltor® 120 (Can); Eltor® (Can); Neofed® [OTC]; PediaCare® Oral; Pseudofrin (Can); Sudafed® [OTC]; Sudafed® 12 Hour [OTC]; Sufedrin® [OTC]; Triaminic® AM Decongestant Formula [OTC]
**Therapeutic Category** Adrenergic Agonist Agent
(Continued)

## pseudoephedrine *(Continued)*

**Use** Temporary symptomatic relief of nasal congestion due to common cold, upper respiratory allergies, and sinusitis; also promotes nasal or sinus drainage

**Usual Dosage** Oral:

Children:

<2 years: 4 mg/kg/day in divided doses every 6 hours
2-5 years: 15 mg every 6 hours; maximum: 60 mg/24 hours
6-12 years: 30 mg every 6 hours; maximum: 120 mg/24 hours

Adults: 60 mg every 6 hours; maximum: 240 mg/24 hours

**Dosage Forms**

Pseudoephedrine hydrochloride:

Capsule: 60 mg
Capsule, timed release: 120 mg
Drops, oral: 7.5 mg/0.8 mL (15 mL)
Liquid: 15 mg/5 mL (120 mL); 30 mg/5 mL (120 mL, 240 mL, 473 mL)
Syrup: 15 mg/5 mL (118 mL)
Tablet: 30 mg, 60 mg
Tablet, timed release: 120 mg

Pseudoephedrine sulfate:

Extended release: 120 mg, 240 mg

**pseudoephedrine and acetaminophen** *see* acetaminophen and pseudoephedrine *on page 6*

**pseudoephedrine and acrivastine** *see* acrivastine and pseudoephedrine *on page 11*

## pseudoephedrine and dextromethorphan

(soo doe e FED rin & deks troe meth OR fan)

**U.S./Canadian Brand Names** Balminil DM D (Can); Benylin DM-D; Drixoral® Cough & Congestion Liquid Caps [OTC]; Koffex DM-D (Can); Novahistex® DM; Novahistine® DM; Robitussin® Childrens Cough & Cold; Vicks® 44D Cough & Head Congestion; Vicks® 44 Non-Drowsy Cold & Cough Liqui-Caps [OTC]

**Therapeutic Category** Antitussive/Decongestant

**Use** Temporary symptomatic relief of nasal congestion due to common cold, upper respiratory allergies, and sinusitis; also promotes nasal or sinus drainage; symptomatic relief of coughs caused by minor viral upper respiratory tract infections or inhaled irritants; most effective for a chronic nonproductive cough

**Usual Dosage** Adults: Oral: 1 capsule every 6 hours

**Dosage Forms**

Capsule: Pseudoephedrine hydrochloride 60 mg and dextromethorphan hydrobromide 30 mg

Liquid: Pseudoephedrine hydrochloride 20 mg and dextromethorphan hydrobromide 10 mg per 5 mL

## pseudoephedrine and ibuprofen

(soo doe e FED rin & eye byoo PROE fen)

**U.S./Canadian Brand Names** Advil® Cold & Sinus Caplets [OTC]; Dimetapp® Sinus Caplets [OTC]; Dristan® Sinus Caplets [OTC]; Motrin® IB Sinus [OTC]; Sine-Aid® IB [OTC]

**Therapeutic Category** Decongestant/Analgesic

**Use** Temporary symptomatic relief of nasal congestion due to common cold, upper respiratory allergies, and sinusitis; also promotes nasal or sinus drainage; sinus headaches and pains

**Usual Dosage** Adults: Oral: 1-2 caplets every 4-6 hours

**Dosage Forms** Caplet: Pseudoephedrine hydrochloride 30 mg and ibuprofen 200 mg

**Pseudofrin (Can)** *see* pseudoephedrine *on previous page*

**Pseudo-Gest Plus® Tablet [OTC]** *see* chlorpheniramine and pseudoephedrine *on page 130*

**pseudomonic acid A** *see* mupirocin *on page 402*

**Psorcon™** *see* diflorasone *on page 185*

**psoriGel® [OTC]** *see* coal tar *on page 149*

**Psorion® Topical** *see* betamethasone (topical) *on page 78*

**P&S® Shampoo [OTC]** *see* salicylic acid *on page 535*

## psyllium (SIL i yum)

**Synonyms** plantago seed; plantain seed

**U.S./Canadian Brand Names** Effer-Syllium® [OTC]; Fiberall® Powder [OTC]; Fiberall® Wafer [OTC]; Hydrocil® [OTC]; Konsyl® [OTC]; Konsyl-D® [OTC]; Metamucil® [OTC]; Metamucil® Instant Mix [OTC]; Modane® Bulk [OTC]; Novo-Mucilax (Can); Perdiem® Plain [OTC]; Reguloid® [OTC]; Serutan® [OTC]; Syllact® [OTC]; V-Lax® [OTC]

**Therapeutic Category** Laxative

**Use** Treatment of chronic atonic or spastic constipation and in constipation associated with rectal disorders; management of irritable bowel syndrome

**Usual Dosage** Oral:

Children 6-11 years: ½ to 1 rounded teaspoonful 1-3 times/day

Adults: 1-2 rounded teaspoonfuls or 1-2 packets 1-4 times/day

**Dosage Forms**

Granules: 4.03 g per rounded teaspoon (100 g, 250 g); 2.5 g per rounded teaspoon

Powder: Psyllium 50% and dextrose 50% (6.5 g, 325 g, 420 g, 480 g, 500 g)

Powder:

Effervescent: 3 g/dose (270 g, 480 g); 3.4 g/dose (single-dose packets)

Psyllium hydrophilic: 3.4 g per rounded teaspoon (210 g, 300 g, 420 g, 630 g)

Squares, chewable: 1.7 g, 3.4 g

Wafers: 3.4 g

**P.T.E.-4®** *see* trace metals *on page 598*

**P.T.E.-5®** *see* trace metals *on page 598*

**pteroylglutamic acid** *see* folic acid *on page 262*

**PTU** *see* propylthiouracil *on page 505*

**Pulmicort Respules™** *see* budesonide *on page 89*

**Pulmicort® Turbuhaler®** *see* budesonide *on page 89*

**Pulmozyme®** *see* dornase alfa *on page 201*

**Puralube® Tears Solution [OTC]** *see* artificial tears *on page 53*

**Purge® [OTC]** *see* castor oil *on page 112*

**Puri-Clens™ [OTC]** *see* methylbenzethonium chloride *on page 383*

**purified protein derivative** *see* tuberculin tests *on page 612*

**Purinethol®** *see* mercaptopurine *on page 373*

**P-V-Tussin®** *see* hydrocodone, phenylephrine, pyrilamine, phenindamine, chlorpheniramine, and ammonium chloride *on page 302*

**$P_xE_x$® Ophthalmic** *see* pilocarpine and epinephrine *on page 471*

## pyrantel pamoate (pi RAN tel PAM oh ate)

**U.S./Canadian Brand Names** Ascarel® [OTC]; Combantrin™ (Can); Pamix® [OTC]; Pin-X® [OTC]; Reese's® Pinworm Medicine [OTC]

**Therapeutic Category** Anthelmintic

**Use** Roundworm (*Ascaris lumbricoides*), pinworm (*Enterobius vermicularis*), and hookworm (*Ancylostoma duodenale* and *Necator americanus*) infestations, and trichostrongyliasis

(Continued)

## pyrantel pamoate *(Continued)*

**Usual Dosage** Children and Adults: Oral:

Roundworm, pinworm, or trichostrongyliasis: 11 mg/kg administered as a single dose; maximum dose is 1 g; dosage should be repeated in 2 weeks for pinworm infection

Hookworm: 11 mg/kg/day once daily for 3 days

**Dosage Forms**

Suspension, oral: 144 mg/mL (30 mL, 60 mL, 240 mL)

Tablet: 180 mg

## pyrazinamide (peer a ZIN a mide)

**Synonyms** pyrazinoic acid amide

**U.S./Canadian Brand Names** Tebrazid™ (Can)

**Therapeutic Category** Antitubercular Agent

**Use** In combination with other antituberculosis agents in the treatment of *Mycobacterium* tuberculosis infection (especially useful in disseminated and meningeal tuberculosis); CDC currently recommends a 3 or 4 multidrug regimen which includes pyrazinamide, rifampin, INH, and at times ethambutol or streptomycin for the treatment of tuberculosis

**Usual Dosage** Oral:

Children: 15-30 mg/kg/day in divided doses every 12-24 hours; daily dose not to exceed 2 g

Adults: 15-30 mg/kg/day in 3-4 divided doses; maximum daily dose: 2 g/day

**Dosage Forms** Tablet: 500 mg

**pyrazinoic acid amide** *see* pyrazinamide *on this page*

**Pyrecot® [OTC]** *see* acetaminophen *on page 3*

**Pyregesic® [OTC]** *see* acetaminophen *on page 3*

**Pyregesic-C®** *see* acetaminophen and codeine *on page 4*

## pyrethrins (pye RE thrins)

**U.S./Canadian Brand Names** A-200™ Shampoo [OTC]; Barc™ Liquid [OTC]; End Lice® Liquid [OTC]; Lice-Enz® Shampoo [OTC]; Pronto® Shampoo [OTC]; Pyrinex® Pediculicide Shampoo [OTC]; Pyrinyl II® Liquid [OTC]; Pyrinyl Plus® Shampoo [OTC]; R & C® Shampoo [OTC]; RID® Mousse [OTC]; RID® Shampoo [OTC]; Tisit® Blue Gel [OTC]; Tisit® Liquid [OTC]; Tisit® Shampoo [OTC]; Triple X® Liquid [OTC]

**Therapeutic Category** Scabicides/Pediculicides

**Use** Treatment of *Pediculus humanus* infestations

**Usual Dosage** Application of pyrethrins: Topical:

Apply enough solution to completely wet infested area, including hair

Allow to remain on area for 10 minutes

Wash and rinse with large amounts of warm water

Use fine-toothed comb to remove lice and eggs from hair

Shampoo hair to restore body and luster

Treatment may be repeated if necessary once in a 24-hours period

Repeat treatment in 7-10 days to kill newly hatched lice

**Dosage Forms**

Gel, topical: Pyrethrins 0.3% and piperonyl butoxide 3% with petroleum distillate 1.2% (30 g, 480 g)

Liquid, topical: Pyrethrins 0.18% and piperonyl butoxide 2.2% with petroleum distillate 5.52% (60 mL); pyrethrins 0.2% and piperonyl butoxide 2% with deodorized kerosene 0.8% (60 mL, 120 mL); pyrethrins 0.3% and piperonyl butoxide 2% (60 mL, 118 mL); pyrethrins 0.3% and piperonyl butoxide 3% (60 mL, 120 mL, 240 mL)

Mousse: Pyrethrins 0.33% and piperonyl butoxide 4% (5.5 oz)

Shampoo: Pyrethrins 0.2% and piperonyl butoxide 2% with deodorized kerosene 0.8% (118 mL); pyrethrins 0.3% and piperonyl butoxide 3% (60 mL, 118 mL); pyrethrins 0.33% and piperonyl butoxide 4% (60 mL, 120 mL)

**Pyridiate®** *see* phenazopyridine *on page 463*

**2-pyridine aldoxime methochloride** *see* pralidoxime *on page 489*

**Pyridium®** *see* phenazopyridine *on page 463*

**Pyridium Plus®** ***(Discontinued)*** *see page 750*

## pyridostigmine (peer id oh STIG meen)

**U.S./Canadian Brand Names** Mestinon® Injection; Mestinon® Oral; Regonol® Injection

**Therapeutic Category** Cholinergic Agent

**Use** Symptomatic treatment of myasthenia gravis by improving muscle strength; reversal of effects of nondepolarizing neuromuscular blocking agents

**Usual Dosage** Normally, sustained-release dosage form is used at bedtime for patients who complain of morning weakness

Myasthenia gravis:
- Oral:
  - Children: 7 mg/kg/day in 5-6 divided doses
  - Adults: Initial: 60 mg 3 times/day with maintenance dose ranging from 60 mg to 1.5 g/day; sustained-release formulation should be dosed at least every 6 hours (usually 12-24 hours)
- I.M., I.V.:
  - Children: 0.05-0.15 mg/kg/dose (maximum single dose: 10 mg)
  - Adults: 2 mg every 2-3 hours or 1/30th of oral dose

Reversal of nondepolarizing neuromuscular blocker: I.M., I.V.:
- Children: 0.1-0.25 mg/kg/dose preceded by atropine
- Adults: 10-20 mg preceded by atropine

**Dosage Forms**

Injection, as bromide: 5 mg/mL (2 mL, 5 mL)
Syrup, as bromide (raspberry flavor): 60 mg/5 mL (480 mL)
Tablet, as bromide: 60 mg

## pyridoxine (peer i DOKS een)

**Synonyms** vitamin $B_6$

**Therapeutic Category** Vitamin, Water Soluble

**Use** Prevent and treat vitamin $B_6$ deficiency, pyridoxine-dependent seizures in infants, treatment of drug-induced deficiency (eg, isoniazid or hydralazine)

**Usual Dosage**

Pyridoxine-dependent Infants:
- Oral: 2-100 mg/day
- I.M., I.V.: 10-100 mg

Dietary deficiency: Oral:
- Children: 5-10 mg/24 hours for 3 weeks
- Adults: 10-20 mg/day for 3 weeks

Drug-induced neuritis (eg, isoniazid, hydralazine, penicillamine, cycloserine): Oral treatment:
- Children: 10-50 mg/24 hours; prophylaxis: 1-2 mg/kg/24 hours
- Adults: 100-200 mg/24 hours; prophylaxis: 10-100 mg/24 hours

For the treatment of seizures and/or coma from acute isoniazid toxicity, a dose of pyridoxine hydrochloride equal to the amount of INH ingested can be administered I.M./I.V. in divided doses together with other anticonvulsants

**Dosage Forms**

Injection, as hydrochloride: 100 mg/mL (10 mL, 30 mL)
Tablet, as hydrochloride: 25 mg, 50 mg, 100 mg
Tablet, as hydrochloride, extended release: 100 mg

## pyrimethamine (peer i METH a meen)

**U.S./Canadian Brand Names** Daraprim®

**Therapeutic Category** Folic Acid Antagonist (Antimalarial)

(Continued)

## pyrimethamine *(Continued)*

**Use** Prophylaxis of malaria due to susceptible strains of plasmodia; used in conjunction with quinine and sulfadoxine for the treatment of uncomplicated attacks of chloroquine-resistant *P. falciparum* malaria; used in conjunction with fast-acting schizonticide to initiate transmission control and suppression cure; synergistic combination with sulfadiazine in treatment of toxoplasmosis

**Usual Dosage** Oral:

Malaria chemoprophylaxis:

Children: 0.5 mg/kg once weekly; not to exceed 25 mg/dose **or**

Children:

<4 years: 6.25 mg once weekly

4-10 years: 12.5 mg once weekly

Children >10 years and Adults: 25 mg once weekly

Dosage should be continued for all age groups for at least 6-10 weeks after leaving endemic areas

Chloroquine-resistant *P. falciparum* malaria (when used in conjunction with quinine and sulfadiazine):

Children:

<10 kg: 6.25 mg/day once daily for 3 days

10-20 kg: 12.5 mg/day once daily for 3 days

20-40 kg: 25 mg/day once daily for 3 days

Adults: 25 mg twice daily for 3 days

Toxoplasmosis (with sulfadiazine or trisulfapyrimidines):

Children: 1 mg/kg/day divided into 2 equal daily doses; decrease dose after 2-4 days by 50%, continue for about 1 month; used with 100 mg sulfadiazine/kg/day divided every 6 hours; **or** 2 mg/kg/day divided every 12 hours for 3 days followed by 1 mg/kg/day once daily for 4 weeks

Adults: 50-75 mg/day together with 1-4 g of a sulfonamide for 1-3 weeks depending on patient's tolerance and response

**Dosage Forms** Tablet: 25 mg

**Pyrinex® Pediculicide Shampoo [OTC]** *see* pyrethrins *on page 510*

**Pyrinyl II® Liquid [OTC]** *see* pyrethrins *on page 510*

**Pyrinyl Plus® Shampoo [OTC]** *see* pyrethrins *on page 510*

## pyrithione zinc (peer i THYE one zingk)

**U.S./Canadian Brand Names** DHS Zinc® [OTC]; Head & Shoulders® [OTC]; Sebulon® Shampoo [OTC]; Theraplex Z® [OTC]; Zincon® Shampoo [OTC]; ZNP® Bar [OTC]

**Therapeutic Category** Antiseborrheic Agent, Topical

**Use** Relieves the itching, irritation and scalp flaking associated with dandruff and/or seborrheal dermatitis of the scalp

**Usual Dosage** Topical: Shampoo hair twice weekly, wet hair, apply to scalp and massage vigorously, rinse and repeat

**Dosage Forms**

Bar: 2% (119 g)

Shampoo: 1% (120 mL); 2% (120 mL, 180 mL, 240 mL, 360 mL)

**Q-Gesic® [OTC]** *see* acetaminophen and phenyltoloxamine *on page 5*

**Q-Naftate® [OTC]** *see* tolnaftate *on page 595*

**Q-Pap® [OTC]** *see* acetaminophen *on page 3*

**Q-Pap® Children's [OTC]** *see* acetaminophen *on page 3*

## quazepam (KWAY ze pam)

**U.S./Canadian Brand Names** Doral®

**Therapeutic Category** Benzodiazepine

**Controlled Substance** C-IV

**Use** Short-term treatment of insomnia

**Usual Dosage** Adults: Oral: Initial: 15 mg at bedtime; in some patients the dose may be reduced to 7.5 mg after a few nights

**Dosage Forms** Tablet: 7.5 mg, 15 mg

**Quelicin®** *see* succinylcholine *on page 560*

**Quenalog®** *see* nystatin and triamcinolone *on page 433*

**Questran®** *see* cholestyramine resin *on page 134*

**Questran® Light** *see* cholestyramine resin *on page 134*

**Questran® Tablet *(Discontinued)*** *see page 750*

## quetiapine (kwe TYE a peen)

**U.S./Canadian Brand Names** Seroquel®

**Therapeutic Category** Antipsychotic Agent

**Use** Management of psychotic disorders; this antipsychotic drug belongs to a new chemical class, the dibenzothiazepine derivatives

**Usual Dosage** Adults: Oral: 25-100 mg 2-3 times/day

**Dosage Forms** Tablet, as fumarate: 25 mg, 100 mg, 200 mg, 300 mg

**Quibron®** *see* theophylline and guaifenesin *on page 583*

**Quibron®-T** *see* theophylline *on page 581*

**Quibron®-T/SR** *see* theophylline *on page 581*

**Quiess® Injection *(Discontinued)*** *see page 750*

**Quinaglute® Dura-Tabs®** *see* quinidine *on next page*

**Quinalan®** *see* quinidine *on next page*

**quinalbarbitone** *see* secobarbital *on page 539*

**Quinamm® *(Discontinued)*** *see page 750*

## quinapril (KWIN a pril)

**U.S./Canadian Brand Names** Accupril®

**Therapeutic Category** Angiotensin-Converting Enzyme (ACE) Inhibitor

**Use** Treatment of hypertension, either alone or in combination with other antihypertensive agents

**Usual Dosage** Adults: Oral: Initial: 10 mg once daily, adjust according to blood pressure response at peak and trough blood levels; in general, the normal dosage range is 40-80 mg/day

**Dosage Forms** Tablet, as hydrochloride: 5 mg, 10 mg, 20 mg, 40 mg

## quinapril and hydrochlorothiazide *(Canada only)*

(KWIN a pril & hye droe klor oh THYE a zide)

**U.S./Canadian Brand Names** Accuretic® (Can)

**Therapeutic Category** Angiotensin-Converting Enzyme (ACE) Inhibitor; Diuretic, Thiazide

**Use** Treatment of essential hypertension when combination therapy is appropriate

**Usual Dosage** Dosage must be individualized; the fixed combination is not for initial therapy; the dose should be determined by titration of the individual components

**Dosage Forms** Tablet: Quinapril hydrochloride 10 mg and hydrochlorothiazide 12.5 mg; quinapril hydrochloride 20 mg and hydrochlorothiazide 12.5 mg; quinapril hydrochloride 20 mg and hydrochlorothiazide 25 mg

**Quinidex® Extentabs®** *see* quinidine *on next page*

## quinidine (KWIN i deen)

**U.S./Canadian Brand Names** Quinaglute® Dura-Tabs®; Quinalan®; Quinidex® Extentabs®; Quinora®; Biquin Durules® (Can)

**Therapeutic Category** Antiarrhythmic Agent, Class I-A

**Use** Prophylaxis after cardioversion of atrial fibrillation and/or flutter to maintain normal sinus rhythm; also used to prevent reoccurrence of paroxysmal supraventricular tachycardia, paroxysmal A-V junctional rhythm, paroxysmal ventricular tachycardia, paroxysmal atrial fibrillation, and atrial or ventricular premature contractions; also has activity against *Plasmodium falciparum* malaria

**Usual Dosage Note:** Dosage expressed in terms of the salt: 267 mg of quinidine gluconate = 275 mg of quinidine polygalacturonate = 200 mg of quinidine sulfate

Children: Test dose for idiosyncratic reaction (sulfate, oral or gluconate, I.M.): 2 mg/kg or 60 mg/m$^2$

Oral (quinidine sulfate): 15-60 mg/kg/day in 4-5 divided doses or 6 mg/kg every 4-6 hours (AMA 1991); usual 30 mg/kg/day or 900 mg/m$^2$/day administered in 5 daily doses

I.V. **not** recommended (quinidine gluconate): 2-10 mg/kg/dose every 3-6 hours as needed

Adults: Test dose: 200 mg administered several hours before full dosage (to determine possibility of idiosyncratic reaction)

Oral (sulfate): 100-600 mg/dose every 4-6 hours; begin at 200 mg/dose and titrate to desired effect

Oral (gluconate): 324-972 mg every 8-12 hours

Oral (polygalacturonate): 275 mg every 8-12 hours

I.M.: 400 mg/dose every 4-6 hours

I.V.: 200-400 mg/dose diluted and administered at a rate ≤10 mg/minute

**Dosage Forms**

Quinidine gluconate:

Injection: 80 mg/mL (10 mL)

Tablet, sustained release: 324 mg

Quinidine sulfate:

Tablet: 200 mg, 300 mg

Tablet, sustained action: 300 mg

## quinine (KWYE nine)

**U.S./Canadian Brand Names** Quinine-Odan™ (Can)

**Therapeutic Category** Antimalarial Agent

**Use** Suppression or treatment of chloroquine-resistant *P. falciparum* malaria (inactive against sporozoites, pre-erythrocytic or exoerythrocytic forms of plasmodia); treatment of *Babesia microti* infection

**Usual Dosage** Oral (parenteral dosage form may be obtained from Centers for Disease Control if needed):

Children: Chloroquine-resistant malaria and babesiosis: 25 mg/kg/day in divided doses every 8 hours for 7 days; maximum: 650 mg/dose

Adults:

Chloroquine-resistant malaria: 650 mg every 8 hours for 7 days in conjunction with another agent

Babesiosis: 650 mg every 6-8 hours for 7 days

**Dosage Forms**

Capsule, as sulfate: 64.8 mg, 65 mg, 200 mg, 300 mg, 325 mg

Tablet, as sulfate: 162.5 mg, 260 mg

**Quinine-Odan™ (Can)** *see* quinine *on this page*

**quinol** *see* hydroquinone *on page 305*

**Quinora®** *see* quinidine *on this page*

**Quintasa® (Can)** *see* mesalamine *on page 374*

## quinupristin and dalfopristin (kwi NYOO pris tin & dal FOE pris tin)

**Synonyms** pristinamycin; RP59500

**U.S./Canadian Brand Names** Synercid®

**Therapeutic Category** Antibiotic, Streptogramin

**Use** Treatment of serious or life-threatening infections associated with vancomycin-resistant *Enterococcus faecium* bacteremia; treatment of complicated skin and skin structure infections caused by methcillin-susceptible *Staphylococcus aureus* or *Streptococcus pyogenes*

Investigational use: Has been studied in the treatment of a variety of infections caused by *Enterococcus faecium* (not *E. fecalis*) including vancomycin-resistant strains. May also be effective in the treatment of serious infections caused by *Staphylococcus* species including those resistant to methicillin.

**Usual Dosage** Adults: I.V.:

Vancomycin-resistant *Enterococcus faecium:* 7.5 mg/kg every 8 hours

Complicated skin and skin structure infection: 7.5 mg/kg every 12 hours

**Dosage adjustment in renal impairment:** No adjustment required in renal failure, hemodialysis or peritoneal dialysis

**Dosage adjustment in hepatic impairment:** Pharmacokinetic data suggest dosage adjustment may be necessary, however, specific recommendations have not been proposed

Elderly: No dosage adjustment is required

**Dosage Forms** Powder for injection: 500 mg (350 mg dalfopristin and 150 mg quinupristin)

**Quiphile® *(Discontinued)*** *see page 750*

**Quixin™ Ophthalmic** *see* levofloxacin *on page 346*

**QVAR™** *see* beclomethasone *on page 68*

**Q-vel® *(Discontinued)*** *see page 750*

## rabeprazole (ra BE pray zole)

**Synonyms** pariprazole

**U.S./Canadian Brand Names** AcipHex™

**Therapeutic Category** Gastric Acid Secretion Inhibitor

**Use** Short-term (4-8 weeks) treatment of erosive or ulcerative gastroesophageal reflux disease (GERD); maintenance therapy in erosive or ulcerative GERD; short-term (up to 4 weeks) treatment of duodenal ulcers; long-term treatment of pathological hypersecretory conditions, including Zollinger-Ellison syndrome

**Usual Dosage** Adults and Elderly:

GERD: 20 mg once daily for 4-8 weeks; maintenance: 20 mg once daily

Duodenal ulcer: 20 mg/day after breakfast for 4 weeks

Hypersecretory conditions: 60 mg once daily; dose may need to be adjusted as necessary. Doses as high as 100 mg and 60 mg twice daily have been used.

**Dosage Forms** Tablet, delayed release: 20 mg

## rabies immune globulin (human)

(RAY beez i MYUN GLOB yoo lin HYU man)

**Synonyms** RIG

**U.S./Canadian Brand Names** Bayrab®; Imogam® Rabies-HT

**Therapeutic Category** Immune Globulin

**Use** Passive immunity to rabies for postexposure prophylaxis of individuals exposed to the virus

**Usual Dosage** Children and Adults: I.M.: 20 units/kg in a single dose (RIG should always be administered in conjunction with rabies vaccine (HDCV)) (infiltrate $^1/_2$ of the dose locally around the wound; administer the remainder I.M.)

**Dosage Forms** Injection: 150 units/mL (2 mL, 10 mL)

## rabies virus vaccine (RAY beez VYE rus vak SEEN)

**Synonyms** HDCV; HDRS

**U.S./Canadian Brand Names** Imovax® Rabies I.D. Vaccine; Imovax® Rabies Vaccine

**Therapeutic Category** Vaccine, Inactivated Virus

**Use** Pre-exposure rabies immunization for high risk persons; postexposure antirabies immunization along with local treatment and immune globulin

**Usual Dosage**

Pre-exposure prophylaxis: Two 1 mL doses I.M. or I.D. one week apart, third dose 3 weeks after second dose. If exposure continues, booster doses can be administered every 2 years, or an antibody titer determined and a booster dose administered if the titer is inadequate.

Postexposure prophylaxis: All postexposure treatment should begin with immediate cleansing of the wound with soap and water. Persons not previously immunized as above: Rabies immune globulin 20 units/kg body weight, half infiltrated at bite site if possible, remainder I.M.; and 5 doses of rabies vaccine, 1 mL I.M., one each on days 0, 3, 7, 14, 28.

Persons who have previously received postexposure prophylaxis with rabies vaccine, received a recommended I.M. or I.D. pre-exposure series of rabies vaccine or have a previously documented rabies antibody titer considered adequate: Two doses of rabies vaccine, 1 mL I.M., one each on days 0 and 3

**Dosage Forms** Injection:

I.M. (HDCV): Rabies antigen 2.5 units/mL (1 mL)

Intradermal: Rabies antigen 0.25 units/mL (1 mL)

## radiological/contrast media (ionic)

**U.S./Canadian Brand Names** Anatrast®; Angio Conray®; Angiovist®; Baricon®; Barobag®; Baro-CAT®; Baroflave®; Barosperse®; Bar-Test®; Bilopaque®; Cholebrine®; Cholografin® Meglumine; Conray®; Cystografin®; Dionosil Oily®; Enecat®; Entrobar®; Epi-C®; Ethiodol®; Flo-Coat®; Gastrografin®; HD 85®; HD 200 Plus®; Hexabrix™; Hypaque-Cysto®; Hypaque® Meglumine; Hypaque® Sodium; Liquid Barosperse®; Liquipake®; Lymphazurin®; Magnevist®; MD-Gastroview®; Oragrafin® Calcium; Oragrafin® Sodium; Perchloracap®; Prepcat®; Reno-M-30®; Reno-M-60®; Reno-M-DIP®; Renovue®-65; Renovue®-DIP; Sinografin®; Telepaque®; Tomocat®; Tonopaque®; Urovist Cysto®; Urovist® Meglumine; Urovist® Sodium 300; Vascoray®

**Therapeutic Category** Radiopaque Agents

**Dosage Forms**

**Oral cholecystographic agents**:

Iocetamic acid: Tablet (Cholebrine®): 750 mg

Iopanoic acid: Tablet (Telepaque®): 500 mg

Ipodate calcium: Granules for oral suspension (Oragrafin® Calcium): 3 g

Ipodate sodium: Capsule (Bilivist®, Oragrafin® Sodium): 500 mg

Tyropanoate sodium: Capsule (Bilopaque®): 750 mg

**GI contrast agents**: **Barium sulfate**:

Paste (Anatrast®): 100% (500 g)

Powder:

- Baroflave®: 100%
- Baricon®, HD 200 Plus®: 98%
- Barosperse®, Tonopaque®: 95%

Suspension:

- Baro-CAT®, Prepcat®: 1.5%
- Enecat®, Tomocat®: 5%
- Entrobar®: 50%
- Liquid Barasperse®: 60%
- HD 85®: 85%
- Barobag®: 97%
- Flo-Coat®, Liquipake®: 100%
- Epi-C®: 150%

Tablet (Bar-Test®): 650 mg

**Parenteral agents**: Injection:
 **Diatrizoate meglumine**:
  Hypaque® Meglumine
  Reno-M-DIP®
  Urovist® Meglumine
  Angiovist® 282
  Hypaque® Meglumine
  Reno-M-60®
 **Diatrizoate sodium**:
  Hypaque® Sodium
  Hypaque® Sodium
  Urovist® Sodium 300
 **Gadopentetate dimeglumine**: Magnevist®
 **Iodamide meglumine**:
  Renovue®-DIP
  Renovue®-65
 **Iodipamide meglumine**: Cholografin® meglumine
 **Iothalamate meglumine**:
  Conray® 30
  Conray® 43
  Conray®
 **Iothalamate sodium**:
  Angio Conray®
  Conray® 325
  Conray® 400
 **Diatrizoate meglumine and diatrizoate sodium**:
  Angiovist® 292
  Angiovist® 370
  Hypaque-76®
  Hypaque-M®, 75%
  Hypaque-M®, 90%
  MD-60®
  MD-76®
  Renografin-60®
  Renografin-76®
  Renovist® II
  Renovist®
 **Iothalamate meglumine and iothalamate sodium**:
  Vascoray®
  Hexabrix™

**Miscellaneous agents**: (**NOT** for intravascular use, for instillation into various cavities)
 **Diatrizoate meglumine**: Urogenital solution, sterile:
  Crystografin®
  Crystografin® Dilute
  Hypaque-Cysto®
  Reno-M-30®
  Urovist Cysto®
 **Diatrizoate meglumine and diatrizoate sodium**: Solution, oral or rectal:
  Gastrografin®
  MD-Gastroview®
 **Diatrizoate sodium**:
  Solution, oral or rectal (Hypaque® sodium oral)
  Solution, urogenital (Hypaque® sodium 20%)
 **Iothalamate meglumine**: Solution, urogenital:
  Cysto-Conray®
  Cysto-Conray® II

**Diatrizoate meglumine and iodipamide meglumine**:
 Injection, urogenital for intrauterine instillation (Sinografin®)
(Continued)

## radiological/contrast media (ionic) *(Continued)*

**Ethiodized oil**: Injection (Ethiodol®)
**Propyliodone**: Suspension (Dionosil Oily®)
**Isosulfan blue**: Injection (Lymphazurin® 1%)
**Potassium perchlorate**: Capsule (Perchloracap®): 200 mg

## radiological/contrast media (non-ionic)

**U.S./Canadian Brand Names** Amipaque®; Isovue®; Omnipaque®; Optiray®
**Therapeutic Category** Radiopaque Agents
**Dosage Forms** **Parenteral agents**: Injection:
**Iohexol**: Omnipaque®: 140 mg/mL; 180 mg/mL; 210 mg/mL; 240 mg/mL; 300 mg/mL; 350 mg/mL
**Iopamidol**:
Isovue-128®
Isovue-200®
Isovue-M 200®
Isovue-300®
Isovue-M 300®
Isovue-370®
**Ioversol**:
Optiray® 160
Optiray® 240
Optiray® 320
**Metrizamide**: Amipaque®

**R-albuterol** *see* levalbuterol *on page 343*

## raloxifene (ral OX i feen)

**U.S./Canadian Brand Names** Evista®
**Therapeutic Category** Selective Estrogen Receptor Modulator (SERM)
**Use** Prevention and treatment of osteoporosis in postmenopausal women
**Usual Dosage** Adults: Oral: 1 tablet daily, may be administered any time of the day without regard to meals
**Dosage Forms** Tablet, as hydrochloride: 60 mg

## raltitrexed *(Canada only)* (ral ti TREX ed)

**U.S./Canadian Brand Names** Tomudex® (Can)
**Therapeutic Category** Antineoplastic Agent
**Use** Undergoing clinical trials for a variety of neoplasms, including breast, colorectal nonsmall cell lung, ovarian, and pancreatic cancers
**Usual Dosage** Refer to individual protocols
I.V.: 3 mg/m$^2$ every 3 weeks
**Dosage Forms** Powder for injection, lyophilized: 2 mg

## ramipril (ra MI pril)

**U.S./Canadian Brand Names** Altace™
**Therapeutic Category** Angiotensin-Converting Enzyme (ACE) Inhibitor
**Use** Treatment of hypertension, alone or in combination with thiazide diuretics; congestive heart failure immediately after myocardial infarction
**Usual Dosage** Adults: Oral: 2.5-5 mg once daily
**Dosage Forms** Capsule: 1.25 mg, 2.5 mg, 5 mg, 10 mg

**Ramses® [OTC]** *see* nonoxynol 9 *on page 424*

## ranitidine bismuth citrate (ra NI ti deen BIZ muth SIT rate)

**Synonyms** RBC
**U.S./Canadian Brand Names** Tritec®

**Therapeutic Category** Gastrointestinal Agent, Gastric or Duodenal Ulcer Treatment

**Use** In combination with clarithromycin for the treatment of active duodenal ulcer associated with *H. pylori* infection; not to be used alone for the treatment of active duodenal ulcer

**Usual Dosage** Adults: Oral: 400 mg twice daily for 4 weeks (28 days) in conjunction with clarithromycin 500 mg 3 times/day for first 2 weeks

**Dosage Forms** Tablet: 400 mg (ranitidine 162 mg, trivalent bismuth 128 mg, and citrate 110 mg)

## ranitidine hydrochloride (ra NI ti deen hye droe KLOR ide)

**U.S./Canadian Brand Names** Alti-Ranitidine (Can); Apo®-Ranitidine (Can); Gen-Ranitidine (Can); Novo-Ranidine (Can); Nu-Ranit (Can); Zantac®; Zantac® 75 [OTC]

**Therapeutic Category** Histamine $H_2$ Antagonist

**Use** Short-term treatment of active duodenal ulcers and benign gastric ulcers; long-term prophylaxis of duodenal ulcer and gastric hypersecretory states; gastroesophageal reflux (GER)

**Usual Dosage**

Children:

Oral: 1.5-2 mg/kg/dose every 12 hours

I.M., I.V.: 0.75-1.5 mg/kg/dose every 6-8 hours, maximum daily dose: 400 mg

Continuous infusion: 0.1-0.25 mg/kg/hour (preferred for stress ulcer prophylaxis in patients with concurrent maintenance I.V.s or TPNs)

Adults:

Short-term treatment of ulceration: 150 mg/dose twice daily or 300 mg at bedtime

Prophylaxis of recurrent duodenal ulcer: 150 mg at bedtime

Gastric hypersecretory conditions: Oral: 150 mg twice daily, up to 600 mg /day

I.M., I.V.: 50 mg/dose every 6-8 hours (dose not to exceed 400 mg/day)

**Dosage Forms**

Capsule (GELdose™): 150 mg, 300 mg

Granules, effervescent (EFFERdose™): 150 mg

Infusion, preservative free, in NaCl 0.45%: 1 mg/mL (50 mL)

Injection: 25 mg/mL (2 mL, 6 mL, 10 mL, 40 mL)

Syrup (peppermint flavor): 15 mg/mL (473 mL)

Tablet: 75 mg [OTC]; 150 mg, 300 mg

Tablet, effervescent (EFFERdose™): 150 mg

## rapacuronium (ra pa kyoo ROE nee um)

**U.S./Canadian Brand Names** Raplon™

**Therapeutic Category** Neuromuscular Blocker Agent, Nondepolarizing

**Use** Adjunct to general anesthesia to facilitate tracheal intubation; to provide skeletal muscle relaxation during surgical procedures; does not relieve pain

**Usual Dosage** I.V. (do not administer I.M.):

Children 1 month to 12 years: Initial: 2 mg/kg. Repeat dosing is not recommended in pediatric patients.

Children 13-17 years: Clinicians should consider the physical maturity, height and weight of the patient in determining the dose. Adults (1.5 mg/kg), pediatric (2 mg/kg) and Cesarean section (2.5 mg/kg) dosing recommendations may serve as a general guideline in determining an intubating dose in this age group.

Adults: Tracheal Intubation:

Initial: Short surgical procedures: 1.5 mg/kg; Cesarean section: 2.5 mg/kg

Repeat dosing: Up to three maintenance doses of 0.5 mg/kg, administered at 25% recovery of control T1 may be administered. **Note:** The duration of neuromuscular blockade increases with each additional dose.

Elderly: No dosing adjustment is recommended in geriatric patients

**Dosage Forms** Powder for injection: 100 mg (5 mL); 200 mg (10 mL)

**Rapamune®** *see* sirolimus *on page 546*

**Raplon™** *see* rapacuronium *on this page*

**Remeron® SolTab™** *see* mirtazapine *on page 395*

**Remicade®** *see* infliximab *on page 318*

## remifentanil (rem i FEN ta nil)

**U.S./Canadian Brand Names** Ultiva™

**Therapeutic Category** Analgesic, Narcotic

**Use** Analgesic for use during general anesthesia for continued analgesia

**Usual Dosage** Adults: I.V. continuous infusion:

During induction: 0.5-1 mcg/kg/minute

During maintenance:

With nitrous oxide (66%): 0.4 mcg/kg/minute (range: 0.1-2 mcg/kg/min)

With isoflurane: 0.25 mcg/kg/minute (range: 0.05-2 mcg/kg/min)

With propofol: 0.25 mcg/kg/minute (range: 0.05-2 mcg/kg/min)

Continuation as an analgesic in immediate postoperative period: 0.1 mcg/kg/minute (range: 0.025-0.2 mcg/kg/min)

**Dosage Forms** Powder for injection, lyophilized: 1 mg, 2 mg, 5 mg

**Reminyl®** *see* galantamine *on page 268*

**Renacidin®** *see* citric acid bladder mixture *on page 140*

**Renagel®** *see* sevelamer *on page 542*

**Renedil® (Can)** *see* felodipine *on page 242*

**Renese®** *see* polythiazide *on page 482*

**Reno-M-30®** *see* radiological/contrast media (ionic) *on page 516*

**Reno-M-60®** *see* radiological/contrast media (ionic) *on page 516*

**Reno-M-DIP®** *see* radiological/contrast media (ionic) *on page 516*

**Renoquid® *(Discontinued)*** *see page 750*

**Renormax®** *see* spirapril *on page 556*

**Renova® Cream** *see* tretinoin (topical) *on page 600*

**Renovue®-65** *see* radiological/contrast media (ionic) *on page 516*

**Renovue®-DIP** *see* radiological/contrast media (ionic) *on page 516*

**Rentamine®** *see* chlorpheniramine, ephedrine, phenylephrine, and carbetapentane *on page 130*

**ReoPro®** *see* abciximab *on page 2*

## repaglinide (re PAG li nide)

**U.S./Canadian Brand Names** GlucoNorm® (Can); Prandin™

**Therapeutic Category** Hypoglycemic Agent, Oral

**Use** As an adjunct to diet and exercise to lower blood glucose on noninsulin-dependent (Type 2) diabetes patients

**Usual Dosage** Oral: Adults: 0.5-4 mg before each meal

Oral hypoglycemic-naive individuals or those with HbA1c levels <8%: Initial: 0.5 mg before each meal; for other patients, the starting dose is 1-2 mg before each meal

Dose can be adjusted (by prescribers) up to 4 mg before each meal. If a meal is skipped, the patient should also skip the repaglinide dose.

**Dosage Forms** Tablet: 0.5 mg, 1 mg, 2 mg

**Repan®** *see* butalbital compound and acetaminophen *on page 93*

**Reposans-10® Oral *(Discontinued)*** *see page 750*

**Rep-Pred® *(Discontinued)*** *see page 750*

**Repronex®** *see* menotropins *on page 371*

**Requip®** *see* ropinirole *on page 532*

**Resa® *(Discontinued)*** *see page 750*

**Resaid®** ***(Discontinued)*** *see page 750*

**Rescaps-D® S.R. Capsule** ***(Discontinued)*** *see page 750*

**Rescon Liquid** ***(Discontinued)*** *see page 750*

**Rescriptor®** *see* delavirdine *on page 169*

**Rescula®** *see* unoprostone *on page 616*

**Resectisol® Irrigation Solution** *see* mannitol *on page 364*

## reserpine (re SER peen)

**Therapeutic Category** Rauwolfia Alkaloid

**Use** Management of mild to moderate hypertension

**Usual Dosage** Adults: Oral: 0.1-0.5 mg/day in 1-2 doses

**Dosage Forms** Tablet: 0.1 mg, 0.25 mg

**Respa-1st®** *see* guaifenesin and pseudoephedrine *on page 283*

**Respa®-DM** *see* guaifenesin and dextromethorphan *on page 282*

**Respa-GF®** *see* guaifenesin *on page 281*

**Respaire®-60 SR** *see* guaifenesin and pseudoephedrine *on page 283*

**Respaire®-120 SR** *see* guaifenesin and pseudoephedrine *on page 283*

**Respbid®** *see* theophylline *on page 581*

**RespiGam™** *see* respiratory syncytial virus immune globulin (intravenous) *on this page*

## respiratory syncytial virus immune globulin (intravenous)

(RES peer rah tor ee sin SISH al VYE rus i MYUN GLOB yoo lin in tra VEE nus)

**Synonyms** RSV-IGIV

**U.S./Canadian Brand Names** RespiGam™

**Therapeutic Category** Immune Globulin

**Use** Prevention of serious lower respiratory infection caused by respiratory syncytial virus (RSV) in children <24 months of age with bronchopulmonary dysplasia (BPD) or a history of premature birth (≤35 weeks gestation)

**Usual Dosage** I.V.: 750 mg/kg/month according to the following infusion schedule: 1.5 mL/kg/hour for 15 minutes, then at 3 mL/kg/hour for the next 15 minutes if the clinical condition does not contraindicate a higher rate, and finally, administer at 6 mL/kg/hour until completion of dose

**Dosage Forms** Injection: 2500 mg RSV immunoglobulin/50 mL vial

**Restall® Injection** *see* hydroxyzine *on page 308*

**Restoril®** *see* temazepam *on page 572*

**Retavase™** *see* reteplase *on this page*

## reteplase (RE ta plase)

**Synonyms** recombinant plasminogen activator; r-PA

**U.S./Canadian Brand Names** Retavase™

**Therapeutic Category** Fibrinolytic Agent

**Use** Management of acute myocardial infarction

**Usual Dosage** Adults: I.V.: Given as two (2) bolus doses of 10 units each over a period of 2 minutes (second dose given 30 minutes after the initiation of the first dose)

**Dosage Forms** Powder for injection, lyophilized: 10.8 units [reteplase 18.8 mg]

**Retin-A® Micro Topical** *see* tretinoin (topical) *on page 600*

**Retin-A® Topical** *see* tretinoin (topical) *on page 600*

**retinoic acid** *see* tretinoin (topical) *on page 600*

**Retrovir®** *see* zidovudine *on page 638*

**Reversol®** *see* edrophonium *on page 210*

**Revex®** *see* nalmefene *on page 407*

**Rēv-Eyes™** *see* dapiprazole *on page 165*

**ReVia®** *see* naltrexone *on page 408*

**Revitalose-C-1000® (Can)** *see* ascorbic acid *on page 54*

**Rexigen Forte®** ***(Discontinued)*** *see page 750*

**Rezulin®** ***(Discontinued)*** *see page 750*

**rFVIIa** *see* factor VIIa (recombinant) *on page 239*

**R-Gel®** ***(Discontinued)*** *see page 750*

**R-Gen®** ***(Discontinued)*** *see page 750*

**R-Gene®** *see* arginine *on page 52*

**RGM-CSF** *see* sargramostim *on page 537*

**r-hCG** *see* chorionic gonadotropin (recombinant) *on page 136*

**Rheaban® [OTC]** *see* attapulgite *on page 60*

**Rheomacrodex®** *see* dextran *on page 177*

**Rhesonativ® Injection** ***(Discontinued)*** *see page 750*

**Rheumatrex®** *see* methotrexate *on page 380*

**rhIL-11** *see* oprelvekin *on page 437*

**Rhinalar® (Can)** *see* flunisolide *on page 253*

**Rhinall® Nasal Solution [OTC]** *see* phenylephrine *on page 467*

**Rhinatate® Tablet** *see* chlorpheniramine, pyrilamine, and phenylephrine *on page 132*

**Rhindecon®** ***(Discontinued)*** *see page 750*

**Rhinocort®** *see* budesonide *on page 89*

**Rhinocort® Aqua™** *see* budesonide *on page 89*

**Rhinolar®** ***(Discontinued)*** *see page 750*

**Rhinosyn-DMX® [OTC]** *see* guaifenesin and dextromethorphan *on page 282*

**Rhinosyn® Liquid [OTC]** *see* chlorpheniramine and pseudoephedrine *on page 130*

**Rhinosyn-PD® Liquid [OTC]** *see* chlorpheniramine and pseudoephedrine *on page 130*

**Rhinosyn-X® Liquid [OTC]** *see* guaifenesin, pseudoephedrine, and dextromethorphan *on page 285*

**Rho®-Clonazepam (Can)** *see* clonazepam *on page 145*

**Rhodacine® (Can)** *see* indomethacin *on page 317*

## $Rh_o$(D) immune globulin (intramuscular)

(ar aych oh (dee) i MYUN GLOB yoo lin IN tra MUS kyoo ler)

**U.S./Canadian Brand Names** BayRho-D®; MICRhoGAM™; RhoGAM™

**Therapeutic Category** Immune Globulin

**Use** Prevent isoimmunization in Rh-negative individuals exposed to Rh-positive blood during delivery of an Rh-positive infant, as a result of an abortion, following amniocentesis or abdominal trauma, or following a transfusion accident; to prevent hemolytic disease of the newborn if there is a subsequent pregnancy with an Rh-positive fetus

**Usual Dosage** Adults: I.M.:

Obstetrical usage: 1 vial (300 mcg) prevents maternal sensitization if fetal packed red blood cell volume that has entered the circulation is <15 mL; if it is more, administer additional vials. The number of vials = RBC volume of the calculated fetomaternal hemorrhage divided by 15 mL

(Continued)

## $Rh_0$(D) immune globulin (intramuscular) *(Continued)*

Postpartum prophylaxis: 300 mcg within 72 hours of delivery

Antepartum prophylaxis: 300 mcg at approximately 26-28 weeks gestation; followed by 300 mcg within 72 hours of delivery if infant is Rh-positive

Following miscarriage, abortion, or termination of ectopic pregnancy at up to 13 weeks of gestation: 50 mcg ideally within 3 hours, but may be administered up to 72 hours after; if pregnancy has been terminated at 13 or more weeks of gestation, administer 300 mcg

**Dosage Forms**

Injection: Each package contains one single dose 300 mcg of $Rh_0$ (D) immune globulin

Injection, microdose: Each package contains one single dose of microdose, 50 mcg of $Rh_0$ (D) immune globulin

## $Rh_0$(D) immune globulin (intravenous-human)

(ar aych oh (dee) i MYUN GLOB yoo lin in tra VEE nus-HYU man)

**Synonyms** RhoIGIV

**U.S./Canadian Brand Names** WinRho SD®; WinRho SDF®

**Therapeutic Category** Immune Globulin

**Use**

Prevention of Rh isoimmunization in nonsensitized Rho(D) antigen-negative women within 7 hours after spontaneous or induced abortion, amniocentesis, chorionic villus sampling, ruptured tubal pregnancy, abdominal trauma, transplacental hemorrhage, or in the normal course of pregnancy unless the blood type of the fetus or father is known to be Rho(D) antigen-negative

Suppression of Rh isoimmunization in Rho(D) antigen-negative female children and female adults in their childbearing years transfused with Rho(D) antigen-positive RBCs or blood components containing Rho(D) antigen-positive RBCs

Treatment of idiopathic thrombocytopenic purpura (ITP) in nonsplenectomized Rho(D) antigen-positive patients

**Usual Dosage**

Prevention of Rh isoimmunization:

I.V.: 1500 units (300 mcg) at 28 weeks gestation or immediately after amniocentesis if <34 weeks gestation or after chorionic villus sampling; repeat this dose every 12 weeks during the pregnancy, 600 units (120 mcg) at delivery (within 72 hours) and after invasive intrauterine procedures such as abortion, amniocentesis, or any other manipulation if at >34 weeks gestation. **Note:** If the Rh status of the baby is not known at 72 hours, administer Rho(D) immune globulin to the mother at 72 hours after delivery. If >72 hours have elapsed, do not withhold Rho(D) immune globulin, but administer as soon as possible, up to 28 days after delivery.

I.M.: Reconstitute vial with 1.25 mL and administer as above

Transfusion: Administer within 72 hours after exposure for treatment of incompatible blood transfusions or massive fetal hemorrhage as follows:

I.V.: 3000 units (600 mcg) every 8 hours until the total dose is administered (45 units [9 mcg] of Rh+ blood/mL blood; 90 units [18 mcg] Rh+ red cells/mL cells)

I.M.: 6000 units [1200 mcg] every 12 hours until the total dose is administered (60 units [12 mcg] of Rh+ blood/mL blood; 120 units [24 mcg] Rh+ red cells/mL cells)

Treatment of ITP: I.V.: Initial: 25-50 mcg/kg depending on the patient's Hg concentration; maintenance: 25-60 mcg/kg depending on the clinical response

**Dosage Forms** Injection: 600 units [120 mcg], 1500 units [300 mcg] with 2.5 mL diluent; 5000 units [1000 units] with 8.5 mL diluent

**Rhodis™ (Can)** *see* ketoprofen *on page 334*

**Rhodis-EC™ (Can)** *see* ketoprofen *on page 334*

**RhoGAM™** *see* $Rh_0$(D) immune globulin (intramuscular) *on previous page*

**RhoIGIV** *see* $Rh_0$(D) immune globulin (intravenous-human) *on this page*

**Rho®-Loperamide (Can)** *see* loperamide *on page 354*

**Rho®-Metformin (Can)** *see* metformin *on page 377*

**Rho®-Sotalol (Can)** *see* sotalol *on page 555*

**Rhotral (Can)** *see* acebutolol *on page 3*

**Rhotrimine® (Can)** *see* trimipramine *on page 608*

**Rhovail® (Can)** *see* ketoprofen *on page 334*

**Rhovane® (Can)** *see* zopiclone *(Canada only) on page 641*

**Rhoxal-famotidine (Can)** *see* famotidine *on page 240*

**Rhoxal-minocycline (Can)** *see* minocycline *on page 394*

**Rhoxal-timolol (Can)** *see* timolol *on page 591*

**Rhoxal-valproic (Can)** *see* valproic acid and derivatives *on page 620*

**RHUEPO-α** *see* epoetin alfa *on page 218*

**Rhulicaine® [OTC]** *see* benzocaine *on page 72*

**Rhuli® Cream *(Discontinued)*** *see page 750*

## ribavirin (rye ba VYE rin)

**Synonyms** RTCA; tribavirin

**U.S./Canadian Brand Names** Virazole® Aerosol

**Therapeutic Category** Antiviral Agent

**Use** Treatment of patients with respiratory syncytial virus (RSV) infections; specially indicated for treatment of severe lower respiratory tract RSV infections in patients with an underlying compromising condition (prematurity, bronchopulmonary dysplasia and other chronic lung conditions, congenital heart disease, immunodeficiency, immunosuppression), and recent transplant recipients; may also be used in other viral infections including influenza A and B and adenovirus

**Usual Dosage** Infants, Children, and Adults:

Aerosol inhalation: Use with Viratek® small particle aerosol generator (SPAG-2) at a concentration of 20 mg/mL (6 g reconstituted with 300 mL of sterile water without preservatives)

Aerosol only: 12-18 hours/day for 3 days, up to 7 days in length

**Dosage Forms** Powder for aerosol: 6 g (100 mL)

## riboflavin (RYE boe flay vin)

**Synonyms** lactoflavin; vitamin $B_2$; vitamin G

**Therapeutic Category** Vitamin, Water Soluble

**Use** Prevent riboflavin deficiency and treat ariboflavinosis

**Usual Dosage** Oral:

Riboflavin deficiency:

- Children: 2.5-10 mg/day in divided doses
- Adults: 5-30 mg/day in divided doses

Recommended daily allowance: Adults:

- Male: 1.4-4.8 mg
- Female: 1.2-1.3 mg

**Dosage Forms** Tablet: 25 mg, 50 mg, 100 mg

**Ridactate®** *see* calcium lactate *on page 100*

**Rid-A-Pain®** *see* capsaicin *on page 104*

**Rid-A-Pain® Dental [OTC]** *see* benzocaine *on page 72*

**Rid-A-Pain-HP®** *see* capsaicin *on page 104*

**Ridaura®** *see* auranofin *on page 60*

**Ridifed® [OTC]** *see* triprolidine and pseudoephedrine *on page 609*

**RID® Mousse [OTC]** *see* pyrethrins *on page 510*

**RID® Shampoo [OTC]** *see* pyrethrins *on page 510*

## rifabutin (rif a BYOO tin)

**Synonyms** ansamycin

**U.S./Canadian Brand Names** Mycobutin®

**Therapeutic Category** Antibiotic, Miscellaneous

**Use** Prevention of disseminated *Mycobacterium avium* complex (MAC) in patients with advanced HIV infection; utilized in multiple drug regimens for treatment of MAC

**Usual Dosage** Oral:

Children: Efficacy and safety of rifabutin have not been established in children; a limited number of HIV-positive children with MAC (n=22) have been given rifabutin for MAC prophylaxis; doses of 5 mg/kg/day have been useful

Adults: 300 mg once daily; for patients who experience gastrointestinal upset, rifabutin can be administered 150 mg twice daily with food

**Dosage Forms** Capsule: 150 mg

**Rifadin® Injection** *see* rifampin *on this page*

**Rifadin® Oral** *see* rifampin *on this page*

**Rifamate®** *see* rifampin and isoniazid *on this page*

**rifampicin** *see* rifampin *on this page*

## rifampin (RIF am pin)

**Synonyms** rifampicin

**U.S./Canadian Brand Names** Rifadin® Injection; Rifadin® Oral; Rimactane® Oral; Rofact™ (Can)

**Therapeutic Category** Antibiotic, Miscellaneous

**Use** In combination with other antitubercular drugs for the treatment of active tuberculosis; eliminate meningococci from asymptomatic carriers; prophylaxis in contacts of patients with *Haemophilus influenzae* type B infection; used in combination with other anti-infectives in the treatment of staphylococcal infections

**Usual Dosage** Oral (I.V. infusion dose is the same as for the oral route):

Tuberculosis:

Children: 10-20 mg/kg/day in divided doses every 12-24 hours

Adults: 10 mg/kg/day; maximum: 600 mg/day

American Thoracic Society and CDC currently recommend twice weekly therapy as part of a short-course regimen which follows 1-2 months of daily treatment of uncomplicated pulmonary tuberculosis in the compliant patient

Children: 10-20 mg/kg/dose (up to 600 mg) twice weekly under supervision to ensure compliance

Adults: 10 mg/kg (up to 600 mg) twice weekly

*H. influenzae* prophylaxis:

Infants and Children: 20 mg/kg/day every 24 hours for 4 days

Adults: 600 mg every 24 hours for 4 days

Meningococcal prophylaxis:

<1 month: 10 mg/kg/day in divided doses every 12 hours

Infants and Children: 20 mg/kg/day in divided doses every 12 hours for 2 days

Adults: 600 mg every 12 hours for 2 days

Nasal carriers of *Staphylococcus aureus*: Adults: 600 mg/day for 5-10 days in combination with other antibiotics

**Dosage Forms**

Capsule: 150 mg, 300 mg

Powder for injection: 600 mg (contains a sulfite)

## rifampin and isoniazid (RIF am pin & eye soe NYE a zid)

**U.S./Canadian Brand Names** Rifamate®

**Therapeutic Category** Antibiotic, Miscellaneous

**Use** Management of active tuberculosis; see individual monographs for additional information

**Usual Dosage** Oral: 2 capsules/day

**Dosage Forms** Capsule: Rifampin 300 mg and isoniazid 150 mg

## rifampin, isoniazid, and pyrazinamide

(RIF am pin , eye soe NYE a zid, & peer a ZIN a mide)

**U.S./Canadian Brand Names** Rifater®

**Therapeutic Category** Antibiotic, Miscellaneous

**Use** Management of active tuberculosis

**Usual Dosage** Adults: Oral: Patients weighing:

≤44 kg: 4 tablets

45-54 kg: 5 tablets

≥55 kg: 6 tablets

Doses should be administered in a single daily dose

**Dosage Forms** Tablet: Rifampin 120 mg, isoniazid 50 mg, and pyrazinamide 300 mg

## rifapentine (RIF a pen teen)

**U.S./Canadian Brand Names** Priftin®

**Therapeutic Category** Antitubercular Agent

**Use** Treatment of pulmonary tuberculosis (indication is based on the 6-month follow-up treatment outcome observed in controlled clinical trial). Rifapentine must always be used in conjunction with at least one other antituberculosis drug to which the isolate is susceptible; it may also be necessary to add a third agent (either streptomycin or ethambutol) until susceptibility is known.

**Usual Dosage**

Children: No dosing information available

Adults: **Rifapentine should not be used alone**; initial phase should include a 3- to 4-drug regimen

Intensive phase of short-term therapy: 600 mg (four 150 mg tablets) given weekly (every 72 hours); following the intensive phase, treatment should continue with rifapentine 600 mg once weekly for 4 months in combination with INH or appropriate agent for susceptible organisms

**Dosage Forms** Tablet, film-coated: 150 mg

**Rifater®** *see* rifampin, isoniazid, and pyrazinamide *on this page*

**rIFN-A** *see* interferon alfa-2a *on page 321*

**RIG** *see* rabies immune globulin (human) *on page 515*

**rIL-11** *see* oprelvekin *on page 437*

**Rilutek®** *see* riluzole *on this page*

## riluzole (RIL yoo zole)

**Synonyms** 2-amino-6-trifluoromethoxy-benzothiazole; RP54274

**U.S./Canadian Brand Names** Rilutek®

**Therapeutic Category** Glutamate Inhibitor

**Use** Treatment of amyotrophic lateral sclerosis (ALS), also known as Lou Gehrig's disease

**Usual Dosage** Adults: Oral: 50 mg twice daily

**Dosage Forms** Tablet: 50 mg

**Rimactane® Oral** *see* rifampin *on previous page*

**Ri-Mag®** *see* magaldrate and simethicone *on page 360*

## rimantadine (ri MAN ta deen)

**U.S./Canadian Brand Names** Flumadine®

**Therapeutic Category** Antiviral Agent

**Use** Prophylaxis (adults and children) and treatment (adults) of influenza A viral infection

(Continued)

## rimantadine *(Continued)*

**Usual Dosage** Oral:

Prophylaxis:

Children <10 years: 5 mg/kg administered once daily

Children >10 years and Adults: 100 mg twice daily

Treatment: Adults: 100 mg twice daily

**Dosage Forms**

Syrup, as hydrochloride: 50 mg/5 mL (240 mL)

Tablet, as hydrochloride: 100 mg

## rimexolone (ri MEKS oh lone)

**U.S./Canadian Brand Names** Vexol® Ophthalmic Suspension

**Therapeutic Category** Adrenal Corticosteroid

**Use** Treatment of inflammation after ocular surgery and the treatment of anterior uveitis

**Usual Dosage** Children >2 years and Adults: Ophthalmic: Instill 1-2 drops into conjunctival sac every hour during day, every 2 hours at night until favorable response is obtained, then use 1 drop every 4 hours; for mild to moderate inflammation, instill 1-2 drops into conjunctival sac 2-4 times/day

**Dosage Forms** Suspension, ophthalmic: 1% (5 mL, 10 mL)

**Rimso®-50** *see* dimethyl sulfoxide *on page 189*

**Riobin® *(Discontinued)*** *see page 750*

**Riopan® [OTC]** *see* magaldrate *on page 360*

**Riopan Plus® [OTC]** *see* magaldrate and simethicone *on page 360*

**Riphenidate® (Can)** *see* methylphenidate *on page 384*

## risedronate (ris ED roe nate)

**U.S./Canadian Brand Names** Actonel™

**Therapeutic Category** Bisphosphonate Derivative

**Use** Treatment of hypercalcemia associated with malignancy, osteolytic bone lesions of multiple myeloma; also used in postmenopausal osteoporosis; primary hyperparathyroidism and Paget's disease (moderate to severe)

**Usual Dosage** Adults: Oral: 30 mg once daily for 2 months

**Dosage Forms** Tablet, as sodium: 5 mg, 30 mg

**Risperdal®** *see* risperidone *on this page*

## risperidone (ris PER i done)

**U.S./Canadian Brand Names** Risperdal®

**Therapeutic Category** Antipsychotic Agent, Benzisoxazole

**Use** Management of psychotic disorders (eg, schizophrenia)

**Usual Dosage** Oral: Recommended starting dose: 1 mg twice daily; slowly increase to the optimum range of 4-8 mg/day; daily dosages >10 mg does not appear to confer any additional benefit, and the incidence of extrapyramidal reactions is higher than with lower doses

**Dosage Forms**

Solution, oral: 1 mg/mL (30 mL)

Tablet: 0.25 mg, 0.5 mg, 1 mg, 2 mg, 3 mg, 4 mg

**Ritalin®** *see* methylphenidate *on page 384*

**Ritalin-SR®** *see* methylphenidate *on page 384*

**Ritifed® [OTC]** *see* triprolidine and pseudoephedrine *on page 609*

## ritodrine (RI toe dreen)

**U.S./Canadian Brand Names** Yutopar®

**Therapeutic Category** Adrenergic Agonist Agent

**Use** Inhibit uterine contraction in preterm labor

**Usual Dosage** Adults:

Oral: Start 30 minutes before stopping I.V. infusion; 10 mg every 2 hours for 24 hours, then 10-20 mg every 4-6 hours up to 120 mg/day. Continue treatment as long as it is desirable to prolong pregnancy.

I.V.: 50-100 mcg/minute; increase by 50 mcg/minute every 10 minutes; continue for 12 hours after contractions have stopped

**Dosage Forms** Ritodrine hydrochloride:

Injection: 10 mg/mL (5 mL); 15 mg/mL (10 mL)

Tablet: 10 mg

## ritonavir (rye TON a veer)

**U.S./Canadian Brand Names** Norvir®

**Therapeutic Category** Antiviral Agent

**Use** Treatment of HIV, especially advanced cases; usually is used as part of triple or double therapy with other nucleoside and protease inhibitors

**Usual Dosage** Adults: Oral: 600 mg twice daily with meals

**Dosage Forms**

Capsule: 100 mg

Solution: 80 mg/mL (240 mL)

**Rituxan®** *see* rituximab *on this page*

## rituximab (ri TUK si mab)

**Synonyms** anti-CD20 monoclonal antibodies; C2B8 monoclonal antibody; Pan-B antibodies

**U.S./Canadian Brand Names** Rituxan®

**Therapeutic Category** Antineoplastic Agent

**Use** Treatment of patients with relapsed or refractory low-grade or follicular, CD20 positive, B-cell non-Hodgkin's lymphoma

**Usual Dosage** Adults: I.V.: 375 mg/m$^2$ given as an I.V. infusion once weekly for 4 doses (days 1, 8, 15, and 22); may be administered in an outpatient setting; **do not administer as an intravenous push or bolus**

**Dosage Forms** Injection: 10 mg/mL (10 mL, 50 mL)

**Riva-Loperamide (Can)** *see* loperamide *on page 354*

**Riva-Lorazepam (Can)** *see* lorazepam *on page 356*

**Riva-Naproxen (Can)** *see* naproxen *on page 409*

**Rivanase AQ (Can)** *see* beclomethasone *on page 68*

**Riva-Norfloxacin (Can)** *see* norfloxacin *on page 425*

## rivastigmine (ri va STIG meen)

**Synonyms** ENA 713; SDZ ENA 713

**U.S./Canadian Brand Names** Exelon®

**Therapeutic Category** Acetylcholinesterase Inhibitor; Cholinergic Agent

**Use** Mild to moderate dementia from Alzheimer's disease

**Usual Dosage** Adults: Oral: Initial: 1.5 mg twice daily to start; if dose is tolerated for at least 2 weeks then it may be increased to 3 mg twice daily; increases to 4.5 mg twice daily and 6 mg twice daily should only be attempted after at least 2 weeks at the previous dose; maximum dose: 6 mg twice daily. If adverse events such as nausea, vomiting, abdominal pain, or loss of appetite occur, the patient should be instructed to discontinue treatment for several doses then restart at the same or next lower dosage level; antiemetics have been used to control GI symptoms.

(Continued)

## rivastigmine *(Continued)*

**Dosage adjustment in renal impairment:** Dosage adjustments are not recommended, however, titrate the dose to the individual's tolerance.

**Dosage adjustment in hepatic impairment:** Clearance is significantly reduced in mild to moderately impaired patients. Although dosage adjustments are not recommended, use lowest possible dose and titrate according to individual's tolerance. May consider waiting >2 weeks between dosage adjustments.

Elderly: Clearance is significantly lower in patients older than 60 years of age, but dosage adjustments are not recommended. Titrate dose to individual's tolerance.

**Dosage Forms**

Capsule: 1.5 mg, 3 mg, 4.5 mg, 6 mg

Solution, oral: 2 mg/mL (120 mL)

**Rivotril® (Can)** *see* clonazepam *on page 145*

## rizatriptan (rye za TRIP tan)

**U.S./Canadian Brand Names** Maxalt®; Maxalt-MLT™

**Therapeutic Category** Antimigraine Agent; Serotonin Agonist

**Use** Acute treatment of migraine with or without aura

**Usual Dosage** Oral: 10-20 mg, repeat after 2 hours if significant relief is not attained

**Dosage Forms** Tablet, as benzoate:

Maxalt®: 5 mg, 10 mg

Maxalt-MLT™ (orally disintegrating): 5 mg, 10 mg

**rLFN-α2** *see* interferon alfa-2b *on page 321*

**RMS® Rectal** *see* morphine sulfate *on page 400*

**Ro 11-1163** *see* moclobemide *(Canada only) on page 397*

**Robafen® AC** *see* guaifenesin and codeine *on page 282*

**Robafen® CF *(Discontinued)*** *see page 750*

**Robafen DM® [OTC]** *see* guaifenesin and dextromethorphan *on page 282*

**Robaxin®** *see* methocarbamol *on page 380*

**Robaxisal®** *see* methocarbamol and aspirin *on page 380*

**Robicillin® Tablet *(Discontinued)*** *see page 750*

**Robinul®** *see* glycopyrrolate *on page 278*

**Robinul® Forte** *see* glycopyrrolate *on page 278*

**Robitet® *(Discontinued)*** *see page 750*

**Robitussin® [OTC]** *see* guaifenesin *on page 281*

**Robitussin® A-C** *see* guaifenesin and codeine *on page 282*

**Robitussin-CF® *(Discontinued)*** *see page 750*

**Robitussin® Childrens Cough & Cold** *see* pseudoephedrine and dextromethorphan *on page 508*

**Robitussin® Cough Calmers [OTC]** *see* dextromethorphan *on page 178*

**Robitussin® Cough & Cold (Can)** *see* guaifenesin, pseudoephedrine, and dextromethorphan *on page 285*

**Robitussin®-DAC** *see* guaifenesin, pseudoephedrine, and codeine *on page 284*

**Robitussin®-DM [OTC]** *see* guaifenesin and dextromethorphan *on page 282*

**Robitussin-PE® [OTC]** *see* guaifenesin and pseudoephedrine *on page 283*

**Robitussin® Pediatric [OTC]** *see* dextromethorphan *on page 178*

**Robitussin® Severe Congestion Liqui-Gels® [OTC]** *see* guaifenesin and pseudoephedrine *on page 283*

**Rocaltrol®** *see* calcitriol *on page 96*

**Rocephin®** *see* ceftriaxone *on page 118*

## rocuronium (roe kyoor OH nee um)

**U.S./Canadian Brand Names** Zemuron™

**Therapeutic Category** Skeletal Muscle Relaxant

**Use** Produces skeletal muscle relaxation during surgery after induction of general anesthesia, increases pulmonary compliance during assisted mechanical respiration, facilitates endotracheal intubation

**Usual Dosage** I.V.:

Children:

Initial: 0.6 mg/kg under halothane anesthesia produce excellent to good intubating conditions within 1 minute and will provide a median time of 41 minutes of clinical relaxation in children 3 months to 1 year of age, and 27 minutes in children 1-12 years

Maintenance: 0.075-0.125 mg/kg administered upon return of $T_1$ to 25% of control provides clinical relaxation for 7-10 minutes

Adults:

Tracheal intubation:

Initial: 0.6 mg/kg is expected to provide approximately 31 minutes of clinical relaxation under opioid/nitrous oxide/oxygen anesthesia with neuromuscular block sufficient for intubation attained in 1-2 minutes; lower doses (0.45 mg/kg) may be used to provide 22 minutes of clinical relaxation with median time to neuromuscular block of 1-3 minutes; maximum blockade is achieved in <4 minutes

Maximum: 0.9-1.2 mg/kg may be administered during surgery under opioid/nitrous oxide/oxygen anesthesia without adverse cardiovascular effects and is expected to provide 58-67 minutes of clinical relaxation; neuromuscular blockade sufficient for intubation is achieved in <2 minutes with maximum blockade in <3 minutes

Maintenance: 0.1, 0.15, and 0.2 mg/kg administered at 25% recovery of control $T_1$ (defined as 3 twitches of train-of-four) provides a median of 12, 17, and 24 minutes of clinical duration under anesthesia

Rapid sequence intubation: 0.6-1.2 mg/kg in appropriately premedicated and anesthetized patients with excellent or good intubating conditions within 2 minutes

Continuous infusion: Initial: 0.01-0.012 mg/kg/minute only after early evidence of spontaneous recovery of neuromuscular function is evident

**Dosage Forms** Injection, as bromide: 10 mg/mL (5 mL, 10 mL)

**Rofact™ (Can)** *see* rifampin *on page 526*

## rofecoxib (roe fe COX ib)

**U.S./Canadian Brand Names** Vioxx®

**Therapeutic Category** Nonsteroidal Anti-inflammatory Drug (NSAID), COX-2 Selective

**Use** Relief of the signs and symptoms of osteoarthritis; management of acute pain in adults; treatment of primary dysmenorrhea

**Usual Dosage** Adult: Oral:

Osteoarthritis: 12.5 mg once daily; may be increased to a maximum of 25 mg once daily

Acute pain and management of dysmenorrhea: 50 mg once daily as needed (use for longer than 5 days has not been studied)

**Dosage Forms**

Suspension, oral: 12.5 mg/5 mL (150 mL); 25 mg/5 mL (150 mL)

Tablet: 12.5 mg, 25 mg, 50 mg

**Roferon-A®** *see* interferon alfa-2a *on page 321*

**Rogaine® Topical** *see* minoxidil *on page 394*

**Rogitine® (Can)** *see* phentolamine *on page 466*

**Rolaids® [OTC]** *see* dihydroxyaluminum sodium carbonate *on page 187*

**Rolaids® Calcium Rich [OTC]** *see* calcium carbonate *on page 97*

**Rolatuss® Plain Liquid** *see* chlorpheniramine and phenylephrine *on page 129*

**Romazicon®** *see* flumazenil *on page 252*

**Romycin® Solution *(Discontinued)*** *see page 750*

**Rondamine-DM® Drops** *see* carbinoxamine, pseudoephedrine, and dextromethorphan *on page 108*

**Rondec®-DM** *see* carbinoxamine, pseudoephedrine, and dextromethorphan *on page 108*

**Rondec® Drops** *see* carbinoxamine and pseudoephedrine *on page 107*

**Rondec® Filmtab®** *see* carbinoxamine and pseudoephedrine *on page 107*

**Rondec® Syrup** *see* carbinoxamine and pseudoephedrine *on page 107*

**Rondec-TR®** *see* carbinoxamine and pseudoephedrine *on page 107*

**Rondomycin® Capsule *(Discontinued)*** *see page 750*

## ropinirole (roe PIN i role)

**U.S./Canadian Brand Names** Requip®

**Therapeutic Category** Anti-Parkinson's Agent

**Use** Treatment of idiopathic Parkinson's disease; in patients with early Parkinson's disease who were not receiving concomitant levodopa therapy as well as in patients with advanced disease on concomitant levodopa

**Usual Dosage** Adults: Oral: Dosage should be increased to achieve a maximum therapeutic effect, balanced against the principal side effects of nausea, dizziness, somnolence, and dyskinesia

Recommended starting dose: 0.25 mg 3 times/day; based on individual patient response, the dosage should be titrated with weekly increments

Week 1: 0.25 mg 3 times/day; total daily dose: 0.75 mg

Week 2: 0.5 mg 3 times/day; total daily dose: 1.5 mg

Week 3: 0.75 mg 3 times/day; total daily dose: 2.25 mg

Week 4: 1 mg 3 times/day; total daily dose: 3 mg

After week 4, if necessary, daily dosage may be increased by 1.5 mg/day on a weekly basis up to a dose of 9 mg/day, and then by up to 3 mg/day weekly to a total of 24 mg/day

**Dosage Forms** Tablet, as hydrochloride: 0.25 mg, 0.5 mg, 1 mg, 2 mg, 5 mg

## ropivacaine (roe PIV a kane)

**U.S./Canadian Brand Names** Naropin™

**Therapeutic Category** Local Anesthetic

**Use** Production of local or regional anesthesia for surgery, postoperative pain management and obstetrical procedures by infiltration anesthesia and nerve block anesthesia

**Usual Dosage** Administer the smallest dose and concentration required to produce the desired result

**Dosage Forms**

Infusion, as hydrochloride: 2 mg/mL (100 mL, 200 mL)

Injection, as hydrochloride (single dose): 2 mg/mL (20 mL); 5 mg/mL (30 mL); 7.5 mg/mL (10 mL, 20 mL); 10 mg/mL (10 mL, 20 mL)

## rosiglitazone (roe si GLI ta zone)

**U.S./Canadian Brand Names** Avandia®

**Therapeutic Category** Hypoglycemic Agent, Oral; Thiazolidinedione Derivative

**Use**

Type 2 diabetes, monotherapy: Improve glycemic control as an adjunct to diet and exercise

Type 2 diabetes, combination therapy: In combination with metformin when diet, exercise and metformin alone or diet, exercise and rosiglitazone alone do not result in adequate glycemic control.

**Usual Dosage** Adults: Oral: Initial: 4 mg daily as a single daily dose or in divided doses twice daily. If response is inadequate after 12 weeks of treatment, the dosage may be increased to 8 mg daily as a single daily dose or in divided doses twice daily.

**Dosage Forms** Tablet: 2 mg, 4 mg, 8 mg

**RotaShield® *(Discontinued)*** *see page 750*

**Rovamycine® (Can)** *see* spiramycin *(Canada only) on page 556*

**Rowasa® Rectal** *see* mesalamine *on page 374*

**Roxanol™ Oral** *see* morphine sulfate *on page 400*

**Roxanol SR™ Oral** *see* morphine sulfate *on page 400*

**Roxanol-T™** *see* morphine sulfate *on page 400*

**Roxicet® 5/500** *see* oxycodone and acetaminophen *on page 444*

**Roxicodone™** *see* oxycodone *on page 443*

**Roxilox™** *see* oxycodone and acetaminophen *on page 444*

**Roxiprin® *(Discontinued)*** *see page 750*

**Roychlor® (Can)** *see* potassium chloride *on page 485*

**RP54274** *see* riluzole *on page 527*

**RP59500** *see* quinupristin and dalfopristin *on page 515*

**r-PA** *see* reteplase *on page 522*

**RSV-IGIV** *see* respiratory syncytial virus immune globulin (intravenous) *on page 522*

**R-Tannamine® Tablet** *see* chlorpheniramine, pyrilamine, and phenylephrine *on page 132*

**R-Tannate® Tablet** *see* chlorpheniramine, pyrilamine, and phenylephrine *on page 132*

**RTCA** *see* ribavirin *on page 525*

**RU-486** *see* mifepristone *on page 393*

**RU-38486** *see* mifepristone *on page 393*

## rubella and mumps vaccines, combined

(rue BEL a & mumpz vak SEENS, kom BINED)

**U.S./Canadian Brand Names** Biavax® II

**Therapeutic Category** Vaccine, Live Virus

**Use** Promote active immunity to rubella and mumps by inducing production of antibodies

**Usual Dosage** Children >12 months and Adults: 1 vial in outer aspect of the upper arm

**Dosage Forms** Injection (mixture of 2 viruses):

1. Wistar RA 27/3 strain of rubella virus
2. Jeryl Lynn (B level) mumps strain grown cell cultures of chick embryo

## rubella virus vaccine (live) (rue BEL a VYE rus vak SEEN live)

**Synonyms** German measles vaccine

**U.S./Canadian Brand Names** Meruvax® II

**Therapeutic Category** Vaccine, Live Virus

**Use** Provide vaccine-induced immunity to rubella

**Usual Dosage** S.C.: 1000 $TCID_{50}$ of rubella

**Dosage Forms** Injection, single dose: 1000 $TCID_{50}$ (Wistar RA 27/3 Strain)

**rubeola vaccine** *see* measles virus vaccine (live) *on page 367*

**Rubex®** *see* doxorubicin *on page 203*

**rubidomycin** *see* daunorubicin hydrochloride *on page 167*

**Rubramin-PC®** *see* cyanocobalamin *on page 158*

**Rufen® *(Discontinued)*** *see page 750*

**Rum-K®** *see* potassium chloride *on page 485*

**Ru-Tuss® *(Discontinued)*** *see page 750*

**Ru-Tuss® DE** *see* guaifenesin and pseudoephedrine *on page 283*

**Ru-Tuss® Expectorant [OTC]** *see* guaifenesin, pseudoephedrine, and dextromethorphan *on page 285*

**Ru-Vert-M®** *see* meclizine *on page 367*

**Rylosol® (Can)** *see* sotalol *on page 555*

**Rymed®** *see* guaifenesin and pseudoephedrine *on page 283*

**Rymed-TR® *(Discontinued)*** *see page 750*

**Ryna-C® Liquid** *see* chlorpheniramine, pseudoephedrine, and codeine *on page 132*

**Ryna-CX®** *see* guaifenesin, pseudoephedrine, and codeine *on page 284*

**Ryna® Liquid [OTC]** *see* chlorpheniramine and pseudoephedrine *on page 130*

**Rynatan® Extended Release** *see* azatadine and pseudoephedrine *on page 61*

**Rynatan® Pediatric Suspension** *see* chlorpheniramine, pyrilamine, and phenylephrine *on page 132*

**Rynatan® Tablet** *see* chlorpheniramine, pyrilamine, and phenylephrine *on page 132*

**Rynatuss® Pediatric Suspension** *see* chlorpheniramine, ephedrine, phenylephrine, and carbetapentane *on page 130*

**Rythmodan® (Can)** *see* disopyramide *on page 195*

**Rythmodan®-LA (Can)** *see* disopyramide *on page 195*

**Rythmol®** *see* propafenone *on page 502*

**Sabin vaccine** *see* poliovirus vaccine, live, trivalent, oral *on page 480*

**Sabril® (Can)** *see* vigabatrin *(Canada only)* *on page 627*

## sacrosidase (sak RO se dase)

**U.S./Canadian Brand Names** Sucraid™

**Therapeutic Category** Enzyme

**Use** An enzyme replacement therapy for the treatment of the genetically determined sucrase deficiency, which is part of congenital sucrase-isomaltase deficiency (CSID)

**Usual Dosage** Oral:

<15 kg: 1 mL [8500 int. units] (one full measuring scoop or 22 drops) per meal or snack

>15 kg: 2 mL [17,000 int. units] (two full measuring scoops or 44 drops) per meal or snack

It is recommended that approximately half of the dosage be taken at the beginning of each meal or snack, and the remainder be taken at the end of each meal or snack.

The beverage or infant formula should be served cold or at room temperature; the beverage or infant formula should not be warmed or heated before or after addition of sacrosidase

**Dosage Forms** Solution, oral: 8500 int. units/mL (118 mL)

**Safe Tussin® 30 [OTC]** *see* guaifenesin and dextromethorphan *on page 282*

**Saizen®** *see* human growth hormone *on page 296*

**Salacid® Ointment** *see* salicylic acid *on next page*

**Sal-Acid® Plaster** *see* salicylic acid *on next page*

**Salagen® Oral** *see* pilocarpine *on page 471*

**Salazopyrin® (Can)** *see* sulfasalazine *on page 565*

**salbutamol** *see* albuterol *on page 16*

**Saleto-200® [OTC]** *see* ibuprofen *on page 311*

**Saleto-400®** *see* ibuprofen *on page 311*

**Salflex®** *see* salsalate *on next page*

**Salgesic®** ***(Discontinued)*** *see page 750*

**salicylazosulfapyridine** *see* sulfasalazine *on page 565*

## salicylic acid (sal i SIL ik AS id)

**U.S./Canadian Brand Names** Clear Away® Disc [OTC]; Freezone® Solution [OTC]; Gordofilm® Liquid; Mediplast® Plaster [OTC]; Occlusal®-HP Liquid; Panscol® Lotion [OTC]; Panscol® Ointment [OTC]; PediaPatch Transdermal Patch [OTC]; P&S® Shampoo [OTC]; Salacid® Ointment; Sal-Acid® Plaster; Trans-Plantar® Transdermal Patch [OTC]; Trans-Ver-Sal® Transdermal Patch [OTC]; Vergogel® Gel [OTC]; Verukan® Solution

**Therapeutic Category** Keratolytic Agent

**Use** Topically for its keratolytic effect in controlling seborrheic dermatitis or psoriasis of body and scalp, dandruff, and other scaling dermatoses; to remove warts, corns, calluses; also used in the treatment of acne

**Usual Dosage**

Shampoo: Apply to scalp and allow to remain for a few minutes, then rinse, initially use every day or every other day; 2 treatments/week are usually sufficient to maintain control

Topical: Apply to affected area and place under occlusion at night; hydrate skin for at least 5 minutes before use

**Dosage Forms**

Cream: 2% (30 g)
Disk: 40%
Gel: 5% (60 g); 6% (30 g); 17% (7.5 g)
Liquid: 13.6% (9.3 mL); 17% (9.3 mL, 13.5 mL, 15 mL); 16.7% (15 mL)
Lotion: 3% (120 mL)
Ointment: 3% (90 g)
Patch, transdermal: 15% (20 mm); 40% (20 mm)
Plaster: 40%
Soap: 2% (97.5 g)
Strip: 40%

## salicylic acid and lactic acid (sal i SIL ik AS id & LAK tik AS id)

**U.S./Canadian Brand Names** Duofilm® Solution

**Therapeutic Category** Keratolytic Agent

**Use** Treatment of benign epithelial tumors such as warts

**Usual Dosage** Topical: Apply a thin layer directly to wart once daily (may be useful to apply at bedtime and wash off in morning)

**Dosage Forms** Solution, topical: Salicylic acid 16.7% and lactic acid 16.7% in flexible collodion (15 mL)

## salicylic acid and propylene glycol

(sal i SIL ik AS id & PROE pi leen GLYE cole)

**U.S./Canadian Brand Names** Keralyt® Gel

**Therapeutic Category** Keratolytic Agent

**Use** Removal of excessive keratin in hyperkeratotic skin disorders, including various ichthyosis, keratosis palmaris and plantaris and psoriasis; may be used to remove excessive keratin in dorsal and plantar hyperkeratotic lesions

**Usual Dosage** Topical: Apply to area at night after soaking region for at least 5 minutes to hydrate area, and place under occlusion; medication is washed off in morning

**Dosage Forms** Gel, topical: Salicylic acid 6% and propylene glycol 60% in ethyl alcohol 19.4% with hydroxypropyl methylcellulose and water (30 g)

**SalineX® [OTC]** *see* sodium chloride *on page 549*

**Salivart® Solution [OTC]** *see* saliva substitute *on this page*

## saliva substitute (sa LYE va SUB stee tute)

**U.S./Canadian Brand Names** Entertainer's Secret® Spray [OTC]; Moi-Stir® Solution [OTC]; Moi-Stir® Swabsticks [OTC]; Mouthkote® Solution [OTC]; Optimoist® Solution [OTC]; Salivart® Solution [OTC]; Salix® Lozenge [OTC]

**Therapeutic Category** Gastrointestinal Agent, Miscellaneous

**Use** Relief of dry mouth and throat in xerostomia

**Usual Dosage** Use as needed

**Dosage Forms**

Lozenge: 100s

Solution: 60 mL, 75 mL, 120 mL, 180 mL, 240 mL

Swabstix: 3s

**Salix® Lozenge [OTC]** *see* saliva substitute *on this page*

**Salk vaccine** *see* poliovirus vaccine (inactivated) *on page 480*

## salmeterol (sal ME te role)

**U.S./Canadian Brand Names** Serevent®; Serevent® Diskus®

**Therapeutic Category** Adrenergic Agonist Agent

**Use** Maintenance treatment of asthma; prevention of bronchospasm in patients >12 years of age with reversible obstructive airway disease, including patients with symptoms of nocturnal asthma who require regular treatment with inhaled, short-acting $beta_2$ agonists; prevention of exercise-induced bronchospasm

**Usual Dosage**

Inhalation: 42 mcg (2 puffs) twice daily (12 hours apart) for maintenance and prevention of symptoms of asthma

Prevention of exercise-induced asthma: 42 mcg (2 puffs) 30-60 minutes prior to exercise; additional doses should not be used for 12 hours

**Dosage Forms**

Inhaler: 21 mcg/metered inhalation

Powder for inhalation, oral (Serevent® Diskus®): 50 mcg [46 mcg/inhalation] (60 doses)

## *Salmonella typhi* Vi capsular polysaccharide vaccine *(Canada only)* (sal mo NEL la TI fi vi CAP su lar po le SAK ar ide VAK seen)

**U.S./Canadian Brand Names** Typherix™ (Can)

**Therapeutic Category** Vaccine

**Use** For active immunization against typhoid fever in persons 2 years of age and older.

**Usual Dosage** One dose administered I.M. ensures protection for at least 3 years. The vaccine must be given at least 2 weeks prior to travel to endemic areas.

**Dosage Forms** Injection: Vi polysaccharide vaccine of *S. typhi* 25 mcg (0.5 mL)

**Salmonine®** ***(Discontinued)*** *see page 750*

**Salofalk® (Can)** *see* mesalamine *on page 374*

## salsalate (SAL sa late)

**Synonyms** disalicylic acid

**U.S./Canadian Brand Names** Amigesic®; Argesic®-SA; Disalcid®; Mono-Gesic®; Salflex®

**Therapeutic Category** Analgesic, Non-narcotic; Antipyretic; Nonsteroidal Anti-inflammatory Drug (NSAID)

**Use** Treatment of minor pain or fever; rheumatoid arthritis, osteoarthritis, and related inflammatory conditions

**Usual Dosage** Adults: Oral: 1 g 2-4 times/day

**Dosage Forms**
Capsule: 500 mg
Tablet: 500 mg, 750 mg

**Salsitab®** ***(Discontinued)*** *see page 750*

**salt** *see* sodium chloride *on page 549*

**Sal-Tropine™ Oral** *see* atropine *on page 58*

**Saluron®** *see* hydroflumethiazide *on page 304*

**Salutensin®** ***(Discontinued)*** *see page 750*

**Salutensin-Demi®** ***(Discontinued)*** *see page 750*

**Sandimmune®** *see* cyclosporine *on page 160*

**Sandoglobulin®** *see* immune globulin (intravenous) *on page 315*

**Sandomigran® (Can)** *see* pizotifen *(Canada only)* *on page 475*

**Sandomigran DS® (Can)** *see* pizotifen *(Canada only)* *on page 475*

**Sandostatin®** *see* octreotide *on page 433*

**Sandostatin LAR®** *see* octreotide *on page 433*

**SangCya™** ***(Discontinued)*** *see page 750*

**Sani-Supp® Suppository [OTC]** *see* glycerin *on page 277*

**Sanorex®** ***(Discontinued)*** *see page 750*

**Sansert®** *see* methysergide *on page 387*

**Santyl®** *see* collagenase *on page 152*

## saquinavir (sa KWIN a veer)

**U.S./Canadian Brand Names** Fortovase®; Invirase®

**Therapeutic Category** Antiviral Agent

**Use** Treatment of advanced HIV infection, used in combination with older nucleoside analog medications

**Usual Dosage** Adults: Oral:
Fortovase®: Six 200 mg (1200 mg) capsules 3 times/day within 2 hours after a meal
Invirase®: Three 200 mg (600 mg) capsules 3 times/day within 2 hours after a full meal

**Dosage Forms**
Capsule (hard) as mesylate (Invirase®): 200 mg
Capsule (soft) (Fortovase®): 200 mg

**Sarafem™** *see* fluoxetine *on page 256*

## sargramostim (sar GRAM oh stim)

**Synonyms** GM-CSF; granulocyte-macrophage colony-stimulating factor; RGM-CSF

**U.S./Canadian Brand Names** Leukine™

**Therapeutic Category** Colony-Stimulating Factor

**Use** Myeloid reconstitution after autologous bone marrow transplantation; to accelerate myeloid recovery in patients with non-Hodgkin's lymphoma, Hodgkin's lymphoma, and acute lymphoblastic leukemia undergoing autologous BMT; following induction chemotherapy in patients with acute myelogenous leukemia to shorten time to neutrophil recovery

**Usual Dosage**
Children and Adults: I.V. infusion over ≥2 hours or S.C.
Existing clinical data suggest that starting GM-CSF between 24 and 72 hours subsequent to chemotherapy may provide optimal neutrophil recover; continue therapy until the occurrence of an absolute neutrophil count of 10,000/µL after the neutrophil nadir
**The available data suggest that rounding the dose to the nearest vial size may enhance patient convenience and reduce costs without clinical detriment**
(Continued)

## sargramostim *(Continued)*

**Myeloid reconstitution after peripheral stem cell, allogeneic or autologous bone marrow transplant:** I.V.: 250 mcg/m²/day for 21 days to begin 2-4 hours after the marrow infusion on day 0 of autologous bone marrow transplant or ≥24 hours after chemotherapy or 12 hours after last dose of radiotherapy

If a severe adverse reaction occurs, reduce or temporarily discontinue the dose until the reaction abates

If blast cells appear or progression of the underlying disease occurs, disrupt treatment

Interrupt or reduce the dose by half if ANC is >20,000 cells/mm³

Patients should not receive sargramostim until the postmarrow infusion ANC is <500 cells/mm³

**Neutrophil recovery following chemotherapy in AML:** I.V.: 250 mcg/m²/day over a 4-hour period starting ~day 11 or 4 days following the completion of induction chemotherapy, if day 10 bone marrow is hypoblastic with <5% blasts

If a second cycle of chemotherapy is necessary, administer ~4 days after the completion of chemotherapy if the bone marrow is hypoblastic with <5% blasts

Continue sargramostim until ANC is >1500 cells/mm³ for consecutive days or a maximum of 42 days

Discontinue sargramostim immediately if leukemic regrowth occurs

If a severe adverse reaction occurs, reduce the dose by 50% or temporarily discontinue the dose until the reaction abates

**Mobilization of peripheral blood progenitor cells:** I.V.: 250 mcg/m²/day over 24 hours or S.C. once daily

Continue the same dose through the period of PBPC collection

The optimal schedule for PBPC collection has not been established (usually begun by day 5 and performed daily until protocol specified targets are achieved)

If WBC >50,000 cells/mm³, reduce the dose by 50%

If adequate numbers of progenitor cells are not collected, consider other mobilization therapy

**Postperipheral blood progenitor cell transplantation:** I.V.: 250 mcg/m²/day over 24 hours or S.C. once daily beginning immediately following infusion of progenitor cells and continuing until ANC is >1500 for 3 consecutive days is attained

**BMT failure or engraftment delay:** I.V.: 250 mcg/m²/day for 14 days as a 2-hour infusion

The dose can be repeated after 7 days off therapy if engraftment has not occurred

If engraftment still has not occurred, a third course of 500 mcg/m²/day for 14 days may be tried after another 7 days off therapy; if there is still no improvement, it is unlikely that further dose escalation will be beneficial

If a severe adverse reaction occurs, reduce or temporarily discontinue the dose until the reaction abates

If blast cells appear or disease progression occurs, discontinue treatment

**Dosage Forms** Injection: 250 mcg, 500 mcg

**Sarna [OTC]** *see* camphor, menthol, and phenol *on page 102*

**Sarna® HC (Can)** *see* hydrocortisone (topical) *on page 304*

**S.A.S.™ (Can)** *see* sulfasalazine *on page 565*

**Sastid® Plain Therapeutic Shampoo and Acne Wash [OTC]** *see* sulfur and salicylic acid *on page 566*

**Scabene®** ***(Discontinued)*** *see page 750*

**Scalpicin® Topical** *see* hydrocortisone (topical) *on page 304*

**Scheinpharm™ Amoxicillin (Can)** *see* amoxicillin *on page 35*

**Scheinpharm Cefaclor (Can)** *see* cefaclor *on page 113*

**Sclavo - PPD® Solution** ***(Discontinued)*** *see page 750*

**Sclavo Test - PPD®** ***(Discontinued)*** *see page 750*

**Scleromate™** *see* morrhuate sodium *on page 401*

**Scopace® Tablet** *see* scopolamine *on this page*

## scopolamine (skoe POL a meen)

**Synonyms** hyoscine

**U.S./Canadian Brand Names** Buscopan® (Can); Isopto® Hyoscine; Scopace® Tablet; Transderm Scop®; Transderm-V® (Can)

**Therapeutic Category** Anticholinergic Agent

**Use** Preoperative medication to produce amnesia and decrease salivary and respiratory secretions; to produce cycloplegia and mydriasis; treatment of iridocyclitis; prevention of motion sickness; prevention of nausea/vomiting associated with anesthesia or opiate analgesia (patch)

**Usual Dosage**

Preoperatively:

Children: I.M., S.C.: 6 mcg/kg/dose (maximum: 0.3 mg/dose) or 0.2 mg/m$^2$ may be repeated every 6-8 hours **or** alternatively:

4-7 months: 0.1 mg

7 months to 3 years: 0.15 mg

3-8 years: 0.2 mg

8-12 years: 0.3 mg

Adults: I.M., I.V., S.C.: 0.3-0.65 mg; may be repeated every 4-6 hours

Motion sickness: Transdermal: Children >12 years and Adults: Apply 1 disc behind the ear at least 4 hours prior to exposure and every 3 days as needed

Ophthalmic:

Refraction:

Children: Instill 1 drop of 0.25% to eye(s) twice daily for 2 days before procedure

Adults: Instill 1-2 drops of 0.25% to eye(s) 1 hour before procedure

Iridocyclitis:

Children: Instill 1 drop of 0.25% to eye(s) up to 3 times/day

Adults: Instill 1-2 drops of 0.25% to eye(s) up to 4 times/day

**Dosage Forms**

Disc, transdermal: 1.5 mg/disc (4's)

Injection, as hydrobromide: 0.3 mg/mL (1 mL); 0.4 mg/mL (0.5 mL, 1 mL); 0.86 mg/mL (0.5 mL); 1 mg/mL (1 mL)

Solution, ophthalmic, as hydrobromide: 0.25% (5 mL, 15 mL)

Tablet: 0.4 mg

**Scot-Tussin® [OTC]** *see* guaifenesin *on page 281*

**Scot-Tussin DM® Cough Chasers [OTC]** *see* dextromethorphan *on page 178*

**Scot-Tussin® Senior Clear [OTC]** *see* guaifenesin and dextromethorphan *on page 282*

**SDZ ENA 713** *see* rivastigmine *on page 529*

**SeaMist® [OTC]** *see* sodium chloride *on page 549*

**Seba-Gel®** *see* benzoyl peroxide *on page 74*

**Sebizon®** *see* sulfacetamide *on page 562*

**Sebulex® Shampoo (Can)** *see* sulfur and salicylic acid *on page 566*

**Sebulon® Shampoo [OTC]** *see* pyrithione zinc *on page 512*

## secobarbital (see koe BAR bi tal)

**Synonyms** quinalbarbitone

**U.S./Canadian Brand Names** Seconal™

**Therapeutic Category** Barbiturate

**Controlled Substance** C-II

**Use** Short-term treatment of insomnia and as preanesthetic agent

**Usual Dosage** Oral:

Children: Preoperative sedation: 2-6 mg/kg (maximum 100 mg)

(Continued)

## secobarbital *(Continued)*

Adults:

Hypnotic: 100 mg

Preoperative sedation: 200-300 mg 1-2 hours before surgery

**Dosage Forms** Capsule, as sodium: 100 mg

**Seconal™** *see* secobarbital *on previous page*

**Secran®** *see* vitamin (multiple/oral) *on page 632*

## secretin (SEE kre tin)

**U.S./Canadian Brand Names** Secretin-Ferring Powder

**Therapeutic Category** Diagnostic Agent

**Use** Diagnosis of Zollinger-Ellison syndrome, chronic pancreatic dysfunction, and some hepatobiliary diseases such as obstructive jaundice resulting from cancer or stones in the biliary tract

**Usual Dosage** I.V.:

Pancreatic function: 1 CU/kg slow I.V. injection over 1 minute

Zollinger-Ellison: 2 CU/kg slow I.V. injection over 1 minute

**Dosage Forms** Powder for injection: 75 units (10 mL)

**Secretin-Ferring Powder** *see* secretin *on this page*

**Sectral®** *see* acebutolol *on page 3*

**Sedapap-10®** *see* butalbital compound and acetaminophen *on page 93*

**Selax® (Can)** *see* docusate *on page 197*

**Seldane®** ***(Discontinued)*** *see page 750*

**Seldane-D®** ***(Discontinued)*** *see page 750*

**Selectol®** ***(Discontinued)*** *see page 750*

## selegiline (seh LEDGE ah leen)

**Synonyms** deprenyl; *l*-deprenyl

**U.S./Canadian Brand Names** Apo®-Selegiline (Can); Atapryl®; Eldepryl®; Gen-Selegiline (Can); Novo-Selegiline (Can); Nu-Selegiline (Can); Selpak®

**Therapeutic Category** Anti-Parkinson's Agent; Dopaminergic Agent (Anti-Parkinson's)

**Use** Adjunct in the management of Parkinsonian patients in which levodopa/carbidopa therapy is deteriorating

**Unlabeled uses:** Early Parkinson's disease, Alzheimer's disease

**Usual Dosage** Adults: Oral: 5 mg twice daily

**Dosage Forms**

Capsule, as hydrochloride: 5 mg

Tablet: 5 mg

## selenium sulfide (se LEE nee um SUL fide)

**U.S./Canadian Brand Names** Dandrex® [OTC]; Exsel® Shampoo; Selsun Blue® Shampoo [OTC]; Selsun® Shampoo; Versel® (Can)

**Therapeutic Category** Antiseborrheic Agent, Topical

**Use** Treat itching and flaking of the scalp associated with dandruff; to control scalp seborrheic dermatitis; treatment of tinea versicolor

**Usual Dosage** Topical:

Dandruff, seborrhea: Massage 5-10 mL into wet scalp, leave on scalp 2-3 minutes, rinse thoroughly and repeat application; shampoo twice weekly for 2 weeks initially, then use once every 1-4 weeks as indicated depending upon control

Tinea versicolor: Apply the 2.5% lotion to affected area and lather with small amounts of water; leave on skin for 10 minutes, then rinse thoroughly; apply every day for 7 days

**Dosage Forms** Shampoo: 1% (120 mL, 210 mL, 240 mL, 330 mL); 2.5% (120 mL)

**Sele-Pak®** *see* trace metals *on page 598*

**Selepen®** *see* trace metals *on page 598*

**Selestoject®** ***(Discontinued)*** *see page 750*

**Selpak®** *see* selegiline *on previous page*

**Selsun Blue® Shampoo [OTC]** *see* selenium sulfide *on previous page*

**Selsun® Shampoo** *see* selenium sulfide *on previous page*

**Semicid® [OTC]** *see* nonoxynol 9 *on page 424*

**Semprex®-D** *see* acrivastine and pseudoephedrine *on page 11*

## senna (SEN na)

**U.S./Canadian Brand Names** Black Draught® [OTC]; Correctol® [OTC]; Fletcher's® Castoria® [OTC]; Gentlax® [OTC]; Innerclean® [OTC]; Laxagel® [OTC]; Senokot® [OTC]; Swiss Kriss® [OTC]; Uni Cenna® [OTC]; X-Prep® Liquid [OTC]

**Therapeutic Category** Laxative

**Use** Short-term treatment of constipation; evacuate the colon for bowel or rectal examinations

**Usual Dosage**

Children:

Oral:

>6 years: 10-20 mg/kg/dose at bedtime; maximum daily dose: 872 mg

6-12 years, >27 kg: 1 tablet at bedtime, up to 4 tablets/day **or** $^1/_2$ teaspoonful of granules (326 mg/tsp) at bedtime (up to 2 teaspoonfuls/day)

Liquid:

2-5 years: 5-10 mL at bedtime

6-15 years: 10-15 mL at bedtime

Suppository: $^1/_2$ at bedtime

Syrup:

1 month to 1 year: 1.25-2.5 mL at bedtime up to 5 mL/day

1-5 years: 2.5-5 mL at bedtime up to 10 mL/day

5-10 years: 5-10 mL at bedtime up to 20 mL/day

Adults:

Granules (326 mg/teaspoon): 1 teaspoonful at bedtime, not to exceed 2 teaspoonfuls twice daily

Liquid: 15-30 mL with meals and at bedtime

Suppository: 1 at bedtime, may repeat once in 2 hours

Syrup: 2-3 teaspoonfuls at bedtime, not to exceed 30 mL/day

Tablet: 187 mg: 2 tablets at bedtime, not to exceed 8 tablets/day

Tablet: 374 mg: 1 at bedtime, up to 4/day; 600 mg: 2 tablets at bedtime, up to 3 tablets/day

**Dosage Forms**

Granules: 326 mg/teaspoonful

Liquid: 7% [70 mg/mL] (130 mL, 360 mL); 6.5% [65 mg/mL] (75 mL, 150 mL)

Suppository, rectal: 652 mg

Syrup: 218 mg/5 mL (60 mL, 240 mL)

Tablet: 187 mg, 217 mg, 600 mg

**Senokot® [OTC]** *see* senna *on this page*

**Senolax®** ***(Discontinued)*** *see page 750*

**Sensorcaine®** *see* bupivacaine *on page 90*

**Sensorcaine®-MPF** *see* bupivacaine *on page 90*

**Septa® Topical Ointment [OTC]** *see* bacitracin, neomycin, and polymyxin B *on page 65*

**Septisol®** ***(Discontinued)*** *see page 750*

**Septra®** *see* sulfamethoxazole and trimethoprim *on page 564*

**Septra® DS** *see* sulfamethoxazole and trimethoprim *on page 564*

**Ser-A-Gen®** *see* hydralazine, hydrochlorothiazide, and reserpine *on page 298*

**Ser-Ap-Es®** ***(Discontinued)*** *see page 750*

**Serax®** *see* oxazepam *on page 441*

**Serc® (Can)** *see* betahistine *(Canada only) on page 77*

**Serentil®** *see* mesoridazine *on page 375*

**Serevent®** *see* salmeterol *on page 536*

**Serevent® Diskus®** *see* salmeterol *on page 536*

## sermorelin acetate (ser moe REL in AS e tate )

**U.S./Canadian Brand Names** Geref®

**Therapeutic Category** Diagnostic Agent

**Use** Evaluate ability of the somatotroph of the pituitary gland to secrete growth hormone

**Usual Dosage** I.V. (in a single dose in the morning following an overnight fast):

Children or subjects <50 kg: Draw venous blood samples for GH determinations 15 minutes before and immediately prior to administration, then administer 1 mcg/kg followed by a 3 mL normal saline flush, draw blood samples again for GH determinations

Adults or subjects >50 kg: Determine the number of ampules needed based on a dose of 1 mcg/kg, draw venous blood samples for GH determinations 15 minutes before and immediately prior to administration, then administer 1 mcg/kg followed by a 3 mL normal saline flush, draw blood samples again for GH determinations

**Dosage Forms** Powder for injection, lyophilized: 50 mcg, 500 mcg, 1000 mcg

**Seromycin® Pulvules®** *see* cycloserine *on page 160*

**Serophene®** *see* clomiphene *on page 145*

**Seroquel®** *see* quetiapine *on page 513*

**Serostim®** *see* human growth hormone *on page 296*

**Serpalan®** ***(Discontinued)*** *see page 750*

**Serpasil®** ***(Discontinued)*** *see page 750*

**Serpatabs®** ***(Discontinued)*** *see page 750*

## sertraline (SER tra leen)

**U.S./Canadian Brand Names** Apo®-Sertraline (Can); Novo-Sertraline (Can); Zoloft®

**Therapeutic Category** Antidepressant, Selective Serotonin Reuptake Inhibitor

**Use** Treatment of major depression; pediatric obsessive-compulsive disorder; also being studied for use in obesity

**Usual Dosage** Oral: Initial: 50 mg/day as a single dose, dosage may be increased at intervals of at least 1 week to a maximum recommended dosage of 200 mg/day

**Dosage Forms**

Oral concentrate, as hydrochloride: 20 mg/mL (60 mL)

Tablet, as hydrochloride: 25 mg, 50 mg, 100 mg

**Serutan® [OTC]** *see* psyllium *on page 509*

**Serzone®** *see* nefazodone *on page 412*

## sevelamer (se VEL a mer)

**U.S./Canadian Brand Names** Renagel®

**Therapeutic Category** Phosphate Binder

**Use** Reduction of serum phosphorous in patients with end-stage renal disease

**Usual Dosage** Adults: Oral: 2-4 capsules 3 times/day with meals; the initial dose may be based on serum phosphorous:

(Phosphorous: Initial dose)

>6.0 and <7.5: 2 capsules 3 times/day
>7.5 and <9.0: 3 capsules 3 times/day
≥9.0: 4 capsules 3 times/day

Dosage should be adjusted based on serum phosphorous concentration, with a goal of lowering to <6.0 mg/dL; maximum daily dose studied was 30 capsules/day

**Dosage Forms**
Capsule: 403 mg
Tablet: 400 mg, 800 mg

## sevoflurane (see voe FLOO rane)

**U.S./Canadian Brand Names** Sevorane™ (Can); Ultane®

**Therapeutic Category** General Anesthetic

**Use** General induction and maintenance of anesthesia (inhalation)

**Usual Dosage** Surgical levels of anesthesia can usually be obtained with concentrations of 0.5% to 3%

**Dosage Forms** Liquid for inhalation: 250 mL

**Sevorane™ (Can)** *see* sevoflurane *on this page*

**Shur-Seal® [OTC]** *see* nonoxynol 9 *on page 424*

**Sibelium® (Can)** *see* flunarizine *(Canada only) on page 253*

**Siblin® *(Discontinued)*** *see page 750*

## sibutramine (si BYOO tra meen)

**U.S./Canadian Brand Names** Meridia™

**Therapeutic Category** Anorexiant

**Use** Management of obesity, including weight loss and maintenance of weight loss, and should be used in conjunction with a reduced calorie diet

**Usual Dosage** Adults ≥16 years: Initial: 10 mg once daily; after 4 weeks may titrate up to 15 mg once daily as needed and tolerated

**Dosage Forms** Capsule, as hydrochloride monohydrate: 5 mg, 10 mg, 15 mg

**Silace-C® [OTC]** *see* docusate and casanthranol *on page 198*

**Siladryl® Oral [OTC]** *see* diphenhydramine *on page 191*

**Silafed® [OTC]** *see* triprolidine and pseudoephedrine *on page 609*

**Silafed® Syrup [OTC]** *see* triprolidine and pseudoephedrine *on page 609*

**Silain® *(Discontinued)*** *see page 750*

**Silaminic® Cold Syrup *(Discontinued)*** *see page 750*

**Silaminic® Expectorant *(Discontinued)*** *see page 750*

**Silapap® Children's [OTC]** *see* acetaminophen *on page 3*

**Silapap® Infant's [OTC]** *see* acetaminophen *on page 3*

## sildenafil (sil DEN a fil)

**Synonyms** UK 92480

**U.S./Canadian Brand Names** Viagra®

**Therapeutic Category** Phosphodiesterase Enzyme Inhibitor

**Use** Effective in most men with erectile dysfunction (ED), the medical term for impotence, which is associated with a broad range of physical or psychological medical conditions.

**Usual Dosage** Oral: Adults: 50 mg taken one hour before sexual activity; individuals may need more (100 mg) or less (25 mg) and dosing should be determined by a physician depending on effectiveness and side effects. The drug should not be used more than once daily.

**Dosage Forms** Tablet, as citrate: 25 mg, 50 mg, 100 mg

**Sildicon-E® *(Discontinued)*** *see page 750*

**Silphen® Cough [OTC]** *see* diphenhydramine *on page 191*

**Silphen DM® [OTC]** *see* dextromethorphan *on page 178*

**Siltussin® [OTC]** *see* guaifenesin *on page 281*

**Siltussin-CF®** ***(Discontinued)*** *see page 750*

**Siltussin DM® [OTC]** *see* guaifenesin and dextromethorphan *on page 282*

**Silvadene®** *see* silver sulfadiazine *on this page*

## silver nitrate (SIL ver NYE trate)

**Synonyms** $AgNO_3$

**Therapeutic Category** Topical Skin Product

**Use** Prevention of gonococcal ophthalmia neonatorum; cauterization of wounds and sluggish ulcers, removal of granulation tissue and warts

**Usual Dosage**

Neonates: Ophthalmic: Instill 2 drops immediately after birth into conjunctival sac of each eye as a single dose; do not irrigate eyes following instillation of eye drops

Children and Adults:

Sticks: Apply to mucous membranes and other moist skin surfaces only on area to be treated 2-3 times/week for 2-3 weeks

Topical solution: Apply a cotton applicator dipped in solution on the affected area 2-3 times/week for 2-3 weeks

**Dosage Forms**

Applicator, topical: 75% with potassium nitrate 25% (6")

Ointment, topical: 10% (30 g)

Solution:

Ophthalmic: 1% (wax ampuls)

Topical: 10% (30 mL); 25% (30 mL); 50% (30 mL)

## silver sulfadiazine (SIL ver sul fa DYE a zeen)

**U.S./Canadian Brand Names** Dermazin™ (Can); Flamazine® (Can); Silvadene®; SSD® AF; SSD® Cream; Thermazene®

**Therapeutic Category** Antibacterial, Topical

**Use** Adjunct in the prevention and treatment of infection in second and third degree burns

**Usual Dosage** Children and Adults: Topical: Apply once or twice daily with a sterile gloved hand; apply to a thickness of $^1/_{16}$"; burned area should be covered with cream at all times

**Dosage Forms** Cream, topical: 1% [10 mg/g] (20 g, 50 g, 100 g, 400 g, 1000 g)

## simethicone (sye METH i kone)

**Synonyms** activated dimethicone; activated methylpolysiloxane

**U.S./Canadian Brand Names** Anti-Gas® [OTC]; Flatulex® [OTC]; Gas Relief® [OTC]; Gas-X® [OTC]; Maalox Anti-Gas® [OTC]; Mylanta Gas® [OTC]; Mylicon® [OTC]; Ovol® (Can); Phazyme® [OTC]

**Therapeutic Category** Antiflatulent

**Use** Relieve flatulence, functional gastric bloating, and postoperative gas pains

**Usual Dosage** Oral:

Infants: 20 mg 4 times/day

Children <12 years: 40 mg 4 times/day

Children >12 years and Adults: 40-120 mg after meals and at bedtime as needed, not to exceed 500 mg/day

**Dosage Forms**

Capsule: 125 mg

Drops, oral: 40 mg/0.6 mL (30 mL)

Tablet: 50 mg, 60 mg, 95 mg

Chewable: 40 mg, 80 mg, 125 mg

**Simplet® [OTC]** *see* acetaminophen, chlorpheniramine, and pseudoephedrine *on page 6*

**Simron® [OTC]** *see* ferrous gluconate *on page 246*

**Simulect®** *see* basiliximab *on page 67*

## simvastatin (SIM va stat in)

**U.S./Canadian Brand Names** Zocor®

**Therapeutic Category** HMG-CoA Reductase Inhibitor

**Use** Adjunct to dietary therapy to decrease elevated serum total and LDL cholesterol concentrations in primary hypercholesterolemia; lowering elevated triglyceride levels

**Usual Dosage** Adults: Oral: Start with 5-10 mg/day as a single bedtime dose; starting dose of 5 mg/day should be considered for patients with LDL-C of ≤190 mg/dL and for the elderly; patients with LDL-C levels >190 mg/dL should be started on 10 mg/day; adjustments of dosage should be made at intervals of 4 weeks or more; maximum recommended dose: 40 mg/day

**Dosage Forms** Tablet: 5 mg, 10 mg, 20 mg, 40 mg, 80 mg

**Sinarest® 12 Hour Nasal Solution** *see* oxymetazoline *on page 444*

**Sinarest® Nasal Solution [OTC]** *see* phenylephrine *on page 467*

**Sinarest® Sinus [OTC]** *see* acetaminophen, chlorpheniramine, and pseudoephedrine *on page 6*

## sincalide (SIN ka lide)

**Synonyms** C8-CCK; OP-CCK

**U.S./Canadian Brand Names** Kinevac®

**Therapeutic Category** Diagnostic Agent

**Use** Postevacuation cholecystography; gallbladder bile sampling; stimulate pancreatic secretion for analysis

**Usual Dosage** Adults: I.V.:

Contraction of gallbladder: 0.02 mcg/kg over 30 seconds to 1 minute, may repeat in 15 minutes a 0.04 mcg/kg dose

Pancreatic function: 0.02 mcg/kg over 30 minutes

**Dosage Forms** Injection: 5 mcg

**Sine-Aid® IB [OTC]** *see* pseudoephedrine and ibuprofen *on page 508*

**Sine-Aid®, Maximum Strength [OTC]** *see* acetaminophen and pseudoephedrine *on page 6*

**Sinemet®** *see* carbidopa and levodopa *on page 107*

**Sine-Off® [OTC]** *see* acetaminophen, chlorpheniramine, and pseudoephedrine *on page 6*

**Sine-Off® Maximum Strength [OTC]** *see* acetaminophen and pseudoephedrine *on page 6*

**Sinequan® Oral** *see* doxepin *on page 202*

**Sinex® Long-Acting [OTC]** *see* oxymetazoline *on page 444*

**Singlet® [OTC]** *see* acetaminophen, chlorpheniramine, and pseudoephedrine *on page 6*

**Singulair®** *see* montelukast *on page 399*

**Sinografin®** *see* radiological/contrast media (ionic) *on page 516*

**Sintrom® (Can)** *see* nicoumalone *(Canada only) on page 419*

**Sinubid®** ***(Discontinued)*** *see page 750*

**Sinufed® Timecelles®** *see* guaifenesin and pseudoephedrine *on page 283*

**Sinumed® [OTC]** *see* acetaminophen, chlorpheniramine, and pseudoephedrine *on page 6*

**Sinumist®-SR Capsulets®** *see* guaifenesin *on page 281*

**Sinupan®** *see* guaifenesin and phenylephrine *on page 283*

**Sinus® [OTC]** *see* acetaminophen, chlorpheniramine, and pseudoephedrine *on page 6*

**Sinus Maximum Strength [OTC]** *see* acetaminophen and pseudoephedrine *on page 6*

**Sinus-Relief® Maximum Relief [OTC]** *see* acetaminophen and pseudoephedrine *on page 6*

**Sinustab® [OTC]** *see* acetaminophen and pseudoephedrine *on page 6*

**Sinutab® Maximum Strength [OTC]** *see* acetaminophen, chlorpheniramine, and pseudoephedrine *on page 6*

**Sinutab® Regular Strength [OTC]** *see* acetaminophen and pseudoephedrine *on page 6*

## sirolimus (sir OH li mus)

**U.S./Canadian Brand Names** Rapamune®

**Therapeutic Category** Immunosuppressant Agent

**Use** Prophylaxis of organ rejection in patients receiving renal transplants, in combination with cyclosporin and corticosteroids

**Unlabeled use:** Prophylaxis of organ rejection in solid organ transplant patients in combination with tacrolimus and corticosteroids

**Usual Dosage** Oral:

Adults ≥40 kg: Loading dose: For *de novo* transplant recipients, a loading dose of 3 times the daily maintenance dose should be administered on day 1 of dosing. Maintenance dose: 2 mg/day. Doses should be taken 4 hours after cyclosporine, and should be taken consistently either with or without food.

Children ≥13 years or Adults <40 kg: Loading dose: 3 mg/m$^2$ (day 1); followed by a maintenance of 1 mg/m$^2$/day.

**Dosage Forms**

Solution, oral: 1 mg/mL (1 mL, 2 mL, 5 mL, 60 mL, 150 mL)

Tablet: 1 mg

**SK** *see* streptokinase *on page 558*

**Skelaxin®** *see* metaxalone *on page 377*

**Skelex®** ***(Discontinued)*** *see page 750*

**Skelid®** *see* tiludronate *on page 590*

**SKF 104864** *see* topotecan *on page 596*

## skin test antigens, multiple (skin test AN tee gens, MUL ti pul)

**U.S./Canadian Brand Names** Multitest CMI®

**Therapeutic Category** Diagnostic Agent

**Use** Detection of nonresponsiveness to antigens by means of delayed hypersensitivity skin testing

**Usual Dosage** Select only test sites that permit sufficient surface area and subcutaneous tissue to allow adequate penetration of all 8 points, avoid hairy areas

Press loaded unit into the skin with sufficient pressure to puncture the skin and allow adequate penetration of all points, maintain firm contact for at least five seconds, during application the device should not be "rocked" back and forth and side to side without removing any of the test heads from the skin sites

If adequate pressure is applied it will be possible to observe:

1. The puncture marks of the nine tines on each of the eight test heads
2. An imprint of the circular platform surrounding each test head
3. Residual antigen and glycerin at each of the eight sites

If any of the above three criteria are not fully followed, the test results may not be reliable

Reading should be done in good light, read the test sites at both 24 and 48 hours, the largest reaction recorded from the two readings at each test site should be used; if two readings are not possible, a single 48 hour is recommended

A positive reaction from any of the seven delayed hypersensitivity skin test antigens is **induration of ≥2 mm** providing there is no induration at the negative control site; the size of the induration reactions with this test may be smaller than those obtained with other intradermal procedures

**Dosage Forms** Individual carton containing one preloaded skin test antigen for cellular hypersensitivity

**Sleep-eze 3® Oral [OTC]** *see* diphenhydramine *on page 191*

**Sleepinal® [OTC]** *see* diphenhydramine *on page 191*

**Sleepwell 2-nite® [OTC]** *see* diphenhydramine *on page 191*

**Slim-Mint® [OTC]** *see* benzocaine *on page 72*

**Sloan's Liniment®** *see* capsaicin *on page 104*

**Slo-bid™** *see* theophylline *on page 581*

**Slo-Niacin® [OTC]** *see* niacin *on page 417*

**Slo-Phyllin®** *see* theophylline *on page 581*

**Slo-Phyllin® GG** *see* theophylline and guaifenesin *on page 583*

**Slo-Salt®** ***(Discontinued)*** *see page 750*

**Slow FE® [OTC]** *see* ferrous sulfate *on page 247*

**Slow-K®** *see* potassium chloride *on page 485*

**Slow-Mag® [OTC]** *see* magnesium chloride *on page 361*

**Slow-Trasicor® (Can)** *see* oxprenolol *(Canada only) on page 442*

**smelling salts** *see* ammonia spirit (aromatic) *on page 34*

**SMX-TMP** *see* sulfamethoxazole and trimethoprim *on page 564*

**snake (pit vipers) antivenin** *see* antivenin (*Crotalidae*) polyvalent *on page 45*

**Snaplets-EX®** ***(Discontinued)*** *see page 750*

**sodium 2-mercaptoethane sulfonate** *see* mesna *on page 375*

## sodium acetate (SOW dee um AS e tate)

**Therapeutic Category** Alkalinizing Agent; Electrolyte Supplement, Oral

**Use** Sodium salt replacement; correction of acidosis through conversion of acetate to bicarbonate

**Usual Dosage** Sodium acetate is metabolized to bicarbonate on an equimolar basis outside the liver; administer in large volume I.V. fluids as a sodium source. Refer to sodium bicarbonate monograph.

Maintenance electrolyte requirements of sodium in parenteral nutrition solutions:

Daily requirements: 3-4 mEq/kg/24 hours or 25-40 mEq/1000 kcal/24 hours

Maximum: 100-150 mEq/24 hours

**Dosage Forms** Injection: 2 mEq/mL (20 mL, 50 mL); 4 mEq/mL (50 mL)

**sodium acid carbonate** *see* sodium bicarbonate *on next page*

## sodium ascorbate (SOW dee um a SKOR bate)

**Therapeutic Category** Vitamin, Water Soluble

**Use** Prevention and treatment of scurvy and to acidify the urine; large doses may decrease the severity of "colds"

**Usual Dosage** Oral, I.V.:

Children:

Scurvy: 100-300 mg/day in divided doses for at least 2 weeks

Urinary acidification: 500 mg every 6-8 hours

(Continued)

## sodium ascorbate *(Continued)*

Dietary supplement: 35-45 mg/day
Adults:
Scurvy: 100-250 mg 1-2 times/day for at least 2 weeks
Urinary acidification: 4-12 g/day in divided doses
Dietary supplement: 50-60 mg/day
Prevention and treatment of cold: 1-3 g/day

**Dosage Forms**

Crystals: 1020 mg per 1/4 teaspoonful [ascorbic acid 900 mg]
Injection: 250 mg/mL [ascorbic acid 222 mg/mL] (30 mL); 562.5 mg/mL [ascorbic acid 500 mg/mL] (1 mL, 2 mL)
Tablet: 585 mg [ascorbic acid 500 mg]

## sodium bicarbonate (SOW dee um bye KAR bun ate)

**Synonyms** baking soda; $NaHCO_3$; sodium acid carbonate; sodium hydrogen carbonate

**U.S./Canadian Brand Names** Neut®

**Therapeutic Category** Alkalinizing Agent; Antacid; Electrolyte Supplement, Oral

**Use** Management of metabolic acidosis; antacid; alkalinize urine; stabilization of acid base status in cardiac arrest, and treatment of life-threatening hyperkalemia

**Usual Dosage**

Cardiac arrest (patient should be adequately ventilated before administering $NaHCO_3$):
Infants: Use 1:1 dilution of 1 mEq/mL $NaHCO_3$ or use 0.5 mEq/mL $NaHCO_3$ at a dose of 1 mEq/kg slow IVP initially; may repeat with 0.5 mEq/kg in 10 minutes one time or as indicated by the patient's acid-base status. Rate of administration should not exceed 10 mEq/minute.
Children and Adults: IVP: 1 mEq/kg initially; may repeat with 0.5 mEq/kg in 10 minutes one time or as indicated by the patient's acid-base status
Metabolic acidosis: Dosage should be based on the following formula if blood gases and pH measurements are available:
Infants and Children: $HCO_3$-(mEq) = 0.3 x weight (kg) x base deficit (mEq/L) **or** $HCO_3$-(mEq) = 0.5 x weight (kg) x (24 - serum $HCO_3$-) (mEq/L)
Adults: $HCO_3$-(mEq) = 0.2 x weight (kg) x base deficit (mEq/L) **or** $HCO_3$-(mEq) = 0.5 x weight (kg) x (24 - serum $HCO_3$-) (mEq/L)
If acid-base status is not available: Dose for older Children and Adults: 2-5 mEq/kg I.V. infusion over 4-8 hours; subsequent doses should be based on patient's acid-base status
Chronic renal failure: Oral: Children: 1-3 mEq/kg/day
Renal tubular acidosis: Oral:
Distal:
Children: 2-3 mEq/kg/day
Adults: 1 mEq/kg/day
Proximal: Children: Initial: 5-10 mEq/kg/day; maintenance: Increase as required to maintain serum bicarbonate in the normal range
Urine alkalinization: Oral:
Children: 1-10 mEq (84-840 mg)/kg/day in divided doses; dose should be titrated to desired urinary pH
Adults: Initial: 48 mEq (4 g), then 12-24 mEq (1-2 g) every 4 hours; dose should be titrated to desired urinary pH; doses up to 16 g/day have been used

**Dosage Forms**

Injection: 4% [40 mg/mL = 2.4 mEq/5 mL] (5 mL); 4.2% [42 mg/mL = 5 mEq/10 mL] (10 mL); 7.5% [75 mg/mL = 8.92 mEq/10 mL] (10 mL, 50 mL); 8.4% [84 mg/mL = 10 mEq/10 mL] (10 mL, 50 mL)
Powder: 120 g, 480 g
Tablet: 300 mg [3.6 mEq]; 325 mg [3.8 mEq]; 520 mg [6.3 mEq]; 600 mg [7.3 mEq]; 650 mg [7.6 mEq]

**sodium cellulose phosphate** *see* cellulose sodium phosphate *on page 119*

## sodium chloride (SOW dee um KLOR ide)

**Synonyms** NaCl; normal saline; salt

**U.S./Canadian Brand Names** Adsorbonac® Ophthalmic [OTC]; Afrin® Saline Mist [OTC]; AK-NaCl® [OTC]; Ayr® Nasal [OTC]; Breathe Free® [OTC]; Dristan® Saline Spray [OTC]; HuMIST® Nasal Mist [OTC]; Hydrasense® (Can); Muro 128® Ophthalmic [OTC]; Muroptic-5® [OTC]; NaSal™ [OTC]; Nasal Moist® [OTC]; Ocean Nasal Mist [OTC]; Pretz® [OTC]; SalineX® [OTC]; SeaMist® [OTC]

**Therapeutic Category** Electrolyte Supplement, Oral; Lubricant, Ocular

**Use** Prevention of muscle cramps and heat prostration; restoration of sodium ion in hyponatremia; restore moisture to nasal membranes; reduction of corneal edema

**Usual Dosage**

Newborn electrolyte requirement:

Premature: 2-8 mEq/kg/24 hours

Term:

0-48 hours: 0-2 mEq/kg/24 hours

>48 hours: 1-4 mEq/kg/24 hours

Children: I.V.: Hypertonic solutions (>0.9%) should only be used for the initial treatment of acute serious symptomatic hyponatremia; maintenance: 3-4 mEq/kg/day; maximum: 100-150 mEq/day; dosage varies widely depending on clinical condition

Replacement: Determined by laboratory determinations mEq

Sodium deficiency (mEq/kg) = [% dehydration (L/kg)/100 x 70 (mEq/L) = [0.6 (L/kg) x (140 - serum sodium) (mEq/L)]

Nasal: Use as often as needed

Adults:

GI irrigant: 1-3 L/day by intermittent irrigation

Heat cramps: Oral: 0.5-1 g with full glass of water, up to 4.8 g/day

Replacement I.V.: Determined by laboratory determinations mEq

Sodium deficiency (mEq/kg) = [% dehydration (L/kg)/100 x 70 (mEq/L)] + [0.6 (L/kg) x (140 - serum sodium) (mEq/L)]

To correct acute, serious hyponatremia: mEq sodium = (desired sodium (mEq/L) - actual sodium (mEq/L) x 0.6 x wt (kg)); for acute correction use 125 mEq/L as the desired serum sodium; acutely correct serum sodium in 5 mEq/L/dose increments; more gradual correction in increments of 10 mEq/L/day is indicated in the asymptomatic patient

Chloride maintenance electrolyte requirement in parenteral nutrition: 2-4 mEq/kg/24 hours or 25-40 mEq/1000 kcals/24 hours; maximum: 100-150 mEq/24 hours

Sodium maintenance electrolyte requirement in parenteral nutrition: 3-4 mEq/kg/24 hours or 25-40 mEq/1000 kcals/24 hours; maximum: 100-150 mEq/24 hours.

Nasal: Use as often as needed

Ophthalmic:

Ointment: Apply once daily or more often

Solution: Instill 1-2 drops into affected eye(s) every 3-4 hours

Abortifacient: 20% (250 mL) administered by transabdominal intra-amniotic instillation

**Dosage Forms**

Drops, nasal: 0.9% with dropper

Injection: 0.2% (3 mL); 0.45% (3 mL, 5 mL, 500 mL, 1000 mL); 0.9% (1 mL, 2 mL, 3 mL, 4 mL, 5 mL, 10 mL, 20 mL, 25 mL, 30 mL, 50 mL, 100 mL, 130 mL, 150 mL, 250 mL, 500 mL, 1000 mL); 3% (500 mL); 5% (500 mL); 20% (250 mL); 23.4% (30 mL, 100 mL)

Injection:

Admixtures: 50 mEq (20 mL); 100 mEq (40 mL); 625 mEq (250 mL)

Bacteriostatic: 0.9% (30 mL)

Concentrated: 14.6% (20 mL, 40 mL, 200 mL); 23.4% (10 mL, 20 mL, 30 mL)

Irrigation: 0.45% (500 mL, 1000 mL, 1500 mL); 0.9% (250 mL, 500 mL, 1000 mL, 1500 mL, 2000 mL, 3000 mL, 4000 mL)

Ointment, ophthalmic (Muro 128®): 5% (3.5 g)

Solution:

Inhalation: 0.9% (3 mL)

Irrigation: 0.9% (1000 mL, 2000 mL)

(Continued)

## sodium chloride *(Continued)*

Nasal: 0.4% (15 mL, 50 mL); 0.6% (15 mL); 0.65% (20 mL, 45 mL, 50 mL)
Ophthalmic (Adsorbonac®): 2% (15 mL); 5% (15 mL, 30 mL)
Tablet: 650 mg, 1 g, 2.25 g
Enteric coated: 1 g
Slow release: 600 mg

## sodium citrate and potassium citrate mixture

(SOW dee um SIT rate & poe TASS ee um SIT rate MIKS chur)

**U.S./Canadian Brand Names** Polycitra®

**Therapeutic Category** Alkalinizing Agent

**Use** Conditions where long-term maintenance of an alkaline urine is desirable as in control and dissolution of uric acid and cystine calculi of the urinary tract

**Usual Dosage** Oral:
Children: 5-15 mL diluted in water after meals and at bedtime
Adults: 15-30 mL diluted in water after meals and at bedtime

**Dosage Forms** Syrup: Sodium citrate 500 mg, potassium citrate 550 mg, with citric acid 334 mg per 5 mL [sodium 1 mEq, potassium 1 mEq, bicarbonate 2 mEq]

**sodium edetate** *see* edetate disodium *on page 210*

**sodium ethacrynate** *see* ethacrynic acid *on page 229*

**sodium fusidate** *see* fusidic acid *(Canada only) on page 267*

## sodium hyaluronate (SOW dee um hye al yoor ON nate)

**Synonyms** hyaluronic acid

**U.S./Canadian Brand Names** Biolon®; Cystistat® (Can); Eyestil® (Can); Hyalgan®; Provisc®; Suplasyn® (Can); Vitrax®

**Therapeutic Category** Ophthalmic Agent, Viscoelastic

**Use** Surgical aid in cataract extraction, intraocular implantation, corneal transplant, glaucoma filtration, and retinal attachment surgery

**Usual Dosage** Depends upon procedure (slowly introduce a sufficient quantity into eye)

**Dosage Forms**
Injection (Hyalgan®): 10 mg/mL (2 mL)
Liquid:
Biolon®: 10 mg/mL (0.5 mL, 1 mL)
Provisc®: 10 mg/mL (0.4 mL, 0.55 mL, 0.85 mL)
Vitrax®: 30 mg/mL (0.65 mL)

**sodium hyaluronate-chrondroitin sulfate** *see* chondroitin sulfate-sodium hyaluronate *on page 135*

**sodium hydrogen carbonate** *see* sodium bicarbonate *on page 548*

## sodium hypochlorite solution

(SOW dee um hye poe KLOR ite soe LOO shun)

**Synonyms** Dakin's solution; modified Dakin's solution

**Therapeutic Category** Disinfectant

**Use** Treatment of athlete's foot (0.5%); wound irrigation (0.5%); to disinfect utensils and equipment (5%)

**Usual Dosage** Topical irrigation

**Dosage Forms**
Solution: 5% (4000 mL)
Modified Dakin's solution:
Full strength: 0.5% (1000 mL)
Half strength: 0.25% (1000 mL)
Quarter strength: 0.125% (1000 mL)

## sodium lactate (SOW dee um LAK tate)

**Therapeutic Category** Alkalinizing Agent

**Use** Source of bicarbonate for prevention and treatment of mild to moderate metabolic acidosis

**Usual Dosage** Dosage depends on degree of acidosis

**Dosage Forms** Injection:

1.87 g/100 mL [sodium 16.7 mEq and lactate 16.7 mEq per 100 mL] (1000 mL)
560 mg/mL [sodium 5 mEq sodium and lactate 5 mEq per mL] (10 mL)

**sodium nitroferricyanide** *see* nitroprusside *on page 423*

**Sodium P.A.S.® *(Discontinued)*** *see page 750*

**sodium-pca and lactic acid** *see* lactic acid and sodium-PCA *on page 337*

## sodium phenylacetate and sodium benzoate
(SOW dee um fen il AS e tate & SOW dee um BENZ oh ate)

**U.S./Canadian Brand Names** Ucephan®

**Therapeutic Category** Ammonium Detoxicant

**Use** Adjunctive therapy to prevent/treat hyperammonemia in patients with urea cycle enzymopathy involving partial or complete deficiencies of carbamoyl-phosphate synthetase, ornithine transcarbamoylase or argininosuccinate synthetase

**Usual Dosage** Infants and Children: Oral: 2.5 mL (250 mg sodium benzoate and 250 mg sodium phenylacetate)/kg/day divided 3-6 times/day; total daily dose should not exceed 100 mL

**Dosage Forms** Solution: Sodium phenylacetate 100 mg and sodium benzoate 100 mg per mL (100 mL)

## sodium phenylbutyrate (SOW dee um fen il BYOO ti rate)

**Synonyms** ammonapse

**U.S./Canadian Brand Names** Buphenyl®

**Therapeutic Category** Miscellaneous Product

**Use** Adjunctive therapy in the chronic management of patients with urea cycle disorder involving deficiencies of carbamoylphosphate synthetase, ornithine transcarbamylase, or argininosuccinic acid synthetase

**Usual Dosage**

Powder: Patients weighing <20 kg: 450-600 mg/kg/day or 9.9-13 g/m$^2$/day, administered in equally divided amounts with each meal or feeding, 4-6 times/day; safety and efficacy of doses >20 g/day have not been established

Tablet: Children >20 kg and Adults: 450-600 mg/kg/day or 9.9-13 g/m$^2$/day, administered in equally divided amounts with each meal; safety and efficacy of doses >20 g/day have not been established

**Dosage Forms**

Powder: 3.2 g [sodium phenylbutyrate 3 g] per teaspoon (500 mL, 950 mL); 9.1 g [sodium phenylbutyrate 8.6 g] per **tablespoon** (500 mL, 950 mL)

Tablet: 500 mg

## sodium phosphates (SOW dee um FOS fates)

**U.S./Canadian Brand Names** Fleet® Enema [OTC]; Fleet® Phospho®-Soda [OTC]

**Therapeutic Category** Electrolyte Supplement, Oral; Laxative

**Use** Source of phosphate in large volume I.V. fluids; short-term treatment of constipation (oral/rectal) and to evacuate the colon for rectal and bowel exams; treatment and prevention of hypophosphatemia

**Usual Dosage**

Normal requirements elemental phosphate: Oral:

0-6 months: 240 mg
6-12 months: 360 mg
1-10 years: 800 mg
>10 years: 1200 mg

(Continued)

## sodium phosphates *(Continued)*

Pregnancy lactation: Additional 400 mg/day

Treatment:

It is difficult to provide concrete guidelines for the treatment of severe hypophosphatemia because the extent of total body deficits and response to therapy are difficult to predict. Aggressive doses of phosphate may result in a transient serum elevation followed by redistribution into intracellular compartments or bone tissue. It is recommended that repletion of severe hypophosphatemia (<1 mg/dL in adults) be done I.V. because large doses of oral phosphate may cause diarrhea and intestinal absorption may be unreliable

**Pediatric I.V. phosphate repletion:**

Children: 0.25-0.5 mmol/kg **administer over 4-6 hours and repeat if symptomatic hypophosphatemia persists**; to assess the need for further phosphate administration: obtain serum inorganic phosphate after administration of the first dose and base further doses on serum levels and clinical status

**Adult I.V. phosphate repletion:**

Initial dose: 0.08 mmol/kg if recent uncomplicated hypophosphatemia

Initial dose: 0.16 mmol/kg if prolonged hypophosphatemia with presumed total body deficits; increase dose by 25% to 50% if patient symptomatic with severe hypophosphatemia

Severe hypophosphatemia:

High-dose = 0.36 mmol/kg over 6 hours; use if serum $PO_4$ <0.5 mg/dL

Adults: 0.15-0.3 mmol/kg/dose over 12 hours, may repeat as needed to achieve desired serum level

**With orders for I.V. phosphate, there is considerable confusion associated with the use of millimoles (mmol) versus milliequivalents (mEq) to express the phosphate requirement.** Because inorganic phosphate exists as monobasic and dibasic anions, with the mixture of valences is dependent on pH, ordering by mEq amounts is unreliable and may lead to large dosing errors. In addition, I.V. phosphate is available in the sodium and potassium salt; therefore, the content of these cations must be considered when ordering phosphate. The most reliable method of ordering I.V. phosphate is by millimoles, then specifying the potassium or sodium salt. For example, an order for 15 mmol of phosphate as potassium phosphate in one liter of normal saline would also provide 22 mEq of potassium.

Phosphate maintenance electrolyte requirement in parenteral nutrition: 2 mmol/kg/24 hours or 35 mmol/kcal/24 hours; Maximum: 15-30 mmol/24 hours

Maintenance:

Children: 0.5-1.5 mmol/kg/24 hours I.V. **or** 2-3 mmol/kg/24 hours orally in divided doses

Adults: 15-30 mmol/24 hours I.V. **or** 50-150 mmol/24 hours orally in divided doses

Laxative (Fleet®): Rectal:

Children 2-12 years: 67.5 mL (1/2 bottle) as a single dose, may repeat

Children ≥12 years and Adults: 133 mL enema as a single dose, may repeat

Laxative (Fleet® Phospho®-Soda): Oral:

Children:

5-9 years: 5 mL as a single dose

10-12 years: 10 mL as a single dose

Children ≥12 years and Adults: 20-30 mL as a single dose

### Dosage Forms

Enema: Sodium phosphate 6 g and sodium biphosphate 16 g/100 mL (67.5 mL pediatric enema unit, 135 mL adult enema unit)

Injection: Phosphate 3 mmol and sodium 4 mEq per mL (5 mL, 10 mL, 15 mL, 30 mL, 50 mL)

Solution, oral: Sodium phosphate 18 g and sodium biphosphate 48 g/100 mL (45 mL, 90 mL, 273 mL)

## sodium polystyrene sulfonate

(SOW dee um pol ee STYE reen SUL fon ate)

**U.S./Canadian Brand Names** Kayexalate®; Kionex™; PMS-Sodium Polystyrene Sulfonate (Can); SPS®

**Therapeutic Category** Antidote

**Use** Treatment of hyperkalemia

**Usual Dosage**

Children:

Oral: 1 g/kg/dose every 6 hours

Rectal: 1 g/kg/dose every 2-6 hours (In small children and infants employ lower doses by using the practical exchange ratio of 1 mEq potassium/g of resin as the basis for calculation)

Adults:

Oral: 15 g (60 mL) 1-4 times/day

Rectal: 30-50 g every 6 hours

**Dosage Forms** Oral or rectal:

Powder for suspension: 454 g

Suspension: 1.25 g/5 mL with sorbitol 33% and alcohol 0.3% (60 mL, 120 mL, 200 mL, 500 mL)

## sodium salicylate (SOW dee um sa LIS i late)

**Therapeutic Category** Analgesic, Non-narcotic; Antipyretic

**Use** Treatment of minor pain or fever; arthritis

**Usual Dosage** Adults: Oral: 325-650 mg every 4 hours

**Dosage Forms** Tablet, enteric coated: 325 mg, 650 mg

**Sodium Sulamyd®** *see* sulfacetamide *on page 562*

## sodium tetradecyl (SOW dee um tetra DEK il)

**U.S./Canadian Brand Names** Sotradecol®; Trombovar® (Can)

**Therapeutic Category** Sclerosing Agent

**Use** Treatment of small, uncomplicated varicose veins of the lower extremities; endoscopic sclerotherapy in the management of bleeding esophageal varices

**Usual Dosage** I.V.: 0.5-2 mL of 1% (5-20 mg) for small veins; 0.5-2 mL of 3% (15-60 mg) for medium or large veins

**Dosage Forms** Injection, as sulfate: 1% [10 mg/mL] (2 mL); 3% [30 mg/mL] (2 mL)

## sodium thiosulfate (SOW dee um thye oh SUL fate)

**U.S./Canadian Brand Names** Versiclear™

**Therapeutic Category** Antidote; Antifungal Agent

**Use**

Parenteral: Used alone or with sodium nitrite or amyl nitrite in cyanide poisoning or arsenic poisoning; reduce the risk of nephrotoxicity associated with cisplatin therapy; local infiltration (in diluted form) of selected chemotherapy extravasation

Topical: Treatment of tinea versicolor

**Usual Dosage** I.V.:

Cyanide and nitroprusside antidote:

Children <25 kg: 50 mg/kg after receiving 4.5-10 mg/kg sodium nitrite; a half dose of each may be repeated if necessary

Children >25 kg and Adults: 12.5 g after 300 mg of sodium nitrite; a half dose of each may be repeated if necessary

Cyanide poisoning: Dose should be based on determination as with nitrite, at rate of 2.5-5 mL/minute to maximum of 50 mL

**Dosage Forms**

Injection: 100 mg/mL (10 mL); 250 mg/mL (50 mL)

Lotion: 25% with salicylic acid 1% and isopropyl alcohol 10% (120 mL, 180 mL)

**Sofarin®** ***(Discontinued)*** *see page 750*

**SoFlax™ (Can)** *see* docusate *on page 197*

**Sofra-Tulle® (Can)** *see* framycetin *(Canada only) on page 266*

**Solagé™ Topical Solution** *see* mequinol and tretinoin *on page 373*

**Solaquin® [OTC]** *see* hydroquinone *on page 305*

**Solaquin Forte®** *see* hydroquinone *on page 305*

**Solarcaine® [OTC]** *see* benzocaine *on page 72*

**Solatene®** ***(Discontinued)*** *see page 750*

**Solfoton®** ***(Discontinued)*** *see page 750*

**Solganal®** *see* aurothioglucose *on page 60*

**soluble fluorescein** *see* fluorescein sodium *on page 254*

**Solu-Cortef®** *see* hydrocortisone (systemic) *on page 303*

**Solugel® (Can)** *see* benzoyl peroxide *on page 74*

**Solu-Medrol® Injection** *see* methylprednisolone *on page 385*

**Solurex L.A.®** *see* dexamethasone (systemic) *on page 174*

**Soma®** *see* carisoprodol *on page 110*

**Soma® Compound** *see* carisoprodol and aspirin *on page 110*

**Soma® Compound w/Codeine** *see* carisoprodol, aspirin, and codeine *on page 110*

## somatostatin *(Canada only)* (soe mat oh STA tin)

**U.S./Canadian Brand Names** Stilamin® (Can)

**Therapeutic Category** Variceal Bleeding (Acute) Agent

**Use** For the symptomatic treatment of acute bleeding from esophageal varices. Other treatment options for long-term management of the condition may be considered if necessary, once initial control has been established.

**Usual Dosage** Slow 250 mcg I.V. bolus injection over 3 to 5 minutes, followed by a continuous infusion at a rate of 250 mcg/hr until bleeding from the varices has stopped (usually within 12 to 24 hours). Once bleeding has been controlled, it is recommended that the infusion be continued for at least another 48 to 72 hours, or out to a maximum of 120 hours to prevent recurrent bleeding.

**Dosage Forms** Injection: 250 mcg, 3 mg

**somatrem** *see* human growth hormone *on page 296*

**somatropin** *see* human growth hormone *on page 296*

**Sominex® Oral [OTC]** *see* diphenhydramine *on page 191*

**Sominex® Pain Relief Formula [OTC]** *see* acetaminophen and diphenhydramine *on page 5*

**Somnol® (Can)** *see* flurazepam *on page 259*

**Sonata®** *see* zaleplon *on page 637*

**Sopalamine/3B Plus C (Can)** *see* vitamin (multiple/oral) *on page 632*

## sorbitol (SOR bi tole)

**U.S./Canadian Brand Names** Arlex®

**Therapeutic Category** Genitourinary Irrigant; Laxative

**Use** Humectant; sweetening agent; hyperosmotic laxative; facilitate the passage of sodium polystyrene sulfonate or a charcoal-toxin complex through the intestinal tract

**Usual Dosage** Hyperosmotic laxative (as single dose, at infrequent intervals):

Children 2-11 years:

Oral: 2 mL/kg (as 70% solution)

Rectal enema: 30-60 mL as 25% to 30% solution

Children >12 years and Adults:

Oral: 30-150 mL (as 70% solution)

Rectal enema: 120 mL as 25% to 30% solution

Adjunct to sodium polystyrene sulfonate: 15 mL as 70% solution orally until diarrhea occurs (10-20 mL/2 hours) or 20-100 mL as an oral vehicle for the sodium polystyrene sulfonate resin

When administered with charcoal: Oral:

Children: 4.3 mL/kg of 35% sorbitol with 1 g/kg of activated charcoal

Adults: 4.3 mL/kg of 70% sorbitol with 1 g/kg of activated charcoal

**Dosage Forms**

Liquid: 480 mL, 3840 mL, 28,800 mL

Solution: 70%

Solution, genitourinary irrigation: 3% (1500 mL, 3000 mL); 3.3% (2000 mL)

**Sorbitrate®** *see* isosorbide dinitrate *on page 328*

**Soriatane®** *see* acitretin *on page 10*

**Sotacor® (Can)** *see* sotalol *on this page*

## sotalol (SOE ta lole)

**U.S./Canadian Brand Names** Alti-Sotalol (Can); Apo®-Sotalol (Can); Betapace®; Gen-Sotalol (Can); Novo-Sotalol (Can); Nu-Sotalol (Can); PMS-Sotalol (Can); Rho®-Sotalol (Can); Rylosol® (Can); Sotacor® (Can)

**Therapeutic Category** Antiarrhythmic Agent, Class II; Antiarrhythmic Agent, Class III

**Use** Treatment of ventricular arrhythmias

**Usual Dosage** Adults: Oral: Initial: 80 mg twice daily; may be increased to 240-320 mg/day and up to 480-640 mg/day in patients with life-threatening refractory ventricular arrhythmias

**Dosage Forms** Tablet, as hydrochloride: 80 mg, 120 mg, 160 mg, 240 mg

**Sotradecol®** *see* sodium tetradecyl *on page 553*

**Soyacal®** *see* fat emulsion *on page 241*

**Soyalac® [OTC]** *see* nutritional formula, enteral/oral *on page 432*

**Span-FF® [OTC]** *see* ferrous fumarate *on page 246*

## sparfloxacin (spar FLOKS a sin)

**U.S./Canadian Brand Names** Zagam®

**Therapeutic Category** Quinolone

**Use** Treatment of adult patients with community acquired pneumonia caused by susceptible strains of *Chlamydia pneumoniae*, *Haemophilus influenzae*, *Haemophilus parainfluenzae*, *Moraxella catarrhalis*, *Mycoplasma pneumoniae*, or *Streptococcus pneumoniae* and acute bacterial exacerbations of acute bronchitis caused by susceptible strains of *Chlamydia pneumoniae*, *Enterobacter cloacae*, *Haemophilus influenzae*, *Haemophilus parainfluenzae*, *Klebsiella pneumoniae*, *Moraxella catarrhalis*, *Staphylococcus aureus*, or *Streptococcus pneumoniae*

**Usual Dosage** Adults: Oral: 400 mg on day 1, then 200 mg/day for the next 9 days (11 tablets total). In patients with creatinine clearance <50 mL/minute, administer 400 mg on day 1, then begin 200 mg every 48 hours on day 3 for a total of 9 days (6 tablets total).

**Dosage Forms** Tablet: 200 mg

**Sparine®** ***(Discontinued)*** *see page 750*

**Spasmoban (Can)** *see* dicyclomine *on page 183*

**Spasmoject®** ***(Discontinued)*** *see page 750*

**Spasmolin®** *see* hyoscyamine, atropine, scopolamine, and phenobarbital *on page 310*

**Spec-T® [OTC]** *see* benzocaine *on page 72*

**Spectazole™** *see* econazole *on page 209*

## spectinomycin (spek ti noe MYE sin)

**U.S./Canadian Brand Names** Trobicin®

**Therapeutic Category** Macrolide (Antibiotic)

**Use** Treatment of uncomplicated gonorrhea (ineffective against syphilis)

**Usual Dosage** I.M.:

Children:

<45 kg: 40 mg/kg/dose 1 time

≥45 kg: See adult dose

Children >8 years who are allergic to penicillins/cephalosporins may be treated with oral tetracycline

Adults: 2 g deep I.M. or 4 g where antibiotic resistance is prevalent 1 time; 4 g (10 mL) dose should be administered as 2-5 mL injections

**Dosage Forms** Injection, as hydrochloride: 2 g

**Spectrobid® Tablet *(Discontinued)*** *see page 750*

**Spectro Gram "2"™ (Can)** *see* chlorhexidine gluconate *on page 126*

**Spectrum™ Forte 29 (Can)** *see* vitamin (multiple/oral) *on page 632*

**Spherulin®** *see* coccidioidin skin test *on page 150*

## spiramycin *(Canada only)* (speer a MYE sin)

**U.S./Canadian Brand Names** Rovamycine® (Can)

**Therapeutic Category** Antibiotic, Macrolide

**Use** Treatment of infections of the respiratory tract, buccal cavity, skin and soft tissues due to susceptible organisms. *N. gonorrheae*: as an alternate choice of treatment for gonorrhea in patients allergic to the penicillins. Before treatment of gonorrhea, the possibility of concomitant infection due to *T. pallidum* should be excluded.

**Usual Dosage** Oral:

Children: The usual daily dosage is based on 150,000 units/kg body weight in 2 or 3 divided doses

Adults: 6,000,000-9,000,000 units per 24 hours, in 2 divided doses; in severe infections, the daily dosage may be increased to 12,000,000-15,000,000 units per day

Gonorrhea: 12,000,000-13,500000 units in a single dose.

**Dosage Forms** Capsule: 250 [750,000 units]; 500 [1,500,000 units]

## spirapril (SPYE ra pril)

**U.S./Canadian Brand Names** Renormax®

**Therapeutic Category** Angiotensin-Converting Enzyme (ACE) Inhibitor

**Use** Management of mild to severe hypertension

**Usual Dosage** Adults: Oral: 12 mg/day in 1-2 divided doses

**Dosage Forms** Tablet: 3 mg, 6 mg, 12 mg, 24 mg

**Spironazide® *(Discontinued)*** *see page 750*

## spironolactone (speer on oh LAK tone)

**U.S./Canadian Brand Names** Aldactone®; Novo-Spiroton (Can)

**Therapeutic Category** Diuretic, Potassium Sparing

**Use** Management of edema associated with excessive aldosterone excretion; hypertension; primary hyperaldosteronism; hypokalemia; treatment of hirsutism

**Usual Dosage** Oral:

Children: 1.5-3.5 mg/kg/day in divided doses every 6-24 hours

Diagnosis of primary aldosteronism: 125-375 mg/m$^2$/day in divided doses

Vaso-occlusive disease: 7.5 mg/kg/day in divided doses twice daily (non-FDA approved dose)

Adults:

Edema, hypertension, hypokalemia: 25-200 mg/day in 1-2 divided doses

Diagnosis of primary aldosteronism: 100-400 mg/day in 1-2 divided doses

**Dosage Forms** Tablet: 25 mg, 50 mg, 100 mg

**Spirozide®** ***(Discontinued)*** *see page 750*

**Sporanox®** *see* itraconazole *on page 330*

**Sportscreme® [OTC]** *see* triethanolamine salicylate *on page 605*

**Sportsmed®** *see* capsaicin *on page 104*

**SPS®** *see* sodium polystyrene sulfonate *on page 553*

**SRC® Expectorant** *see* hydrocodone, pseudoephedrine, and guaifenesin *on page 302*

**SSD® AF** *see* silver sulfadiazine *on page 544*

**SSD® Cream** *see* silver sulfadiazine *on page 544*

**SSKI®** *see* potassium iodide *on page 487*

**ST1571** *see* imatinib *on page 313*

**Stadol®** *see* butorphanol *on page 94*

**Stadol® NS** *see* butorphanol *on page 94*

**Staflex® [OTC]** *see* acetaminophen and phenyltoloxamine *on page 5*

**Stagesic®** *see* hydrocodone and acetaminophen *on page 300*

**Stahist®** ***(Discontinued)*** *see page 750*

## stanozolol (stan OH zoe lole)

**U.S./Canadian Brand Names** Winstrol®

**Therapeutic Category** Anabolic Steroid

**Controlled Substance** C-III

**Use** Prophylactic use against angioedema

**Usual Dosage**

Children: Acute attacks:

<6 years: 1 mg/day

6-12 years: 2 mg/day

Adults: Oral: Initial: 2 mg 3 times/day, may then reduce to a maintenance dose of 2 mg/day or 2 mg every other day after 1-3 months

**Dosage Forms** Tablet: 2 mg

**Staphcillin®** ***(Discontinued)*** *see page 750*

**Starlix®** *see* nateglinide *on page 411*

**Starnoc® (Can)** *see* zaleplon *on page 637*

**Statex® (Can)** *see* morphine sulfate *on page 400*

**Staticin® Topical** *see* erythromycin (ophthalmic/topical) *on page 222*

**Statobex®** ***(Discontinued)*** *see page 750*

## stavudine (STAV yoo deen)

**Synonyms** d4T

**U.S./Canadian Brand Names** Zerit®

**Therapeutic Category** Antiviral Agent

**Use** Treatment of advanced HIV infection in patients who experience intolerance, toxicity, resistance, or HIV disease progression with either zidovudine or didanosine therapy; active against most zidovudine-resistant strains; in adults, stavudine used alone in patients with 50-500 CD4 cells/mm$^3$ and at least 6 months previous treatment with zidovudine was more effective than continued zidovudine in preventing disease progression and death

**Usual Dosage** Oral:

Children 7 months to 15 years: 1-2 mg/kg/day divided twice daily

(Continued)

## stavudine *(Continued)*

Adults: 0.5-1 mg/kg/day **or**

<60 kg: 30 mg every 12 hours

≥60 kg: 40 mg every 12 hours

If peripheral neuropathy or elevations in liver enzymes occur, stavudine should be discontinued; once adverse effects resolve, reinitiate therapy at a lower dose of 20 mg every 12 hours (for ≥60 kg patients) or 15 mg every 12 hours (for <60 kg patients)

**Dosage Forms**

Capsule: 15 mg, 20 mg, 30 mg, 40 mg

Powder for oral solution: 1 mg/mL (200 mL)

**S-T Cort® Topical** *see* hydrocortisone (topical) *on page 304*

**Stelazine®** *see* trifluoperazine *on page 605*

**Stemetil® (Can)** *see* prochlorperazine *on page 497*

**Stemex®** ***(Discontinued)*** *see page 750*

**Stilamin® (Can)** *see* somatostatin *(Canada only) on page 554*

**stilbestrol** *see* diethylstilbestrol *on page 184*

**Stilphostrol®** *see* diethylstilbestrol *on page 184*

**Stimate™** *see* desmopressin acetate *on page 172*

**St Joseph® Adult Chewable Aspirin [OTC]** *see* aspirin *on page 55*

**St. Joseph® Cough Suppressant [OTC]** *see* dextromethorphan *on page 178*

**St. Joseph® Measured Dose Nasal Solution [OTC]** *see* phenylephrine *on page 467*

**Stop® [OTC]** *see* fluoride *on page 255*

**Streptase®** *see* streptokinase *on this page*

## streptokinase (strep toe KYE nase)

**Synonyms** SK

**U.S./Canadian Brand Names** Kabikinase®; Streptase®

**Therapeutic Category** Fibrinolytic Agent

**Use** Thrombolytic agent used in treatment of recent severe or massive deep vein thrombosis, pulmonary emboli, myocardial infarction, and occluded arteriovenous cannulas

**Usual Dosage** I.V.:

Children: Safety and efficacy not established; limited studies have used: 3500-4000 units/kg over 30 minutes followed by 1000-1500 units/kg/hour; clotted catheter: 25,000 units, clamp for 2 hours then aspirate contents and flush with normal saline

Adults (best results are realized if used within 5-6 hours of myocardial infarction; antibodies to streptokinase remain for 3-6 months after initial dose, use another thrombolytic enzyme, ie, urokinase, if thrombolytic therapy is indicated):

**Guidelines for Acute Myocardial Infarction (AMI):**

1.5 million units infused over 60 minutes. Monitor for the first few hours for signs of anaphylaxis or allergic reaction. **Infusion should be slowed if lowering of 25 mm Hg in blood pressure or terminated if asthmatic symptoms appear.** Begin heparin 5000-10,000 unit bolus followed by 1000 units/hour approximately 3-4 hours after completion of streptokinase infusion or when PTT is <100 seconds.

**Guidelines for Acute Pulmonary Embolism (APE):**

3 million unit dose; administer 250,000 units over 30 minutes followed by 100,000 units/hour for 24 hours. Monitor for the first few hours for signs of anaphylaxis or allergic reaction. **Infusion should be slowed if blood pressure is lowered by 25 mm Hg or if asthmatic symptoms appear**. Begin heparin 1000 units/hour approximately 3-4 hours after completion of streptokinase infusion or when PTT is <100 seconds.

Thromboses: 250,000 units to start, then 100,000 units/hour for 24-72 hours depending on location

Cannula occlusion: 250,000 units into cannula, clamp for 2 hours, then aspirate contents and flush with normal saline. **Not recommended**

**Dosage Forms** Powder for injection: 250,000 units, 750,000 units, 1,500,000 units

## streptomycin (strep toe MYE sin)

**Therapeutic Category** Antibiotic, Aminoglycoside; Antitubercular Agent

**Use** Combination therapy of active tuberculosis; used in combination with other agents for treatment of streptococcal or enterococcal endocarditis, mycobacterial infections, plague, tularemia, and brucellosis. Streptomycin is indicated for persons from endemic areas of drug-resistant *Mycobacterium tuberculosis* or who are HIV infected.

**Usual Dosage** Intramuscular (may also be given intravenous piggyback):

Tuberculosis therapy: **Note:** A four-drug regimen (isoniazid, rifampin, pyrazinamide and either streptomycin or ethambutol) is preferred for the initial, empiric treatment of TB. When the drug susceptibility results are available, the regimen should be altered as appropriate.

**Patients with TB and without HIV infection:**

**OPTION 1:**

Isoniazid resistance rate <4%: Administer daily isoniazid, rifampin, and pyrazinamide for 8 weeks followed by isoniazid and rifampin daily or directly observed therapy (DOT) 2-3 times/week for 16 weeks

If isoniazid resistance rate is not documented, ethambutol or streptomycin should also be administered until susceptibility to isoniazid or rifampin is demonstrated. Continue treatment for at least 6 months or 3 months beyond culture conversion.

**OPTION 2:** Administer daily isoniazid, rifampin, pyrazinamide, and either streptomycin or ethambutol for 2 weeks followed by DOT 2 times/week administration of the same drugs for 6 weeks, and subsequently, with isoniazid and rifampin DOT 2 times/week administration for 16 weeks

**OPTION 3:** Administer isoniazid, rifampin, pyrazinamide, and either ethambutol or streptomycin by DOT 3 times/week for 6 months

**Patients with TB and with HIV infection:** Administer any of the above OPTIONS 1, 2 or 3, however, treatment should be continued for a total of 9 months and at least 6 months beyond culture conversion

**Note:** Some experts recommend that the duration of therapy should be extended to 9 months for patients with disseminated disease, miliary disease, disease involving the bones or joints, or tuberculosis lymphadenitis

Children:

Daily therapy: 20-30 mg/kg/day (maximum: 1 g/day)

Directly observed therapy (DOT): Twice weekly: 25-30 mg/kg (maximum: 1.5 g)

DOT: 3 times/week: 25-30 mg/kg (maximum: 1 g)

Adults:

Daily therapy: 15 mg/kg/day (maximum: 1 g)

Directly observed therapy (DOT): Twice weekly: 25-30 mg/kg (maximum: 1.5 g)

DOT: 3 times/week: 25-30 mg/kg (maximum: 1 g)

Enterococcal endocarditis: 1 g every 12 hours for 2 weeks, 500 mg every 12 hours for 4 weeks in combination with penicillin

Streptococcal endocarditis: 1 g every 12 hours for 1 week, 500 mg every 12 hours for 1 week

Tularemia: 1-2 g/day in divided doses for 7-10 days or until patient is afebrile for 5-7 days

Plague: 2-4 g/day in divided doses until the patient is afebrile for at least 3 days

Elderly: 10 mg/kg/day, not to exceed 750 mg/day; dosing interval should be adjusted for renal function; some authors suggest not to give more than 5 days/week or give as 20-25 mg/kg/dose twice weekly

**Dosage Forms** Injection, as sulfate: 1 g

**streptozocin** (strep toe ZOE sin)

**U.S./Canadian Brand Names** Zanosar®

**Therapeutic Category** Antineoplastic Agent

**Use** Treat metastatic islet cell carcinoma of the pancreas, carcinoid tumor and syndrome, Hodgkin's disease, palliative treatment of colorectal cancer

**Usual Dosage** Children and Adults: I.V.: 500 mg/m$^2$ for 5 days every 6 weeks until optimal benefit or toxicity occurs; or may be administered in single dose 1000 mg/m$^2$ at weekly intervals for 2 doses, then increased to 1500 mg/m$^2$ weekly; the median total dose to onset of response is about 2000 mg/m$^2$ and the median total dose to maximum response is about 4000 mg/m$^2$

**Dosage Forms** Injection: 1 g

**Sterapred®** *see* prednisone *on page 493*

**Stresstabs® 600 Advanced Formula Tablets [OTC]** *see* vitamin (multiple/oral) *on page 632*

**Stromectol®** *see* ivermectin *on page 330*

**strong iodine solution** *see* potassium iodide *on page 487*

**strontium-89** (STRON shee um-atey nine)

**U.S./Canadian Brand Names** Metastron®

**Therapeutic Category** Radiopharmaceutical

**Use** Relief of bone pain in patients with skeletal metastases

**Usual Dosage** Adults: I.V.: 148 megabecquerel (4 millicurie) administered by slow I.V. injection over 1-2 minutes or 1.5-2.2 megabecquerel (40-60 microcurie)/kg; repeated doses are generally not recommended at intervals <90 days

**Dosage Forms** Injection, as chloride: 10.9-22.6 mg/mL [148 megabecquerel, 4 millicurie] (10 mL)

**Stuartnatal® 1 + 1** *see* vitamin (multiple/prenatal) *on page 632*

**Stuart Prenatal® [OTC]** *see* vitamin (multiple/prenatal) *on page 632*

**Sublimaze® Injection** *see* fentanyl *on page 244*

**succimer** (SUKS i mer)

**U.S./Canadian Brand Names** Chemet®

**Therapeutic Category** Chelating Agent

**Use** Treatment of lead poisoning in children with blood levels >45 mcg/dL. It is not indicated for prophylaxis of lead poisoning in a lead-containing environment.

**Usual Dosage** Children and Adults: Oral: 30 mg/kg/day in divided doses every 8 hours for an additional 5 days followed by 20 mg/kg/day for 14 days

**Dosage Forms** Capsule: 100 mg

**succinate mafenide acetate** *see* mafenide *on page 360*

**succinylcholine** (suks in il KOE leen)

**Synonyms** suxamethonium

**U.S./Canadian Brand Names** Anectine® Chloride; Anectine® Flo-Pack®; Quelicin®

**Therapeutic Category** Skeletal Muscle Relaxant

**Use** Produces skeletal muscle relaxation in procedures of short duration such as endotracheal intubation or endoscopic exams

**Usual Dosage** I.M., I.V.:

Children: 1-2 mg/kg

Intermittent: Initial: 1 mg/kg/dose one time; maintenance: 0.3-0.6 mg/kg every 5-10 minutes as needed

Adults: 0.6 mg/kg (range: 0.3-1.1 mg/kg) over 10-30 seconds, up to 150 mg total dose

Maintenance: 0.04-0.07 mg/kg every 5-10 minutes as needed

Continuous infusion: 2.5 mg/minute (or 0.5-10 mg/minute); dilute to concentration of 1-2 mg/mL in $D_5W$ or NS

**Note:** Pretreatment with atropine may reduce occurrence of bradycardia

**Dosage Forms** Injection, as chloride: 20 mg/mL (5 mL, 10 mL); 50 mg/mL (10 mL); 100 mg/mL (10 mL)

**Sucostrin®** ***(Discontinued)*** *see page 750*

**Sucraid™** *see* sacrosidase *on page 534*

## sucralfate (soo KRAL fate)

**Synonyms** aluminum sucrose sulfate, basic

**U.S./Canadian Brand Names** Apo®-Sucralfate (Can); Carafate®; Novo-Sucralate (Can); Nu-Sucralfate (Can); PMS-Sucralfate (Can); Sulcrate® (Can)

**Therapeutic Category** Gastrointestinal Agent, Gastric or Duodenal Ulcer Treatment

**Use** Short-term management of duodenal ulcers; gastric ulcers; suspension may be used topically for treatment of stomatitis due to cancer chemotherapy or other causes of esophageal and gastric erosions

**Usual Dosage**

Children: Dose not established, doses of 40-80 mg/kg/day divided every 6 hours have been used

Stomatitis: Oral: 2.5-5 mL (1 g/10 mL suspension), swish and spit or swish and swallow 4 times/day

Adults:

Duodenal ulcer treatment: Oral: 1 g 4 times/day, 1 hour before meals or food and at bedtime for 4-8 weeks, or alternatively 2 g twice daily

Duodenal ulcer maintenance therapy: Oral: 1 g twice daily

Stomatitis: Oral: 1 g/10 mL suspension, swish and spit or swish and swallow 4 times/day

**Dosage Forms**

Suspension, oral: 1 g/10 mL (10 mL, 414 mL, 420 mL)

Tablet: 1 g

**Sucrets® [OTC]** *see* dyclonine *on page 208*

**Sucrets® Cough Calmers [OTC]** *see* dextromethorphan *on page 178*

**Sucrets® Sore Throat [OTC]** *see* hexylresorcinol *on page 294*

**Sudafed® [OTC]** *see* pseudoephedrine *on page 507*

**Sudafed® 12 Hour [OTC]** *see* pseudoephedrine *on page 507*

**Sudafed® Children** ***(Discontinued)*** *see page 750*

**Sudafed® Cold & Cough Liquid Caps [OTC]** *see* guaifenesin, pseudoephedrine, and dextromethorphan *on page 285*

**Sudafed® Cough** ***(Discontinued)*** *see page 750*

**Sudafed Plus® Liquid** ***(Discontinued)*** *see page 750*

**Sudafed® Plus Tablet [OTC]** *see* chlorpheniramine and pseudoephedrine *on page 130*

**Sudafed® Severe Cold Formula [OTC]** *see* acetaminophen, dextromethorphan, and pseudoephedrine *on page 7*

**Sudafed® Sinus [OTC]** *see* acetaminophen and pseudoephedrine *on page 6*

**Sudogest® Sinus Maximum Strength [OTC]** *see* acetaminophen and pseudoephedrine *on page 6*

**Sufedrin® [OTC]** *see* pseudoephedrine *on page 507*

**Sufenta®** *see* sufentanil *on next page*

## sufentanil (soo FEN ta nil)

**U.S./Canadian Brand Names** Sufenta®

**Therapeutic Category** Analgesic, Narcotic; General Anesthetic

**Controlled Substance** C-II

**Use** Analgesia; analgesia adjunct; anesthetic agent

**Usual Dosage** I.V.:

Children <12 years: 10-25 mcg/kg with 100% $O_2$, maintenance: 25-50 mcg as needed (total dose of up to 1-2 mcg/kg)

Adults: Dose should be based on body weight. **Note:** In obese patients (ie, >20% above ideal body weight), use lean body weight to determine dosage

1-2 mcg/kg with $N_2O/O_2$ for endotracheal intubation; maintenance: 10-25 mcg as needed

2-8 mcg/kg with $N_2O/O_2$ more complicated major surgical procedures; maintenance: 10-50 mcg as needed

8-30 mcg/kg with 100% $O_2$ and muscle relaxant produces sleep; at doses of ≥8 mcg/kg maintains a deep level of anesthesia; maintenance: 10-50 mcg as needed

**Dosage Forms** Injection, as citrate: 50 mcg/mL (1 mL, 2 mL, 5 mL)

**Sular®** *see* nisoldipine *on page 421*

**sulbactam and ampicillin** *see* ampicillin and sulbactam *on page 39*

## sulconazole (sul KON a zole)

**U.S./Canadian Brand Names** Exelderm® Topical

**Therapeutic Category** Antifungal Agent

**Use** Treatment of superficial fungal infections of the skin, including tinea cruris, tinea corporis, tinea versicolor and possibly tinea pedis

**Usual Dosage** Topical: Apply once or twice daily for 4-6 weeks

**Dosage Forms**

Cream, as nitrate: 1% (15 g, 30 g, 60 g)

Solution, as nitrate, topical: 1% (30 mL)

**Sulcrate® (Can)** *see* sucralfate *on previous page*

**Sulf-10®** *see* sulfacetamide *on this page*

## sulfabenzamide, sulfacetamide, and sulfathiazole

(sul fa BENZ a mide, sul fa SEE ta mide, & sul fa THYE a zole)

**Synonyms** triple sulfa

**U.S./Canadian Brand Names** V.V.S.®

**Therapeutic Category** Antibiotic, Vaginal

**Use** Treatment of *Haemophilus vaginalis* vaginitis

**Usual Dosage** Adults: Vaginal:

Cream: Insert 1 applicatorful in vagina twice daily for 4-6 days; dosage may then be decreased to $^1/_2$ to $^1/_4$ of an applicatorful twice daily

Tablet: Insert 1 intravaginally twice daily for 10 days

**Dosage Forms**

Cream, vaginal: Sulfabenzamide 3.7%, sulfacetamide 2.86%, and sulfathiazole 3.42% (78 g with applicator, 90 g, 120 g)

Tablet, vaginal: Sulfabenzamide 184 mg, sulfacetamide 143.75 mg, and sulfathiazole 172.5 mg (20 tablets/box with vaginal applicator)

## sulfacetamide (sul fa SEE ta mide)

**U.S./Canadian Brand Names** AK-Sulf®; Bleph®-10; Carmol® Scalp; Cetamide®; Diosulf™ (Can); Klaron®; Ocu-Sul®; Sebizon®; Sodium Sulamyd®; Sulf-10®

**Therapeutic Category** Antibiotic, Ophthalmic

**Use** Treatment and prophylaxis of conjunctivitis, corneal ulcers, and other superficial ocular infections due to susceptible organisms; adjunctive treatment with systemic sulfonamides for therapy of trachoma

**Usual Dosage** Children >2 months and Adults: Ophthalmic:
Ointment: Apply to lower conjunctival sac 1-4 times/day and at bedtime
Solution: 1-2 drops every 2-3 hours in the lower conjunctival sac during the waking hours and less frequently at night

**Dosage Forms** Sulfacetamide sodium:
Lotion: 10% (60 mL, 85 g)
Ointment, ophthalmic: 10% (3.5 g)
Solution, ophthalmic: 10% (5 mL, 15 mL); 15% (15 mL); 30% (15 mL)

## sulfacetamide and phenylephrine (sul fa SEE ta mide & fen il EF rin)

**U.S./Canadian Brand Names** Vasosulf® Ophthalmic

**Therapeutic Category** Antibiotic, Ophthalmic

**Use** Treatment of conjunctivitis, corneal ulcer, and other superficial ocular infections due to susceptible microorganisms; adjunctive in systemic sulfonamide therapy

**Usual Dosage** Ophthalmic: Instill 1-3 drops in lower conjunctival sac every 3-4 hours

**Dosage Forms** Solution, ophthalmic: Sulfacetamide sodium 15% and phenylephrine hydrochloride 0.125% (5 mL, 15 mL)

## sulfacetamide and prednisolone (sul fa SEE ta mide & pred NIS oh lone)

**U.S./Canadian Brand Names** AK-Cide® Ophthalmic; Blephamide® Ophthalmic; Cetapred® Ophthalmic; Dioptimyd® (Can); Isopto® Cetapred® Ophthalmic; Metimyd® Ophthalmic; Vasocidin® Ophthalmic

**Therapeutic Category** Antibiotic/Corticosteroid, Ophthalmic

**Use** Steroid-responsive inflammatory ocular conditions where infection is present or there is a risk of infection; ophthalmic suspension may be used as an otic preparation

**Usual Dosage** Children >2 and Adults: Ophthalmic:
Ointment: Apply to lower conjunctival sac 1-4 times/day
Solution: Instill 1-3 drops every 2-3 hours while awake

**Dosage Forms**
Ointment, ophthalmic:
AK-Cide®, Metimyd®, Vasocidin®: Sulfacetamide sodium 10% and prednisolone acetate 0.5% (3.5 g)
Blephamide®: Sulfacetamide sodium 10% and prednisolone acetate 0.2% (3.5 g)
Cetapred®: Sulfacetamide sodium 10% and prednisolone acetate 0.25% (3.5 g)
Suspension, ophthalmic: Sulfacetamide sodium 10% and prednisolone sodium phosphate 0.25% (5 mL)
Suspension, ophthalmic:
AK-Cide®, Metimyd®: Sulfacetamide sodium 10% and prednisolone acetate 0.5% (5 mL)
Blephamide®: Sulfacetamide sodium 10% and prednisolone acetate 0.2% (2.5 mL, 5 mL, 10 mL)
Isopto® Cetapred®: Sulfacetamide sodium 10% and prednisolone acetate 0.25% (5 mL, 15 mL)
Vasocidin®: Sulfacetamide sodium 10% and prednisolone sodium phosphate: 0.25% (5 mL, 10 mL)

## sulfacetamide sodium and fluorometholone

(sul fa SEE ta mide SOW dee um & flure oh METH oh lone)

**U.S./Canadian Brand Names** FML-S® Ophthalmic Suspension

**Therapeutic Category** Antibiotic/Corticosteroid, Ophthalmic

**Use** Steroid-responsive inflammatory ocular conditions where infection is present or there is a risk of infection

**Usual Dosage** Children >2 months and Adults: Ophthalmic: Instill 1-3 drops every 2-3 hours while awake

**Dosage Forms** Suspension, ophthalmic: Sulfacetamide sodium 10% and fluorometholone 0.1% (5 mL, 10 mL)

**Sulfacet-R® Topical** *see* sulfur and sulfacetamide *on page 566*

## sulfadiazine (sul fa DYE a zeen)

**Therapeutic Category** Sulfonamide

**Use** Adjunctive treatment in toxoplasmosis; treatment of urinary tract infections and nocardiosis; rheumatic fever prophylaxis in penicillin-allergic patient; uncomplicated attack of malaria

**Usual Dosage** Oral:

Congenital toxoplasmosis:

Newborns and Children <2 months: 100 mg/kg/day divided every 6 hours in conjunction with pyrimethamine 1 mg/kg/day once daily and supplemental folinic acid 5 mg every 3 days for 6 months

Children >2 months: 25-50 mg/kg/dose 4 times/day

Toxoplasmosis:

Children: 120-150 mg/kg/day, maximum dose: 6 g/day; divided every 6 hours in conjunction with pyrimethamine 2 mg/kg/day divided every 12 hours for 3 days followed by 1 mg/kg/day once daily (maximum: 25 mg/day) with supplemental folinic acid

Adults: 2-8 g/day divided every 6 hours in conjunction with pyrimethamine 25 mg/day and with supplemental folinic acid

**Dosage Forms** Tablet: 500 mg

## sulfadoxine and pyrimethamine (sul fa DOKS een & peer i METH a meen)

**U.S./Canadian Brand Names** Fansidar®

**Therapeutic Category** Antimalarial Agent

**Use** Treatment of *Plasmodium falciparum* malaria in patients in whom chloroquine resistance is suspected; malaria prophylaxis for travelers to areas where chloroquine-resistant malaria is endemic

**Usual Dosage** Children and Adults: Oral:

Treatment of acute attack of malaria: A single dose of the following number of Fansidar® tablets is used in sequence with quinine or alone:

2-11 months: 1/4 tablet
1-3 years: 1/2 tablet
4-8 years: 1 tablet
9-14 years: 2 tablets
>14 years: 3 tablets

Malaria prophylaxis: A single dose should be carried for self-treatment in the event of febrile illness when medical attention is not immediately available:

2-11 months: 1/4 tablet
1-3 years: 1/2 tablet
4-8 years: 1 tablet
9-14 years: 2 tablets
>14 years and Adults: 3 tablets

**Dosage Forms** Tablet: Sulfadoxine 500 mg and pyrimethamine 25 mg

**Sulfa-Gyn®** ***(Discontinued)*** *see page 750*

**Sulfalax® [OTC]** *see* docusate *on page 197*

**Sulfamethoprim®** ***(Discontinued)*** *see page 750*

## sulfamethoxazole and trimethoprim

(sul fa meth OKS a zole & trye METH oh prim)

**Synonyms** co-trimoxazole; SMX-TMP; TMP-SMX

**U.S./Canadian Brand Names** Apo®-Sulfatrim (Can); Bactrim™; Bactrim™ DS; Novo-Trimel (Can); Nu-Cotrimox (Can); Septra®; Septra® DS; Sulfatrim®; Sulfatrim® DS

**Therapeutic Category** Sulfonamide

**Use** Treatment of urinary tract infections caused by susceptible *E. coli*, *Klebsiella*, *Enterobacter*, *Proteus mirabilis*, *Proteus* (indole positive); acute otitis media due to amoxicillin-resistant *H. influenzae*, *S. pneumoniae*, and *M. catarrhalis*; acute exacerbations of chronic bronchitis; prophylaxis and treatment of *Pneumocystis carinii* pneumonitis

(PCP); treatment of susceptible shigellosis, typhoid fever, *Nocardia asteroides* infection, and *Xanthomonas maltophilia* infection; the I.V. preparation is used for treatment of *Pneumocystis carinii* pneumonitis, *Shigella*, and severe urinary tract infections

**Usual Dosage** Oral, I.V. (dosage recommendations are based on the trimethoprim component):

Children >2 months:

Mild to moderate infections: 6-12 mg TMP/kg/day in divided doses every 12 hours

Serious infection/*Pneumocystis*: 15-20 mg TMP/kg/day in divided doses every 6 hours

Urinary tract infection prophylaxis: 2 mg TMP/kg/dose daily

Prophylaxis of *Pneumocystis*: 5-10 mg TMP/kg/day or 150 mg TMP/$m^2$/day in divided doses every 12 hours 3 days/week; dose should not exceed 320 mg trimethoprim and 1600 mg sulfamethoxazole 3 days/week; Mon, Tue, Wed

Adults: Urinary tract infection/chronic bronchitis: 1 double strength tablet every 12 hours for 10-14 days

**Dosage Forms** 5:1 ratio (SMX:TMP) remains constant in all dosage forms

Injection: Sulfamethoxazole 80 mg and trimethoprim 16 mg per mL (5 mL, 10 mL, 20 mL, 30 mL, 50 mL)

Suspension, oral: Sulfamethoxazole 200 mg and trimethoprim 40 mg per 5 mL (20 mL, 100 mL, 150 mL, 200 mL, 480 mL)

Tablet: Sulfamethoxazole 400 mg and trimethoprim 80 mg

Tablet, double strength: Sulfamethoxazole 800 mg and trimethoprim 160 mg

**Sulfamylon® Topical** *see* mafenide *on page 360*

## sulfanilamide (sul fa NIL a mide)

**U.S./Canadian Brand Names** AVC™ Cream; AVC™ Suppository

**Therapeutic Category** Antifungal Agent

**Use** Treatment of vulvovaginitis caused by *Candida albicans*

**Usual Dosage** Vaginal: 1 applicatorful once or twice daily continued through 1 complete menstrual cycle

**Dosage Forms**

Cream, vaginal (AVC™, Vagitrol®): 15% [150 mg/g] (120 g with applicator)

Suppository, vaginal (AVC™): 1.05 g (16s)

## sulfasalazine (sul fa SAL a zeen)

**Synonyms** salicylazosulfapyridine

**U.S./Canadian Brand Names** Alti-Sulfasalazine (Can); Azulfidine®; Azulfidine® EN-tabs®; Salazopyrin® (Can); S.A.S.™ (Can)

**Therapeutic Category** 5-Aminosalicylic Acid Derivative

**Use** Management of ulcerative colitis; treatment of active Crohn's disease

**Usual Dosage** Oral:

Children >2 years:

Initial: 40-60 mg/kg/day divided every 4-6 hour

Maintenance dose: 20-30 mg/kg/day divided every 6 hours, up to a maximum of 2 g/day

Adults:

Initial: 3-4 g/day divided every 4-6 hours

Maintenance dose: 2 g/day divided every 6 hours

**Dosage Forms**

Tablet: 500 mg

Tablet, enteric coated: 500 mg

**Sulfatrim®** *see* sulfamethoxazole and trimethoprim *on previous page*

**Sulfatrim® DS** *see* sulfamethoxazole and trimethoprim *on previous page*

**Sulfa-Trip®** ***(Discontinued)*** *see page 750*

## sulfinpyrazone (sul fin PEER a zone)

**U.S./Canadian Brand Names** Anturane®; Apo®-Sulfinpyraz (Can); Nu-Sulfinpyrazone (Can)

**Therapeutic Category** Uricosuric Agent

**Use** Treatment of chronic gouty arthritis and intermittent gouty arthritis

**Usual Dosage** Oral: 200 mg twice daily

**Dosage Forms**

Capsule: 200 mg

Tablet: 100 mg

## sulfisoxazole (sul fi SOKS a zole)

**Synonyms** sulphafurazole

**U.S./Canadian Brand Names** Gantrisin® Pediatric Suspension; Truxazole® Tablet

**Therapeutic Category** Sulfonamide

**Use** Treatment of uncomplicated urinary tract infections, otitis media, *Chlamydia*; nocardiosis; treatment of acute pelvic inflammatory disease in prepubertal children

**Usual Dosage**

Children >2 months: Oral: 75 mg/kg stat, 120-150 mg/kg/day in divided doses every 4-6 hours; not to exceed 6 g/day

Pelvic inflammatory disease: 100 mg/kg/day in divided doses every 6 hours; used in combination with ceftriaxone

*Chlamydia trachomatis*: 100 mg/kg/day divided every 6 hours

Adults: Oral: 2-4 g stat, 4-8 g/day in divided doses every 4-6 hours

**Dosage Forms**

Suspension, oral, pediatric, as acetyl (raspberry flavor): 500 mg/5 mL (480 mL)

Tablet: 500 mg

## sulfisoxazole and phenazopyridine

(sul fi SOKS a zole & fen az oh PEER i deen)

**Therapeutic Category** Sulfonamide

**Use** Treatment of urinary tract infections and nocardiosis

**Usual Dosage** Oral: 4-6 tablets to start, then 2 tablets 4 times/day for 2 days, then continue with sulfisoxazole only

**Dosage Forms** Tablet: Sulfisoxazole 500 mg and phenazopyridine 50 mg

## sulfur and salicylic acid (SUL fur & sal i SIL ik AS id)

**U.S./Canadian Brand Names** Aveeno® Cleansing Bar [OTC]; Fostex® [OTC]; Meted® Shampoo (Can); Pernox® [OTC]; Sastid® Plain Therapeutic Shampoo and Acne Wash [OTC]; Sebulex® Shampoo (Can)

**Therapeutic Category** Antiseborrheic Agent, Topical

**Use** Therapeutic shampoo for dandruff and seborrheal dermatitis; acne skin cleanser

**Usual Dosage** Children and Adults: Topical:

Shampoo: Initial: Use daily or every other day; 1-2 treatments/week will usually maintain control

Soap: Use daily or every other day

**Dosage Forms**

Cake: Sulfur 2% and salicylic acid 2% (123 g)

Cleanser: Sulfur 2% and salicylic acid 1.5% (60 mL, 120 mL)

Shampoo: Micropulverized sulfur 2% and salicylic acid 2% (120 mL, 240 mL)

Soap: Micropulverized sulfur 2% and salicylic acid 2% (113 g)

Wash: Sulfur 1.6% and salicylic acid 1.6% (75 mL)

## sulfur and sulfacetamide (SUL fur & sul fa SEE ta mide)

**U.S./Canadian Brand Names** Novacet® Topical; Sulfacet-R® Topical

**Therapeutic Category** Antiseborrheic Agent, Topical

**Use** Aid in the treatment of acne vulgaris, acne rosacea and seborrheic dermatitis

**Usual Dosage** Topical: Apply in a thin film 1-3 times/day

**Dosage Forms** Lotion, topical: Sulfur colloid 5% and sulfacetamide sodium 10% (30 mL)

## sulindac (sul IN dak)

**U.S./Canadian Brand Names** Apo®-Sulin (Can); Clinoril®; Novo-Sundac (Can); Nu-Sulindac (Can)

**Therapeutic Category** Analgesic, Non-narcotic; Nonsteroidal Anti-inflammatory Drug (NSAID)

**Use** Management of inflammatory disease, rheumatoid disorders; acute gouty arthritis

**Usual Dosage** Oral:

Children: Dose not established

Adults: 150-200 mg twice daily; not to exceed 400 mg/day

**Dosage Forms** Tablet: 150 mg, 200 mg

**sulphafurazole** *see* sulfisoxazole *on previous page*

**Sultrin™** ***(Discontinued)*** *see page 750*

**Sumacal® [OTC]** *see* glucose polymers *on page 276*

## sumatriptan succinate (SOO ma trip tan SUKS i nate)

**U.S./Canadian Brand Names** Imitrex®

**Therapeutic Category** Antimigraine Agent

**Use** Acute treatment of migraine with or without aura

**Unlabeled use:** Cluster headaches

**Usual Dosage** Adults:

Oral: 25 mg (taken with fluids); maximum recommended dose is 100 mg. If a satisfactory response has not been obtained at 2 hours, a second dose of up to 100 mg may be given. Efficacy of this second dose has not been examined. If a headache returns, additional doses may be taken at intervals of at least 2 hours up to a daily maximum of 300 mg. There is no evidence that an initial dose of 100 mg provides substantially greater relief than 25 mg.

Intranasal: Single dose of 5, 10, or 20 mg administered in one nostril; a 10 mg dose may be achieved by administration of a single 5 mg dose in each nostril; if headache returns, the dose may be repeated once after 2 hours, not to exceed a total daily dose of 40 mg

S.C.: 6 mg; a second injection may be administered at least 1 hour after the initial dose, but not more than two injections in a 24-hour period

**Dosage Forms**

Injection: 12 mg/mL (0.5 mL, 2 mL)

Spray, nasal: 5 mg (100 mcL); 20 mg (100 mcL)

Tablet: 25 mg, 50 mg

**Summer's Eve® Medicated Douche [OTC]** *see* povidone-iodine *on page 489*

**Sumycin® Oral** *see* tetracycline *on page 579*

**Sun-Benz (Can)** *see* benzydamine *(Canada only) on page 75*

**Supac® [OTC]** *see* acetaminophen, aspirin, and caffeine *on page 6*

**Superchar®** ***(Discontinued)*** *see page 750*

**Superchar® With Sorbitol** ***(Discontinued)*** *see page 750*

**Supeudol® (Can)** *see* oxycodone *on page 443*

**Suphedrine® Severe Cold [OTC]** *see* acetaminophen, dextromethorphan, and pseudoephedrine *on page 7*

**Suphedrin® Sinus Maximum Strength [OTC]** *see* acetaminophen and pseudoephedrine *on page 6*

**Suplasyn® (Can)** *see* sodium hyaluronate *on page 550*

**Supprelin™** *see* histrelin *on page 295*

**Suppress® [OTC]** *see* dextromethorphan *on page 178*

**Suprane®** *see* desflurane *on page 171*

**Suprax®** *see* cefixime *on page 115*

**Suprefact® (Can)** *see* buserelin *on page 91*

**Suprefact® Depot (Can)** *see* buserelin *on page 91*

**Surbex® [OTC]** *see* vitamin B complex *on page 630*

**Surbex-T® Filmtabs® [OTC]** *see* vitamin B complex with vitamin C *on page 630*

**Surbex® With C Filmtabs® [OTC]** *see* vitamin B complex with vitamin C *on page 630*

**Surfak® [OTC]** *see* docusate *on page 197*

**Surgam® (Can)** *see* tiaprofenic acid *(Canada only) on page 589*

**Surgam® SR (Can)** *see* tiaprofenic acid *(Canada only) on page 589*

**Surgicel®** *see* cellulose, oxidized *on page 119*

**Surital® *(Discontinued)*** *see page 750*

**Surmontil®** *see* trimipramine *on page 608*

**Survanta®** *see* beractant *on page 76*

**Sus-Phrine®** *see* epinephrine *on page 216*

**Sustaire® *(Discontinued)*** *see page 750*

**Sustiva™** *see* efavirenz *on page 211*

**suxamethonium** *see* succinylcholine *on page 560*

**Sween Cream® [OTC]** *see* methylbenzethonium chloride *on page 383*

**Swim-Ear® Otic [OTC]** *see* boric acid *on page 84*

**Swiss Kriss® [OTC]** *see* senna *on page 541*

**Syllact® [OTC]** *see* psyllium *on page 509*

**Symadine® *(Discontinued)*** *see page 750*

**Symmetrel® Capsule *(Discontinued)*** *see page 750*

**Symmetrel® Syrup** *see* amantadine *on page 28*

**Symmetrel® Tablet** *see* amantadine *on page 28*

**Synacol® CF [OTC]** *see* guaifenesin and dextromethorphan *on page 282*

**Synacort® Topical** *see* hydrocortisone (topical) *on page 304*

**synacthen** *see* cosyntropin *on page 156*

**Synacthen Depot (Can)** *see* cosyntropin *on page 156*

**Synagis®** *see* palivizumab *on page 446*

**Synalar-HP® Topical *(Discontinued)*** *see page 750*

**Synalar® Topical** *see* fluocinolone *on page 253*

**Synalgos®-DC** *see* dihydrocodeine compound *on page 186*

**Synarel®** *see* nafarelin *on page 406*

**Synercid®** *see* quinupristin and dalfopristin *on page 515*

**Synflex® (Can)** *see* naproxen *on page 409*

**Synflex® DS (Can)** *see* naproxen *on page 409*

**Synkayvite® *(Discontinued)*** *see page 750*

**Synphasic® (Can)** *see* ethinyl estradiol and norethindrone *on page 232*

**synthetic lung surfactant** *see* colfosceril palmitate *on page 152*

**Synthroid®** *see* levothyroxine *on page 348*

**Syntocinon® Nasal *(Discontinued)*** *see page 750*

**Syprine®** *see* trientine *on page 604*

**Syracol-CF® [OTC]** *see* guaifenesin and dextromethorphan *on page 282*

**Sytobex®** *see* cyanocobalamin *on page 158*

**$t_3$/$t_4$ liotrix** *see* liotrix *on page 352*

**$t_3$ thyronine** *see* liothyronine *on page 351*

**$t_4$ thyroxine** *see* levothyroxine *on page 348*

**222® Tablets (Can)** *see* aspirin and codeine *on page 56*

**282® Tablets (Can)** *see* aspirin and codeine *on page 56*

**292® Tablets (Can)** *see* aspirin and codeine *on page 56*

**624® Tablets (Can)** *see* propoxyphene *on page 503*

**Tabron® *(Discontinued)*** *see page 750*

**Tac™-3 Injection** *see* triamcinolone (systemic) *on page 602*

**Tac™-40 Injection** *see* triamcinolone (systemic) *on page 602*

**Tacaryl® *(Discontinued)*** *see page 750*

**TACE® *(Discontinued)*** *see page 750*

## tacrine (TAK reen)

**Synonyms** tetrahydroaminoacrine; THA

**U.S./Canadian Brand Names** Cognex®

**Therapeutic Category** Acetylcholinesterase Inhibitor; Cholinergic Agent

**Use** Treatment of Alzheimer's disease

**Usual Dosage** Adults: Oral: 40 mg/day

**Dosage Forms** Capsule, as hydrochloride: 10 mg, 20 mg, 30 mg, 40 mg

## tacrolimus (ta KROE li mus)

**Synonyms** FK506

**U.S./Canadian Brand Names** Protopic® Topical: Prograf®

**Therapeutic Category** Immunosuppressant Agent

**Use**

Oral/injection: Potent immunosuppressive drug used in liver or kidney transplant recipients

Topical: Moderate to severe atopic dermatitis in patients not responsive to conventional therapy or when conventional therapy is not appropriate

**Unlabeled use:** Potent immunosuppressive drug used in heart, lung, small bowel transplant recipients; immunosuppressive drug for peripheral stem cell/bone marrow transplantation

**Usual Dosage**

Initial: I.V. continuous infusion: 0.1 mg/kg/day until the tolerance of oral intake

Oral: Usually 3-4 times the I.V. dose, or 0.3 mg/kg/day in divided doses every 12 hours

**Dosage Forms**

Capsule: 0.5 mg, 1 mg, 5 mg

Injection, with alcohol and surfactant: 5 mg/mL (1 mL)

Ointment: 0.03% (30 g, 60 g); 0.1% (30 g, 60g)

**Tactinal® [OTC]** *see* acetaminophen *on page 3*

**Tactinal® Children's [OTC]** *see* acetaminophen *on page 3*

**Tactinal® Extra Strength [OTC]** *see* acetaminophen *on page 3*

**Tagamet®** *see* cimetidine *on page 137*

**Tagamet-HB® [OTC]** *see* cimetidine *on page 137*

**Talacen®** *see* pentazocine compound *on page 459*

**Talwin®** *see* pentazocine *on page 458*

**Talwin® Compound** *see* pentazocine compound *on page 459*

**Talwin® NX** *see* pentazocine *on page 458*

**Tambocor™** *see* flecainide *on page 250*

**Tamiflu™** *see* oseltamivir *on page 439*

**Tamine®** ***(Discontinued)*** *see page 750*

**Tamofen® (Can)** *see* tamoxifen *on this page*

## tamoxifen (ta MOKS i fen)

**U.S./Canadian Brand Names** Apo®-Tamox (Can); Gen-Tamoxifen (Can); Nolvadex®; Novo-Tamoxifen (Can); PMS-Tamoxifen (Can); Tamofen® (Can)

**Therapeutic Category** Antineoplastic Agent

**Use** Palliative or adjunctive treatment of advanced breast cancer in postmenopausal women

**Usual Dosage** Oral: 10-20 mg twice daily

**Dosage Forms** Tablet, as citrate: 10 mg, 20 mg

## tamsulosin (tam SOO loe sin)

**U.S./Canadian Brand Names** Flomax®

**Therapeutic Category** Alpha-Adrenergic Blocking Agent

**Use** Treatment of signs and symptoms of benign prostatic hyperplasia (BPH)

**Usual Dosage** Oral: Adults: 0.4 mg once daily approximately 30 minutes after the same meal each day

**Dosage Forms** Capsule, as hydrochloride: 0.4 mg

**Tanac® [OTC]** *see* benzocaine *on page 72*

**Tanoral® Tablet** *see* chlorpheniramine, pyrilamine, and phenylephrine *on page 132*

**Tantum™ (Can)** *see* benzydamine *(Canada only) on page 75*

**Tao®** *see* troleandomycin *on page 610*

**Tapazole®** *see* methimazole *on page 379*

**Tarabine® PFS** *see* cytarabine *on page 162*

**Taractan®** ***(Discontinued)*** *see page 750*

**Targretin®** *see* bexarotene *on page 79*

**Tarka®** *see* trandolapril and verapamil *on page 598*

**Taro-Atenol® (Can)** *see* atenolol *on page 56*

**Taro-Carbamazepine (Can)** *see* carbamazepine *on page 105*

**Taro-Desoximetasone (Can)** *see* desoximetasone *on page 173*

**Tasmar®** *see* tolcapone *on page 595*

**TAT** *see* tetanus antitoxin *on page 577*

**Tavist®** *see* clemastine *on page 141*

**Tavist®-1 [OTC]** *see* clemastine *on page 141*

**Tavist-D®** ***(Discontinued)*** *see page 750*

**Taxol®** *see* paclitaxel *on page 446*

**Taxotere®** *see* docetaxel *on page 197*

## tazarotene (taz AR oh teen)

**U.S./Canadian Brand Names** Tazorac®

**Therapeutic Category** Keratolytic Agent

**Use** Topical treatment of facial acne vulgaris; topical treatment of stable plaque psoriasis of up to 20% body surface area involvement

**Usual Dosage** Children >12 years and Adults: Topical:

Acne: Cleanse the face gently. After the skin is dry, apply a thin film of tazarotene (2 mg/cm$^2$) once daily, in the evening, to the skin where the acne lesions appear. Use enough to cover the entire affected area. Tazarotene was investigated ≤12 weeks during clinical trials for acne.

Psoriasis: Apply tazarotene once daily, in the evening, to psoriatic lesions using enough (2 mg/cm$^2$) to cover only the lesion with a thin film to no more than 20% of body surface area. If a bath or shower is taken prior to application, dry the skin before applying the gel. Because unaffected skin may be more susceptible to irritation, avoid application of tazarotene to these areas. Tazarotene was investigated for up to 12 months during clinical trials for psoriasis.

### Dosage Forms

Cream, topical: 0.05% (60 g); 0.1% (15 g, 30 g)

Gel, topical: 0.05% (30 g, 100 g); 0.1% (30 g, 100 g)

**Tazicef®** *see* ceftazidime *on page 117*

**Tazidime®** *see* ceftazidime *on page 117*

**Tazocin® (Can)** *see* piperacillin and tazobactam sodium *on page 473*

**Tazorac®** *see* tazarotene *on previous page*

**3TC** *see* lamivudine *on page 339*

**T-Caine® Lozenge *(Discontinued)*** *see page 750*

**3TC® (Can)** *see* lamivudine *on page 339*

**TCN** *see* tetracycline *on page 579*

**Td** *see* diphtheria and tetanus toxoid *on page 192*

**Tear Drop® Solution [OTC]** *see* artificial tears *on page 53*

**TearGard® Ophthalmic Solution [OTC]** *see* artificial tears *on page 53*

**Teargen® Ophthalmic Solution [OTC]** *see* artificial tears *on page 53*

**Tearisol® Solution [OTC]** *see* artificial tears *on page 53*

**Tears Naturale® Free Solution [OTC]** *see* artificial tears *on page 53*

**Tears Naturale® II Solution [OTC]** *see* artificial tears *on page 53*

**Tears Naturale® Solution [OTC]** *see* artificial tears *on page 53*

**Tears Plus® Solution [OTC]** *see* artificial tears *on page 53*

**Tears Renewed® Solution [OTC]** *see* artificial tears *on page 53*

**Tebamide® *(Discontinued)*** *see page 750*

**Tebrazid™ (Can)** *see* pyrazinamide *on page 510*

**Tecnal (Can)** *see* butalbital compound and aspirin *on page 93*

**Tecnal C (Can)** *see* butalbital compound and codeine *on page 93*

**Teczem®** *see* enalapril and diltiazem *on page 213*

**Tedral® *(Discontinued)*** *see page 750*

**Teejel® (Can)** *see* choline salicylate *on page 135*

**Tega-Vert® Oral** *see* dimenhydrinate *on page 188*

**Tegison®** *see* etretinate *on page 237*

**Tegopen® *(Discontinued)*** *see page 750*

**Tegretol®** *see* carbamazepine *on page 105*

**Tegretol®-XR** *see* carbamazepine *on page 105*

**Tegrin®-HC Topical [OTC]** *see* hydrocortisone (topical) *on page 304*

**Teladar® Topical** *see* betamethasone (topical) *on page 78*

**Telepaque®** *see* radiological/contrast media (ionic) *on page 516*

**Teline® *(Discontinued)*** *see page 750*

## telmisartan (tel mi SAR tan)

**U.S./Canadian Brand Names** Micardis®

**Therapeutic Category** Angiotensin II Antagonist

**Use** Treatment of hypertension alone or in combination with other antihypertensives

**Usual Dosage** Adults: Oral: The usual starting dose is 40 mg once daily. Blood pressure response is dose-related over the range of 20 mg-80 mg/day; when additional antihypertensive effects are needed beyond that achieved with 80 mg/day, a diuretic may be added.

**Dosage Forms** Tablet: 20 mg, 40 mg, 80 mg

## telmisartan and hydrochlorothiazide

(tel mi SAR tan & hye droe klor oh THYE a zide)

**U.S./Canadian Brand Names** Micardis® HCT

**Therapeutic Category** Angiotensin II Antagonist Combination; Antihypertensive Agent, Combination

**Use** Treatment of hypertension; combination product should not be used for initial therapy

**Usual Dosage** Adults: Oral: Replacement therapy: Combination product can be substituted for individual titrated agents. Initiation of combination therapy when monotherapy has failed to achieve desired effects:

**Patients currently on telmisartan:** Initial dose if blood pressure is not currently controlled on monotherapy of 80 mg telmisartan: Telmisartan 80 mg/hydrochlorothiazide 12.5 mg once daily; may titrate up to telmisartan 160 mg/hydrochlorothiazide 25 mg if needed

**Patients currently on HCTZ:** Initial dose if blood pressure is not currently controlled on monotherapy of 25 mg once daily, or is controlled and experiencing hypokalemia: Telmisartan 80 mg/hydrochlorothiazide 12.5 mg once daily; may titrate up to telmisartan 160 mg/hydrochlorothiazide 25 mg if blood pressure remains uncontrolled after 2-4 weeks of therapy

**Dosage Forms** Tablet: Telmisartan 40 mg and hydrochlorothiazide 12.5 mg; telmisartan 80 mg and hydrochlorothiazide 12.5 mg

**Temaril® *(Discontinued)*** *see page 750*

## temazepam (te MAZ e pam)

**U.S./Canadian Brand Names** Apo®-Temazepam (Can); Gen-Temazepam (Can); Novo-Temazepam (Can); Nu-Temazepam (Can); PMS-Temazepam (Can); Restoril®

**Therapeutic Category** Benzodiazepine

**Controlled Substance** C-IV

**Use** Treatment of anxiety and as an adjunct in the treatment of depression; also may be used in the management of panic attacks; transient insomnia and sleep latency

**Usual Dosage** Adults: Oral: 15-30 mg at bedtime

**Dosage Forms** Capsule: 7.5 mg, 15 mg, 30 mg

**Temazin® Cold Syrup *(Discontinued)*** *see page 750*

**Temodal™ (Can)** *see* temozolomide *on this page*

**Temodar®** *see* temozolomide *on this page*

**Temovate®** *see* clobetasol *on page 143*

**Temovate E®** *see* clobetasol *on page 143*

## temozolomide (te mo ZOLE oh mide)

**U.S./Canadian Brand Names** Temodal™ (Can); Temodar®

**Therapeutic Category** Antineoplastic Agent

**Use** Treatment of adult patients with refractory (first relapse) anaplastic astrocytoma who have experienced disease progression on nitrosourea and procarbazine

**Unlabeled use:** Glioma, first relapse/advanced metastatic malignant melanoma

**Usual Dosage** The dosage is adjusted according to nadir neutrophil and platelet counts of previous cycle and counts at the time of the next cycle.

Adults: Initial dose: 150 mg/m$^2$ once daily for 5 consecutive days per 28-day treatment cycle

Measure day 22 ANC and platelets. Measure day 29 ANC and platelets. Based on lowest counts at either day 22 or day 29:

On day 22 or day 29, if ANC <1,000/µL or the platelet count is <50,000/µL, postpone therapy until ANC >1,500/µL and platelet count >100,000/µL. Reduce dose by 50 mg/m$^2$ for subsequent cycle.

If ANC 1,000-1,500/µL or platelets 50,000-100,000/µL, postpone therapy until ANC >1,500/µL and platelet count >100,000/µL; maintain initial dose.

If ANC >1,500/µL (on day 22 and day 29) and platelet count >100,000/µL, increase dose to, or maintain dose at 200 mg/m$^2$/day for 5 for subsequent cycle.

**Dosage Forms** Capsule: 5 mg, 20 mg, 100 mg, 250 mg

**Tempra® 1 [OTC]** *see* acetaminophen *on page 3*

**Tempra® 2 [OTC]** *see* acetaminophen *on page 3*

## tenecteplase (ten EK te plase)

**U.S./Canadian Brand Names** TNKase™

**Therapeutic Category** Thrombolytic Agent

**Use** Reduce mortality associated with acute myocardial infarction

**Usual Dosage** I.V.:

Adult: Recommended total dose should not exceed 50 mg and is based on patient's weight; administer as a bolus over 5 seconds

If patient's weight:

<60 kg, dose: 30 mg

≥60 to <70 kg, dose: 35 mg

≥70 to <80 kg, dose: 40 mg

≥80 to <90 kg, dose: 45 mg

≥90 kg, dose: 50 mg

All patients received 150-325 mg of aspirin as soon as possible and then daily. Intravenous heparin was initiated as soon as possible and PTT was maintained between 50-70 seconds.

**Dosage Forms** Powder for injection, lyophilized (recombinant): 50 mg

**Tenex®** *see* guanfacine *on page 286*

## teniposide (ten i POE side)

**Synonyms** EPT; VM-26

**U.S./Canadian Brand Names** Vumon®

**Therapeutic Category** Antineoplastic Agent

**Use** Treatment of Hodgkin's and non-Hodgkin's lymphomas, acute lymphocytic leukemia, bladder carcinoma and neuroblastoma

**Usual Dosage** I.V.:

Children: 130 mg/m$^2$/week, increasing to 150 mg/m$^2$ after 3 weeks and to 180 mg/m$^2$ after 6 weeks

Adults: 50-180 mg/m$^2$ once or twice weekly for 4-6 weeks

**Dosage Forms** Injection: 10 mg/mL (5 mL)

**Ten-K®** *see* potassium chloride *on page 485*

**Tenolin (Can)** *see* atenolol *on page 56*

**Tenoretic®** *see* atenolol and chlorthalidone *on page 57*

**Tenormin®** *see* atenolol *on page 56*

**Tensilon®** *see* edrophonium *on page 210*

**Tension® [OTC]** *see* acetaminophen and phenyltoloxamine *on page 5*

**Tenuate®** *see* diethylpropion *on page 184*

**Tenuate® Dospan®** *see* diethylpropion *on page 184*

**Tepanil®** ***(Discontinued)*** *see page 750*

**Tepanil® TenTabs®** ***(Discontinued)*** *see page 750*

**Tequin®** *see* gatifloxacin *on page 269*

**Terak® Ophthalmic Ointment** *see* oxytetracycline and polymyxin B *on page 446*

**Terazol® Vaginal** *see* terconazole *on next page*

## terazosin (ter AY zoe sin)

**U.S./Canadian Brand Names** Alti-Terazosin (Can); Apo®-Terazosin (Can); Hytrin®; Novo-Terazosin (Can); Nu-Terazosin (Can)

**Therapeutic Category** Alpha-Adrenergic Blocking Agent

**Use** Management of mild to moderate hypertension; considered a step 2 drug in stepped approach to hypertension; benign prostate hypertrophy

**Usual Dosage** Adults: Oral: 1 mg; slowly increase dose to achieve desired blood pressure, up to 20 mg/day

**Dosage Forms**

Capsule: 1 mg, 2 mg, 5 mg, 10 mg

Tablet: 1 mg, 2 mg, 5 mg, 10 mg

## terbinafine (oral) (TER bin a feen OR al)

**U.S./Canadian Brand Names** Lamisil® Oral

**Therapeutic Category** Antifungal Agent

**Use** Treatment of onychomycosis infections of the toenail or fingernail

**Usual Dosage** Adults: Oral:

Fingernail onychomycosis: 250 mg once daily for 6 weeks

Toenail onychomycosis: 250 mg once daily for 12 weeks

**Dosage Forms** Tablet: 250 mg

## terbinafine (topical) (TER bin a feen TOP i kal)

**U.S./Canadian Brand Names** Lamisil® Cream

**Therapeutic Category** Antifungal Agent

**Use** Topical antifungal for the treatment of tinea pedis (athlete's foot), tinea cruris (jock itch), and tinea corporis (ring worm); tinea versicolor (lotion)

**Unlabeled use:** Cutaneous candidiasis

**Usual Dosage** Adults: Topical:

Athlete's foot: Apply to affected area twice daily for at least 1 week, not to exceed 4 weeks

Ringworm and jock itch: Apply to affected area once or twice daily for at least 1 week, not to exceed 4 weeks

**Dosage Forms**

Cream: 1% (15 g, 30 g)

Lotion: 1%

## terbutaline (ter BYOO ta leen)

**U.S./Canadian Brand Names** Brethine®

**Therapeutic Category** Adrenergic Agonist Agent

**Use** Bronchodilator in reversible airway obstruction and bronchial asthma

**Usual Dosage**

Children <6 years:

Oral: Initial: 0.05 mg/kg/dose 3 times/day, increased gradually as required; maximum: 0.15 mg/kg/dose 3-4 times/day or a total of 5 mg/24 hours

S.C.: 0.005-0.01 mg/kg/dose to a maximum of 0.3 mg/dose every 15-20 minutes for 3 doses

Inhalation nebulization dose: 0.06 mg/kg; maximum: 8 mg
Inhalation: 0.3 mg/kg/dose up to maximum of 10 mg/dose every 4-6 hours
Children >6 years and Adults:
Oral:
6-15 years: 2.5 mg every 6 hours 3 times/day; not to exceed 7.5 mg in 24 hours
>15 years: 5 mg/dose every 6 hours 3 times/day; if side effects occur, reduce dose to 2.5 mg every 6 hours; not to exceed 15 mg in 24 hours
S.C.: 0.25 mg/dose repeated in 15-30 minutes for one time only; a total dose of 0.5 mg should not be exceeded within a 4-hour period

**Dosage Forms**
Injection, as sulfate: 1 mg/mL (1 mL)
Tablet, as sulfate: 2.5 mg, 5 mg

## terconazole (ter KONE a zole)

**Synonyms** triaconazole
**U.S./Canadian Brand Names** Terazol® Vaginal
**Therapeutic Category** Antifungal Agent
**Use** Local treatment of vulvovaginal candidiasis
**Usual Dosage** Vaginal: 1 applicatorful in vagina at bedtime for 7 consecutive days
**Dosage Forms**
Cream, vaginal: 0.4% (45 g); 0.8% (20 g)
Suppository, vaginal: 80 mg (3s)

## teriparatide (ter i PAR a tide)

**U.S./Canadian Brand Names** Parathar™
**Therapeutic Category** Diagnostic Agent
**Use** Diagnosis of hypocalcemia in either hypoparathyroidism or pseudohypoparathyroidism
**Usual Dosage** I.V.:
Children ≥3 years: 3 units/kg up to 200 units
Adults: 200 units over 10 minutes
**Dosage Forms** Powder for injection: 200 units hPTH activity (10 mL)

**terpin hydrate** ***(Discontinued)*** *see page 750*

**terpin hydrate and codeine** ***(Discontinued)*** *see page 750*

**Terra-Cortril® Ophthalmic Suspension** ***(Discontinued)*** *see page 750*

**Terramycin® I.M. Injection** *see* oxytetracycline *on page 445*

**Terramycin® Ophthalmic Ointment** *see* oxytetracycline and polymyxin B *on page 446*

**Terramycin® Oral** ***(Discontinued)*** *see page 750*

**Terramycin® w/Polymyxin B Ophthalmic Ointment** *see* oxytetracycline and polymyxin B *on page 446*

**Tesamone® Injection** *see* testosterone *on next page*

**Teslac®** *see* testolactone *on next page*

**TESPA** *see* thiotepa *on page 587*

**Tessalon® Perles** *see* benzonatate *on page 74*

**Tes-Tape®** ***(Discontinued)*** *see page 750*

**Testoderm®** *see* testosterone *on next page*

**Testoderm® TTS** *see* testosterone *on next page*

**Testoderm® with Adhesive** *see* testosterone *on next page*

**testolactone** (tes toe LAK tone)

**U.S./Canadian Brand Names** Teslac®

**Therapeutic Category** Androgen

**Use** Palliative treatment of advanced disseminated breast carcinoma

**Usual Dosage** Adults: Females: Oral: 250 mg 4 times/day for at least 3 months; desired response may take as long as 3 months

**Dosage Forms** Tablet: 50 mg

**Testomar®** *see* yohimbine *on page 636*

**Testopel® Pellet** *see* testosterone *on this page*

**testosterone** (tes TOS ter one)

**Synonyms** aqueous testosterone

**U.S./Canadian Brand Names** Androderm® Transdermal System; AndroGel®; Andro-L.A.® Injection; Andropository® Injection; Delatest® Injection; Delatestryl® Injection; depAndro® Injection; Depotest® Injection; Depo®-Testosterone Injection; Duratest® Injection; Durathate® Injection; Everone® Injection; Histerone® Injection; Tesamone® Injection; Testoderm®; Testoderm® TTS; Testoderm® with Adhesive; Testopel® Pellet

**Therapeutic Category** Androgen

**Controlled Substance** C-III

**Use** Androgen replacement therapy in the treatment of delayed male puberty; male hypogonadism

**Usual Dosage**

Children: I.M.:

Male hypogonadism:

Initiation of pubertal growth: 40-50 mg/m$^2$/dose (cypionate or enanthate ester) monthly until the growth rate falls to prepubertal levels

Terminal growth phase: 100 mg/m$^2$/dose (cypionate or enanthate ester) monthly until growth ceases

Maintenance virilizing dose: 100 mg/m$^2$/dose (cypionate or enanthate ester) twice monthly

Delayed puberty: 40-50 mg/m$^2$/dose monthly (cypionate or enanthate ester) for 6 months

Adults: Inoperable breast cancer: I.M.: 200-400 mg every 2-4 weeks

Male: Short-acting formulations: Testosterone Aqueous/Testosterone Propionate (in oil): I.M.:

Androgen replacement therapy: 10-50 mg 2-3 times/week

Male hypogonadism: 40-50 mg/m$^2$/dose monthly until the growth rate falls to prepubertal levels (~5 cm/year); during terminal growth phase: 100 mg/m$^2$/dose monthly until growth ceases; maintenance virilizing dose: 100 mg/m$^2$/dose twice monthly or 50-400 mg/dose every 2-4 weeks

Male: Long-acting formulations: Testosterone enanthate (in oil)/testosterone cypionate (in oil): I.M.:

Male hypogonadism: 50-400 mg every 2-4 weeks

Male with delayed puberty: 50-200 mg every 2-4 weeks for a limited duration

Male ≥18 years: Transdermal: Primary hypogonadism **or** hypogonadotropic hypogonadism:

Testoderm®: Apply 6 mg patch daily to scrotum (if scrotum is inadequate, use a 4 mg daily system)

Testoderm-TTS®: Apply 5 mg patch daily to clean, dry area of skin on the arm, back or upper buttocks. **Do not apply Testoderm-TTS® to the scrotum**.

Androderm®: Apply 2 systems nightly to clean, dry area on the back, abdomen, upper arms, or thighs for 24 hours for a total of 5 mg/day

AndroGel®: Males >18 years of age: 5 g (to deliver 50 mg of testosterone) applied once daily (preferably in the morning) to clean, dry, intact skin of the shoulder and upper arms and/or abdomen. Upon opening the packet(s), the entire contents should be squeezed into the palm of the hand and immediately applied to the application site(s). Application sites should be allowed to dry for a few minutes prior to dressing. Hands should be washed with soap and water after application. **Do not apply AndroGel® to the genitals**.

**Dosage Forms**

Injection:

Aqueous suspension: 25 mg/mL (10 mL, 30 mL); 50 mg/mL (10 mL, 30 mL); 100 mg/mL (10 mL, 30 mL)

In oil, as cypionate: 100 mg/mL (1 mL, 10 mL); 200 mg/mL (1 mL, 10 mL)

In oil, as enanthate: 100 mg/mL (1 mL, 5 mL, 10 mL); 200 mg/mL (1 mL, 5 mL, 10 mL)

In oil, as propionate: 100 mg/mL (10 mL, 30 mL)

Pellet: 75 mg (1 pellet per vial)

Transdermal system:

Androderm®: 2.5 mg/day; 5 mg/day

Testoderm®: 4 mg/day; 6 mg/day

Testoderm-TTS®: 5 mg/day

Transdermal gel: AndroGel®: 1%: 50 mg (5 g gel); 75 mg (7.5 g gel)

**Testred®** *see* methyltestosterone *on page 386*

**tetanus and diphtheria toxoid** *see* diphtheria and tetanus toxoid *on page 192*

## tetanus antitoxin (TET a nus an tee TOKS in)

**Synonyms** TAT

**Therapeutic Category** Antitoxin

**Use** Tetanus prophylaxis or treatment of active tetanus only when tetanus immune globulin (TIG) is not available

**Usual Dosage**

Prophylaxis: I.M., S.C.:

Children <30 kg: 1500 units

Children and Adults >30 kg: 3000-5000 units

Treatment: Children and Adults: Inject 10,000-40,000 units into wound; administer 40,000-100,000 units I.V.

**Dosage Forms** Injection, equine: Not less than 400 units/mL (12.5 mL, 50 mL)

## tetanus immune globulin (human)

(TET a nus i MYUN GLOB yoo lin HYU man)

**Synonyms** TIG

**U.S./Canadian Brand Names** BayTet™

**Therapeutic Category** Immune Globulin

**Use** Passive immunization against tetanus; tetanus immune globulin is preferred over tetanus antitoxin for treatment of active tetanus; part of the management of an unclean, nonminor wound in a person whose history of previous receipt of tetanus toxoid is unknown or who has received less than three doses of tetanus toxoid

**Usual Dosage** I.M.:

Prophylaxis of tetanus:

Children: 4 units/kg; some recommend administering 250 units to small children

Adults: 250 units

Treatment of tetanus:

Children: 500-3000 units; some should infiltrate locally around the wound

Adults: 3000-6000 units

**Dosage Forms** Injection: 250 units/mL

## tetanus toxoid (adsorbed) (TET a nus TOKS oyd ad SORBED)

**Therapeutic Category** Toxoid

**Use** Active immunization against tetanus

**Usual Dosage** Adults: I.M.:

Primary immunization: 0.5 mL; repeat 0.5 mL at 4-8 weeks after first dose and at 6-12 months after second dose

Routine booster doses are recommended only every 5-10 years

(Continued)

## tetanus toxoid (adsorbed) *(Continued)*

**Dosage Forms** Injection, adsorbed:

Tetanus 5 Lf units per 0.5 mL dose (0.5 mL, 5 mL)
Tetanus 10 Lf units per 0.5 mL dose (0.5 mL, 5 mL)

## tetanus toxoid (fluid) (TET a nus TOKS oyd FLOO id)

**Synonyms** tetanus toxoid plain

**Therapeutic Category** Toxoid

**Use** Active immunization against tetanus in adults and children

**Usual Dosage** Inject 3 doses of 0.5 mL I.M. or S.C. at 4- to 8-week intervals with fourth dose administered only 6-12 months after third dose

**Dosage Forms** Injection, fluid:

Tetanus 4 Lf units per 0.5 mL dose (7.5 mL)
Tetanus 5 Lf units per 0.5 mL dose (0.5 mL, 7.5 mL)

**tetanus toxoid plain** *see* tetanus toxoid (fluid) *on this page*

## tetrabenazine *(Canada only)* (tet ra BENZ a zeen)

**U.S./Canadian Brand Names** Nitoman® (Can)

**Therapeutic Category** Monoamine Depleting Agent

**Use** Treatment of hyperkinetic movement disorders such as Huntington's chorea, hemiballismus, senile chorea, tic and Gilles de la Tourette's syndrome and tardive dyskinesia; not indicated for the treatment of levodopa-induced dyskinetic/choreiform movements; should only be used by (or in consultation with) physicians who are experienced in the treatment of hyperkinetic movement disorders.

**Usual Dosage** Oral:

Children: No adequately controlled clinical studies have been performed in children. Limited clinical experience suggests that treatment should be started at approximately half the adult dose, and titrated slowly and carefully according to tolerance and individual response.

Adults: Initial starting dose: 12.5 mg 2-3 times/day is recommended. This can be increased by 12.5 mg/day every 3-5 days until the maximal tolerated and effective dose is reached for the individual, and may have to be up/down titrated depending on individual tolerance. In most cases the maximal tolerated dose will be 25 mg 3 times/day. In very rare cases, a 200 mg dose has been reached (the maximum recommended dose in some publications). If there is no improvement at the maximal tolerated dose in 7 days, it is unlikely that Nitoman® will be of benefit to the patient, either by increasing the dose or by extending the duration of treatment.

Elderly and debilitated patients: No adequately controlled clinical studies have been performed in the elderly and/or debilitated patients. Clinical experience suggests that a reduced initial and maintenance dose should be used. Parkinsonian-like adverse reactions are relatively common in these patients and may be dose-limiting.

**Dosage Forms** Tablet: 25 mg

## tetracaine (TET ra kane)

**Synonyms** amethocaine

**U.S./Canadian Brand Names** Ametop™ (Can); Pontocaine®

**Therapeutic Category** Local Anesthetic

**Use** Local anesthesia in the eye for various diagnostic and examination purposes; spinal anesthesia; topical anesthesia for local skin disorders; local anesthesia for mucous membranes

**Usual Dosage**

Children: Safety and efficacy have not been established

Adults:

Ophthalmic (not for prolonged use):

Ointment: Apply ½" to 1" to lower conjunctival fornix

Solution: Instill 1-2 drops

Spinal anesthesia 1% solution:
Subarachnoid injection: 5-20 mg
Saddle block: 2-5 mg; a 1% solution should be diluted with equal volume of CSF before administration
Topical mucous membranes (2% solution): Apply as needed; dose should not exceed 20 mg
Topical for skin: Apply to affected areas as needed

**Dosage Forms**
Cream, as hydrochloride: 1% (28 g)
Injection, as hydrochloride: 1% [10 mg/mL] (2 mL)
Injection, as hydrochloride, with dextrose 6%: 0.2% [2 mg/mL] (2 mL); 0.3% [3 mg/mL] (5 mL)
Ointment, as hydrochloride:
Ophthalmic: 0.5% [5 mg/mL] (3.75 g)
Topical: 0.5% [5 mg/mL] (28 g)
Powder for injection, as hydrochloride: 20 mg
Solution, as hydrochloride:
Ophthalmic: 0.5% [5 mg/mL] (1 mL, 2 mL, 15 mL, 59 mL)
Topical: 2% [20 mg/mL] (30 mL, 118 mL)

## tetracaine and dextrose (TET ra kane & DEKS trose)

**U.S./Canadian Brand Names** Pontocaine® With Dextrose
**Therapeutic Category** Local Anesthetic
**Use** Spinal anesthesia (saddle block)
**Usual Dosage** Dose varies with procedure, depth of anesthesia, duration desired, and physical condition of patient
**Dosage Forms** Injection: Tetracaine hydrochloride 0.2% and dextrose 6% (2 mL); tetracaine hydrochloride 0.3% and dextrose 6% (5 mL)

**TetraCap®** *see* tetracycline *on this page*

**TetraCon®** *see* tetracycline *on this page*

**tetracosactide** *see* cosyntropin *on page 156*

## tetracycline (tet ra SYE kleen)

**Synonyms** TCN
**U.S./Canadian Brand Names** Apo®-Tetra® (Can); BrodSpec®; EmTet-500®; Novo-Tetra (Can); Nu-Tetra (Can); Sumycin® Oral; TetraCap®; TetraCon®; Topicycline® Topical; Westmycin®
**Therapeutic Category** Antibiotic, Ophthalmic; Antibiotic, Topical; Tetracycline Derivative

**Use**
Children, Adolescents, and Adults: Treatment of Rocky mountain spotted fever caused by susceptible Rickettsia or brucellosis
Adolescents and Adults: Presumptive treatment of chlamydial infection in patients with gonorrhea
Older Children, Adolescents, and Adults: Treatment of Lyme disease, mycoplasmal disease or *Legionella*

**Usual Dosage**
Children >8 years:
Oral: 25-50 mg/kg/day in divided doses every 6 hours; not to exceed 3 g/day
Ophthalmic:
Suspension: Instill 1-2 drops 2-4 times/day or more often as needed
Ointment: Instill every 2-12 hours
Adults:
Oral: 250-500 mg/dose every 6 hours
Ophthalmic:
Suspension: Instill 1-2 drops 2-4 times/day or more often as needed
Ointment: Instill every 2-12 hours
(Continued)

**tetracycline** *(Continued)*

Topical: Apply to affected areas 1-4 times/day

**Dosage Forms**

Capsule, as hydrochloride: 100 mg, 250 mg, 500 mg
Ointment:
Ophthalmic: 1% [10 mg/mL] (3.5 g)
Topical, as hydrochloride: 3% [30 mg/mL] (14.2 g, 30 g)
Solution, topical: 2.2 mg/mL (70 mL)
Suspension:
Ophthalmic: 1% [10 mg/mL] (0.5 mL, 1 mL, 4 mL)
Oral, as hydrochloride: 125 mg/5 mL (60 mL, 480 mL)
Tablet, as hydrochloride: 250 mg, 500 mg

**tetrahydroaminoacrine** *see* tacrine *on page 569*

**tetrahydrocannabinol** *see* dronabinol *on page 205*

## tetrahydrozoline (tet ra hye DROZ a leen)

**Synonyms** tetryzoline

**U.S./Canadian Brand Names** Eyesine® Ophthalmic [OTC]; Eye-Zine® [OTC]; Geneye® Ophthalmic [OTC]; Murine® Plus Ophthalmic [OTC]; Optigene® Ophthalmic [OTC]; Tetrasine® Extra Ophthalmic [OTC]; Tetrasine® Ophthalmic [OTC]; Tyzine® Nasal; Visine® [OTC]; Visine® Clear Ophthalmic [OTC]; Visine® Eye Ophthalmic [OTC]

**Therapeutic Category** Adrenergic Agonist Agent

**Use** Symptomatic relief of nasal congestion and conjunctival congestion

**Usual Dosage**

Nasal congestion:
Children 2-6 years: Instill 2-3 drops of 0.05% solution every 4-6 hours as needed
Children >6 years and Adults: Instill 2-4 drops or 0.1% spray nasal mucosa every 4-6 hours as needed
Conjunctival congestion: Adults: Instill 1-2 drops in each eye 2-3 times/day

**Dosage Forms** Solution, as hydrochloride:
Nasal: 0.05% (15 mL); 0.1% (30 mL, 473 mL)
Ophthalmic: 0.05% (15 mL)

**Tetralan®** ***(Discontinued)*** *see page 750*

**Tetram®** ***(Discontinued)*** *see page 750*

**Tetramune®** *see* diphtheria, tetanus toxoids, whole-cell pertussis, and *Haemophilus* B conjugate vaccine *on page 194*

**Tetrasine® Extra Ophthalmic [OTC]** *see* tetrahydrozoline *on this page*

**Tetrasine® Ophthalmic [OTC]** *see* tetrahydrozoline *on this page*

**tetryzoline** *see* tetrahydrozoline *on this page*

**Teveten®** *see* eprosartan *on page 218*

**Texacort® Topical** *see* hydrocortisone (topical) *on page 304*

**TG** *see* thioguanine *on page 585*

**6-TG** *see* thioguanine *on page 585*

**T/Gel® [OTC]** *see* coal tar *on page 149*

**T-Gen®** ***(Discontinued)*** *see page 750*

**T-Gesic®** *see* hydrocodone and acetaminophen *on page 300*

**THA** *see* tacrine *on page 569*

## thalidomide (tha LI doe mide)

**U.S./Canadian Brand Names** Thalomid®

**Therapeutic Category** Immunosuppressant Agent

**Use** Treatment or prevention of graft-versus-host reactions after bone marrow transplantation; in aphthous ulceration in HIV-positive patients; reactional lepromatous or erythema nodosum leprosy; Langerhans cell histiocytosis, Behçet's syndrome; hypnotic agent; also may be effective in rheumatoid arthritis, discoid lupus, and erythema multiforme; useful in type 2 lepra reactions, but not type 1; can assist in healing mouth ulcers in AIDS patients

**Usual Dosage**

Leprosy: Up to 400 mg/day; usual maintenance dose: 50-100 mg/day

Behçet's syndrome: 100-400 mg/day

Graft-vs-host reactions:

Children: 3 mg/kg 4 times/day

Adults: 100-1600 mg/day; usual initial dose: 200 mg 4 times/day for use up to 700 days

AIDS-related aphthous stomatitis: 200 mg twice daily for 5 days, then 200 mg/day for up to 8 weeks

Discoid lupus erythematosus: 100-400 mg/day; maintenance dose: 25-50 mg

**Dosage Forms** Capsule: 50 mg

**Thalitone®** *see* chlorthalidone *on page 133*

**Thalomid®** *see* thalidomide *on previous page*

**THAM®** *see* tromethamine *on page 611*

**THC** *see* dronabinol *on page 205*

**Theelin® Aqueous Injection *(Discontinued)*** *see page 750*

**Theo-24®** *see* theophylline *on this page*

**Theobid® *(Discontinued)*** *see page 750*

**Theobid® Jr Duracaps® *(Discontinued)*** *see page 750*

**Theochron®** *see* theophylline *on this page*

**Theoclear-80® *(Discontinued)*** *see page 750*

**Theoclear®-L.A. *(Discontinued)*** *see page 750*

**Theocon®** *see* theophylline and guaifenesin *on page 583*

**Theo-Dur®** *see* theophylline *on this page*

**Theo-Dur® Sprinkle® *(Discontinued)*** *see page 750*

**Theolair™** *see* theophylline *on this page*

**Theolate®** *see* theophylline and guaifenesin *on page 583*

**Theomar G.G.®** *see* theophylline and guaifenesin *on page 583*

**Theo-Organidin® *(Discontinued)*** *see page 750*

## theophylline (thee OF i lin)

**U.S./Canadian Brand Names** Aerolate III®; Aerolate JR®; Aerolate SR®; Apo®-Theo LA (Can); Elixophyllin®; Novo-Theophyl SR (Can); Quibron®-T; Quibron®-T/SR; Respbid®; Slo-bid™; Slo-Phyllin®; Theo-24®; Theochron®; Theo-Dur®; Theolair™; T-Phyl®; Uni-Dur®; Uniphyl®

**Therapeutic Category** Theophylline Derivative

**Use** Treatment of symptoms and reversible airway obstruction due to chronic asthma, chronic bronchitis, or COPD; for treatment of idiopathic apnea of prematurity in neonates

**Usual Dosage**

Apnea: Dosage should be determined by plasma level monitoring; each 0.5 mg/kg of theophylline administered as a loading dose will result in a 1 mcg/mL increase in serum theophylline concentration

Loading dose: 5 mg/kg; dilute dose in 1-hour I.V. fluid via syringe pump over 1 hour

Maintenance: 2 mg/kg every 8-12 hours or 1-3 mg/kg/dose every 8-12 hours; administer I.V. push 1 mL/minute (2 mg/minute)

(Continued)

## theophylline *(Continued)*

Treatment of acute bronchospasm in older patients: (>6 months of age): Loading dose (in patients not currently receiving theophylline): 6 mg/kg (based on aminophylline) administered I.V. over 20-30 minutes; 4.7 mg/kg (based on theophylline) administered I.V. over 20-30 minutes; administration rate should not exceed 20 mg (1 mL)/minute (theophylline) or 25 mg (1 mL)/minute (aminophylline)

Approximate maintenance dosage for treatment of acute bronchospasm:

Children:

6 months to 9 years: 1.2 mg/kg/hour (aminophylline); 0.95 mg/kg/hour (theophylline)

9-16 years and young adult smokers: 1 mg/kg/hour (aminophylline); 0.79 mg/kg/hour (theophylline)

Adults (healthy, nonsmoking): 0.7 mg/kg/hour (aminophylline); 0.55 mg/kg/hour (theophylline)

Older patients and patients with cor pulmonale: 0.6 mg/kg/hour (aminophylline); 0.47 mg/kg/hour (theophylline)

Patients with CHF or liver failure: 0.5 mg/kg/hour (aminophylline); 0.39 mg/kg/hour (theophylline)

Chronic therapy: Slow clinical titration is generally preferred

Initial dose: 16 mg/kg/24 hours or 400 mg/24 hours, whichever is less

Increasing dose: The above dosage may be increased in ~25% increments at 2- to 3-day intervals so long as the drug is tolerated or until the maximum dose is reached; monitor serum levels

Exercise caution in younger children who cannot complain of minor side effects, older adults, and those with cor pulmonale; CHF or liver disease may have unusually low dosage requirements

### Dosage Forms

Capsule:

Immediate release: 100 mg, 200 mg

Timed release:

8-12 hours (Aerolate®): 65 mg [III]; 130 mg [JR], 260 mg [SR]

8-12 hours (Slo-bid™): 50 mg, 75 mg, 100 mg, 125 mg, 200 mg, 300 mg

8-12 hours (Slo-Phyllin® Gyrocaps®): 60 mg, 125 mg, 250 mg

24 hours (Theo-24®): 100 mg, 200 mg, 300 mg

Elixir (Elixophyllin®): 80 mg/15 mL (15 mL, 30 mL, 480 mL, 4000 mL)

Infusion, in $D_5W$: 0.4 mg/mL (1000 mL); 0.8 mg/mL (500 mL, 1000 mL); 1.6 mg/mL (250 mL, 500 mL); 2 mg/mL (100 mL); 3.2 mg/mL (250 mL); 4 mg/mL (50 mL, 100 mL);

Solution, oral:

Theolair™: 80 mg/15 mL (15 mL, 18.75 mL, 30 mL, 480 mL)

Syrup:

Slo-Phyllin®: 80 mg/15 mL (15 mL, 30 mL, 500 mL)

Tablet: Immediate release:

Slo-Phyllin®: 100 mg, 200 mg

Theolair™: 125 mg, 250 mg

Quibron®-T: 300 mg

Tablet:

Controlled release (Theo-X®): 100 mg, 200 mg, 300 mg

Timed release:

12-24 hours: 100 mg, 200 mg, 300 mg, 450 mg

8-12 hours (Quibron®-T/SR): 300 mg

8-12 hours (Respbid®): 250 mg, 500 mg

8-12 hours (T-Phyl®): 200 mg

12-24 hours (Theochron®): 100 mg, 200 mg, 300 mg

8-24 hours (Theo-Dur®): 100 mg, 200 mg, 300 mg, 450 mg

24 hours (Theolair™-SR): 200 mg, 300 mg, 500 mg

24 hours (Uni-Dur®, Uniphyl®): 400 mg, 600 mg

**theophylline and guaifenesin** (thee OF i lin & gwye FEN e sin)

**U.S./Canadian Brand Names** Elixophyllin-GG®; Neoasma®; Quibron®; Slo-Phyllin® GG; Theocon®; Theolate®; Theomar G.G.®

**Therapeutic Category** Theophylline Derivative

**Use** Symptomatic treatment of bronchospasm associated with bronchial asthma, chronic bronchitis and pulmonary emphysema

**Usual Dosage** Adults: Oral: 1-2 capsules every 6-8 hours

**Dosage Forms**

Capsule: Theophylline 150 mg and guaifenesin 90 mg
Elixir: Theophylline 150 mg and guaifenesin 90 mg per 15 mL (480 mL)
Liquid: Theophylline 100 mg and guaifenesin 100 mg per 15 mL (480 mL)
Syrup: Theophylline 150 mg and guaifenesin 90 mg per 15 mL (480 mL)
Tablet: Theophylline 125 mg and guaifenesin 100mg

**theophylline, ephedrine, and hydroxyzine**
(thee OF i lin, e FED rin, & hye DROKS i zeen)

**Therapeutic Category** Theophylline Derivative

**Use** Possibly effective for controlling bronchospastic disorders

**Usual Dosage** Oral:

Children:
2-5 years: 1/2 tablet 2-4 times/day or 2.5 mL 3-4 times/day
>5 years: 1/2 tablet 2-4 times/day or 5 mL 3-4 times/day
Adults: 1 tablet 2-4 times/day

**Dosage Forms**

Syrup, dye free: Theophylline 32.5 mg, ephedrine 6.25 mg, and hydroxyzine 2.5 mg per 5 mL
Tablet: Theophylline 130 mg, ephedrine 25 mg, and hydroxyzine 10 mg

**theophylline ethylenediamine** *see* aminophylline *on page 31*

**Theo-Sav® *(Discontinued)*** *see page 750*

**Theospan®-SR *(Discontinued)*** *see page 750*

**Theostat-80® *(Discontinued)*** *see page 750*

**Theovent® *(Discontinued)*** *see page 750*

**Theo-X® *(Discontinued)*** *see page 750*

**Therabid® [OTC]** *see* vitamin (multiple/oral) *on page 632*

**Thera-Combex® H-P Kapseals® [OTC]** *see* vitamin B complex with vitamin C *on page 630*

**TheraCys®** *see* BCG vaccine *on page 68*

**Theraflu® [OTC]** *see* acetaminophen, dextromethorphan, and pseudoephedrine *on page 7*

**Theraflu® Flu & Cold [OTC]** *see* acetaminophen, chlorpheniramine, and pseudoephedrine *on page 6*

**Theraflu® Flu Cold & Cough [OTC]** *see* acetaminophen, dextromethorphan, and pseudoephedrine *on page 7*

**Thera-Flur®** *see* fluoride *on page 255*

**Thera-Flur-N®** *see* fluoride *on page 255*

**Theragen®** *see* capsaicin *on page 104*

**Theragen HP®** *see* capsaicin *on page 104*

**Theragran® [OTC]** *see* vitamin (multiple/oral) *on page 632*

**Theragran® Hematinic®** *see* vitamin (multiple/oral) *on page 632*

**Theragran® Liquid [OTC]** *see* vitamin (multiple/oral) *on page 632*

**Theragran-M® [OTC]** *see* vitamin (multiple/oral) *on page 632*

**Thera-Hist® Syrup *(Discontinued)*** *see page 750*

**Theramine® Expectorant *(Discontinued)*** *see page 750*

**Therapatch Warm®** *see* capsaicin *on page 104*

**Theraplex Z® [OTC]** *see* pyrithione zinc *on page 512*

**Thermazene®** *see* silver sulfadiazine *on page 544*

## thiabendazole (thye a BEN da zole)

**Synonyms** tiabendazole

**U.S./Canadian Brand Names** Mintezol®

**Therapeutic Category** Anthelmintic

**Use** Treatment of strongyloidiasis, cutaneous larva migrans, visceral larva migrans, dracunculosis, trichinosis, and mixed helminthic infections

**Usual Dosage** Children and Adults: Oral: 50 mg/kg/day divided every 12 hours (maximum dose: 3 g/day)

Strongyloidiasis: For 2 consecutive days

Cutaneous larva migrans: For 2-5 consecutive days

Visceral larva migrans: For 5-7 consecutive days

Trichinosis: For 2-4 consecutive days

Dracunculosis: 50-75 mg/kg/day divided every 12 hours for 3 days

**Dosage Forms**

Suspension, oral: 500 mg/5 mL (120 mL)

Tablet, chewable (orange flavor): 500 mg

**Thiacide® *(Discontinued)*** *see page 750*

**thiamazole** *see* methimazole *on page 379*

## thiamine (THYE a min)

**Synonyms** aneurine; thiaminium; vitamin $B_1$

**U.S./Canadian Brand Names** Betaxin® (Can)

**Therapeutic Category** Vitamin, Water Soluble

**Use** Treatment of thiamine deficiency including beriberi, Wernicke's encephalopathy syndrome, and peripheral neuritis associated with pellagra; alcoholic patients with altered sensorium; various genetic metabolic disorders

**Usual Dosage** Dietary supplement (depends on caloric or carbohydrate content of the diet):

Infants: 0.3-0.5 mg/day

Children: 0.5-1 mg/day

Adults: 1-2 mg/day

**Note:** The above doses can be found as a combination in multivitamin preparations

Children:

Noncritically ill thiamine deficiency: Oral: 10-50 mg/day in divided doses every day for 2 weeks followed by 5-10 mg/day for one month

Beriberi: I.M.: 10-25 mg/day for 2 weeks, then 5-10 mg orally every day for one month (oral as therapeutic multivitamin)

Adults:

Wernicke's encephalopathy: I.M., I.V.: 50 mg as a single dose, then 50 mg I.M. every day until normal diet resumed

Noncritically ill thiamine deficiency: Oral: 10-50 mg/day in divided doses

Beriberi: I.M., I.V.: 10-30 mg 3 times/day for 2 weeks, then switch to 5-10 mg orally every day for one month (oral as therapeutic multivitamin)

**Dosage Forms**

Injection, as hydrochloride: 100 mg/mL (1 mL, 2 mL, 10 mL, 30 mL); 200 mg/mL (30 mL)

Tablet, as hydrochloride: 50 mg, 100 mg, 250 mg, 500 mg

Tablet, as hydrochloride, enteric coated: 20 mg

**thiaminium** *see* thiamine *on this page*

## thiethylperazine (thye eth il PER a zeen)

**U.S./Canadian Brand Names** Torecan® Injection; Torecan® Tablet

**Therapeutic Category** Phenothiazine Derivative

**Use** Relief of nausea and vomiting

**Usual Dosage** Children >12 years and Adults:

Oral, I.M.: 10 mg 1-3 times/day as needed

I.V. and S.C. routes of administration are not recommended

**Dosage Forms**

Injection, as maleate: 5 mg/mL (2 mL)

Tablet, as maleate: 10 mg

## thimerosal (thye MER oh sal)

**U.S./Canadian Brand Names** Mersol® [OTC]; Merthiolate® [OTC]

**Therapeutic Category** Antibacterial, Topical

**Use** Organomercurial antiseptic with sustained bacteriostatic and fungistatic activity

**Usual Dosage** Apply 1-3 times/day

**Dosage Forms**

Liquid: 0.1% [1 mg/mL = 1:1000] (30 mL)

Solution, topical: 0.1% [1 mg/mL = 1:1000] (120 mL, 480 mL, 4000 mL)

Spray, antiseptic: 0.1% [1 mg/mL = 1:1000] with alcohol 2% (90 mL)

Swab: 2% (10s)

Tincture: 0.1% [1 mg/mL = 1:1000] with alcohol 50% (120 mL, 480 mL, 4000 mL)

## thioguanine (thye oh GWAH neen)

**Synonyms** 2-amino-6-mercaptopurine; TG; 6-TG; 6-thioguanine; tioguanine

**U.S./Canadian Brand Names** Lanvis® (Can)

**Therapeutic Category** Antineoplastic Agent

**Use** Remission induction in acute myelogenous (nonlymphocytic) leukemia; treatment of chronic myelogenous leukemia and acute lymphocytic leukemia

**Usual Dosage** Refer to individual protocols. Oral:

Infants <3 years: Combination drug therapy for acute nonlymphocytic leukemia: 3.3 mg/kg/day in divided doses twice daily for 4 days

Children and Adults: 2-3 mg/kg/day calculated to nearest 20 mg or 75-200 mg/m$^2$/day in 1-2 divided doses for 5-7 days or until remission is attained

**Dosage Forms** Tablet, scored: 40 mg

**6-thioguanine** *see* thioguanine *on this page*

**Thiola™** *see* tiopronin *on page 592*

## thiopental (thye oh PEN tal)

**U.S./Canadian Brand Names** Pentothal® Sodium

**Therapeutic Category** Barbiturate

**Controlled Substance** C-III

**Use** Induction of anesthesia; adjunct for intubation in head injury patients; control of convulsive states; treatment of elevated intracranial pressure

**Usual Dosage** I.V.:

Induction anesthesia:

- Infants: 5-8 mg/kg
- Children 1-12 years: 5-6 mg/kg
- Adults: 3-5 mg/kg

Maintenance anesthesia:

- Children: 1 mg/kg as needed
- Adults: 25-100 mg as needed

Increased intracranial pressure: Children and Adults: 1.5-5 mg/kg/dose; repeat as needed to control intracranial pressure

Seizures:

- Children: 2-3 mg/kg/dose, repeat as needed

(Continued)

## thiopental *(Continued)*

Adults: 75-250 mg/dose, repeat as needed

**Rectal administration:** (Patient should be NPO for no less than 3 hours prior to administration)

**Suggested initial doses of thiopental rectal suspension are:**

<3 months: 15 mg/kg/dose

>3 months: 25 mg/kg/dose

**Note:** The age of a premature infant should be adjusted to reflect the age that the infant would have been if full-term (eg, an infant, now age 4 months, who was 2 months premature should be considered to be a 2-month old infant).

Doses should be rounded downward to the nearest 50 mg increment to allow for accurate measurement of the dose

Inactive or debilitated patients and patients recently medicated with other sedatives, (eg, chloral hydrate, meperidine, chlorpromazine, and promethazine), may require smaller doses than usual

**If the patient is not sedated within 15-20 minutes, a single repeat dose of thiopental can be administered; the single repeat doses are:**

<3 months of age: <7.5 mg/kg/dose

>3 months of age: 15 mg/kg/dose

Adults weighing >90 kg should not receive >3 g as a total dose (initial plus repeat doses)

Children weighing >34 kg should not receive >1 g as a total dose (initial plus repeat doses)

Neither adults nor children should receive more than one course of thiopental rectal suspension (initial dose plus repeat dose) per 24-hour period

**Dosage Forms**

Injection, as sodium: 250 mg, 400 mg, 500 mg, 1 g, 2.5 g, 5 g

Suspension, rectal, as sodium: 400 mg/g (2 g)

**Thioplex®** *see* thiotepa *on next page*

## thioproperazine *(Canada only)* (thye oh pro PER a zeen)

**U.S./Canadian Brand Names** Majeptil® (Can)

**Therapeutic Category** Neuroleptic Agent

**Use** All types of acute and chronic schizophrenia, including those which did not respond to the usual neuroleptics; manic syndromes.

**Usual Dosage** Initial treatment: Adults: It is recommended to start treatment at a low dosage of about 5 mg/day in a single dose or in divided doses. This initial dosage is gradually increased by the same amount every 2-3 days until the usual effective dosage of 30-40 mg/day is reached. In some cases, higher dosages of 90 mg or more per day, are necessary to control the psychotic manifestations.

Children >10 years of age: Start treatment with a daily dosage of 1-3 mg following the method of treatment described for adults

Maintenance therapy: Adults and Children: Dosage should be reduced gradually to the lowest effective level, which may be as low as a few mg per day and maintained as long as necessary

**Dosage Forms** Tablet, as mesylate: 10 mg

## thioridazine (thye oh RID a zeen)

**U.S./Canadian Brand Names** Apo®-Thioridazine (Can); Mellaril®

**Therapeutic Category** Phenothiazine Derivative

**Use** Management of psychotic disorders; depressive neurosis; dementia in elderly; severe behavioral problems in children

**Usual Dosage** Oral:

Children >2 years: Range: 0.5-3 mg/kg/day in 2-3 divided doses; usual: 1 mg/kg/day; maximum: 3 mg/kg/day

Behavior problems: Initial: 10 mg 2-3 times/day, increase gradually

Severe psychoses: Initial: 25 mg 2-3 times/day, increase gradually

Adults:

Psychoses: Initial: 50-100 mg 3 times/day with gradual increments as needed and tolerated; maximum daily dose: 800 mg/day in 2-4 divided doses

Depressive disorders, dementia: Initial: 25 mg 3 times/day; maintenance dose: 20-200 mg/day

**Dosage Forms**

Concentrate, as hydrochloride, oral: 30 mg/mL (120 mL); 100 mg/mL (3.4 mL, 120 mL)

Tablet, as hydrochloride: 10 mg, 15 mg, 25 mg, 50 mg, 100 mg, 150 mg, 200 mg

## thiotepa (thye oh TEP a)

**Synonyms** TESPA; triethylenethiophosphoramide; TSPA

**U.S./Canadian Brand Names** Thioplex®

**Therapeutic Category** Antineoplastic Agent

**Use** Treatment of superficial tumors of the bladder; palliative treatment of adenocarcinoma of breast or ovary; lymphomas and sarcomas; meningeal neoplasms; control pleural, pericardial or peritoneal effusions caused by metastatic tumors; high-dose regimens with autologous bone marrow transplantation

**Usual Dosage** Refer to individual protocols

Children: Sarcomas: I.V.: 25-65 mg/m$^2$ as a single dose every 21 days

Adults:

I.M., I.V., S.C.: 8 mg/m$^2$ daily for 5 days or 30-60 mg/m$^2$ once per week

High-dose therapy for bone marrow transplant: I.V.: 500 mg/m$^2$

Intracavitary: 0.6-0.8 mg/kg or 60 mg in 60 mL SWI instilled into the bladder at 1- to 4-week intervals

Intrathecal: Doses of 1-10 mg/m$^2$ administered 1-2 times/week

**Dosage Forms** Powder for injection: 15 mg

## thiothixene (thye oh THIKS een)

**Synonyms** tiotixene

**U.S./Canadian Brand Names** Navane® Capsule

**Therapeutic Category** Thioxanthene Derivative

**Use** Management of psychotic disorders

**Usual Dosage**

Children <12 years: 0.25 mg/kg/24 hours in divided doses (dose not well established)

Children >12 years and Adults: Mild to moderate psychosis: 2 mg 3 times/day, up to 20-30 mg/day; more severe psychosis: Initial: 5 mg 2 times/day, may increase gradually, if necessary; maximum: 60 mg/day

Hemodialysis: Not dialyzable (0% to 5%)

**Dosage Forms** Capsule: 1 mg, 2 mg, 5 mg, 10 mg, 20 mg

**Thorazine®** *see* chlorpromazine *on page 132*

**Thrombate III™** *see* antithrombin III *on page 45*

**Thrombinar®** ***(Discontinued)*** *see page 750*

## thrombin (topical) (THROM bin TOP i kal)

**U.S./Canadian Brand Names** Thrombogen®

**Therapeutic Category** Hemostatic Agent

**Use** Hemostasis whenever minor bleeding from capillaries and small venules is accessible

**Usual Dosage** Use 1000-2000 units/mL of solution where bleeding is profuse; apply powder directly to the site of bleeding or on oozing surfaces; use 100 units/mL for bleeding from skin or mucosal surfaces

**Dosage Forms** Powder: 1000 units, 5000 units, 10,000 units, 20,000 units, 50,000 units

**Thrombogen®** *see* thrombin (topical) *on this page*

**Thrombostat®** ***(Discontinued)*** *see page 750*

**Thymoglobulin®** *see* antithymocyte globulin (rabbit) *on page 45*

**Thypinone®** ***(Discontinued)*** *see page 750*

**Thyrar®** ***(Discontinued)*** *see page 750*

**Thyrel® TRH** *see* protirelin *on page 506*

**Thyrogen®** *see* thyrotropin alpha *on this page*

## thyroid (THYE royd)

**Synonyms** desiccated thyroid; thyroid extract

**U.S./Canadian Brand Names** Armour® Thyroid; Westhroid®

**Therapeutic Category** Thyroid Product

**Use** Replacement or supplemental therapy in hypothyroidism

**Usual Dosage** Adults: Oral: Start at 30 mg/day and titrate by 30 mg/day in increments of 2- to 3-week intervals; usual maintenance dose: 60-120 mg/day

**Dosage Forms** Tablet: 15 mg, 30 mg, 32.4 mg, 60 mg, 64.8 mg, 65 mg, 90 mg, 120 mg, 129.6 mg, 130 mg, 180 mg, 194.4 mg, 240 mg, 300 mg

**thyroid extract** *see* thyroid *on this page*

**thyroid-stimulating hormone** *see* thyrotropin *on this page*

**Thyroid Strong®** ***(Discontinued)*** *see page 750*

**Thyrolar®** *see* liotrix *on page 352*

## thyrotropin (thye roe TROE pin)

**Synonyms** thyroid-stimulating hormone; TSH

**U.S./Canadian Brand Names** Thytropar®

**Therapeutic Category** Diagnostic Agent

**Use** Diagnostic aid to determine subclinical hypothyroidism or decreased thyroid reserve, to differentiate between primary and secondary hypothyroidism and between primary hypothyroidism and euthyroidism in patients receiving thyroid replacement

**Usual Dosage** I.M., S.C.: 10 units/day for 1-3 days; follow by a radioiodine study 24 hours past last injection, no response in thyroid failure, substantial response in pituitary failure

**Dosage Forms** Injection: 10 units

## thyrotropin alpha (thye roe TROE pin AL fa)

**Synonyms** human thyroid-stimulating hormone

**U.S./Canadian Brand Names** Thyrogen®

**Therapeutic Category** Diagnostic Agent

**Use** As an adjunctive diagnostic tool for serum thyroglobulin (Tg) testing with or without radioiodine imaging in the follow-up of patients with well-differentiated thyroid cancer

Potential clinical uses:

1. Patients with an undetectable Tg on thyroid hormone suppressive therapy to exclude the diagnosis of residual or recurrent thyroid cancer
2. Patients requiring serum Tg testing and radioiodine imaging who are unwilling to undergo thyroid hormone withdrawal testing and whose treating physician believes that use of a less sensitive test is justified
3. Patients who are either unable to mount an adequate endogenous TSH response to thyroid hormone withdrawal or in whom withdrawal is medically contraindicated

**Usual Dosage** Children >16 years and Adults: I.M.: 0.9 mg every 24 hours for 2 doses or every 72 hours for 3 doses. For radioiodine imaging, radioiodine administration should be given 24 hours following the final Thyrogen® injection. Scanning should be performed 48 hours after radioiodine administration (72 hours after the final injection of Thyrogen®).

**Dosage Forms** Kits containing two 1.1 mg vials (>4 int. units) of Thyrogen® and two 10 mL vials of sterile water for injection

**Thyrox®** *see* levothyroxine *on page 348*

**Thytropar®** *see* thyrotropin *on this page*

**tiabendazole** *see* thiabendazole *on page 584*

## tiagabine (tye AG a bene)

**U.S./Canadian Brand Names** Gabitril®

**Therapeutic Category** Anticonvulsant

**Use** Adjunctive therapy in adults and children 12 years and older in the treatment of partial seizures

**Usual Dosage** Children >12 years and Adults: Oral: Initial: 4 mg, once daily; the total daily dose may be increased in 4 mg increments beginning the second week of therapy; thereafter, the daily dose may be increased by 4-8 mg/day until clinical response is achieved, up to a maximum of 32 mg/day; the total daily dose at higher levels should be given in divided doses, 2-4 times/day

**Dosage Forms** Tablet, as hydrochloride: 2 mg, 4 mg, 12 mg, 16 mg

**Tiamate®** *see* diltiazem *on page 187*

**Tiamol® (Can)** *see* fluocinonide *on page 254*

## tiaprofenic acid *(Canada only)* (tye ah PRO fen ik AS id)

**U.S./Canadian Brand Names** Albert® Tiafen (Can); Apo®-Tiaprofenic (Can); Novo-Tiaprofenic (Can); Nu-Tiaprofenic (Can); PMS-Tiaprofenic (Can); Surgam® (Can); Surgam® SR (Can)

**Therapeutic Category** Nonsteroidal Anti-inflammatory Drug (NSAID)

**Use** Relief of signs and symptoms of rheumatoid arthritis and osteoarthritis (degenerative joint disease)

**Usual Dosage** Adults: Oral:

Tablet:

Rheumatoid arthritis: Usual initial and maintenance dose: 600 mg/day in 3 divided doses; some patients may do well on 300 mg twice daily; maximum daily dose: 600 mg

Osteoarthritis: Usual initial and maintenance dose: 600 mg/day in 2 or 3 divided doses; in rare instances patients may be maintained on 300 mg/day in divided doses; maximum daily dose: 600 mg

Extended release capsule:

Rheumatoid arthritis or osteoarthritis: Initial and maintenance dose: 2 sustained release capsules of 300 mg once daily; Surgam® SR capsules should be swallowed whole

**Dosage Forms**

Capsule, sustained release: 300 mg

Tablet: 200 mg, 300 mg

**Tiazac®** *see* diltiazem *on page 187*

**Ticar®** *see* ticarcillin *on this page*

## ticarcillin (tye kar SIL in)

**U.S./Canadian Brand Names** Ticar®

**Therapeutic Category** Penicillin

**Use** Treatment of infections such as septicemia, acute and chronic respiratory tract infections, skin and soft tissue infections, and urinary tract infections due to susceptible strains of *Pseudomonas*, *Proteus*, *Escherichia coli*, and *Enterobacter*

**Usual Dosage** I.V. (ticarcillin is generally administered I.M. only for the treatment of uncomplicated urinary tract infections):

Infants and Children: 200-300 mg/kg/day in divided doses every 4-6 hours; maximum dose: 24 g/day

Adults: 1-4 g every 4-6 hours

**Dosage Forms** Powder for injection, as disodium: 3 g, 20 g

## ticarcillin and clavulanate potassium

(tye kar SIL in & klav yoo LAN ate poe TASS ee um)

**Synonyms** ticarcillin and clavulanic acid

**U.S./Canadian Brand Names** Timentin®

**Therapeutic Category** Penicillin

**Use** Treatment of infections caused by susceptible organisms involving the lower respiratory tract, urinary tract, skin and skin structures, bone and joint, and septicemia. Clavulanate expands activity of ticarcillin to include beta-lactamase producing strains of *S. aureus*, *H. influenzae*, *Moraxella catarrhalis*, *B. fragilis*, *Klebsiella*, and *Proteus* species

**Usual Dosage** I.V.:

Children: 200-300 mg of ticarcillin/kg/day in divided doses every 4-6 hours

Adults: 3.1 g (ticarcillin 3 g plus clavulanic acid 0.1 g) every 4-6 hours; maximum: 18-24 g/day; for urinary tract infections: 3.1 g every 6-8 hours

**Dosage Forms**

Infusion, premixed (frozen): Ticarcillin disodium 3 g and clavulanate potassium 0.1 g (100 mL)

Powder for injection: Ticarcillin disodium 3 g and clavulanate potassium 0.1 g (3.1 g, 31 g)

**ticarcillin and clavulanic acid** *see* ticarcillin and clavulanate potassium *on this page*

**TICE® BCG** *see* BCG vaccine *on page 68*

**Ticlid®** *see* ticlopidine *on this page*

## ticlopidine (tye KLOE pi deen)

**U.S./Canadian Brand Names** Alti-Ticlopidine (Can); Apo®-Ticlopidine (Can); Gen-Ticlopidine (Can); Nu-Ticlopidine (Can); Ticlid®

**Therapeutic Category** Antiplatelet Agent

**Use** Platelet aggregation inhibitor that reduces the risk of thrombotic stroke in patients who have had a stroke or stroke precursors

**Usual Dosage** Adults: Oral: 1 tablet twice daily with food

**Dosage Forms** Tablet, as hydrochloride: 250 mg

**Ticon®** ***(Discontinued)*** *see page 750*

**TIG** *see* tetanus immune globulin (human) *on page 577*

**Tigan®** *see* trimethobenzamide *on page 607*

**Tiject-20®** ***(Discontinued)*** *see page 750*

**Tikosyn™** *see* dofetilide *on page 198*

**Tilade® Inhalation Aerosol** *see* nedocromil (inhalation) *on page 411*

## tiludronate (tye LOO droe nate)

**Synonyms** tiludronic acid

**U.S./Canadian Brand Names** Skelid®

**Therapeutic Category** Bisphosphonate Derivative

**Use** Paget's disease of the bone

**Usual Dosage** Adults: Oral: 400 mg/day (2 tablets) [tiludronic acid]

**Dosage Forms** Tablet, as disodium: 240 mg [tiludronic acid 200 mg]; dosage is expressed in terms of tiludronic acid.

**tiludronic acid** *see* tiludronate *on this page*

**Tim-Ak (Can)** *see* timolol *on next page*

**Timecelles® [OTC]** *see* ascorbic acid *on page 54*

**Timentin®** *see* ticarcillin and clavulanate potassium *on this page*

## timolol (TYE moe lole)

**U.S./Canadian Brand Names** Apo®-Timol (Can); Apo®-Timop (Can); Blocadren® Oral; Gen-Timolol (Can); Novo-Timol (Can); Nu-Timolol (Can); PMS-Timolol (Can); Rhoxal-timolol (Can); Tim-Ak (Can); Timoptic® Ophthalmic; Timoptic-XE® Ophthalmic

**Therapeutic Category** Beta-Adrenergic Blocker

**Use** Ophthalmic dosage form used to treat elevated intraocular pressure such as glaucoma or ocular hypertension; orally for treatment of hypertension and angina and for prevention of myocardial infarction and migraine headaches

**Usual Dosage**

Children and Adults: Ophthalmic: Initial: 0.25% solution, instill 1 drop twice daily; increase to 0.5% solution if response not adequate; decrease to 1 drop/day if controlled; do not exceed 1 drop twice daily of 0.5% solution

Adults: Oral:

Hypertension: Initial: 10 mg twice daily, increase gradually every 7 days, usual dosage: 20-40 mg/day in 2 divided doses; maximum: 60 mg/day

Prevention of myocardial infarction: 10 mg twice daily initiated within 1-4 weeks after infarction

Migraine headache: Initial: 10 mg twice daily, increase to maximum of 30 mg/day

**Dosage Forms**

Timolol hemihydrate:

Solution, ophthalmic (Betimol®): 0.25% (2.5 mL, 5 mL, 10 mL, 15 mL); 0.5% (2.5 mL, 5 mL, 10 mL, 15 mL)

Timolol maleate:

Gel, ophthalmic (Timoptic-XE®): 0.25% (2.5 mL, 5 mL); 0.5% (2.5 mL, 5 mL)

Solution, ophthalmic (Timoptic®): 0.25% (2.5 mL, 5 mL, 10 mL, 15 mL); 0.5% (2.5 mL, 5 mL, 10 mL, 15 mL)

Solution, ophthalmic, preservative free, single use (Timoptic® OcuDose®): 0.25%, 0.5%

Tablet (Blocadren®): 5 mg, 10 mg, 20 mg

**Timoptic® Ophthalmic** *see* timolol *on this page*

**Timoptic-XE® Ophthalmic** *see* timolol *on this page*

**Tinactin® [OTC]** *see* tolnaftate *on page 595*

**Tinamar® [OTC]** *see* tolnaftate *on page 595*

**TinBen® [OTC]** *see* benzoin *on page 74*

**TinCoBen® [OTC]** *see* benzoin *on page 74*

**Tindal® *(Discontinued)*** *see page 750*

**Tine Test PPD** *see* tuberculin tests *on page 612*

**Ting® [OTC]** *see* tolnaftate *on page 595*

**Tinver® *(Discontinued)*** *see page 750*

## tinzaparin (tin ZA pa rin)

**U.S./Canadian Brand Names** Innohep®

**Therapeutic Category** Anticoagulant

**Use** Treatment of acute symptomatic deep vein thrombosis, with or without pulmonary embolism, in conjunction with warfarin sodium

**Usual Dosage** S.C.:

Adults: 175 anti-Xa int. units/kg of body weight once daily. Warfarin sodium should be started when appropriate. Administer tinzaparin for at least 6 days and until patient is adequately anticoagulated with warfarin.

Note: To calculate the volume of solution to administer per dose: Volume to be administered (mL) = patient weight (kg) x 0.00875 mL/kg (may be rounded off to the nearest 0.05 mL)

**Dosage Forms** Injection: 20,000 anti-Xa int. units/mL (2 mL vial)

**tioconazole** (tye oh KONE a zole)

**U.S./Canadian Brand Names** GyneCure™ (Can); Monistat® 1 [OTC]; Trosyd™ AF (Can); Trosyd™ J (Can); Vagistat®-1 Vaginal [OTC]

**Therapeutic Category** Antifungal Agent

**Use** Local treatment of vulvovaginal candidiasis

**Usual Dosage** Vaginal: Insert 1 applicatorful in vagina, just prior to bedtime, as a single dose

**Dosage Forms** Cream, vaginal: 6.5% with applicator (4.6 g)

**tioguanine** *see* thioguanine *on page 585*

**tiopronin** (tye oh PROE nin)

**U.S./Canadian Brand Names** Thiola™

**Therapeutic Category** Urinary Tract Product

**Use** Prevention of kidney stone (cystine) formation in patients with severe homozygous cystinuric who have urinary cystine >500 mg/day who are resistant to treatment with high fluid intake, alkali, and diet modification, or who have had adverse reactions to penicillamine

**Usual Dosage** Adults: Initial: 800 mg/day; average dose: 1000 mg/day

**Dosage Forms** Tablet: 100 mg

**tiotixene** *see* thiothixene *on page 587*

**tirofiban** (tye roe FYE ban)

**U.S./Canadian Brand Names** Aggrastat®

**Therapeutic Category** Antiplatelet Agent

**Use** In combination with heparin, is indicated for the treatment of acute coronary syndrome, including patients who are to be managed medically and those undergoing PTCA or atherectomy. In this setting, it has been shown to decrease the rate of a combined endpoint of death, new myocardial infarction or refractory ischemia/repeat cardiac procedure.

**Usual Dosage** Adults: I.V.: Initial rate of 0.4 mcg/kg/minute for 30 minutes and then continued at 0.1 mcg/kg/minute

**Dosage Forms**

Injection for solution: 250 mcg/mL (50 mL)

Injection, premixed bags: 50 mcg/mL (250 mL)

**Ti-Screen® [OTC]** *see* methoxycinnamate and oxybenzone *on page 382*

**Tisit® Blue Gel [OTC]** *see* pyrethrins *on page 510*

**Tisit® Liquid [OTC]** *see* pyrethrins *on page 510*

**Tisit® Shampoo [OTC]** *see* pyrethrins *on page 510*

**Tisseel® VH Fibrin Sealant Kit** *see* fibrin sealant kit *on page 248*

**tissue plasminogen activator, recombinant** *see* alteplase *on page 24*

**Titralac® Plus Liquid [OTC]** *see* calcium carbonate and simethicone *on page 98*

**Ti-U-Lac® HC (Can)** *see* urea and hydrocortisone *on page 617*

**tizanidine** (tye ZAN i deen)

**U.S./Canadian Brand Names** Zanaflex®

**Therapeutic Category** $Alpha_2$-Adrenergic Agonist Agent

**Use** Intermittent management of increased muscle tone associated with spasticity (eg, multiple sclerosis, spinal cord injury)

**Usual Dosage** Adults: Oral: Initial: 4 mg every 6-8 hours, not to exceed 3 doses/day or 36 mg in a 24-hour period; doses may be increased at 2 mg or 4 mg increments with single doses not exceeding 12 mg

**Dosage Forms** Tablet, as hydrochloride: 2 mg, 4 mg

**TMP** *see* trimethoprim *on page 607*

**TMP-SMX** *see* sulfamethoxazole and trimethoprim *on page 564*

**TNKase™** *see* tenecteplase *on page 573*

**TOBI™ Inhalation Solution** *see* tobramycin *on this page*

**TobraDex® Ophthalmic** *see* tobramycin and dexamethasone *on this page*

## tobramycin (toe bra MYE sin)

**U.S./Canadian Brand Names** AKTob® Ophthalmic; Nebcin® Injection; PMS-Tobramycin (Can); TOBI™ Inhalation Solution; Tobrex® Ophthalmic; Tomycine®

**Therapeutic Category** Aminoglycoside (Antibiotic); Antibiotic, Ophthalmic

**Use** Treatment of documented or suspected infections caused by susceptible gram-negative bacilli including *Pseudomonas aeruginosa*; infection with a nonpseudomonal enteric bacillus which is more sensitive to tobramycin than gentamicin based on susceptibility tests; susceptible organisms in lower respiratory tract infections, septicemia; intra-abdominal, skin, bone, and urinary tract infections; empiric therapy in cystic fibrosis and immunocompromised patients; used topically to treat superficial ophthalmic infections caused by susceptible bacteria

**Usual Dosage** Dosage should be based on an estimate of ideal body weight

Infants and Children: I.M., I.V.: 2.5 mg/kg/dose every 8 hours

**Note:** Some patients may require larger or more frequent doses if serum levels document the need (ie, cystic fibrosis or febrile granulocytopenic patients)

Adults: I.M., I.V.: 3-5 mg/kg/day in 3 divided doses

Children and Adults:

Renal dysfunction: 2.5 mg/kg (2-3 serum level measurements should be obtained after the initial dose to measure the half-life in order to determine the frequency of subsequent doses)

Ophthalmic: 1-2 drops every 4 hours; apply ointment 2-3 times/day; for severe infections apply ointment every 3-4 hours, or 2 drops every 30-60 minutes initially, then reduce to less frequent intervals

**Dosage Forms**

Injection, as sulfate: 10 mg/mL (2 mL, 6 mL, 8 mL); 40 mg/mL (1 mL, 2 mL, 30 mL, 50 mL)

Ointment, ophthalmic: 0.3% (3.5 g)

Powder for injection: 40 mg/mL (1.2 g vials)

Solution, inhalation (TOBI™): 60 mg/mL (5 mL)

Solution, ophthalmic: 0.3% (5 mL)

AKTob®, Tobrex®: 0.3% (5 mL)

## tobramycin and dexamethasone (toe bra MYE sin & deks a METH a sone)

**U.S./Canadian Brand Names** TobraDex® Ophthalmic

**Therapeutic Category** Antibiotic/Corticosteroid, Ophthalmic

**Use** Treatment of external ocular infection caused by susceptible gram-negative bacteria and steroid responsive inflammatory conditions of the palpebral and bulbar conjunctiva, lid, cornea, and anterior segment of the globe

**Usual Dosage** Ophthalmic: Adults:

Ointment: Apply 1.25 cm (½") every 3-4 hours to 2-3 times/day

Suspension: Instill 1-2 drops every 4-6 hours (first 24-48 hours may increase frequency to every 2 hours until signs of clinical improvement are seen); apply every 30-60 minutes for severe infections

**Dosage Forms**

Ointment, ophthalmic: Tobramycin 0.3% and dexamethasone 0.1% (3.5 g)

Suspension, ophthalmic: Tobramycin 0.3% and dexamethasone 0.1% (2.5 mL, 5 mL)

**Tobrex® Ophthalmic** *see* tobramycin *on this page*

## tocainide (toe KAY nide)

**U.S./Canadian Brand Names** Tonocard®

**Therapeutic Category** Antiarrhythmic Agent, Class I-B

**Use** Suppress and prevent symptomatic ventricular arrhythmias

**Usual Dosage** Adults: Oral: 1200-1800 mg/day in 3 divided doses

**Dosage Forms** Tablet, as hydrochloride: 400 mg, 600 mg

## tocophersolan (toe kof er SOE lan)

**Synonyms** TPGS

**U.S./Canadian Brand Names** Liqui-E®

**Therapeutic Category** Vitamin, Fat Soluble

**Use** Treatment of vitamin E deficiency resulting from malabsorption due to prolonged cholestatic hepatobiliary disease

**Usual Dosage** Dietary supplement: Oral: 15 mg (400 units) every day

**Dosage Forms** Liquid: 26.6 units/mL

**Tofranil®** *see* imipramine *on page 314*

**Tofranil-PM®** *see* imipramine *on page 314*

## tolazamide (tole AZ a mide)

**U.S./Canadian Brand Names** Tolinase®

**Therapeutic Category** Antidiabetic Agent, Oral

**Use** Adjunct to diet for the management of mild to moderately severe, stable, noninsulin-dependent (type 2) diabetes mellitus

**Usual Dosage** Adults: Oral: 100-1000 mg/day

**Dosage Forms** Tablet: 100 mg, 250 mg, 500 mg

## tolazoline (tole AZ oh leen)

**Synonyms** benzazoline

**U.S./Canadian Brand Names** Priscoline®

**Therapeutic Category** Alpha-Adrenergic Blocking Agent

**Use** Persistent pulmonary hypertension of the newborn (PPHN), also known as persistent fetal circulation (PFC); peripheral vasospastic disorders

**Usual Dosage**

Neonates: Initial: I.V.: 1-2 mg/kg over 10-15 minutes via scalp vein or upper extremity; maintenance: 1-2 mg/kg/hour; use lower maintenance doses in patients with decreased renal function. Also used in neonates for acute vasospasm "cath toes" at 0.25 mg/kg/hour (no load)

Adults: Peripheral vasospastic disorder: I.M., I.V., S.C.: 10-50 mg 4 times/day

**Dosage Forms** Injection, as hydrochloride: 25 mg/mL (4 mL)

## tolbutamide (tole BYOO ta mide)

**U.S./Canadian Brand Names** Apo®-Tolbutamide (Can); Orinase® Diagnostic Injection; Tol-Tab®

**Therapeutic Category** Antidiabetic Agent, Oral

**Use** Adjunct to diet for the management of mild to moderately severe, stable, noninsulin-dependent (type 2) diabetes mellitus

**Usual Dosage** Adults:

Oral: 250-2000 mg/day

I.V. bolus: 20 mg/kg

**Dosage Forms**

Injection, diagnostic, as sodium: 1 g (20 mL)

Tablet: 500 mg

## tolcapone (TOLE ka pone)

**U.S./Canadian Brand Names** Tasmar®

**Therapeutic Category** Anti-Parkinson's Agent

**Use** Adjunct to levodopa and carbidopa for the treatment of signs and symptoms of idiopathic Parkinson's disease

**Usual Dosage** Adults: Oral: Initial: 100 mg 3 times/day, may increase to 200 mg 3 times/day

**Dosage Forms** Tablet: 100 mg, 200 mg

**Tolectin®** *see* tolmetin *on this page*

**Tolectin® DS** *see* tolmetin *on this page*

**Tolinase®** *see* tolazamide *on previous page*

## tolmetin (TOLE met in)

**U.S./Canadian Brand Names** Novo-Tolmetin (Can); Tolectin®; Tolectin® DS

**Therapeutic Category** Analgesic, Non-narcotic; Nonsteroidal Anti-inflammatory Drug (NSAID)

**Use** Treatment of inflammatory and rheumatoid disorders, including juvenile rheumatoid arthritis

**Usual Dosage** Oral:

Children ≥2 years: Anti-inflammatory: Initial: 20 mg/kg/day in 3 divided doses, then 15-30 mg/kg/day in 3 divided doses; maximum dose: 30 mg/kg/day

Adults: 400 mg 3 times/day; usual dose: 600 mg to 1.8 g/day; maximum: 2 g/day

**Dosage Forms**

Capsule, as sodium: 400 mg

Tablet, as sodium: 200 mg, 600 mg

## tolnaftate (tole NAF tate)

**U.S./Canadian Brand Names** Aftate® [OTC]; Blis-To-Sol® [OTC]; D-Care® [OTC]; Fungi-Gard® [OTC]; NP-27® [OTC]; Pitrex (Can); Podactin® [OTC]; Q-Naftate® [OTC]; Tinactin® [OTC]; Tinamar® [OTC]; Ting® [OTC]; Tolnaftin® [OTC]

**Therapeutic Category** Antifungal Agent

**Use** Treatment of tinea pedis, tinea cruris, tinea corporis, tinea manuum caused by *Trichophyton rubrum*, *T. mentagrophytes*, *T. tonsurans*, *M. canis*, *M. audouinii*, and *E. floccosum*; also effective in the treatment of tinea versicolor infections due to *Malassezia furfur*

**Usual Dosage** Children and Adults: Topical: Wash and dry affected area; apply 1-2 drops of solution or a small amount of cream or powder and rub into the affected areas twice daily for 2-4 weeks

**Dosage Forms**

Aerosol, topical:

- Liquid: 1% (59.2 mL, 90 mL, 120 mL)
- Powder: 1% (56.7 g, 100 g, 105 g, 150 g)

Cream: 1% (15 g, 30 g)

Gel, topical: 1% (15 g)

Powder, topical: 1% (45 g, 90 g)

Solution, topical: 1% (10 mL)

**Tolnaftin® [OTC]** *see* tolnaftate *on this page*

**Tol-Tab®** *see* tolbutamide *on previous page*

## tolterodine (tole TER oh dine)

**U.S./Canadian Brand Names** Detrol™; Detrol® LA

**Therapeutic Category** Anticholinergic Agent

**Use** Treatment of patients with an overactive bladder with symptoms of urinary frequency, urgency, or urge incontinence

(Continued)

## tolterodine *(Continued)*

**Usual Dosage**

Children: Safety and efficacy in pediatric patients have not been established

Adults: Treatment of overactive bladder: Oral:

Immediate release tablet: 2 mg twice daily; the dose may be lowered to 1 mg twice daily based on individual response and tolerability

Dosing adjustment in patients concurrently taking CYP3A4 inhibitors: 1 mg twice daily

Extended release capsule: 4 mg once a day; dose may be lowered to 2 mg daily based on individual response and tolerability

Dosing adjustment in patients concurrently taking CYP3A4 inhibitors: 2 mg daily

Elderly: Safety and efficacy in patients >64 years was found to be similar to that in younger patients; no dosage adjustment is needed based on age

**Dosage Forms** As tartrate:

Capsule, extended release: 2 mg, 4 mg

Tablet: 1 mg, 2 mg

**Tolu-Sed® DM [OTC]** *see* guaifenesin and dextromethorphan *on page 282*

**Tomocat®** *see* radiological/contrast media (ionic) *on page 516*

**Tomudex® (Can)** *see* raltitrexed *(Canada only) on page 518*

**Tomycine®** *see* tobramycin *on page 593*

**Tonocard®** *see* tocainide *on page 594*

**Tonopaque®** *see* radiological/contrast media (ionic) *on page 516*

**Topamax®** *see* topiramate *on this page*

**Topamax® Sprinkle** *see* topiramate *on this page*

**Topicort®** *see* desoximetasone *on page 173*

**Topicort®-LP** *see* desoximetasone *on page 173*

**Topicycline® Topical** *see* tetracycline *on page 579*

## topiramate (toe PYE ra mate)

**U.S./Canadian Brand Names** Topamax®; Topamax® Sprinkle

**Therapeutic Category** Anticonvulsant

**Use** Adjunctive therapy for partial onset seizures in adults

**Usual Dosage**

Adults: Initial: 25-50 mg/day; titrate in increments of 25-50 mg per week until an effective daily dose is reached; the daily dose may be increased by 25 mg at weekly intervals for the first 4 weeks; thereafter, the daily dose may be increased by 25-50 mg weekly to an effective daily dose (usually at least 400 mg); usual maximum dose: 1600 mg/day

**Note:** A more rapid titration schedule has been previously recommended (ie, 50 mg/week), and may be attempted in some clinical situations; however, this may reduce the patient's ability to tolerate topiramate.

Children 2-16 years: Partial seizures (adjunctive therapy): Initial dose titration should begin at 25 mg (or less, based on a range of 1-3 mg/kg/day) nightly for the first week. Dosage may be increased in increments of 1-3 mg/kg/day (administered in two divided doses) at 1- or 2-week intervals to a total daily dose of 5-9 mg/kg/day.

**Dosage Forms**

Capsule (Topamax® Sprinkles): 15 mg, 25 mg

Tablet: 25 mg, 100 mg, 200 mg

**Toposar® Injection** *see* etoposide *on page 236*

## topotecan (toe poe TEE kan)

**Synonyms** hycamptamine; SKF 104864

**U.S./Canadian Brand Names** Hycamtin™

**Therapeutic Category** Antineoplastic Agent

**Use** Metastatic carcinoma of the ovary after failure of initial or subsequent chemotherapy; experimentally in childhood solid tumors and leukemia resistant to standard therapies; treatment of small cell lung cancer sensitive disease after failure of first-line chemotherapy (sensitive disease is defined as disease responding to chemotherapy but subsequently progressing at least 60 days or at least 90 days after chemotherapy)

**Usual Dosage**

Children: A phase I study in pediatric patients by CCSG determined the recommended phase II dose to be 5.5 mg/m$^2$ as a 24-hour continuous infusion

Adults: Most phase II studies currently utilize topotecan at 1.5-2.0 mg/m$^2$/day for 5 days, repeated every 21-28 days. Alternative dosing regimens evaluated in phase I studies have included 21-day continuous infusion (recommended phase II dose: 0.53-0.7 mg/m$^2$/day) and weekly 24-hour infusions (recommended phase II dose: 1.5 mg/m$^2$/week).

Dose modifications: Dosage modification may be required for toxicity

**Dosage Forms** Powder for injection, as hydrochloride, lyophilized: 4 mg (base)

**Toprol XL®** *see* metoprolol *on page 388*

**Topsyn® (Can)** *see* fluocinonide *on page 254*

**TOPV** *see* poliovirus vaccine, live, trivalent, oral *on page 480*

**Toradol®** *see* ketorolac tromethamine *on page 334*

**Torecan® Injection** *see* thiethylperazine *on page 585*

**Torecan® Suppository *(Discontinued)*** *see page 750*

**Torecan® Tablet** *see* thiethylperazine *on page 585*

## toremifene (TORE em i feen)

**Synonyms** FC1157a

**U.S./Canadian Brand Names** Fareston®

**Therapeutic Category** Antineoplastic Agent

**Use** Treatment of advanced breast cancer; management of desmoid tumors and endometrial carcinoma

**Usual Dosage** Refer to individual protocols

Adults: Oral: 60 mg once daily, generally continued until disease progression is observed

**Dosage Forms** Tablet, as citrate: 60 mg

**Tornalate®** *see* bitolterol *on page 82*

## torsemide (TOR se mide)

**U.S./Canadian Brand Names** Demadex®

**Therapeutic Category** Diuretic, Loop

**Use** Management of edema associated with congestive heart failure and hepatic or renal disease; used alone or in combination with antihypertensives in treatment of hypertension

**Usual Dosage** Adults:

Oral: 5-10 mg once daily; if ineffective, may double dose until desired effect is achieved

I.V.: 10-20 mg/dose repeated in 2 hours as needed with a doubling of the dose with each succeeding dose until desired diuresis is achieved

Continues to be effective in patients with cirrhosis, no apparent change in dose is necessary

**Dosage Forms**

Injection: 10 mg/mL (2 mL, 5 mL)

Tablet: 5 mg, 10 mg, 20 mg, 100 mg

**Totacillin® *(Discontinued)*** *see page 750*

**Totacillin-N® *(Discontinued)*** *see page 750*

**Touro Ex®** *see* guaifenesin *on page 281*

**Touro LA®** *see* guaifenesin and pseudoephedrine *on page 283*

**t-PA** *see* alteplase *on page 24*

**T-Painol® [OTC]** *see* acetaminophen *on page 3*

**T-Painol® Extra Strength [OTC]** *see* acetaminophen *on page 3*

**TPGS** *see* tocophersolan *on page 594*

**T-Phyl®** *see* theophylline *on page 581*

**Trace-4®** *see* trace metals *on this page*

## trace metals (trase MET als)

**Synonyms** chromium injection; copper injection; manganese injection; molybdenum injection; neonatal trace metals; zinc injection

**U.S./Canadian Brand Names** Chroma-Pak®; Iodopen®; Molypen®; M.T.E.-4®; M.T.E.-5®; M.T.E.-6®; MulTE-PAK-4®; MulTE-PAK-5®; Neotrace-4®; PedTE-PAK-4®; Pedtrace-4®; P.T.E.-4®; P.T.E.-5®; Sele-Pak®; Selepen®; Trace-4®; Zinca-Pak®

**Therapeutic Category** Trace Element

**Use** Prevent and correct trace metal deficiencies

**Dosage Forms**

Chromium: Injection: 4 mcg/mL, 20 mcg/mL
Copper: Injection: 0.4 mg/mL, 2 mg/mL
Manganese: Injection: 0.1 mg/mL (as chloride or sulfate salt)
Molybdenum: Injection: 25 mcg/mL
Selenium: Injection: 40 mcg/mL
Zinc: Injection: 1 mg/mL (sulfate); 1 mg/mL (chloride); 5 mg/mL (sulfate)

**Tracrium®** *see* atracurium *on page 58*

**Tral®** ***(Discontinued)*** *see page 750*

## tramadol (TRA ma dole)

**U.S./Canadian Brand Names** Ultram®

**Therapeutic Category** Analgesic, Non-narcotic

**Use** Relief of moderate to moderately severe pain

**Usual Dosage** Adults: Oral: 50-100 mg every 4-6 hours, not to exceed 400 mg/day

**Dosage Forms** Tablet, as hydrochloride: 50 mg

**Trandate®** *see* labetalol *on page 336*

## trandolapril (tran DOE la pril)

**U.S./Canadian Brand Names** Mavik®

**Therapeutic Category** Angiotensin-Converting Enzyme (ACE) Inhibitor

**Use** Management of hypertension alone or in combination with other antihypertensive agents

**Unlabeled use:** As a class, ACE inhibitors are recommended in the treatment of systolic congestive heart failure

**Usual Dosage** Adults:

Non-Black patients: 0.5-1 mg for those not receiving diuretics; increase dose at 0.5-1 mg increments at 1- to 2-week intervals; maximum dose: 4 mg/day

Black patients: Initiate doses of 1-2 mg; maximum dose: 4 mg/day

**Dosage Forms** Tablet: 1 mg, 2 mg, 4 mg

## trandolapril and verapamil (tran DOE la pril & ver AP a mil)

**U.S./Canadian Brand Names** Tarka®

**Therapeutic Category** Antihypertensive Agent, Combination

**Use** Combination drug for the treatment of hypertension

**Usual Dosage** Dose is individualized

**Dosage Forms** Tablet, extended release:

Trandolapril (immediate release) 1 mg and verapamil hydrochloride (sustained release) 240 mg

Trandolapril (immediate release) 2 mg and verapamil hydrochloride (sustained release) 180 mg
Trandolapril (immediate release) 2 mg and verapamil hydrochloride (sustained release) 240 mg
Trandolapril (immediate release) 4 mg and verapamil hydrochloride (sustained release) 240 mg

## tranexamic acid (tran eks AM ik AS id)

**U.S./Canadian Brand Names** Cyklokapron®
**Therapeutic Category** Antihemophilic Agent
**Use** Short-term use (2-8 days) in hemophilia patients during and following tooth extraction to reduce or prevent hemorrhage
**Usual Dosage** Children and Adults: I.V.: 10 mg/kg immediately before surgery, then 25 mg/kg/dose orally 3-4 times/day for 2-8 days
Alternatively:
Oral: 25 mg/kg 3-4 times/day beginning 1 day prior to surgery
I.V.: 10 mg/kg 3-4 times/day in patients who are unable to take oral
**Dosage Forms**
Injection: 100 mg/mL (10 mL)
Tablet: 500 mg

**transamine** *see* tranylcypromine *on this page*

**Transdermal-NTG® Patch** *see* nitroglycerin *on page 422*

**Transderm-Nitro® Patch** *see* nitroglycerin *on page 422*

**Transderm Scop®** *see* scopolamine *on page 539*

**Transderm-V® (Can)** *see* scopolamine *on page 539*

**Trans-Plantar® Transdermal Patch [OTC]** *see* salicylic acid *on page 535*

**Trans-Ver-Sal® Transdermal Patch [OTC]** *see* salicylic acid *on page 535*

**Tranxene®** *see* clorazepate *on page 147*

## tranylcypromine (tran il SIP roe meen)

**Synonyms** transamine
**U.S./Canadian Brand Names** Parnate®
**Therapeutic Category** Antidepressant, Monoamine Oxidase Inhibitor
**Use** Symptomatic treatment of depressed patients refractory to or intolerant to tricyclic antidepressants or electroconvulsive therapy; has a more rapid onset of therapeutic effect than other MAO inhibitors, but causes more severe hypertensive reactions
**Usual Dosage** Adults: Oral: 10 mg twice daily, increase by 10 mg increments at 1- to 3-week intervals; maximum: 60 mg/day
**Dosage Forms** Tablet, as sulfate: 10 mg

**Trasicor® (Can)** *see* oxprenolol *(Canada only) on page 442*

## trastuzumab (tras TU zoo mab)

**U.S./Canadian Brand Names** Herceptin®
**Therapeutic Category** Antineoplastic Agent
**Use** Treatment of patients with metastatic breast cancer whose tumors overexpress the HER2 protein
**Usual Dosage** Adults: I.V.:
Loading dose: 4 mg/kg over 90 minutes; do not administer as an I.V. bolus or I.V. push
Maintenance dose: 2 mg/kg once weekly (may be infused over 30 minutes if prior infusions are well tolerated)
**Dosage Forms** Powder for injection: 440 mg

**Trasylol®** *see* aprotinin *on page 50*

**Travase®** ***(Discontinued)*** *see page 750*

## trazodone (TRAZ oh done)

**U.S./Canadian Brand Names** Alti-Trazodone (Can); Apo®-Trazodone (Can); Desyrel®; Gen-Trazodone (Can); Novo-Trazodone (Can); Nu-Trazodone (Can); PMS-Trazodone (Can); Trazorel (Can)

**Therapeutic Category** Antidepressant, Triazolopyridine

**Use** Treatment of depression

**Usual Dosage** Oral:

Adolescents: Initial: 25-50 mg/day; increase to 100-150 mg/day in divided doses

Adults: Initial: 150 mg/day in 3 divided doses (may increase by 50 mg/day every 3-7 days); maximum: 600 mg/day

**Dosage Forms** Tablet, as hydrochloride: 50 mg, 100 mg, 150 mg, 300 mg

**Trazorel (Can)** *see* trazodone *on this page*

**Trecator®-SC** *see* ethionamide *on page 234*

**Trelstar™ Depot** *see* triptorelin *on page 610*

**Tremytoine® (Can)** *see* phenytoin *on page 468*

**Trendar® [OTC]** *see* ibuprofen *on page 311*

**Trental®** *see* pentoxifylline *on page 460*

## tretinoin (oral) (TRET i noyn oral)

**Synonyms** all-*trans*-retinoic acid

**U.S./Canadian Brand Names** Vesanoid®

**Therapeutic Category** Antineoplastic Agent

**Use** Acute promyelocytic leukemia (APL): Induction of remission in patients with APL, French American British (FAB) classification M3 (including the M3 variant), characterized by the presence of the t(15;17) translocation or the presence of the PML/RARα gene who are refractory to or who have relapsed from anthracycline chemotherapy, or for whom anthracycline-based chemotherapy is contraindicated. Tretinoin is for the induction of remission only. All patients should receive an accepted form of remission consolidation or maintenance therapy for APL after completion of induction therapy with tretinoin.

**Usual Dosage** Oral:

Children: There are limited clinical data on the pediatric use of tretinoin. Of 15 pediatric patients (age range: 1-16 years) treated with tretinoin, the incidence of complete remission was 67%. Safety and efficacy in pediatric patients <1 year of age have not been established. Some pediatric patients experience severe headache and pseudotumor cerebri, requiring analgesic treatment and lumbar puncture for relief. Increased caution is recommended. Consider dose reduction in children experiencing serious or intolerable toxicity; however, the efficacy and safety of tretinoin at doses <45 mg/m$^2$/day have not been evaluated.

Adults: 45 mg/m$^2$/day administered as two evenly divided doses until complete remission is documented. Discontinue therapy 30 days after achievement of complete remission or after 90 days of treatment, whichever occurs first. If after initiation of treatment the presence of the t(15;17) translocation is not confirmed by cytogenetics or by polymerase chain reaction studies and the patient has not responded to tretinoin, consider alternative therapy.

**Note:** Tretinoin is for the induction of remission only. Optimal consolidation or maintenance regimens have not been determined. All patients should, therefore, receive a standard consolidation or maintenance chemotherapy regimen for APL after induction therapy with tretinoin unless otherwise contraindicated.

**Dosage Forms** Capsule: 10 mg

## tretinoin (topical) (TRET i noyn TOP i kal)

**Synonyms** retinoic acid; vitamin A acid

**U.S./Canadian Brand Names** Altinac™ Cream; Avita®; Rejuva-A® (Can); Renova® Cream; Retin-A® Micro Topical; Retin-A® Topical

**Therapeutic Category** Retinoic Acid Derivative

**Use** Treatment of acne vulgaris, photodamaged skin, and some skin cancers

**Usual Dosage** Children >12 years and Adults: Topical: Apply once daily before retiring; if stinging or irritation develop, decrease frequency of application

**Dosage Forms**

Cream

Altinac™: 0.025% (20 g, 45 g); 0.05% (20 g, 45 g); 0.1% (20 g, 45 g)

Avita®: 0.025% (20 g, 45 g)

Retin-A®: 0.025% (20 g, 45 g); 0.05% (20 g, 45 g); 0.1% (20 g, 45 g)

Cream, emollient (Renova®): 0.02% (40 g); 0.05% (20 g, 40 g, 60 g)

Gel, topical (Retin-A®): 0.01% (15 g, 45 g); 0.025% (15 g, 45 g)

Gel, topical (Retin-A® Micro): 0.1% (20 g, 45 g)

Liquid, topical (Retin-A®): 0.05% (28 mL)

## triacetin (trye a SEE tin)

**Synonyms** glycerol triacetate

**U.S./Canadian Brand Names** Myco-Nail® [OTC]

**Therapeutic Category** Antifungal Agent

**Use** Fungistat for athlete's foot and other superficial fungal infections

**Usual Dosage** Topical: Apply twice daily, cleanse areas with dilute alcohol or mild soap and water before application; continue treatment for 7 days after symptoms have disappeared

**Dosage Forms** Liquid: 25% (30 mL)

**Triacet™ Topical** *see* triamcinolone (topical) *on next page*

**triacetyloleandomycin** *see* troleandomycin *on page 610*

**Triacin® [OTC]** *see* triprolidine and pseudoephedrine *on page 609*

**Triacin-C®** *see* triprolidine, pseudoephedrine, and codeine *on page 609*

**triaconazole** *see* terconazole *on page 575*

**Triacting® Sore Throat Formula [OTC]** *see* acetaminophen, dextromethorphan, and pseudoephedrine *on page 7*

**Triad®** *see* butalbital compound and acetaminophen *on page 93*

**Triaderm (Can)** *see* triamcinolone (topical) *on next page*

**Triafed® [OTC]** *see* triprolidine and pseudoephedrine *on page 609*

**Triam-A® Injection** *see* triamcinolone (systemic) *on next page*

## triamcinolone (inhalation, nasal)

(trye am SIN oh lone in hil LA shun, NAY sal)

**U.S./Canadian Brand Names** Nasacort®; Nasacort® AQ

**Therapeutic Category** Corticosteroid, Topical

**Use** Symptoms of seasonal and perennial allergic rhinitis

**Usual Dosage** Children >12 years and Adults: Intranasal: 2 sprays in each nostril once daily; may increase after 4-7 days up to 4 sprays once daily or 1 spray 4 times/day in each nostril

**Dosage Forms**

Aerosol, nasal: 55 mcg per actuation (15 mL)

Spray, nasal: 55 mcg per actuation in aqueous base (16.5 g)

## triamcinolone (inhalation, oral) (trye am SIN oh lone in hil LA shun, OR al)

**U.S./Canadian Brand Names** Azmacort® Oral Inhaler

**Therapeutic Category** Adrenal Corticosteroid

**Use** Asthma

**Usual Dosage**

Children 6-12 years: Inhalation: 1-2 inhalations 3-4 times/day, not to exceed 12 inhalations/day

(Continued)

## triamcinolone (inhalation, oral) *(Continued)*

Children >12 years and Adults: Oral inhalation: 2 inhalations 3-4 times/day, not to exceed 16 inhalations/day

**Dosage Forms** Aerosol: Oral inhalation: 100 mcg/metered spray (2 oz)

## triamcinolone (systemic) (trye am SIN oh lone sis TEM ik)

**U.S./Canadian Brand Names** Amcort® Injection; Aristocort® Forte Injection; Aristocort® Intralesional Injection; Aristocort® Oral; Aristospan® Intra-articular Injection; Aristospan® Intralesional Injection; Atolone® Oral; Kenacort® Oral; Kenaject® Injection; Kenalog® Injection; Tac™-3 Injection; Tac™-40 Injection; Triam-A® Injection; Triam Forte® Injection; Triamonide® Injection; Tri-Kort® Injection; Trilog® Injection; Trilone® Injection; Trisoject® Injection

**Therapeutic Category** Adrenal Corticosteroid

**Use** Severe inflammation or immunosuppression

**Usual Dosage** In general, single I.M. dose of 4-7 times oral dose will control patient from 4-7 days up to 3-4 weeks

Children 6-12 years:
- I.M.: Acetonide or hexacetonide: 0.03-0.2 mg/kg at 1- to 7-day intervals

Children >12 years and Adults:
- Oral: 4-100 mg/day
- I.M.: Acetonide or hexacetonide: 60 mg (of 40 mg/mL), additional 20-100 mg doses (usual: 40-80 mg) may be administered when signs and symptoms recur, best at 6-week intervals to minimize HPA suppression
- Intra-articularly, intrasynovially, intralesionally: 2.5-40 mg as diacetate salt or acetonide salt, dose may be repeated when signs and symptoms recur
- Intra-articularly: Hexacetonide: 2-20 mg every 3-4 weeks as hexacetonide salt
- Intralesional (use 10 mg/mL): Diacetate or acetonide: 1 mg/injection site, may be repeated one or more times/week depending upon patients response; maximum; 30 mg at any one time; may use multiple injections if they are more than 1 cm apart
- Intra-articular, intrasynovial, and soft-tissue injection (use 10 mg/mL or 40 mg/mL): Diacetate or acetonide: 2.5-40 mg depending upon location, size of joints, and degree of inflammation; repeat when signs and symptoms recur
- Sublesionally (as acetonide): Up to 1 mg per injection site and may be repeated one or more times weekly; multiple sites may be injected if they are 1 cm or more apart, not to exceed 30 mg

**Dosage Forms**

Syrup: 2 mg/5 mL (120 mL); 4 mg/5 mL (120 mL)

Tablet: 1 mg, 2 mg, 4 mg, 8 mg

Triamcinolone acetonide:
- Injection: 10 mg/mL (5 mL); 40 mg/mL (1 mL, 5 mL, 10 mL)

Triamcinolone diacetate: Injection: 25 mg/mL (5 mL); 40 mg/mL (1 mL, 5 mL, 10 mL)

Triamcinolone hexacetonide: Injection: 5 mg/mL (5 mL); 20 mg/mL (1 mL, 5 mL)

## triamcinolone (topical) (trye am SIN oh lone TOP i kal)

**U.S./Canadian Brand Names** Aristocort® A Topical; Aristocort® Topical; Delta-Tritex® Topical; Flutex® Topical; Kenalog® in Orabase®; Kenalog® Topical; Kenonel® Topical; Triacet™ Topical; Triaderm (Can)

**Therapeutic Category** Corticosteroid, Topical

**Use** Severe inflammation or immunosuppression; nasal spray for symptoms of seasonal and perennial allergic rhinitis

**Usual Dosage** Children >12 years and Adults: Topical: Apply a thin film 2-3 times/day. Therapy should be discontinued when control is achieved. If no improvement is seen, reassessment of diagnosis may be necessary.

**Dosage Forms**

Aerosol, topical: 0.2 mg/2 second spray (23 g, 63 g)

Cream: 0.025% (15 g, 60 g, 80 g, 240 g, 454 g); 0.1% (15 g, 30 g, 60 g, 80 g, 90 g, 120 g, 240 g); 0.5% (15 g, 20 g, 30 g, 240 g)
Lotion: 0.025% (60 mL); 0.1% (15 mL, 60 mL)
Ointment, oral: 0.1% (5 g)
Ointment, topical: 0.025% (15 g, 30 g, 60 g, 80 g, 120 g, 454 g); 0.1% (15 g, 30 g, 60 g, 80 g, 120 g, 240 g, 454 g); 0.5% (15 g, 20 g, 30 g, 240 g)

**Triam Forte® Injection** *see* triamcinolone (systemic) *on previous page*

**Triaminic® Allergy Tablet *(Discontinued)*** *see page 750*

**Triaminic® AM Decongestant Formula [OTC]** *see* pseudoephedrine *on page 507*

**Triaminic® Cold Tablet *(Discontinued)*** *see page 750*

**Triaminic® Expectorant *(Discontinued)*** *see page 750*

**Triaminicol® Multi-Symptom Cold Syrup *(Discontinued)*** *see page 750*

**Triaminic® Oral Infant Drops *(Discontinued)*** *see page 750*

**Triaminic® Syrup *(Discontinued)*** *see page 750*

**Triamonide® Injection** *see* triamcinolone (systemic) *on previous page*

## triamterene (trye AM ter een)

**U.S./Canadian Brand Names** Dyrenium®

**Therapeutic Category** Diuretic, Potassium Sparing

**Use** Alone or in combination with other diuretics to treat edema and hypertension; decreases potassium excretion caused by kaliuretic diuretics

**Usual Dosage** Oral:
Children: 2-4 mg/kg/day in 1-2 divided doses; maximum: 300 mg/day
Adults: 100-300 mg/day in 1-2 divided doses; maximum: 300 mg/day

**Dosage Forms** Capsule: 50 mg, 100 mg

**triamterene and hydrochlorothiazide** *see* hydrochlorothiazide and triamterene *on page 299*

**Triapin®** *see* butalbital compound and acetaminophen *on page 93*

**Triatec-8® (Can)** *see* acetaminophen and codeine *on page 4*

**Triatec-8® Strong (Can)** *see* acetaminophen and codeine *on page 4*

**Triatec-30® (Can)** *see* acetaminophen and codeine *on page 4*

**Triavil®** *see* amitriptyline and perphenazine *on page 33*

**Triavil® 4-50 *(Discontinued)*** *see page 750*

**Triaz®** *see* benzoyl peroxide *on page 74*

## triazolam (trye AY zoe lam)

**U.S./Canadian Brand Names** Apo®-Triazo (Can); Gen-Triazolam (Can); Halcion®

**Therapeutic Category** Benzodiazepine

**Controlled Substance** C-IV

**Use** Short-term treatment of insomnia

**Usual Dosage** Oral (onset of action is rapid, patient should be in bed when taking medication):
Children <18 years: Dosage not established
Adults: 0.125-0.25 mg at bedtime

**Dosage Forms** Tablet: 0.125 mg, 0.25 mg

**tribavirin** *see* ribavirin *on page 525*

**Tri-Chlor®** *see* trichloroacetic acid *on next page*

**trichlormethiazide** (trye klor meth EYE a zide)
**U.S./Canadian Brand Names** Aquacot®; Naqua®
**Therapeutic Category** Diuretic, Thiazide
**Use** Management of mild to moderate hypertension; treatment of edema in congestive heart failure and nephrotic syndrome
**Usual Dosage** Oral:
Children >6 months: 0.07 mg/kg/24 hours or 2 mg/m$^2$/24 hours
Adults: 1-4 mg/day
**Dosage Forms** Tablet: 2 mg, 4 mg

**trichloroacetaldehyde monohydrate** *see* chloral hydrate *on page 124*

**trichloroacetic acid** (trye klor oh a SEE tik AS id)
**U.S./Canadian Brand Names** Tri-Chlor®
**Therapeutic Category** Keratolytic Agent
**Use** Debride callous tissue
**Usual Dosage** Apply to verruca, cover with bandage for 5-6 days, remove verruca, reapply as needed
**Dosage Forms** Liquid: 80% (15 mL)

***Trichophyton* skin test** (trye koe FYE ton skin test)
**U.S./Canadian Brand Names** Dermatophytin®
**Therapeutic Category** Diagnostic Agent
**Use** Assess cell-mediated immunity
**Usual Dosage** 0.1 mL intradermally, examine reaction site in 24-48 hours; induration of ≥5 mm in diameter is a positive reaction
**Dosage Forms** Injection:
Diluted: 1:30 V/V (5 mL)
Undiluted: 5 mL

**Tri-Clear® Expectorant *(Discontinued)*** *see page 750*

**TriCor®** *see* fenofibrate *on page 243*

**Tricosal®** *see* choline magnesium trisalicylate *on page 135*

**Tridesilon® Topical** *see* desonide *on page 173*

**Tridil® Injection** *see* nitroglycerin *on page 422*

**Tridione® *(Discontinued)*** *see page 750*

**Tridione® Suppository *(Discontinued)*** *see page 750*

**trientine** (TRYE en teen)
**U.S./Canadian Brand Names** Syprine®
**Therapeutic Category** Chelating Agent
**Use** Treatment of Wilson's disease in patients intolerant to penicillamine
**Usual Dosage** Oral (administer on an empty stomach):
Children <12 years: 500-750 mg/day in divided doses 2-4 times/day; maximum: 1.5 g/day
Adults: 750-1250 mg/day in divided doses 2-4 times/day; maximum daily dose: 2 g
**Dosage Forms** Capsule, as hydrochloride: 250 mg

**triethanolamine polypeptide oleate-condensate**
(trye eth a NOLE a meen pol i PEP tide OH lee ate-KON den sate)
**U.S./Canadian Brand Names** Cerumenex® Otic
**Therapeutic Category** Otic Agent, Cerumenolytic
**Use** Removal of ear wax (cerumen)
**Usual Dosage** Children and Adults: Otic: Fill ear canal, insert cotton plug; allow to remain 15-30 minutes; flush ear with lukewarm water

**Dosage Forms** Solution, otic: 10% (6 mL, 12 mL)

## triethanolamine salicylate (trye eth a NOLE a meen sa LIS i late)

**U.S./Canadian Brand Names** Antiphlogistine Rub A-535 No Odour (Can); Myoflex® [OTC]; Sportscreme® [OTC]

**Therapeutic Category** Analgesic, Topical

**Use** Relief of pain of muscular aches, rheumatism, neuralgia, sprains, arthritis on intact skin

**Usual Dosage** Topical: Apply to area as needed

**Dosage Forms** Cream: 10% in a nongreasy base

**triethylenethiophosphoramide** *see* thiotepa *on page 587*

**Tri-Fed® [OTC]** *see* triprolidine and pseudoephedrine *on page 609*

**Trifed-C® *(Discontinued)*** *see page 750*

## trifluoperazine (trye floo oh PER a zeen)

**U.S./Canadian Brand Names** Apo®-Trifluoperazine (Can); Stelazine®

**Therapeutic Category** Phenothiazine Derivative

**Use** Treatment of psychoses and management of anxiety

**Usual Dosage**

Children 6-12 years: Psychoses:

Oral: Hospitalized or well supervised patients: Initial dose: 1 mg 1-2 times/day, gradually increase until symptoms are controlled or adverse effects become troublesome; maximum: 15 mg/day

I.M.: 1 mg twice daily

Adults:

Psychoses:

Outpatients: Oral: 1-2 mg twice daily

Hospitalized or well supervised patients: Initial dose: 2-5 mg twice daily with optimum response in the 15-20 mg/day range; do not exceed 40 mg/day

I.M.: 1-2 mg every 4-6 hours as needed up to 10 mg/24 hours maximum

Nonpsychotic anxiety: Oral: 1-2 mg twice daily; maximum: 6 mg/day; therapy for anxiety should not exceed 12 weeks; do not exceed 6 mg/day for longer than 12 weeks when treating anxiety; agitation, jitteriness or insomnia may be confused with original neurotic or psychotic symptoms

**Dosage Forms**

Concentrate, oral, as hydrochloride: 10 mg/mL (60 mL)

Injection, as hydrochloride: 2 mg/mL (10 mL)

Tablet, as hydrochloride: 1 mg, 2 mg, 5 mg, 10 mg

**trifluorothymidine** *see* trifluridine *on this page*

## triflupromazine (trye floo PROE ma zeen)

**U.S./Canadian Brand Names** Vesprin®

**Therapeutic Category** Phenothiazine Derivative

**Use** Treatment of psychoses, nausea, vomiting, and intractable hiccups

**Usual Dosage**

Children: I.M.: 0.2-0.25 mg/kg

Adults:

I.M.: 5-15 mg every 4 hours

I.V.: 1 mg

**Dosage Forms** Injection, as hydrochloride: 10 mg/mL (10 mL); 20 mg/mL (1 mL)

## trifluridine (trye FLURE i deen)

**Synonyms** $f_3t$; trifluorothymidine

**U.S./Canadian Brand Names** Viroptic® Ophthalmic

**Therapeutic Category** Antiviral Agent

(Continued)

**trifluridine** *(Continued)*

**Use** Treatment of primary keratoconjunctivitis and recurrent epithelial keratitis caused by herpes simplex virus types I and II

**Usual Dosage** Adults: Ophthalmic: Instill 1 drop into affected eye every 2 hours while awake, to a maximum of 9 drops/day, until re-epithelialization of corneal ulcer occurs; then use 1 drop every 4 hours for another 7 days; do **not** exceed 21 days of treatment

**Dosage Forms** Solution, ophthalmic: 1% (7.5 mL)

**triglycerides, medium chain** *see* medium chain triglycerides *on page 368*

## trihexyphenidyl (trye heks ee FEN i dil)

**Synonyms** benzhexol

**U.S./Canadian Brand Names** Apo®-Trihex (Can); Artane®

**Therapeutic Category** Anticholinergic Agent; Anti-Parkinson's Agent

**Use** Adjunctive treatment of Parkinson's disease; also used in treatment of drug-induced extrapyramidal effects and acute dystonic reactions

**Usual Dosage** Oral:

Parkinsonism: Initial: Administer 1-2 mg the first day; increase by 2 mg increments at intervals of 3-5 days, until a total of 6-10 mg is administered daily. Many patients derive maximum benefit from a total daily dose of 6-10 mg; however, postencephalitic patients may require a total daily dose of 12-15 mg in 3-4 divided doses

Concomitant use with levodopa: 3-6 mg/day in divided doses is usually adequate

Drug-induced extrapyramidal disorders: Start with a single 1 mg dose; daily dosage usually ranges between 5-15 mg in 3-4 divided doses

**Dosage Forms**

Elixir, as hydrochloride: 2 mg/5 mL (480 mL)

Tablet, as hydrochloride: 2 mg, 5 mg

**TriHIBit®** *see* diphtheria, tetanus toxoids, and acellular pertussis vaccine and *Haemophilus* b conjugate vaccine *on page 193*

**Tri-Immunol®** *see* diphtheria, tetanus toxoids, and whole-cell pertussis vaccine *on page 193*

**Tri-K®** *see* potassium acetate, potassium bicarbonate, and potassium citrate *on page 484*

**TRIKOF-D®** ***(Discontinued)*** *see page 750*

**Tri-Kort® Injection** *see* triamcinolone (systemic) *on page 602*

**Trilafon®** *see* perphenazine *on page 462*

**Trileptal®** *see* oxcarbazepine *on page 441*

**Tri-Levlen®** *see* ethinyl estradiol and levonorgestrel *on page 232*

**Trilisate®** *see* choline magnesium trisalicylate *on page 135*

**Trilog® Injection** *see* triamcinolone (systemic) *on page 602*

**Trilone® Injection** *see* triamcinolone (systemic) *on page 602*

**Trimazide®** ***(Discontinued)*** *see page 750*

## trimebutine *(Canada only)* (trye me BYOO teen)

**U.S./Canadian Brand Names** Modulon® (Can)

**Therapeutic Category** Antispasmodic Agent, Gastrointestinal

**Use** For the treatment and relief of symptoms associated with the irritable bowel syndrome (spastic colon). In postoperative paralytic ileus in order to accelerate the resumption of the intestinal transit following abdominal surgery.

**Usual Dosage** Adults:

Parenteral: Dosage should be individually tailored according to response, but the total parenteral daily dose should not exceed 300 mg. The usual adult dose is 50-100 mg 3 times daily, administered as an I.M. injection, as a 3-minute I.V. injection, or as a 60-minute I.V. infusion (in $D_5W$ or NS), until resumption of intestinal motility.

Tablets: Up to 600 mg daily in divided doses. It may be administered as two 100 mg tablets 3 times daily before meals or one 200 mg tablet 3 times daily before meals.

**Dosage Forms**

Injection, as maleate: 10 mg/mL (5 mL)

Tablet, as maleate: 100 mg, 200 mg

## trimeprazine *(Canada only)* (trye MEP re zeen)

**U.S./Canadian Brand Names** Panectyl® (Can)

**Therapeutic Category** Antihistamine

**Use** Perennial and seasonal allergic rhinitis and other allergic symptoms including urticaria

**Usual Dosage** Oral:

Children:

6 months to 3 years: 1.25 mg at bedtime or 3 times/day if needed

>3 years: 2.5 mg at bedtime or 3 times/day if needed

>6 years: 5 mg/day

Adults: 2.5 mg 4 times/day

**Dosage Forms** Tablet, as tartrate: 2.5 mg, 5 mg

## trimethobenzamide (trye meth oh BEN za mide)

**U.S./Canadian Brand Names** Benzacot®; Tigan®

**Therapeutic Category** Anticholinergic Agent; Antiemetic

**Use** Control of nausea and vomiting (especially for long-term antiemetic therapy)

**Usual Dosage** Rectal use: Contraindicated in neonates and premature infants

Children:

Oral, rectal: 15-20 mg/kg/day or 400-500 mg/m$^2$/day divided into 3-4 doses

I.M.: Not recommended

Adults:

Oral: 250 mg 3-4 times/day

I.M., rectal: 200 mg 3-4 times/day

**Dosage Forms**

Capsule, as hydrochloride: 100 mg, 250 mg

Injection, as hydrochloride: 100 mg/mL (2 mL, 20 mL)

Suppository, rectal, as hydrochloride: 100 mg, 200 mg

## trimethoprim (trye METH oh prim)

**Synonyms** TMP

**U.S./Canadian Brand Names** Primsol®; Proloprim®; Trimpex®

**Therapeutic Category** Antibiotic, Miscellaneous

**Use** Treatment and prophylaxis of urinary tract infections; in combination with other agents for treatment of *Pneumocystis carinii* pneumonia; otitis media in children

**Usual Dosage** Adults: Oral: 100 mg every 12 hours or 200 mg every 24 hours

**Dosage Forms**

Solution, oral, as base: 50 mg/5 mL

Tablet: 100 mg, 200 mg

## trimethoprim and polymyxin B (trye METH oh prim & pol i MIKS in bee)

**U.S./Canadian Brand Names** Polytrim® Ophthalmic

**Therapeutic Category** Antibiotic, Ophthalmic

**Use** Treatment of surface ocular bacterial conjunctivitis and blepharoconjunctivitis

**Usual Dosage** Ophthalmic: Instill 1-2 drops in eye(s) every 4-6 hours

**Dosage Forms** Solution, ophthalmic: Trimethoprim sulfate 1 mg and polymyxin B sulfate 10,000 units per mL (10 mL)

**trimethylpsoralen** *see* trioxsalen *on next page*

**trimetrexate glucuronate** (tri me TREKS ate gloo KYOOR oh nate)

**U.S./Canadian Brand Names** Neutrexin®

**Therapeutic Category** Antibiotic, Miscellaneous

**Use** Alternative therapy for the treatment of moderate-to-severe *Pneumocystis carinii* pneumonia (PCP) in immunocompromised patients, including patients with acquired immunodeficiency syndrome (AIDS), who are intolerant of, or are refractory to, co-trimoxazole therapy or for whom co-trimoxazole is contraindicated

**Usual Dosage** Adults: I.V.: 45 mg/m$^2$ once daily over 60 minutes for 21 days; it is necessary to reduce the dose in patients with liver dysfunction, although no specific recommendations exist

**Dosage Forms** Powder for injection: 25 mg, 200 mg

**trimipramine** (trye MI pra meen)

**U.S./Canadian Brand Names** Apo®-Trimip (Can); Novo-Tripramine (Can); Nu-Trimipramine (Can); Rhotrimine® (Can); Surmontil®

**Therapeutic Category** Antidepressant, Tricyclic (Tertiary Amine)

**Use** Treatment of various forms of depression, often in conjunction with psychotherapy

**Usual Dosage** Oral: 50-150 mg/day as a single bedtime dose

**Dosage Forms** Capsule, as maleate: 25 mg, 50 mg, 100 mg

**Trimox®** *see* amoxicillin *on page 35*

**Trimox® 500 mg *(Discontinued)*** *see page 750*

**Trimpex®** *see* trimethoprim *on previous page*

**Trinalin® Repetabs®** *see* azatadine and pseudoephedrine *on page 61*

**Tri-Nefrin® Extra Strength Tablet *(Discontinued)*** *see page 750*

**Tri-Norinyl®** *see* ethinyl estradiol and norethindrone *on page 232*

**Triofed® Syrup *(Discontinued)*** *see page 750*

**Triostat™ Injection** *see* liothyronine *on page 351*

**Triotann® Tablet** *see* chlorpheniramine, pyrilamine, and phenylephrine *on page 132*

**trioxsalen** (trye OKS a len)

**Synonyms** trimethylpsoralen

**U.S./Canadian Brand Names** Trisoralen®

**Therapeutic Category** Psoralen

**Use** In conjunction with controlled exposure to ultraviolet light or sunlight for repigmentation of idiopathic vitiligo; increasing tolerance to sunlight with albinism; enhance pigmentation

**Usual Dosage** Children >12 years and Adults: Oral: 10 mg/day as a single dose, 2-4 hours before controlled exposure to UVA or sunlight

**Dosage Forms** Tablet: 5 mg

**Tripedia®** *see* diphtheria, tetanus toxoids, and acellular pertussis vaccine *on page 193*

**tripelennamine** (tri pel EN a meen)

**Therapeutic Category** Antihistamine

**Use** Perennial and seasonal allergic rhinitis and other allergic symptoms including urticaria

**Usual Dosage** Oral:

Infants and Children: 5 mg/kg/day in 4-6 divided doses, up to 300 mg/day maximum

Adults: 25-50 mg every 4-6 hours, extended release tablets 100 mg morning and evening up to 100 mg every 8 hours

**Dosage Forms** Tablet, as hydrochloride: 50 mg

**Triphasil®** *see* ethinyl estradiol and levonorgestrel *on page 232*

**Triphed® [OTC]** *see* triprolidine and pseudoephedrine *on this page*

**Tri-Phen-Chlor® *(Discontinued)*** *see page 750*

**Triphenyl® Expectorant *(Discontinued)*** *see page 750*

**Triphenyl® Syrup *(Discontinued)*** *see page 750*

**Triple Antibiotic® Topical** *see* bacitracin, neomycin, and polymyxin B *on page 65*

**triple sulfa** *see* sulfabenzamide, sulfacetamide, and sulfathiazole *on page 562*

**Triple X® Liquid [OTC]** *see* pyrethrins *on page 510*

**Tri-P® Oral Infant Drops *(Discontinued)*** *see page 750*

**Triposed® Syrup [OTC]** *see* triprolidine and pseudoephedrine *on this page*

**Triposed® Tablet [OTC]** *see* triprolidine and pseudoephedrine *on this page*

## triprolidine and pseudoephedrine

(trye PROE li deen & soo doe e FED rin)

**U.S./Canadian Brand Names** Act-A-Med® [OTC]; Actanol® [OTC]; Actedril® [OTC]; Actifed® Tablet [OTC]; Allerfed® [OTC]; Allerfrim® [OTC]; Allerphed® Syrup [OTC]; Altafed® [OTC]; Aphedrid™ [OTC]; Aprodine® Syrup [OTC]; Aprodine® Tablet [OTC]; Biofed-PE® [OTC]; Cenafed® Plus Tablet [OTC]; Genac® Tablet [OTC]; Histafed® [OTC]; Hista-Tabs® [OTC]; Pseudocot-T® [OTC]; Ridifed® [OTC]; Ritifed® [OTC]; Silafed® [OTC]; Silafed® Syrup [OTC]; Triacin® [OTC]; Triafed® [OTC]; Tri-Fed® [OTC]; Triphed® [OTC]; Triposed® Syrup [OTC]; Triposed® Tablet [OTC]; Tri-Pseudafed® [OTC]; Tri-Pseudo® [OTC]; Tri-Sofed® [OTC]; Trisudex® [OTC]; Tri-Sudo® [OTC]; Uni-Fed® [OTC]; Vi-Sudo® [OTC]

**Therapeutic Category** Antihistamine/Decongestant Combination

**Use** Temporary relief of nasal congestion, running nose, sneezing, itching of nose or throat and itchy, watery eyes due to common cold, hay fever or other upper respiratory allergies

**Usual Dosage** May dose according to **pseudoephedrine** component (4 mg/kg/day in divided doses 3-4 times/day) Oral:

Children:
- 4 months to 2 years: 1.25 mL 3-4 times/day
- 2-4 years: 2.5 mL 3-4 times/day
- 4-6 years: 3.75 mL 3-4 times/day
- 6-12 years: 5 mL or 1/2 tablet 3-4 times/day, not to exceed 2 tablets/day

Children >12 years and Adults: 10 mL or 1 tablet 3-4 times/day, not to exceed 4 tablets/day

**Dosage Forms**

Capsule: Triprolidine hydrochloride 2.5 mg and pseudoephedrine hydrochloride 60 mg
- Extended release: Triprolidine hydrochloride 5 mg and pseudoephedrine hydrochloride 120 mg

Syrup: Triprolidine hydrochloride 1.25 mg and pseudoephedrine hydrochloride 30 mg per 5 mL

Tablet: Triprolidine hydrochloride 2.5 mg and pseudoephedrine hydrochloride 60 mg

## triprolidine, pseudoephedrine, and codeine

(trye PROE li deen, soo doe e FED rin, & KOE deen)

**U.S./Canadian Brand Names** Aprodine® w/C; CoActifed® (Can); Cotridin® (Can); Triacin-C®

**Therapeutic Category** Antihistamine/Decongestant/Antitussive

**Controlled Substance** C-V

**Use** Symptomatic relief of cough

**Usual Dosage** Oral:

Children:
- 2-6 years: 2.5 mL 4 times/day

(Continued)

## triprolidine, pseudoephedrine, and codeine *(Continued)*

7-12 years: 5 mL 4 times/day

Children >12 years and Adults: 10 mL 4 times/day

**Dosage Forms** Syrup: Triprolidine hydrochloride 1.25 mg, pseudoephedrine hydrochloride 30 mg, and codeine phosphate 10 mg per 5 mL with alcohol 4.3%

**Tri-Pseudafed® [OTC]** *see* triprolidine and pseudoephedrine *on previous page*

**Tri-Pseudo® [OTC]** *see* triprolidine and pseudoephedrine *on previous page*

**Triptil® (Can)** *see* protriptyline *on page 507*

**TripTone® Caplets® [OTC]** *see* dimenhydrinate *on page 188*

## triptorelin (trip toe REL in)

**U.S./Canadian Brand Names** Trelstar™ Depot

**Therapeutic Category** Luteinizing Hormone-Releasing Hormone Analog

**Use** Palliative treatment of advanced prostate cancer as an alternative to orchiectomy or estrogen administration

**Usual Dosage** I.M.: Adults: 3.75 mg once monthly

**Dosage Forms** Powder for injection, depot, as pamoate: 3.75 mg

**Triquilar® (Can)** *see* ethinyl estradiol and levonorgestrel *on page 232*

**tris buffer** *see* tromethamine *on next page*

**Trisenox™** *see* arsenic trioxide *on page 53*

**tris(hydroxymethyl)aminomethane** *see* tromethamine *on next page*

**Tri-Sofed® [OTC]** *see* triprolidine and pseudoephedrine *on previous page*

**Trisoject® Injection** *see* triamcinolone (systemic) *on page 602*

**Trisoralen®** *see* trioxsalen *on page 608*

**Tri-Statin® II Topical *(Discontinued)*** *see page 750*

**Trisudex® [OTC]** *see* triprolidine and pseudoephedrine *on previous page*

**Tri-Sudo® [OTC]** *see* triprolidine and pseudoephedrine *on previous page*

**Tri-Tannate Plus®** *see* chlorpheniramine, ephedrine, phenylephrine, and carbetapentane *on page 130*

**Tri-Tannate® Tablet** *see* chlorpheniramine, pyrilamine, and phenylephrine *on page 132*

**Tritec®** *see* ranitidine bismuth citrate *on page 518*

**Trivagizole 3™ [OTC]** *see* clotrimazole *on page 147*

**Tri-Vi-Flor®** *see* vitamin (multiple/pediatric) *on page 632*

**Tri-Vi-Sol® [OTC]** *see* vitamin (multiple/pediatric) *on page 632*

**Trixaicin®** *see* capsaicin *on page 104*

**Trixaicin HP®** *see* capsaicin *on page 104*

**Trizivir™** *see* abacavir, lamivudine, and zidovudine *on page 2*

**Trobicin®** *see* spectinomycin *on page 556*

**Trocaine® [OTC]** *see* benzocaine *on page 72*

**Trocal® [OTC]** *see* dextromethorphan *on page 178*

**Trofan® *(Discontinued)*** *see page 750*

**Trofan DS® *(Discontinued)*** *see page 750*

## troleandomycin (troe lee an doe MYE sin)

**Synonyms** triacetyloleandomycin

**U.S./Canadian Brand Names** Tao®

**Therapeutic Category** Macrolide (Antibiotic)

**Use** Adjunct in the treatment of severe corticosteroid-dependent asthma due to its steroid-sparing properties; obsolete antibiotic with spectrum of activity similar to erythromycin

**Usual Dosage** Oral:

Children: 25-40 mg/kg/day divided every 6 hours

Adjunct in corticosteroid-dependent asthma: 14 mg/kg/day in divided doses every 6-12 hours not to exceed 250 mg every 6 hours; dose is tapered to once daily then alternate day dosing

Adults: 250-500 mg 4 times/day

**Dosage Forms** Capsule: 250 mg

**Trombovar® (Can)** *see* sodium tetradecyl *on page 553*

## tromethamine (troe METH a meen)

**Synonyms** tris buffer; tris(hydroxymethyl)aminomethane

**U.S./Canadian Brand Names** THAM®

**Therapeutic Category** Alkalinizing Agent

**Use** Correction of metabolic acidosis associated with cardiac bypass surgery or cardiac arrest; to correct excess acidity of stored blood that is preserved with acid citrate dextrose (ACD); to prime the pump-oxygenator during cardiac bypass surgery; indicated in severe metabolic acidosis in patients in whom sodium or carbon dioxide elimination is restricted [eg, infants needing alkalinization after receiving maximum sodium bicarbonate (8-10 mEq/kg/24 hours)]

**Usual Dosage** Dose depends on buffer base deficit; when deficit is known: tromethamine mL of 0.3 M solution = body weight (kg) x base deficit (mEq/L); when base deficit is not known: 3-6 mL/kg/dose I.V. (1-2 mEq/kg/dose)

Metabolic acidosis with cardiac arrest:

I.V.: 3.5-6 mL/kg (1-2 mEq/kg/dose) into large peripheral vein; 500-1000 mL if needed in adults

I.V. continuous drip: Infuse slowly by syringe pump over 3-6 hours

Excess acidity of ACD priming blood: 14-70 mL of 0.3 molar solution added to each 500 mL of blood

**Dosage Forms** Injection: 18 g [0.3 molar = 36 mL/mL] (500 mL)

**Tronolane® [OTC]** *see* pramoxine *on page 490*

**Tropicacyl®** *see* tropicamide *on this page*

## tropicamide (troe PIK a mide)

**Synonyms** bistropamide

**U.S./Canadian Brand Names** Diotrope® (Can); Mydral®; Mydriacyl®; Ocu-Tropic®; Tropicacyl®

**Therapeutic Category** Anticholinergic Agent

**Use** Short-acting mydriatic used in diagnostic procedures; as well as preoperatively and postoperatively; treatment of some cases of acute iritis, iridocyclitis, and keratitis

**Usual Dosage** Children and Adults: Ophthalmic:

Cycloplegia: 1-2 drops (1%); may repeat in 5 minutes

Mydriasis: 1-2 drops (0.5%) 15-20 minutes before exam; may repeat every 30 minutes as needed

**Dosage Forms** Solution, ophthalmic: 0.5% (2 mL, 15 mL); 1% (2 mL, 3 mL, 15 mL)

**Trosyd™ AF (Can)** *see* tioconazole *on page 592*

**Trosyd™ J (Can)** *see* tioconazole *on page 592*

## trovafloxacin (TROE va flox a sin)

**Synonyms** alatrofloxacin; CP-99,219-27

**U.S./Canadian Brand Names** Trovan®

**Therapeutic Category** Antibiotic, Quinolone

(Continued)

## trovafloxacin *(Continued)*

**Use Should be used only in life- or limb-threatening infections**

Treatment of nosocomial pneumonia, community-acquired pneumonia, complicated intra-abdominal infections, gynecologic/pelvic infections, complicated skin and skin structure infections

**Usual Dosage** Adults:

Nosocomial pneumonia: I.V.: 300 mg single dose followed by 200 mg/day orally for a total duration of 10-14 days

Community-acquired pneumonia: Oral, I.V.: 200 mg/day for 7-14 days

Complicated intra-abdominal infections, including postsurgical infections/gynecologic and pelvic infections: I.V.: 300 mg as a single dose followed by 200 mg/day orally for a total duration of 7-14 days

Skin and skin structure infections, complicated, including diabetic foot infections: Oral, I.V.: 200 mg/day for 10-14 days

**Dosage Forms**

Injection, as mesylate (alatrofloxacin): 5 mg/mL (40 mL, 60 mL)

Tablet, as mesylate (trovafloxacin): 100 mg, 200 mg

**Trovan®** *see* trovafloxacin *on previous page*

**Trusopt®** *see* dorzolamide *on page 201*

**Truxazole® Tablet** *see* sulfisoxazole *on page 566*

**Truxcillin VK®** *see* penicillin V potassium *on page 457*

## trypsin, balsam Peru, and castor oil

(TRIP sin, BAL sam pe RUE, & KAS tor oyl)

**U.S./Canadian Brand Names** Granulex

**Therapeutic Category** Protectant, Topical

**Use** Treatment of decubitus ulcers, varicose ulcers, debridement of eschar, dehiscent wounds and sunburn

**Usual Dosage** Topical: Apply a minimum of twice daily or as often as necessary

**Dosage Forms** Aerosol, topical: Trypsin 0.1 mg, balsam Peru 72.5 mg, and castor oil 650 mg per 0.82 mL (60 g, 120 g)

**Tryptacin®** ***(Discontinued)*** *see page 750*

**Trysul®** ***(Discontinued)*** *see page 750*

**TSH** *see* thyrotropin *on page 588*

**TSPA** *see* thiotepa *on page 587*

**T-Stat® Topical** *see* erythromycin (ophthalmic/topical) *on page 222*

## tuberculin tests (too BER kyoo lin tests)

**Synonyms** Mantoux; old tuberculin; PPD; purified protein derivative

**U.S./Canadian Brand Names** Aplisol®; Aplitest®; Tine Test PPD; Tubersol®

**Therapeutic Category** Diagnostic Agent

**Use** Skin test in diagnosis of tuberculosis, to aid in assessment of cell-mediated immunity; routine tuberculin testing is recommended at 12 months of age and at every 1-2 years thereafter, before the measles vaccination

**Usual Dosage** Children and Adults: Intradermally: 0.1 mL approximately 4" below elbow; use 1/4" to 1/2" or 26- or 27-gauge needle; significant reactions are ≥5 mm in diameter

**Dosage Forms** Injection:

First test strength: 1 TU/0.1 mL (1 mL)

Intermediate test strength: 5 TU/0.1 mL (1 mL, 5 mL, 10 mL)

Second test strength: 250 TU/0.1 mL (1 mL)

Tine: 5 TU each test

**Tubersol®** *see* tuberculin tests *on this page*

**tubocurarine** (too boe kyoor AR een)

**Synonyms** *d*-tubocurarine

**Therapeutic Category** Skeletal Muscle Relaxant

**Use** Adjunct to anesthesia to induce skeletal muscle relaxation

**Usual Dosage** Children and Adults: I.V.: 0.2-0.4 mg/kg as a single dose; maintenance: 0.04-0.2 mg/kg/dose as needed to maintain paralysis

Alternative adult dose: 6-9 mg once daily, then 3-4.5 mg as needed to maintain paralysis

**Dosage Forms** Injection, as chloride: 3 mg/mL [3 units/mL] (5 mL, 10 mL, 20 mL)

**Tucks® [OTC]** *see* witch hazel *on page 635*

**Tucks® Cream *(Discontinued)*** *see page 750*

**Tuinal®** *see* amobarbital and secobarbital *on page 35*

**Tums® [OTC]** *see* calcium carbonate *on page 97*

**Tums® E-X Extra Strength Tablet [OTC]** *see* calcium carbonate *on page 97*

**Tums® Extra Strength Liquid [OTC]** *see* calcium carbonate *on page 97*

**Tusal® *(Discontinued)*** *see page 750*

**Tusibron® [OTC]** *see* guaifenesin *on page 281*

**Tusibron-DM® [OTC]** *see* guaifenesin and dextromethorphan *on page 282*

**Tussafed® Drops** *see* carbinoxamine, pseudoephedrine, and dextromethorphan *on page 108*

**Tussafin® Expectorant** *see* hydrocodone, pseudoephedrine, and guaifenesin *on page 302*

**Tuss-Allergine® Modified T.D. Capsule *(Discontinued)*** *see page 750*

**Tussar® SF Syrup** *see* guaifenesin, pseudoephedrine, and codeine *on page 284*

**Tuss-DM® [OTC]** *see* guaifenesin and dextromethorphan *on page 282*

**Tussigon®** *see* hydrocodone and homatropine *on page 301*

**Tussionex®** *see* hydrocodone and chlorpheniramine *on page 300*

**Tussi-Organidin® *(Discontinued)*** *see page 750*

**Tussi-Organidin® DM *(Discontinued)*** *see page 750*

**Tussi-Organidin® DM NR** *see* guaifenesin and dextromethorphan *on page 282*

**Tussi-Organidin® NR** *see* guaifenesin and codeine *on page 282*

**Tuss-LA®** *see* guaifenesin and pseudoephedrine *on page 283*

**Tusso-DM® *(Discontinued)*** *see page 750*

**Tussogest® Extended Release Capsule *(Discontinued)*** *see page 750*

**Tuss-Ornade® *(Discontinued)*** *see page 750*

**Tusstat® Syrup** *see* diphenhydramine *on page 191*

**Twice-A-Day® Nasal Solution [OTC]** *see* oxymetazoline *on page 444*

**Twilite® Oral [OTC]** *see* diphenhydramine *on page 191*

**Twin-K®** *see* potassium citrate and potassium gluconate *on page 487*

**Twinrix®** *see* hepatitis A inactivated and hepatitis B (recombinant) vaccine *on page 291*

**Two-Dyne®** *see* butalbital compound and acetaminophen *on page 93*

**Tycolene® [OTC]** *see* acetaminophen *on page 3*

**Tylenol® [OTC]** *see* acetaminophen *on page 3*

**Tylenol® Allergy Sinus [OTC]** *see* acetaminophen, chlorpheniramine, and pseudoephedrine *on page 6*

**Tylenol® Allergy Sinus (Can)** *see* acetaminophen, chlorpheniramine, and pseudoephedrine *on page 6*

**Tylenol® Arthritis [OTC]** *see* acetaminophen *on page 3*

**Tylenol® Children's [OTC]** *see* acetaminophen *on page 3*

**Tylenol® Cold [OTC]** *see* acetaminophen, dextromethorphan, and pseudoephedrine *on page 7*

**Tylenol® Cold (Can)** *see* acetaminophen, chlorpheniramine, and pseudoephedrine *on page 6*

**Tylenol® Cold Children's [OTC]** *see* acetaminophen, chlorpheniramine, and pseudoephedrine *on page 6*

**Tylenol® Cold Effervescent Medication Tablet *(Discontinued)*** *see page 750*

**Tylenol® Cold Infants [OTC]** *see* acetaminophen and pseudoephedrine *on page 6*

**Tylenol® Cold Plus Cough Infants' [OTC]** *see* acetaminophen, dextromethorphan, and pseudoephedrine *on page 7*

**Tylenol® Extra Strength [OTC]** *see* acetaminophen *on page 3*

**Tylenol® Flu Maximum Strength [OTC]** *see* acetaminophen, dextromethorphan, and pseudoephedrine *on page 7*

**Tylenol® Infants [OTC]** *see* acetaminophen *on page 3*

**Tylenol® Infants Original [OTC]** *see* acetaminophen *on page 3*

**Tylenol® Junior Strength [OTC]** *see* acetaminophen *on page 3*

**Tylenol® PM Strength [OTC]** *see* acetaminophen and diphenhydramine *on page 5*

**Tylenol® Severe Allergy [OTC]** *see* acetaminophen and diphenhydramine *on page 5*

**Tylenol® Sinus Children's [OTC]** *see* acetaminophen and pseudoephedrine *on page 6*

**Tylenol® Sinus, Maximum Strength [OTC]** *see* acetaminophen and pseudoephedrine *on page 6*

**Tylenol® Sore Throat [OTC]** *see* acetaminophen *on page 3*

**Tylenol® With Codeine** *see* acetaminophen and codeine *on page 4*

**Tylex® [OTC]** *see* acetaminophen *on page 3*

**Tylex® Extra Strength [OTC]** *see* acetaminophen *on page 3*

**Tylophen® [OTC]** *see* acetaminophen *on page 3*

**Tylox®** *see* oxycodone and acetaminophen *on page 444*

**Tyltabs® [OTC]** *see* acetaminophen *on page 3*

**Tyltabs® Allergy Sinus [OTC]** *see* acetaminophen, chlorpheniramine, and pseudoephedrine *on page 6*

**Tyltabs® Children's [OTC]** *see* acetaminophen *on page 3*

**Tyltabs® Extra Strength [OTC]** *see* acetaminophen *on page 3*

**Tyltabs® PM [OTC]** *see* acetaminophen and diphenhydramine *on page 5*

**Typherix™ (Can)** *see Salmonella typhi* Vi capsular polysaccharide vaccine *(Canada only) on page 536*

**Typhim Vi®** *see* typhoid vaccine *on this page*

## typhoid vaccine (TYE foid vak SEEN)

**Synonyms** typhoid vaccine live oral Ty21a

**U.S./Canadian Brand Names** Typhim Vi®; Vivotif Berna™ Oral

**Therapeutic Category** Vaccine, Inactivated Bacteria

**Use** Promotes active immunity to typhoid fever for patients exposed to typhoid carrier or foreign travel to typhoid fever endemic area

**Usual Dosage**

Oral: Adults:

Primary immunization: 1 capsule on alternate days (day 1, 3, 5, and 7)

Booster immunization: Repeat full course of primary immunization every 5 years

S.C.:

Children 6 months to 10 years: 0.25 mL; repeat in ≥4 weeks (total immunization is 2 doses)

Children >10 years and Adults: 0.5 mL; repeat dose in ≥4 weeks (total immunization is 2 doses)

Booster: 0.25 mL every 3 years for children 6 months to 10 years and 0.5 mL every 3 years for adults and children >10 years

**Dosage Forms**

Capsule, enteric coated (Vivotif Berna™): Viable *S. typhi* Ty21a colony-forming units 2-6 x $10^9$ and nonviable *S. typhi* Ty21a colony-forming units 50 x $10^9$ with sucrose, ascorbic acid, amino acid mixture, lactose and magnesium stearate

Injection, suspension (H-P): Heat- and phenol-inactivated, killed Ty-2 strain of *S. typhi* organisms; provides 8 units/mL, ≤1 billion/mL and ≤35 mcg nitrogen/mL (5 mL, 10 mL)

Injection (Typhim Vi®): Purified Vi capsular polysaccharide 25 mcg/0.5 mL (0.5 mL)

Powder for suspension (AKD): 8 units/mL ≤1 billion/mL, acetone inactivated dried (50 doses)

**typhoid vaccine live oral Ty21a** *see* typhoid vaccine *on previous page*

**Tyrodone® Liquid** *see* hydrocodone and pseudoephedrine *on page 301*

**Tyzine® Nasal** *see* tetrahydrozoline *on page 580*

**U-90152S** *see* delavirdine *on page 169*

**UAA®** *see* methenamine, phenyl salicylate, atropine, hyoscyamine, benzoic acid, and methylene blue *on page 379*

**UAD Otic®** *see* neomycin, polymyxin B, and hydrocortisone *on page 415*

**UCB-P071** *see* cetirizine *on page 121*

**Ucephan®** *see* sodium phenylacetate and sodium benzoate *on page 551*

**U-Cort™ Topical** *see* hydrocortisone (topical) *on page 304*

**UK** *see* urokinase *on page 618*

**UK-68-798** *see* dofetilide *on page 198*

**UK 92480** *see* sildenafil *on page 543*

**Ulcerease® [OTC]** *see* phenol *on page 465*

**Ulcidine® (Can)** *see* famotidine *on page 240*

**ULR-LA®** ***(Discontinued)*** *see page 750*

**Ultane®** *see* sevoflurane *on page 543*

**Ultiva™** *see* remifentanil *on page 521*

**Ultradol™ (Can)** *see* etodolac *on page 236*

**Ultralente® U** ***(Discontinued)*** *see page 750*

**Ultram®** *see* tramadol *on page 598*

**Ultra Mide® Topical** *see* urea *on page 617*

**Ultramop™ (Can)** *see* methoxsalen *on page 381*

**Ultraquin® (Can)** *see* hydroquinone *on page 305*

**Ultrase®** *see* pancrelipase *on page 448*

**Ultrase® MT12** *see* pancrelipase *on page 448*

**Ultrase® MT18** *see* pancrelipase *on page 448*

**Ultrase® MT20** *see* pancrelipase *on page 448*

**Ultrase® MT24 *(Discontinued)*** *see page 750*

**Ultra Tears® Solution [OTC]** *see* artificial tears *on page 53*

**Ultravate™** *see* halobetasol *on page 288*

**Unasyn®** *see* ampicillin and sulbactam *on page 39*

## undecylenic acid and derivatives (un de sil EN ik AS id & dah RIV ah tivs)

**Synonyms** zinc undecylenate

**U.S./Canadian Brand Names** Desenex® Foot & Sneaker [OTC]; Undex-25% [OTC]

**Therapeutic Category** Antifungal Agent

**Use** Treatment of athlete's foot (tinea pedis), ringworm (except nails and scalp), prickly heat, jock itch (tinea cruris), diaper rash and other minor skin irritations due to superficial dermatophytes

**Usual Dosage** Children and Adults: Topical: Apply as needed twice daily after cleansing the affected area for 2-4 weeks

**Dosage Forms**

Ointment, topical: 28 g, 60 g, 454 g

Spray, topical: 90 mL

**Undex-25% [OTC]** *see* undecylenic acid and derivatives *on this page*

**Unguentine® [OTC]** *see* benzocaine *on page 72*

**Uni-Bent® Cough Syrup** *see* diphenhydramine *on page 191*

**Unicap® [OTC]** *see* vitamin (multiple/oral) *on page 632*

**Uni Cenna® [OTC]** *see* senna *on page 541*

**Uni-Decon® *(Discontinued)*** *see page 750*

**Uni-Dur®** *see* theophylline *on page 581*

**Uni-Fed® [OTC]** *see* triprolidine and pseudoephedrine *on page 609*

**Unipen® *(Discontinued)*** *see page 750*

**UniPerr® [OTC]** *see* acetaminophen and phenyltoloxamine *on page 5*

**Uniphyl®** *see* theophylline *on page 581*

**Unipres® *(Discontinued)*** *see page 750*

**Uni-Pro® [OTC]** *see* ibuprofen *on page 311*

**Uniretic™** *see* moexipril and hydrochlorothiazide *on page 397*

**Unison® w/Pain Relief [OTC]** *see* acetaminophen and diphenhydramine *on page 5*

**Unithroid®** *see* levothyroxine *on page 348*

**Unitrol® *(Discontinued)*** *see page 750*

**Uni-Tussin® [OTC]** *see* guaifenesin *on page 281*

**Uni-tussin® DM [OTC]** *see* guaifenesin and dextromethorphan *on page 282*

**Univasc®** *see* moexipril *on page 397*

**Univol® (Can)** *see* aluminum hydroxide and magnesium hydroxide *on page 27*

**Unna's boot** *see* zinc gelatin *on page 639*

**Unna's paste** *see* zinc gelatin *on page 639*

## unoprostone (yoo noe PROS tone)

**U.S./Canadian Brand Names** Rescula®

**Therapeutic Category** Ophthalmic Agent, Miscellaneous

**Use** To lower intraocular pressure (IOP) in patients with open-angle glaucoma or ocular hypertension; should be used in patients who are not tolerant of, or failed treatment with other IOP-lowering medications

**Usual Dosage** Ophthalmic: Adults: Instill 1 drop into affected eye(s) twice daily
**Dosage Forms** Solution, ophthalmic: 0.15% (5 mL)

**Urabeth® *(Discontinued)*** *see page 750*

**Uracel® *(Discontinued)*** *see page 750*

**Urasal® (Can)** *see* methenamine *on page 379*

## urea (yoor EE a)

**Synonyms** carbamide

**U.S./Canadian Brand Names** Amino-Cerv™ Vaginal Cream; Aquacare® Topical [OTC]; Carmol® Topical [OTC]; Gormel® Creme [OTC]; Lanaphilic® Topical [OTC]; Nutraplus® Topical [OTC]; Rea-Lo® [OTC]; Ultra Mide® Topical; Ureacin®-20 Topical [OTC]; Ureaphil® Injection; Uremol® (Can); Urisec® (Can)

**Therapeutic Category** Diuretic, Osmotic; Topical Skin Product

**Use** Reduce intracranial pressure and intraocular pressure (30%); promotes hydration and removal of excess keratin in hyperkeratotic conditions and dry skin; mild cervicitis

**Usual Dosage**

Children: I.V. slow infusion:
- <2 years: 0.1-0.5 g/kg
- >2 years: 0.5-1.5 g/kg

Adults:
- I.V. infusion: 1-1.5 g/kg by slow infusion (1-2½ hours); maximum: 120 g/24 hours
- Topical: Apply 1-3 times/day
- Vaginal: 1 applicatorful in vagina at bedtime for 2-4 weeks

**Dosage Forms**

Cream:
- Topical: 2% [20 mg/mL] (75 g); 10% [100 mg/mL] (75 g, 90 g, 454 g); 20% [200 mg/mL] (45 g, 75 g, 90 g, 454 g); 30% [300 mg/mL] (60 g, 454 g); 40% (30 g)
- Vaginal: 8.34% [83.4 mg/g] (82.5 g)

Injection: 40 g/150 mL

Lotion: 2% (240 mL); 10% (180 mL, 240 mL, 480 mL); 15% (120 mL, 480 mL); 25% (180 mL)

## urea and hydrocortisone (yoor EE a & hye droe KOR ti sone)

**U.S./Canadian Brand Names** Carmol-HC® Topical; Ti-U-Lac® HC (Can); Uremol®-HC (Can)

**Therapeutic Category** Corticosteroid, Topical

**Use** Inflammation of corticosteroid-responsive dermatoses

**Usual Dosage** Topical: Apply thin film and rub in well 1-4 times/day. Therapy should be discontinued when control is achieved. If no improvement is seen, reassessment of diagnosis may be necessary.

**Dosage Forms** Cream, topical: Urea 10% and hydrocortisone acetate 1% in a water-washable vanishing cream base (30 g)

**Ureacin®-20 Topical [OTC]** *see* urea *on this page*

**Ureacin®-40 Topical *(Discontinued)*** *see page 750*

**urea peroxide** *see* carbamide peroxide *on page 106*

**Ureaphil® Injection** *see* urea *on this page*

**Urecholine®** *see* bethanechol *on page 79*

**Uremol® (Can)** *see* urea *on this page*

**Uremol®-HC (Can)** *see* urea and hydrocortisone *on this page*

**Urex®** *see* methenamine *on page 379*

**Uridon Modified®** *see* methenamine, phenyl salicylate, atropine, hyoscyamine, benzoic acid, and methylene blue *on page 379*

**Urisec® (Can)** *see* urea *on this page*

**Urised®** *see* methenamine, phenyl salicylate, atropine, hyoscyamine, benzoic acid, and methylene blue *on page 379*

**Urispas®** *see* flavoxate *on page 250*

**Uristat® [OTC]** *see* phenazopyridine *on page 463*

**Uri-Tet® *(Discontinued)*** *see page 750*

**Uritin®** *see* methenamine, phenyl salicylate, atropine, hyoscyamine, benzoic acid, and methylene blue *on page 379*

**Urobak® *(Discontinued)*** *see page 750*

**Urobiotic-25® *(Discontinued)*** *see page 750*

**Urocit®-K** *see* potassium citrate *on page 486*

**Urodine® *(Discontinued)*** *see page 750*

**Urodol® [OTC]** *see* phenazopyridine *on page 463*

**Urofemme® [OTC]** *see* phenazopyridine *on page 463*

## urofollitropin (yoor oh fol li TROE pin)

**U.S./Canadian Brand Names** Fertinex®; Fertinorm® HP (Can); Metrodin®

**Therapeutic Category** Ovulation Stimulator

**Use** Induction of ovulation in patients with polycystic ovarian disease and to stimulate the development of multiple oocytes

**Usual Dosage** Adults: Female: S.C.: 75 units/day for 7-12 days, used with hCG may repeat course of treatment 2 more times

**Dosage Forms** Injection: 0.83 mg [75 units FSH activity] (2 mL); 1.66 mg [150 units FSH activity]

**Urogesic®** *see* phenazopyridine *on page 463*

## urokinase (yoor oh KIN ase)

**Synonyms** UK

**U.S./Canadian Brand Names** Abbokinase®

**Therapeutic Category** Fibrinolytic Agent

**Use** Treatment of recent severe or massive deep vein or arterial thrombosis, pulmonary emboli, and occluded arteriovenous cannulas

**Usual Dosage**

Children and Adults: Deep vein thrombosis: I.V.: Loading: 4400 units/kg over 10 minutes, then 4400 units/kg/hour for 12 hours

Adults:

Myocardial infarction: Intracoronary: 750,000 units over 2 hours (6000 units/minute over up to 2 hours)

Occluded I.V. catheters:

5000 units (use only Abbokinase® Open Cath) in each lumen over 1-2 minutes, leave in lumen for 1-4 hours, then aspirate; may repeat with 10,000 units in each lumen if 5000 units fails to clear the catheter; **do not infuse into the patient**; volume to instill into catheter is equal to the volume of the catheter

I.V. infusion: 200 units/kg/hour in each lumen for 12-48 hours at a rate of at least 20 mL/hour

Dialysis patients: 5000 units is administered in each lumen over 1-2 minutes; leave urokinase in lumen for 1-2 days, then aspirate

Clot lysis (large vessel thrombi): Loading: I.V.: 4400 units/kg over 10 minutes, increase to 6000 units/kg/hour; maintenance: 4400-6000 units/kg/hour adjusted to achieve clot lysis or patency of affected vessel; doses up to 50,000 units/kg/hour have been used. **Note:** Therapy should be initiated as soon as possible after diagnosis of thrombi and continued until clot is dissolved (usually 24-72 hours).

Acute pulmonary embolism: Three treatment alternatives: 3 million unit dosage

Alternative 1: 12-hour infusion: 4400 units/kg (2000 units/lb) bolus over 10 minutes followed by 4400 units/kg/hour (2000 units/lb); begin heparin 1000 units/hour approximately 3-4 hours after completion of urokinase infusion or when PTT is <100 seconds

Alternative 2: 2-hour infusion: 1 million unit bolus over 10 minutes followed by 2 million units over 110 minutes; begin heparin 1000 units/hour approximately 3-4 hours after completion of urokinase infusion or when PTT is <100 seconds

Alternative 3: Bolus dose only: 15,000 units/kg over 10 minutes; begin heparin 1000 units/hour approximately 3-4 hours after completion of urokinase infusion or when PTT is <100 seconds

**Dosage Forms**

Powder for injection: 250,000 units

Powder for injection, catheter clear: 5000 units, 9000 units

**Uro-KP-Neutral®** *see* potassium phosphate and sodium phosphate *on page 488*

**Urolene Blue®** *see* methylene blue *on page 384*

**Uro-Mag® [OTC]** *see* magnesium oxide *on page 362*

**Uromitexan™ (Can)** *see* mesna *on page 375*

**Uroplus® DS *(Discontinued)*** *see page 750*

**Uroplus® SS *(Discontinued)*** *see page 750*

**Urovist Cysto®** *see* radiological/contrast media (ionic) *on page 516*

**Urovist® Meglumine** *see* radiological/contrast media (ionic) *on page 516*

**Urovist® Sodium 300** *see* radiological/contrast media (ionic) *on page 516*

**Urso®** *see* ursodiol *on this page*

**ursodeoxycholic acid** *see* ursodiol *on this page*

## ursodiol (ER soe dye ole)

**Synonyms** ursodeoxycholic acid

**U.S./Canadian Brand Names** Actigall™; Urso®

**Therapeutic Category** Gallstone Dissolution Agent

**Use** Gallbladder stone dissolution

**Usual Dosage** Oral: 8-10 mg/kg/day in 2-3 divided doses

**Dosage Forms**

Capsule: 300 mg

Tablet: 250 mg

**Uticort® *(Discontinued)*** *see page 750*

**Uvadex® Injection** *see* methoxsalen *on page 381*

**Vagifem®** *see* estradiol *on page 224*

**Vagistat®-1 Vaginal [OTC]** *see* tioconazole *on page 592*

**Vagitrol® *(Discontinued)*** *see page 750*

## valacyclovir (val ay SYE kloe veer)

**U.S./Canadian Brand Names** Valtrex®

**Therapeutic Category** Antiviral Agent

**Use** Treatment of herpes zoster (shingles) in immunocompetent patients; once daily therapy for the suppression of genital herpes

**Usual Dosage** Adults: Oral: 1000 mg 3 times/day for 7 days

**Dosage Forms** Tablet: 500 mg, 1000 mg

**Valadol® *(Discontinued)*** *see page 750*

**Valergen® Injection *(Discontinued)*** *see page 750*

**Valertest No.1®** *see* estradiol and testosterone *on page 226*

**Valisone® Topical** *see* betamethasone (topical) *on page 78*

**Valium® Injection** *see* diazepam *on page 179*

**Valium® Oral** *see* diazepam *on page 179*

**Valmid® Capsule *(Discontinued)*** *see page 750*

**Valorin® [OTC]** *see* acetaminophen *on page 3*

**Valorin® Extra [OTC]** *see* acetaminophen *on page 3*

**Valpin® 50 *(Discontinued)*** *see page 750*

## valproic acid and derivatives (val PROE ik AS id & dah RIV ah tives)

**Synonyms** dipropylacetic acid; DPA; 2-propylpentanoic acid; 2-propylvaleric acid

**U.S./Canadian Brand Names** Alti-Valproic (Can); Apo®-Divalproex (Can); Apo®-Valproic (Can); Depacon™; Depakene®; Depakote® Delayed Release; Depakote® ER; Deproic® (Can); Epival® (Can); Gen-Valproic (Can); Novo-Divalproex® (Can); Nu-Divalproex® (Can); Nu-Valproic (Can); PMS-Valproic Acid (Can); Rhoxal-valproic (Can)

**Therapeutic Category** Anticonvulsant

**Use**

Mania associated with bipolar disorder (Depakote®)

Migraine prophylaxis (Depakote®, Depakote® ER)

Monotherapy and adjunctive therapy in the treatment of patients with complex partial seizures that occur either in isolation or in association with other types of seizures (Depacon™, Depakote®)

Sole and adjunctive therapy of simple and complex absence seizures (Depacon™, Depakene®, Depakote®)

Adjunctively in patients with multiple seizure types that include absence seizures (Depacon™, Depakene®)

**Unlabeled use:** Behavior disorders in Alzheimer's disease

**Usual Dosage**

Seizures:

Children >10 years and Adults:

Oral: Initial: 10-15 mg/kg/day in 1-3 divided doses; increase by 5-10 mg/kg/day at weekly intervals until therapeutic levels are achieved; maintenance: 30-60 mg/kg/day in 2-3 divided doses. Adult usual dose: 1000-2500 mg/day

Children receiving more than one anticonvulsant (ie, polytherapy) may require doses up to 100 mg/kg/day in 3-4 divided doses

I.V.: Administer as a 60-minute infusion (≤20 mg/minute) with the same frequency as oral products; switch patient to oral products as soon as possible

Rectal: Dilute syrup 1:1 with water for use as a retention enema; loading dose: 17-20 mg/kg one time; maintenance: 10-15 mg/kg/dose every 8 hours

Mania: Adults: Oral: 750 mg/day in divided doses; dose should be adjusted as rapidly as possible to desired clinical effect; a loading dose of 20 mg/kg may be used; maximum recommended dosage: 60 mg/kg/day

Migraine prophylaxis: Adults: Oral:

Extended release tablets: 500 mg once daily for 7 days, then increase to 1000 mg once daily; adjust dose based on patient response; usual dosage range 500-1000 mg/day

Delayed release tablets: 250 mg twice daily; adjust dose based on patient response, up to 1000 mg/day

**Dosage Forms**

Capsule, sprinkle, as divalproex sodium (Depakote® Sprinkle®): 125 mg

Capsule, as valproic acid (Depakene®): 250 mg

Injection, as sodium valproate (Depacon™): 100 mg/mL (5 mL)

Syrup, as sodium valproate (Depakene®): 250 mg/5 mL (5 mL, 50 mL, 480 mL)

Tablet, delayed release, as divalproex sodium (Depakote®): 125 mg, 250 mg, 500 mg

Tablet, extended release, as divalproex sodium (Depakote® ER): 500 mg

**Valrelease® *(Discontinued)*** *see page 750*

**valrubicin** (val ru BYE cin)

**U.S./Canadian Brand Names** Valstar™

**Therapeutic Category** Antineoplastic Agent, Anthracycline

**Use** Intravesical therapy of BCG-refractory carcinoma *in situ* of the urinary bladder

**Usual Dosage** Adults: Intravesical: 800 mg once weekly for 6 weeks

**Dosage Forms** Injection: 40 mg/mL (5 mL)

**valsartan** (val SAR tan)

**U.S./Canadian Brand Names** Diovan™

**Therapeutic Category** Angiotensin II Antagonist

**Use** Treatment of hypertension alone or in combination with other antihypertensives

**Usual Dosage** Adults: Oral: 80 mg/day; may be increased to 160 mg if needed (maximal effects observed in 4-6 weeks)

**Dosage Forms** Capsule: 80 mg, 160 mg

**valsartan and hydrochlorothiazide**
(val SAR tan & hye droe klor oh THYE a zide)

**U.S./Canadian Brand Names** Diovan HCT™

**Therapeutic Category** Angiotensin II Antagonist Combination; Diuretic, Thiazide

**Use** Treatment of hypertension

**Usual Dosage** Adults: Oral: Dose is individualized

**Dosage Forms** Tablet: Valsartan 80 mg and hydrochlorothiazide 12.5 mg; valsartan 160 mg and hydrochlorothiazide 12.5 mg

**Valstar™** *see* valrubicin *on this page*

**Valtrex®** *see* valacyclovir *on page 619*

**Vamate® Oral *(Discontinued)*** *see page 750*

**Vanatrip®** *see* amitriptyline *on page 33*

**Vancenase® AQ 84 mcg** *see* beclomethasone *on page 68*

**Vancenase® AQ Inhaler** *see* beclomethasone *on page 68*

**Vancenase® Nasal Inhaler** *see* beclomethasone *on page 68*

**Vanceril® 84 mcg Double Strength** *see* beclomethasone *on page 68*

**Vanceril® Oral Inhaler** *see* beclomethasone *on page 68*

**Vancocin® Injection** *see* vancomycin *on this page*

**Vancocin® Oral** *see* vancomycin *on this page*

**Vancoled® Injection** *see* vancomycin *on this page*

**vancomycin** (van koe MYE sin)

**U.S./Canadian Brand Names** Lyphocin® Injection; Vancocin® Injection; Vancocin® Oral; Vancoled® Injection

**Therapeutic Category** Antibiotic, Miscellaneous

**Use** Treatment of patients with the following infections or conditions: treatment of infections due to documented or suspected methicillin-resistant *S. aureus* or beta-lactam resistant coagulase-negative *Staphylococcus*; treatment of serious or life-threatening infections (ie, endocarditis, meningitis, osteomyelitis) due to documented or suspected staphylococcal or streptococcal infections in patients who are allergic to penicillins and/or cephalosporins; empiric therapy of infections associated with central lines, VP shunts, hemodialysis shunts, vascular grafts, prosthetic heart valves; used orally for staphylococcal enterocolitis or for antibiotic-associated pseudomembranous colitis produced by *C. difficile*

**Usual Dosage** I.V. (initial dosage recommendation):

Infants >1 month and Children: 40 mg/kg/day in divided doses every 6 hours

Infants >1 month and Children with staphylococcal central nervous system infection: 60 mg/kg/day in divided doses every 6 hours

(Continued)

## vancomycin *(Continued)*

Adults: With normal renal function: 0.5 g every 6 hours or 1 g every 12 hours

Intrathecal:
Children: 5-20 mg/day
Adults: 20 mg/day

Oral:
Children: 10-50 mg/kg/day in divided doses every 6-8 hours; not to exceed 2 g/day
Adults: 0.5-2 g/day in divided doses every 6-8 hours

Pseudomembranous colitis produced by *C. difficile*:
Children: 40 mg/kg/day in divided doses, added to fluids
Adults: 500 mg to 2 g/day administered in 3 or 4 divided doses for 7-10 days

**Dosage Forms**
Capsule, as hydrochloride: 125 mg, 250 mg
Powder for oral solution, as hydrochloride: 1 g, 10 g
Powder for injection, as hydrochloride: 500 mg, 1 g, 2 g, 5 g, 10 g

**Vanex-LA®** ***(Discontinued)*** *see page 750*

**Vaniqa™ Cream** *see* eflornithine *on page 211*

**Vanoxide-HC®** *see* benzoyl peroxide and hydrocortisone *on page 75*

**Vanquish® [OTC]** *see* acetaminophen, aspirin, and caffeine *on page 6*

**Vanseb-T® Shampoo** ***(Discontinued)*** *see page 750*

**Vansil™** ***(Discontinued)*** *see page 750*

**Vantin®** *see* cefpodoxime *on page 116*

**Vaponefrin® [OTC]** *see* epinephrine *on page 216*

**VAQTA®** *see* hepatitis A vaccine *on page 292*

## varicella virus vaccine (var i SEL a VYE rus vak SEEN)

**Synonyms** chicken pox vaccine; varicella-zoster virus (VZV) vaccine

**U.S./Canadian Brand Names** Varivax®

**Therapeutic Category** Vaccine, Live Virus

**Use** The American Association of Pediatrics recommends that the chickenpox vaccine should be given to all healthy children between 12 months and 18 years; children between 12 months and 13 years who have not been immunized or who have not had chickenpox should receive 1 vaccination while children 13-18 years of age require 2 vaccinations 4-8 weeks apart; the vaccine has been added to the childhood immunization schedule for infants 12-28 months of age and children 11-12 years of age who have not been vaccinated previously or who have not had the disease; it is recommended to be given with the measles, mumps, and rubella (MMR) vaccine

**Usual Dosage** S.C.:
Children 12 months to 12 years: 0.5 mL
Children 12 years to Adults: 2 doses of 0.5 mL separated by 4-8 weeks

**Dosage Forms** Powder for injection, lyophilized powder, preservative free: 1350 plaque forming units (PFU)/0.5 mL (0.5 mL single-dose vials)

## varicella-zoster immune globulin (human)

(var i SEL a-ZOS ter i MYUN GLOB yoo lin HYU man)

**Synonyms** VZIG

**Therapeutic Category** Immune Globulin

**Use** Passive immunization of susceptible immunodeficient patients after exposure to varicella; most effective if begun within 96 hours of exposure

**VZIG supplies are limited, restrict administration to those meeting the following criteria:**

**One of the following underlying illnesses or conditions:**
Neoplastic disease (eg, leukemia or lymphoma)

Congenital or acquired immunodeficiency

Immunosuppressive therapy with steroids, antimetabolites or other immunosuppressive treatment regimens

Newborn of mother who had onset of chickenpox within 5 days before delivery or within 48 hours after delivery

Premature (≥28 weeks gestation) whose mother has no history of chickenpox

Premature (<28 weeks gestation or ≤1000 g VZIG) regardless of maternal history

**One of the following types of exposure to chickenpox or zoster patient(s):**

Continuous household contact

Playmate contact (>1 hour play indoors)

Hospital contact (in same 2-4 bedroom or adjacent beds in a large ward or prolonged face-to-face contact with an infectious staff member or patient)

Susceptible to varicella-zoster

Age of <15 years; administer to immunocompromised adolescents and adults and to other older patients on an individual basis

An acceptable alternative to VZIG prophylaxis is to treat varicella, if it occurs, with high-dose I.V. acyclovir

**Usual Dosage** High-risk susceptible patients who are exposed again more than 3 weeks after a prior dose of VZIG should receive another full dose; there is no evidence VZIG modifies established varicella-zoster infections.

I.M.: Administer by deep injection in the gluteal muscle or in another large muscle mass. Inject 125 units/10 kg (22 lb); maximum dose: 625 units (5 vials); minimum dose: 125 units; do not administer fractional doses. Do not inject I.V.

**Dosage Forms** Injection: 125 units of antibody in single dose vials; 625 units of antibody

**varicella-zoster virus (VZV) vaccine** *see* varicella virus vaccine *on previous page*

**Varivax®** *see* varicella virus vaccine *on previous page*

**Vascor®** *see* bepridil *on page 76*

**Vascoray®** *see* radiological/contrast media (ionic) *on page 516*

**Vaseretic® 10-25** *see* enalapril and hydrochlorothiazide *on page 214*

**Vasocidin® Ophthalmic** *see* sulfacetamide and prednisolone *on page 563*

**VasoClear® Ophthalmic [OTC]** *see* naphazoline *on page 409*

**Vasocon-A® [OTC] Ophthalmic** *see* naphazoline and antazoline *on page 409*

**Vasocon Regular® Ophthalmic** *see* naphazoline *on page 409*

**Vasodilan®** *see* isoxsuprine *on page 329*

## vasopressin (vay soe PRES in)

**Synonyms** antidiuretic hormone (ADH); 8-arginine vasopressin

**U.S./Canadian Brand Names** Pitressin®; Pressyn® (Can)

**Therapeutic Category** Hormone, Posterior Pituitary

**Use** Treatment of diabetes insipidus; prevention and treatment of postoperative abdominal distention; differential diagnosis of diabetes insipidus; adjunct in the treatment of acute massive hemorrhage of GI tract or esophageal varices

**Usual Dosage**

Diabetes insipidus:

I.M., S.C.:

Children: 2.5-5 units 2-4 times/day as needed

Adults: 5-10 units 2-4 times/day as needed (dosage range 5-60 units/day)

Intranasal: Administer on cotton pledget or nasal spray

Abdominal distention Adults: I.M.: 5 mg stat, 10 mg every 3-4 hours

GI hemorrhage: I.V.: Administer in a peripheral vein; dilute aqueous in NS or $D_5W$ to 0.1-1 unit/mL and infuse at 0.2-0.4 unit/minute and progressively increase to 0.9 unit/minute if necessary; I.V. infusion administration requires the use of an infusion pump and should be administered in a peripheral line to minimize adverse reactions on coronary arteries

(Continued)

## vasopressin *(Continued)*

**Dosage Forms** Injection, aqueous: 20 pressor units/mL (0.5 mL, 1 mL, 10 mL)

**Vasosulf® Ophthalmic** *see* sulfacetamide and phenylephrine *on page 563*

**Vasotate® Otic** *see* acetic acid *on page 8*

**Vasotec® I.V.** *see* enalapril *on page 213*

**Vasotec® Oral** *see* enalapril *on page 213*

**Vasoxyl® *(Discontinued)*** *see page 750*

**Va-Zone®** *see* acetaminophen, isometheptene, and dichloralphenazone *on page 8*

**V-Cillin K® *(Discontinued)*** *see page 750*

**VCR** *see* vincristine *on page 628*

**V-Dec-M®** *see* guaifenesin and pseudoephedrine *on page 283*

**Vectrin®** *see* minocycline *on page 394*

## vecuronium (ve KYOO roe nee um)

**Synonyms** ORG NC 45

**U.S./Canadian Brand Names** Norcuron®

**Therapeutic Category** Skeletal Muscle Relaxant

**Use** Adjunct to anesthesia, to facilitate endotracheal intubation, and provide skeletal muscle relaxation during surgery or mechanical ventilation

**Usual Dosage** I.V.:

Infants >7 weeks to 1 year: Initial: 0.08-0.1 mg/kg/dose; maintenance: 0.05-0.1 mg/kg/ every hour as needed

Children >1 year and Adults: Initial: 0.08-0.1 mg/kg/dose; maintenance: 0.05-0.1 mg/kg/ every hour as needed; may be administered as a continuous infusion at 0.1 mg/kg/hour

**Note:** Children may require slightly higher initial doses and slightly more frequent supplementation

**Dosage Forms** Powder for injection:

With diluent: 10 mg (10 mL)

Without diluent: 10 mg (10 mL); 20 mg (20 mL)

**Veetids®** *see* penicillin V potassium *on page 457*

**Velban®** *see* vinblastine *on page 627*

**Velosef®** *see* cephradine *on page 121*

**Velosulin® BR Human (Buffered)** *see* insulin preparations *on page 319*

**Velosulin® Human Iletin® (Can)** *see* insulin preparations *on page 319*

**Velsar® Injection *(Discontinued)*** *see page 750*

## venlafaxine (VEN la faks een)

**U.S./Canadian Brand Names** Effexor®; Effexor-XR®

**Therapeutic Category** Antidepressant, Phenethylamine

**Use** Treatment of depression

**Usual Dosage** Adults: Oral:

Capsule: One capsule daily

Tablet: 75 mg/day, administered in 2 or 3 divided doses, taken with food; dose may be increased in 75 mg/day increments at intervals of at least 4 days, up to 225-375 mg/ day

**Dosage Forms**

Capsule, extended release: 37.5 mg, 75 mg, 150 mg

Tablet: 25 mg, 37.5 mg, 50 mg, 75 mg, 100 mg, 150 mg

**Venofer®** *see* iron sucrose *on page 326*

**Venoglobulin®-I** *see* immune globulin (intravenous) *on page 315*

**Venoglobulin®-S** *see* immune globulin (intravenous) *on page 315*

**Ventolin®** *see* albuterol *on page 16*

**Ventolin® HFA** *see* albuterol *on page 16*

**Ventolin Rotacaps®** *see* albuterol *on page 16*

**VePesid®** *see* etoposide *on page 236*

## verapamil (ver AP a mil)

**Synonyms** iproveratril

**U.S./Canadian Brand Names** Alti-Verapamil (Can); Apo®-Verap (Can); Calan®; Calan® SR; Chronovera® (Can); Covera-HS®; Gen-Verapamil (Can); Isoptin®; Isoptin® SR; Novo-Veramil (Can); Nu-Verap (Can); Verelan®; Verelan® PM

**Therapeutic Category** Antiarrhythmic Agent, Class IV; Calcium Channel Blocker

**Use** Angina, hypertension; I.V. for supraventricular tachyarrhythmias (PSVT, atrial fibrillation, atrial flutter)

**Usual Dosage**

Children: I.V.:

0-1 year: 0.1-0.2 mg/kg/dose, repeated after 30 minutes as needed

1-16 years: 0.1-0.3 mg/kg over 2-3 minutes; maximum: 5 mg/dose, may repeat dose once in 30 minutes if adequate response not achieved; maximum for second dose: 10 mg/dose

Children: Oral (dose not well established):

4-8 mg/kg/day in 3 divided doses **or** 1-5 years: 40-80 mg every 8 hours

>5 years: 80 mg every 6-8 hours

Adults:

Oral: 240-480 mg/24 hours divided 3-4 times/day

I.V.: 5-10 mg (0.075-0.15 mg/kg); may repeat 10 mg (0.15 mg/kg) 15-30 minutes after the initial dose if needed and if patient tolerated initial dose

**Dosage Forms**

Capsule, as hydrochloride, sustained release: 120 mg, 180 mg, 240 mg, 360 mg

Verelan®: 120 mg, 180 mg, 240 mg, 360 mg

Verelan® PM: 100 mg, 200 mg, 300 mg

Injection, as hydrochloride: 2.5 mg/mL (2 mL, 4 mL)

Isoptin®: 2.5 mg/mL (2 mL, 4 mL)

Tablet, as hydrochloride: 40 mg, 80 mg, 120 mg

Calan®, Isoptin®: 40 mg, 80 mg, 120 mg

Tablet, as hydrochloride, sustained release: 180 mg, 240 mg

Calan® SR, Isoptin® SR: 120 mg, 180 mg, 240 mg

Covera-HS®: 180 mg, 240 mg

**Verazinc® Oral [OTC]** *see* zinc sulfate *on page 639*

**Vercyte® *(Discontinued)*** *see page 750*

**Verelan®** *see* verapamil *on this page*

**Verelan® PM** *see* verapamil *on this page*

**Vergogel® Gel [OTC]** *see* salicylic acid *on page 535*

**Vergon® [OTC]** *see* meclizine *on page 367*

**Vermizine® *(Discontinued)*** *see page 750*

**Vermox®** *see* mebendazole *on page 367*

**Verr-Canth™ *(Discontinued)*** *see page 750*

**Verrex-C&M® *(Discontinued)*** *see page 750*

**Verrusol® *(Discontinued)*** *see page 750*

**Versacaps®** *see* guaifenesin and pseudoephedrine *on page 283*

**Versed®** *see* midazolam *on page 391*

**Versel® (Can)** *see* selenium sulfide *on page 540*

**Versiclear™** *see* sodium thiosulfate *on page 553*

## verteporfin (ver te POR fin)

**U.S./Canadian Brand Names** Visudyne™

**Therapeutic Category** Ophthalmic Agent

**Use** Treatment of age-related macular degeneration in patients with classic subfoveal choroidal neovascularization

**Usual Dosage** Therapy is a two-step process; first the infusion of verteporfin, then the activation of verteporfin with a nonthermal diode laser

Adults: I.V.: 6 mg/m$^2$ body surface area

**Dosage Forms** Powder for injection: 2 mg/mL (7.5 mL)

**Verukan® Solution** *see* salicylic acid *on page 535*

**Vesanoid®** *see* tretinoin (oral) *on page 600*

**Vesprin®** *see* triflupromazine *on page 605*

**Vexol® Ophthalmic Suspension** *see* rimexolone *on page 528*

**V-Gan® Injection *(Discontinued)*** *see page 750*

**Viagra®** *see* sildenafil *on page 543*

**Vibazine® *(Discontinued)*** *see page 750*

**Vibramycin®** *see* doxycycline *on page 204*

**Vibra-Tabs®** *see* doxycycline *on page 204*

**Vicks® 44D Cough & Head Congestion** *see* pseudoephedrine and dextromethorphan *on page 508*

**Vicks® 44E [OTC]** *see* guaifenesin and dextromethorphan *on page 282*

**Vicks® 44 Non-Drowsy Cold & Cough Liqui-Caps [OTC]** *see* pseudoephedrine and dextromethorphan *on page 508*

**Vicks® Children's Chloraseptic® [OTC]** *see* benzocaine *on page 72*

**Vicks® Chloraseptic® Sore Throat [OTC]** *see* benzocaine *on page 72*

**Vicks® Dayquil® [OTC]** *see* acetaminophen, dextromethorphan, and pseudoephedrine *on page 7*

**Vicks® DayQuil® Allergy Relief 4 Hour Tablet *(Discontinued)*** *see page 750*

**Vicks® Dayquil® Multi-Symptom [OTC]** *see* acetaminophen, dextromethorphan, and pseudoephedrine *on page 7*

**Vicks® DayQuil® Sinus Pressure & Congestion Relief *(Discontinued)*** *see page 750*

**Vicks Formula 44® [OTC]** *see* dextromethorphan *on page 178*

**Vicks Formula 44® Pediatric Formula [OTC]** *see* dextromethorphan *on page 178*

**Vicks® Pediatric Formula 44E [OTC]** *see* guaifenesin and dextromethorphan *on page 282*

**Vicks® Sinex® Nasal Solution [OTC]** *see* phenylephrine *on page 467*

**Vicks® Vatronol® *(Discontinued)*** *see page 750*

**Vicodin®** *see* hydrocodone and acetaminophen *on page 300*

**Vicodin® ES** *see* hydrocodone and acetaminophen *on page 300*

**Vicon-C® [OTC]** *see* vitamin B complex with vitamin C *on page 630*

**Vicon Forte®** *see* vitamin (multiple/oral) *on page 632*

**Vicon® Plus [OTC]** *see* vitamin (multiple/oral) *on page 632*

**Vicoprofen®** *see* hydrocodone and ibuprofen *on page 301*

## vidarabine (vye DARE a been)

**Synonyms** adenine arabinoside; ARA-A; arabinofuranosyladenine

**U.S./Canadian Brand Names** Vira-A® Ophthalmic

**Therapeutic Category** Antiviral Agent

**Use** Treatment of acute keratoconjunctivitis and epithelial keratitis due to herpes simplex virus; herpes simplex encephalitis; neonatal herpes simplex virus infections; disseminated varicella-zoster in immunosuppressed patients

**Usual Dosage** Children and Adults: Ophthalmic: Keratoconjunctivitis: ½" of ointment in lower conjunctival sac 5 times/day every 3 hours while awake until complete re-epithelialization has occurred, then twice daily for an additional 7 days

**Dosage Forms** Ointment, ophthalmic, as monohydrate: 3% [30 mg/mL = 28 mg/mL base] (3.5 g)

**Vi-Daylin® [OTC]** *see* vitamin (multiple/pediatric) *on page 632*

**Vi-Daylin/F®** *see* vitamin (multiple/pediatric) *on page 632*

**Videx®** *see* didanosine *on page 183*

## vigabatrin *(Canada only)* (vye GA ba trin)

**Synonyms** GVG; MDL-71754

**U.S./Canadian Brand Names** Sabril® (Can)

**Therapeutic Category** Anticonvulsant

**Use** Partial/secondary generalized seizures; useful for spasticity or tardive dyskinesia

**Usual Dosage**

Initial dose: 1-2 g/day then titrate to maintenance dose of 2-4 g/day in 1-2 divided doses (lower initial doses in the elderly, patients with renal insufficiency, or patients with psychiatric illnesses)

Infantile spasm: 50-200 mg/kg/day

Spasticity: 2-3 g/day

Tardive dyskinesia: 2-8 g/day

**Dosage Forms**

Sachet: 500 mg (50s)

Tablet: 500 mg

## vinblastine (vin BLAS teen)

**Synonyms** vincaleukoblastine; VLB

**U.S./Canadian Brand Names** Alkaban-AQ®; Velban®

**Therapeutic Category** Antineoplastic Agent

**Use** Palliative treatment of Hodgkin's disease; advanced testicular germinal-cell cancers; non-Hodgkin's lymphoma, histiocytosis, and choriocarcinoma

**Usual Dosage** Refer to individual protocol. Varies depending upon clinical and hematological response. Administer at intervals of at least 7 days and only after leukocyte count has returned to at least 4000/mm$^3$; maintenance therapy should be titrated according to leukocyte count. Dosage should be reduced in patients with recent exposure to radiation therapy or chemotherapy; single doses in these patients should not exceed 5.5 mg/m$^2$.

Children and Adults: I.V.: 4-12 mg/m$^2$ every 7-10 days **or** 5-day continuous infusion of 1.4-1.8 mg/m$^2$/day **or** 0.1-0.5 mg/kg/week

**Dosage Forms**

Injection, as sulfate: 1 mg/mL (10 mL)

Powder for injection, as sulfate: 10 mg

**vincaleukoblastine** *see* vinblastine *on this page*

**Vincasar® PFS™** *see* vincristine *on next page*

**vincristine** (vin KRIS teen)

**Synonyms** LCR; leurocristine; VCR

**U.S./Canadian Brand Names** Oncovin®; Vincasar® PFS™

**Therapeutic Category** Antineoplastic Agent

**Use** Treatment of leukemias, Hodgkin's disease, neuroblastoma, malignant lymphomas, Wilms' tumor, and rhabdomyosarcoma

**Usual Dosage** Refer to individual protocol as dosages vary with protocol used. Adjustments are made depending upon clinical and hematological response and upon adverse reactions.

Children: I.V.:
$\leq$10 kg or BSA <1 m$^2$: 0.05 mg/kg once weekly
2 mg/m$^2$; may repeat every week
Adults: I.V.: 0.4-1.4 mg/m$^2$, up to 2 mg maximum; may repeat every week

**Dosage Forms** Injection, as sulfate: 1 mg/mL (1 mL, 2 mL, 5 mL)

**vinorelbine** (vi NOR el been)

**U.S./Canadian Brand Names** Navelbine®

**Therapeutic Category** Antineoplastic Agent

**Use** Treatment of nonsmall cell lung cancer (as a single agent or in combination with cisplatin)

**Unlabeled use:** Breast cancer, ovarian carcinoma (cisplatin-resistant), Hodgkin's disease

**Usual Dosage** Varies depending upon clinical and hematological response (refer to individual protocols)

Adults: I.V.: 30 mg/m$^2$ every 7 days

**Dosage adjustment in hematological toxicity (based on granulocyte counts):**
Granulocytes $\geq$1500 cells/mm$^3$ on day of treatment: Administer 30 mg/m$^2$
Granulocytes 1000-1499 cells/mm$^3$ on day of treatment: Administer 15 mg/m$^2$
Granulocytes <1000 cells/mm$^3$ on day of treatment: Do not administer. Repeat granulocyte count in one week; if 3 consecutive doses are held because granulocyte count is <1000 cells/mm$^3$, discontinue vinorelbine

For patients who, during treatment, have experienced fever or sepsis while granulocytopenic or had 2 consecutive weekly doses held due to granulocytopenia, subsequent doses of vinorelbine should be:
22.5 mg/m$^2$ for granulocytes $\geq$1,500 cells/mm$^3$
11.25 mg/m$^2$ for granulocytes 1000-1499 cells/mm$^3$

**Dosage Forms** Injection, as tartrate: 10 mg/mL (1 mL, 5 mL)

**Vioform®** ***(Discontinued)*** *see page 750*

**Vioform® Hydrocortisone (Can)** *see* clioquinol and hydrocortisone *on page 143*

**Vioform®-Hydrocortisone Topical** ***(Discontinued)*** *see page 750*

**Viokase®** *see* pancrelipase *on page 448*

**viosterol** *see* ergocalciferol *on page 220*

**Vioxx®** *see* rofecoxib *on page 531*

**Vira-A® Ophthalmic** *see* vidarabine *on previous page*

**Viracept®** *see* nelfinavir *on page 412*

**Viramune®** *see* nevirapine *on page 417*

**Virazole® Aerosol** *see* ribavirin *on page 525*

**Virilon®** *see* methyltestosterone *on page 386*

**Viroptic® Ophthalmic** *see* trifluridine *on page 605*

**Viscoat®** *see* chondroitin sulfate-sodium hyaluronate *on page 135*

**Visine® [OTC]** *see* tetrahydrozoline *on page 580*

**Visine® Clear Ophthalmic [OTC]** *see* tetrahydrozoline *on page 580*

**Visine® Eye Ophthalmic [OTC]** *see* tetrahydrozoline *on page 580*

**Visine® L.R. Ophthalmic [OTC]** *see* oxymetazoline *on page 444*

**Visken®** *see* pindolol *on page 472*

**Vistacon-50® Injection *(Discontinued)*** *see page 750*

**Vistacot® Injection** *see* hydroxyzine *on page 308*

**Vistaject-25® *(Discontinued)*** *see page 750*

**Vistaject-50® *(Discontinued)*** *see page 750*

**Vistaquel® Injection *(Discontinued)*** *see page 750*

**Vistaril®** *see* hydroxyzine *on page 308*

**Vistaril® Injection *(Discontinued)*** *see page 750*

**Vistazine® Injection *(Discontinued)*** *see page 750*

**Vistide®** *see* cidofovir *on page 137*

**Vi-Sudo® [OTC]** *see* triprolidine and pseudoephedrine *on page 609*

**Visudyne™** *see* verteporfin *on page 626*

**Vita-C® [OTC]** *see* ascorbic acid *on page 54*

**VitaCarn® Oral** *see* levocarnitine *on page 345*

**Vital HN® [OTC]** *see* nutritional formula, enteral/oral *on page 432*

## vitamin A (VYE ta min aye)

**Synonyms** oleovitamin A

**U.S./Canadian Brand Names** Aquasol A®; Del-Vi-A®; Palmitate-A® 5000 [OTC]

**Therapeutic Category** Vitamin, Fat Soluble

**Use** Treatment and prevention of vitamin A deficiency; supplementation in patients with measles

**Usual Dosage**

RDA:
- 0-3 years: 400 mcg*
- 4-6 years: 500 mcg*
- 7-10 years: 700 mcg*
- >10 years: 800-1000 mcg*
- *mcg retinol equivalent (0.3 mcg retinol = 1 unit vitamin A)

Supplementation in measles: Children: Oral:
- <1 year: 100,000 units/day for 2 days
- >1 year: 200,000 units/day for 2 days

Severe deficiency with xerophthalmia:
- Children 1-8 years:
  - Oral: 5000-10,000 units/kg/day for 5 days or until recovery occurs
  - I.M.: 5000-15,000 units/day for 10 days
- Children >8 years and Adults:
  - Oral: 500,000 units/day for 3 days, then 50,000 units/day for 14 days, then 10,000-20,000 units/day for 2 months
  - I.M.: 50,000-100,000 units/day for 3 days, 50,000 units/day for 14 days

Deficiency (without corneal changes): Oral:
- Infants <1 year: 10,000 units/kg/day for 5 days, then 7500-15,000 units/day for 10 days
- Children 1-8 years: 5000-10,000 units/kg/day for 5 days, then 17,000-35,000 units/day for 10 days
- Children >8 years and Adults: 100,000 units/day for 3 days then 50,000 units/day for 14 days

Malabsorption syndrome (prophylaxis): Children >8 years and Adults: Oral: 10,000-50,000 units/day of water miscible product

(Continued)

## vitamin A *(Continued)*

Dietary supplement: Oral:
Infants up to 6 months: 1500 units/day
Children:
6 months to 3 years: 1500-2000 units/day
4-6 years: 2500 units/day
7-10 years: 3300-3500 units/day
Children >10 years and Adults: 4000-5000 units/day

**Dosage Forms**
Capsule: 10,000 units [OTC], 25,000 units, 50,000 units
Drops, oral (water miscible) [OTC]: 5000 units/0.1 mL (30 mL)
Injection: 50,000 units/mL (2 mL)
Tablet [OTC]: 5000 units

**vitamin A acid** *see* tretinoin (topical) *on page 600*

## vitamin A and vitamin D (VYE ta min aye & VYE ta min dee)

**Synonyms** cod liver oil
**U.S./Canadian Brand Names** A and D™ Ointment [OTC]
**Therapeutic Category** Protectant, Topical
**Use** Temporary relief of discomfort due to chapped skin, diaper rash, minor burns, abrasions, as well as irritations associated with ostomy skin care
**Usual Dosage**
Oral, oil: Dietary supplement: 2.5 mL/day
Topical: Apply locally with gentle massage as needed
**Dosage Forms** Ointment, topical: In a lanolin-petrolatum base (60 g)

**vitamin $B_1$** *see* thiamine *on page 584*

**vitamin $B_2$** *see* riboflavin *on page 525*

**vitamin $B_3$** *see* niacin *on page 417*

**vitamin $B_5$** *see* pantothenic acid *on page 450*

**vitamin $B_6$** *see* pyridoxine *on page 511*

**vitamin $B_{12}$** *see* cyanocobalamin *on page 158*

**vitamin $B_{12a}$** *see* hydroxocobalamin *on page 306*

## vitamin B complex (VYE ta min bee KOM pleks)

**U.S./Canadian Brand Names** Apatate® [OTC]; Gevrabon® [OTC]; Lederplex® [OTC]; Lipovite® [OTC]; Mega B® [OTC]; Megaton™ [OTC]; Mucoplex® [OTC]; NeoVadrin® B Complex [OTC]; Orexin® [OTC]; Surbex® [OTC]
**Therapeutic Category** Vitamin, Water Soluble
**Usual Dosage** Dosage is usually 1 tablet or capsule/day; please refer to package insert
**Dosage Forms**
Capsule
Solution: 5 mL, 360 mL

## vitamin B complex with vitamin C

(VYE ta min bee KOM pleks with VYE ta min see)

**U.S./Canadian Brand Names** Allbee® With C [OTC]; Surbex-T® Filmtabs® [OTC]; Surbex® With C Filmtabs® [OTC]; Thera-Combex® H-P Kapseals® [OTC]; Vicon-C® [OTC]
**Therapeutic Category** Vitamin, Water Soluble
**Use** Supportive nutritional supplementation in conditions in which water-soluble vitamins are required like GI disorders, chronic alcoholism, pregnancy, severe burns, and recovery from surgery
**Usual Dosage** Adults: Oral: 1 tablet/capsule daily
**Dosage Forms** Actual vitamin content may vary slightly depending on product used

Tablet/capsule: Vitamin $B_1$ 10-15 mg, vitamin $B_2$ 10 mg, vitamin $B_3$ 100 mg, vitamin $B_5$ 20 mg, vitamin $B_6$ 2-5 mg, vitamin $B_{12}$ 6-10 mg, vitamin C 300-500 mg

## vitamin B complex with vitamin C and folic acid

(VYE ta min bee KOM pleks with VYE ta min see & FOE lik AS id)

**U.S./Canadian Brand Names** Berocca®; Nephrocaps®

**Therapeutic Category** Vitamin, Water Soluble

**Use** Supportive nutritional supplementation in conditions in which water-soluble vitamins are required like GI disorders, chronic alcoholism, pregnancy, severe burns, and recovery from surgery

**Usual Dosage** Adults: Oral: 1 capsule/day

**Dosage Forms** Capsule

**vitamin C** *see* ascorbic acid *on page 54*

**Vitamin C Drops [OTC]** *see* ascorbic acid *on page 54*

**vitamin $D_2$** *see* ergocalciferol *on page 220*

## vitamin E (VYE ta min ee)

**Synonyms** *d*-alpha tocopherol; *dl*-alpha tocopherol

**U.S./Canadian Brand Names** Amino-Opti-E® [OTC]; Aquasol E® [OTC]; E-Complex-600® [OTC]; E-Vitamin® [OTC]; Vita-Plus® E Softgels® [OTC]; Vitec® [OTC]; Vite E® Creme [OTC]

**Therapeutic Category** Vitamin, Fat Soluble; Vitamin, Topical

**Use** Prevention and treatment of vitamin E deficiency

**Usual Dosage**

RDA: Oral:

Premature Infants ≤3 months: 25 units/day

Infants:

≤6 months: 4.5 units/day

6-12 months: 6 units/day

Children:

1-3 years: 9 units/day

4-10 years: 10.5 units/day

Adults >11 years:

Female: 12 units/day

Male: 15 units/day

Prevention of vitamin E deficiency: Neonates, premature, low birthweight (results in normal levels within 1 week): Oral: 25-50 units/24 hours until 6-10 weeks of age or 125-150 units/kg total in 4 doses on days 1, 2, 7, and 8 of life

Vitamin E deficiency treatment: Adults: Oral: 50-200 units/24 hours for 2 weeks

Topical: Apply a thin layer over affected areas as needed

**Dosage Forms**

Capsule: 100 units, 200 units, 330 mg, 400 units, 500 units, 600 units, 1000 units

Capsule, water miscible: 73.5 mg, 147 mg, 165 mg, 330 mg, 400 units

Cream: 50 mg/g (15 g, 30 g, 60 g, 75 g, 120 g, 454 g)

Drops, oral: 50 mg/mL (12 mL, 30 mL)

Liquid, topical: 10 mL, 15 mL, 30 mL, 60 mL

Lotion: 120 mL

Oil: 15 mL, 30 mL, 60 mL

Ointment, topical: 30 mg/g (45 g, 60 g)

Tablet: 200 units, 400 units

**vitamin G** *see* riboflavin *on page 525*

**vitamin $K_1$** *see* phytonadione *on page 470*

## vitamin (multiple/injectable)

**U.S./Canadian Brand Names** M.V.C.® 9 + 3; M.V.I.®-12; M.V.I.® Concentrate; M.V.I.® Pediatric

**Therapeutic Category** Vitamin

**Usual Dosage** I.V.:

Children:

≤5 kg: 10 mL/1000 mL TPN (M.V.I.® Pediatric)

5.1 kg to 11 years: 5 mL/one TPN bag/day (M.V.I.® Pediatric)

Children >11 years and Adults: 5 mL of vials 1 and 2 (M.V.I.®-12)/one TPN bag/day

**Dosage Forms** See Multivitamins table.

## vitamin (multiple/oral) (VYE ta mins, MUL ti pul/OR al)

**U.S./Canadian Brand Names** Becotin® Pulvules®; Cefol® Filmtab®; Eldercaps® [OTC]; Icaps® (Can); Infantol® (Can); Maltlevol® (Can); NeoVadrin® [OTC]; Niferex®-PN; Ocuvite™ (Can); Orifer® F (Can); Penta/3B® Plus (Can); Prenavite® Forte (Can); Secran®; Sopalamine/3B Plus C (Can); Spectrum™ Forte 29 (Can); Stresstabs® 600 Advanced Formula Tablets [OTC]; Therabid® [OTC]; Theragran® [OTC]; Theragran® Hematinic®; Theragran® Liquid [OTC]; Theragran-M® [OTC]; Unicap® [OTC]; Vicon Forte®; Vicon® Plus [OTC]

**Therapeutic Category** Vitamin

**Use** Dietary supplement

**Usual Dosage** Adults: Oral: 1 tablet/day or 5 mL/day liquid

**Dosage Forms** See Multivitamins table.

## vitamin (multiple/pediatric)

**Synonyms** children's vitamins; multivitamins/fluoride

**U.S./Canadian Brand Names** Adeflor®; ADEKs® Pediatric Drops; LKV-Drops® [OTC]; Multi Vit® Drops [OTC]; Poly-Vi-Flor®; Poly-Vi-Sol® [OTC]; Tri-Vi-Flor®; Tri-Vi-Sol® [OTC]; Vi-Daylin® [OTC]; Vi-Daylin/F®

**Therapeutic Category** Vitamin

**Use** Nutritional supplement, vitamin deficiency

**Usual Dosage** Oral: 0.6 mL or 1 mL/day; please refer to package insert

**Dosage Forms** See Multivitamins table.

## vitamin (multiple/prenatal)

**Synonyms** prenatal vitamins

**U.S./Canadian Brand Names** Chromagen® OB [OTC]; Materna®; Natabec® [OTC]; Natabec® FA [OTC]; Natabec® Rx; Natalins® [OTC]; Natalins® Rx; Pramet® FA; Pramilet® FA; Prenavite® [OTC]; Stuartnatal® 1 + 1; Stuart Prenatal® [OTC]

**Therapeutic Category** Vitamin

**Use** Nutritional supplement, vitamin deficiency

**Usual Dosage** Oral: 1 tablet or capsule daily; please refer to package insert

**Dosage Forms** See Multivitamins table.

**Vitaneed™ [OTC]** *see* nutritional formula, enteral/oral *on page 432*

**Vita-Plus® E Softgels® [OTC]** *see* vitamin E *on previous page*

**Vitec® [OTC]** *see* vitamin E *on previous page*

**Vite E® Creme [OTC]** *see* vitamin E *on previous page*

**Vitoxapap® [OTC]** *see* acetaminophen and phenyltoloxamine *on page 5*

**Vitrasert®** *see* ganciclovir *on page 269*

**Vitravene™** *see* fomivirsen *on page 264*

**Vitrax®** *see* sodium hyaluronate *on page 550*

**Vivactil®** *see* protriptyline *on page 507*

**Viva-Drops® Solution [OTC]** *see* artificial tears *on page 53*

## Multivitamin Products Available

| Product | Content Given Per | A IU | D IU | E IU | C mg | FA mg | $B_1$ mg | $B_2$ mg | $B_3$ mg | $B_6$ mg | $B_{12}$ mcg | Other |
|---|---|---|---|---|---|---|---|---|---|---|---|---|
| Theragran® | 5 mL liquid | 10,000 | 400 | | 200 | | 10 | 10 | 100 | 4.1 | 5 | $B_5$ 21.4 mg |
| Vi-Daylin® | 1 mL drops | 1500 | 400 | 4.1 | 35 | | 0.5 | 0.6 | 8 | 0.4 | 1.5 | Alcohol <0.5% |
| Vi-Daylin® Iron | 1 mL | 1500 | 400 | 4.1 | 35 | | 0.5 | 0.6 | 8 | 0.4 | | Fe 10 mg |
| Albee® with C | tablet | | | | 300 | | 15 | 10.2 | | 5 | | Niacinamide 50 mg, pantothenic acid 10 mg |
| Vitamin B complex | tablet | | | | | 400 mcg | 1.5 | 1.7 | | 2 | 6 | Niacinamide 20 mg |
| Hexavitamin | cap/tab | 5000 | 400 | | 75 | | 2 | 3 | 20 | | | |
| Iberet-Folic-500® | tablet | | | | 500 | 0.8 | 6 | 6 | 30 | 5 | 25 | $B_5$ 10 mg, Fe 105 mg |
| Stuartnatal® 1+1 | tablet | 4000 | 400 | 11 | 120 | 1 | 1.5 | 3 | 20 | 10 | 12 | Cu, Zn 25 mg, Fe 65 mg, Ca 200 mg |
| Theragran-M® | tablet | 5000 | 400 | 30 | 90 | 0.4 | 3 | 3.4 | 30 | 3 | 9 | Cl, Cr, I, K, $B_5$ 10 mg, Mg, Mn, Mo, P, Se, Zn 15 mg, Fe 27 mg, biotin 30 mcg, beta-carotene 1250 IU |
| Vi-Daylin® | tablet | 2500 | 400 | 15 | 60 | 0.3 | 1.05 | 1.2 | 13.5 | 1.05 | 4.5 | |
| M.V.I.®-12 injection | 5 mL | 3300 | 200 | 10 | 100 | 0.4 | 3 | 3.6 | 40 | 4 | 5 | $B_5$ 15 mg, biotin 60 mcg |
| M.V.I.®-12 unit vial | 20 mL | | | | | | | | | | | |
| M.V.I.® pediatric powder | 5 mL | 2300 | 400 | 7 | 80 | 0.14 | 1.2 | 1.4 | 17 | 1 | 1 | $B_5$ 5 mg, biotin 20 mcg, vitamin K 200 mcg |

**Vivelle™ Transdermal** *see* estradiol *on page 224*

**Vivol® (Can)** *see* diazepam *on page 179*

**Vivonex® [OTC]** *see* nutritional formula, enteral/oral *on page 432*

**Vivonex® T.E.N. [OTC]** *see* nutritional formula, enteral/oral *on page 432*

**Vivotif Berna™ Oral** *see* typhoid vaccine *on page 614*

**V-Lax® [OTC]** *see* psyllium *on page 509*

**VLB** *see* vinblastine *on page 627*

**VM-26** *see* teniposide *on page 573*

**Vofenal™ (Can)** *see* diclofenac *on page 181*

**Volmax®** *see* albuterol *on page 16*

**Voltaren® Ophthalmic** *see* diclofenac *on page 181*

**Voltaren® Oral** *see* diclofenac *on page 181*

**Voltaren Rapide® (Can)** *see* diclofenac *on page 181*

**Voltaren®-XR Oral** *see* diclofenac *on page 181*

**Vontrol®** ***(Discontinued)*** *see page 750*

**VōSol® HC Otic** *see* acetic acid, propylene glycol diacetate, and hydrocortisone *on page 9*

**VōSol® Otic** *see* acetic acid *on page 8*

**VP-16** *see* etoposide *on page 236*

**Vumon®** *see* teniposide *on page 573*

**V.V.S.®** *see* sulfabenzamide, sulfacetamide, and sulfathiazole *on page 562*

**Vytone® Topical** *see* iodoquinol and hydrocortisone *on page 324*

**VZIG** *see* varicella-zoster immune globulin (human) *on page 622*

## warfarin (WAR far in)

**U.S./Canadian Brand Names** Coumadin®

**Therapeutic Category** Anticoagulant

**Use** Prophylaxis and treatment of venous thromboembolic disorders; prevention of arterial thromboembolism in patients with prosthetic heart valves or atrial fibrillation; prevention of death, venous thromboembolism, and recurrent MI after acute MI

**Usual Dosage**

Oral:

Infants and Children: 0.05-0.34 mg/kg/day; infants <12 months of age may require doses at or near the high end of this range; consistent anticoagulation may be difficult to maintain in children <5 years of age

Adults: 5-15 mg/day for 2-5 days, then adjust dose according to results of prothrombin time; usual maintenance dose ranges from 2-10 mg/day

I.V. (administer as a slow bolus injection): 2-5 mg/day

**Dosage Forms**

Powder for injection, as sodium, lyophilized: 5 mg

Tablet, as sodium: 1 mg, 2 mg, 2.5 mg, 3 mg, 4 mg, 5 mg, 6 mg, 7.5 mg, 10 mg

**Wartec® (Can)** *see* podofilox *on page 479*

**4-Way® Long Acting Nasal Solution [OTC]** *see* oxymetazoline *on page 444*

**Wehamine® Injection** ***(Discontinued)*** *see page 750*

**Wehdryl®** ***(Discontinued)*** *see page 750*

**Welchol™** *see* colesevelam *on page 152*

**Wellbutrin®** *see* bupropion *on page 91*

**Wellbutrin® SR** *see* bupropion *on page 91*

**Wellcovorin®** *see* leucovorin *on page 343*

**Wesprin® Buffered *(Discontinued)*** *see page 750*

**Westcort® Topical** *see* hydrocortisone (topical) *on page 304*

**Westhroid®** *see* thyroid *on page 588*

**Westmycin®** *see* tetracycline *on page 579*

**Whitfield's Ointment [OTC]** *see* benzoic acid and salicylic acid *on page 73*

**Wigraine®** *see* ergotamine *on page 221*

**Winks® [OTC]** *see* diphenhydramine *on page 191*

**Winpred™ (Can)** *see* prednisone *on page 493*

**WinRho SD®** *see* $Rh_0$(D) immune globulin (intravenous-human) *on page 524*

**WinRho SDF®** *see* $Rh_0$(D) immune globulin (intravenous-human) *on page 524*

**Winstrol®** *see* stanozolol *on page 557*

## witch hazel (witch HAY zel)

**Synonyms** hamamelis water

**U.S./Canadian Brand Names** Tucks® [OTC]; Preparation H® Cleansing Pads (Can)

**Therapeutic Category** Astringent

**Use** After-stool wipe to remove most causes of local irritation; temporary management of vulvitis, pruritus ani and vulva; help relieve the discomfort of simple hemorrhoids, anorectal surgical wounds, and episiotomies

**Usual Dosage** Apply to anorectal area as needed

**Dosage Forms**

Cream: 50% (40 g)
Gel: 50% with glycerin (19.8 g)
Pads: 50% with glycerin 10%, and benzalkonium chloride 0.003% (40s, 100s)

**Wolfina® *(Discontinued)*** *see page 750*

**wood sugar** *see* d-xylose *on page 208*

**Wyamine® Sulfate** *see* mephentermine *on page 372*

**Wyamycin S® *(Discontinued)*** *see page 750*

**Wycillin®** *see* penicillin G procaine *on page 457*

**Wydase®** *see* hyaluronidase *on page 297*

**Wygesic®** *see* propoxyphene and acetaminophen *on page 504*

**Wymox®** *see* amoxicillin *on page 35*

**Wytensin®** *see* guanabenz *on page 285*

**Xalatan®** *see* latanoprost *on page 341*

**Xanax®** *see* alprazolam *on page 22*

**Xeloda®** *see* capecitabine *on page 103*

**Xenical®** *see* orlistat *on page 438*

**Xiral®** *see* chlorpheniramine, pseudoephedrine, and methscopolamine *on page 132*

**Xopenex™** *see* levalbuterol *on page 343*

**X-Prep® Liquid [OTC]** *see* senna *on page 541*

**X-Seb® T [OTC]** *see* coal tar and salicylic acid *on page 149*

**Xylocaine® HCl I.V. Injection for Cardiac Arrhythmias** *see* lidocaine *on page 348*

**Xylocaine® Oral** *see* lidocaine *on page 348*

**Xylocaine® Topical Ointment** *see* lidocaine *on page 348*

**Xylocaine® Topical Solution** *see* lidocaine *on page 348*

**Xylocaine® Topical Spray** *see* lidocaine *on page 348*

**Xylocaine® With Epinephrine** *see* lidocaine and epinephrine *on page 349*

**Xylocard® (Can)** *see* lidocaine *on page 348*

## xylometazoline (zye loe met AZ oh leen)

**U.S./Canadian Brand Names** Otrivin® Nasal [OTC]; Decongest (Can)

**Therapeutic Category** Adrenergic Agonist Agent

**Use** Symptomatic relief of nasal and nasopharyngeal mucosal congestion

**Usual Dosage**

Children <12 years: 2-3 drops (0.05%) in each nostril every 8-10 hours

Children >12 years and Adults: 2-3 drops or sprays (0.1%) in each nostril every 8-10 hours

**Dosage Forms** Solution, nasal, as hydrochloride: 0.05% [0.5 mg/mL] (20 mL); 0.1% [1 mg/mL] (15 mL, 20 mL)

**Xylo-Pfan® [OTC]** *see* d-xylose *on page 208*

**Yasmin®** *see* ethinyl estradiol and drospirenone *on page 231*

**Yeast-Gard® Medicated Douche** *see* povidone-iodine *on page 489*

## yellow fever vaccine (YEL oh FEE ver vak SEEN)

**U.S./Canadian Brand Names** YF-VAX®

**Therapeutic Category** Vaccine, Live Virus

**Use** Active immunization against yellow fever

**Usual Dosage** Single-dose S.C.: 0.5 mL

**Dosage Forms** Injection: Not less than 5.04 $Log_{10}$ Plaque Forming Units (PFU); Not less than 25.2 $Log_{10}$ Plaque Forming Units (PFU)

**yellow mercuric oxide** *see* mercuric oxide *on page 374*

**YF-VAX®** *see* yellow fever vaccine *on this page*

**Yocon®** *see* yohimbine *on this page*

**Yodoxin®** *see* iodoquinol *on page 324*

## yohimbine (yo HIM bine)

**U.S./Canadian Brand Names** Actibine®; Aphrodyne™; Testomar®; Yocon®; Yohimex™

**Therapeutic Category** Miscellaneous Product

**Use** No FDA sanctioned indications

**Usual Dosage** Adults: Oral: 1 tablet 3 times/day

**Dosage Forms** Tablet, as hydrochloride: 5.4 mg

**Yohimex™** *see* yohimbine *on this page*

**Yutopar®** *see* ritodrine *on page 529*

**Zaditen® (Can)** *see* ketotifen *on page 335*

**Zaditor™** *see* ketotifen *on page 335*

## zafirlukast (za FIR loo kast)

**U.S./Canadian Brand Names** Accolate®

**Therapeutic Category** Leukotriene Receptor Antagonist

**Use** Prophylaxis and chronic treatment of asthma in adults and children ≥7 years of age

**Usual Dosage**

Children <7 years: Safety and effectiveness has not been established

Children 7-11 years: 10 mg twice daily

Adults: Oral: 20 mg twice daily; administer 1 hour before food or 2 hours after food

**Dosage Forms** Tablet: 10 mg, 20 mg

**Zagam®** *see* sparfloxacin *on page 555*

**zalcitabine** (zal SITE a been)

**Synonyms** ddC; dideoxycytidine

**U.S./Canadian Brand Names** Hivid®

**Therapeutic Category** Antiviral Agent

**Use** Treatment of HIV infections as monotherapy (in patients intolerant to zidovudine or with disease progression while on zidovudine) or in combination with zidovudine in patients with advanced HIV disease (adult CD4 cell count of 150-300 cells/mm$^3$)

**Usual Dosage** Oral:

Safety and efficacy in children <13 years of age have not been established

Adults (dosed in combination with zidovudine): Daily dose: 0.750 mg every 8 hours, administered together with 200 mg of zidovudine (ie, total daily dose: 2.25 mg of zalcitabine and 600 mg of zidovudine)

**Dosage Forms** Tablet: 0.375 mg, 0.75 mg

**zaleplon** (ZAL e plon)

**U.S./Canadian Brand Names** Sonata®; Starnoc® (Can)

**Therapeutic Category** Hypnotic, Nonbenzodiazepine (Pyrazolopyrimidine)

**Use** Short-term treatment of insomnia

**Usual Dosage**

Adults: Oral: 10 mg at bedtime (range: 5-20 mg)

Elderly: 5 mg at bedtime

**Dosage Forms** Capsule: 5 mg, 10 mg

**Zanaflex®** *see* tizanidine *on page 592*

**zanamivir** (za NA mi veer)

**U.S./Canadian Brand Names** Relenza®

**Therapeutic Category** Antiviral Agent

**Use** Treatment of uncomplicated acute illness due to influenza virus in adults and adolescents 12 years of age or older. Treatment should only be initiated in patients who have been symptomatic for no more than 2 days.

**Usual Dosage** Adolescents ≥12 years and Adults: 2 Inhalations: (10 mg total) twice daily for 5 days. Two doses should be taken on the first day of dosing, regardless of interval, while doses should be spaced by approximately 12 hours on subsequent days.

**Dosage Forms** Powder, for inhalation: 5 mg per blister

**Zanosar®** *see* streptozocin *on page 560*

**Zantac®** *see* ranitidine hydrochloride *on page 519*

**Zantac® 75 [OTC]** *see* ranitidine hydrochloride *on page 519*

**Zantryl®** ***(Discontinued)*** *see page 750*

**ZapZyt® [OTC]** *see* benzoyl peroxide *on page 74*

**Zarontin®** *see* ethosuximide *on page 234*

**Zaroxolyn®** *see* metolazone *on page 387*

**Zartan®** ***(Discontinued)*** *see page 750*

**Zeasorb-AF®** ***(Discontinued)*** *see page 750*

**Zeasorb-AF® Powder [OTC]** *see* miconazole *on page 390*

**Zebeta®** *see* bisoprolol *on page 82*

**Zebrax®** ***(Discontinued)*** *see page 750*

**Zebutal®** *see* butalbital compound and acetaminophen *on page 93*

**Zefazone®** ***(Discontinued)*** *see page 750*

**Zemplar™** *see* paricalcitol *on page 451*

**Zemuron™** *see* rocuronium *on page 531*

**Zenapax®** *see* daclizumab *on page 164*

**Zephiran® [OTC]** *see* benzalkonium chloride *on page 72*

**Zephrex®** *see* guaifenesin and pseudoephedrine *on page 283*

**Zephrex LA®** *see* guaifenesin and pseudoephedrine *on page 283*

**Zerit®** *see* stavudine *on page 557*

**Zestoretic®** *see* lisinopril and hydrochlorothiazide *on page 353*

**Zestril®** *see* lisinopril *on page 352*

**Zetar® [OTC]** *see* coal tar *on page 149*

**Zetran®** ***(Discontinued)*** *see page 750*

**Ziac™** *see* bisoprolol and hydrochlorothiazide *on page 82*

**Ziagen®** *see* abacavir *on page 2*

## zidovudine (zye DOE vyoo deen)

**Synonyms** azidothymidine; AZT; compound S

**U.S./Canadian Brand Names** Apo®-Zidovudine (Can); Novo-AZT (Can); Retrovir®

**Therapeutic Category** Antiviral Agent

**Use** Management of patients with HIV infections who have had at least one episode of *Pneumocystis carinii* pneumonia or who have CD4 cell counts (cells/mm$^3$) of ≤500 in children >6 years and adults, <750 in children 2-6 years, <1000 in children 1-2 years, and <1750 for children <1 year; patients who have HIV-related symptoms or who are asymptomatic with abnormal laboratory values indicating HIV-related immunosuppression; prevention of maternal-fetal HIV transmission

**Usual Dosage**

Children 3 months to 12 years:
- Oral: 90-180 mg/m$^2$/dose every 6 hours; maximum: 200 mg every 6 hours
- I.V. continuous infusion: 0.5-1.8 mg/kg/hour
- I.V. intermittent infusion: 100 mg/m$^2$/dose every 6 hours

Adults:
- Oral:
  - Asymptomatic infection: 100 mg every 4 hours while awake (500 mg/day)
  - Symptomatic HIV infection: Initial: 200 mg every 4 hours (1200 mg/day), then after 1 month, 100 mg every 4 hours (600 mg/day)
- I.V.: 1-2 mg/kg/dose every 4 hours

**Dosage Forms**

Capsule: 100 mg
Injection: 10 mg/mL (20 mL)
Syrup (strawberry flavor): 50 mg/5 mL (240 mL)
Tablet: 300 mg

## zidovudine and lamivudine (zye DOE vyoo deen & la MI vyoo deen)

**Synonyms** AZT + 3TC

**U.S./Canadian Brand Names** Combivir®

**Therapeutic Category** Antiviral Agent

**Use** Combivir® given twice a day, provides an alternative regimen to lamivudine 150 mg twice a day plus zidovudine 600 mg per day in divided doses; this drug form reduces capsule/tablet intake for these two drugs to two per day instead of up to eight

**Usual Dosage** Children >12 years and Adults: Oral: One tablet twice daily

**Dosage Forms** Tablet: Zidovudine 300 mg and lamivudine 150 mg

**Zilactin®-B Medicated [OTC]** *see* benzocaine *on page 72*

## zileuton (zye LOO ton)

**U.S./Canadian Brand Names** Zyflo™

**Therapeutic Category** 5-Lipoxygenase Inhibitor

**Use** Prophylaxis and chronic treatment of asthma in adults and children ≥12 years of age

**Usual Dosage** Children ≥12 years and Adults: Oral: 1 tablet 4 times/day, may be taken with meals and at bedtime

**Dosage Forms** Tablet: 600 mg

**Zinacef® Injection** *see* cefuroxime *on page 118*

**Zinca-Pak®** *see* trace metals *on page 598*

**Zincate® Oral** *see* zinc sulfate *on this page*

## zinc chloride (zingk KLOR ide)

**Therapeutic Category** Trace Element

**Use** Cofactor for replacement therapy to different enzymes helps maintain normal growth rates, normal skin hydration and senses of taste and smell

**Usual Dosage** Clinical response may not occur for up to 6-8 weeks

Supplemental to I.V. solutions:

Premature Infants <1500 g, up to 3 kg: 300 mcg/kg/day

Full-term Infants and Children ≤5 years: 100 mcg/kg/day

Adults:

Stable with fluid loss from small bowel: 12.2 mg zinc/liter TPN or 17.1 mg zinc/kg (added to 1000 mL I.V. fluids) of stool or ileostomy output

Metabolically stable: 2.5-4 mg/day, add 2 mg/day for acute catabolic states

**Dosage Forms** Injection: 1 mg/mL (10 mL)

**Zincfrin® Ophthalmic [OTC]** *see* phenylephrine and zinc sulfate *on page 468*

## zinc gelatin (zingk JEL ah tin)

**Synonyms** Unna's boot; Unna's paste

**U.S./Canadian Brand Names** Gelucast®

**Therapeutic Category** Protectant, Topical

**Use** Protectant and to support varicosities and similar lesions of the lower limbs

**Usual Dosage** Apply externally as an occlusive boot

**Dosage Forms** Bandage: 3" x 10 yards, 4" x 10 yards

**zinc injection** *see* trace metals *on page 598*

**Zincon® Shampoo [OTC]** *see* pyrithione zinc *on page 512*

## zinc oxide (zingk OKS ide)

**Synonyms** Lassar's zinc paste

**Therapeutic Category** Topical Skin Product

**Use** Protective coating for mild skin irritations and abrasions; soothing and protective ointment to promote healing of chapped skin, diaper rash

**Usual Dosage** Infants, Children, and Adults: Topical: Apply several times daily to affected area

**Dosage Forms**

Ointment, topical: 20% in white ointment (480 g)

Paste, topical: 25% in white petrolatum (480 g)

## zinc oxide, cod liver oil, and talc (zingk OKS ide, kod LIV er oyl, & talk)

**U.S./Canadian Brand Names** Desitin® [OTC]

**Therapeutic Category** Protectant, Topical

**Use** Relief of diaper rash, superficial wounds and burns, and other minor skin irritations

**Usual Dosage** Topical: Apply thin layer as needed

**Dosage Forms** Ointment, topical: Zinc oxide, cod liver oil and talc in a petrolatum and lanolin base (30 g, 60 g, 120 g, 240 g, 270 g)

## zinc sulfate (zingk SUL fate)

**U.S./Canadian Brand Names** Eye-Sed® Ophthalmic [OTC]; Orazinc® Oral [OTC]; Verazinc® Oral [OTC]; Zincate® Oral

(Continued)

## zinc sulfate *(Continued)*

**Therapeutic Category** Electrolyte Supplement, Oral

**Use** Zinc supplement (oral and parenteral); may improve wound healing in those who are deficient

**Usual Dosage**

RDA: Oral:

Birth to 6 months: 3 mg elemental zinc/day

6-12 months: 5 mg elemental zinc/day

1-10 years: 10 mg elemental zinc/day

≥11 years: 15 mg elemental zinc/day

Zinc deficiency: Oral:

Infants and Children: 0.5-1 mg elemental zinc/kg/day divided 1-3 times/day; somewhat larger quantities may be needed if there is impaired intestinal absorption or an excessive loss of zinc

Adults: 110-220 mg zinc sulfate (25-50 mg elemental zinc)/dose 3 times/day

**Dosage Forms**

Capsule: 110 mg [elemental zinc 25 mg]; 220 mg [elemental zinc 50 mg]

Injection: 1 mg/mL (10 mL, 30 mL); 4 mg/mL (10 mL); 5 mg/mL (5 mL, 10 mL, 50 mL)

Tablet: 66 mg [elemental zinc 15 mg]; 200 mg [elemental zinc 46 mg]

**zinc undecylenate** *see* undecylenic acid and derivatives *on page 616*

**Zinecard®** *see* dexrazoxane *on page 176*

**Zithromax®** *see* azithromycin *on page 62*

**Zithromax® Z-PAK®** *see* azithromycin *on page 62*

**ZNP® Bar [OTC]** *see* pyrithione zinc *on page 512*

**Zocor®** *see* simvastatin *on page 545*

**Zofran®** *see* ondansetron *on page 436*

**Zofran® ODT** *see* ondansetron *on page 436*

**Zoladex® Implant** *see* goserelin *on page 280*

**zoledronate** *see* zoledronic acid *on this page*

## zoledronic acid (ZOE le dron ik AS id)

**Synonyms** CGP-42446; zoledronate

**U.S./Canadian Brand Names** Zometa®

**Therapeutic Category** Bisphosphonate Derivative

**Use** Treatment of cancer-associated hypercalcemia; prevention of skeletal events in patients with osteolytic metastatic lesions

**Usual Dosage** I.V.: Adults: Hypercalcemia of malignancy (albumin-corrected serum calcium ≥12 mg/dL): 4 mg (maximum) given as a single dose infused over **no less than 15 minutes**; patients should be adequately hydrated prior to treatment (restoring urine output to ~2 L/day). Monitor serum calcium and wait at least 7 days before considering retreatment. Dosage adjustment may be needed in patients with decreased renal function following treatment.

**Dosage Forms** Powder for injection: 4 mg [as monohydrate 4.264 mg]

**Zolicef®** *see* cefazolin *on page 114*

## zolmitriptan (zohl mi TRIP tan)

**Synonyms** 311C90

**U.S./Canadian Brand Names** Zomig®

**Therapeutic Category** Antimigraine Agent; Serotonin Agonist

**Use** Acute treatment of adult migraine, with or without auras.

**Usual Dosage** Adults: Oral: Single doses of 1, 2.5, or 5 mg are effective in reducing symptoms of a migraine attack. Patients should be started at a dose of 2.5 mg or lower since the incidence of side effects increases somewhat with dose. If the headache returns, the dose may be repeated after 2 hours but **not to exceed** 10 mg within a 24-hour period.

**Dosage Forms** Tablet: 2.5 mg, 5 mg

**Zoloft®** *see* sertraline *on page 542*

## zolpidem (zole PI dem)

**U.S./Canadian Brand Names** Ambien™

**Therapeutic Category** Hypnotic, Nonbarbiturate

**Use** Short-term treatment of insomnia

**Usual Dosage** Adults: Oral: 10 mg immediately before bedtime

**Dosage Forms** Tablet, as tartrate: 5 mg, 10 mg

**Zolyse®** ***(Discontinued)*** *see page 750*

**Zometa®** *see* zoledronic acid *on previous page*

**Zomig®** *see* zolmitriptan *on previous page*

**Zonalon® Topical Cream** *see* doxepin *on page 202*

**Zone-A Forte®** *see* pramoxine and hydrocortisone *on page 490*

**Zonegran™** *see* zonisamide *on this page*

## zonisamide (zoe NIS a mide)

**U.S./Canadian Brand Names** Zonegran™

**Therapeutic Category** Anticonvulsant, Sulfonamide

**Use** Adjunct treatment of partial seizures in adults with epilepsy

**Usual Dosage**

Children >16 years and Adults: Oral: For the adjunctive treatment of partial seizures, initial dose is 100 mg/day. Dose may be increased to 200 mg/day after 2 weeks. Further dosage increases to 300 mg and 400 mg/day can then be made with a minimum of 2 weeks between adjustments, in order to reach steady state at each dosage level. Doses of up to 600 mg/day have been studied, however, there is no evidence of increased response with doses above 400 mg/day.

**Dosage Forms** Capsule: 100 mg

## zopiclone *(Canada only)* (ZOE pi clone)

**U.S./Canadian Brand Names** Apo®-Zopiclone (Can); Gen-Zopiclone (Can); Imovane® (Can); Nu-Zopiclone (Can); Rhovane® (Can)

**Therapeutic Category** Hypnotic

**Use** Treatment of insomnia (to be used <28-day duration)

**Usual Dosage** Oral: 7.5 mg 30-60 minutes before bedtime

**Dosage Forms** Tablet: 7.5 mg

**ZORprin®** *see* aspirin *on page 55*

**Zostrix® [OTC]** *see* capsaicin *on page 104*

**Zostrix High Potency®** *see* capsaicin *on page 104*

**Zostrix®-HP [OTC]** *see* capsaicin *on page 104*

**Zostrix Sports®** *see* capsaicin *on page 104*

**Zosyn™** *see* piperacillin and tazobactam sodium *on page 473*

**Zovia™** *see* ethinyl estradiol and ethynodiol diacetate *on page 232*

**Zovirax®** *see* acyclovir *on page 12*

## zuclopenthixol *(Canada only)* (zoo kloe pen THIX ol)

**U.S./Canadian Brand Names** Clopixol-Acuphase® (Can); Clopixol® (Can); Clopixol® Depot (Can)

(Continued)

## zuclopenthixol *(Canada only)* *(Continued)*

**Therapeutic Category** Antipsychotic Agent

**Use** Schizophrenia, bipolar disorder, psychoses; usually useful in agitated states

**Usual Dosage**

Oral: Zuclopenthixol hydrochloride: Initial: 20-30 mg/day in divided doses; usual maintenance dose: 20-75 mg/day; maximum daily dose: 150 mg

I.M.:

Zuclopenthixol acetate: 50-150 mg; may be repeated in 2-3 days; no more than 4 injections should be given in the course of treatment; maximum dose during course of treatment: 400 mg

Zuclopenthixol decanoate: 100 mg by deep I.M. injection; additional doses of 100-200 mg (I.M.) may be given over the following 1-4 weeks; maximum weekly dose: 600 mg

**Dosage Forms**

Injection:

Acuphase, as acetate: 50 mg/mL [zuclopenthixol 42.5 mg/mL] (1 mL, 2 mL)

Depot, as decanoate: 200 mg/mL [zuclopenthixol 144.4 mg/mL] (10 mL)

Tablet, as dihydrochloride: 10 mg, 25 mg, 40 mg

**Zyban™** *see* bupropion *on page 91*

**Zyban™ 100 mg *(Discontinued)*** *see page 750*

**Zydone®** *see* hydrocodone and acetaminophen *on page 300*

**Zyflo™** *see* zileuton *on page 638*

**Zyloprim®** *see* allopurinol *on page 21*

**Zymase®** *see* pancrelipase *on page 448*

**Zyprexa®** *see* olanzapine *on page 434*

**Zyprexa® Zydis®** *see* olanzapine *on page 434*

**Zyrtec®** *see* cetirizine *on page 121*

**Zyrtec-D 12 Hour™** *see* cetirizine and pseudoephedrine *on page 122*

**Zyvox™** *see* linezolid *on page 351*

# APPENDIX

APPENDIX

# ABBREVIATIONS & SYMBOLS COMMONLY USED IN MEDICAL ORDERS

| Abbreviation | From | Meaning |
|---|---|---|
| μg | | microgram |
| μmol | | micromole |
| °C | | degrees Celsius (Centigrade) |
| < | | less than |
| > | | greater than |
| ≤ | | less than or equal to |
| ≥ | | greater than or equal to |
| $\overline{aa}$, aa | ana | of each |
| AA | | Alcoholics Anonymous |
| ABG | | arterial blood gas |
| ac | ante cibum | before meals or food |
| ACE | | angiotensin-converting enzyme |
| ACLS | | adult cardiac life support |
| ad | ad | to, up to |
| a.d. | aurio dextra | right ear |
| ADH | | antidiuretic hormone |
| ADHD | | attention-deficit/hyperactivity disorder |
| ADLs | | activities of daily living |
| ad lib | ad libitum | at pleasure |
| AED | | antiepileptic drug |
| AIMS | | Abnormal Involuntary Movement Scale |
| a.l. | aurio laeva | left ear |
| ALL | | acute lymphoblastic leukemia |
| ALT | | alanine aminotransferase (was SGPT) |
| AM | ante meridiem | morning |
| AML | | acute myeloblastic leukemia |
| amp | | ampul |
| amt | | amount |
| ANA | | antinuclear antibodies |
| ANC | | absolute neutrophil count |
| ANL | | acute nonlymphoblastic leukemia |
| aq | aqua | water |
| aq. dest. | aqua destillata | distilled water |
| APTT | | activated partial thromboplastin time |
| a.s. | aurio sinister | left ear |
| ASA (class I-IV) | | classification of surgical patients according to their baseline health (eg, healthy ASA and II or increased severity of illness ASA III or IV) |
| ASAP | | as soon as possible |
| AST | | aspartate aminotransferase (was SGOT) |
| a.u. | aures utrae | each ear |
| AUC | | area under the curve |
| A-V | | atrial-ventricular |
| BDI | | Beck Depression Inventory |
| bid | bis in die | twice daily |
| bm | | bowel movement |
| BMT | | bone marrow transplant |
| bp | | blood pressure |
| BPRS | | Brief Psychiatric Rating Scale |
| BSA | | body surface area |
| BUN | | blood urea nitrogen |
| c | cong | a gallon |
| $\bar{c}$ | cum | with |
| cal | | calorie |
| cAMP | | cyclic adenosine monophosphate |
| cap | capsula | capsule |
| CBC | | complete blood count |
| CBT | | cognitive behavioral therapy |

*(continued)*

| Abbreviation | From | Meaning |
|---|---|---|
| cc | | cubic centimeter |
| CGI | | Clinical Global Impression |
| CHF | | congestive heart failure |
| CI | | cardiac index |
| CIV | | continuous I.V. infusion |
| $Cl_{cr}$ | | creatinine clearance |
| cm | | centimeter |
| CNS | | central nervous system |
| comp | compositus | compound |
| cont | | continue |
| COPD | | chronic obstructive pulmonary disease |
| CSF | | cerebral spinal fluid |
| CT | | computed tomography |
| CVA | | cerebral vascular accident |
| CVP | | central venous pressure |
| d | dies | day |
| $D_5W$ | | dextrose 5% in water |
| $D_{10}W$ | | dextrose 10% in water |
| d/c | | discontinue |
| DIC | | disseminated intravascular coagulation |
| dil | dilue | dilute |
| disp | dispensa | dispense |
| div | divide | divide |
| DNA | | deoxyribonucleic acid |
| DSM-IV | | Diagnostic and Statistical Manual |
| DTs | | delirium tremens |
| dtd | dentur tales doses | give of such a dose |
| DVT | | deep vein thrombosis |
| ECT | | electroconvulsive therapy |
| EEG | | electroencephalogram |
| EKG | | electrocardiogram |
| elix, el | elixir | elixir |
| emp | | as directed |
| EPS | | extrapyramidal side effects |
| ESR | | erythrocyte sedimentation rate |
| E.T. | | endotracheal |
| et | et | and |
| ex aq | | in water |
| f, ft | fac, fiat, fiant | make, let be made |
| FDA | | Food and Drug Administration |
| $FEV_1 1$ | | forced expiratory volume |
| FVC | | forced vital capacity |
| g | gramma | gram |
| G-6-PD | | glucose-6-phosphate dehydrogenase |
| GA | | gestational age |
| GABA | | gamma-aminobutyric acid |
| GAD | | generalized anxiety disorder |
| GAF | | Global Assessment of Functioning Scale |
| GE | | gastroesophageal |
| GI | | gastrointestinal |
| GITS | | gastrointestinal therapeutic system |
| gr | granum | grain |
| gtt | gutta | a drop |
| GU | | genitourinary |
| h | hora | hour |
| HAM-A | | Hamilton Anxiety Scale |
| HAM-D | | Hamilton Depression Scale |
| HIV | | human immunodeficiency virus |
| HPLC | | high performance liquid chromatography |
| hs | hora somni | at bedtime |
| IBW | | ideal body weight |

*(continued)*

| Abbreviation | From | Meaning |
|---|---|---|
| ICP | | intracranial pressure |
| IgG | | immune globulin G |
| I.M. | | intramuscular |
| INR | | international normalized ratio |
| I.O. | | intraosseous |
| I & O | | input and output |
| IOP | | intraocular pressure |
| I.T. | | intrathecal |
| IU | | international unit |
| I.V. | | intravenous |
| IVH | | intraventricular hemorrhage |
| IVP | | intravenous push |
| JRA | | juvenile rheumatoid arthritis |
| kcal | | kilocalorie |
| kg | | kilogram |
| KIU | | kallikrein inhibitor unit |
| L | | liter |
| LAMM | | L-α-acetyl methadol |
| LDH | | lactate dehydrogenase |
| LE | | lupus erythematosus |
| liq | liquor | a liquor, solution |
| LP | | lumbar puncture |
| M | misce | mix |
| MADRS | | Montgomery Asbery Depression Rating Scale |
| MAOIs | | monoamine oxidase inhibitors |
| MAP | | mean arterial pressure |
| mcg | | microgram |
| MDEA | | 3.4-methylene-dioxy amphetamine |
| m. dict | more dictor | as directed |
| MDMA | | 3,4-methylene-dioxy methamphetamine |
| mEq | | milliequivalent |
| mg | | milligram |
| MI | | myocardial infarction |
| min | | minute |
| mixt | mixtura | a mixture |
| mL | | milliliter |
| mm | | millimeter |
| MMSE | | Mini-Mental State Examination |
| mo | | month |
| mOsm | | milliosmols |
| MPPP | | l-methyl-4-proprionoxy-4-phenyl pyridine |
| MR | | mental retardation |
| MRI | | magnetic resonance image |
| ND | | nasoduodenal |
| NF | | National Formulary |
| ng | | nanogram |
| NMS | | neuroleptic malignant syndrome |
| no. | numerus | number |
| noc | nocturnal | in the night |
| non rep | non repetatur | do not repeat, no refills |
| NPO | | nothing by mouth |
| NSAID | | nonsteroidal anti-inflammatory drug |
| O, Oct | octarius | a pint |
| OCD | | obsessive-compulsive disorder |
| o.d. | oculus dexter | right eye |
| o.l. | oculus laevus | left eye |
| O.R. | | operating room |
| o.s. | oculus sinister | left eye |
| OTC | | over-the-counter (nonprescription) |
| o.u. | oculo uterque | each eye |
| PALS | | pediatric advanced life support |

*(continued)*

| Abbreviation | From | Meaning |
|---|---|---|
| PANSS | | Positive and Negative Symptom Scale |
| pc, post cib | post cibos | after meals |
| PCA | | postconceptional age |
| PCP | | *Pneumocystis carinii* pneumonia |
| PCWP | | pulmonary capillary wedge pressure |
| PDA | | patent ductus arteriosus |
| per | | through or by |
| PM | post meridiem | afternoon or evening |
| PNA | | postnatal age |
| P.O. | per os | by mouth |
| P.R. | per rectum | rectally |
| prn | pro re nata | as needed |
| PSVT | | paroxysmal supraventricular tachycardia |
| PT | | prothrombin time |
| PTT | | partial thromboplastin time |
| PTSD | | post-traumatic stress disorder |
| PUD | | peptic ulcer disease |
| pulv | pulvis | a powder |
| PVC | | premature ventricular contraction |
| q | | every |
| qad | quoque alternis die | every other day |
| qd | | every day |
| qh | quiaque hora | every hour |
| qid | quater in die | four times a day |
| qod | | every other day |
| qs | quantum sufficiat | a sufficient quantity |
| qs ad | | a sufficient quantity to make |
| qty | | quantity |
| qv | quam volueris | as much as you wish |
| Rx | recipe | take, a recipe |
| RAP | | right atrial pressure |
| REM | | rapid eye movement |
| rep | repetatur | let it be repeated |
| $\bar{s}$ | sine | without |
| S-A | | sino-atrial |
| sa | secundum artem | according to art |
| sat | sataratus | saturated |
| S.C. | | subcutaneous |
| $S_{cr}$ | | serum creatinine |
| SIADH | | syndrome of inappropriate antidiuretic hormone |
| sig | signa | label, or let it be printed |
| S.L. | | sublingual |
| SLE | | systemic lupus erythematosus |
| sol | solutio | solution |
| solv | | dissolve |
| $\overline{ss}$, ss | semis | one-half |
| sos | si opus sit | if there is need |
| SSRIs | | selective serotonin reuptake inhibitors |
| stat | statim | at once, immediately |
| supp | suppositorium | suppository |
| SVR | | systemic vascular resistance |
| SVT | | supraventricular tachycardia |
| SWI | | sterile water for injection |
| syr | syrupus | syrup |
| tab | tabella | tablet |
| tal | | such |
| TCA | | tricyclic antidepressant |
| TD | | tardive dyskinesia |
| tid | ter in die | three times a day |
| tr, tinct | tincture | tincture |
| trit | | triturate |

*(continued)*

| Abbreviation | From | Meaning |
|---|---|---|
| tsp | | teaspoonful |
| TT | | thrombin time |
| u.d., ut dict | ut dictum | as directed |
| ULN | | upper limits of normal |
| ung | unguentum | ointment |
| USAN | | United States Adopted Names |
| USP | | United States Pharmacopeia |
| UTI | | urinary tract infection |
| $V_d$ | | volume of distribution |
| $V_{dss}$ | | volume of distribution at steady-state |
| v.o. | | verbal order |
| w.a. | | while awake |
| x3 | | 3 times |
| x4 | | 4 times |
| y | | year |
| YBOC | | Yale Brown Obsessive-Compulsive Scale |
| YMRS | | Young Mania Rating Scale |

# NORMAL LABORATORY VALUES FOR ADULTS*

## CHEMISTRY

| | | |
|---|---|---|
| **Chemistry, Routine** | | |
| Albumin | | 3.5-5.0 g/dL |
| Bilirubin, conjugated | | 0-0.2 mg/dL |
| Bilirubin, total | | 0.2-1.2 mg/dL |
| Blood urea nitrogen | | 8-23 mg/dL |
| Calcium | | 8.4-10.3 mg/dL |
| Creatinine | | 0.5-1.2 mg/dL |
| Glucose | | 65-110 mg/dL |
| Phosphorus | | 2.8-4.5 mg/dL |
| Protein, total | | 6.0-8.0 g/dL |
| Uric acid | male | 3.5-7.2 mg/dL |
| | female | 2.6-6.5 mg/dL |
| **Electrolytes** | | |
| Chlorides | | 100-110 mEq/L |
| $CO_2$ | | 23-31 mEq/L |
| Potassium | | 3.5-5.0 mEq/L |
| Sodium | | 136-146 mEq/L |
| Anion gap | | 5-14 mEq/L |
| **Enzymes** | | |
| Alkaline phosphatase | male | 34-110 units/L |
| | female | 24-100 units/L |
| ALT | | 5-35 units/L |
| AST | | 5-35 units/L |
| CPK | male | 0-206 units/L |
| | female | 0-175 units/L |
| LDH | | 50-200 units/L |
| **Thyroid Function** | | |
| FTI (free thyroxine index) | | 4.5-12.0 |
| $T_3$ resin uptake | | 25%-35% |
| $T_3$ (tri-iodothyronine) by RIA | | 70-200 ng/dL |
| $T_4$ (thyroxine) by RIA | | 4.0-11.0 μg/dL |
| **Others** | | |
| Ammonia, plasma | | 20-60 μg/dL |
| Amylase, serum | | 44-128 units/L |
| Calcium, ionized | | 4.6-5.2 mg/dL |
| Cholesterol | | 140-230 mg/dL |
| Iron, serum | | 50-170 μg/dL |
| Lactate, serum | | 1.4-3.9 mEq/L |
| Lipase | | 10-208 units/L |
| Magnesium | | 1.5-2.5 mg/dL |
| Oncotic pressure | | 22-28 mm Hg |
| Osmolality | | 280-300 mOsm/kg |
| Serum ferritin | male | 25-400 ng/mL |
| | female | 10-150 ng/mL |
| TIBC | | 270-390 μg/dL |
| Triglycerides | | 50-150 mg/dL |

*The normal ranges for laboratory values vary with different age groups, and may change as new methodologies for the lab tests are used. These values are current for adults (age 17 years or older). **Note:** Normal laboratory values may differ according to laboratory, institution, and analytical technique.

## HEMATOLOGY

| Test | | Range |
|---|---|---|
| Hematocrit | male | 40%-52% |
| | female | 35%-47% |
| Hemoglobin | male | 13.5-17.5 g/dL |
| | female | 11.5-16.0 g/dL |
| MCH | | 27-34 pg |
| MCV | | 82-100 fL |
| Platelet count | | 150-450 $10^3/mm^3$ |
| RBC count | male | 4.5-5.9 $10^6/mm^3$ |
| | female | 4.0-4.9 $10^6/mm^3$ |
| Reticulocyte count | | 0.5%-1.5% |
| Sed rate (Westergren) | male | 0-10 mm/h |
| | female | 0-20 mm/h |
| WBC count | | 4.5-11.0 $10^3/mm^3$ |
| WBC differential | | |
| bands | | 2%-8% |
| basophils | | 0%-2% |
| eosinophils | | 0%-4% |
| lymphocytes | | 20%-45% |
| monocytes | | 2%-8% |
| neutrophils | | 40%-70% |

## BLOOD GASES

| | Arterial | Venous |
|---|---|---|
| Base excess | -3.0 to +3.0 mEq/L | -5.0 to +5.0 mEq/L |
| $HCO_3$ | 18-25 mEq/L | 18-25 mEq/L |
| $O_2$ saturation | 90%-98% | 60%-85% |
| $pCO_2$ | 34-45 mm Hg | 35-52 mm Hg |
| pH | 7.35-7.45 | 7.32-7.42 |
| $pO_2$ | 80-95 mm Hg | 30-48 mm Hg |
| $TCO_2$ | 23-29 mEq/L | 24-30 mEq/L |

**Weight/Volume Equivalents**

| | |
|---|---|
| 1 mg/dL = 10 μg/mL | 1 ppm = 1 mg/L |
| 1 mg/dL = 1 mg% | 1 μg/mL = 1 mg/L |

# NORMAL LABORATORY VALUES FOR CHILDREN

## CHEMISTRY

| Test | Age | Value |
|---|---|---|
| Albumin | 0-1 y | 2-4 g/dL |
| | 1 y - adult | 3.5-5.5 g/dL |
| Ammonia | newborn | 90-150 µg/dL |
| | child | 40-120 µg/dL |
| | adult | 18-54 µg/dL |
| Amylase | newborn | 0-60 units/L |
| | adult | 30-110 units/L |
| Bilirubin, conjugated, direct | newborn | <1.5 mg/dL |
| | 1 mo - adult | 0-0.5 mg/dL |
| Bilirubin, total | 0-3 d | 2-10 mg/dL |
| | 1 mo - adult | 0-1.5 mg/dL |
| Bilirubin, unconjugated, indirect | | 0.6-10.5 mg/dL |
| Calcium | newborn | 7-12 mg/dL |
| | 0-2 y | 8.8-11.2 mg/dL |
| | 2 y - adult | 9-11 mg/dL |
| Calcium, ionized, whole blood | | 4.4-5.4 mg/dL |
| Carbon dioxide, total | | 23-33 mEq/L |
| Chloride | | 95-105 mEq/L |
| Cholesterol | newborn | 45-170 mg/dL |
| | 0-1 y | 65-175 mg/dL |
| | 1-20 y | 120-230 mg/dL |
| Creatinine | 0-1 y | ≤0.6 mg/dL |
| | 1 y - adult | 0.5-1.5 mg/dL |
| Glucose | newborn | 30-90 mg/dL |
| | 0-2 y | 60-105 mg/dL |
| | child - adult | 70-110 mg/dL |
| Iron | newborn | 110-270 µg/dL |
| | infant | 30-70 µg/dL |
| | child | 55-120 µg/dL |
| | adult | 70-180 µg/dL |
| Iron binding | newborn | 59-175 µg/dL |
| | infant | 100-400 µg/dL |
| | adult | 250-400 µg/dL |
| Lactic acid, lactate | | 2-20 mg/dL |
| Lead, whole blood | | <30 µg/dL |
| Lipase | child | 20-140 units/L |
| | adult | 0-190 units/L |
| Magnesium | | 1.5-2.5 mEq/L |
| Osmolality, serum | | 275-296 mOsm/kg |
| Osmolality, urine | | 50-1400 mOsm/kg |

## Chemistry *(continued)*

| Test | Age/Sex | Normal Range |
|---|---|---|
| Phosphorus | newborn | 4.2-9 mg/dL |
| | 6 wk - 19 mo | 3.8-6.7 mg/dL |
| | 18 mo - 3 y | 2.9-5.9 mg/dL |
| | 3-15 y | 3.6-5.6 mg/dL |
| | >15 y | 2.5-5 mg/dL |
| Potassium, plasma | newborn | 4.5-7.2 mEq/L |
| | 2 d - 3 mo | 4-6.2 mEq/L |
| | 3 mo - 1 y | 3.7-5.6 mEq/L |
| | 1-16 y | 3.5-5 mEq/L |
| Protein, total | 0-2 y | 4.2-7.4 g/dL |
| | >2 y | 6-8 g/dL |
| Sodium | | 136-145 mEq/L |
| Triglycerides | infant | 0-171 mg/dL |
| | child | 20-130 mg/dL |
| | adult | 30-200 mg/dL |
| Urea nitrogen, blood | 0-2 y | 4-15 mg/dL |
| | 2 y - adult | 5-20 mg/dL |
| Uric acid | male | 3-7 mg/dL |
| | female | 2-6 mg/dL |

## ENZYMES

| Test | Age/Sex | Normal Range |
|---|---|---|
| Alanine aminotransferase (ALT) (SGPT) | 0-2 mo | 8-78 units/L |
| | >2 mo | 8-36 units/L |
| Alkaline phosphatase (ALKP) | newborn | 60-130 units/L |
| | 0-16 y | 85-400 units/L |
| | >16 y | 30-115 units/L |
| Aspartate aminotransferase (AST) (SGOT) | infant | 18-74 units/L |
| | child | 15-46 units/L |
| | adult | 5-35 units/L |
| Creatine kinase (CK) | infant | 20-200 units/L |
| | child | 10-90 units/L |
| | adult male | 0-206 units/L |
| | adult female | 0-175 units/L |
| Lactate dehydrogenase (LDH) | newborn | 290-501 units/L |
| | 1 mo - 2 y | 110-144 units/L |
| | >16 y | 60-170 units/L |

## BLOOD GASES

| | Arterial | Capillary | Venous |
|---|---|---|---|
| pH | 7.35-7.45 | 7.35-7.45 | 7.32-7.42 |
| $pCO_2$ (mm Hg) | 35-45 | 35-45 | 38-52 |
| $pO_2$ (mm Hg) | 70-100 | 60-80 | 24-48 |
| $HCO_3$ (mEq/L) | 19-25 | 19-25 | 19-25 |
| $TCO_2$ (mEq/L) | 19-29 | 19-29 | 23-33 |
| $O_2$ saturation (%) | 90-95 | 90-95 | 40-70 |
| Base excess (mEq/L) | -5 to +5 | -5 to +5 | -5 to +5 |

## THYROID FUNCTION TESTS

| | | |
|---|---|---|
| $T_4$ (thyroxine) | 1-7 d | 10.1-20.9 μg/dL |
| | 8-14 d | 9.8-16.6 μg/dL |
| | 1 mo - 1 y | 5.5-16 μg/dL |
| | >1 y | 4-12 μg/dL |
| FTI | 1-3 d | 9.3-26.6 |
| | 1-4 wk | 7.6-20.8 |
| | 1-4 mo | 7.4-17.9 |
| | 4-12 mo | 5.1-14.5 |
| | 1-6 y | 5.7-13.3 |
| | >6 y | 4.8-14 |
| $T_3$ by RIA | newborn | 100-470 ng/dL |
| | 1-5 y | 100-260 ng/dL |
| | 5-10 y | 90-240 ng/dL |
| | 10 y - adult | 70-210 ng/dL |
| $T_3$ uptake | | 35%-45% |
| TSH | cord | 3-22 μU/mL |
| | 1-3 d | <40 μU/mL |
| | 3-7 d | <25 μU/mL |
| | >7 d | 0-10 μU/mL |

# APPENDIX

## HEMATOLOGY VALUES

### Complete Blood Count

| | Hgb (g/dL) | Hct (%) | MCV (fL) | MCH (pg) | MCHC (%) | RBC (x $10^6$/mm$^3$) | RDW | PLTS (x $10^3$/mm$^3$) |
|---|---|---|---|---|---|---|---|---|
| 0-3 d | 15.0-20.0 | 45-61 | 95-115 | 31-37 | 29-37 | 4.0-5.9 | <18.0 | 250-450 |
| 1-2 wk | 12.5-18.5 | 39-57 | 86-110 | 28-36 | 28-38 | 3.6-5.5 | <17.0 | 250-450 |
| 1-6 mo | 10.0-13.0 | 29-42 | 74-96 | 25-35 | 30-36 | 3.1-4.3 | <16.5 | 300-700 |
| 7 mo - 2 y | 10.5-13.0 | 33-38 | 70-84 | 23-30 | 31-37 | 3.7-4.9 | <16.0 | 250-600 |
| 2-5 y | 11.5-13.0 | 34-39 | 75-87 | 24-30 | 31-37 | 3.9-5.0 | <15.0 | 250-550 |
| 5-8 y | 11.5-14.5 | 35-42 | 77-95 | 25-33 | 31-37 | 4.0-4.9 | <15.0 | 250-550 |
| 13-18 y | 12.0-15.2 | 36-47 | 78-96 | 25-35 | 31-37 | 4.5-5.1 | <14.5 | 150-450 |
| Adult male | 13.5-16.5 | 41-50 | 80-100 | 26-34 | 31-37 | 4.5-5.9 | <14.5 | 150-450 |
| Adult female | 12.0-15.0 | 36-45 | 80-100 | 26-34 | 31-37 | 4.0-4.9 | <14.5 | 150-450 |

### WBC and Differential

| | WBC (x $10^3$/mm$^3$) | Segs | Bands | Eos | Basos | Lymphs | Atypical Lymphs | Monos | # of NRBCs |
|---|---|---|---|---|---|---|---|---|---|
| 0-3 d | 9.0-35.0 | 32-62 | 10-18 | 0-2 | 0-1 | 19-29 | 0-8 | 5-7 | 0-2 |
| 1-2 wk | 5.0-20.0 | 14-34 | 6-14 | 0-2 | 0-1 | 36-45 | 0-8 | 6-10 | 0 |
| 1-6 mo | 6.0-17.5 | 13-33 | 4-12 | 0-3 | 0-1 | 41-71 | 0-8 | 4-7 | 0 |
| 7 mo - 2 y | 6.0-17.0 | 15-35 | 5-11 | 0-3 | 0-1 | 45-76 | 0-8 | 3-6 | 0 |
| 2-5 y | 5.5-15.5 | 23-45 | 5-11 | 0-3 | 0-1 | 35-65 | 0-8 | 3-6 | 0 |
| 5-8 y | 5.0-14.5 | 32-54 | 5-11 | 0-3 | 0-1 | 28-48 | 0-8 | 3-6 | 0 |
| 13-18 y | 4.5-13.0 | 34-64 | 5-11 | 0-3 | 0-1 | 25-45 | 0-8 | 3-6 | 0 |
| Adults | 4.5-11.0 | 35-66 | 5-11 | 0-3 | 0-1 | 24-44 | 0-8 | 3-6 | 0 |

| | |
|---|---|
| Sedimentation rate, Westergren | |
| Child | 0-20 mm/h |
| Adult male | 0-15 mm/h |
| Adult female | 0-20 mm/h |
| Sedimentation rate, Wintrobe | |
| Child | 0-13 mm/h |
| Adult male | 0-10 mm/h |
| Adult female | 0-15 mm/h |
| Reticulocyte count | |
| Newborn | 2%-6% |
| 1-6 mo | 0%-2.8% |
| Adult | 0.5%-1.5% |

# APOTHECARY/METRIC CONVERSIONS

## Liquid Measures

Basic equivalent: 1 fluid ounce = 30 mL

Examples:

| | | | |
|---|---|---|---|
| 1 gallon | 3800 mL | 4 fluid oz | 120 mL |
| 1 quart | 960 mL | 15 minims | 1 mL |
| 1 pint | 480 mL | 10 minims | 0.6 mL |
| 8 fluid oz | 240 mL | | |

| | |
|---|---|
| 1 gallon | 128 fluid ounces |
| 1 quart | 32 fluid ounces |
| 1 pint | 16 fluid ounces |

## Approximate Household Equivalents

1 teaspoonful . . . . 5 mL 1 tablespoonful . . . 15 mL

## Weights

Basic equivalents:

1 oz = 30 g 15 gr = 1 g

Examples:

| | | | |
|---|---|---|---|
| 4 oz | 120 g | 1 gr | 60 mg |
| 2 oz | 60 g | $^1/_{100}$ gr | 600 mcg |
| 10 gr | 600 mg | $^1/_{150}$ gr | 400 mcg |
| 7 $^1/_2$ gr | 500 mg | $^1/_{200}$ gr | 300 mcg |
| 16 oz | 1 pound | | |

## Metric Conversions

Basic equivalents:

1 g . . . . . . . . 1000 mg 1 mg . . . . . . . . . 1000 mcg

Examples:

| | | | |
|---|---|---|---|
| 5 g | 5000 mg | 5 mg | 5000 mcg |
| 0.5 g | 500 mg | 0.5 mg | 500 mcg |
| 0.05 g | 50 mg | 0.05 mg | 50 mcg |

## Exact Equivalents

| | |
|---|---|
| 1 g = 15.43 grains | 0.1 mg = $^1/_{600}$ gr |
| 1 milliliter (mL) = 16.23 minims | 0.12 mg = $^1/_{500}$ gr |
| 1 minim = 0.06 milliliter | 0.15 mg = $^1/_{400}$ gr |
| 1 gr = 64.8 milligrams | 0.2 mg = $^1/_{300}$ gr |
| 1 oz = 28.35 grams | 0.5 mg = $^1/_{120}$ gr |
| 1 lb = 453.6 grams | 0.8 mg = $^1/_{80}$ gr |
| 1 kg = 2.2 pounds | 1 mg = $^1/_{65}$ gr |

## Solids*

$^1/_4$ grain = 15 mg
$^1/_2$ grain = 30 mg
1$^1/_2$ grain = 100 mg
5 grains = 300 mg
10 grains = 600 mg

*Use exact equivalents for compounding and calculations requiring a high degree of accuracy.

## POUNDS/KILOGRAMS CONVERSION

**1 pound = 0.45359 kilograms**
**1 kilogram = 2.2 pounds**

| lb | = kg | lb | = kg | lb | = kg |
|---|---|---|---|---|---|
| 1 | 0.45 | 70 | 31.75 | 140 | 63.50 |
| 5 | 2.27 | 75 | 34.02 | 145 | 65.77 |
| 10 | 4.54 | 80 | 36.29 | 150 | 68.04 |
| 15 | 6.80 | 85 | 38.56 | 155 | 70.31 |
| 20 | 9.07 | 90 | 40.82 | 160 | 72.58 |
| 25 | 11.34 | 95 | 43.09 | 165 | 74.84 |
| 30 | 13.61 | 100 | 45.36 | 170 | 77.11 |
| 35 | 15.88 | 105 | 47.63 | 175 | 79.38 |
| 40 | 18.14 | 110 | 49.90 | 180 | 81.65 |
| 45 | 20.41 | 115 | 52.16 | 185 | 83.92 |
| 50 | 22.68 | 120 | 54.43 | 190 | 86.18 |
| 55 | 24.95 | 125 | 56.70 | 195 | 88.45 |
| 60 | 27.22 | 130 | 58.91 | 200 | 90.72 |
| 65 | 29.48 | 135 | 61.24 | | |

## TEMPERATURE CONVERSION

**Centigrade to Fahrenheit = (°C x 9/5) + 32 = °F**
**Fahrenheit to Centigrade = (°F - 32) x 5/9 = °C**

| °C | = °F | °C | = °F | °C | = °F |
|---|---|---|---|---|---|
| 100.0 | 212.0 | 39.0 | 102.2 | 36.8 | 98.2 |
| 50.0 | 122.0 | 38.8 | 101.8 | 36.6 | 97.9 |
| 41.0 | 105.8 | 38.6 | 101.5 | 36.4 | 97.5 |
| 40.8 | 105.4 | 38.4 | 101.1 | 36.2 | 97.2 |
| 40.6 | 105.1 | 38.2 | 100.8 | 36.0 | 96.8 |
| 40.4 | 104.7 | 38.0 | 100.4 | 35.8 | 96.4 |
| 40.2 | 104.4 | 37.8 | 100.1 | 35.6 | 96.1 |
| 40.0 | 104.0 | 37.6 | 99.7 | 35.4 | 95.7 |
| 39.8 | 103.6 | 37.4 | 99.3 | 35.2 | 95.4 |
| 39.6 | 103.3 | 37.2 | 99.0 | 35.0 | 95.0 |
| 39.4 | 102.9 | 37.0 | 98.6 | 0 | 32.0 |
| 39.2 | 102.6 | | | | |

# ACQUIRED IMMUNODEFICIENCY SYNDROME (AIDS) — LAB TESTS AND APPROVED DRUGS FOR HIV INFECTION AND AIDS-RELATED CONDITIONS

This list of tests is not intended in any way to suggest patterns of physician's orders, nor is it complete. These tests may support possible clinical diagnoses or rule out other diagnostic possibilities. Each laboratory test relevant to AIDS is listed and weighted. Two symbols (**) indicate that the test is diagnostic, that is, documents the diagnosis if the expected is found. A single symbol (*) indicates a test frequently used in the diagnosis or management of the disease. The other listed tests are useful on a selective basis with consideration of clinical factors and specific aspects of the case.

Acid-Fast Stain
Acid-Fast Stain, Modified, *Nocardia* Species
Antimicrobial Susceptibility Testing, Fungi
Antimicrobial Susceptibility Testing, Mycobacteria
Arthropod Identification
Babesiosis Serological Test
Bacteremia Detection, Buffy Coat Micromethod
Bacterial Culture, Blood
Bacterial Culture, Bronchoscopy Specimen
Bacterial Culture, Sputum
Bacterial Culture, Stool
Bacterial Culture, Throat
Bacterial Culture, Urine, Clean Catch
Beta$_2$-Microglobulin
Blood and Fluid Precautions, Specimen Collection
Bronchial Washings Cytology
Bronchoalveolar Lavage Cytology
Brushings Cytology
*Candida* Antigen
Candidiasis Serologic Test
Cat Scratch Disease Serology
CD4/CD8 Enumeration
Cerebrospinal Fluid Cytology
Cryptococcal Antigen Titer
*Cryptosporidium* Diagnostic Procedures
Cytomegalic Inclusion Disease Cytology
Cytomegalovirus Antibody
Cytomegalovirus Antigen Detection
Cytomegalovirus Culture
Cytomegalovirus DNA Detection
Darkfield Examination, Syphilis
Electron Microscopy
Folic Acid, Serum
Fungal Culture, Biopsy or Body Fluid
Fungal Culture, Blood
Fungal Culture, Cerebrospinal Fluid
Fungal Culture, Sputum
Fungal Culture, Stool
Fungal Culture, Urine
Hemoglobin $A_2$
Hepatitis B Surface Antigen
Herpes Cytology
Herpes Simplex Virus Antigen Detection
Herpes Simplex Virus Culture
Histopathology
Histoplasmosis Antibody

Histoplasmosis Antigen
**HIV-1/HIV-2 Serology
HTLV-I/II Antibody
*Human Immunodeficiency Virus Culture
*Human Immunodeficiency Virus DNA Amplification
India Ink Preparation
Inhibitor, Lupus, Phospholipid Type
KOH Preparation
Leishmaniasis Serological Test
Leukocyte Immunophenotyping
Lymphocyte Transformation Test
Microsporidia Diagnostic Procedures
Mycobacteria by DNA Probe
Mycobacterial Culture, Biopsy or Body Fluid
Mycobacterial Culture, Cerebrospinal Fluid
Mycobacterial Culture, Cutaneous and Subcutaneous Tissue
Mycobacterial Culture, Sputum
Mycobacterial Culture, Stool
*Neisseria gonorrhoeae* Culture and Smear
*Nocardia* Culture
Ova and Parasites, Stool
*p24 Antigen
Platelet Count
*Pneumocystis carinii* Preparation
*Pneumocystis* Immunofluorescence
Polymerase Chain Reaction
Red Blood Cell Indices
Risks of Transfusion
Skin Biopsy
Sputum Cytology
Toxoplasmosis Serology
VDRL, Serum
Viral Culture
Viral Culture, Blood
Viral Culture, Body Fluid
Viral Culture, Central Nervous System Symptoms
Viral Culture, Dermatological Symptoms
Viral Culture, Tissue
Virus, Direct Detection by Fluorescent Antibody
White Blood Count

**Approved Drugs for HIV/AIDS or AIDS-related Conditions**

abacavir (Ziagen®)
Treatment of HIV-1 in adults and children
alitretinoin (Panretin™)
Topical treatment of lesions in patients with AIDS-related Kaposi's sarcoma
amphotericin B lipid complex (Abelcet®, Ambisome®)
Treatment of aspergillosis
amprenavir (Agenerase®)
Treatment of HIV-1 in adults and children
atovaquone (Mepron®)
Treatment of mild to moderate *Pneumocystis carinii* pneumonia in patients who are intolerant to Bactrim® or Septra®
azithromycin (Zithromax®)
Prevention of *Mycobacterium avium* complex (MAC) in persons with advanced HIV infection
cidofovir (Vistide®)
Treatment of AIDS-related cytomegalovirus retinitis

clarithromycin (Biaxin®, Klacid®)
Treatment of disseminated mycobacterial infections due to *Mycobacterium avium-intracellulare* complex (MAC); approved for prophylaxis of disseminated MAC in patients with advanced HIV infection

daunorubicin-liposomal (DaunoXome®)
Treatment of advanced HIV-related Kaposi's sarcoma

delavirdine mesylate (Rescriptor®)
In combination with appropriate antiretrovirals when therapy is warranted for treatment of HIV infection

didanosine (Videx®)
Treatment of adult and pediatric patients with advanced HIV who are intolerant to or deteriorating on AZT; approved for treatment of adult and pediatric patients with advanced HIV previously treated with AZT; approved for treatment of HIV infection when antiretroviral therapy is warranted

doxorubicin hydrochloride-liposomal (Doxil®)
Treatment of Kaposi's sarcoma in AIDS patients who are intolerant to or have disease progression on prior combination chemotherapy

dronabinol (Marinol®)
Treatment of anorexia associated with weight loss in patients with AIDS

efavirenz (Sustiva®)
Treatment of HIV and AIDS

erythropoietin (Epogen®, Procrit®)
Treatment of anemia related to AZT therapy in HIV infection

famciclovir (Famvir®)
Treatment of recurrent mucocutaneous herpes simplex infections in HIV-infected patients at a dose of 500 mg twice daily

filgrastim [G-CSF] (Neupogen®)
Treatment of neutropenia due to chemotherapy for cancers, including lymphomas and Kaposi's sarcoma

fluconazole (Diflucan®)
Treatment of oropharyngeal and esophageal candidiasis and for treatment of cryptococcal meningitis; approved for treatment of pediatric patients with cryptococcal meningitis and *candida* infections

fomivirsen sodium intravitreal injection (Vitravene®)
Local treatment of cytomegalovirus (CMV) retinitis in patients with AIDS who are intolerant of or have a contraindication to other treatment(s) for CMV retinitis or who were insufficiently responsive to previous treatment(s) for CMV retinitis

foscarnet (Foscavir®)
Treatment of CMV retinitis in patients with AIDS; approved for the treatment of acyclovir-resistant herpes simplex virus

ganciclovir - I.V., oral (Cytovene®)
Treatment of CMV retinitis in immunocompromised patients; oral approved for maintenance therapy for CMV retinitis in some patients; approved for prophylaxis of CMV disease

ganciclovir [DHPG] - implant (Vitrasert®)
Treatment of CMV retinitis in patients with AIDS

immune globulin - I.V. (Gamimune N®)
Prevention of bacterial infections in pediatric HIV infection

indinavir sulfate (Crixivan®)
For use alone or in combination with nucleoside analogues for treatment of HIV infection in adults

interferon alfa-2a (Roferon-A®)
Treatment of AIDS-related Kaposi's sarcoma in selected patients

interferon alfa-2b (Intron-A®)
Treatment of adult AIDS-related Kaposi's sarcoma in selected patients; approved for treatment of chronic non-A, non-B hepatitis

interferon alfa-n3 (Alferon N®)
Treatment of *Condyloma acuminata* (genital warts)

itraconazole (Sporanox®)
  Treatment of histoplasmosis, blastomycosis, and aspergillosis in immunocompromised and nonimmunocompromised patients
ketoconazole (Nizoral®)
  Treatment of histoplasmosis, blastomycosis, and candidiasis
lamivudine [3TC] (Epivir®)
  Combination use with AZT as a treatment option for HIV infection in adults and pediatric patients ≥3 months of age
lopinavir and ritonavir (Kaletra™)
  Treatment of HIV
megestrol acetate (Megace®, Ovaban®)
  Treatment of anorexia, cachexia, or unexplained significant weight loss in patients with AIDS
nelfinavir mesylate (Viracept®)
  Treatment of HIV infection when antiretroviral therapy is warranted in adults and pediatrics ≥2 years of age
nevirapine (Viramune®)
  Combination use with nucleoside analogues for treatment of HIV-infected adults experiencing clinical and/or immunologic deterioration
pentamidine - I.M., I.V. (Pentam® 300)
  Treatment of *Pneumocystis carinii* pneumonia
pentamidine - aerosolized (NebuPent®)
  Prevention of *Pneumocystis carinii* pneumonia
pyrimethamine [with sulfonamide] (Daraprim®; Fansidar® when combined with sulfadoxine)
  Treatment of toxoplasmosis
rifabutin (Ansamycin®, Mycobutin®)
  Prevention of *Mycobacterium avium* complex in patients with advanced HIV
ritonavir (Norvir®)
  For use alone or in combination with nucleoside analogues for treatment of HIV infection
saquinavir mesylate (Invirase®)
  Combination use with nucleoside analogues for treatment of advanced HIV infection in selected patients
sargramostim [GM-CSF] (Leukine®)
  Treatment of cancer patients with lymphomas or leukemia who are receiving bone marrow transplants
somatropin rDNA (Serostim®)
  Treatment of AIDS-wasting and cachexia
stavudine [d4T] (Zerit®)
  Treatment of adults with advanced HIV infection who are intolerant to or deteriorating on approved therapies; approved for treatment of adults with advanced HIV infection who have undergone prolonged treatment with AZT; approved for the treatment of pediatrics with HIV infection who have undergone prolonged prior AZT therapy
sulfamethoxazole (Bactrim® when combined with trimethoprim; Septra® when combined trimethoprim)
  Treatment of *Pneumocystis carinii* pneumonia (PCP); approved for prevention of PCP
trimethoprim (Bactrim® when combined with sulfamethoxazole; Septra® when combined with sulfamethoxazole)
  Treatment of *Pneumocystis carinii* pneumonia (PCP); approved for prevention of PCP
trimetrexate (with leucovorin) [TMTX] (Neutrexin®)
  Treatment of moderate to severe *Pneumocystis carinii* pneumonia when intolerant or refractory to TMP/SMX or when TMP/SMX is contraindicated
zalcitabine [ddC] (Hivid®)
  Combination use with AZT for treatment of selected patients with advanced HIV

disease; approved for monotherapy treatment of advanced HIV for patients ≥13 years of age who are intolerant to or have disease progression on AZT

zidovudine [AZT] (Retrovir®)

Treatment of adult AIDS or symptomatic HIV and CD4 ≤200; approved for treatment of adult HIV infection and CD4 ≤500; approved for treatment of pediatric HIV infection (3 months to 12 years of age); approved for prevention of perinatal transmission in HIV-positive pregnant women between 14 and 34 weeks gestation and in newborns of HIV-positive mothers

zidovudine and lamivudine (Combivir®)

Combination of AZT (zidovudine) and 3TC (lamivudine) for treating AIDS and HIV infection

## Drugs Being Studied in HIV/AIDS Clinical Trials

A-007 [antineoplastic]
ABT-378 (new name: lopinavir) [protease inhibitor]
acetaminophen (Tylenol®, Panadol®) [analgesic, antipyretic]
acetylcysteine (Mucomyst®, Respaire®) [antiretroviral, mycolytic]
acitretin (Soriatane®) [antipsoriatic]
ACT (activated cellular therapy) [other/HIV]
acyclovir (Zovirax®) [antiviral]
aldesleukin (Proleukin®) [immunomodulator, antineoplastic]
alitretinoin (Panretin®) [retinoic acid]
AL 721 [antiviral]
ALVAC-HIV gp 160 MN (vCP125) [vaccine]
ALVAC-HIV MN120TMG (vCP205) [vaccine]
ALVAC-HIV MN120TMGNP (vCP300) [vaccine]
ALVAC-RG rabies glycoprotein (vCP65) [vaccine]
allopurinol (Zyloprim®) [xanthine oxidase inhibitor]
aluminum hydroxide (Amphogel®) [adjuvant, immunostimulant]
alvircept sudotox (CD4-*Pseudomonas* exotoxin) [immunomodulator, antiretroviral]
amikacin sulfate (Kanamycin®) [antibacterial]
amikasin (MiKasome) [no data]
aminosalicylic acid [antibacterial]
amitriptyline hydrochloride (Elavil®) [antidepressant, analgesic]
amoxicillin (Amoxil®) [antimicrobial]
amphotericin B (Fungizone®) [antifungal]
ampligen (Atvogen®) [antiretroviral, immunomodulator]
anti-HIV immune serum globulin (HIVIG®) [immunomodulator]
anti-Rh antibodies (Anti-D) [immunomodulator]
APL 400-003 [vaccine]
AS-101 (ammonium trichlorotellurate) [immunomodulator]
atevirdine mesylate (U-87201E) [antiretroviral]
azidodideoxyuridine (AzdU) [antiretroviral]
BCH 10652 [reverse transcriptase inhibitor/HIV]
beclomethasone dipropionate (Beclovent®) [anti-inflammatory]
benzimidavir (1263W94) [CMV-DNA inhibitor/CMV]
benztropine mesylate (Cogentin®) [anticholinergic, antiparkinsonian]
bis-POM PMEA [antiretroviral]
bleomycin (Blenoxane®) [antineoplastic]
BMS 232 [protease inhibitor]
BMS 232632 [protease azapeptide inhibitor/HIV]
BMS 234475 [second generation protease inhibitor/HIV]
BMS 234475/CGP-61755 [other/HIV]
butyldeoxynojirimicin (SC-48334) [antiretroviral]
calanolide A [antiviral]
capreomycin sulfate (Caprocin®) [antibacterial]
CD4 antigen [antiretroviral]
CD4-IgG [antiretroviral, immunomodulator]

ceftriaxone sodium (Rocephin®) [antimicrobial]
cefuroxime axetil (Ceftin®) [antibiotic]
chimeric anti-TNF monoclonal antibody (Chimeric A2) [immunomodulator]
chlorhexidine gluconate (Peridex®, Hibiclens®) [topical antibacterial, antimicrobial]
cidofovir gel (Forvade®) [antiviral/genital herpes]
cimetidine (Tagamet®) [immunomodulator, histamine receptor antagonist]
ciprofloxacin (Cipro®) [antibacterial]
CI-0694 (Sulfasim®) [immunomodulator]
clavulanate potassium [antibacterial]
clindamycin (Cleocin®) [antibacterial]
clofazimine (Lamprene®) [antimicrobial, antileprotic]
clotrimazole (Lotrimin®, Mycelex®, FemCare®) [antifungal]
*Cryptosporidium* immune whey protein (bovine anticryptosporidium immunoglobulin) [antidiarrheal]
CS-92 [nucleoside reverse transcriptase inhibitor/HIV]
CTL [gene therapy/HIV]
curdlan sulfate [antiviral]
cyclophosphamide (Cytoxan®) [antineoplastic, immunosuppressant]
cycloserine (Seromycin®) [antibacterial]
cysteamine (MEA; mercaptoethylamine) [antiretroviral, antiurolithic]
cytarabine (Cytosar-U®) [antimetabolite, antineoplastic, antiviral, immunosuppressant]
cytolin [nontoxic AIDS monoclonal antibody/HIV]
cytomegalovirus immune globulin intravenous (human) (CytoGam®) [immunomodulator]
dacarbazine [antineoplastic]
DAPD [purine dioxolane nucleoside/HIV]
dapsone [antibacterial]
delavirdine mesylate (U-90152) [antiretroviral]
deoxy-fluorothymidine (FDT) [antiretroviral]
dexamethasone (Decadron®) [anti-inflammatory, immunomodulator, antineoplastic]
dextran sulfate [antiretroviral]
diclazuril [antiprotozoal]
dideoxyadenosine (ddA) [antiretroviral]
diethylhomospermine (DEHSPM) [antidiarrheal]
dinitrochlorobenzene (DNCB) [contact allergen, immunomodulator]
disulfiram (Antabuse®) [alcohol abuse deterrent, immunomodulator, antiretroviral]
ditiocarb sodium (Imuthiol®) [immunomodulator, chelator]
DMP-266 [non-nucleoside reverse transcriptase inhibitor/HIV]
DMP-450 [second generation protease inhibitor/HIV]
doxorubicin (Adriamycin®, Rubex®) [antineoplastic]
emtricitabine (Coviracil) [nucleoside analog]
env 2-3 [vaccine]
ethambutol hydrochloride (Myambutol®) [antibacterial]
ethionamide [antibacterial]
etoposide (VePesid®) [antineoplastic]
F105 human monoclonal antibody [immunomodulator]
fiacitabine (FIAC) [antiviral]
fialuridine (FIAU) [antiviral]
flucytosine (Ancobon®) [antifungal]
fluorouracil (5-FU) [antineoplastic]
G3139 [antisense compound/nonhodgkin's lymphoma]
GEM 132 [hybrid antisense oligonucleotide/CMV retinitis]
glutamic acid (Feracid®) [gastric acidifier]
gp-160 (MicroGeneSys®, VaxSyn®) [vaccine]
gp-160 vaccine (Immuno-AG) [vaccine]
guaifenesin (Robitussin®) [expectorant]
GW275175 [CMV-DNA maturation inhibitor/CMV retinitis]

HBY 097 [antiretroviral]
hepatitis B vaccine (Engerix-B®, Recombivax HB®) [vaccine]
heptavalent pneumococcal conjugate vaccine [vaccine]
HIV p17/p24: Ty-VLP [vaccine]
HIV-1 C4-V3 polyvalent peptide vaccine [vaccine]
HIVAC-1e [vaccine]
hydroxyurea (Hydrea®) [anticancer drug]
hypericin (VIMRyxn®) [antiretroviral]
ibuprofen (Advil®; Motrin®; Nuprin®) [nonsteroidal anti-inflammatory]
ifosfamide [antineoplastic]
imipramine hydrochloride (Tofranil®) [antidepressant]
inosine pranobex (Isoprinosine®) [antiviral, immunostimulant, antiretroviral]
insulin-like growth factor (Somatomedin C®) [immunomodulator]
interferon alfa-n1 (Wellferon®) [antineoplastic, antiviral, immunomodulator]
interferon alfa-n3 (Alferon N®) [antineoplastic, antiviral, immunomodulator]
interferon beta (Betaseron®) [antineoplastic, antiviral, immunomodulator, antiretroviral]
interferon gamma (Actimmune®) [antineoplastic, antiviral, immunomodulator]
interleukin-3 (IL-3) [immunomodulator, hematopoietic]
interleukin-4 (IL-4) [immunomodulator, antineoplastic]
interleukin-10 (IL-10) [immunomodulator]
interleukin-12 (IL-12) [antiviral]
iodenosine (f-dda) [purine-based reverse transcriptase inhibitor/HIV]
ISIS 13312 [second generation antisense compound/CMV retinitis]
ISIS 2922 [antiviral]
isoniazid (INH) [antibacterial]
isotretinoin (Accutane®) [keratolytic]
ketoconazole (Nizoral®) [antifungal, antineoplastic, antiadrenal]
keyhole-limpet hemocyanin [immunomodulator]
kynostatin 272 (KNI-272®) [protease inhibitor, antiretroviral]
L-756,423 [protease inhibitor]
lentinan [immunomodulator, antineoplastic]
letrazuril [antiprotozoal]
leucovorin calcium (Wellcovorin®) [antianemic, antidote for folic acid antagonists]
levamisole [immunomodulator]
levocarnitine [antihyperlipoproteinemic]
levofloxacin [antimicrobial, antiretroviral]
liposome - encapsulated monophosphoryl lipid A [adjuvant, immunostimulant]
Liposyn® III (I.V. fat emulsion 2%) [nutritional support]
Liposyn® II (I.V. fat emulsion 20%) [nutritional support]
lobucavir [antiviral]
lodenosine (F-ddA) [nucleoside analog type drug similar to ddI]
lymphocytes, activated [immunomodulator]
L-697, 639 [antiretroviral]
L-697, 661 [antiretroviral]
magnesium sulfate [electrolyte replenisher, anticonvulsant, laxative]
MDL 28574 [antiretroviral]
MDX-240 [virus-specific bispecific antibody/HIV]
memantine [NMDA receptor antagonist/neuroprotective agent/dementia]
methadone hydrochloride (Dolophine®) [detoxification maintenance, narcotic analgesic]
methotrexate (MTX) [antineoplastic, folic acid antagonist, anti-inflammatory]
methoxsalen (Oxsoralen-ultra®) [photochemotherapeutic]
methylprednisolone (Medrol®) [anti-inflammatory, immunosuppressant]
mexiletine hydrochloride (Mexitil®) [analgesic, antiarrhythmic]
MF59 [adjuvant, immunostimulant]
microparticulate monovalent HIV-1 peptide vaccine [vaccine]
mitoguazone dihydrochloride (MGBG) [antineoplastic]

mitoxantrone hydrochloride (Novantrone®) [antineoplastic]
MKC-442 [antiviral-NNRTI]
monophosphoryl lipid A [adjuvant, immunostimulant]
MTP-PE/MF59 [immunostimulant, adjuvant emulsion]
multikine [immunotherapeutic agent/HIV]
multivalent HIV-1 peptide immunogen [vaccine]
n-docosanol (Lidakol®) [antiviral]
nimodipine (Nimotop®) [calcium channel blocker, vasodilator]
nitazoxanide (NTZ) [antiparasitic]
nystatin (Mycostatin®) [antifungal]
octreotide acetate (Sandostatin®) [antidiarrheal]
OPC 14117 [antioxidant]
oxandrolone (Oxandrin®) [steroid]
oxazepam (Serax®) [anxiolytic, minor tranquilizer]
P3C541b lipopeptide [vaccine]
paclitaxel (Taxol®) [antineoplastic]
paromomycin sulfate (Humatin®) [antibiotic, amebicidal, anthelmintic]
PCLUS [vaccine]
penicillin G [antibacterial]
pentosan polysulfate sodium [antineoplastic, antiviral, anticoagulant, anti-inflammatory,antiretroviral]
pentoxifylline (Trental®) [vasodilator, hemorrheologic]
peptide T [antiretroviral, immunomodulator]
phenylhydrazone [antiviral/HIV]
piritrexim isethionate [antifolate, antineoplastic, antiproliferative, antiprotozoal]
PMEA [antiretroviral]
pneumococcal vaccine polyvalent [vaccine]
polyethylene glycolated IL-2 (PEG IL-2) [immunomodulator]
polymyxin B sulfate/bacitracin zinc ointment (Bacitracin®, Polysporin®) [antibacterial]
prednisone [glucocorticoid]
primaquine [antimalarial]
probenecid (Benemid®) [renal tubular blocker, uricosuric]
probucol (Panavir®) [antiviral]
pseudoephedrine (Sudafed®) [decongestant, sympathomimetic]
pyrazinamide [antibacterial]
pyridoxine hydrochloride (vitamin $B_6$) [vitamin (coenzyme)]
QS-21 [adjuvant, immunostimulant]
quinine [antimalarial, neuromuscular]
ranitidine hydrochloride (Zantac®) [histamine receptor antagonist, immunomodulator]
recombinant p24 vaccine [vaccine]
rgp 120/HIV-1IIIB [vaccine]
rgp 120/HIV-1MN [vaccine]
rgp 120/HIV 1MN monovalent octameric V3 peptide (SynVac®) [vaccine]
rgp 120/HIV-1SF2 [vaccine]
ribavirin (Virazole®) [antiviral, antiretroviral]
rifalazil (PA-1648) [rifampin derivative]
rifampin (Rifadin®, Rimactane®) [antibacterial]
RMP-7 [antifungal]
RO 24-7429 [antiretroviral, *tat* inhibitor]
*Saccharomyces boulardii* [antidiarrheal]
SC-49483 [antiretroviral]
SC-52151 [protease inhibitor, antiretroviral]
SCH 39304 [antifungal]
selegiline hydrochloride (Deprenyl®) [MAO inhibitor, antidyskinetic, antiparkinsonian]
sevirumab (human monoclonal antibody to cytomegalovirus) [antiviral, immunomodulator]
smallpox vaccine (Dryvax®) [vaccine]

sorivudine (Brovavir®) [antiviral]
SP-303T [antiviral]
sparfloxacin (Zagam®) [antibacterial]
spiramycin [antibacterial, antiprotozoal]
streptomycin sulfate [antibacterial]
SU5416 [angiogenesis inhibitor/HIV]
sulfadiazine [antibacterial]
sulfadoxine (Fansidar® when combined with pyrimethamine) [antibacterial]
syntex adjuvant formulation [adjuvant, immunostimulant]
T1249 [fusion inhibitor]
T20 [fusion inhibitor]
TAT antagonist [antiviral]
TBC-3B [vaccine]
tecogalan sodium (SP-PG) [angiogenesis inhibitor]
tenofovir dipivoxil (PMPA) [nucleotide inhibitor]
thalidomide (Synovir®) [immunomodulator, sedative, hypnotic]
thioctic acid [antioxidant]
threonyl muramyl dipeptide [adjuvant, immunostimulant]
thymic humoral factor (THF) [immunomodulator]
thymosin alpha 1 [immunomodulator]
thymopentin (Timunox®) [immunomodulator]
tipranavir [protease inhibitor]
TNP-470 [antineoplastic]
tretinoin (Atragen®) [liposomal all-transretinoic acid]
trichosanthin (GLQ 223) [antiretroviral, immunosuppressant]
trifluridine (ophthalmic) [antiviral]
tuberculin purified protein derivative (PPD) [diagnostic aid]
tumor necrosis factor (TNF) [antineoplastic, antiretroviral]
tumor necrosis factor soluble receptor - immunoadhesion complex [immunomodulator]
valacyclovir hydrochloride (Valtrex®) [antiviral]
valganciclovir (Cymeval®) [antiviral/CMV retinitis]
valproic acid (Depakene®) [anticonvulsant]
varicella virus vaccine live (Varivax®) [vaccine]
vesnarinone (OPC-8212) [antiretroviral, cardiotonic]
vidarabine [antiviral]
vinblastine sulfate (Velban®) [antineoplastic]
vincristine (Oncovin®) [antineoplastic]
virulizin [macrophage activator/HIV and lymphomas]
WF10 [antiretroviral]
wobenzym [immunomodulator]
WR 6026 [antiprotozoal]
zidovudine/didanosine (Sciptene®) [heterodimer/HIV]
524W91 [antiretroviral]
882C87 [antiviral]
935U83 [antiretroviral]

# CANCER CHEMOTHERAPY ACRONYMS

| Acronyms | Used for |
|---|---|
| 7 + 3 | Leukemia — acute myeloid leukemia, induction |
| ABP | Lymphoma — non-Hodgkin's |
| ABC-P | Multiple myeloma |
| ABDIC | Lymphoma — Hodgkin's |
| ABVD | Lymphoma — Hodgkin's |
| AC | Sarcoma — bony sarcoma |
| AC | Breast cancer |
| AC (DC) | Multiple myeloma |
| ACE | Lung cancer — small cell |
| ACe | Breast cancer |
| ACMF | Breast cancer |
| ACOMLA | Lymphoma — non-Hodgkin's |
| ADOC | Thymoma (malignant) |
| AVM | Breast cancer |
| m-BACOD | Lymphoma — non-Hodgkin's |
| BACOP | Lymphoma — non-Hodgkin's |
| BAP | Multiple myeloma |
| BAPP | Thymoma (malignant) |
| BCDT | Malignant melanoma |
| BCNU-DAG | Brain tumors |
| B-CMF | Head and neck cancer |
| BCVM | Cervical cancer |
| BCP | Multiple myeloma |
| BEP | Genitourinary cancer — testicular, induction, good risk |
| BHD | Malignant melanoma<br>Breast cancer |
| BMC | Head and neck cancer |
| B-MOPP | Lymphoma — Hodgkin's |
| BMVL | Head and neck cancer |
| BOMP | Cervical cancer |
| BVCPP | Lymphoma — Hodgkin's |
| CAF | Breast cancer |
| CAFVP | Breast cancer |
| CAM | Genitourinary cancer — prostate |
| CAMP | Lung cancer — non-small cell |
| CAP | Genitourinary cancer — bladder<br>Head and neck cancer<br>Lung cancer — non-small cell<br>Adrenal cortical cancer<br>Endometrial cancer |
| CAP-BOP | Lymphoma — non-Hodgkin's |
| CAP-M | Genitourinary cancer — bladder |
| CBM | Head and neck cancer |
| CC | Ovarian cancer — epithelial |
| CCCP | Multiple myeloma |
| CCNU-VP | Lymphoma — Hodgkin's |
| CCVPP | Lymphoma — Hodgkin's |
| CD | Leukemia — acute nonlymphoblastic, consolidation<br>Ewing's sarcoma<br>Genitourinary cancer — prostate |
| CDC | Ovarian cancer — epithelial |
| CDF | Genitourinary cancer — prostate |

| Acronyms | Used for |
|---|---|
| CE | Adrenal cortical cancer |
| CF | Head and neck cancer |
| CFM | Breast cancer |
| CFPT | Breast cancer |
| CHAP | Ovarian cancer — epithelial |
| CHL + PRED | Leukemia — chronic lymphocytic leukemia |
| CHOP | Lymphoma — non-Hodgkin's |
| CHOP-B (Yale) | Lymphoma — non-Hodgkin's |
| CHOP-Bleo | Lymphoma — non-Hodgkin's |
| CHOP (P) | Lymphoma — non-Hodgkin's |
| CHOR | Lung cancer — small cell |
| CISCA | Gastric cancer<br>Genitourinary cancer — bladder |
| Cladribine (2-CdA) | Leukemia — chronic lymphocytic leukemia |
| CMB | Cervical cancer |
| CMC-High Dose | Lung cancer — small cell |
| CMF | Breast cancer |
| CMFP | Breast cancer |
| CMFVP (Cooper's) | Breast cancer |
| C-MOPP | Lymphoma — non-Hodgkin's |
| CMV | Genitourinary cancer — bladder |
| COB | Head and neck cancer |
| CODE | Lung cancer — small cell |
| COPE | Lung cancer — small cell |
| COLP | Thymoma (malignant) |
| COM | Colon cancer |
| COMF | Colon cancer |
| COP-BLAM | Lymphoma — non-Hodgkin's |
| COP-BLAM III | Lymphoma — non-Hodgkin's |
| COP-BLAM IV | Lymphoma — non-Hodgkin's |
| COP | Lymphoma — non-Hodgkin's |
| COP-BLAM | Lymphoma — non-Hodgkin's |
| COPP (or "C" MOPP) | Lymphoma — non-Hodgkin's |
| CP | Ovarian cancer — epithelial |
| CV | Lung cancer — non-small cell |
| CVB | Esophageal cancer |
| CVI | Lung cancer — non-small cell |
| CVM | Gestational trophoblastic disease |
| CVP | Leukemia — chronic lymphocytic leukemia<br>Lymphoma — non-Hodgkin's |
| CYADIC | Sarcoma — soft tissue |
| CYVADIC | Sarcoma — bony sarcoma<br>Sarcoma — soft tissue |
| DAFS | Carcinoid (malignant) |
| DAT | Leukemia — acute myeloid leukemia, induction<br>Breast cancer |
| DC | Multiple myeloma |
| DHAP | Lymphoma — non-Hodgkin's |
| DMC | Gestational trophoblastic cancer |
| DS | Genitourinary cancer — prostate |
| DTIC-ACTD | Malignant melanoma |
| DVP | Leukemia — acute lymphoblastic, induction |
| DVPA | Leukemia — acute lymphoblastic, induction |
| ELF | Gastric cancer |

# APPENDIX

| Acronyms | Used for |
|---|---|
| EMA-CO | Gestational trophoblastic disease |
| FAC | Breast cancer |
| FAC-S | Carcinoid (malignant) |
| FAM | Gastric cancer<br>Lung cancer — non-small cell<br>Pancreatic cancer |
| FAME | Gastric cancer |
| FAMTX | Gastric cancer |
| FAP | Gastric cancer |
| FAP-2 | Pancreatic cancer |
| FCE | Gastric cancer |
| F-CL | Colon cancer |
| FDC | Gastric cancer |
| FL | Genitourinary cancer — prostate |
| FLe | Colon cancer |
| Fludarabine | Leukemia — chronic lymphocytic leukemia |
| FMS (SMF) | Pancreatic cancer |
| FMV | Colon cancer |
| FOAM | Breast cancer |
| FOMi | Lung cancer — non-small cell |
| FOMi/CAP | Lung cancer — non-small cell |
| 5FU/LDLF | Colon cancer |
| FU/HU | Colon cancer |
| FU/LV | Colon cancer |
| 5FU Hurt | Head and neck cancer |
| 5FU/LV (weekly) | Colon cancer |
| FL | Genitourinary cancer — prostate |
| HDAC | Leukemia — acute myeloid leukemia, induction |
| HDMTX | Sarcoma — bony sarcoma |
| IC | Leukemia — acute myeloid leukemia, induction |
| ID | Sarcoma — soft tissue |
| IMAC | Sarcoma — bony sarcoma |
| IMF | Breast cancer |
| IMVP-16 | Lymphoma — non-Hodgkin's |
| LDAC | Leukemia — acute myeloid leukemia, induction |
| L-VAM | Genitourinary cancer — prostate |
| M-2 | Multiple myeloma |
| MAC | Genitourinary cancer — bladder<br>Endometrial cancer |
| MACC | Lung cancer — non-small cell |
| MACOP-B | Lymphoma — non-Hodgkin's |
| MAID | Sarcoma — soft tissue |
| MAP | Head and neck cancer |
| MBC (MBD) | Head and neck cancer<br>Cervical cancer<br>Esophageal cancer |
| MBD | Head and neck cancer |
| MC | Leukemia — acute myeloid leukemia, induction |
| MeCP | Multiple myeloma |
| MF | Head and neck cancer<br>Esophageal cancer |
| MICE (ICE) | Lung cancer — small cell |
| MINE | Lymphoma — non-Hodgkin's |
| MM | Leukemia — acute lymphoblastic, maintenance |

| Acronyms | Used for |
|---|---|
| MMC (MTX + MP + CTX) | Leukemia — acute lymphoblastic, maintenance |
| MOF-STREP | Colon cancer |
| MOP-BAP | Lymphoma — Hodgkin's |
| MOPP | Lymphoma — Hodgkin's |
| MOPP/ABV Hybrid | Lymphoma — Hodgkin's |
| MP | Multiple myeloma |
| m-PFL | Genitourinary cancer — bladder |
| MS | Adrenal cortical cancer |
| MV | Leukemia — acute myeloid leukemia, induction |
| MVAC | Genitourinary cancer — bladder |
| MVPP | Lymphoma — Hodgkin's |
| NFL | Breast cancer |
| PAC (CAP) | Ovarian cancer — epithelial<br>Endometrial cancer |
| PE | Genitourinary cancer — testicular, induction, good risk<br>Lung cancer — small cell |
| PFL | Gastric cancer<br>Head and neck cancer |
| PFL + IFN | Head and neck cancer |
| Pt-FU | Head and neck cancer |
| POCC | Lung cancer — small cell |
| Pro-MACE | Lymphoma — non-Hodgkin's |
| Pro-MACE-CytaBOM | Lymphoma — non-Hodgkin's |
| Pro-MACE-MOPP | Lymphoma — non-Hodgkin's |
| PT | Ovarian cancer — epithelial |
| SC | Carcinoid (malignant) |
| SCAB | Lymphoma — Hodgkin's |
| SD | Pancreatic cancer |
| SF | Carcinoid (malignant) |
| SMF | Pancreatic cancer |
| T-9 | Ewing's sarcoma |
| VAB VI | Genitourinary cancer — testicular, induction, salvage |
| VAC | Ovarian cancer — germ cell<br>Sarcoma — soft tissue Ewing's sarcoma |
| VAC (CAV) (Induction) | Lung cancer — small cell |
| VAD | Leukemia — acute lymphoblastic, induction<br>Multiple myeloma |
| VADRIAC — High Dose | Sarcoma — bony sarcoma |
| VAIE | Sarcoma — bony sarcoma |
| VAM | Breast cancer |
| VAP | Multiple myeloma |
| VATH | Breast cancer |
| VBAP | Multiple myeloma |
| VBC | Malignant melanoma |
| VBP (PVB) | Genitourinary cancer — testicular, induction, salvage |
| VC | Lung cancer — small cell |
| VCAP | Multiple myeloma |
| VDCP | Endometrial cancer |
| VDP | Malignant melanoma |
| VIP | Genitourinary cancer — testicular, induction, poor risk |
| VIP (Einhorn) | Genitourinary cancer — testicular, induction, poor risk |
| VP | Leukemia — acute lymphoblastic, induction |
| VP-L-Asparaginase | Leukemia — acute lymphoblastic, induction |
| Wayne State | Head and neck cancer |

# CANCER CHEMOTHERAPY REGIMENS

## ADULT REGIMENS

### Adenocarcinoma – Unknown Primary

**Carbo-Tax**

Paclitaxel, I.V., 135 mg/m$^2$ over 24 hours, day 1, followed by
Carboplatin dose targeted by Calvert equation to AUC 7.5 I.V.

Repeat cycle every 21 days

**EP**

Cisplatin, I.V., 60-100 mg/m$^2$, day 1
Etoposide, I.V., 80-100 mg/m$^2$, days 1-3

Repeat cycle every 21 days

**FAM**

Fluorouracil, I.V., 600 mg/m$^2$, days 1, 8, 29, 36
Doxorubicin, I.V., 30 mg/m$^2$, days 1, 29
Mitomycin, I.V., 10 mg/m$^2$, day 1

Repeat cycle every 8 weeks

**Paclitaxel/Carboplatin/Etoposide**

Paclitaxel, I.V., 200 mg/m$^2$ over 1 hour, day 1, followed by
Carboplatin dose targeted by Calvert equation to AUC 6 I.V.
Etoposide, P.O., 50 mg/day alternated with 100 mg/day, days 1-10

Repeat cycle every 21 days

### Breast Cancer

Standard adjuvant chemotherapy includes 4 cycles of AC or 6 cycles of CMF ($d_1/d_8$ variety)

**AC**

Doxorubicin, I.V., 60 mg/m$^2$, day 1
Cyclophosphamide, I.V., 400-600 mg/m$^2$, day 1

Repeat cycle every 21 days

**ACe**

Doxorubicin, I.V., 40 mg/m$^2$, day 1
Cyclophosphamide, P.O., 200 mg/m$^2$/day, days 1-3 or 3-6

Repeat cycle every 21-28 days

**CAF**

Cyclophosphamide, P.O., 100 mg/m$^2$, days 1-14 or 600 mg/m$^2$ I.V., day 1
Doxorubicin, I.V., 25 mg/m$^2$, days 1, 8 or 60 mg/m$^2$ I.V., day 1
Fluorouracil, I.V., 500-600 mg/m$^2$, days 1, 8

Repeat cycle every 28 days

**or**

Cyclophosphamide, I.V., 500 mg/m$^2$, day 1
Doxorubicin, I.V., 50 mg/m$^2$, day 1
Fluorouracil, I.V., 500 mg/m$^2$, day 1

Repeat cycle every 21 days

**CFM**

Cyclophosphamide, I.V., 500-600 mg/m$^2$, day 1
Fluorouracil, I.V., 500-600 mg/m$^2$, day 1
Mitoxantrone, I.V., 10-12 mg/m$^2$, day 1

Repeat cycle every 21 days

## Breast Cancer *(continued)*

### CFPT

Cyclophosphamide, I.V., 150 mg/m$^2$, days 1-5
Fluorouracil, I.V., 300 mg/m$^2$, days 1-5
Prednisone, P.O., 10 mg tid, days 1-7
Tamoxifen, P.O., 10 mg bid, days 1-42

Repeat cycle every 42 days

### CMF

Cyclophosphamide, P.O., 100 mg/m$^2$, days 1-14 or 600 mg/m$^2$ I.V., days 1, 8
Methotrexate, I.V., 40 mg/m$^2$, days 1, 8
Fluorouracil, I.V., 600 mg/m$^2$, days 1, 8

Repeat cycle every 28 days

**or**

Cyclophosphamide, I.V., 600 mg/m$^2$, day 1
Methotrexate, I.V., 40 mg/m$^2$, day 1
Fluorouracil, I.V., 400-600 mg/m$^2$, day 1

Repeat cycle every 21 days

### CMFP

Cyclophosphamide, P.O., 100 mg/m$^2$, days 1-14
Methotrexate, I.V., 40-60 mg/m$^2$, days 1, 8
Fluorouracil, I.V., 600-700 mg/m$^2$, days 1, 8
Prednisone, P.O., 40 mg (first 3 cycles only), days 1-14

Repeat cycle every 28 days

### FAC

Fluorouracil, I.V., 500 mg/m$^2$, days 1, 8
Doxorubicin, I.V., 50 mg/m$^2$, day 1
Cyclophosphamide, I.V., 500 mg/m$^2$, day 1

Repeat cycle every 21 days

### IMF

Ifosfamide, I.V., 1.5 g/m$^2$, days 1, 8
Mesna, I.V., 20% of ifosfamide dose, give immediately before and 4 and 8 hours after ifosfamide infusion, days 1, 8
Methotrexate, I.V., 40 mg/m$^2$, days 1, 8
Fluorouracil, I.V., 600 mg/m$^2$, days 1, 8

Repeat cycle every 28 days

### NFL

Mitoxantrone, I.V., 12 mg/m$^2$, day 1
Fluorouracil, I.V., 350 mg/m$^2$, days 1-3, given after leucovorin calcium
Leucovorin calcium, I.V., 300 mg/m$^2$, days 1-3

**or**

Mitoxantrone, I.V., 10 mg/m$^2$, day 1
Fluorouracil, I.V., 1000 mg/m$^2$ continuous infusion, given after leucovorin calcium, days 1-3
Leucovorin calcium, I.V., 100 mg/m$^2$, days 1-3

Repeat cycle every 21 days

### Sequential Dox-CMF

Doxorubicin, I.V., 75 mg/m$^2$, every 21 days for 4 cycles followed by 21- or 28-day CMF for 8 cycles

### Vinorelbine/Doxorubicin

Vinorelbine, I.V., 25 mg/m$^2$, days 1, 8
Doxorubicin, I.V., 50 mg/m$^2$, day 1

Repeat cycle every 21 days

### VATH

Vinblastine, I.V., 4.5 mg/m$^2$, day 1
Doxorubicin, I.V., 45 mg/m$^2$, day 1
Thiotepa, I.V., 12 mg/m$^2$, day 1
Fluoxymesterone, P.O., 10 mg tid, days 1-21

Repeat cycle every 21 days

**Breast Cancer** *(continued)*

**Single-Agent Regimens**

Anastrozole, P.O., 1 mg qd

Capecitabine, P.O., 2500 mg/m$^2$/day, bid regimen, days 1-14, repeat cycle every 21 days

Docetaxel, I.V., 60-100 mg/m$^2$ over 1 hour; patient must be premedicated with dexamethasone 8 mg bid P.O. for 5 days, start 1 day before docetaxel; repeat cycle every 3 weeks

Gemcitabine, I.V., 725 mg/m$^2$ over 30 minutes, weekly for 3 weeks, followed by 1-week rest, repeat cycle every 28 days

Letrozole, P.O., 2.5 mg qd

Megestrol, P.O., 40 mg qid

Paclitaxel, I.V., 175 mg/m$^2$ over 3 hours, every 21 days or 250 mg/m$^2$ over 3-24 hours, every 21 days
Patient must be premedicated with:
Dexamethasone 20 mg P.O., 12 and 6 hours prior
Diphenhydramine 50 mg I.V., 30 minutes prior
Cimetidine 300 mg I.V., or ranitidine 50 mg I.V., 30 minutes prior

Tamoxifen, P.O., 20 mg qd

Toremifene citrate, P.O., 60 mg qd

Vinorelbine, I.V., 30 mg/m$^2$, every 7 days

# Cervical Cancer

**CLD-BOMP**

Bleomycin, I.V., 5 mg continuous infusion, days 1-7
Cisplatin, I.V., 10 mg/m$^2$, day 1, 22
Vincristine, I.V., 0.7 mg/m$^2$, day 7
Mitomycin-C. I.V., 7 mg/m$^2$, day 7

Repeat cycle every 21 days

**MOBP**

Bleomycin, I.V., 30 units/day continuous infusion, days 1, 4
Vincristine, I.V., 0.5 mg/m$^2$, days 1, 4
Mitomycin-C. I.V., 10 mg/m$^2$, day 1
Cisplatin, I.V., 50 mg/m$^2$, days 1, 22

Repeat cycle every 28 days

**Single-Agent Regimen**

Cisplatin, I.V., 50-100 mg/m$^2$, every 21 days

# Colon Cancer

**F-CL**

Fluorouracil, I.V., 375 mg/m$^2$, days 1-5
Leucovorin calcium, I.V., 200 mg/m$^2$, days 1-5

Repeat cycle every 28 days

**or**

Fluorouracil, I.V., 500 mg/m$^2$/week 1 hour after initiating the calcium leucovorin infusion for 6 weeks
Leucovorin calcium, I.V., 500 mg/m$^2$, over 2 hours, weekly for 6 weeks

2-week break, then repeat cycle

**FLe**

Fluorouracil, I.V., 450 mg/m$^2$ for 5 days, then, after a pause of 4 weeks, 450 mg/m$^2$/week for 48 weeks
Levamisole, P.O., 50 mg tid for 3 days, repeated every 2 weeks for 1 year

### Colon Cancer *(continued)*

#### FMV

Fluorouracil, I.V., 10 mg/kg/day, days 1-5
Methyl-CCNU, P.O., 175 mg/m$^2$, day 1
Vincristine, I.V., 1 mg/m$^2$ (max: 2 mg), day 1

Repeat cycle every 35 days

#### FU/LV

Fluorouracil, I.V., 370-400 mg/m$^2$/day, days 1-5
Leucovorin calcium, I.V., 200 mg/m$^2$/day, commence infusion 15 minutes prior to fluorouracil infusion, days 1-5

Repeat cycle every 21 days

**or**

Fluorouracil, I.V., 1000 mg/m$^2$/day by continuous infusion, days 1-4
Leucovorin calcium, I.V., 200 mg/m$^2$/day, days 1-4

Repeat cycle every 28 days

#### Weekly 5FU/LV

Fluorouracil, I.V., 600 mg/m$^2$ over 1 hour given after leucovorin, repeat weekly x 6 then 2-week rest period = 1 cycle, days 1, 8, 15, 22, 29, 36
Leucovorin calcium, I.V., 500 mg/m$^2$ over 2 hours, days 1, 8, 15, 22, 29, 36

Repeat cycle every 56 days

#### 5FU/LDLF

Fluorouracil, I.V., 425 mg/m$^2$/day, days 1-5
Leucovorin calcium, I.V., 20-25 mg/m$^2$/day, days 1-5

Repeat cycle every 28 days

#### Single-Agent Regimens

5-FU, I.V., 1000 mg/m$^2$/day, continuous infusion, days 1-5

Repeat cycle every 21-28 days

Irinotecan, I.V., 125 mg/m$^2$ over 90 minutes every 7 days for 4 cycles or 350 mg/m$^2$ over 30 minutes

Repeat cycle every 21 days

## Endometrial Cancer

#### AP

Doxorubicin, I.V., 60 mg/m$^2$, day 1
Cisplatin, I.V., 60 mg/m$^2$, day 1

Repeat cycle every 21 days

#### Single-Agent Regimens

Doxorubicin, I.V., 40-60 mg/m$^2$, day 1

Repeat cycle every 21-28 days

Medroxyprogesterone, P.O., 200 mg/day

## Gastric Cancer

#### EAP

Etoposide, I.V., 120 mg/m$^2$, days 4, 5, 6
Doxorubicin, I.V., 20 mg/m$^2$, days 1, 7
Cisplatin, I.V., 40 mg/m$^2$, days 2, 8

Repeat cycle every 28 days

#### ELF

Leucovorin calcium, I.V., 300 mg/m$^2$, days 1-3 followed by
Etoposide, I.V., 120 mg/m$^2$, days 1-3 followed by
Fluorouracil, I.V., 500 mg/m$^2$, days 1-3

Repeat cycle every 21-28 days

## Gastric Cancer *(continued)*

### FAM

Fluorouracil, I.V., 600 mg/m$^2$, days 1, 8, 29, 36
Doxorubicin, I.V., 30 mg/m$^2$, days 1, 29
Mitomycin C, I.V., 10 mg/m$^2$, day 1

Repeat cycle every 8 weeks

### FAME

Fluorouracil, I.V., 350 mg/m$^2$, days 1-5, 36-40
Doxorubicin, I.V., 40 mg/m$^2$, days 1, 36
Methyl-CCNU, P.O., 150 mg/m$^2$, day 1

Repeat cycle every 70 days

### FAMTX

Methotrexate, IVPB, 1500 mg/m$^2$, day 1
Fluorouracil, IVPB, 1500 mg/m$^2$ 1 hour after methotrexate, day 1
Leucovorin calcium, P.O., 15 mg/m$^2$ q6h x 48 hours, 24 hours after methotrexate, day 2
Doxorubicin, IVPB, 30 mg/m$^2$, day 15

Repeat cycle every 28 days

### FCE

Fluorouracil, I.V., 900 mg/m$^2$/day continuous infusion, days 1-5
Cisplatin, I.V., 20 mg/m$^2$, days 1-5
Etoposide, I.V., 90 mg/m$^2$, days 1, 3, 5

Repeat cycle every 21 days

### PFL

Cisplatin, I.V., 25 mg/m$^2$ continuous infusion, days 1-5
Fluorouracil, I.V., 800 mg/m$^2$ continuous infusion, days 2-5
Leucovorin calcium, I.V., 500 mg/m$^2$ continuous infusion, days 1-5

Repeat cycle every 28 days

### Single-Agent Regimens

Irinotecan, I.V., over 90 minutes: 125 mg/m$^2$/week; repeat weekly for 4 weeks, then 2-week rest period

**or**

Irinotecan, I.V. over 30-90 minutes: 350 mg/m$^2$; repeat every 21 days

# Genitourinary Cancer

## Bladder

### CAP

Cyclophosphamide, I.V., 400 mg/m$^2$, day 1
Doxorubicin, I.V., 40 mg/m$^2$, day 1
Cisplatin, I.V., 60 mg/m$^2$, day 1

Repeat cycle every 21 days

### CISCA

Cisplatin, I.V., 70-100 mg/m$^2$, day 2
Cyclophosphamide, I.V., 650 mg/m$^2$, day 1
Doxorubicin, I.V., 50 mg/m$^2$, day 1

Repeat cycle every 21-28 days

### CMV

Cisplatin, I.V., 100 mg/m$^2$ over 4 hours, start 12 hours after MTX, day 2
Methotrexate, I.V., 30 mg/m$^2$, days 1, 8
Vinblastine, I.V., 4 mg/m$^2$, days 1, 8

Repeat cycle every 21 days

## Genitourinary Cancer — Bladder *(continued)*

### m-PFL

Methotrexate, I.V., 60 mg/m$^2$, day 1
Cisplatin, I.V., 25 mg/m$^2$ continuous infusion, days 2-6
Fluorouracil, I.V., 800 mg/m$^2$ continuous infusion, days 2-6
Leucovorin calcium, I.V., 500 mg/m$^2$ continuous infusion, days 2-6

Repeat cycle every 28 days for 4 cycles

### MVAC

Methotrexate, I.V., 30 mg/m$^2$, days 1, 15, 22
Vinblastine, I.V., 3 mg/m$^2$, days 2, 15, 22
Doxorubicin, I.V., 30 mg/m$^2$, day 2
Cisplatin, I.V., 70 mg/m$^2$, day 2

Repeat cycle every 28 days

### PC

Paclitaxel, I.V., 200 mg/m$^2$ or 225 mg/m$^2$ over 3 hours, day 1
Carboplatin, I.V., dose targeted by Calvert equation to AUC 5 or 6 after paclitaxel, day 1

Repeat cycle every 21 days

### Single-Agent Regimens

Gemcitabine, I.V., 1200 mg/m$^2$, days 1, 8, 15

Repeat cycle every 28 days

Paclitaxel, I.V., 250 mg/m$^2$ over 24 hours, day 1

Repeat cycle every 21 days

## Ovarian, Epithelial

### Carbo-Tax

Paclitaxel, I.V., 135 mg/m$^2$ over 24 hours, day 1

**or**

175 mg/m$^2$ over 3 hours, day 1, followed by
Carboplatin dose targeted by Calvert equation to AUC 7.5 I.V.

Repeat cycle every 21 days

### CC

Carboplatin, I.V., dose targeted by Calvert equation to AUC 6-7
Cyclophosphamide, I.V., 600 mg/m$^2$, day 1

Repeat cycle every 28 days

### CP

Cyclophosphamide, I.V., 750 mg/m$^2$, day 1
Cisplatin, I.V., 75 mg/m$^2$, day 1

Repeat cycle every 21 days

### CT

Paclitaxel, I.V., 135 mg/m$^2$ over 24 hours, day 1

**or**

175 mg/m$^2$ over 3 hours, day 1, followed by
Cisplatin, I.V., 75 mg/m$^2$

Repeat cycle every 21 days

### PAC (CAP)

Cisplatin, I.V., 50 mg/m$^2$, day 1
Doxorubicin, I.V., 50 mg/m$^2$, day 1
Cyclophosphamide, I.V., 1000 mg/m$^2$, day 1

Repeat cycle every 21 days x 8 cycles

## Genitourinary Cancer — Ovarian, Epithelial *(continued)*

### Single-Agent Regimens

Altretamine, P.O., 260 mg/m$^2$/day, qid for 1-15 days
Repeat cycle every 28 days for 2 cycles, then reassess

Etoposide, I.V., 50-60 mg/m$^2$/day, days 1-21
Repeat cycle every 28 days

Liposomal doxorubicin, I.V., 50 mg/m$^2$, 1-hour infusion, day 1
Repeat cycle every 21 days

Paclitaxel, I.V., 135 mg/m$^2$, over 3 or 24 hours, day 1
Repeat cycle every 21 days for 2 cycles, then reassess

Topotecan, I.V., 1.5 mg/m$^2$, over 30 minutes, days 1-5
Repeat cycle every 21 days for 2 cycles, then reassess

## Ovarian, Germ Cell

### BEP

Bleomycin, I.V., 30 units, days 2, 9, 16
Etoposide, I.V., 100 mg/m$^2$, days 1-5
Cisplatin, I.V., 20 mg/m$^2$, days 1-5
Repeat cycle every 21 days

### VAC

Vincristine, I.V., 1.2-1.5 mg/m$^2$ (max: 2 mg) weekly for 10-12 weeks, or every 2 weeks for 12 doses
Dactinomycin, I.V., 0.3-0.4 mg/m$^2$, days 1-5
Cyclophosphamide, I.V., 150 mg/m$^2$, days 1-5
Repeat every 28 days

## Prostate

### EV

Estramustine, P.O., 200 mg tid, days 1-42
Vinblastine, I.V., 4 mg/m$^2$/week, begin day 1
Repeat cycle every 6 weeks

### FL

Flutamide, P.O., 250 mg tid, days 1-28
Leuprolide acetate, S.C., 1 mg qd, days 1-28
Repeat cycle every 28 days

**or**

Flutamide, P.O., 250 mg tid, days 1-28
Leuprolide acetate depot, I.M., 7.5 mg, day 1
Repeat cycle every 28 days

### FZ

Flutamide, P.O., 250 mg tid
Goserelin acetate, S.C., 3.6 mg implant, every 28 days or goserelin S.C., 10.8 mg depot every 12 weeks

### L-VAM

Leuprolide acetate, S.C., 1 mg qd, days 1-28
Vinblastine, I.V., 1.5 mg/m$^2$/day continuous infusion, days 2-7
Doxorubicin, I.V., 50 mg/m$^2$ continuous infusion, day 1
Mitomycin C, I.V., 10 mg/m$^2$, day 2
Repeat cycle every 28 days

### Mitoxantrone/Prednisone

Mitoxantrone, I.V., 12 mg/m$^2$, day 1
Prednisone, P.O., 5 mg bid
Repeat cycle every 21 days

## Genitourinary Cancer — Prostate *(continued)*

### No Known Acronym

Bicalutamide, P.O., 50 mg/day

Leuprolide acetate depot, I.M., 7.5 mg or goserelin S.C. 3.6 mg implant every 28 days

### PE

Paclitaxel, I.V., 120 mg/m$^2$, days 1-4

Estramustine, P.O., 600 mg qd, 24 hours before paclitaxel

Repeat cycle every 21 days

### Single-Agent Regimens

Estramustine, P.O., 14 mg/kg/day, tid or qid

Goserelin acetate implant, S.C., 3.6 mg every 28 days or 10.8 mg every 12 weeks

Nilutamide, P.O., 300 mg qd, days 1-30, then 150 mg qd in combination with surgical castration; begin on same day or day after castration

Prednisone, P.O., 5 mg bid

## Renal

Interleukin-2 (rIL-2), S.C.
20 million units/m$^2$, days 3-5, weeks 1, 4
5 million units/m$^2$, days 1, 3, 5, weeks 2, 3, 5, 6

**or**

Interferon alfa (rIFN$\alpha$2), S.C.
6 million units/m$^2$, day 1, weeks 1, 4;
6 million units/m$^2$, days 1, 3, 5, weeks 2, 3, 5, 6

Repeat cycle every 8 weeks

### Single-Agent Regimen

Interleukin-2:
High dose: I.V. bolus over 15 minutes, 600,000-720,000 units/kg q8h until toxicity or 14 days; administer 2 courses separated by 7-10 days
Low dose: S.C., 18 million units/day for 5 days, then 9 million units/day for 2 days, then 18 million units/day 3 days/week for 6 weeks

**or**

3 million units/m$^2$/day for 5 days/week, every 2 weeks for 1 month, then every 4 weeks

## Testicular

### EP

Etoposide, I.V., 100 mg/m$^2$, days 1-5

Cisplatin, I.V., 20 mg/m$^2$, days 1-5

Repeat cycle every 21 days

## Testicular, Induction, Good Risk

### BEP

Bleomycin, I.V., 30 units, days 2, 9, 16

Etoposide, I.V., 100 mg/m$^2$, days 1-5

Cisplatin, I.V., 20 mg/m$^2$, days 1-5

Repeat cycle every 21 days

### PVB

Cisplatin, I.V., 20 mg/m$^2$, days 1-5

Vinblastine, I.V., 0.15 mg/kg, days 1, 2

Bleomycin, I.V., 30 units, days 2, 9, 16

Repeat cycle every 21 days

### Testicular, Induction, Poor Risk

**VIP**

Etoposide, I.V., 75 mg/m$^2$, days 1-5
Ifosfamide, I.V., 1.2 g/m$^2$, days 1-5
Cisplatin, I.V., 20 mg/m$^2$, days 1-5
Mesna, I.V., 400 mg/m$^2$, then 1200 mg/m$^2$/day continuous infusion, days 1-5

Repeat cycle every 21 days

**VIP (Einhorn)**

Vinblastine, I.V., 0.11 mg/kg, days 1-2
Ifosfamide, I.V., 1200 mg/m$^2$, days 1-5
Cisplatin, I.V., 20 mg/m$^2$, days 1-5
Mesna, I.V., 400 mg/m$^2$, then 1200 mg/m$^2$/day continuous infusion, days 1-5

Repeat cycle every 21 days

### Testicular, Induction, Salvage

**VAB VI**

Vinblastine, I.V., 4 mg/m$^2$, day 1
Dactinomycin, I.V., 1 mg/m$^2$, day 1
Bleomycin, I.V., 30 units push day 1, then 20 units/m$^2$/day continuous infusion, days 1-3
Cisplatin, I.V., 120 mg/m$^2$, day 4
Cyclophosphamide, I.V., 600 mg/m$^2$, day 1

Repeat cycle every 21 days

**VBP (PVB)**

Vinblastine, I.V., 6 mg/m$^2$, days 1, 2
Bleomycin, I.V., 30 units, days 1, 8, 15, (22)
Cisplatin, I.V., 20 mg/m$^2$, days 1-5

Repeat cycle every 21-28 days

## Gestational Trophoblastic Cancer

**DMC**

Dactinomycin, I.V., 0.37 mg/m$^2$, days 1-5
Methotrexate, I.V., 11 mg/m$^2$, days 1-5
Cyclophosphamide, I.V., 110 mg/m$^2$, days 1-5

Repeat cycle every 21 days

## Head and Neck Cancer

**CAP**

Cyclophosphamide, I.V., 500 mg/m$^2$, day 1
Doxorubicin, I.V., 50 mg/m$^2$, day 1
Cisplatin, I.V., 50 mg/m$^2$, day 1

Repeat cycle every 28 days

**CF**

Carboplatin, I.V., 400 mg/m$^2$, day 1
Fluorouracil, I.V., 1000 mg/m$^2$/day continuous infusion, days 1-5

Repeat cycle every 21-28 days

**COB**

Cisplatin, I.V., 100 mg/m$^2$, day 1
Vincristine, I.V., 1 mg, days 2, 5
Bleomycin, I.V., 30 units/day continuous infusion, days 2-5

Repeat cycle every 21 days

## Head and Neck Cancer *(continued)*

### 5-FU HURT

Hydroxyurea, P.O., 1000 mg q12h x 11 doses; start PM of admission, give 2 hours prior to radiation therapy, days 0-5
Fluorouracil, I.V., 800 $mg/m^2/day$ continuous infusion, start AM after admission, days 1-5
Paclitaxel, I.V., 5-25 $mg/m^2/day$ continuous infusion, start AM after admission; dose escalation study – refer to protocol, days 1-5
G-CSF, S.C., 5 mcg/kg/day, days 6-12, start ≥12 hours after completion of 5-FU infusion

5-7 cycles may be administered

### PFL

Cisplatin, I.V., 100 $mg/m^2$, day 1
Fluorouracil, I.V., 600-800 $mg/m^2/day$ continuous infusion, days 1-5
Leucovorin calcium, I.V., 200-300 $mg/m^2/day$, days 1-5

Repeat cycle every 21 days

### PFL+IFN

Cisplatin, I.V., 100 $mg/m^2$, day 1
Fluorouracil, I.V., 640 $mg/m^2/day$ continuous infusion, days 1-5
Leucovorin calcium, P.O., 100 mg q4h, days 1-5
Interferon alfa-2b, S.C., 2 x $10^6$ $units/m^2$, days 1-6

### Pt-FU

Cisplatin, I.V., 100 $mg/m^2$, day 1
Fluorouracil, I.V., 1000 $mg/m^2/day$ continuous infusion, days 1-5

Repeat cycle every 21 days for 2 cycles

### TIP

Paclitaxel, I.V., 175 $mg/m^2$ 3-hour infusion, day 1
Ifosfamide, I.V., 1000 $mg/m^2$ 2-hour infusion, days 1-3
Mesna, I.V., 400 $mg/m^2$ before ifosfamide and 200 $mg/m^2$ I.V., 4 hours after ifosfamide
Cisplatin, I.V., 60 $mg/m^2$, day 1

Repeat cycle every 21-28 days

### Single-Agent Regimens

Carboplatin, I.V., 300-400 $mg/m^2$, over 2 hours every 21-28 days

Methotrexate, I.V., I.M., 40 $mg/m^2$, bolus day 1; cycle repeated every 7 days for 6 cycles

Cisplatin I.V., 100 $mg/m^2$, every 28 days divided into 1, 2, or 4 equal doses per month

Vinorelbine, I.V., 25-30 $mg/m^2$, repeat weekly

# Leukemia

## Acute Lymphoblastic, Induction

### VAD

Vincristine, I.V., 0.4 mg/day continuous infusion, days 1-4
Doxorubicin, I.V., 12 $mg/m^2/day$ continuous infusion, days 1-4
Dexamethasone, P.O., 40 mg, days 1-4, 9-12, 17-20

### VP

Vincristine, I.V., 2 $mg/m^2/week$ for 4-6 weeks (max: 2 mg)
Prednisone, P.O., 60 $mg/m^2/day$ in divided doses for 4 weeks, taper weeks 5-7

### No Known Acronym

Cyclophosphamide, I.V., 1200 $mg/m^2$, day 1
Daunorubicin, I.V., 45 $mg/m^2$, days 1-3
Prednisone, P.O., 60 $mg/m^2$, days 1-21
Vincristine, I.V., 2 $mg/m^2/week$
L-asparaginase, I.V., 6000 $units/m^2$, 3 times/week

**or**

Pegaspargase, I.M./I.V., 2500 $units/m^2$, every 14 days if patient develops hypersensitivity to native L-asparaginase

## Acute Lymphoblastic, Maintenance

**MM**

Mercaptopurine, P.O., 50-75 mg/m$^2$, days 1-7
Methotrexate, P.O./I.V., 20 mg/m$^2$, day 1

Repeat cycle every 7 days

**MMC (MTX + MP + CTX)***

Methotrexate, I.V., 20 mg/m$^2$/week
Mercaptopurine, P.O., 50 mg/m$^2$/day
Cyclophosphamide, I.V., 200 mg/m$^2$/week

*Continue all 3 drugs until relapse of disease or after 3 years of remission.

## Acute Lymphoblastic, Relapse

**AVDP**

Asparaginase, I.V., 15,000 units/m$^2$, days 1-5, 8-12, 15-19, 22-26
Vincristine, I.V., 2 mg/m$^2$ (max: 2 mg), days 8, 15, 22
Daunorubicin, I.V., 30-60 mg/m$^2$, days 8, 15, 22
Prednisone, P.O., 40 mg/m$^2$, days 8-12, 15-19, 22-26

## Acute Myeloid Leukemia, Induction

**7+3**

Cytarabine, I.V., 100-200 mg/m$^2$/day continuous infusion, days 1-7

**with**

Daunorubicin, I.V., 45 mg/m$^2$, days 1-3

**or**

Idarubicin, I.V., 12 mg/m$^2$, days 1-3

**or**

Mitoxantrone, I.V., 12 mg/m$^2$, days 1-3

**5+2***

Cytarabine, I.V., 100-200 mg/m$^2$/day continuous infusion, days 1-5

**with**

Daunorubicin, I.V., 45 mg/m$^2$, days 1-2

**or**

Mitoxantrone, I.V., 12 mg/m$^2$, days 1-2
*For reinduction

**DAT/DCT**

Daunorubicin, I.V., 60 mg/m$^2$/day, days 1-3
Cytarabine, I.V., 200 mg/m$^2$/day continuous infusion, days 1-5
Thioguanine, P.O., 100 mg/m$^2$ q12h, days 1-5

***Modified DAT (considerations in elderly patients)***

Daunorubicin, I.V., 50 mg/m$^2$, day 1
Cytarabine, S.C., 100 mg/m$^2$/day q12h, days 1-5
Thioguanine, P.O., 100 mg/m$^2$ q12h, days 1-5

**EMA-86**

Etoposide, I.V., 200 mg/m$^2$/day continuous infusion, days 8-10
Mitoxantrone, I.V., 12 mg/m$^2$, days 1-3
Cytarabine, I.V., 500 mg/m$^2$/day continuous infusion, days 1-3, 8-10

**LDAC**

***Considerations in Elderly Patients***

Cytarabine, S.C., 10 mg/m$^2$ bid, days 10-21

**MC**

Mitoxantrone, I.V., 12 mg/m$^2$/day, days 1-3
Cytarabine, I.V., 100-200 mg/m$^2$/day continuous infusion, days 1-7

***Consolidation***

Mitoxantrone, I.V., 12 mg/m$^2$, days 1-2
Cytarabine, I.V., 100 mg/m$^2$ continuous infusion, days 1-5

Repeat cycle every 28 days

## Leukemia — Acute Myeloid Leukemia, Induction *(continued)*

**MV**

Mitoxantrone, I.V., 10 mg/m$^2$/day, days 1-5
Etoposide, I.V., 100 mg/m$^2$/day, days 1-3

### Single-Agent Regimen

All transrelincic acid (ATRA), P.O., 45 mg/m$^2$/day (1 or 2 divided doses) with or without 7+3 induction regimen

## Acute Myeloid Leukemia, Postremission

### Single-Agent Regimens

Cytarabine, I.V., 100 mg/m$^2$/day continuous infusion, days 1-5*; repeat cycle every 28 days
*For patients >60 years of age

Cytarabine (HiDAC), I.V. 3000 mg/m$^2$ over 1-3 hours, every 12 hours, days 1-6

**or**

3000 mg/m$^2$ over 1-3 hours, every 12 hours, days 1, 3, 5. Administer with saline, methylcellulose, or steroid eyedrops OU, every 2-4 hours, beginning with cytarabine and continuing 48-72 hours after last cytarabine dose

Repeat cycle every 28 days

## Acute Nonlymphoblastic, Consolidation

**CD**

Cytarabine, I.V., 3000 mg/m$^2$ q12h, days 1-6
Daunorubicin, I.V., 30 mg/m$^2$/day, days 7-9

## Chronic Lymphocytic Leukemia

**CHL + PRED**

Chlorambucil, P.O., 0.4 mg/kg/day for 1 day every other week
Prednisone, P.O., 100 mg/day for 2 days every other week; adjust dosage according to blood counts every 2 weeks prior to therapy; increase initial dose of 0.4 mg/kg by 0.1 mg/kg every 2 weeks until toxicity or disease control is achieved

**CVP**

Cyclophosphamide, P.O., 400 mg/m$^2$/day, days 1-5
Vincristine, I.V., 1.4 mg/m$^2$ (max: 2 mg), day 1
Prednisone, P.O., 100 mg/m$^2$, days 1-5

Repeat cycle every 21 days

### Single-Agent Regimens

Chlorambucil, P.O., 0.1-0.2 mg/kg/day for 3-6 weeks

**or**

Chlorambucil, P.O., 20-30 mg/m$^2$, day 1

Repeat cycle every 14-28 days

**or**

Chlorambucil, P.O., 0.4 mg/kg/day, for 1 day every other week

**or**

Chlorambucil, P.O., 0.4 mg/kg/day, for 1 day every other day

Cladribine, I.V., 0.1 mg/kg/day continuous infusion, days 1-5 or 1-7

Repeat cycle every 28-35 days

Cyclophosphamide, P.O., 2-4 mg/kg, days 1-10

Repeat cycle every 21-28 days

Fludarabine, I.V., 25-30 mg/m$^2$, days 1-5

Repeat cycle every 28 days

Prednisone,* P.O., 30-60 mg/m$^2$, days 1-5 or 1-7

*Use if patient symptomatic with autoimmune thrombocytopenia or hemolytic anemia.

### Chronic Myelogenous Leukemia

#### Single-Agent Regimens

Busulfan, P.O., 4-8 mg/day for 5-10 weeks (until WBC reduced to 20 x $10^3/\mu L$)

Hydroxyurea, P.O., 2-5 g/day; decrease dose by 1/2 as counts decrease (stop when WBC = 20 x $10^3/\mu L$)

Interferon alfa-2a, S.C., 3-9 million units/day; dose may be adjusted as per response and adverse events.

### Hairy-Cell Leukemia

#### Single-Agent Regimens

Cladribine, I.V., 0.1 mg/kg/day continuous infusion, days 1-7

Administer one cycle

Interferon alfa-2a, S.C., 3 million units, 3 times/week

Pentostatin, I.V., 4 mg/m$^2$, day 1

Repeat cycle every 14 days

## Lung Cancer

### Small Cell

#### CAV/VAC

Cyclophosphamide, I.V., 750-1000 mg/m$^2$, day 1
Doxorubicin, I.V., 50 mg/m$^2$, day 1
Vincristine, I.V., 1.4 mg/m$^2$ (max: 2 mg), day 1

Repeat cycle every 3 weeks

#### CAVE

Cyclophosphamide, I.V., 750 mg/m$^2$, day 1
Doxorubicin, I.V., 50 mg/m$^2$, day 1
Vincristine, I.V., 1.4 mg/m$^2$ (max: 2 mg), day 1
Etoposide, I.V., 60-100 mg/m$^2$, days 1-3

Repeat cycle every 21 days

#### EC

Etoposide, I.V., 100-120 mg/m$^2$, days 1-3
Carboplatin, I.V., 325-400 mg/m$^2$, day 1

Repeat cycle every 28 days

#### EP/PE

Etoposide, I.V., 120 mg/m$^2$, days 1-3
Cisplatin, I.V., 60-120 mg/m$^2$, day 1

Repeat cycle every 21-28 days

#### Single-Agent Regimen

Etoposide, P.O., 50 mg/m$^2$, days 1-21

Repeat cycle every 28 days

Topotecan, I.V., 1.5 mg/m$^2$/day, over 30 minutes, days 1-5

Repeat cycle every 21 days

### Non-small Cell

#### Carbo-Tax

Paclitaxel, I.V., 135 mg/m$^2$ over 24 hours, day 1 **or**
175 mg/m$^2$ over 3 hours, day 1, followed by
Carboplatin dose targeted by Calvert equation to AUC 7.5 I.V.

Repeat cycle every 21 days

### Lung Cancer — Non-small Cell *(continued)*

**EC**

Etoposide, I.V., 100-120 mg/m$^2$, days 1-3

**with**

Carboplatin, I.V., 300-325 mg/m$^2$, day 1

Repeat cycle every 21-28 days

**EP**

Etoposide, I.V., 80 mg/m$^2$, days 1-3
Cisplatin, I.V., 60-100 mg/m$^2$, day 1

Repeat cycle every 21-28 days

**Gemcitabine-Cis**

Gemcitabine, I.V., 1000 mg/m$^2$, days 1, 8, 15
Cisplatin, I.V., 100 mg/m$^2$, day 2 or 15

Repeat cycle every 28 days

**PC**

Paclitaxel, I.V., 175 mg/m$^2$, 3-hour infusion, day 1
Cisplatin, I.V., 80 mg/m$^2$, day 1

Repeat cycle every 21 days

**Vinorelbine-Cis**

Vinorelbine, I.V., 30 mg/m$^2$, every 7 days
Cisplatin, I.V., 120 mg/m$^2$, day 1, 29, then every 6 weeks

**Single-Agent Regimens**

Topotecan, I.V., 1.5 mg/m$^2$/day, over 30 minutes, days 1-5

Repeat cycle every 21 days

Vinorelbine, I.V., 30 mg/m$^2$, every 7 days

## Lymphoma

### Hodgkin's

**ABVD**

Doxorubicin, I.V., 25 mg/m$^2$, days 1, 15
Bleomycin, I.V., 10 units/m$^2$, days 1, 15
Vinblastine, I.V., 6 mg/m$^2$, days 1, 15
Dacarbazine, I.V., 350-375 mg/m$^2$, days 1, 15

Repeat cycle every 28 days

**ChlVPP**

Chlorambucil, P.O., 6 mg/m$^2$ (max: 10 mg/day), days 1-14
Vinblastine, I.V., 6 mg/m$^2$ (max: 10 mg dose), days 1, 8
Procarbazine, P.O., 100 mg/m$^2$ (max: 150 mg/day), days 1-14
Prednisone, P.O., 40 mg/day, days 1-14

Repeat cycle every 28 days

**CVPP**

Lomustine, P.O., 75 mg/m$^2$, day 1
Vinblastine, I.V., 4 mg/m$^2$, days 1, 8
Procarbazine, P.O., 100 mg/m$^2$, days 1-14
Prednisone, P.O., 30 mg/m$^2$, days 1-14 (cycles 1 and 4 only)

Repeat cycle every 28 days

**EVA**

Etoposide, I.V., 100 mg/m$^2$, days 1-3
Vinblastine, I.V., 6 mg/m$^2$, day 1
Doxorubicin, I.V., 50 mg/m$^2$, day 1

Repeat cycle every 28 days

## Lymphoma — Hodgkin's *(continued)*

### MOPP

Mechlorethamine, I.V., 6 mg/m$^2$, days 1, 8
Vincristine, I.V., 1.4 mg/m$^2$ (max: 2.5 mg), days 1, 8
Procarbazine, P.O., 100 mg/m$^2$, days 1-14
Prednisone, P.O., 40 mg/m$^2$, days 1-14

Repeat cycle every 28 days

### MOPP/ABV Hybrid

Mechlorethamine, I.V., 6 mg/m$^2$, day 1
Vincristine, I.V., 1.4 mg/m$^2$, day 1
Procarbazine, P.O., 100 mg/m$^2$, days 1-7
Prednisone, P.O., 40 mg/m$^2$, days 1-14
Doxorubicin, I.V., 35 mg/m$^2$, day 8
Bleomycin, I.V., 10 units/m$^2$, day 8
Vinblastine, I.V., 6 mg/m$^2$, day 8

Repeat cycle every 28 days

### MVPP

Mechlorethamine, I.V., 6 mg/m$^2$, days 1, 8
Vinblastine, I.V., 6 mg/m$^2$, days 1, 8
Procarbazine, P.O., 100 mg/m$^2$, days 1-14
Prednisone, P.O., 40 mg/m$^2$, days 1-14

Repeat cycle every 42 days

### NOVP

Mitoxantrone, I.V., 10 mg/m$^2$, day 1
Vincristine, I.V., 2 mg, day 8
Vinblastine, I.V., 6 mg/m$^2$, day 1
Prednisone, P.O., 100 mg/m$^2$, days 1-5

Repeat cycle every 21 days

### Stanford V*

Mechlorethamine, I.V., 6 mg/m$^2$, day 1
Doxorubicin, I.V., 25 mg/m$^2$, days 1, 15
Vinblastine, I.V., 6 mg/m$^2$, days 1, 15
Vincristine, I.V., 1.4 mg/m$^2$, days 8, 22
Bleomycin, I.V., 5 units/m$^2$, days 8, 22
Etoposide, I.V., 60 mg/m$^2$, days 15, 16
Prednisone, P.O., 40 mg/m$^2$/day, dose tapered over the last 15 days

Repeat cycle every 28 days

*In patients older than 50 years of age, vinblastine dose decreased to 4 mg/m$^2$ and vincristine dose decreased to 1 mg/m$^2$ on weeks 9-12. Concomitant trimethoprim/sulfamethoxazole DS P.O. bid; acyclovir 200 mg P.O. tid; ketoconazole 200 mg P.O. qd; and stool softeners used.

## Non-Hodgkin's

### BACOP

Bleomycin, I.V., 5 units/m$^2$, days 15, 22
Doxorubicin, I.V., 25 mg/m$^2$, days 1, 8
Cyclophosphamide, I.V., 650 mg/m$^2$, days 1, 8
Vincristine, I.V., 1.4 mg/m$^2$ (max: 2 mg), days 1, 8
Prednisone, P.O., 60 mg/m$^2$, days 15-28

Repeat cycle every 28 days

### CHOP

Cyclophosphamide, I.V., 750 mg/m$^2$, day 1
Doxorubicin, I.V., 50 mg/m$^2$, day 1
Vincristine, I.V., 1.4 mg/m$^2$ (max: 2 mg), day 1
Prednisone, P.O., 100 mg/m$^2$, days 1-5

Repeat cycle every 21 days

## Lymphoma — Non-Hodgkin's *(continued)*

### CHOP-Bleo

Cyclophosphamide, I.V., 750 mg/m$^2$, day 1
Doxorubicin, I.V., 50 mg/m$^2$, day 1
Vincristine, I.V., 2 mg, days 1, 5
Prednisone, P.O., 100 mg, days 1-5
Bleomycin, I.V., 15 units, days 1, 5

Repeat cycle every 21-28 days

### CNOP

Cyclophosphamide, I.V., 750 mg/m$^2$, day 1
Mitoxantrone, I.V., 10 mg/m$^2$, day 1
Vincristine, I.V., 1.4 mg/m$^2$, day 1
Prednisone, P.O., 50 mg/m$^2$, days 1-5

Repeat cycle every 21 days

### COMLA

Cyclophosphamide, I.V., 1500 mg/m$^2$, day 1
Vincristine, I.V., 1.4 mg/m$^2$ (max: 2.5 mg), days 1, 8, 15
Methotrexate, I.V., 120 mg/m$^2$, days 22, 29, 36, 43, 50, 57, 64, 71
Leucovorin calcium rescue, P.O., 25 mg/m$^2$, q6h for 4 doses, beginning 24 hours after each methotrexate dose
Cytarabine, I.V., 300 mg/m$^2$, days 22, 29, 36, 43, 50, 57, 64, 71

Repeat cycle every 21 days

### COP

Cyclophosphamide, I.V., 800 mg/m$^2$, day 1
Vincristine, I.V., 1.4 mg/m$^2$ (max: 2 mg), day 1
Prednisone, P.O., 60 mg/m$^2$, days 1-5

Repeat cycle every 21 days

### COP-BLAM

Cyclophosphamide, I.V., 400 mg/m$^2$, day 1
Vincristine, I.V., 1 mg/m$^2$, day 1
Prednisone, P.O., 40 mg/m$^2$, days 1-10
Bleomycin, I.V., 15 mg, day 14
Doxorubicin, I.V., 40 mg/m$^2$, day 1
Procarbazine, P.O., 100 mg/m$^2$, days 1-10

### COPP (or "C" MOPP)

Cyclophosphamide, I.V., 400-650 mg/m$^2$, days 1, 8
Vincristine, I.V., 1.4-1.5 mg/m$^2$ (max: 2 mg), days 1, 8
Procarbazine, P.O., 100 mg/m$^2$, days 1-14
Prednisone, P.O., 40 mg/m$^2$, days 1-14

Repeat cycle every 28 days

### CVP

Cyclophosphamide, P.O., 400 mg/m$^2$, days 1-5
Vincristine, I.V., 1.4 mg/m$^2$ (max: 2 mg), day 1
Prednisone, P.O., 100 mg/m$^2$, days 1-5

Repeat cycle every 21 days

### DHAP*

Dexamethasone, I.V., 10 mg q6h, days 1-4
Cytarabine, I.V., 2 g/m$^2$ q12h x 2 doses, day 2
Cisplatin, I.V., 100 mg/m$^2$ continuous infusion, day 1

Repeat cycle every 21-28 days

*Administer with saline, methylcellulose, or steroid eyedrops OU, every 2-4 hours, beginning with cytarabine and continuing 48-72 hours after last cytarabine dose.

## Lymphoma — Non-Hodgkin's *(continued)*

### ESHAP*

Etoposide, I.V., 60 mg/m$^2$, days 1-4
Cisplatin, I.V., 25 mg/m$^2$/day continuous infusion, days 1-4
Cytarabine, I.V., 2 g/m$^2$, immediately following completion of etoposide and cisplatin therapy
Methylprednisolone, I.V., 500 mg/day, days 1-4

Repeat cycle every 21-28 days

*Administer with saline, methylcellulose, or steroid eyedrops OU, every 2-4 hours, beginning with cytarabine and continuing 48-72 hours after last cytarabine dose.

### IMVP-16

Ifosfamide, I.V., 4 g/m$^2$ continuous infusion over 24 hours, day 1
Mesna, I.V., 800 mg/m$^2$ bolus prior to ifosfamide, then 4 g/m$^2$ continuous infusion over 12 hours concurrent w/ifosfamide; then 2.4 g/m$^2$ continuous infusion over 12 hours after ifosfamide infusion, day 1
Methotrexate, I.V., 30 mg/m$^2$, days 3, 10
Etoposide, I.V., 100 mg/m$^2$, days 1-3

Repeat cycle every 21-28 days

### MACOP-B

Methotrexate, I.V., 400 mg/m$^2$, weeks 2, 6, 10
Doxorubicin, I.V., 50 mg/m$^2$, weeks 1, 3, 5, 7, 9, 11
Cyclophosphamide, I.V., 350 mg/m$^2$, weeks 1, 3, 5, 7, 9, 11
Vincristine, I.V., 1.4 mg/m$^2$ (max: 2 mg), weeks 2, 4, 8, 10, 12
Bleomycin, I.V., 10 units/m$^2$, weeks 4, 8, 12
Prednisone, P.O., 75 mg/day tapered over 15 d, days 1-15
Leucovorin calcium, P.O., 15 mg/m$^2$, q6h x 6 doses 24 hours after methotrexate, weeks 2, 6, 10
Trimethoprim/sulfamethoxazole DS, P.O., tablet, bid, for 12 weeks
Ketoconazole, P.O., 200 mg/day

Administer one cycle

### m-BACOD

Methotrexate, I.V., 200 mg/m$^2$, days 8, 15
Leucovorin calcium, P.O., 10 mg/m$^2$ q6h x 8 doses beginning 24 hours after each methotrexate dose, days 8, 15
Bleomycin, I.V., 4 units/m$^2$, day 1
Doxorubicin, I.V., 45 mg/m$^2$, day 1
Cyclophosphamide, I.V., 600 mg/m$^2$, day 1
Vincristine, I.V., 1 mg/m$^2$, day 1
Dexamethasone, P.O., 6 mg/m$^2$, days 1-5

Repeat cycle every 21 days

### m-BACOS

Methotrexate, I.V., 1 g/m$^2$, day 2
Bleomycin, I.V., 10 units/m$^2$, day 1
Doxorubicin, I.V., 50 mg/m$^2$ continuous infusion, day 1
Cyclophosphamide, I.V., 750 mg/m$^2$, day 1
Vincristine, I.V., 1.4 mg/m$^2$ (max: 2 mg), day 1
Leucovorin calcium rescue, P.O., 15 mg q6h for 8 doses, starting 24 hours after methotrexate
Methylprednisolone, I.V., 500 mg, days 1-3

Repeat cycle every 21-25 days

### MINE

Mesna, I.V., 1.33 g/m$^2$/day concurrent with ifosfamide dose, then 500 mg P.O. 4 hours after each ifosfamide infusion, days 1-3
Ifosfamide, I.V., 1.33 g/m$^2$/day, days 1-3
Mitoxantrone, I.V., 8 mg/m$^2$, day 1
Etoposide, I.V., 65 mg/m$^2$/day, days 1-3

Repeat cycle every 28 days

## Lymphoma — Non-Hodgkin's *(continued)*

### MINE-ESHAP

Mesna, I.V., 1.33 g/m$^2$, administered at same time as ifosfamide, then 500 mg P.O., 4 hours after ifosfamide, days 1-3
Ifosfamide, I.V., 1.33 g/m$^2$, over 1 hour, days 1-3
Mitoxantrone, I.V., 8 mg/m$^2$, day 1
Etoposide, I.V., 65 mg/m$^2$, days 1-3

Repeat cycle every 21 days for 6 cycles, followed by 3-6 cycles of ESHAP

### NOVP

Mitoxantrone, I.V., 10 mg/m$^2$, day 1
Vinblastine, I.V., 6 mg/m$^2$, day 1
Prednisone, P.O., 100 mg, days 1-5
Vincristine, I.V., 2 mg, day 8

Repeat cycle every 21 days

### Pro-MACE

Prednisone, P.O., 60 mg/m$^2$, days 1-14
Methotrexate, I.V., 1.5 g/m$^2$, day 14
Leucovorin calcium, I.V., 50 mg/m$^2$ q6h x 5 doses beginning 24 hours after methotrexate dose, day 14
Doxorubicin, I.V., 25 mg/m$^2$, days 1, 8
Cyclophosphamide, I.V., 650 mg/m$^2$, days 1, 8
Etoposide, I.V., 120 mg/m$^2$, days 1, 8

Repeat cycle every 28 days

### Pro-MACE-CytaBOM

Prednisone, P.O., 60 mg/m$^2$, days 1-14
Doxorubicin, I.V., 25 mg/m$^2$, day 1
Cyclophosphamide, I.V., 650 mg/m$^2$, day 1
Etoposide, I.V., 120 mg/m$^2$, day 1
Cytarabine, I.V., 300 mg/m$^2$, day 8
Bleomycin, I.V., 5 units/m$^2$, day 8
Vincristine, I.V., 1.4 mg/m$^2$ (max: 2 mg), day 8
Methotrexate, I.V., 120 mg/m$^2$, day 8
Leucovorin calcium, P.O., 25 mg/m$^2$ q6h x 4 doses, day 9
Concomitant trimethoprim/sulfamethoxazole DS, P.O., bid

Repeat cycle every 21-28 days

### Single-Agent Regimens

CDA cladribine, S.C., 0.1 mg/kg/day for 5 days or 0.1 mg/kg/day I.V., for 7 days

Repeat cycle every 28 days

Rituximab, I.V., 375 mg/m$^2$, days 1, 8, 15, 22

## Malignant Melanoma

### CVD

Cisplatin, I.V., 20 mg/m$^2$, days 1-5
Vinblastine, I.V., 1.6 mg/m$^2$, days 1-5
Dacarbazine, I.V., 800 mg/m$^2$, day 1

Repeat cycle every 21 days

### CVD + IL-21

Cisplatin, I.V., 20 mg/m$^2$/day, days 1-4
Vinblastine, I.V., 1.6 mg/m$^2$/day, days 1-4
Dacarbazine, I.V., 800 mg/m$^2$, day 1
IL-2, I.V., 9 million units/m$^2$ continuous infusion, days 1-4
Interferon alfa, S.C., 5 million units/m$^2$, every day, days 1-5, 7, 9, 11, 13

Repeat cycle every 21 days

### Malignant Melanoma *(continued)*

**Dacarbazine/Tamoxifen**

Dacarbazine, I.V., 250 mg/m$^2$, days 1-5, every 21 days
Tamoxifen,* P.O., 20 mg/day

**No Known Acronym**

Dacarbazine, I.V., 220 mg/m$^2$, days 1-3, every 21-28 days
Carmustine, I.V., 150 mg/m$^2$, day 1, every 42-56 days
Cisplatin, I.V., 25 mg/m$^2$, days 1-3, every 21-28 days
Tamoxifen,* P.O., 20 mg/day

*Use of tamoxifen is optional.

**Single-Agent Regimens**

Interferon alfa-2b adjuvant therapy, I.M., 20 million units/m$^2$, days 1-30, **then**

10 million units/m$^2$ S.C., 3 times/week for 48 weeks

Interferon alfa-2a, I.M., 20 million units/m$^2$ 3 times/week for 12 weeks

## Multiple Myeloma

**EDAP**

Etoposide, I.V., 100-200 mg/m$^2$, days 1-4
Dexamethasone, P.O./I.V., 40 mg/m$^2$, days 1-5
Cytarabine, 1000 mg, day 5
Cisplatin, I.V., 20 mg continuous infusion, days 1-4

**MP**

Melphalan, P.O., 8-10 mg/m$^2$, days 1-4
Prednisone, P.O., 40-60 mg/m$^2$/day, days 1-4

Repeat cycle every 28-42 days

**M-2**

Vincristine, I.V., 0.03 mg/kg (max: 2 mg), day 1
Carmustine, I.V., 0.5-1 mg/kg, day 1
Cyclophosphamide, I.V., 10 mg/kg, day 1
Melphalan, P.O., 0.25 mg/kg, days 1-4 or 0.1 mg/kg, days 1-7 or 1-10
Prednisone, P.O., 1 mg/kg/day, days 1-7

Repeat cycle every 35-42 days

**VAD**

Vincristine, I.V., 0.4 mg/day continuous infusion, days 1-4
Doxorubicin, I.V., 9 mg/m$^2$/day continuous infusion, days 1-4
Dexamethasone, P.O., 40 mg, days 1-4, 9-12, 17-20

Repeat cycle every 28-35 days

***VAD induction therapy followed by maintenance***
Interferon alfa, S.C., 3 million units/m$^2$, 3 times/week
Prednisone, P.O., 50 mg, 3 times/week, after interferon

**VBAP**

Vincristine, I.V., 1 mg, day 1
Carmustine, I.V., 30 mg/m$^2$, day 1
Doxorubicin, I.V., 30 mg/m$^2$, day 1
Prednisone, P.O., 100 mg, days 1-4

Repeat cycle every 21 days

**VBMCP**

Vincristine, I.V., 1.2 mg/m$^2$, day 1
Carmustine, I.V., 20 mg/m$^2$, day 1
Melphalan, P.O., 8 mg/m$^2$, days 1-4
Cyclophosphamide, I.V., 400 mg/m$^2$, day 1
Prednisone, P.O., 40 mg/m$^2$, days 1-7 all cycles, and 20 mg/m$^2$, days 8-14 first 3 cycles only

Repeat cycle every 35 days

### Multiple Myeloma *(continued)*

**VCAP**

Vincristine, I.V., 1 mg, day 1
Cyclophosphamide, P.O., 100 mg/m$^2$, days 1-4
Doxorubicin, I.V., 25 mg/m$^2$, day 2
Prednisone, P.O., 60 mg/m$^2$, days 1-4

Repeat cycle every 28 days

**Single-Agent Regimens**

Aldesleukin, 600,000-700,000 int. units/kg every 8 hours x 14 doses

Repeat cycle every 14 days

Dexamethasone, P.O., 20 mg/m$^2$ for 4 days beginning on days 1-4, 9-12, and 17-20

Repeat cycle every 35 days

Interferon alfa-2b, S.C., 2 million units/m$^2$, 3 times/week for maintenance therapy in selected patients with significant response to initial chemotherapy treatment

Melphalan, I.V., 90-140 mg/m$^2$

Administer one cycle

## Pancreatic Cancer

**FAM**

Fluorouracil, I.V., 600 mg/m$^2$, days 1, 8, 29, 36
Doxorubicin, I.V., 30 mg/m$^2$, days 1, 29
Mitomycin, I.V., 10 mg/m$^2$, day 1

Repeat cycle every 72 days

**SMF**

Streptozocin, I.V., 1000 mg/m$^2$, days 1, 8, 29, 36
Mitomycin, I.V., 10 mg/m$^2$, day 1
Fluorouracil, I.V., 600 mg/m$^2$, days 1, 8, 29, 36

Repeat cycle every 72 days

**Single-Agent Regimens**

Gemcitabine, I.V., 1000 mg/m$^2$ over 30 minutes once weekly for 7 weeks, followed by a 1-week rest period; subsequent cycles once weekly for 3 consecutive weeks out of every 4 weeks

## Sarcoma

**AC**

Doxorubicin, I.V., 75-90 mg/m$^2$ 96-hour continuous infusion
Cisplatin, I.A./I.V., 90-120 mg/m$^2$, 6 days

Repeat cycle every 28 days

**AD**

Doxorubicin, I.V., 22.5 mg/m$^2$/day continuous infusion, days 1-4
Dacarbazine, I.V., 225 mg/m$^2$/day continuous infusion, days 1-4

Repeat cycle every 21 days

**CYVADIC**

Cyclophosphamide, I.V., 500 mg/m$^2$, day 1
Vincristine, I.V., 1.4 mg/m$^2$, days 1, 5
Doxorubicin, I.V., 50 mg/m$^2$, day 1
Dacarbazine, I.V., 250 mg/m$^2$, days 1-5

Repeat cycle every 21 days

## Sarcoma *(continued)*

### DI

Doxorubicin, I.V., 50 mg/$m^2$ bolus, day 1

Ifosfamide, I.V., 5000 mg/$m^2$/day continuous infusion, following doxorubicin, day 1

Mesna, I.V., 600 mg/$m^2$, bolus before ifosfamide, followed by 2500 mg/$m^2$/day, continuous infusion, for 36 hours

Repeat cycle every 21 days

### HDMTX

Methotrexate, I.V., 8-12 g/$m^2$

Leucovorin calcium, P.O./I.V., 15-25 mg q6h for at least 10 doses beginning 24 hours after methotrexate dose; courses repeated weekly for 2-4 weeks, alternating with various cancer chemotherapy combination regimens

### IE

Etoposide, I.V., 100 mg/$m^2$, days 1-5

Ifosfamide, I.V., 1800 mg/$m^2$, days 1-5

Mesna, I.V., at 20% of ifosfamide dose prior to and 4 and 8 hours after ifosfamide administration

Repeat cycle every 21-28 days

### MAID

Mesna, I.V., 2500 mg/$m^2$/day continuous infusion, days 1-4

Doxorubicin, I.V., 15 mg/$m^2$/day continuous infusion, days 1-4

Ifosfamide, I.V., 2500 mg/$m^2$/day continuous infusion, days 1-3

Dacarbazine, I.V., 250 mg/$m^2$/day continuous infusion, days 1-4

Repeat cycle every 21-28 days

### VAC

Vincristine, I.V., 2 mg/$m^2$/week (max: 2 mg), during weeks 1-12

Dactinomycin, I.V., 0.015 mg/kg (max: 0.5 mg) every 3 months for 5-6 courses, days 1-5

Cyclophosphamide, P.O., 2.5 mg/kg/day for 2 years

### Single-Agent Regimens

Doxorubicin, I.V., 75 mg/$m^2$, day 1

Repeat cycle every 21 days

# PEDIATRIC REGIMENS

Small patients have a large body surface area relative to their kg weight and could possibly be overdosed if a $m^2$ dosing regimen is applied. Therefore, for calculating pediatric doses of chemotherapy agents, as a general rule a child who weighs 30 kg is ~1 $m^2$. **For children weighing <15 kg or with surface area <0.6 $m^2$**, the dose per $m^2$ of an agent listed herein should be divided by 30 and multiplied by the weight of the child (in kg) to obtain the correct dose.

## ALL, Consolidation

### IDMTX/6-MP

Methotrexate, I.V. push, 200 mg/$m^2$, then 800 mg/$m^2$ as a 24-hour infusion

Mercaptopurine, I.V., 200 mg/$m^2$ over 20 minutes, then 800 mg/$m^2$ as an 8-hour infusion

Leucovorin, P.O./I.V., 15 mg/$m^2$ q6h x 9; begin 24 hours after end of methotrexate

## ALL, Continuation

### MTX/6-MP

Methotrexate, I.M., 20 mg/$m^2$/week, during weeks 25-130

Mercaptopurine, P.O., 50 mg/$m^2$/day, during weeks 25-130

### ALL, Continuation *(continued)*

#### MTX/6-MP/VP

Methotrexate, P.O., 20 mg/m$^2$/week
Mercaptopurine, P.O., 75 mg/m$^2$/day
Vincristine, I.V., 1.5 mg/m$^2$ x 1 each month
Prednisone, P.O., 40 mg/m$^2$ x 5 days each month

## ALL, Induction

#### PVD

Prednisone, P.O., 40 mg/m$^2$/day x 28 days
Vincristine, I.V., 1.5 mg/m$^2$/week x 4
Asparaginase, I.M., 5000 int. units/m$^2$ on days 2, 5, 8, 12, 15, 18

#### PVDA

Prednisone, P.O., 40 mg/m$^2$, days 1-28
Vincristine, I.V., 1.5 mg/m$^2$, days 2, 8, 15, 22
Daunorubicin, I.V., 25 mg/m$^2$, days 2, 8, 15, 22
Asparaginase, I.M., 5000 int. units/m$^2$ on days 2, 5, 8, 12, 15, 19

#### TIT (CNS Prophylaxis)

Methotrexate: 1 y: 10 mg; 2 y: 12.5 mg; ≥3 y: 15 mg
Cytarabine: 1 y: 20 mg; 2 y: 25 mg; ≥3 y: 30 mg
Hydrocortisone: 1 y: 10 mg; 2 y: 12.5 mg; ≥3 y: 15 mg

## AML, Induction

#### CA

Cytarabine, I.V., 3 g/m$^2$, q12h for 4 doses
Asparaginase, I.M., 6000 int. units/m$^2$ 3 hours after last dose of cytarabine

#### DA

Daunorubicin, I.V., 45 mg/m$^2$, days 1-3
Cytarabine, I.V., 100 mg/m$^2$/day, continuous infusion, days 1-7

#### DAT

Daunorubicin, I.V., 45 mg/m$^2$/day continuous infusion, days 1-3
Cytarabine, I.V., 100 mg/m$^2$/day continuous infusion, days 1-7
Thioguanine, P.O., 100 mg/m$^2$, days 1-7

#### DAV

Daunorubicin, I.V., 60 mg/m$^2$, days 3, 4, 5
Cytarabine, I.V., 100 mg/m$^2$ continuous infusion, days 1-2, then 30-minute infusion q12h on days 3-8
Etoposide, I.V., 150 mg/m$^2$, days 6, 7, 8

#### HI-CDAZE

Daunorubicin, I.V., 30 mg/m$^2$, days 1-3
Cytarabine, I.V., 3 g/m$^2$, q12h, days 1-4
Etoposide, I.V., 200 mg/m$^2$, days 1-3, 6-8
Azacytidine, I.V., 150 mg/m$^2$, days 3-5, 8-10

## Brain Tumors

#### CDDP/VP

Cisplatin, I.V., 90 mg/m$^2$, day 1
Etoposide, I.V., 150 mg/m$^2$, days 3, 4

Repeat cycle every 21 days

## Brain Tumors *(continued)*

### CDDP/VP-16

Cisplatin, I.V., 90 mg/$m^2$, day 1
Etoposide, I.V., 150 mg/$m^2$, days 3, 4

Repeat cycle every 21 days

### COPE or "Baby Brain I"

**Cycle A:**
Vincristine, I.V., 0.065 mg/kg (max: 1.5 mg), days 1, 8
Cyclophosphamide, I.V., 65 mg/kg, day 1
**Cycle B:**
Cisplatin, I.V., 4 mg/$m^2$, day 1
Etoposide, I.V., 6.5 mg/kg, days 3, 4

Regimens given in alternating 28-day cycles in the sequence AABAAB

### MOP

Mechlorethamine (nitrogen mustard), I.V., 6 mg/$m^2$, days 1, 8
Vincristine, I.V., 1.4 mg/$m^2$, days 1, 8
Procarbazine, P.O., 100 mg/$m^2$, days 1-14

### MOPP

Mechlorethamine (nitrogen mustard), I.V., 3 mg/$m^2$, days 1, 8
Vincristine, I.V., 1.4 mg/$m^2$, days 1, 8
Procarbazine, P.O., 50 mg on day 1, 100 mg on day 2, then 100 mg/$m^2$ on days 3-10
Prednisone, P.O., 40 mg/$m^2$, days 1-10

Repeat cycle every 28 days

### PCV

Procarbazine, P.O., 60 mg/$m^2$, days 8-21
Methyl-CCNU, P.O., 110 mg/$m^2$, day 1
Vincristine, I.V., 1.4 mg/$m^2$, days 8 and 29

### POC

Prednisone, P.O., 40 mg/$m^2$, days 1-14
CCNU, P.O., 100 mg/$m^2$, day 1
Vincristine, I.V., 1.5 mg/$m^2$, days 1, 8, 15

### "8 in 1"

Methylprednisolone, P.O., 300 mg/$m^2$ for 3 doses q6h
Vincristine, I.V., 1.5 mg/$m^2$
Lomustine, P.O., 100 mg/$m^2$
Procarbazine, P.O., 75 mg/$m^2$
Hydroxyurea, P.O., 3000 mg/$m^2$
Cisplatin, I.V., 90 mg/$m^2$
Cytarabine, I.V., 300 mg/$m^2$
Dacarbazine, I.V., 150 mg/$m^2$

Repeat cycle every 14 days

### Single-Agent Regimen

Carboplatin, I.V., 560 mg/$m^2$, every 4 weeks

## Lymphoma

### ABVD

Doxorubicin, I.V., 25 mg/$m^2$, days 1, 15
Bleomycin, I.V., 10 units/$m^2$, days 1, 15
Vinblastine, I.V., 6 mg/$m^2$, days 1, 15
Dacarbazine (DTIC), I.V., 375 mg/$m^2$, days 1, 15

Repeat cycle every 28 days

### Lymphoma *(continued)*

#### CHOP

Cyclophosphamide, I.V., 750 mg/m$^2$, days 1, 22
Doxorubicin, I.V., 40 mg/m$^2$, days 1, 22
Vincristine, I.V., 1.5 mg/m$^2$/week for 6 doses
Prednisone, P.O., 40 mg/m$^2$/day, for 28 days

#### COMP

Cyclophosphamide, I.V., 1.2 g/m$^2$, day 1
Vincristine, I.V., 2 mg/m$^2$, days 3, 10, 17, 24
Methotrexate, I.V., 300 mg/m$^2$, day 12
Prednisone, P.O., 60 mg/m$^2$, days 3-30, then taper for 7 days (max: 60 mg)

#### COPP

Cyclophosphamide, I.V., 500 mg/m$^2$, days 1, 8
Vincristine, I.V., 1.5 mg/m$^2$, days 1, 8
Procarbazine, P.O., 100 mg/m$^2$ (max: 150 mg), days 1-14
Prednisone, P.O., 40 mg/m$^2$, days 1-14

#### MOPP

Mechlorethamine (nitrogen mustard), I.V., 6 mg/m$^2$, days 1, 8
Vincristine, I.V., 1.4 mg/m$^2$, days 1, 8
Procarbazine, P.O., 50 mg, day 1, then 100 mg/m$^2$, days 2-14
Prednisone, P.O., 40 mg/m$^2$, days 1-14 in courses 1 and 4 only

#### OPA

Vincristine, I.V., 1.5 mg/m$^2$, days 1, 8, 15
Prednisone, P.O., 60 mg/m$^2$, days 1-15
Doxorubicin, I.V., 40 mg/m$^2$, days 1, 15

#### OPPA

Vincristine, I.V., 1.5 mg/m$^2$, days 1, 8, 15
Procarbazine, P.O., 100 mg/m$^2$, days 1-15
Prednisone, P.O., 60 mg/m$^2$, days 1-15
Doxorubicin, I.V., 40 mg/m$^2$, days 1, 15

Repeat cycle every 28 days

### Burkitt's Lymphoma

#### Advanced Stage Burkitt's/B-cell ALL

Methotrexate, I.T., 10 mg/m$^2$ at hour 0
Cytarabine, I.T., 50 mg/m$^2$ at hour 0
Cyclophosphamide, I.V., 300 mg/m$^2$ q12h x 6 at hours 0-60
Vincristine, I.V., 1.5 mg/m$^2$ at hour 72
Doxorubicin, I.V., 50 mg/m$^2$ at hour 72

**Followed after hematopoietic recovery by:**

Methotrexate, I.T., 12 mg/m$^2$ at hour 0
Methotrexate, I.V. push, 200 mg/m$^2$, then 800 mg/m$^2$ as a 24-hour infusion from hours 0-24
Cytarabine, I.T., 50 mg/m$^2$ at hour 24
Cytarabine, I.V., 400 mg/m$^2$ over 48 hours from hours 24-72, with escalating doses in succeeding courses
Leucovorin, I.V., 30 mg/m$^2$ at hours 36 and 42, then 3 mg/m$^2$ at hours 54, 66, 78

## Neuroblastoma

#### Cy/A

Cyclophosphamide, P.O., 150 mg/m$^2$/day x 7 days
Doxorubicin, I.V., 35 mg/m$^2$ on day 8

#### Pt/VM

Cisplatin, I.V., 90 mg/m$^2$ over 6 hours
Teniposide, I.V., 100 mg/m$^2$, 48 hours after completion of cisplatin

# Osteosarcoma

### HDMTX

Methotrexate, I.V., 12 g/m$^2$/week for 2-12 weeks
Leucovorin calcium rescue, P.O./I.V., 15 mg/m$^2$ q6h for 10 doses beginning 30 hours after the beginning of the 4-hour methotrexate infusion (serum methotrexate levels must be monitored)

### IFoVP

Ifosfamide, I.V., 1800 mg/m$^2$, days 1-5
Etoposide, I.V., 100 mg/m$^2$, days 1-5
Mesna uroprotection, I.V., 2880 mg/m$^2$, days 1-5

Repeat cycle every 21 days

### MTX-CDDPAdr

Methotrexate, I.V., 12 g/m$^2$/week for 2 weeks
Leucovorin calcium rescue, I.V., 20 mg/m$^2$ q3h for 8 doses beginning 16 hours after completion of methotrexate, then q6h P.O. for 8 doses

**alternating with**

Cisplatin, I.V., 75 mg/m$^2$, day 15 of cycles 1-7, then 120 mg/m$^2$ for cycles 8-10
Doxorubicin, I.V., 25 mg/m$^2$, days 15, 16, 17 of cycles 1-7

# Sarcoma (Bony and Soft Tissue)

### ICE

Ifosfamide, I.V., 1500 mg/m$^2$, days 1-3 (with mesna uroprotection)
Carboplatin, I.V., 635 mg/m$^2$, day 3
Etoposide, I.V., 100 mg/m$^2$, days 1, 2, 3

### Topo/CTX

Cyclophosphamide, I.V., 250 mg/m$^2$ on days 1-5, followed by
Topotecan, I.V., 0.75 mg/m$^2$ on days 1-5

### VACAdr

Vincristine, I.V., 1.5 mg/m$^2$/week for 6 weeks
Cyclophosphamide, I.V., 500 mg/m$^2$/week for 6 weeks
Doxorubicin, I.V., 60 mg/m$^2$, week 6

**6-week rest period, then**

Dactinomycin, I.V., 15 mcg/kg/day, for 5 days, followed 9 days later by
Vincristine + cyclophosphamide as above, given weekly for 5 weeks, and with
Doxorubicin given with the last treatment

**or**

Vincristine, I.V., 1.4 mg/m$^2$, day 1
Doxorubicin, I.V., 50 mg/m$^2$, day 1
Cyclophosphamide, I.V., 750 mg/m$^2$, day 1

### VAC

Vincristine, I.V., 2 mg/m$^2$, day 1
Dactinomycin, I.V., 1 mg/m$^2$, day 1
Cyclophosphamide, I.V., 600 mg/m$^2$, day 1

**or**

Vincristine, I.V., 1.5 mg/m$^2$, day 1
Dactinomycin, I.V., 25 mcg/kg, day 1
Cyclophosphamide, I.V., 1.5 g/m$^2$, day 1

Repeat cycle every 21 days

### VACAdr-IfoVP

Vincristine, I.V., 1.5 mg/m$^2$ (max: 2 mg), weekly
Dactinomycin, I.V., 1.5 mg/m$^2$ (max: 2 mg), every other week
Doxorubicin, I.V., 60 mg/m$^2$ continuous infusion over 24 hours
Cyclophosphamide, I.V., 1-1.5 g/m$^2$
Ifosfamide, I.V., 1.6-2 g/m$^2$, days 1-5
Etoposide, I.V., 150 mg/m$^2$, days 1-5

## Sarcoma (Bony and Soft Tissue) *(continued)*

### VAdrC

Vincristine, I.V., 1.5 mg/m$^2$ (max: 2 mg)
Doxorubicin, I.V., 35-60 mg/m$^2$
Cyclophosphamide, I.V., 500-1500 mg/m$^2$

# Wilms' Tumor

### VAD

Vincristine, I.V., 1.5 mg/m$^2$/week for 10 weeks, then every 3 weeks
Dactinomycin, I.V., 1.5 mg/m$^2$, every 3 weeks, alternating with
Doxorubicin, I.V., 40 mg/m$^2$, every 3 weeks

**or**

Vincristine, I.V., 1.5 mg/m$^2$, every 6 weeks
Dactinomycin, I.V., 15 mcg/kg x 5

**or**

60 mcg/kg I.V. x 1 every 6 weeks ± (add if stage III or IV)
Doxorubicin, I.V., 20 mg/m$^2$, every 6 weeks

# HERBS AND COMMON NATURAL AGENTS

The authors have chosen to include this list of natural products and their reported uses. Due to limited scientific evidence to support these uses, the information provided here is not intended as a cure for any disease, and should not be construed as curative or healing. In addition, the reader is strongly encouraged to seek other references that discuss this information in more detail, and that discuss important issues such as contraindications, warnings, precautions, adverse reactions, and interactions.

## PROPOSED MEDICINAL CLAIMS

| Herb | Reported Uses |
|---|---|
| Acetyl-L-carnitine (ALC) | Alzheimer's disease; depression; diabetic peripheral neuropathy |
| Adrenal extract | Fatigue; stress |
| Aloe (*Aloe supp*) | Healing agent in wounds, minor burns, and other minor skin irritations |
| Alpha-Lipoic acid | Diabetes, diabetic neuropathy; glaucoma; prevention of cataracts; prevention of neurologic disorders, including stroke |
| Androstenedione | Increase strength and muscle mass |
| Aortic extract | Enhancement of the function, structure, and integrity of arteries and veins; helps to protect against various forms of vascular disease, including atherosclerosis, cerebral and peripheral arterial insufficiency, varicose veins, hemorrhoids, and vascular retinopathies such as macular degeneration |
| Arabinoxylane | Decreases chemotherapy-induced leukopenia; immune system enhancement (antiviral and anticancer activity); reported useful in HIV infection |
| Arginine | Helps lower elevated cholesterol; improvement in circulation; increases lean body mass; inflammatory bowel disease; immune enhancement; male infertility; surgery and wound healing; sexual vitality and enhancement |
| Artichoke (*Cynara scolymus*) | Eczema and other dermatologic problems; hepatic protection/stimulation; hypercholesterolemia; improvement in bile flow |
| Ashwagandha (*Withania somnifera*) | Adaptogen; chemotherapy and radiation protection; general tonic; stress, fatigue, nervous exhaustion |
| Astragalus (*Astragalus membranaceus*) [Milk Vetch] | Adaptogen (tonic-enhanced endurance, stamina); improvement in immune function and disease resistance; improvement in tissue oxygenation; support for chemotherapy and radiation |
| Bacopa (*Bacopa monniera*) | Memory enhancement and improvement of cognitive function |
| Beta-Carotene | Cancer prevention; cervical dysplasia; immunostimulant; photoprotection (erythropoietic protoporphyria) |
| Betaine hydrochloride | Digestive aid (hypochlorhydria and achlorhydria) |
| *Bifidobacterium bifidum* (*bifidus*) | Crohn's disease; diarrhea; maintenance of anaerobic microflora in the colon; ulcerative colitis |
| Bilberry (*Vaccinium myrtillus*) | Ophthalmologic disorders (antioxidant) including myopia, diminished acuity, dark adaptation, macular degeneration, night blindness, diabetic retinopathy, cataracts; vascular disorders including varicose veins, capillary permeability/stability, phlebitis |
| Biotin | Brittle nails; diabetes; diabetic neuropathy; seborrheic dermatitis; uncombable hair syndrome |
| Bismuth | Ulcers |
| Bitter melon (*Momordica charantia*) | Antiviral; hypoglycemic, impaired glucose tolerance (IGT) |

*(continued)*

| Herb | Reported Uses |
|---|---|
| Black cohosh (*Cimicifuga racemosa*) | Vasomotor symptoms of menopause; premenstrual syndrome (PMS), mild depression, arthritis |
| Bladderwrack (*Fucus vesiculosus*) | Rich source of iodine, potassium, magnesium, calcium, and iron; hypothyroidism; fibrocystic breast disease |
| Boron | Osteoarthritis; osteoporosis; rheumatoid arthritis |
| Boswellia (*Boswellia serrata*) | Anti-inflammatory; ulcerative colitis, arthritis |
| Branched-chain amino acids (BCAAs) | Muscle development and improvement in lean body mass |
| Bromelain (*Anas comosus*) | Digestive enzyme; proteolytic, anti-inflammatory (arthritis); sinusitis |
| Bupleurum (*Bupleurum falcatum*) | Chronic inflammatory disease; liver support |
| Calcium | Blood pressure regulation; cancer prevention; elevated cholesterol; hypertension; kidney stones; PMS; pregnancy; prevention of osteoporosis |
| Calendula (*Calendula officinalis*) | Antibacterial, antifungal, antiviral, antiprotozoal; vulnerary; wound-healing agent (increases wound healing by stimulating immune system) |
| Caprylic acid | Antifungal/antiyeast; dysbiosis |
| Carnitine | Congestive heart failure (CHF); enhanced athletic performance; hyperlipidemia; male infertility; weight loss |
| Cascara (*Rhamnus persiana*) | Anthranquinone laxative |
| Cat's claw (*Uncaria tomentosa*) | Anti-inflammatory; antimicrobial (antibacterial, antifungal, antiviral); antioxidant; immunosupportive |
| Cayenne (*Capsicum annuum, Capsicum frutescens*) | Cardiovascular circulatory support; digestive stimulant; inflammation and pain (topical) |
| Chamomile, German (*Matricaria chamomilla, Matricaria recutita*) | Carminative, antispasmotic; mild sedative; anxiolytic; mouth rinse and gargle (for oral health); topical anti-inflammatory; uterine tonic |
| Chasteberry (*Vitex agnus-castus*) | Acne vulgaris; corpus luteum insufficiency; hyperprolactinemia and insufficient lactation; menopause; menstrual disorders, including amenorrhea, endometriosis, premenstrual syndrome |
| Chitosan | Weight reduction |
| Chlorophyll | Absorbs and suppresses odors, which makes it useful in breath fresheners, toothpastes, mouthwashes, and deodorants; anti-inflammatory, antioxidant, and wound-healing properties; exhibits bacteriostatic properties; protects against toxins |
| Chondroitin sulfate | Osteoarthritis |
| Chromium | Atherosclerosis; elevated cholesterol; elevated triglycerides; glaucoma; hypoglycemia; type 1 diabetes; type 2 diabetes; weight loss |
| Clove (*Syzygium aromaticum*) | Antiseptic; symptomatic relief of toothache and teething problems |
| Coenzyme $Q_{10}$ | Angina; adjunct in chemotherapy; chronic fatigue syndrome; congestive heart failure (CHF); hypertension; muscular dystrophy; obesity; periodontal disease |
| Coleus (*Coleus forskohlii*) | Asthma, allergies; hypertension, congestive heart failure; eczema; psoriasis |
| Collagen (Type II) | Arthritis; first- and second-degree burns; pressure ulcers, venous stasis ulcers, diabetic ulcers (those resulting from arterial insufficiencies); surgical and traumatic wounds; topical application for wound healing |

*(continued)*

| Herb | Reported Uses |
|---|---|
| Colostrum | Antidiarrheal; antiviral; immunostimulant |
| Conjugated linoleic acid (CLA) | Increases metabolism, decreases body fat |
| Copper | Anemia; osteoporosis; rheumatoid arthritis |
| Cordyceps (*Cordyceps sinensis*) | Adaptogen/tonic (to promote wellness, longevity, and general health); adjunct support for chemotherapy and radiation; antioxidant; enhancement in cellular oxygenation during stress; reduction in symptoms of fatigue; immunomodulatory; enhancement of sexual vitality (males and females); hepatoprotection; improvement in endurance and stamina; support of lung, liver, and kidney function |
| Cranberry (*Vaccinium macrocarpon*) | Prevention of nephrolithiasis; urinary tract infection |
| Creatine | Enhancement of athletic performance (energy production and protein synthesis for muscle building) |
| Cyclo-hispro | Type 2 diabetes |
| Dandelion (*Taraxacum officinale*) | Leaf used as a diuretic; root used for disorders of bile secretion (cholerectic); appetite stimulation; dyspeptic complaints |
| Dehydroepiandrosterone (DHEA) | Antiaging; depression; diabetes; fatigue; lupus |
| Devil's claw (*Harpagophytum procumbens*) | Anti-inflammatory; back pain; osteoarthritis, gout, and other inflammatory conditions |
| Docosahexaenoic acid (DHA) | Alzheimer's disease; attention deficit disorder (ADD) and attention deficit hyperactivity disorder; Crohn's disease; diabetes; eczema, psoriasis; elevated triglycerides; hypertension; rheumatoid arthritis |
| Dong quai (*Angelica sinensis*) | Anemia; hypertension; improvement in energy, particularly in females; menopause, dysmenorrhea, premenstrual syndrome (PMS), and amenorrhea; phytoestrogen |
| Echinacea (*Echinacea purpurea, Echinacea angustifolia*) | Antiviral; arthritis (*E. augustifolia*); immunostimulant (colds and other upper respiratory infection); topical anti-infective (boils, abscesses, tonsillitis) |
| Elder (*Sambucus nigra, Sambucus canadensis*) | Berry used as an antiviral, antioxidant, and for influenza; flower used as an anti-inflammatory, diaphoretic, diuretic, and for colds and influenza |
| Ephedra (*Ephedra sinica*) | Bronchodilator in asthma; decongestant in allergies, sinusitis, hay fever; thermogenic aid in weight loss |
| Evening primrose (*Oenothera blennis*) | Attention deficit disorder (ADD); diabetic neuropathy; eczema, dermatitis, and psoriasis; endometriosis; hyperglycemia; irritable bowel syndrome; multiple sclerosis; omega-G6 fatty acid supplementation; PMS and menopause; rheumatoid arthritis |
| Eyebright (*Euphrasia officinalis*) | Eye fatigue; catarrh of the eyes |
| Fenugreek (*Trigonella foenum-graecum*) | Support of blood sugar regulation |
| Feverfew (*Tanacetum parthenium*) | Anti-inflammatory, rheumatoid arthritis; prevention of migraine headaches |
| Fish oils | Crohn's disease; diabetes; dysmenorrhea; eczema, psoriasis; hypertension; hypertriglyceridemia; memory enhancement; rheumatoid arthritis |
| Flaxseed oil | Source of omega-3 essential fatty acid; integral part of structure of cell walls and cellular membranes; necessary for the transport and oxidation of cholesterol; precursor for prostaglandins |

*(continued)*

| Herb | Reported Uses |
|---|---|
| Folic acid | Alcoholism; anemia; atherosclerosis; cancer prevention (colon and breast); cervical dysplasia; Crohn's disease; depression; gingivitis; osteoporosis; pregnancy (prevention of birth defects) and lactation |
| Garcinia (*Garcinia cambogia*) | Support of pancreas function and glucose regulation; weight reduction protocols |
| Garlic (*Allium sativum*) | Antimicrobial (bacteria and fungi); hypertension; may lower cholesterol and blood fats; mild inhibitor of platelet-activating factor; practitioners should be aware that aged garlic extracts have been reported to improve the antioxidant benefits; support of immune function |
| Ginger (*Zingiber officinale*) | Antiemetic; anti-inflammatory (musculoskeletal); GI distress and dyspepsia |
| Ginkgo (*Ginkgo biloba*) | Alzheimer's disease, dementia; asthma; increase peripheral blood flow (cerebral vascular disease, peripheral vascular insufficiency, impotence, tinnitus, and resistant depression); intermittent claudication; macular degeneration; memory enhancement; sexual dysfunction (antidepressant-induced) |
| Ginseng, Panax (*Panax ginseng*) | Adrenal tonic; enhancement of physical and mental performance; enhancement of energy levels; adaptation to stress; supports immune function; adjunct support for chemotherapy and radiation |
| Ginseng, Siberian (*Eleutherococcus senticosus*) | Adaptogen; beneficial in athletic performance; adaptation to stress (decreased fatigue); support of immune function |
| Glucosamine | Osteoarthritis; rheumatoid arthritis and other inflammatory conditions |
| Glutamine | Adjunct therapy for cancer; adjunct therapy for HIV; alcoholism; catabolic wasting processes; immunosupportive; peptic ulcers; performance enhancement; postsurgical healing; ulcerative colitis and other forms of inflammatory bowel disease |
| Glutathione | Hepatoprotection (alcohol-induced liver damage); immune system support; peptic ulcer disease |
| Golden seal (*Hydrastis canadensis*) | Mucous membrane tonifying (used in inflammation of mucosal membranes); gastritis; antimicrobial (antibacterial/antifungal); bronchitis, cystitis, and infectious diarrhea |
| Gotu kola (*Centella asiatica*) | Hemorrhoids (topical); memory enhancement; psoriasis; support/modulation of connective tissue synthesis; venous insufficiency; wound healing (topical) |
| Grapefruit seed (*Citrus paradisi*) | Antifungal, antibacterial, antiparasitic agent |
| Grape seed (*Vitis vinifera*) | Antioxidant; treatment of allergies, asthma; improve circulation; antiplatelet (blocks aggregation); improve capillary fragility; anti-inflammatory; arterial/venous insufficiency (intermittent claudication, varicose veins) |
| Green tea (*Camellia sinensis*) | Anticarcinogenic activity; antioxidant; support in cancer prevention and cardiovascular disease; chemotherapy and radiation; adjunct support for chemotherapy and radiation; may lower cholesterol; platelet-aggregation inhibitor |
| Ground ivy (*Hedera helix*) | Mucolytic action; upper respiratory congestion and cough |
| Guggul (*Commiphora mukul*) | May lower blood cholesterol levels |
| Gymnema (*Gymnema sylvestre*) | Diabetes, supports regulation of blood sugar levels |
| Hawthorn (*Crataegus oxyacantha*) | Angina, hypotension, hypertension, peripheral vascular disease, tachycardia; cardiotonic; congestive heart failure |
| Hops (*Humulus lupulus*) | Mild sedative and hypnotic |

*(continued)*

| Herb | Reported Uses |
|---|---|
| Horse chestnut (*Aesculus hippocastanum*) | Oral and topical used to treat varicose veins, hemorrhoids, other venous insufficiencies; deep venous thrombosis, lower extremity edema |
| Horsetail (*Equisetum arvense*) | Diuretic; high mineral content (including silicic acid); used to support bone and connective tissue strengthening, including osteoporosis |
| HuperzineA (*Huperzia serrata*) | Acetylcholinesterase inhibitor in senile dementia and Alzheimer's disease |
| Hydroxymethyl butyrate (HMB) | Increases muscle mass during intense exercise |
| 5-Hydroxytryptophan (5-HTP) | Anxiety; depression; fibromyalgia; headache; migraine; obesity; sleep disorders, insomnia (stimulates the production of melatonin) |
| Inositol hexaphosphate (IP-6) | Anticancer agent |
| Iodine | Fibrocystic breast disease; goiter prevention; mucolytic agent |
| Ipriflavone | Prevention of and use in osteoporosis (men and women) |
| Iron | Anemia; menorrhagia; pregnancy; restless legs syndrome |
| Isoflavones (soy) | Cancer prevention; chemotherapy support; decreased bone loss; hypercholesterolemia; menopausal symptoms |
| Kava kava (*Piper methysticum*) | Anxiety; sedation; skeletal muscle relaxation; postischemic episodes |
| *Lactobacillus acidophilus* | Constipation; enhance immunity; hypercholesterolemia; infant diarrhea; lactose intolerance; recolonize the GI tract with beneficial bacteria during and after antibiotic use; vaginal candidiasis |
| Lavender (*Lavendula officinalis*) | Wound-healing agent (topical); minor burns (topical) |
| Lemon balm/Melissa (*Melissa officinalis*) | Antiviral agent (oral herpes virus); sedative agent (in pediatrics) |
| Licorice (*Glycyrrhiza glabra*) | Adrenal insufficiency (licorice); expectorant and antitussive (licorice); GI ulceration (DGL chewable products) |
| Liver extract | Liver tonic |
| Lutein | Cataracts; macular degeneration |
| Lycopene | Atherosclerosis; cancer prevention, especially prostate; macular degeneration |
| Lysine | Angina pectoris; herpes simplex; osteoporosis |
| Magnesium | Asthma; attention deficit hyperactivity disorder; cardiovascular disease; congestive heart failure (CHF); diabetes; epilepsy; fatigue; high blood pressure; kidney stones; migraine headaches; mitral valve prolapse (MVP); muscle cramps; nervousness; osteoporosis; premenstrual syndrome (PMS) |
| Malic acid | Aluminum toxicity; fibromyalgia |
| Manganese | Diabetes; epilepsy; osteoporosis |
| Marshmallow (*Althaea officinalis*) | Mucilaginous, demulcent; peptic ulceration |
| Mastic (*Pistacia lentiscus*) | *H. pylori* inhibitor; peptic ulcer disease |
| Melatonin | Insomnia; recovery from jet lag |
| Methionine | Liver detoxification |
| Methyl sulfonyl methane (MSM) | Analgesic; interstitial cystitis; lupus; osteoarthritis |
| Milk thistle (*Silybum marianum*) | Antidote for Poisoning by Death Cup mushroom; antioxidant, specifically for hepatic cells, liver diseases including acute/chronic hepatitis, jaundice, and stimulation of bile secretion/cholagogue; hepatoprotective, including drug toxicities (ie, phenothiazines, butyrophenones, ethanol, and acetaminophen) |
| Modified citrus pectin (MCP) | Anticancer activity; lowers cholesterol |

*(continued)*

| Herb | Reported Uses |
|---|---|
| Muira puama (*Ptychopetalum olacoides*) | Athletic performance enhancement; increased sexual vitality of males |
| *N*-Acetyl cysteine (NAC) | Acetaminophen toxicity; AIDS; asthma (mucolytic, antioxidant); bronchitis; cardioprotection during chemotherapy; fatigue; heavy metal detoxification; increases glutathione production |
| Nicotinamide adenine dinucleotide (NADH) | Chronic fatigue; Parkinson's disease; stamina and energy |
| Olive leaf (*Olea europaea*) | Antibiotic, antifungal, antiviral; hypoglycemic activity; antihypertensive activity |
| Pancreatic extract | Digestive disturbances; food allergies; celiac disease; anti-inflammatory; immune complex diseases; adjunct support for cancer therapy |
| Para-Aminobenzoic acid (PABA) | Peyronie's disease; scleroderma; vitiligo |
| Parsley (*Petroselinum crispum*) | Halitosis; antibacterial, antifungal |
| Passion flower (*Passiflora spp*) | Sedative |
| Peppermint (*Mentha piperita*) | Carminative, spasmolytic; irritable bowel syndrome |
| Phenylalanine | Reward deficiency syndrome in the treatment of addiction; depression; pain relief; vitiligo |
| Phosphatidyl choline (PC) | Alcohol-induced liver damage; Alzheimer's disease (may benefit some individuals); gallstones; hepatitis |
| Phosphatidyl serine (PS) | Alzheimer's disease; depression; memory enhancement |
| Potassium | Cardiac arrhythmias; congestive heart failure (CHF); hypertension; kidney stones |
| Pregnenolone | Arthritis; improved mental performance; natural precursor for the production of DHEA, cortisol, progesterone, estrogens, and testosterone in the body |
| Progesterone | Endometriosis; menopause symptoms; osteoporosis; PMS symptoms; prevention of breast cancer |
| Psyllium (*Plantago ovata, Plantago isphagula*) | Bulk-forming laxative (containing 10% to 30% mucilage) |
| Pygeum (*Pygeum africanum, Prunus africana*) | Symptoms associated with benign prostatic hyperplasia (BPH) |
| Pyruvate | Enhancement of athletic performance; obesity and weight loss |
| Quercetin | Allergies; atherosclerosis; cataracts; peptic ulcer |
| Red clover (*Trifolium pratense*) | Liquid extract used for liver detoxification and kidney detoxification; menopausal symptoms; proprietary extract contains 4 phytoestrogens |
| Red yeast rice (*Monascus purpureus*) | Hypercholesterolemic agent; may lower triglycerides and LDL cholesterol and raise HDL cholesterol |
| Rehmannia (*Rehmannia glutinosa*) | Immunosuppressive agent in rheumatoid arthritis |
| Reishi (*Ganoderma lucidum*) | Immunomodulation, fatigue, and hemo- and radioprotection, antihypertensive, anticonvulsive |
| SAMe (S-adenosyl methionine) | Cardiovascular disease; depression; fibromyalgia; insomnia; liver disease; osteoarthritis; rheumatoid arthritis |
| Saw palmetto (*Serenoa repens*) | Benign prostatic hyperplasia (BPH) |

*(continued)*

| Herb | Reported Uses |
|---|---|
| Schisandra (*Schizandra chinensis*) | Adaptogen/health tonic; hepatic protection and detoxification; adjunct support for chemotherapy and radiation; increased endurance, stamina, and work performance |
| Selenium | AIDS; atherosclerosis; bronchial asthma; cancer prevention; cardiomyopathy; cataracts; chemotherapy/radiation support; eczema |
| Senna (*Cassia senna*) | Anthraquinone laxative |
| Shark cartilage | Cancer therapy; osteoarthritis, rheumatoid arthritis |
| Spleen extract | Support following removal of the spleen or for individuals with weak spleen function |
| Stinging nettle (*Urtica dioica*) | Leaf used for allergic rhinitis; leaf increases uric acid excretion; root used for benign prostatic hyperplasia (BPH) |
| St John's wort (*Hypericum perforatum*) | Antiviral activity in increased doses; antibacterial, anti-inflammatory; used topically for minor wounds and infections; may be used topically for bruises, muscle soreness, and sprains; mild to moderate depression, melancholia, and anxiety |
| Taurine | Congestive heart failure (CHF); diabetes; epilepsy; hypertension |
| Tea tree (*Melaleuca alternifolia*) | **Not for ingestion**; as an antifungal, antibacterial; mouthwash for dental and oral health; burns, cuts, scrapes, insect bites |
| Thyme (*Thymus vulgaris*) | Antifungal; coughs and upper respiratory congestion |
| Thymus extract | Immunostimulant |
| Thyroid extract | Fatigue; immune support |
| Tocotrienols | Heart disease, high cholesterol; cancer prevention; protection from ultraviolet light, protection of the skin |
| Tribulus (*Tribulus terrestris*) | Steroidal properties (enhancement of athletic performance, increased sexual vitality) |
| Turmeric (*Curcuma longa*) | Antioxidant; anti-inflammatory; antirheumatic, used in arthritic problems; may lower blood lipid levels |
| Tylophora (*Tylophora asthmatica*) | Allergies; used in bronchial asthma |
| Tyrosine | Alzheimer's disease; depression; hypothyroidism; phenylketonuria (PKU); substance abuse |
| Uva-Ursi (*Arctostaphylos uva-ursi*) | Urinary tract infections and kidney stone prevention |
| Valerian (*Valeriana officinalis*) | Sedative or hypnotic; nervous tension during PMS, menopause; restless motor syndromes and muscle spasms |
| Vanadium | Type 1 diabetes; type 2 diabetes |
| Vinpocetine | Enhanced cognitive function; increased brain function (cerebral metabolic enhancing agent) |
| Vitamin A (Retinol) | Acne; AIDS; cancer prevention; cervical dysplasia; Crohn's disease; measles; menorrhagia; night blindness; PMS; ulcerative colitis |
| Vitamin $B_1$ (Thiamine) | Alcoholism; Alzheimer's disease; anemia (megaloblastic); congestive heart failure (CHF); diabetes; insomnia; neurological conditions (Bell's palsy, trigeminal neuralgia, sciatica, sensory neuropathies); psychiatric illness |
| Vitamin $B_2$ | Cataracts; depression; migraine |
| Vitamin $B_3$ | Acne vulgaris (4% niacinamide topical gel); cataracts; hyperlipidemia (hypercholesterolemia, hypertriglyceridemia); impaired glucose tolerance; intermittent claudication; osteoarthritis; prevention of myocardial infarction; Raynaud's syndrome; rheumatoid arthritis; schizophrenia; type 1 diabetes of recent onset; type 2 diabetes |
| Vitamin $B_5$ (Pantothenic acid) | Adrenal support; allergies; arthritis; constipation; hyperlipidemia (pantethine, but not pantothenic acid, lowers cholesterol and triglycerides); rheumatoid arthritis; surgery and wound healing |

*(continued)*

| Herb | Reported Uses |
|---|---|
| Vitamin $B_6$ (Pyridoxine) | Arthritis; asthma; autism; cardiovascular disease; carpal tunnel syndrome; depression associated with oral contraceptives; diabetic neuropathy; epilepsy, $B_6$-dependant; kidney stones; MSG sensitivity; nausea and vomiting in pregnancy; peptic ulcers; PMS |
| Vitamin $B_{12}$ (Cobalamin) | AIDS; atherosclerosis (due to homocysteine elevation); bronchial asthma; Crohn's disease; depression; diabetic neuropathy; male infertility; memory loss; multiple sclerosis; pernicious anemia; sulfite sensitivity |
| Vitamin B complex-25 | See individual B vitamins |
| Vitamin C | AIDS; allergies; asthma; atherosclerosis; cancer; cataracts; cervical dysplasia; common cold; Crohn's disease; diabetes; gingivitis; immune enhancement; Parkinson's disease; peptic ulcer; sunburn; wound healing |
| Vitamin D | Crohn's disease; epilepsy during anticonvulsant therapy; hearing loss; osteoporosis; psoriasis; rickets; scleroderma |
| Vitamin E | Alzheimer's disease; atherosclerosis; Benign prostatic hyperplasia (BPH); cancer prevention; cataracts; cervical dysplasia; diabetes; dyslipidemias; lupus; osteoarthritis; peptic ulcer; peripheral circulation; PMS; prevention of myocardial infarction; rheumatoid arthritis; sunburn |
| Vitamin K | Osteoporosis; synthesis of blood clotting factors |
| White oak (*Quercus alba*) | Soothing agent in mild inflammation of the throat and mouth |
| White willow (*Salix alba*) | Antipyretic; anti-inflammatory; reducing fever and in arthritic complaints |
| Wild yam (*Dioscorea villosa*) | Contains steroidal precursors and used in female vitality, however, conversion to progesterone in the body is poor |
| Yohimbe (*Pausinystalia yohimbe*) | May increase sexual vitality in men and women; male erectile dysfunction |
| Zinc | Acne; apthous ulcers; benign prostatic hyperplasia (BPH); common cold; Crohn's disease; diabetes; diaper rash; gastric ulcer healing; immune function; macular degeneration; male sexual vitality; osteoporosis; skin conditions, eczema; wound healing |

# SOUND-ALIKE COMPARISON LIST

The following list contains over 2000 pairs of sound-alike drugs accompanied by a subjective pronunciation of each drug name. Any such list can only suggest possible pronunciation or enunciation miscues and is by no means meant to be exhaustive.

New or rarely used drugs are likely to cause the most problems related to interpretation. Healthcare workers should be made aware of the existence of both drugs in a sound-alike pair in order to avoid (or minimize) the potential for error. Drug companies attempt to avoid naming different drugs with similar-sounding names; however, mix-ups do occur. Reading current drug advertisements, professional literature, and drug handbooks is a good way to avert or surely lessen such sound-alike drug errors at all levels of the healthcare industry.

| Drug Name | Pronunciation |
|---|---|
| Accolate® | (ak′ cue late) |
| Accutane® | (ak′ yu tane) |
| Accolate® | (ak′ cue late) |
| Accupril® | (ak′ yu pril) |
| Accubron® | (ak′ cue bron) |
| Accutane® | (ak′ yu tane) |
| Accupril® | (ak′ cue pril) |
| Accolate® | (ak′ cue late) |
| Accupril® | (ak′ cue pril) |
| Accutane® | (ak′ yu tane) |
| Accupril® | (ak′ cue pril) |
| Aciphex™ | (a′ si fecks) |
| Accupril® | (ak′ cue pril) |
| Monopril® | (mon′ oh pril) |
| Accutane® | (ak′ yu tane) |
| Accubron® | (ak′ cue bron) |
| Accutane® | (ak′ yu tane) |
| Accolate® | (ak′ cue late) |
| Accutane® | (ak′ yu tane) |
| Accupril® | (ak′ cue pril) |
| Acephen® | (a′ ce fen) |
| Aciphex™ | (a′ si fecks) |
| acetazolamide | (ah set ah zole′ ah mide) |
| acetohexamide | (ah set oh heks′ ah mide) |
| acetohexamide | (ah set oh heks′ ah mide) |
| acetazolamide | (ah set ah zole′ ah mide) |
| Achromycin® | (ak roe mye′ sin) |
| Adriamycin™ | (ade rya mye′ sin) |
| Achromycin® | (ak roe mye′ sin) |
| actinomycin | (ak ti noe mye′ sin) |
| Aciphex™ | (a′ si fecks) |
| Accupril® | (ak′ cue pril) |
| Aciphex™ | (a′ si fecks) |
| Acephen® | (a′ ce fen) |
| Acthar® | (ac′ thar) |
| Acular® | (ac′ yu lar) |
| Actidose® | (ac′ ti dose) |
| Actos® | (ac′ tose) |
| actinomycin | (ak ti noe mye′ sin) |
| Achromycin® | (ak roe mye′ sin) |
| Actos® | (ac′ tose) |
| Actidose® | (ac′ ti dose) |
| Acular® | (ac′ yu lar) |
| Acthar® | (ac′ thar) |
| adapalene | (ah dap′ ah lene) |
| Adapin® | (ad′ ah pin) |
| Adapin® | (ad′ ah pin) |
| adapalene | (ah dap′ ah lene) |
| Adapin® | (ad′ ah pin) |
| Adipex-P® | (ad′ di pex pea) |
| Adapin® | (ad′ ah pin) |
| Ativan® | (at′ tee van) |
| Adderall® | (ad′ der all) |
| Inderal® | (in′ der al) |
| Adipex-P® | (ad′ di pex pea) |
| Adapin® | (ad′ ah pin) |
| Adriamycin™ | (ade rya mye′ sin) |
| Aredia® | (ah red′ de ah) |
| Adriamycin™ | (ade rya mye′ sin) |
| Achromycin® | (ak roe mye′ sin) |
| Adriamycin™ | (ade rya mye′ sin) |
| Idamycin® | (eye da mye′ sin) |
| Aerolone® | (air′ oh lone) |
| Aralen® | (air′ ah len) |
| Afrin® | (aye′ frin or af′ rin) |
| aspirin | (as′ pir in) |
| Afrinol® | (af′ ree nol) |
| Arfonad® | (arr′ foe nad) |
| Aggrastat® | (ag′ gra stat) |
| Aggrenox™ | (ag′ gro noks) |
| Aggrenox™ | (ag′ gro noks) |
| Aggrastat® | (ag′ gra stat) |

| Drug Name | Pronunciation |
|---|---|
| Akarpine® | (ay kar' peen) |
| atropine | (a' troe peen) |
| AK-Mycin® | (aye kay mye' sin) |
| Akne-Mycin® | (ak nee mye' sin) |
| Akne-Mycin® | (ak nee mye' sin) |
| AK-Mycin® | (aye kay mye' sin) |
| AKTob® | (ak' tobe) |
| AK-Trol® | (aye' kay trol) |
| AK-Trol® | (aye' kay trol) |
| AKTob® | (ak' tobe) |
| Albutein® | (al byoo' teen) |
| albuterol | (al byoo' ter ole) |
| albuterol | (al byoo' ter ole) |
| Albutein® | (al byoo' teen) |
| albuterol | (al byoo' ter ole) |
| atenolol | (ah ten' oh lole) |
| Alcaine® | (al' kain) |
| Alcare® | (al' kare) |
| Alcare® | (al' kare) |
| Alcaine® | (al' kain) |
| Aldactazide® | (al dak' ta zide) |
| Aldactone® | (al' dak tone) |
| Aldactone® | (al' dak tone) |
| Aldactazide® | (al dak' ta zide) |
| Aldara™ | (al dar' a) |
| Alora® | (a lor' a) |
| aldesleukin | (al des lu' kin) |
| oprelvekin | (oh prel' ve kin) |
| Aldomet® | (al' doe met) |
| Aldoril® | (al' doe ril) |
| Aldomet® | (al' doe met) |
| Anzemet® | (an' ze met) |
| Aldoril® | (al' doe ril) |
| Aldomet® | (al' doe met) |
| Aldoril® | (al' doe ril) |
| Elavil® | (el' ah vil) |
| Alesse™ | (ah less') |
| Aleve® | (ah leve') |
| Aleve® | (ah leve') |
| Alesse™ | (ah less') |
| Alfenta® | (al fen' tah) |
| Sufenta® | (sue fen' tah) |
| alfentanil | (al fen' ta nil) |
| Anafranil® | (ah naf' ra nil) |
| alfentanil | (al fen' ta nil) |
| fentanyl | (fen' ta nil) |
| alfentanil | (al fen' ta nil) |
| remifentanil | (rem i fen' ta nil) |

| Drug Name | Pronunciation |
|---|---|
| alfentanil | (al fen' ta nil) |
| sufentanil | (sue fen' ta nil) |
| Alferon® | (al' fer on) |
| Alkeran® | (al' ker an) |
| Allegra® | (al leg' ra) |
| Viagra® | (vye ag' ra) |
| Alkeran® | (al' ker an) |
| Alferon® | (al' fer on) |
| Alkeran® | (al' ker an) |
| Leukeran® | (lu' keh ran) |
| Allerest® | (al' e rest) |
| Sinarest® | (sy' na rest) |
| Allergan® | (al' er gan) |
| Auralate® | (ahl' ah late) |
| allopurinol | (al oh pure' i nole) |
| Apresoline® | (aye press' sow leen) |
| Alora® | (a lor' a) |
| Aldara™ | (al dar' a) |
| alprazolam | (al pray' zoe lam) |
| alprostadil | (al pros' ta dil) |
| alprazolam | (al pray' zoe lam) |
| lorazepam | (lor a' ze pam) |
| alprazolam | (al pray' zoe lam) |
| triazolam | (trye ay' zoe lam) |
| alprostadil | (al pros' ta dil) |
| alprazolam | (al pray' zoe lam) |
| Altace™ | (al' tase) |
| alteplase | (al' te place) |
| Altace™ | (al' tase) |
| Amaryl® | (am' ah ril) |
| Altace™ | (al' tase) |
| Amerge® | (ah merge') |
| Altace™ | (al' tase) |
| Artane® | (ar' tane) |
| Altenol® | (al ten' ol) |
| atenolol | (ah ten' oh lole) |
| alteplase | (al' te place) |
| Altace™ | (al' tase) |
| alteplase | (al' te place) |
| anistreplase | (ah nis' tre place) |
| Alupent® | (al' yu pent) |
| Atrovent® | (at' troe vent) |
| amantadine | (ah man' ta deen) |
| ranitidine | (ra ni' ti deen) |
| amantadine | (ah man' ta deen) |
| rimantadine | (ri man' ta deen) |
| Amaryl® | (am' ah ril) |
| Amerge® | (ah merge') |

| Drug Name | Pronunciation |
|---|---|
| Amaryl® | (am′ ah ril) |
| Altace™ | (al′ tase) |
| Amaryl® | (am′ ah ril) |
| Ambenyl® | (am′ ba nil) |
| Amaryl® | (am′ ah ril) |
| Amerge® | (ah merge′) |
| Ambenyl® | (am′ ba nil) |
| Amaryl® | (am′ ah ril) |
| Ambenyl® | (am′ ba nil) |
| Aventyl® | (ah ven′ til) |
| Ambi 10® | (am′ bee ten′) |
| Ambien® | (am′ bee en) |
| Ambien® | (am′ bee en) |
| Ambi 10® | (am′ bee ten′) |
| Amerge® | (ah merge′) |
| Altace™ | (al′ tase) |
| Amerge® | (ah merge′) |
| Amaryl® | (am′ ah ril) |
| Amicar® | (am′ i car) |
| Amikin® | (am′ i kin) |
| Amikin® | (am′ i kin) |
| Amicar® | (am′ i car) |
| amiloride | (ah mil′ oh ride) |
| amiodarone | (ah mee′ oh da rone) |
| amiloride | (ah mil′ oh ride) |
| amlodipine | (am lo′ di pine) |
| aminophylline | (am in off′ i lin) |
| amitriptyline | (ah mee′ trip ti leen) |
| aminophylline | (am in off′ i lin) |
| ampicillin | (am pi sil′ in) |
| amiodarone | (ah mee′ oh da rone) |
| amiloride | (ah mil′ oh ride) |
| amiodarone | (ah mee′ oh da rone) |
| amrinone | (am′ ri none) |
| amitriptyline | (ah mee′ trip ti leen) |
| aminophylline | (am in off′ I lin) |
| amitriptyline | (ah mee trip′ ti leen) |
| imipramine | (im ip′ ra meen) |
| amitriptyline | (ah mee trip′ ti leen) |
| nortriptyline | (nor trip′ ti leen) |
| amlodipine | (am lo′ di pine) |
| amiloride | (ah mil′ oh ride) |
| amoxapine | (ah moks′ ah peen) |
| amoxicillin | (a moks i sil′ in) |
| amoxapine | (ah moks′ ah peen) |
| Amoxil® | (ay moks′ il) |
| amoxicillin | (a moks i sil′ in) |
| amoxapine | (ah moks′ ah peen) |
| amoxicillin | (a moks i sil′ in) |
| Amoxil® | (ay moks′ il) |
| amoxicillin | (a moks i sil′ in) |
| Atarax® | (at′ ah raks) |
| Amoxil® | (ay moks′ il) |
| amoxapine | (ah moks′ ah peen) |
| Amoxil® | (ay moks′ il) |
| amoxicillin | (a moks i sil′ in) |
| ampicillin | (am pi sil′ in) |
| aminophylline | (am in off′ i lin) |
| amrinone | (am′ ri none) |
| amiodarone | (ah mee′ oh da rone) |
| Anafranil® | (ah naf′ ra nil) |
| alfentanil | (al fen′ ta nill) |
| Anafranil® | (ah naf′ ra nil) |
| enalapril | (e nal′ ah pril) |
| Anafranil® | (ah naf′ ra nil) |
| nafarelin | (naf′ ah re lin) |
| Anaprox® | (an′ ah prox) |
| Anaspaz® | (an′ ah spaz) |
| Anaprox® | (an′ ah prox) |
| Avapro® | (ah′ va pro) |
| Anaspaz® | (an′ ah spaz) |
| Anaprox® | (an′ ah prox) |
| Anaspaz® | (an′ ah spaz) |
| Antispas® | (an′ te spaz) |
| Ancobon® | (an′ coe bon) |
| Oncovin® | (on′ coe vin) |
| anisindione | (ah nis in dy′ one) |
| anisotropine | (an iss oh troe′ peen) |
| anisotropine | (an iss oh troe′ peen) |
| anisindione | (ah nis in dy′ one) |
| anistreplase | (ah nis′ tre place) |
| alteplase | (al′ te place) |
| Ansaid® | (an′ said) |
| Asacol® | (as′ ah col) |
| Ansaid® | (an′ said) |
| Axid® | (aks′ id) |
| Ansaid® | (an′ said) |
| Axsain® | (aks′ ane) |
| Antabuse® | (an ta byoose′) |
| Anturane® | (ann′ chu rane) |
| Antispas® | (an′ te spaz) |
| Anaspaz® | (an′ ah spaz) |
| Antril® | (an′ trill) |
| enalapril | (e nal′ ah pril) |
| Anturane® | (ann′ chu rane) |
| Antabuse® | (an ta byoose′) |

| Drug Name | Pronunciation |
|---|---|
| Anturane® | (ann' chu rane) |
| Artane® | (ar' tane) |
| Anusol® | (an' yu sol) |
| Aquasol® | (ah' kwa sol) |
| Anusol® | (an' yu sol) |
| Anusol-HC® | (an' yu sol aych cee) |
| Anusol® | (an' yu sol) |
| Aplisol® | (ap' lee sol) |
| Anusol-HC® | (an' yu sol aych cee) |
| Anusol® | (an' yu sol) |
| Anzemet® | (an' ze met) |
| Aldomet® | (al' doe met) |
| Aphrodyne® | (af' roe dine) |
| Aprodine® | (ap' roe dine) |
| Aplisol® | (ap' lee sol) |
| Anusol® | (an' yu sol) |
| Aplisol® | (ap' lee sol) |
| Aplitest® | (ap' le test) |
| Aplisol® | (ap' lee sol) |
| A.P.L.® | (aye pee el') |
| Aplitest® | (ap' le test) |
| Aplisol® | (ap' lee sol) |
| A.P.L.® | (aye pee el') |
| Aplisol® | (ap' lee sol) |
| Apresoline® | (aye press' sow leen) |
| allopurinol | (al oh pure' i nole) |
| Apresoline® | (aye press' sow leen) |
| Priscoline® | (pris' coe leen) |
| Aprodine® | (ap' roe dine) |
| Aphrodyne® | (af' roe dine) |
| Aquasol® | (ah' kwa sol) |
| Anusol® | (an' yu sol) |
| AquaTar® | (ah' kwa tar) |
| Aquatag® | (ah' kwa tag) |
| Aquatag® | (ah' kwa tag) |
| AquaTar® | (ah' kwa tar) |
| ara-C | (ah ra cee') |
| Arasine® | (ah ra seen') |
| Aralen® | (air' ah len) |
| Aerolone® | (air' oh lone) |
| Aramine® | (air' ah meen) |
| Arasine® | (ah ra seen') |
| Aramine® | (air' ah meen) |
| Artane® | (ar' tane) |
| Arasine® | (ah ra seen') |
| ara-C | (ah ra cee') |
| Arasine® | (ah ra seen') |
| Aramine® | (air' ah meen) |

| Drug Name | Pronunciation |
|---|---|
| Aredia® | (ah red' de ah) |
| Adriamycin® | (ade rya mye' sin) |
| Arfonad® | (arr' foe nad) |
| Afrinol® | (af' ree nol) |
| Aricept® | (ar' e cept) |
| Ascriptin® | (ah srip' tin) |
| Artane® | (ar' tane) |
| Altace® | (al' tase) |
| Artane® | (ar' tane) |
| Anturane® | (an' chu rane) |
| Artane® | (ar' tane) |
| Aramine® | (air' ah meen) |
| Asacol® | (as' ah col) |
| Ansaid® | (an' said) |
| Asacol® | (as' ah col) |
| Os-Cal® | (os' cal) |
| Ascriptin® | (ah srip' tin) |
| Aricept® | (ar' e cept) |
| asparaginase | (ah spir' ah ji nase) |
| pegaspargase | (peg as' par jase) |
| aspirin | (as' pir in) |
| Afrin® | (aye' frin or af' rin) |
| Atarax® | (at' ah raks) |
| Ativan® | (at' tee van) |
| Atarax® | (at' ah raks) |
| amoxicillin | (a moks i sil' in) |
| Atgam® | (at' gam) |
| ratgam | (rat' gam) |
| atenolol | (ah ten' oh lole) |
| albuterol | (al byoo' ter ole) |
| atenolol | (ah ten' oh lole) |
| Altenol® | (al ten' ol) |
| atenolol | (ah ten' oh lole) |
| timolol | (tye' moe lole) |
| atenolol | (ah ten' oh lole) |
| Tylenol® | (tye' le nole) |
| Atgam® | (at' gam) |
| Ativan® | (at' tee van) |
| Ativan® | (at' tee van) |
| Adapin® | (ad' ah pin) |
| Ativan® | (at' tee van) |
| Atarax® | (at' ah raks) |
| Ativan® | (at' tee van) |
| Atgam® | (at' gam) |
| Ativan® | (at' tee van) |
| ATnativ® | (aye tee nay' tif) |
| Ativan® | (at' tee van) |
| Avitene® | (aye' va teen) |

| Drug Name | Pronunciation |
|---|---|
| ATnativ® | (aye tee nay′ tif) |
| Ativan® | (at′ tee van) |
| atropine | (a′ troe peen) |
| Akarpine® | (ay kar′ peen) |
| Atrovent® | (at′ troe vent) |
| Alupent® | (al′ yu pent) |
| Atrovent® | (at′ troe vent) |
| Natru-Vent® | (nay′ tru vent) |
| Attenuvax® | (at ten′ yu vaks) |
| Meruvax® | (mur′ yu vaks) |
| Augmentin® | (aug men′ tin) |
| Azulfidine® | (ay zul′ fi deen) |
| Auralate® | (ahl′ ah late) |
| Allergan® | (al′ er gan) |
| Auralgan® | (ah ral′ gan) |
| Larylgan® | (la ril′ gan) |
| Auralgan® | (ah ral′ gan) |
| Ophthalgan® | (opp thal′ gan) |
| Avalide® | (av′ ah lide) |
| Avandia® | (ah van′ de a) |
| Avandia® | (ah van′ de a) |
| Avalide® | (av′ ah lide) |
| Avandia® | (ah van′ de a) |
| Coumadin® | (ku′ ma din) |
| Avandia® | (ah van′ de a) |
| Prandin™ | (pran′ din) |
| Avapro | (ah′ va pro) |
| Anaprox® | (an′ ah prox) |
| Aventyl® | (ah ven′ til) |
| Ambenyl® | (am′ ba nil) |
| Aventyl® | (ah ven′ til) |
| Bentyl® | (ben′ till) |
| Avitene® | (aye′ va teen) |
| Ativan® | (at′ tee van) |
| Axid® | (aks′ id) |
| Ansaid® | (an′ said) |
| Axsain® | (aks′ ane) |
| Ansaid® | (an′ said) |
| azatadine | (ah za′ ta deen) |
| azathioprine | (ay za thye′ oh preen) |
| azathioprine | (ay za thye′ oh preen) |
| azatadine | (ah za′ ta deen) |
| azathioprine | (ay za thye′ oh preen) |
| azidothymidine | (ay zi doe thy′ mi dine) |
| azathioprine | (ay za thye′ oh preen) |
| Azulfidine® | (ay zul′ fi deen) |
| azidothymidine | (ay zi doe thy′ mi dine) |
| azathioprine | (ay za thye′ oh preen) |

| Drug Name | Pronunciation |
|---|---|
| azithromycin | (az ith roe mye′ sin) |
| erythromycin | (er ith roe mye′ sin) |
| Azulfidine® | (ay zul′ fi deen) |
| azathioprine | (ay za thye′ oh preen) |
| Azulfidine® | (ay zul′ fi deen) |
| Augmentin® | (aug men′ tin) |
| bacitracin | (bas i tray′ sin) |
| Bactrim® | (bak′ trim) |
| bacitracin | (bas i tray′ sin) |
| Bactroban® | (bak′ troe ban) |
| baclofen | (bak′ loe fen) |
| Bactroban® | (bak′ troe ban) |
| baclofen | (bak′ loe fen) |
| Beclovent® | (bec′ lo vent) |
| Bactine® | (bak′ teen) |
| Bactrim® | (bak′ trim) |
| Bactrim® | (bak′ trim) |
| bacitracin | (bas i tray′ sin) |
| Bactrim® | (bak′ trim) |
| Bactine® | (bak′ teen) |
| Bactroban® | (bak′ troe ban) |
| baclofen | (bak′ loe fen) |
| Bactroban® | (bak′ troe ban) |
| bacitracin | (bas i tray′ sin) |
| Banophen® | (ban′ oh fen) |
| Barophen® | (bear′ oh fen) |
| Barophen® | (bear′ oh fen) |
| Banophen® | (ban′ oh fen) |
| Beclovent® | (bec′ lo vent) |
| baclofen | (bak′ loe fen) |
| Beminal® | (bem′ eh nall) |
| Benemid® | (ben′ ah mid) |
| Benadryl® | (ben′ ah drill) |
| benazepril | (ban ay′ ze pril) |
| Benadryl® | (ben′ ah drill) |
| Bentyl® | (ben′ till) |
| Benadryl® | (ben′ ah drill) |
| Benylin® | (ben′ eh lin) |
| Benadryl® | (ben′ ah drill) |
| Caladryl® | (kal′ ah drill) |
| benazepril | (ban ay′ ze pril) |
| Benadryl® | (ben′ ah drill) |
| Benemid® | (ben′ ah mid) |
| Beminal® | (bem′ eh nall) |
| Benoxyl® | (ben ox′ ill) |
| Brevoxyl® | (brev ox′ il) |
| Benoxyl® | (ben ox′ ill) |
| Peroxyl® | (per ox′ ill) |

| Drug Name | Pronunciation |
|---|---|
| Bentyl® | (ben′ till) |
| Aventyl® | (ah ven′ til) |
| Bentyl® | (ben′ till) |
| Benadryl® | (ben′ ah drill) |
| Bentyl® | (ben′ till) |
| Bontril® | (bon′ trill) |
| Bentyl® | (ben′ till) |
| Cantil® | (can′ til) |
| Bentyl® | (ben′ til) |
| Proventil® | (pro ven′ till) |
| Bentyl® | (ben′ til) |
| Trental® | (tren′ tal) |
| Benylin® | (ben′ eh lin) |
| Benadryl® | (ben′ ah drill) |
| Benylin® | (ben′ eh lin) |
| Ventolin® | (ven′ tow lin) |
| Benza® | (ben′ zah) |
| Benzac® | (ben′ zak) |
| Benzac® | (ben′ zak) |
| Benza® | (ben′ zah) |
| benztropine | (benz′ troe peen) |
| bromocriptine | (broe moe krip′ teen) |
| Bepridil® | (be′ pri dil) |
| Prepidil® | (pre′ pi dil) |
| Betadine® | (bay′ ta deen) |
| Betagan® | (bay′ ta gan) |
| Betagan® | (bay′ ta gan) |
| Betadine® | (bay′ ta deen) |
| Betagan® | (bay′ ta gan) |
| Betagen® | (bay′ ta gen) |
| Betagen® | (bay′ ta gen) |
| Betagan® | (bay′ ta gan) |
| Betagen® | (bay′ ta gen) |
| Betoptic® | (bay top′ ik) |
| betaxolol | (be taks′ oh lol) |
| labetalol | (la bet′ ah lole) |
| Betoptic® | (bay top′ ik) |
| Betagen® | (bay′ ta gen) |
| Bicillin® | (bye sil′ lin) |
| Wycillin® | (wye sil′ lin) |
| bleomycin | (blee oh mye′ sin) |
| Cleocin® | (klee′ oh sin) |
| Bleph®-10 | (blef ten′) |
| Blephamide® | (blef′ ah mide) |
| Blephamide® | (blef′ ah mide) |
| Bleph®-10 | (blef ten′) |
| Bontril® | (bon′ trill) |
| Bentyl® | (ben′ till) |

| Drug Name | Pronunciation |
|---|---|
| Borofax® | (boroe′ faks) |
| Boropak® | (boroe′ pak) |
| Boropak® | (boroe′ pak) |
| Borofax® | (boroe′ faks) |
| Brevibloc® | (brev′ i block) |
| Brevital® | (brev′ i tall) |
| Brevital® | (brev′ i tall) |
| Brevibloc® | (brev′ i block) |
| Brevoxyl® | (brev ox′ il) |
| Benoxyl® | (ben ox′ ill) |
| brimonidine | (bri moe′ ni deen) |
| bromocriptine | (broe moe krip′ teen) |
| Bromfed® | (brom′ fed) |
| Bromphen® | (brom′ fen) |
| bromocriptine | (broe moe krip′ teen) |
| benztropine | (benz′ troe peen) |
| bromocriptine | (broe moe krip′ teen) |
| brimonidine | (bri moe′ ni deen) |
| Bromphen® | (brom′ fen) |
| Bromfed® | (brom′ fed) |
| bumetanide | (byoo met′ ah nide) |
| Buminate® | (byoo′ mi nate) |
| Bumex® | (byoo′ mex) |
| Buprenex® | (byoo′ pre nex) |
| Bumex® | (byoo′ mex) |
| Permax® | (per′ max) |
| Buminate® | (byoo′ mi nate) |
| bumetanide | (byoo met′ ah nide) |
| bupivacaine | (byoo piv′ ah kane) |
| mepivacaine | (me piv′ ah kane) |
| bupivacaine | (byoo piv′ ah kane) |
| ropivacaine | (roe piv′ a kane) |
| Buprenex® | (byoo′ pre nex) |
| Bumex® | (byoo′ mex) |
| bupropion | (byoo proe′ pee on) |
| buspirone | (byoo spye′ rone) |
| buspirone | (byoo spye′ rone) |
| bupropion | (byoo proe′ pee on) |
| busalfan | (byoo sul′ fan) |
| Butalan® | (byoo′ ta lan) |
| butabarbital | (byoo ta bar′ bi tal) |
| butalbital | (byoo tal′ bi tal) |
| Butalan® | (byoo′ ta lan) |
| busalfan | (byoo sul′ fan) |
| butalbital | (byoo tal′ bi tal) |
| butabarbital | (byoo ta bar′ bi tal) |
| Byclomine® | (bye′ clo meen) |
| Bydramine® | (bye′ dra meen) |

| Drug Name | Pronunciation |
|---|---|
| Byclomine® | (bye′ clo meen) |
| Hycomine® | (hye′ coe meen) |
| Bydramine® | (bye′ dra meen) |
| Byclomine® | (bye′ clo meen) |
| Bydramine® | (bye′ dra meen) |
| Hydramyn® | (hye′ dra min) |
| Cafergot® | (kaf′ er got) |
| Carafate® | (care′ ah fate) |
| Caladryl® | (kal′ ah drill) |
| Benadryl® | (ben′ ah drill) |
| Caladryl® | (kal′ ah drill) |
| calamine | (kal′ ah mine) |
| calamine | (kal′ ah mine) |
| Caladryl® | (kal′ ah drill) |
| Calan® | (kal′ an) |
| Colace® | (ko′ lace) |
| calcifediol | (kal si fe dye′ ole) |
| calcitriol | (kal si trye′ ole) |
| Calciferol® | (kal si′ fer ole) |
| calcitriol | (kal si trye′ ole) |
| calcitonin | (kal si toe′ nin) |
| calcitriol | (kal si trye′ ole) |
| calcitriol | (kal si trye′ ole) |
| calcifediol | (kal si fe dye′ ole) |
| calcitriol | (kal si trye′ ole) |
| Calciferol® | (kal si′ fer ole) |
| calcitriol | (kal si trye′ ole) |
| calcitonin | (kal si toe′ nin) |
| calcium glubionate | (kal′ see um gloo bye′ oh nate) |
| calcium gluconate | (kal′ see um gloo′ koe nate) |
| calcium gluconate | (kal′ see um gloo′ koe nate) |
| calcium glubionate | (kal′ see um gloo bye′ oh nate) |
| Cantil® | (can′ til) |
| Bentyl® | (ben′ till) |
| Capastat® | (kap′ ah stat) |
| Cepastat® | (sea′ pa stat) |
| Capital® | (kap′ i tal) |
| Capitrol® | (kap′ i trol) |
| Capitrol® | (kap′ i trol) |
| Capital® | (kap′ i tal) |
| Capitrol® | (kap′ i trol) |
| captopril | (kap′ toe pril) |
| captopril | (kap′ toe pril) |
| Capitrol® | (kap′ i trol) |
| captopril | (kap′ toe pril) |
| carvedilol | (kar′ ve dil ole) |
| Carafate® | (care′ ah fate) |
| Cafergot® | (kaf′ er got) |
| carboplatin | (kar′ boe pla tin) |
| cisplatin | (sis′ pla tin) |
| Cardene SR® | (kar′ deen ess are) |
| Cardizem SR® | (kar′ di zem ess are) |
| Cardene® | (kar′ deen) |
| Cardizem® | (kar′ di zem) |
| Cardene® | (kar′ deen) |
| Cardura® | (kar dur′ ah) |
| Cardene® | (kar′ deen) |
| codeine | (koe′ deen) |
| Cardiem | (car′ dee em) |
| Cardizem® | (kar′ di zem) |
| Cardizem® | (kar′ di zem) |
| Cardiem | (car′ dee em) |
| Cardizem® | (kar′ di zem) |
| Cardene® | (kar′ deen) |
| Cardizem CD® | (kar′ di zem see dee) |
| Cardizem SR® | (kar′ di zem ess are) |
| Cardizem SR® | (kar′ di zem ess are) |
| Cardene SR® | (kar′ deen ess are) |
| Cardizem SR® | (kar′ di zem ess are) |
| Cardizem CD® | (kar′ di zem see dee) |
| Cardura® | (kar dur′ ah) |
| Cardene® | (kar′ deen) |
| Cardura® | (kar dur′ ah) |
| Cordarone® | (kor da rone′) |
| Cardura® | (kar dur′ ah) |
| Cordran® | (kor′ dran) |
| Cardura® | (kar dur′ ah) |
| Coumadin® | (ku′ ma din) |
| Cardura® | (kar dur′ ah) |
| Ridaura® | (ri dur′ ah) |
| carteolol | (kar′ tee oh lole) |
| carvedilol | (kar′ ve dil ole) |
| Cartia® XT | (car′ te ah xt) |
| Procardia XL® | (pro car′ dee ah xl) |
| carvedilol | (kar′ ve dil ole) |
| captopril | (kap′ toe pril) |
| carvedilol | (kar′ ve dil ole) |
| carteolol | (kar′ tee oh lole) |
| Cataflam® | (kat′ ah flam) |
| Catapres® | (kat′ ah pres) |
| Catapres® | (kat′ ah pres) |
| Cataflam® | (kat′ ah flam) |

| Drug Name | Pronunciation |
|---|---|
| Catapres®<br>Cetapred® | (kat′ ah pres)<br>(see′ ta pred) |
| Catapres®<br>Combipres® | (kat′ ah pres)<br>(kom′ bee pres) |
| cefaclor<br>cephalexin | (sef′ ah klor)<br>(sef ah leks′ in) |
| cefamandole<br>cefmetazole | (sef ah man′ dole)<br>(sef met′ ah zole) |
| cefazolin<br>cephalexin | (sef a′ zoe lin)<br>(sef ah leks′ in) |
| cefazolin<br>cephalothin | (sef a′ zoe lin)<br>(sef a′ loe thin) |
| cefazolin<br>cefprozil | (sef a′ zoe lin)<br>(sef proe′ zil) |
| cefmetazole<br>cefamandole | (sef met′ ah zole)<br>(sef ah man′ dole) |
| Cefobid®<br>cefonicid | (se′ foh bid)<br>(se fon′ i sid) |
| Cefol®<br>Cefzil® | (cee′ fol)<br>(sef′ zil) |
| cefonicid<br>Cefobid® | (se fon′ i sid)<br>(se′ foh bid) |
| Cefotan®<br>Ceftin® | (se′ foh tan)<br>(sef′ tin) |
| cefotaxime<br>cefoxitin | (sef oh taks′ eem)<br>(se fox′ i tin) |
| cefotaxime<br>ceftizoxime | (sef oh taks′ eem)<br>(sef ti zoks′ eem) |
| cefotaxime<br>cefuroxime | (sef oh taks′ eem)<br>(se fyoor oks′ eem) |
| cefotetan<br>Ceftin® | (sef′ oh tee tan)<br>(sef′ tin) |
| cefoxitin<br>cefotaxime | (se fox′ i tin)<br>(sef oh taks′ eem) |
| cefoxitin<br>Cytoxan® | (se foks′ i tin)<br>(sy toks′ an) |
| cefprozil<br>cefazolin | (sef proe′ zil)<br>(sef a′ zoe lin) |
| cefprozil<br>cefuroxime | (sef proe′ zil)<br>(se fyoor oks′ eem) |
| ceftazidime<br>ceftizoxime | (sef′ tay zi deem)<br>(sef ti zoks′ eem) |
| Ceftin®<br>Cefotan® | (sef′ tin)<br>(se′ foh tan) |
| Ceftin®<br>cefotetan | (sef′ tin)<br>(sef′ oh tee tan) |
| Ceftin®<br>Cefzil® | (sef′ tin)<br>(sef′ zil) |

| Drug Name | Pronunciation |
|---|---|
| Ceftin®<br>Cipro® | (sef′ tin)<br>(ceh′ pro) |
| ceftizoxime<br>cefotaxime | (sef ti zoks′ eem)<br>(sef oh taks′ eem) |
| ceftizoxime<br>ceftazidime | (sef ti zoks′ eem)<br>(sef′ tay zi deem) |
| cefuroxime<br>cefotaxime | (se fyoor oks′ eem)<br>(sef oh taks′ eem) |
| cefuroxime<br>cefprozil | (se fyoor oks′ eem)<br>(sef proe′ zil) |
| cefuroxime<br>deferoxamine | (se fyoor oks′ eem)<br>(de fer oks′ ah meen) |
| ceftizoxime<br>cefuroxime | (sef ti zoks′ eem)<br>(se fyoor oks′ eem) |
| cefuroxime<br>ceftizoxime | (se fyoor oks′ eem)<br>(sef ti zoks′ eem) |
| Cefzil®<br>Cefol® | (sef′ zil)<br>(cee′ fol) |
| Cefzil®<br>Ceftin® | (sef′ zil)<br>(sef′ tin) |
| Cefzil®<br>Kefzol® | (sef′ zil)<br>(kef′ zol) |
| Celebrex®<br>Celexa® | (sel′ ah brex)<br>(se lex′ a) |
| Celebrex®<br>cerebra | (sel′ ah brex)<br>(cer′ eh bra) |
| Celebrex®<br>Cerebyx® | (sel′ ah brex)<br>(ser′ e bix) |
| Celexa®<br>Celebrex® | (se lex′ a)<br>(sel′ ah brex) |
| Celexa®<br>cerebra | (se lex′ a)<br>(cer′ eh bra) |
| Celexa®<br>Cerebyx® | (se lex′ a)<br>(ser′ e bix) |
| Celexa®<br>Zyprexa® | (se lex′ a)<br>(zye preks′ a) |
| Cenestin®<br>Senexon® | (se nes′ tin)<br>(sen′ e son) |
| Centoxin®<br>Cytoxan® | (sen toks′ in)<br>(sy toks′ an) |
| Cepastat®<br>Capastat® | (sea′ pa stat)<br>(kap′ ah stat) |
| cephalexin<br>cefaclor | (sef ah leks′ in)<br>(sef′ ah klor) |
| cephalexin<br>cefazolin | (sef ah leks′ in)<br>(sef a′ zoe lin) |
| cephalexin<br>cephalothin | (sef ah leks′ in)<br>(sef a′ loe thin) |

| Drug Name | Pronunciation |
|---|---|
| cephalexin | (sef ah leks′ in) |
| ciprofloxacin | (sip ro floks′ a sin) |
| cephalothin | (sef a′ loe thin) |
| cefazolin | (sef a′ zoe lin) |
| cephalothin | (sef a′ loe thin) |
| cephalexin | (sef ah leks′ in) |
| cephapirin | (sef ah pye′ rin) |
| cephradine | (sef′ ra deen) |
| cephradine | (sef′ ra deen) |
| cephapirin | (sef ah pye′ rin) |
| Ceptaz® | (sep′ taz) |
| Septra® | (sep′ trah) |
| cerebra | (cer′ eh bra) |
| Celebrex® | (sel′ ah brex) |
| cerebra | (cer′ eh bra) |
| Celexa® | (se lex′ a) |
| Cerebyx® | (ser′ e bix) |
| Celebrex® | (sel′ ah brex) |
| Cerebyx® | (ser′ e bix) |
| Celexa® | (se lex′ a) |
| Cerebyx® | (ser′ e bix) |
| Cerezyme® | (ser′ e zime) |
| Cerezyme® | (ser′ e zime) |
| Cerebyx® | (ser′ e bix) |
| Cetaphil® | (see′ ta fill) |
| Cetapred® | (see′ ta pred) |
| Cetapred® | (see′ ta pred) |
| Catapres® | (kat′ ah pres) |
| Cetapred® | (see′ ta pred) |
| Cetaphil® | (see′ ta fill) |
| chlorambucil | (klor am′ byoo sil) |
| Chloromycetin® | (klor oh my see′ tin) |
| Chloromycetin® | (klor oh my see′ tin) |
| chlorambucil | (klor am′ byoo sil) |
| Chloromycetin® | (klor oh my see′ tin) |
| Chlor-Trimeton® | (klor try′ me ton) |
| chlorpromazine | (klor proe′ ma zeen) |
| prochlorperazine | (proe klor per′ ah zeen) |
| chlorpromazine | (klor proe′ ma zeen) |
| promethazine | (proe meth′ ah zeen) |
| chlorpromazine | (klor proe′ ma zeen) |
| chlorpropamide | (klor proe′ pa mide) |
| chlorpropamide | (klor proe′ pa mide) |
| chlorpromazine | (klor proe′ ma zeen) |
| Chlor-Trimeton® | (klor try′ me ton) |
| Chloromycetin® | (klor oh my see′ tin) |
| Cidex® | (sy′ decks) |
| Lidex® | (ly′ decks) |
| Ciloxan® | (sy loks′ an) |
| cinoxacin | (sin oks′ ah sin) |
| Ciloxan® | (sy loks′ an) |
| Cytoxan® | (sy toks′ an) |
| cimetidine | (sye met′ i deen) |
| simethicone | (sye meth′i kone) |
| cinoxacin | (sin oks′ ah sin) |
| Ciloxan® | (sy loks′ an) |
| Cipro® | (ceh′ pro) |
| Ceftin® | (sef′ tin) |
| ciprofloxacin | (sip ro floks′ a sin) |
| cephalexin | (sef ah leks′ in) |
| cisplatin | (sis′ pla tin) |
| carboplatin | (kar′ boe pla tin) |
| Citracal® | (sit′ tra cal) |
| Citrucel® | (sit′ tru cel) |
| Citrucel® | (sit′ tru cel) |
| Citracal® | (sit′ tra cal) |
| clarithromycin | (kla rith′ roe mye sin) |
| erythromycin | (er ith roe mye′ sin) |
| Cleocin® | (klee′ oh sin) |
| bleomycin | (blee oh mye′ sin) |
| Cleocin® | (klee′ oh sin) |
| Clinoril® | (klin′ oh rill) |
| Cleocin® | (klee′ oh sin) |
| Lincocin® | (link′ oh sin) |
| Clinoril® | (klin′ oh rill) |
| Cleocin® | (klee′ oh sin) |
| Clinoril® | (klin′ oh rill) |
| Clozaril® | (klo′ zah rill) |
| Clinoril® | (klin′ oh rill) |
| Oruvail® | (or′ yu vale) |
| Clinoxide® | (klin ox′ ide) |
| Clipoxide® | (kleh pox′ ide) |
| Clipoxide® | (kleh pox′ ide) |
| Clinoxide® | (klin ox′ ide) |
| Clocort® | (klo′ kort) |
| Cloderm® | (klo′ derm) |
| Cloderm® | (klo′ derm) |
| Clocort® | (klo′ kort) |
| clofazimine | (kloe fa′ zi meen) |
| clonazepam | (kloe na′ ze pam) |
| clofazimine | (kloe fa′ zi meen) |
| clozapine | (kloe′ za peen) |
| clofibrate | (kloe fye′ brate) |
| clorazepate | (klor az′ ah pate) |
| Clomid® | (klo′ mid) |
| clonidine | (kloe′ ni deen) |

| Drug Name | Pronunciation |
|---|---|
| clomiphene<br>clomipramine | (kloe′ mi feen)<br>(kloe mi′ pra meen) |
| clomiphene<br>clonidine | (kloe′ mi feen)<br>(kloe′ ni deen) |
| clomipramine<br>clomiphene | (kloe mi′ pra meen)<br>(kloe′ mi feen) |
| clomipramine<br>desipramine | (kloe mi′ pra meen)<br>(des ip′ ra meen) |
| clomipramine<br>Norpramin® | (kloe mi′ pra meen)<br>(nor′ pra min) |
| clonazepam<br>clofazimine | (kloe na′ ze pam)<br>(kloe fa′ zi meen) |
| clonazepam<br>clonidine | (kloe na′ ze pam)<br>(kloe′ ni deen) |
| clonazepam<br>clorazepate | (kloe na′ ze pam)<br>(klor az′ ah pate) |
| clonazepam<br>Klonopin™ | (kloe na′ ze pam)<br>(klon′ oh pin) |
| clonazepam<br>lorazepam | (kloe na′ ze pam)<br>(lor a′ ze pam) |
| clonidine<br>Clomid® | (kloe′ ni deen)<br>(klo′ mid) |
| clonidine<br>clomiphene | (kloe′ ni deen)<br>(kloe′ mi feen) |
| clondine<br>clonazepam | (kloe′ ni deen)<br>(kloe na′ ze pam) |
| clonidine<br>clozapine | (kloe′ ni deen)<br>(kloe′ za peen) |
| clonidine<br>Klonopin™ | (kloe′ ni deen)<br>(klon′ oh pin) |
| clonidine<br>Loniten® | (kloe′ ni deen)<br>(lon′ eh ten) |
| clonidine<br>quinidine | (kloe′ ni deen)<br>(kwin′ i deen) |
| clorazepate<br>clofibrate | (klor az′ ah pate)<br>(kloe fye′ brate) |
| clorazepate<br>clonazepam | (klor az′ ah pate)<br>(kloe na′ ze pam) |
| clotrimazole<br>co-trimoxazole | (kloe trim′ ah zole)<br>(koe-trye moks′ ah zole) |
| clozapine<br>clonidine | (kloe′ za peen)<br>(kloe′ ni deen) |
| Clozaril®<br>Clinoril® | (klo′ zah rill)<br>(klin′ oh rill) |
| Colace®<br>Calan® | (ko′ lace)<br>(kal′ an) |
| Co-Lav®<br>Colax® | (koe′ lav)<br>(koe′ laks) |

| Drug Name | Pronunciation |
|---|---|
| co-trimoxazole<br>clotrimazole | (koe-trye moks′ ah zole)<br>(kloe trim′ ah zole) |
| CodAphen®<br>Codafed® | (kod′ ah fen)<br>(kode′ ah fed) |
| Codafed®<br>CodAphen® | (kode′ ah fed)<br>(kod′ ah fen) |
| codeine<br>Cardene® | (koe′ deen)<br>(kar′ deen) |
| codeine<br>Cophene® | (koe′ deen)<br>(koe′ feen) |
| codeine<br>Cordran® | (koe′ deen)<br>(kor′ dran) |
| codeine<br>iodine | (koe′ deen)<br>(eye′ oh dyne) |
| codeine<br>Lodine® | (koe′ deen)<br>(low′ deen) |
| Cognex®<br>Corgard® | (kog′ neks)<br>(kor′ gard) |
| Colace®<br>Calan® | (ko′ lace)<br>(kal′ an) |
| Colax®<br>Co-Lav® | (koe′ laks)<br>(koe′ lav) |
| Colestid®<br>colistin | (koe les′ tid)<br>(koe lis′ tin) |
| colistin<br>Colestid® | (koe lis′ tin)<br>(koe les′ tid) |
| Combipres®<br>Catapres® | (kom′ bee pres)<br>(kat′ ah pres) |
| Combivent®<br>Combivir® | (kom′ bi vent)<br>(kom′ bi veer) |
| Combivir®<br>Combivent® | (kom′ bi veer)<br>(kom′ bi vent) |
| Combivir®<br>Epivir® | (kom′ bi veer)<br>(ep′ ih vir) |
| Compazine®<br>Coumadin® | (kom′ pah zeen)<br>(ku′ ma din) |
| Cophene®<br>codeine | (koe′ feen)<br>(koe′ deen) |
| Cordarone®<br>Cardura® | (kor da rone′)<br>(kar dur′ ah) |
| Cordarone®<br>Cordran® | (kor da rone′)<br>(kor′ dran) |
| Cordran®<br>Cardura® | (kor′ dran)<br>(kar dur′ ah) |
| Cordran®<br>codeine | (kor′ dran)<br>(koe′ deen) |
| Cordran®<br>Cordarone® | (kor′ dran)<br>(kor da rone′) |

| Drug Name | Pronunciation |
|---|---|
| Corgard® | (kor′ gard) |
| Cognex® | (kog′ neks) |
| Cortef® | (kor′ tef) |
| Lortab® | (lor′ tab) |
| cortisone | (kor′ ti sone) |
| Cortizone® | (kor′ ti zone) |
| Cortizone® | (kor′ ti zone) |
| cortisone | (kor′ ti sone) |
| Coumadin® | (ku′ ma din) |
| Avandia® | (ah van′ de a) |
| Coumadin® | (ku′ ma din) |
| Cardura® | (kar dur′ ah) |
| Coumadin® | (ku′ ma din) |
| Compazine® | (kom′ pah zeen) |
| Coumadin® | (ku′ ma din) |
| Kemadrin® | (kem′ ah drin) |
| Covera® | (co ver′ ah) |
| Provera® | (pro ver′ ah) |
| Cozaar® | (koe′ zar) |
| Hyzaar® | (hi′ zar) |
| Cozaar® | (koe′ zar) |
| Zocor® | (zoe′ cor) |
| Cutivate™ | (kyu′ te vate) |
| Ultravate® | (ul′ trah vate) |
| cyclobenzaprine | (sye kloe ben′ za preen) |
| cycloserine | (sye kloe ser′ een) |
| cyclobenzaprine | (sye kloe ben′ za preen) |
| cyproheptadine | (si proe hep′ ta deen) |
| cyclophosphamide | (sye kloe fos′ fa mide) |
| cyclosporine | (sye′ kloe spor een) |
| cycloserine | (sye kloe ser′ een) |
| cyclosporine | (sye′ kloe spor een) |
| cycloserine | (sye kloe ser′ een) |
| cyclobenzaprine | (sye kloe ben′ za preen) |
| cyclosporine | (sye′ kloe spor een) |
| cyclophosphamide | (sye kloe fos′ fa mide) |
| cyclosporine | (sye′ kloe spor een) |
| cycloserine | (sye kloe ser′ een) |
| cyclosporine | (sye′ kloe spor een) |
| Cyklokapron® | (sye kloe kay′ pron) |
| Cyklokapron® | (sye kloe kay′ pron) |
| cyclosporine | (sye′ kloe spor een) |
| cyproheptadine | (si proe hep′ ta deen) |
| cyclobenzaprine | (sye kloe ben′ za preen) |
| cytarabine | (sye tare′ ah been) |
| Cytosar® | (sye′ to sar) |
| cytarabine | (sye tare′ ah been) |
| Cytoxan® | (sy toks′ an) |
| cytarabine | (sye tare′ ah been) |
| vidarabine | (vye dare′ ah been) |
| CytoGam® | (sy′ to gam) |
| Cytoxan® | (sy toks′ an) |
| Cytosar® | (sye′ to sar) |
| Cytovene® | (sye′ toe veen) |
| Cytosar® | (sye′ to sar) |
| Cytoxan® | (sy toks′ an) |
| Cytosar® | (sye′ to sar) |
| cytarabine | (sye tare′ ah been) |
| Cytosar-U® | (sye′ to sar u) |
| Neosar® | (ne′ oh sar) |
| Cytotec® | (sye′ toe tek) |
| Cytoxan® | (sye tox′ an) |
| Cytotec® | (sye′ toe tek) |
| Sytobex® | (sye′ toe beks) |
| Cytovene® | (sye′ toe veen) |
| Cytosar® | (sye′ to sar) |
| Cytoxan® | (sy toks′ an) |
| cefoxitin | (se foks′ i tin) |
| Cytoxan® | (sy toks′ an) |
| Centoxin® | (sen toks′ in) |
| Cytoxan® | (sy toks′ an) |
| Ciloxan® | (sy loks′ an) |
| Cytoxan® | (sy toks′ an) |
| cytarabine | (sye tare′ ah been) |
| Cytoxan® | (sy toks′ an) |
| CytoGam® | (sy′ to gam) |
| Cytoxan® | (sy toks′ an) |
| Cytosar® | (sye′ to sar) |
| Cytoxan® | (sye tox′ an) |
| Cytotec® | (sye′ toe tek) |
| dacarbazine | (da kar′ ba zeen) |
| Dicarbosil® | (dye kar′ bow sil) |
| dacarbazine | (da kar′ ba zeen) |
| procarbazine | (proe kar′ ba zeen) |
| Dacriose® | (dak′ ree ose) |
| Danocrine® | (dan′ oh crin) |
| dactinomycin | (dak ti noe mye′ sin) |
| daunorubicin | (daw noe roo′ bi sin) |
| Dalmane® | (dal′ mane) |
| Demulen® | (dem′ yu len) |
| Dalmane® | (dal′ mane) |
| Dialume® | (dy′ ah lume) |
| danazol | (da′ na zole) |
| Dantrium® | (dan′ tree um) |
| Danocrine® | (dan′ oh crin) |
| Dacriose® | (dak′ ree ose) |

| Drug Name | Pronunciation |
|---|---|
| Dantrium® | (dan′ tree um) |
| danazol | (da′ na zole) |
| dapsone | (dap′ sone) |
| Diprosone® | (dip′ ro sone) |
| Daranide® | (dare′ ah nide) |
| Daraprim® | (dare′ ah prim) |
| Daraprim® | (dare′ ah prim) |
| Daranide® | (dare′ ah nide) |
| Darvocet-N® | (dar′ voh set en) |
| Darvon-N® | (dar′ von en) |
| Darvon-N® | (dar′ von en) |
| Darvocet-N® | (dar′ voh set en) |
| Darvon® | (dar′ von) |
| Devrom® | (dev′ rom) |
| Darvon® | (dar′ von) |
| Diovan® | (dye oh′ van) |
| daunorubicin | (daw noe roo′ bi sin) |
| dactinomycin | (dak ti noe mye′ sin) |
| daunorubicin | (daw noe roo′ bi sin) |
| doxorubicin | (dox oh roo′ bi sin) |
| Daypro® | (day′ pro) |
| Diupres® | (dye′ yu press) |
| Decadron® | (dek′ ah dron) |
| Percodan® | (per′ koe dan) |
| Deconal® | (dek′ oh nal) |
| Deconsal® | (dek′ on sal) |
| Deconsal® | (dek′ on sal) |
| Deconal® | (dek′ oh nal) |
| deferoxamine | (de fer oks′ ah meen) |
| cefuroxime | (se fyoor oks′ eem) |
| Delacort® | (del′ ah kort) |
| Delcort® | (del′ kort) |
| Delcort® | (del′ kort) |
| Delacort® | (del′ ah kort) |
| Delfen® | (del′ fen) |
| Delsym® | (del′ sim) |
| Delsym® | (del′ sim) |
| Delfen® | (del′ fen) |
| Delsym® | (del′ sim) |
| Desyrel® | (des′ e rell) |
| Demadex® | (dem′ ah deks) |
| Denorex® | (den′ oh reks) |
| Demerol® | (dem′ eh rol) |
| Demulen® | (dem′ yu len) |
| Demerol® | (dem′ eh rol) |
| Desyrel® | (des′ e rell) |
| Demerol® | (dem′ eh rol) |
| dicumarol | (dye koo′ ma role) |
| Demerol® | (dem′ eh rol) |
| Dilaudid® | (dye law′ did) |
| Demerol® | (dem′ eh rol) |
| Dymelor® | (dye′ meh lor) |
| Demerol® | (dem′ eh rol) |
| Pamelor® | (pam′ meh lor) |
| Demulen® | (dem′ yu len) |
| Dalmane® | (dal′ mane) |
| Demulen® | (dem′ yu len) |
| Demerol® | (dem′ eh rol) |
| Denavir™ | (den′ ah vir) |
| indinavir | (in din′ a veer) |
| Denorex® | (den′ oh reks) |
| Demadex® | (dem′ ah deks) |
| Depakene® | (dep′ ah keen) |
| Depakote® | (dep′ ah kote) |
| Depakote® | (dep′ ah kote) |
| Depakene® | (dep′ ah keen) |
| Depakote® | (dep′ ah kote) |
| Senokot® | (sen′ oh kot) |
| Depen® | (dee′ pen) |
| Endal® | (en′ dal) |
| DepoCyt® | (de′ po set) |
| Depoject® | (de′ po ject) |
| Depo-Estradiol® | (dep′ oh es tra dye′ ole) |
| Depo-Testadiol® | (dep′ oh tes ta dye′ ole) |
| Depogen® | (dep′ oh jen) |
| Depoject® | (dep′ oh ject) |
| Depoject® | (de′ po ject) |
| DepoCyt® | (de′ po set) |
| Depoject® | (dep′ oh ject) |
| Depogen® | (dep′ oh jen) |
| Depo-Medrol® | (dep′ oh med′ role) |
| Solu-Medrol® | (sol′ yu med′ role) |
| Depo-Testadiol® | (dep′ oh tes ta dye′ ole) |
| Depotestogen® | (dep oh tes′ tow gen) |
| Depo-Testadiol® | (dep′ oh tes ta dye′ ole) |
| Depo-Estradiol® | (dep′oh es tra dye′ ole) |
| Depotestogen® | (dep oh tes′ tow gen) |
| Depo-Testadiol® | (dep′ oh tes ta dye′ ole) |
| Dermacort® | (der′ ma kort) |
| DermiCort® | (der′ meh kort) |
| Dermatop® | (der′ ma top) |
| DermiCort® | (der′ meh kort) |
| Dermatop® | (der′ ma top) |
| Dimetapp® | (di meh′ tap) |
| DermiCort® | (der′ meh kort) |
| Dermacort® | (der′ ma kort) |

| Drug Name | Pronunciation |
|---|---|
| DermiCort® | (der′ meh kort) |
| Dermatop® | (der′ ma top) |
| DES® | (dee ee ess) |
| E.E.S.® | (ee ee ess) |
| deserpidine | (de ser′ pi deen) |
| desipramine | (des ip′ ra meen) |
| Desferal® | (des′ fer al) |
| Disophrol® | (dye′ so frol) |
| Desferal® | (des′ fer al) |
| desflurane | (des flu′ rane) |
| Desferal® | (des′ fer al) |
| DexFerrum® | (deks′ fer rum) |
| desflurane | (des flu′ rane) |
| Desferal® | (des′ fer al) |
| desipramine | (des ip′ ra meen) |
| clomipramine | (kloe mi′ pra meen) |
| desipramine | (des ip′ ra meen) |
| deserpidine | (de ser′ pi deen) |
| desipramine | (des ip′ ra meen) |
| diphenhydramine | (dye fen hye′ dra meen) |
| desipramine | (des ip′ ra meen) |
| disopyramide | (dye soe peer′ ah mide) |
| desipramine | (des ip′ ra meen) |
| imipramine | (im ip′ ra meen) |
| desipramine | (des ip′ ra meen) |
| nortriptyline | (nor trip′ ti leen) |
| desoximetasone | (des ox i met′ ah sone) |
| dexamethasone | (deks ah meth′ ah sone) |
| Desoxyn® | (de soks′ in) |
| digitoxin | (di ji toks′ in) |
| Desoxyn® | (de soks′ in) |
| digoxin | (di joks′ in) |
| Desyrel® | (des′ e rell) |
| Delsym® | (del′ sim) |
| Desyrel® | (des′ e rell) |
| Demerol® | (dem′ eh rol) |
| Desyrel® | (des′ e rell) |
| Zestril® | (zes′ trill) |
| Devrom® | (dev′ rom) |
| Darvon® | (dar′ von) |
| dexamethasone | (deks ah meth′ ah sone) |
| desoximetasone | (des ox i met′ ah sone) |
| Dexatrim® | (deks′ ah trim) |
| Dextran® | (deks′ tran) |
| Dexatrim® | (deks′ ah trim) |
| Excedrin® | (eks sed′ drin) |
| DexFerrum® | (deks′ fer rum) |
| Desferal® | (des′ fer al) |

| Drug Name | Pronunciation |
|---|---|
| Dextran® | (deks′ tran) |
| Dexatrim® | (deks′ ah trim) |
| Diaβeta® | (dye ah bay′ tah) |
| Diabinese® | (dye ab′ beh neese) |
| Diaβeta® | (dye ah bay′ tah) |
| Zebeta® | (ze′ bay tah) |
| Diabinese® | (dye ab′ beh neese) |
| Dialume® | (dy′ ah lume) |
| Diabinese® | (dye ab′ beh neese) |
| Diaβeta® | (dye ah bay′ tah) |
| Dialume® | (dy′ ah lume) |
| Dalmane® | (dal′ mane) |
| Dialume® | (dy′ ah lume) |
| Diabinese® | (dye ab′ beh neese) |
| Diamox® | (dye′ ah moks) |
| Dobutrex® | (doe byoo′ treks) |
| Diamox® | (dye′ ah moks) |
| Trimox® | (trye′ moks) |
| diazepam | (dye az′ ah pam) |
| Ditropan® | (di troe′ pan) |
| diazepam | (dye az′ ah pam) |
| diazoxide | (dye az oks′ ide) |
| diazepam | (dye az′ ah pam) |
| lorazepam | (lor a′ ze pam) |
| diazoxide | (dye az oks′ ide) |
| diazepam | (dye az′ ah pam) |
| diazoxide | (dye az oks′ ide) |
| Dyazide® | (dye′ ah zide) |
| Dicarbosil® | (dye kar′ bow sil) |
| dacarbazine | (da kar′ ba zeen) |
| diclofenac | (dye kloe′ fen ak) |
| Diflucan® | (dye flu′ can) |
| diclofenac | (dye kloe′ fen ak) |
| Duphalac® | (du′ fa lak) |
| dicumarol | (dye koo′ ma role) |
| Demerol® | (dem′ eh rol) |
| dicyclomine | (dye sye′ kloe meen) |
| diphenhydramine | (dye fen hye′ dra meen) |
| dicyclomine | (dye sye′ kloe meen) |
| dyclonine | (dye′ kloe neen) |
| Diflucan® | (dye flu′ can) |
| diclofenac | (dye kloe′ fen ak) |
| Diflucan® | (dye flu′ can) |
| Diprivan® | (dye′ pri van) |
| digitoxin | (di ji tox′ in) |
| digoxin | (di jox′ in) |
| digoxin | (di joks′ in) |
| Desoxyn® | (de soks′ in) |

| Drug Name | Pronunciation |
|---|---|
| digoxin | (di jox′ in) |
| digitoxin | (di ji tox′ in) |
| digoxin | (di jox′ in) |
| doxepin | (doks′ e pin) |
| Dilantin® | (dye lan′ tin) |
| Dilaudid® | (dye law′ did) |
| Dilantin® | (dye lan′ tin) |
| diltiazem | (dil tye′ ah zem) |
| Dilantin® | (dye lan′ tin) |
| Dipentum® | (dye pen′ tum) |
| Dilaudid® | (dye law′ did) |
| Demerol® | (dem′ eh rol) |
| Dilaudid® | (dye law′ did) |
| Dilantin® | (dye lan′ tin) |
| Dilomine® | (dy′ lo meen) |
| Dyclone® | (dye′ klone) |
| diltiazem | (dil tye′ ah zem) |
| Dilantin® | (dye lan′ tin) |
| dimenhydrinate | (dye men hye′ dri nate) |
| diphenhydramine | (dye fen hye′ dra meen) |
| Dimetabs® | (di meh′ tabs) |
| Dimetapp® | (di meh′ tap) |
| Dimetane® | (dye′ meh tane) |
| Dimetapp® | (di meh′ tap) |
| Dimetapp® | (di meh′ tap) |
| Dermatop® | (der′ ma top) |
| Dimetapp® | (di meh′ tap) |
| Dimetabs® | (di meh′ tabs) |
| Dimetapp® | (di meh′ tap) |
| Dimetane® | (dye′ meh tane) |
| Dioval® | (dy′ oh val) |
| Diovan® | (dye oh′ van) |
| Diovan® | (dye oh′ van) |
| Darvon® | (dar′ von) |
| Diovan® | (dye oh′ van) |
| Dioval® | (dy′ oh val) |
| Diovan® | (dye oh′ van) |
| Zyban™ | (zy′ ban) |
| Dipentum® | (dye pen′ tum) |
| Dilantin® | (dye lan′ tin) |
| diphenhydramine | (dye fen hye′ dra meen) |
| desipramine | (des ip′ ra meen) |
| diphenhydramine | (dye fen hye′ dra meen) |
| dicyclomine | (dye sye′ kloe meen) |
| diphenhydramine | (dye fen hye′ dra meen) |
| dimenhydrinate | (dye men hye′ dri nate) |
| Diphenatol® | (dye fen′ ah tol) |
| diphenidiol | (dye fen′ i dole) |

| Drug Name | Pronunciation |
|---|---|
| diphenidiol | (dye fen′ i dole) |
| Diphenatol® | (dye fen′ ah tol) |
| Diprivan® | (dye′ pri van) |
| Diflucan® | (dye flu′ can) |
| Diprivan® | (dip′ riv an) |
| Ditropan® | (di troe′ pan) |
| Diprosone® | (dip′ ro sone) |
| dapsone | (dap′ sone) |
| dipyridamole | (dye peer id′ ah mole) |
| disopyramide | (dye soe peer′ ah mide) |
| Disophrol® | (dye′ so frol) |
| Desferal® | (des′ fer al) |
| Disophrol® | (dye′ so frol) |
| Isuprel® | (eye′ sue prel) |
| Disophrol® | (dye′ so frol) |
| Stilphostrol® | (stil phos′ trol) |
| disopyramide | (dye soe peer′ ah mide) |
| desipramine | (des ip′ ra meen) |
| disopyramide | (dye soe peer′ ah mide) |
| dipyridamole | (dye peer id′ ah mole) |
| Ditropan® | (di troe′ pan) |
| diazepam | (dye az′ ah pam) |
| Ditropan® | (di troe′ pan) |
| Diprivan® | (dip′ riv an) |
| Diupres® | (dye′ yu press) |
| Daypro® | (day′ pro) |
| dobutamine | (doe byoo′ ta meen) |
| dopamine | (doe′ pa meen) |
| Dobutrex® | (doe byoo′ treks) |
| Diamox® | (dye′ ah moks) |
| docusate | (dok′ yoo sate) |
| Doxinate® | (dox′ eh nate) |
| Dolobid® | (dol′ ah bid) |
| Slo-Bid® | (slo′ bid) |
| Donnagel® | (don′ ah jel) |
| Donnatal® | (don′ ah tall) |
| Donnapine® | (don′ ah peen) |
| Donnazyme® | (don′ ah zime) |
| Donnatal® | (don′ ah tall) |
| Donnagel® | (don′ ah jel) |
| Donnazyme® | (don′ ah zime) |
| Donnapine® | (don′ ah peen) |
| dopamine | (doe′ pa meen) |
| dobutamine | (doe byoo′ ta meen) |
| dopamine | (doe′ pa meen) |
| Dopram® | (doe′ pram) |
| Dopram® | (doe′ pram) |
| dopamine | (doe′ pa meen) |

| Drug Name | Pronunciation |
|---|---|
| doxacurium | (doks ah kyoo′ ri um) |
| doxapram | (doks′ ah pram) |
| doxacurium | (doks ah kyoo′ ri um) |
| doxorubicin | (doks oh roo′ bi sin) |
| doxapram | (doks′ ah pram) |
| doxacurium | (doks ah kyoo′ ri um) |
| doxapram | (doks′ ah pram) |
| doxazosin | (doks aye′ zoe sin) |
| doxapram | (doks′ ah pram) |
| doxepin | (doks′ e pin) |
| doxapram | (doks′ ah pram) |
| doxorubicin | (doks oh roo′bi sin) |
| doxazosin | (doks aye′ zoe sin) |
| doxapram | (doks′ ah pram) |
| doxazosin | (doks aye′ zoe sin) |
| doxorubicin | (doks oh roo′ bi sin) |
| doxazosin | (doks aye′ zoe sin) |
| doxepin | (doks′ e pin) |
| doxepin | (doks′ e pin) |
| digoxin | (di joks′ in) |
| doxepin | (doks′ e pin) |
| doxazosin | (doks aye′ zoe sin) |
| doxepin | (doks′ e pin) |
| doxapram | (doks′ ah pram) |
| doxepin | (doks′ e pin) |
| Doxidan® | (dox′ e dan) |
| doxepin | (doks′ e pin) |
| doxycycline | (doks i sye′ kleen) |
| Doxidan® | (dox′ e dan) |
| doxepin | (doks′ e pin) |
| Doxil® | (doks′ il) |
| Paxil® | (paks′ il) |
| Doxinate® | (dox′ eh nate) |
| docusate | (dok′ yoo sate) |
| doxorubicin | (doks oh roo′ bi sin) |
| dactinomycin | (dak ti noe mye′ sin) |
| doxorubicin | (doks oh roo′ bi sin) |
| daunorubicin | (daw noe roo′ bi sin) |
| doxorubicin | (doks oh roo′ bi sin) |
| doxacurium | (doks ah kyoo′ ri um) |
| doxorubicin | (doks oh roo′ bi sin) |
| doxapram | (doks′ ah pram) |
| doxorubicin | (doks oh roo′ bi sin) |
| doxazosin | (doks aye′ zoe sin) |
| doxorubicin | (doks oh roo′ bi sin) |
| idarubicin | (eye da roo′ bi sin) |
| doxycycline | (doks i sye′ kleen) |
| doxepin | (doks′ e pin) |

| Drug Name | Pronunciation |
|---|---|
| Drisdol® | (dris′ doll) |
| Drysol® | (dry′ sol) |
| dronabinol | (droe nab′ i nol) |
| droperidol | (droe per′ i dole) |
| droperidol | (droe per′ i dole) |
| dronabinol | (droe nab′ i nol) |
| Drysol® | (dry′ sol) |
| Drisdol® | (dris′ doll) |
| Duo-Cyp® | (du′ oh sip) |
| DuoCet™ | (du′ oh set) |
| DuoCet™ | (du′ oh set) |
| Duo-Cyp® | (du′ oh sip) |
| Duphalac® | (du′ fa lak) |
| diclofenac | (dye kloe′ fen ak) |
| Dyazide® | (dye′ ah zide) |
| diazoxide | (dye az oks′ ide) |
| Dyazide® | (dye′ ah zide) |
| Dynacin® | (dye′ na sin) |
| Dyazide® | (dye′ ah zide) |
| Thiazide® | (thye′ ah zide) |
| dyclonine | (dye′ kloe neen) |
| dicyclomine | (dye sye′ kloe meen) |
| Dymelor® | (dye′ meh lor) |
| Demerol® | (dem′ eh rol) |
| Dymelor® | (dye′ meh lor) |
| Pamelor® | (pam′ meh lor) |
| Dynabac® | (dye′ na bac) |
| DynaCirc® | (dye′ na sirk) |
| Dynabac® | (dye′ na bac) |
| Dynapen® | (dye′ na pen) |
| Dynacin® | (dye′ na sin) |
| DynaCirc® | (dye′ na sirk) |
| Dynacin® | (dye′ na sin) |
| Dyazide® | (dye′ ah zide) |
| Dynacin® | (dye′ na sin) |
| Dynapen® | (dye′ na pen) |
| DynaCirc® | (dye′ na sirk) |
| Dynabac® | (dye′ na bac) |
| DynaCirc® | (dye′ na sirk) |
| Dynacin® | (dye′ na sin) |
| Dynapen® | (dye′ na pen) |
| Dynabac® | (dye′ na bac) |
| Dynapen® | (dye′ na pen) |
| Dynacin® | (dye′ na sin) |
| Dyrenium® | (dye ren′ e um) |
| Pyridium® | (pye rid′ dee um) |
| Echogen® | (ek′ oh jen) |
| Epogen® | (ee′ poe jen) |

| Drug Name | Pronunciation |
|---|---|
| Ecotrin® | (eh′ ko trin) |
| Akineton® | (ah kin′ eh ton) |
| Ecotrin® | (eh′ ko trin) |
| Edecrin® | (ed′ eh crin) |
| Ecotrin® | (eh′ ko trin) |
| Epogen® | (ee′ poe jen) |
| Edecrin® | (ed′ eh crin) |
| Ecotrin® | (eh′ ko trin) |
| Edecrin® | (ed′ eh crin) |
| Eulexin® | (yu leks′ in) |
| E.E.S.® | (ee ee ess) |
| DES® | (dee ee ess) |
| Efudex® | (ef′ yu deks) |
| Eurax® | (yoor′ aks) |
| Elase® | (e′ lase) |
| Ellence® | (el′ lens) |
| Elavil® | (el′ ah vil) |
| Aldoril® | (al′ doe ril) |
| Elavil® | (el′ ah vil) |
| Eldepryl® | (el′ de pril) |
| Elavil® | (el′ ah vil) |
| Equanil® | (eh′ kwa nil) |
| Elavil® | (el′ ah vil) |
| Mellaril® | (mel′ la ril) |
| Elavil® | (el′ ah vil) |
| Oruvail® | (or′ yu vale) |
| Eldepryl® | (el′ de pril) |
| Elavil® | (el′ ah vil) |
| Eldepryl® | (el′ de pril) |
| enalapril | (e nal′ ah pril) |
| Eldopaque Forte® | (el′ do pak for′ tay) |
| Eloquin® Forte® | (el′ do kwin for′ tay) |
| Eloquin® Forte® | (el′ do kwin for′ tay) |
| Eldopaque Forte® | (el′ do pak for′ tay) |
| Elixicon® | (eh lix′ i con) |
| Elocon® | (ee′ lo con) |
| Ellence® | (el′ lens) |
| Elase® | (e′ lase) |
| Elmiron® | (el′ mi ron) |
| Imuran® | (im′ yu ran) |
| Elocon® | (ee′ lo con) |
| Elixicon® | (eh lix′ i con) |
| Emcyt® | (em′ sit) |
| Eryc® | (err′ ik) |
| emetine | (em′ eh teen) |
| Emetrol® | (em′ eh trol) |
| Emetrol® | (em′ eh trol) |
| emetine | (em′ eh teen) |

| Drug Name | Pronunciation |
|---|---|
| Empirin® | (em′ pir in) |
| Enduron® | (en′ du ron) |
| enalapril | (e nal′ ah pril) |
| Anafranil® | (ah naf′ ra nil) |
| enalapril | (e nal′ ah pril) |
| Antril® | (an′ trill) |
| enalapril | (e nal′ ah pril) |
| Eldepryl® | (el′ de pril) |
| enalapril | (e nal′ ah pril) |
| nafarelin | (naf′ ah re lin) |
| enalapril | (e nal′ ah pril) |
| ramipril | (ra mi′ pril) |
| encainide | (en′ kay nide) |
| flecainide | (fle kay′ nide) |
| Endal® | (en′ dal) |
| Depen® | (dee′ pen) |
| Endal® | (en′ dal) |
| Intal® | (in′ tal) |
| Enduron® | (en′ du ron) |
| Empirin® | (em′ pir in) |
| Enduron® | (en′ du ron) |
| Imuran® | (im′ yu ran) |
| Enduron® | (en′ du ron) |
| Inderal® | (in′ der al) |
| Enduronyl® | (en dur′ oh nil) |
| Inderal® | (in′ der al) |
| Enduronyl® Forte | (en dur′ oh nil for′ tay) |
| Inderal® 40 | (in′ der al for′ tee) |
| enflurane | (en′ floo rane) |
| isoflurane | (eye soe flure′ ane) |
| Entex® | (en′ teks) |
| Tenex® | (ten′ eks) |
| ephedrine | (e fed′ rin) |
| Epifrin® | (ep′ eh frin) |
| EpiPen® | (ep′ eh pen) |
| Epifrin® | (ep′ eh frin) |
| Epifrin® | (ep′ eh frin) |
| ephedrine | (e fed′ rin) |
| Epifrin® | (ep′ eh frin) |
| EpiPen® | (ep′ eh pen) |
| Epinal® | (ep′ eh nal) |
| Epitol® | (ep′ eh tol) |
| Epitol® | (ep′ eh tol) |
| Epinal® | (ep′ eh nal) |
| Epivir® | (ep′ ih vir) |
| Combivir® | (kom′ bi veer) |
| Epogen® | (ee′ poe jen) |
| Echogen® | (ek′ oh jen) |

| Drug Name | Pronunciation |
|---|---|
| Equanil® | (eh′ kwa nil) |
| Elavil® | (el′ ah vil) |
| Erex® | (err′ eks) |
| Urex® | (yur′ eks) |
| Eryc® | (err′ ik) |
| Emcyt® | (em′ sit) |
| Eryc® | (err′ ik) |
| Ery-Tab® | (air′ ee tab) |
| Ery-Tab® | (air′ ee tab) |
| Eryc® | (err′ ik) |
| Erythrocin® | (ee rith′ roe sin) |
| Ethmozine® | (eth′ mo zeen) |
| erythromycin | (er ith roe mye′ sin) |
| azithromycin | (az ith roe mye′ sin) |
| erythromycin | (er ith roe mye′ sin) |
| clarithromycin | (kla rith′ roe mye sin) |
| Esidrix® | (es′ eh driks) |
| Lasix® | (lay′ siks) |
| Esimil® | (es′ eh mil) |
| Estinyl® | (es′ teh nil) |
| Esimil® | (es′ eh mil) |
| F.M.L.® | (ef em el) |
| Esimil® | (es′ eh mil) |
| Ismelin® | (is′ meh lin) |
| Eskalith® | (es′ ka lith) |
| Estratest® | (es′ tra test) |
| esmolol | (es′ moe lol) |
| Osmitrol® | (os′ mi trol) |
| Estinyl® | (es′ teh nil) |
| Esimil® | (es′ eh mil) |
| Estraderm® | (es′ tra derm) |
| Testoderm® | (tes′ toh derm) |
| Estratab® | (es′ tra tab) |
| Estratest® | (es′ tra test) |
| Estratest® | (es′ tra test) |
| Eskalith® | (es′ ka lith) |
| Estratest® | (es′ tra test) |
| Estratab® | (es′ tra tab) |
| Estratest® | (es′ tra test) |
| Estratest HS® | (es′ tra test aych ess) |
| Estratest HS® | (es′ tra test aych ess) |
| Estratest® | (es′ tra test) |
| Ethamolin® | (ath am′ oh lin) |
| ethanol | (eth′ e nol) |
| ethanol | (eth′ e nol) |
| Ethamolin® | (ath am′ oh lin) |
| ethanol | (eth′ e nol) |
| Ethyol® | (eth′ e ole) |

| Drug Name | Pronunciation |
|---|---|
| Ethmozine® | (eth′ mo zeen) |
| Erythrocin® | (ee rith′ roe sin) |
| ethosuximide | (eth oh sux′ i mide) |
| methsuximide | (meth sux′ i mide) |
| Ethyol® | (eth′ e ole) |
| ethanol | (eth′ e nol) |
| etidocaine | (e ti′ doe kane) |
| etidronate | (e ti droe′ nate) |
| etidronate | (e ti droe′ nate) |
| etidocaine | (e ti′ doe kane) |
| etidronate | (e ti droe′ nate) |
| etomidate | (e tom′ i date) |
| etidronate | (e ti droe′ nate) |
| etretinate | (e tret′ i nate) |
| etomidate | (e tom′ i date) |
| etidronate | (e ti droe′ nate) |
| etretinate | (e tret′ i nate) |
| etidronate | (e ti droe′ nate) |
| Eulexin® | (yu leks′ in) |
| Edecrin® | (ed′ eh crin) |
| Eulexin® | (yu leks′ in) |
| Eurax® | (yoor′ aks) |
| Eurax® | (yoor′ aks) |
| Efudex® | (ef′ yu deks) |
| Eurax® | (yoor′ aks) |
| Eulexin® | (yu leks′ in) |
| Eurax® | (yoor′ aks) |
| Serax® | (sear′ aks) |
| Eurax® | (yoor′ aks) |
| Urex® | (yur′ eks) |
| Excedrin® | (eks sed′ drin) |
| Dexatrim® | (deks′ ah trim) |
| Factrel® | (fak′ trel) |
| Sectral® | (sek′ tral) |
| fenoprofen | (fen oh proe′ fen) |
| flurbiprofen | (flure bi′ proe fen) |
| fentanyl | (fen′ ta nil) |
| alfentanil | (al fen′ ta nil) |
| fentanyl citrate | (fen′ ta nil sit′ rate) |
| sufentanil citrate | (sue fen′ ta nil sit′ rate) |
| Feosol® | (fee′ oh sol) |
| Feostat® | (fee′ oh stat) |
| Feosol® | (fee′ oh sol) |
| Fer-In-Sol® | (fehr′ in sol) |
| Feosol® | (fee′ oh sol) |
| Festal® | (fes′ tal) |
| Feosol® | (fee′ oh sol) |
| Fluosol® | (flu′ oh sol) |

| Drug Name | Pronunciation |
|---|---|
| Feostat® | (fee' oh stat) |
| Feosol® | (fee' oh sol) |
| Fer-In-Sol® | (fehr' in sol) |
| Feosol® | (fee' oh sol) |
| Ferralet® | (fer' ah let) |
| Ferrlecit® | (fer' le set) |
| Ferrlecit® | (fer' le set) |
| Ferralet® | (fer' ah let) |
| Festal® | (fes' tal) |
| Feosol® | (fee' oh sol) |
| Feverall™ | (fee' ver all) |
| Fiberall® | (fye' ber all) |
| Fiberall® | (fye' ber all) |
| Feverall™ | (fee' ver all) |
| Fioricet® | (fee oh' reh set) |
| Fiorinal® | (fee or' reh nal) |
| Fioricet® | (fee oh' reh set) |
| Lorcet® | (lor' set) |
| Fiorinal® | (fee or' reh nal) |
| Fioricet® | (fee oh' reh set) |
| Fiorinal® | (fee or' reh nal) |
| Florical® | (flor' eh kal) |
| Fiorinal® | (fee or' reh nal) |
| Florinef® | (flor' eh nef) |
| flecainide | (fle kay' nide) |
| encainide | (en' kay nide) |
| Flexeril® | (fleks' eh ril) |
| Floxin® | (floks' in) |
| Flexeril® | (fleks' eh ril) |
| Hectoral™ | (hek' to ral) |
| Flexon® | (fleks' on) |
| Floxin® | (floks' in) |
| Flomax® | (flo' maks) |
| Fosamax® | (fos' ah maks) |
| Flomax® | (flo' maks) |
| Volmax® | (vol' maks) |
| Florical® | (flor' eh kal) |
| Fiorinal® | (fee or' reh nal) |
| Florinef® | (flor' eh nef) |
| Fiorinal® | (fee or' reh nal) |
| Floxin® | (floks' in) |
| Flexeril® | (fleks' eh ril) |
| Floxin® | (floks' in) |
| Flexon® | (fleks' on) |
| flucytosine | (floo sye' toe seen) |
| fluorouracil | (flure oh yoor' ah sil) |
| Fludara® | (floo dare' ah) |
| FUDR® | (ef yu dee are) |

| Drug Name | Pronunciation |
|---|---|
| fludarabine | (floo dare' ah been) |
| Flumadine® | (floo' ma deen) |
| Flumadine® | (floo' ma deen) |
| fludarabine | (floo dare' ah been) |
| flunisolide | (floo nis' oh lide) |
| fluocinonide | (floo oh sin' oh nide) |
| fluocinolone | (floo oh sin' oh lone) |
| fluocinonide | (floo oh sin' oh nide) |
| fluocinonide | (floo oh sin' oh nide) |
| flunisolide | (floo nis' oh lide) |
| fluocinonide | (floo oh sin' oh nide) |
| fluocinolone | (floo oh sin' oh lone) |
| fluorouracil | (flure oh yoor' ah sil) |
| flucytosine | (floo sye' toe seen) |
| Fluosol® | (flu' oh sol) |
| Feosol® | (fee' oh sol) |
| flurazepam | (flure az' e pam) |
| temazepam | (te maz' e pam) |
| flurbiprofen | (flure bi' proe fen) |
| fenoprofen | (fen oh proe' fen) |
| F.M.L.® | (ef em el) |
| Esimil® | (es' eh mil) |
| folic acid | (foe' lik as' id) |
| folinic acid | (foe lin' ik as' id) |
| folinic acid | (foe lin' ik as' id) |
| folic acid | (foe' lik as' id) |
| Fortovase® | (for' to vase) |
| Invirase® | (in' vir ase) |
| Fosamax® | (fos' ah maks) |
| Flomax™ | (flo' maks) |
| fosinopril | (foe sin' oh pril) |
| lisinopril | (lyse in' oh pril) |
| Fostex® | (fos' teks) |
| pHisoHex® | (fye' so heks) |
| FUDR® | (ef yu dee are) |
| Fludara® | (floo dare' ah) |
| Fulvicin® | (ful' vi sin) |
| Furacin® | (fur' ah sin) |
| Furacin® | (fur' ah sin) |
| Fulvicin® | (ful' vi sin) |
| furosemide | (fyoor oh' se mide) |
| torsemide | (tor' se mide) |
| Gantrisin® | (gan' tri sin) |
| Gastrosed™ | (gas' troe sed) |
| Garamycin® | (gar ah mye' sin) |
| kanamycin | (kan ah mye' sin) |
| Garamycin® | (gar ah mye' sin) |
| Terramycin® | (tehr ah mye' sin) |

| Drug Name | Pronunciation |
|---|---|
| Gastrosed™ | (gas′ troe sed) |
| Gantrisin® | (gan′ tri sin) |
| Genapap® | (gen′ ah pap) |
| Genapax® | (gen′ ah paks) |
| Genapax® | (gen′ ah paks) |
| Genapap® | (gen′ ah pap) |
| Gengraf™ | (gen′ graf) |
| Prograf® | (pro′ graf) |
| gentamicin | (jen ta mye′ sin) |
| kanamycin | (kan ah mye′ sin) |
| Glaucon® | (glow′ kon) |
| glucagon | (gloo′ ka gon) |
| glipizide | (glip′ i zide) |
| glyburide | (glye′ byoo ide) |
| glucagon | (gloo′ ka gon) |
| Glaucon® | (glow′ kon) |
| Glucophage® | (glue′ co faagsch) |
| Glutofac® | (glue′ toe fak) |
| Glucophage® | (glue′ co faagsch) |
| Glucotrol® | (glue′ co trol) |
| Glucotrol® | (glue′ co trol) |
| Glucophage® | (glue′ co faagsch) |
| Glucotrol® | (glue′ co trol) |
| glyburide | (glye′ byoo ide) |
| glutethimide | (gloo teth′ i mide) |
| guanethidine | (gwahn eth′ i deen) |
| Glutofac® | (glue′ toe fak) |
| Glucophage® | (glue′ co faagsch) |
| Glutofac® | (glue′ toe fak) |
| Glutose® | (glue′ tose) |
| Glutose® | (glue′ tose) |
| Glutofac® | (glue′ toe fak) |
| glyburide | (glye′ byoo ide) |
| glipizide | (glip′ i zide) |
| glyburide | (glye′ byoo ide) |
| Glucotrol® | (glue′ co trol) |
| Glycotuss® | (glye′ co tuss) |
| Glytuss® | (glye′ tuss) |
| Glytuss® | (glye′ tuss) |
| Glycotuss® | (glye′ co tuss) |
| gonadorelin | (goe nad oh rel′ in) |
| gonadotropin | (goe nad′ oh troe pin) |
| gonadorelin | (goe nad oh rel′ in) |
| guanadrel | (gwahn′ ah drel) |
| gonadotropin | (goe nad′ oh troe pin) |
| gonadorelin | (goe nad oh rel′ in) |
| Granulex® | (gran′ u lecks) |
| Regranex® | (re gra′ neks) |
| guaifenesin | (gwye fen′ e sin) |
| guanfacine | (gwahn′ fa seen) |
| guanabenz | (gwahn′ ah benz) |
| guanadrel | (gwahn′ ah drel) |
| guanabenz | (gwahn′ ah benz) |
| guanfacine | (gwahn′ fa seen) |
| guanadrel | (gwahn′ ah drel) |
| gonadorelin | (goe nad oh rel′ in) |
| guanadrel | (gwahn′ ah drel) |
| guanabenz | (gwahn′ ah benz) |
| guanethidine | (gwahn eth′ i deen) |
| glutethimide | (gloo teth′ i mide) |
| guanethidine | (gwahn eth′ i deen) |
| guanidine | (gwahn′ i deen) |
| guanfacine | (gwahn′ fa seen) |
| guanabenz | (gwahn′ ah benz) |
| guanfacine | (gwahn′ fa seen) |
| guaifenesin | (gwye fen′ e sin) |
| guanfacine | (gwahn′ fa seen) |
| guanidine | (gwahn′ i deen) |
| guanidine | (gwahn′ i deen) |
| guanethidine | (gwahn eth′ i deen) |
| guanidine | (gwahn′ i deen) |
| guanfacine | (gwahn′ fa seen) |
| halcinonide | (hal sin′ oh nide) |
| Halcion® | (hal′ cee on) |
| Halcion® | (hal′ cee on) |
| halcinonide | (hal sin′ oh nide) |
| Halcion® | (hal′ cee on) |
| Haldol® | (hal′ dol) |
| Haldol® | (hal′ dol) |
| Halenol® | (hal′ e nol) |
| Haldol® | (hal′ dol) |
| Halog® | (hay′ log) |
| Haldol® | (hal′ dol) |
| Halotestin® | (hay lo tes′ tin) |
| Haldol® | (hal′ dol) |
| Stadol® | (stay′ dol) |
| Halenol® | (hal′ e nol) |
| Haldol® | (hal′ dol) |
| Halfan® | (hal′ fan) |
| Halfprin® | (haf′ prin) |
| Halfprin® | (haf′ prin) |
| Halfan® | (hal′ fan) |
| Halfprin® | (haf′ prin) |
| Haltran® | (hal′ tran) |
| Halog® | (hay′ log) |
| Haldol® | (hal′ dol) |

| Drug Name | Pronunciation |
|---|---|
| Halog® | (hay′ log) |
| Mycolog® | (mye′ co log) |
| haloperidol | (ha loe per′ i dole) |
| Halotestin® | (hay lo tes′ tin) |
| Halotestin® | (hay lo tes′ tin) |
| Haldol® | (hal′ dol) |
| Halotestin® | (hay lo tes′ tin) |
| haloperidol | (ha loe per′ i dole) |
| Halotestin® | (hay lo tes′ tin) |
| halothane | (ha′ loe thane) |
| Halotestin® | (hay lo tes′ tin) |
| Halotussin® | (hay lo tus′ sin) |
| Halotussin® | (hay lo tus′ sin) |
| Halotestin® | (hay lo tes′ tin) |
| Haltran® | (hal′ tran) |
| Halfprin® | (haf′ prin) |
| Hectoral™ | (hek′ to ral) |
| Flexeril® | (fleks′ eh ril) |
| Hemoccult® | (he′ mo cult) |
| Seracult® | (ser′ a cult) |
| heparin | (hep′ a rin) |
| Hespan® | (hes′ pan) |
| Herceptin® | (her cep′ tin) |
| Perceptin™ | (per cep′ tin) |
| Hespan® | (hes′ pan) |
| heparin | (hep′ a rin) |
| Hespan® | (hes′ pan) |
| Histaspan® | (his′ ta span) |
| Hexadrol® | (heks′ ah drol) |
| Hexalol® | (heks′ ah lole) |
| Hexadrol® | (heks′ ah drol) |
| hexatol | (heks′ ah tol) |
| Hexadrol® | (heks′ ah drol) |
| labetalol | (la bet′ ah lole) |
| Hexalol® | (heks′ ah lole) |
| Hexadrol® | (heks′ ah drol) |
| hexatol | (heks′ ah tol) |
| Hexadrol® | (heks′ ah drol) |
| hexatol | (heks′ ah tol) |
| labetalol | (la bet′ ah lole) |
| Histaspan® | (his′ ta span) |
| Hespan® | (hes′ pan) |
| Hycamtin® | (hye cam′ tin) |
| Hycomine® | (hye′ co meen) |
| Hycodan® | (hye′ co dan) |
| Hycomine® | (hye′ co meen) |
| Hycodan® | (hye′ co dan) |
| Vicodin® | (vye′ co din) |

| Drug Name | Pronunciation |
|---|---|
| Hycomine® | (hye′ coe meen) |
| Byclomine® | (bye′ clo meen) |
| Hycomine® | (hye′ co meen) |
| Hycamtin® | (hye cam′ tin) |
| Hycomine® | (hye′ co meen) |
| Hycodan® | (hye′ co dan) |
| Hycomine® | (hye′ co meen) |
| Vicodin® | (vye′ co din) |
| Hydergine® | (hye′ der geen) |
| Hydramyn® | (hye′ dra min) |
| hydralazine | (hye dral′ ah zeen) |
| hydroxyzine | (hye drox′ i zeen) |
| Hydramyn® | (hye′ dra min) |
| Hydergine® | (hye′ der geen) |
| Hydramyn® | (hye′ dra min) |
| Bydramine® | (bye′ dra meen) |
| Hydrocet® | (hye′ dro set) |
| Hydrocil® | (hye′ dro sil) |
| Hydrocil® | (hye′ dro sil) |
| Hydrocet® | (hye′ dro set) |
| hydrochlorothiazide | (hye droe klor oh thye′ ah zide) |
| hydroflumethiazide | (hye droe floo meth eye′ ah zide) |
| hydrocodone | (hye droe koe′ done) |
| hydrocortisone | (hye droe kor′ ti sone) |
| hydrocortisone | (hye droe kor′ ti sone) |
| hydrocodone | (hye droe koe′ done) |
| hydrocortisone | (hye droe kor′ ti sone) |
| hydroxychloroquine | (hye droks ee klor′ oh kwin) |
| hydroflumethiazide | (hye droe floo meth eye′ ah zide) |
| hydrochlorothiazide | (hye droe klor oh thye′ ah zide) |
| hydromorphone | (hye droe mor′ fone) |
| morphine | (mor′ feen) |
| hydroxychloroquine | (hye droks ee klor′ oh kwin) |
| hydrocortisone | (hye droe kor′ ti sone) |
| hydroxyprogesterone | (hye droks ee proe jes′ te rone) |
| medroxyprogesterone | (me droks′ ee proe jes′ te rone) |
| hydroxyurea | (hye drox ee yoor ee′ a) |
| hydroxyzine | (hye drox′ i zeen) |
| hydroxyzine | (hye drox′ i zeen) |
| hydralazine | (hye dral′ ah zeen) |
| hydroxyzine | (hye drox′ i zeen) |
| hydroxyurea | (hye drox ee yoor ee′ a) |

| Drug Name | Pronunciation |
|---|---|
| HyperHep® | (hye′ per hep) |
| Hyperstat® | (hye′ per stat) |
| Hyperstat® | (hye′ per stat) |
| Nitrostat® | (nye′ troe stat) |
| Hytone® | (hye′ tone) |
| Vytone® | (vye′ tone) |
| Hyzaar® | (hi′ zar) |
| Cozaar® | (koe′ zar) |
| Idamycin® | (eye da mye′ sin) |
| Adriamycin™ | (ade rya mye′ sin) |
| idarubicin | (eye byoo proe′ fen) |
| doxorubicin | (doks oh roo′ bi sin) |
| Imdur® | (im′ dure) |
| K-Dur® | (kay′ dure) |
| Imdur® | (im′ dure) |
| Imuran® | (im′ yu ran) |
| Imdur® | (im′ dure) |
| Inderal LA® | (in′ der al el ay) |
| Imferon® | (im′ fer on) |
| interferon | (in ter fer′ on) |
| Imferon® | (im′ fer on) |
| Roferon-A® | (roe fer′ on ay) |
| imipramine | (im ip′ ra meen) |
| amitriptyline | (ah mee trip′ ti leen) |
| imipramine | (im ip′ ra meen) |
| desipramine | (des ip′ ra meen) |
| imipramine | (im ip′ ra meen) |
| Norpramin® | (nor′ pra min) |
| Imuran® | (im′ yu ran) |
| Elmiron® | (el′ mi ron) |
| Imuran® | (im′ yu ran) |
| Enduron® | (en′ du ron) |
| Imuran® | (im′ yu ran) |
| Inderal® | (in′ der al) |
| Imuran® | (im′ yu ran) |
| Imdur® | (im′ dure) |
| Imuran® | (im′ yu ran) |
| Tenormin® | (ten or′ min) |
| Inapsine® | (i nap′ seen) |
| Nebcin® | (neb′ sin) |
| Inderal® | (in′ der al) |
| Adderall® | (ad′ der all) |
| Inderal® | (in′ der al) |
| Enduron® | (en′ du ron) |
| Inderal® | (in′ der al) |
| Enduronyl® | (en dur′ oh nil) |
| Inderal® | (in′ der al) |
| Imuran® | (im′ yu ran) |
| Inderal® | (in′ der al) |
| Inderide® | (in′ der ide) |
| Inderal® | (in′ der al) |
| Isordil® | (eye′ sor dil) |
| Inderal® | (in′ der al) |
| Toradol® | (tor′ ah doll) |
| Inderal® 40 | (in′ der al for′ tee) |
| Enduronyl® Forte | (en dur′ oh nil for′ tay) |
| Inderal LA® | (in′ der al el ay) |
| Imdur® | (im′ dure) |
| Inderide® | (in′ der ide) |
| Inderal® | (in′ der al) |
| indinavir | (in din′ a veer) |
| Denavir™ | (den′ ah vir) |
| Indocin® | (in′ doe sin) |
| Lincocin® | (link′ oh sin) |
| Indocin® | (in′ doe sin) |
| Minocin® | (min′ oh sin) |
| Intal® | (in′ tal) |
| Endal® | (en′ dal) |
| interferon | (in ter fer′ on) |
| Imferon® | (im′ fer on) |
| Invirase® | (in′ vir ase) |
| Fortovase® | (for′ to vase) |
| iodine | (eye′ oh dyne) |
| codeine | (koe′ deen) |
| iodine | (eye′ oh dyne) |
| Lodine® | (low′ deen) |
| iodine | (eye′ oh dyne) |
| lopidine | (low′ pi deen) |
| Ismelin® | (is′ meh lin) |
| Esimil® | (es′ eh mil) |
| Ismelin® | (is′ meh lin) |
| Isuprel® | (eye′ sue prel) |
| Ismelin® | (is′ meh lin) |
| Ritalin® | (ri′ ta lin) |
| isoflurane | (eye soe flure′ ane) |
| enflurane | (en′ floo rane) |
| isoflurane | (eye soe flure′ ane) |
| isoflurophate | (eye soe flure′ oh fate) |
| isoflurophate | (eye soe flure′ oh fate) |
| isoflurane | (eye soe flure′ ane) |
| Isoptin® | (eye sop′ tin) |
| Isopto® Tears | (eye sop′ tow tears) |
| Isopto® Tears | (eye sop′ tow tears) |
| Isoptin® | (eye sop′ tin) |
| Isordil® | (eye′ sor dil) |
| Inderal® | (in′ der al) |

| Drug Name | Pronunciation |
|---|---|
| Isordil® | (eye′ sor dil) |
| Isuprel® | (eye′ sue prel) |
| Isuprel® | (eye′ sue prel) |
| Disophrol® | (dye′ so frol) |
| Isuprel® | (eye′ sue prel) |
| Ismelin® | (is′ meh lin) |
| Isuprel® | (eye′ sue prel) |
| Isordil® | (eye′ sor dil) |
| kanamycin | (kan ah mye′ sin) |
| Garamycin® | (gar ah mye′ sin) |
| kanamycin | (kan ah mye′ sin) |
| gentamicin | (jen ta mye′ sin) |
| Kaochlor® | (kay′ oh klor) |
| K-Lor® | (kay′ lor) |
| kaolin | (kay′ oh lin) |
| Kaon® | (kay′ on) |
| Kaon® | (kay′ on) |
| kaolin | (kay′ oh lin) |
| Kaopectate® | (kay oh pek′ tate) |
| Kayexelate® | (kay eks′ e late) |
| Kayexelate® | (kay eks′ e late) |
| Kaopectate® | (kay oh pek′ tate) |
| K-Dur® | (kay′ dure) |
| Imdur® | (im′ dure) |
| Kefzol® | (kef′ zol) |
| Cefzil® | (sef′ zil) |
| Kemadrin® | (kem′ ah drin) |
| Coumadin® | (ku′ ma din) |
| Kenalog® | (ken′ ah log) |
| Ketalar® | (key′ tah lar) |
| Ketalar® | (key′ tah lar) |
| Kenalog® | (ken′ ah log) |
| Klonopin® | (klon′ oh pin) |
| clonidine | (kloe′ ni deen) |
| Klonopin® | (klon′ oh pin) |
| clonazepam | (kloe na′ ze pam) |
| Klor-Con® | (klor′ kon) |
| K-Lor® | (kay′ lor) |
| K-Lor® | (kay′ lor) |
| Kaochlor® | (kay′ oh klor) |
| K-Lor® | (kay′ lor) |
| Klor-Con® | (klor′ kon) |
| Klotrix® | (klo′ triks) |
| liotrix | (lye′ oh triks) |
| Komex® | (koe′ meks) |
| Koromex® | (kor′ oh meks) |
| Koromex® | (kor′ oh meks) |
| Komex® | (koe′ meks) |

| Drug Name | Pronunciation |
|---|---|
| K-Phos Neutral® | (kay′ fos new′ tral) |
| Neutra-Phos-K® | (new′ tra fos kay) |
| labetalol | (la bet′ ah lole) |
| betaxolol | (be taks′ oh lol) |
| labetalol | (la bet′ ah lole) |
| Hexadrol® | (heks′ ah drol) |
| labetalol | (la bet′ ah lole) |
| hexatol | (heks′ ah tol) |
| Lacrilube® | (lac′ ri lube) |
| Surgilube® | (sur′ gi lube) |
| lactose | (lak′ tose) |
| lactulose | (lak′ tu lose) |
| lactulose | (lak′ tu lose) |
| lactose | (lak′ tose) |
| Lamicel® | (lam′ i cel) |
| Lamisil® | (lam′ eh sil) |
| Lamictal® | (la mic′ tal) |
| Lamisil® | (lam′ eh sil) |
| Lamictal® | (la mic′ tal) |
| Lomotil® | (lo′ mo til) |
| Lamictal® | (la mic′ tal) |
| Ludiomil® | (lu′ de oh mil) |
| Lamisil® | (lam′ eh sil) |
| Lamicel® | (lam′ i cel) |
| Lamisil® | (lam′ eh sil) |
| Lamictal® | (la mic′ tal) |
| Lamisil® | (lam′ eh sil) |
| Lomotil® | (lo′ mo til) |
| lamivudine | (la mi′ vyoo deen) |
| lamotrigine | (la moe′ tri jeen) |
| lamotrigine | (la moe′ tri jeen) |
| lamivudine | (la mi′ vyoo deen) |
| Lanoxin® | (lan oks′ in) |
| Lasix® | (lay′ siks) |
| Lanoxin® | (lan oks′ in) |
| Levoxine® | (lev oks′ een) |
| Lanoxin® | (lan oks′ in) |
| Levoxyl® | (le voks′ ill) |
| Lanoxin® | (lan oks′ in) |
| Levsinex® | (lev′ si neks) |
| Lanoxin® | (lan oks′ in) |
| Lomotil® | (lo′ mo til) |
| Lanoxin® | (lan oks′ in) |
| Lonox® | (lo′ noks) |
| Lanoxin® | (lan oks′ in) |
| Mefoxin® | (me fox′ in) |
| Lanoxin® | (lan oks′ in) |
| Xanax® | (zan′ aks) |

| Drug Name | Pronunciation |
|---|---|
| Larylgan® | (la ril′ gan) |
| Auralgan® | (ah ral′ gan) |
| Lasix® | (lay′ siks) |
| Esidrix® | (es′ eh driks) |
| Lasix® | (lay′ siks) |
| Lanoxin® | (lan oks′ in) |
| Lasix® | (lay′ siks) |
| Lidex® | (lye′ deks) |
| Lasix® | (lay′ siks) |
| Lomotil® | (lo′ mo til) |
| Lasix® | (lay′ siks) |
| Luvox® | (lu′ voks) |
| l-dopa | (l doe′ pa) |
| levodopa | (lee voe doe′ pa) |
| l-dopa | (l doe′ pa) |
| methyldopa | (meth ill doe′ pa) |
| leucovorin | (loo koe vor′ in) |
| Leukeran® | (lu′ keh ran) |
| leucovorin | (loo koe vor′ in) |
| Leukine® | (lu′ keen) |
| Leukeran® | (lu′ keh ran) |
| Alkeran® | (al′ ker an) |
| Leukeran® | (lu′ keh ran) |
| leucovorin | (loo koe vor′ in) |
| Leukeran® | (lu′ keh ran) |
| Leukine® | (lu′ keen) |
| Leukine® | (lu′ keen) |
| leucovorin | (loo koe vor′ in) |
| Leukine® | (lu′ keen) |
| Leukeran® | (lu′ keh ran) |
| Levbid® | (lev′ bid) |
| Lithobid® | (lith′ oh bid) |
| Levbid® | (lev′ bid) |
| Lopid® | (lo′ pid) |
| Levbid® | (lev′ bid) |
| Lorabid® | (lor′ ah bid) |
| levobunolol | (lee voe byoo′ noe lole) |
| levocabastine | (lee′ voe kab as teen) |
| levocabastine | (lee′ voe kab as teen) |
| levobunolol | (lee voe byoo′ noe lole) |
| levocabastine | (lee′ voe kab as teen) |
| levocarnitine | (lee voe kar′ ni teen) |
| levocarnitine | (lee voe kar′ ni teen) |
| levocabastine | (lee voe byoo′ noe lole) |
| levodopa | (lee voe doe′ pa) |
| l-dopa | (l doe′ pa) |
| levodopa | (lee voe doe′ pa) |
| methyldopa | (meth ill doe′ pa) |

| Drug Name | Pronunciation |
|---|---|
| Levophed® | (lee′ voe fed) |
| Levoprome® | (lee′ voe prome) |
| Levoprome® | (lee′ voe prome) |
| Levophed® | (lee′ voe fed) |
| levothyroxine | (lee voe thye rox′ een) |
| liothyronine | (lye oh thye′ roe neen) |
| Levoxine® | (lev oks′ een) |
| Lanoxin® | (lan oks′ in) |
| Levoxine® | (lev oks′ een) |
| Levoxyl® | (le voks′ ill) |
| Levoxine® | (lev oks′ een) |
| Levsin® | (lev′ sin) |
| Levoxyl® | (le voks′ ill) |
| Lanoxin® | (lan oks′ in) |
| Levoxyl® | (le voks′ ill) |
| Levoxine® | (lev oks′ een) |
| Levoxyl® | (le voks′ ill) |
| Luvox® | (lu′ voks) |
| Levsin® | (lev′ sin) |
| Levoxine® | (lev oks′ een) |
| Levsinex® | (lev′ si neks) |
| Lanoxin® | (lan oks′ in) |
| Librax® | (li′ braks) |
| Librium® | (li′ bre um) |
| Librium® | (li′ bre um) |
| Librax® | (li′ braks) |
| Lidex® | (ly′ decks) |
| Cidex® | (sy′ decks) |
| Lidex® | (lye′ deks) |
| Lasix® | (lay′ siks) |
| Lidex® | (lye′ deks) |
| Lidox® | (lye′ dox) |
| Lidex® | (lye′ deks) |
| Videx® | (vye′ deks) |
| Lidex® | (lye′ deks) |
| Wydase® | (wye′ dase) |
| Lidox® | (lye′ dox) |
| Lidex® | (lye′ deks) |
| Lincocin® | (link′ oh sin) |
| Cleocin® | (klee′ oh sin) |
| Lincocin® | (link′ oh sin) |
| Indocin® | (in′ doe sin) |
| Lincocin® | (link′ oh sin) |
| Minocin® | (min′ oh sin) |
| Lioresal® | (lye or′ reh sal) |
| lisinopril | (lyse in′ oh pril) |
| Lioresal® | (lye or′ reh sal) |
| Lotensin® | (lo ten′ sin) |

| Drug Name | Pronunciation |
|---|---|
| liothyronine | (lye oh thye' roe neen) |
| levothyroxine | (lee voe thye rox' een) |
| liotrix | (lye' oh triks) |
| Klotrix® | (klo' triks) |
| lisinopril | (lyse in' oh pril) |
| fosinopril | (foe sin' oh pril) |
| lisinopril | (lyse in' oh pril) |
| Lioresal® | (lye or' reh sal) |
| lisinopril | (lyse in' oh pril) |
| Risperdal® | (ris' per dal) |
| Lithobid® | (lith' oh bid) |
| Levbid® | (lev' bid) |
| Lithobid® | (lith' oh bid) |
| Lithostat® | (lith' oh stat) |
| Lithostat® | (lith' oh stat) |
| Lithobid® | (lith' oh bid) |
| Lodine® | (low' deen) |
| codeine | (koe' deen) |
| Lodine® | (low' deen) |
| iodine | (eye' oh dyne) |
| Lodine® | (low' deen) |
| Lopid® | (lo' pid) |
| Lomodix® | (lo' mo dix) |
| Lovenox® | (lo' ve nox) |
| Lomotil® | (lo' mo til) |
| Lamictal® | (la mic' tal) |
| Lomotil® | (lo' mo til) |
| Lamisil® | (lam' eh sil) |
| Lomotil® | (lo' mo til) |
| Lanoxin® | (lan oks' in) |
| Lomotil® | (lo' mo til) |
| Lasix® | (lay' siks) |
| Loniten® | (lon' eh ten) |
| clonidine | (kloe' ni deen) |
| Loniten® | (lon' eh ten) |
| Lotensin® | (lo ten' sin) |
| Lonox® | (lo' noks) |
| Lanoxin® | (lan oks' in) |
| Lopid® | (lo' pid) |
| Levbid® | (lev' bid) |
| Lopid® | (lo' pid) |
| Lodine® | (low' deen) |
| Lopid® | (lo' pid) |
| Lorabid® | (lor' ah bid) |
| Lopid® | (lo' pid) |
| Slo-bid™ | (slo' bid) |
| Lopressor® | (lo pres' sor) |
| Lopurin® | (lo pure' in) |
| Lopurin® | (lo pure' in) |
| Lopressor® | (lo pres' sor) |
| Lopurin® | (lo pure' in) |
| Lupron® | (lu' pron) |
| Lorabid® | (lor' ah bid) |
| Levbid® | (lev' bid) |
| Lorabid® | (lor' ah bid) |
| Lopid® | (lo' pid) |
| Lorabid® | (lor' ah bid) |
| Lortab® | (lor' tab) |
| Lorabid® | (lor' ah bid) |
| Slo-bid™ | (slo' bid) |
| lorazepam | (lor a' ze pam) |
| alprazolam | (al pray' zoe lam) |
| lorazepam | (lor a' ze pam) |
| clonazepam | (kloe na' ze pam) |
| lorazepam | (lor a' ze pam) |
| diazepam | (dye az' ah pam) |
| lorazepam | (lor a' ze pam) |
| temazepam | (te maz' e pam) |
| Lorcet® | (lor' set) |
| Fioricet® | (fee oh' reh set) |
| Lortab® | (lor' tab) |
| Cortef® | (kor' tef) |
| Lortab® | (lor' tab) |
| Lorabid® | (lor' ah bid) |
| Lortab® | (lor' tab) |
| Luride® | (lure' ide) |
| losartan | (loe sar' tan) |
| valsartan | (val sar' tan) |
| Lotensin® | (lo ten' sin) |
| Lioresal® | (lye or' reh sal) |
| Lotensin® | (lo ten' sin) |
| Loniten® | (lon' eh ten) |
| Lotensin® | (lo ten' sin) |
| lovastatin | (loe' va sta tin) |
| Lotrimin® | (low' tri min) |
| Lotrisone® | (low' tri sone) |
| Lotrimin® | (low' tri min) |
| Otrivin® | (oh' tri vin) |
| Lotrisone® | (low' tri sone) |
| Lotrimin® | (low' tri min) |
| lovastatin | (loe' va sta tin) |
| Lotensin® | (lo ten' sin) |
| Lovenox® | (lo' ve nox) |
| Lomodix® | (lo' mo dix) |
| Loxitane® | (loks' e tane) |
| Soriatane® | (sor' e ah tane) |

| Drug Name | Pronunciation |
|---|---|
| Ludiomil® | (lu′ de oh mil) |
| Lamictal® | (la mic′ tal) |
| Luminal® | (lu′ mi nal) |
| Tuinal® | (tu′ i nal) |
| Lupron® | (lu′ pron) |
| Lopurin® | (lo pure′ in) |
| Lupron® | (lu′ pron) |
| Nuprin® | (nu′ prin) |
| Luride® | (lure′ ide) |
| Lortab® | (lor′ tab) |
| Luvox® | (lu′ voks) |
| Lasix® | (lay′ siks) |
| Luvox® | (lu′ voks) |
| Levoxyl® | (le voks′ ill) |
| Maalox® | (may′ loks) |
| Maox® | (may′ oks) |
| Maalox® | (may′ loks) |
| Monodox® | (mon′ oh doks) |
| Maltsupex® | (malt′ su peks) |
| Manoplax® | (man′ oh plaks) |
| Mandol® | (man′ dole) |
| nadolol | (nay doe′ lole) |
| Manoplax® | (man′ oh plaks) |
| Maltsupex® | (malt′ su peks) |
| Maox® | (may′ oks) |
| Maalox® | (may′ loks) |
| Marcaine® | (mar′ kane) |
| Narcan® | (nar′ kan) |
| Marinol® | (mare′ i nole) |
| Marnal® | (mar′ nal) |
| Marnal® | (mar′ nal) |
| Marinol® | (mare′ i nole) |
| Matulane® | (mat′ chu lane) |
| Modane® | (moe′ dane) |
| Maxidex® | (maks′ i deks) |
| Maxzide® | (maks′ zide) |
| Maxzide® | (maks′ zide) |
| Maxidex® | (maks′ i deks) |
| Mazicon® | (maz′ ih con) |
| mazindol | (may′ zin dole) |
| Mazicon® | (maz′ ih con) |
| Mivacron® | (mi′ va cron) |
| mazindol | (may′ zin dole) |
| Mazicon® | (maz′ ih con) |
| mazindol | (may′ zin dole) |
| mebendazole | (me ben′ da zole) |
| Mebaral® | (meb′ ah ral) |
| Mellaril® | (mel′ ah ril) |
| Mebaral® | (meb′ ah ral) |
| Tegretol® | (teg′ ree tol) |
| mebendazole | (me ben′ da zole) |
| mazindol | (may′ zin dole) |
| mecamylamine | (mek ah mill′ ah meen) |
| mesalamine | (me sal′ ah meen) |
| medroxyprogesterone | (me droks′ ee proe jes′ te rone) |
| hydroxyprogesterone | (hye droks ee proe jes′ te rone) |
| medroxyprogesterone | (me droks′ ee proe jes′ te rone) |
| methylprednisolone | (meth il pred nis′ oh lone) |
| medroxyprogesterone | (me droks′ ee proe jes′ te rone) |
| methyltestosterone | (meth il tes tos′ te rone) |
| Mefoxin® | (me fox′ in) |
| Lanoxin® | (lan oks′ in) |
| Megace® | (me′ gase) |
| Reglan® | (reg′ lan) |
| Mellaril® | (mel′ la ril) |
| Elavil® | (el′ ah vil) |
| Mellaril® | (mel′ ah ril) |
| Mebaral® | (meb′ ah ral) |
| melphalan | (mel′ fa lan) |
| Mephyton® | (meh fye′ ton) |
| melphalan | (mel′ fa lan) |
| Myleran® | (my′ ler an) |
| Mepergan® | (me′ per gan) |
| meprobamate | (me proe ba′ mate) |
| meperidine | (me per′ i deen) |
| meprobamate | (me proe ba′ mate) |
| mephenytoin | (me fen′ i toyn) |
| Mephyton® | (meh fye′ ton) |
| mephenytoin | (me fen′ i toyn) |
| phenytoin | (fen′ i toyn) |
| mephobarbital | (me foe bar′ bi tal) |
| methocarbamol | (meth oh kar′ ba mole) |
| Mephyton® | (meh fye′ ton) |
| melphalan | (mel′ fa lan) |
| Mephyton® | (meh fye′ ton) |
| mephenytoin | (me fen′ i toyn) |
| Mephyton® | (meh fye′ ton) |
| methadone | (meth′ ah done) |
| mepivacaine | (me piv′ ah kane) |
| bupivacaine | (byoo piv′ ah kane) |
| meprobamate | (me proe ba′ mate) |
| Mepergan® | (me′ per gan) |

| Drug Name | Pronunciation |
|---|---|
| meprobamate | (me proe ba′ mate) |
| meperidine | (me per′ i deen) |
| Meruvax® | (mur′ yu vaks) |
| Attenuvax® | (at ten′ yu vaks) |
| mesalamine | (me sal′ ah meen) |
| mecamylamine | (mek ah mill′ ah meen) |
| Mestinon® | (meh′ sti non) |
| Metatensin® | (me ta ten′ sin) |
| metaproterenol | (met ah proe ter′ e nol) |
| metoprolol | (me toe′ proe lole) |
| Metatensin® | (me ta ten′ sin) |
| Mestinon® | (meh′ sti non) |
| metaxalone | (me taks′ ah lone) |
| metolazone | (me tole′ ah zone) |
| methadone | (meth′ ah done) |
| Mephyton® | (meh fye′ ton) |
| methadone | (meth′ ah done) |
| methylphenidate | (meth il fen′ i date) |
| methazolamide | (meth ah zoe′ la mide) |
| methenamine | (meth en′ ah meen) |
| methazolamide | (meth ah zoe′ la mide) |
| metolazone | (me tole′ ah zone) |
| methenamine | (meth en′ ah meen) |
| methazolamide | (meth ah zoe′ la mide) |
| methenamine | (meth en′ ah meen) |
| methionine | (me thye′ oh neen) |
| methicillin | (meth i sill′ in) |
| mezlocillin | (mez loe sill′ in) |
| methionine | (me thye′ oh neen) |
| methenamine | (meth en′ ah meen) |
| methocarbamol | (meth oh kar′ ba mole) |
| mephobarbital | (me foe bar′ bi tal) |
| methotrexate | (meth oh treks′ ate) |
| metolazone | (me tole′ ah zone) |
| methsuximide | (meth sux′ i mide) |
| ethosuximide | (eth oh sux′ i mide) |
| methyldopa | (meth ill doe′ pa) |
| l-dopa | (l doe′ pa) |
| methyldopa | (meth ill doe′ pa) |
| levodopa | (lee voe doe′ pa) |
| methylphenidate | (meth il fen′ i date) |
| methadone | (meth′ ah done) |
| methylprednisolone | (meth il pred nis′ oh lone) |
| medroxyprogesterone | (me droks′ ee proe jes′ te rone) |
| methylprednisolone | (meth il pred nis′ oh lone) |
| prednisone | (pred′ ni sone) |
| methyltestosterone | (meth il tes tos′ te rone) |
| medroxyprogesterone | (me droks′ ee proe jes′ te rone) |
| metoclopramide | (met oh kloe pra′ mide) |
| metolazone | (me tole′ ah zone) |
| metolazone | (me tole′ ah zone) |
| metaxalone | (me taks′ ah lone) |
| metolazone | (me tole′ ah zone) |
| methazolamide | (meth ah zoe′ la mide) |
| metolazone | (me tole′ ah zone) |
| methotrexate | (meth oh treks′ ate) |
| metolazone | (me tole′ ah zone) |
| metoclopramide | (met oh kloe pra′ mide) |
| metolazone | (me tole′ ah zone) |
| metoprolol | (me toe proe′ lole) |
| metolazone | (me tole′ ah zone) |
| minoxidil | (mi nox′ i dill) |
| metoprolol | (me toe′ proe lole) |
| metaproterenol | (met ah proe ter′ e nol) |
| metoprolol | (me toe′ proe lole) |
| metolazone | (me tole′ ah zone) |
| metoprolol | (me toe proe′ lole) |
| misoprostol | (mye soe prost′ ole) |
| metyrapone | (me teer′ ah pone) |
| metyrosine | (me tye′ roe seen) |
| metyrosine | (me tye′ roe seen) |
| metyrapone | (me teer′ ah pone) |
| Mevacor® | (me′ va cor) |
| Mivacron® | (mi′ va cron) |
| Mexitil® | (meks′ i til) |
| Mezlin® | (mes′ lin) |
| Mezlin® | (mes′ lin) |
| Mexitil® | (meks′ i til) |
| mezlocillin | (mez loe sill′ in) |
| methicillin | (meth i sill′ in) |
| Miacalcin® | (my ah cal′ sin) |
| Micatin® | (my′ ca tin) |
| Micatin® | (my′ ca tin) |
| Miacalcin® | (my ah cal′ sin) |
| miconazole | (mi kon′ ah zole) |
| Micronase® | (mye′ croe nase) |
| miconazole | (mi kon′ ah zole) |
| Micronor® | (mye′ croe nor) |
| Micro-K® | (mye′ cro kay) |
| Micronase® | (mye′ croe nase) |
| Micronase® | (mye′ croe nase) |
| Micro-K® | (mye′ cro kay) |
| Micronase® | (mye′ croe nase) |
| Micronor® | (mye′ croe nor) |

| Drug Name | Pronunciation |
|---|---|
| Micronase®<br>miconazole | (mye′ croe nase)<br>(mi kon′ ah zole) |
| Micronor®<br>miconazole | (mye′ croe nor)<br>(mi kon′ ah zole) |
| Micronor®<br>Micronase® | (mye′ croe nor)<br>(mye′ croe nase) |
| Mictrin®<br>Midrin® | (mik′ trin)<br>(mid′ rin) |
| Midrin®<br>Mictrin® | (mid′ rin)<br>(mik′ trin) |
| Midrin®<br>Mydfrin® | (mid′ rin)<br>(mid′ frin) |
| Minizide®<br>Minocin® | (min′ i zide)<br>(min′ oh sin) |
| Minocin®<br>Indocin® | (min′ oh sin)<br>(in′ doe sin) |
| Minocin®<br>Lincocin® | (min′ oh sin)<br>(link′ oh sin) |
| Minocin®<br>Minizide® | (min′ oh sin)<br>(min′ i zide) |
| Minocin®<br>Mithracin® | (min′ oh sin)<br>(mith′ ra sin) |
| Minocin®<br>niacin | (min′ oh sin)<br>(nye′ ah sin) |
| minoxidil<br>metolazone | (mi nox′ i dill)<br>(me tole′ ah zone) |
| minoxidil<br>Monopril® | (mi noks′ i dil)<br>(mon′ oh pril) |
| MiraLax™<br>Mirapex® | (mir′ ah laks)<br>(mir′ ah peks) |
| Mirapex®<br>MiraLax™ | (mir′ ah peks)<br>(mir′ ah laks) |
| misoprostol<br>metoprolol | (mye soe prost′ ole)<br>(me toe proe′ lole) |
| Mithracin®<br>Minocin® | (mith′ ra sin)<br>(min′ oh sin) |
| mitomycin<br>mitoxantrone | (mye toe mye′ sin)<br>(mye toe zan′ trone) |
| mitomycin<br>mitotane | (mye toe mye′ sin)<br>(mye′ toe tane) |
| mitomycin<br>Mutamycin® | (mye toe mye′ sin)<br>(mute ah mye′ sin) |
| mitotane<br>mitomycin | (mye′ toe tane)<br>(mye toe mye′ sin) |
| mitoxantrone<br>mitomycin | (mye toe zan′ trone)<br>(mye toe mye′ sin) |
| Mivacron®<br>Mazicon® | (mi′ va cron)<br>(maz′ ih con) |
| Mivacron®<br>Mevacor® | (mi′ va cron)<br>(me′ va cor) |
| Moban®<br>Mobidin® | (moe′ ban)<br>(moe by′ din) |
| Moban®<br>Modane® | (moe′ ban)<br>(moe′ dane) |
| Mobidin®<br>Moban® | (moe by′ din)<br>(moe′ ban) |
| Mobidin®<br>molindone | (moe by′ din)<br>(moe lin′ done) |
| Modane®<br>Matulane® | (moe′ dane)<br>(mat′ chu lane) |
| Modane®<br>Moban® | (moe′ dane)<br>(moe′ ban) |
| Modane®<br>Mudrane® | (moe′ dane)<br>(mud′ rane) |
| Modicon®<br>Mylicon® | (mod′ i kon)<br>(mye′ li kon) |
| moexipril<br>Monopril® | (mo ex′ i pril)<br>(mon′ oh pril) |
| molindone<br>Mobidin® | (moe lin′ done)<br>(moe by′ din) |
| Monodox®<br>Maalox® | (mon′ oh doks)<br>(may′ loks) |
| Monoket®<br>Monopril® | (mon′ oh ket)<br>(mon′ oh pril) |
| monopril<br>Accupril® | (mon′ oh pril)<br>(ak′ cue pril) |
| Monopril®<br>minoxidil | (mon′ oh pril)<br>(mi noks′ i dil) |
| Monopril®<br>moexipril | (mon′ oh pril)<br>(mo ex′ i pril) |
| Monopril®<br>Monoket® | (mon′ oh pril)<br>(mon′ oh ket) |
| Monopril®<br>ramipril | (mon′ oh pril)<br>(ra mi′ pril) |
| morphine<br>hydromorphone | (mor′ feen)<br>(hye droe mor′ fone) |
| Mudrane®<br>Modane® | (mud′ rane)<br>(moe′ dane) |
| Murocel®<br>Murocoll-2® | (myur′ oh cel)<br>(myur′ oh coll-2) |
| Murocoll-2®<br>Murocel® | (myur′ oh coll-2)<br>(myur′ oh cel) |
| Mutamycin®<br>mitomycin | (mute ah mye′ sin)<br>(mye toe mye′ sin) |
| Myambutol®<br>Nembutal® | (mya am′ byoo tol)<br>(nem′ byoo tal) |

| Drug Name | Pronunciation |
|---|---|
| Mycelex® | (mye′ si leks) |
| Myoflex® | (mye′ oh fleks) |
| Mycifradin® | (mye ce fray′ din) |
| Mycitracin® | (mye ce tray′ sin) |
| Mycitracin® | (mye ce tray′ sin) |
| Mycifradin® | (mye ce fray′ din) |
| Myciguent® | (mye′ ci kwent) |
| Mycitracin® | (mye ce tray′ sin) |
| Mycitracin® | (mye ce tray′ sin) |
| Myciguent® | (mye′ ci kwent) |
| Mycolog® | (mye′ co log) |
| Halog® | (hay′ log) |
| Mydfrin® | (mid′ frin) |
| Midrin® | (mid′ rin) |
| Myleran® | (mye′ leh ran) |
| melphalan | (mel′ fa lan) |
| Myleran® | (mye′ leh ran) |
| Mylicon® | (mye′ li kon) |
| Mylicon® | (mye′ li kon) |
| Modicon® | (mod′ i kon) |
| Mylicon® | (mye′ li kon) |
| Myleran® | (mye′ leh ran) |
| Myoflex® | (mye′ oh fleks) |
| Mycelex® | (mye′ si leks) |
| nadolol | (nay doe′ lole) |
| Mandol® | (man′ dole) |
| nafarelin | (naf′ ah re lin) |
| Anafranil® | (ah naf′ ra nil) |
| nafarelin | (naf′ ah re lin) |
| enalapril | (e nal′ ah pril) |
| Naldecon® | (nal′ dee kon) |
| Nalfon® | (nal′ fon) |
| Nalfon® | (nal′ fon) |
| Naldecon® | (nal′ dee kon) |
| naloxone | (nal ox′ one) |
| naltrexone | (nal treks′ one) |
| naltrexone | (nal treks′ one) |
| naloxone | (nal ox′ one) |
| Naprelan® | (nap′ re lan) |
| Naprosyn® | (na′ pro sin) |
| Naprosyn® | (na′ pro sin) |
| Naprelan® | (na′ pro sin) |
| Naprosyn® | (na′ pro sin) |
| naproxen | (na prox′ en) |
| Naprosyn® | (na′ pro sin) |
| Natacyn® | (na′ ta sin) |
| Naprosyn® | (na′ pro sin) |
| Nebcin® | (neb′ sin) |
| naproxen | (na prox′ en) |
| Naprosyn® | (na′ pro sin) |
| Narcan® | (nar′ kan) |
| Marcaine® | (mar′ kane) |
| Narcan® | (nar′ kan) |
| Norcuron® | (nor′ ku ron) |
| Nardil® | (nar′ dil) |
| Norinyl® | (nor′ eh nil) |
| Nasacort® | (nay′ sa cort) |
| Nasalcrom® | (nay′ sal crome) |
| Nasalcrom® | (nay′ sal crome) |
| Nasacort® | (nay′ sa cort) |
| Nasalcrom® | (nay′ sal crome) |
| Nasalide® | (nay′ sa lide) |
| Nasalide® | (nay′ sa lide) |
| Nasalcrom® | (nay′ sal crome) |
| Nasarel® | (nay′ sa rel) |
| Nizoral® | (nye′ zoh ral) |
| Natacyn® | (na′ ta sin) |
| Naprosyn® | (na′ pro sin) |
| Natru-Vent® | (nay′ tru vent) |
| Atrovent® | (at′ troe vent) |
| Navane® | (nav′ ane) |
| Norvasc® | (nor′ vask) |
| Navane® | (nav′ ane) |
| Nubain® | (nu′ bane) |
| Nebcin® | (neb′ sin) |
| Inapsine® | (i nap′ seen) |
| Nebcin® | (neb′ sin) |
| Naprosyn® | (na′ pro sin) |
| Nebcin® | (neb′ sin) |
| Nubain® | (nu′ bain) |
| nelfinavir | (nel fin′ ah vir) |
| nevirapine | (ne vir′ ah peen) |
| Nembutal® | (nem′ byoo tal) |
| Myambutol® | (mya am′ byoo tol) |
| Neocare® | (ne′ oh care) |
| Neocate® | (ne′ oh cate) |
| Neocate® | (ne′ oh cate) |
| Neocare® | (ne′ oh care) |
| Neoral® | (ne′ oh ral) |
| Neurontin® | (new ron′ tin) |
| Neoral® | (ne′ oh ral) |
| Nizoral® | (nye′ zoh ral) |
| Neosar® | (ne′ oh sar) |
| Cytosar-U® | (sye′ to sar u) |
| Nephrox® | (nef′ roks) |
| Niferex® | (ny′ fen eks) |

| Drug Name | Pronunciation |
|---|---|
| Neptazane® | (nep′ ta zane) |
| Nesacaine® | (nes′ ah kane) |
| Nesacaine® | (nes′ ah kane) |
| Neptazane® | (nep′ ta zane) |
| Neumega® | (new meg′ ah) |
| Neupogen® | (nu′ po gen) |
| Neupogen® | (nu′ po gen) |
| Neumega® | (new meg′ ah) |
| Neupogen® | (nu′ po gen) |
| Nutramigen® | (nu tram′ eh gen) |
| Neurontin® | (new ron′ tin) |
| Neoral® | (ne′ oh ral) |
| Neurontin® | (new ron′ tin) |
| Noroxin® | (nor oks′ in) |
| Neutra-Phos-K® | (new′ tra fos kay) |
| K-Phos Neutral® | (kay′ fos new′ tral) |
| nevirapine | (ne vir′ ah peen) |
| nelfinavir | (nel fin′ ah vir) |
| niacin | (nye′ ah sin) |
| Minocin® | (min′ oh sin) |
| niacin | (nye′ ah sin) |
| Niaspan® | (nye′ ah span) |
| niacinamide | (nye ah sin′ ah mide) |
| nicardipine | (nye kar′ de peen) |
| Niaspan® | (nye′ ah span) |
| niacin | (nye′ ah sin) |
| nicardipine | (nye kar′ de peen) |
| niacinamide | (nye ah sin′ ah mide) |
| nicardipine | (nye kar′ de peen) |
| nifedipine | (nye fed′ i peen) |
| nicardipine | (nye kar′ de peen) |
| nimodipine | (nye moe′ di peen) |
| Nicobid® | (nye′ ko bid) |
| Nitro-Bid® | (nye′ troe bid) |
| NicoDerm® | (nye′ co derm) |
| Nitroderm® | (nye′ tro derm) |
| Nicorette® | (nik′ oh ret) |
| Nordette® | (nor det′) |
| nifedipine | (nye fed′ i peen) |
| nicardipine | (nye kar′ de peen) |
| nifedipine | (nye fed′ i peen) |
| nimodipine | (nye moe′ di peen) |
| nifedipine | (nye fed′ i peen) |
| nisoldipine | (nye′ sole di peen) |
| Niferex® | (ny′ fen eks) |
| Nephrox® | (nef′ roks) |
| Nilstat® | (nil′ stat) |
| Nitrostat® | (nye′ troe stat) |

| Drug Name | Pronunciation |
|---|---|
| Nimbex® | (nim′ beks) |
| Revex® | (rev′ ex) |
| nimodipine | (nye moe′ di peen) |
| nicardipine | (nye kar′ de peen) |
| Nimodipine | (nye moe′ di peen) |
| nifedipine | (nye fed′ i peen) |
| nisoldipine | (nye′ sole di peen) |
| nifedipine | (nye fed′ i peen) |
| Nitro-Bid® | (nye′ troe bid) |
| Nicobid® | (nye′ ko bid) |
| Nitroderm® | (nye′ tro derm) |
| NicoDerm® | (nye′ co derm) |
| Nitroglycerin | (nye troe gli′ ser in) |
| Nitroglyn® | (nye′ troe glin) |
| nitroglycerin | (nye troe gli′ ser in) |
| nitroprusside | (nye troe prus′ ide) |
| Nitroglyn® | (nye′ troe glin) |
| nitroglycerin | (nye troe gli′ ser in) |
| nitroprusside | (nye troe prus′ ide) |
| nitroglycerin | (nye troe gli′ ser in) |
| Nitrostat® | (nye′ troe stat) |
| Hyperstat® | (hye′ per stat) |
| Nitrostat® | (nye′ troe stat) |
| Nilstat® | (nil′ stat) |
| Nitrostat® | (nye′ troe stat) |
| nystatin | (nye stat′ in) |
| Nizoral® | (nye′ zoh ral) |
| Nasarel® | (nay′ sa rel) |
| Nizoral® | (nye′ zoh ral) |
| Neoral® | (ne′ oh ral) |
| Norcuron® | (nor′ ku ron) |
| Narcan® | (nar′ can) |
| Nordette® | (nor det′) |
| Nicorette® | (nik′ oh ret) |
| Norflex® | (nor′ fleks) |
| norfloxacin | (nor floks′ a sin) |
| Norflex® | (nor′ fleks) |
| Noroxin® | (nor oks′ in) |
| norfloxacin | (nor floks′ a sin) |
| Norflex® | (nor′ fleks) |
| norfloxacin | (nor floks′ a sin) |
| Noroxin® | (nor oks′ in) |
| Norgesic 40® | (nor gee′ sik for′ tee) |
| Norgesic Forte® | (nor gee′ sik for′ tay) |
| Norgesic Forte® | (nor gee′ sik for′ tay) |
| Norgesic 40® | (nor gee′ sik for′ tee) |
| Norinyl® | (nor′ eh nil) |
| Nardil® | (nar′ dil) |

| Drug Name | Pronunciation |
|---|---|
| Noroxin® | (nor oks′ in) |
| Neurontin® | (new ron′ tin) |
| Noroxin® | (nor oks′ in) |
| Norflex® | (nor′ fleks) |
| Noroxin® | (nor oks′ in) |
| norfloxacin | (nor floks′ a sin) |
| Norpace® | (nor′ pace) |
| Norpramin® | (nor′ pra min) |
| Norpramin® | (nor′ pra min) |
| clomipramine | (kloe mi′ pra meen) |
| Norpramin® | (nor′ pra min) |
| imipramine | (im ip′ ra meen) |
| Norpramin® | (nor′ pra min) |
| Norpace® | (nor′ pace) |
| Norpramin® | (nor′ pra min) |
| nortriptyline | (nor trip′ ti leen) |
| Norpramin® | (nor′ pra min) |
| Tenormin® | (ten or′ min) |
| nortriptyline | (nor trip′ ti leen) |
| amitriptyline | (ah mee trip′ ti leen) |
| nortriptyline | (nor trip′ ti leen) |
| desipramine | (des ip′ ra meen) |
| nortriptyline | (nor trip′ ti leen) |
| Norpramin® | (nor′ pra min) |
| Norvasc® | (nor′ vask) |
| Navane® | (nav′ ane) |
| Norvasc® | (nor′ vask) |
| Norvir® | (nor′ vir) |
| Norvir® | (nor′ vir) |
| Norvasc® | (nor′ vask) |
| Novacet® | (no′ va set) |
| NovaSeven® | (no′ va se ven) |
| NovaSeven® | (no′ va se ven) |
| Novacet® | (no′ va set) |
| Nubain® | (nu′ bane) |
| Navane® | (nav′ ane) |
| Nubain® | (nu′ bane) |
| Nebcin® | (neb′ sin) |
| Nuprin® | (nu′ prin) |
| Lupron® | (lu′ pron) |
| Nutramigen® | (nu tram′ eh gen) |
| Neupogen® | (nu′ po gen) |
| nystatin | (nye stat′ in) |
| Nitrostat® | (nye′ troe stat) |
| Ocufen® | (ok′ yu fen) |
| Ocuflox® | (ok′ yu floks) |
| Ocufen® | (ok′ yu fen) |
| Ocupress® | (ok′ yu press) |

| Drug Name | Pronunciation |
|---|---|
| Ocuflox® | (ok′ yu floks) |
| Ocufen® | (ok′ yu fen) |
| Ocupress® | (ok′ yu press) |
| Ocufen® | (ok′ yu fen) |
| olanzapine | (oh lan′ za peen) |
| olsalazine | (ole sal′ ah zeen) |
| olsalazine | (ole sal′ ah zeen) |
| olanzapine | (oh lan′ za peen) |
| Oncovin® | (on′ coe vin) |
| Ancobon® | (an′ coe bon) |
| Ophthalgan® | (op thal′ gan) |
| Auralgan® | (ah ral′ gan) |
| Ophthalgan® | (op thal′ gan) |
| Opthetic® | (op thet′ ik) |
| Ophthetic® | (op thet′ ik) |
| Ophthalgan® | (op thal′ gan) |
| oprelvekin | (oh prel′ ve kin) |
| aldesleukin | (al des loo′ kin) |
| oprelvekin | (op rel′ ve kin) |
| Proleukin® | (pro lu′ kin) |
| Optimine® | (op′ ti meen) |
| Optimmune® | (op′ ti mune) |
| Optimmune® | (op′ ti mune) |
| Optimine® | (op′ ti meen) |
| Orabase® | (or′ ah base) |
| Orinase® | (or′ in ase) |
| Orexin® | (or eks′ in) |
| Ornex® | (or′ neks) |
| Orinase® | (or′ in ase) |
| Orabase® | (or′ ah base) |
| Orinase® | (or′ in ase) |
| Ornex® | (or′ neks) |
| Orinase® | (or′ in ase) |
| Tolinase® | (tole′ i nase) |
| Ornex® | (or′ neks) |
| Orexin® | (or eks′ in) |
| Ornex® | (or′ neks) |
| Orinase® | (or′ in ase) |
| Oruvail® | (or′ yu vale) |
| Clinoril® | (klin′ oh rill) |
| Oruvail® | (or′ yu vale) |
| Elavil® | (el′ ah vil) |
| Os-Cal® | (os′ cal) |
| Asacol® | (as′ ah col) |
| Osmitrol® | (os′ mi trol) |
| esmolol | (es′ moe lol) |
| Otrivin® | (oh′ tri vin) |
| Lotrimin® | (low′ tri min) |

| Drug Name | Pronunciation |
|---|---|
| oxazepam | (oks a′ ze pam) |
| quazepam | (kway′ ze pam) |
| oxybutynin | (ok i byoo′ ti nin) |
| OxyContin® | (oks i kon′ tin) |
| oxycodone | (oks i koe′ done) |
| OxyContin® | (oks i kon′ tin) |
| OxyContin® | (oks i kon′ tin) |
| oxybutynin | (ok i byoo′ ti nin) |
| OxyContin® | (oks i kon′ tin) |
| oxycodone | (oks i koe′ done) |
| oxymetazoline | (ox i met az′ oh leen) |
| oxymetholone | (ox i meth′ oh lone) |
| oxymetholone | (ox i meth′ oh lone) |
| oxymetazoline | (ox i met az′ oh leen) |
| oxymetholone | (ox i meth′ oh lone) |
| oxymorphone | (ox i mor′ fone) |
| oxymorphone | (ox i mor′ fone) |
| oxymetholone | (ox i meth′ oh lone) |
| paclitaxel | (pak le taks′ el) |
| paroxetine | (pa roks′ e teen) |
| paclitaxel | (pak le taks′ el) |
| Paxil® | (paks′ ol) |
| Pamelor® | (pam′ meh lor) |
| Demerol® | (dem′ eh rol) |
| Pamelor® | (pam′ meh lor) |
| Dymelor® | (dye′ meh lor) |
| Pamine® | (pa′ meen) |
| Pelamine® | (pel′ ah meen) |
| Panadol® | (pa′ nah dol) |
| pindolol | (pin′ doe lole) |
| Panadol® | (pa′ nah dol) |
| Panafil® | (pan′ ah fill) |
| Panafil® | (pan′ ah fill) |
| Panadol® | (pa′ nah dol) |
| pancreatin | (pan kre′ ah tine) |
| Panretin® | (pan ree′ tin) |
| pancuronium | (pan kyoo roe′ nee um) |
| pipercuronium | (pi pe kur oh′ nee um) |
| Panretin® | (pan ree′ tin) |
| pancreatin | (pan kre′ ah tine) |
| Paraplatin® | (pare ah pla′ tin) |
| Platinol® | (pla′ ti nol) |
| Paregoric® | (pare eh gor′ ik) |
| Percogesic® | (per coe gese′ ik) |
| Parlodel® | (par′ loe dell) |
| pindolol | (pin′ doe lole) |
| Parlodel® | (par′ loe dell) |
| Provera® | (pro ver′ ah) |

| Drug Name | Pronunciation |
|---|---|
| paroxetine | (pa roks′ e teen) |
| paclitaxel | (pak le taks′ el) |
| paroxetine | (pa roks′ e teen) |
| pyridoxine | (peer i dox′ een) |
| Patanol® | (pa′ ta nol) |
| Platinol® | (pla′ ti nol) |
| Paxil® | (paks′ ol) |
| paclitaxel | (pak le taks′ el) |
| Paxil® | (paks′ ol) |
| Plavix® | (plah′ viks) |
| Paxil® | (paks′ ol) |
| Taxol® | (tacks′ ol) |
| Pediapred® | (pe′ de ah pred) |
| Pedia Profen® | (pe′ de ah pro′ fen) |
| Pediapred® | (pe′ de ah pred) |
| Pediazole® | (pe′ de ah zole) |
| Pedia Profen® | (pe′ de ah pro′ fen) |
| Pediapred® | (pe′ de ah pred) |
| Pedia Profen® | (pe′ de ah pro′ fen) |
| Pediazole® | (pe′ de ah zole) |
| Pedia Profen® | (pe′ de ah pro′ fen) |
| Prelone® | (pree′ lone) |
| Pediazole® | (pe′ de ah zole) |
| Pediapred® | (pe′ de ah pred) |
| Pediazole® | (pe′ de ah zole) |
| Pedia Profen® | (pe′ de ah pro′ fen) |
| pegaspargase | (peg as′ par jase) |
| asparaginase | (ah spir′ ah ji nase) |
| Pelamine® | (pel′ ah meen) |
| Pamine® | (pa′ meen) |
| Pelamine® | (pel′ ah meen) |
| pemoline | (pem′ oh leen) |
| pemoline | (pem′ oh leen) |
| Pelamine® | (pel′ ah meen) |
| penicillamine | (pen i sil′ ah meen) |
| penicillin | (pen i sil′ in) |
| penicillin | (pen i sil′ in) |
| penicillamine | (pen i sil′ ah meen) |
| penicillin G potassium | (pen i sil′ in jee poe tass′ ee um) |
| penicillin G procaine | (pen i sil′ in jee proe′ kane) |
| penicillin G procaine | (pen i sil′ in jee proe′ kane) |
| penicillin G potassium | (pen i sil′ in jee poe tass′ ee um) |
| pentobarbital | (pen toe bar′ bi tal) |
| phenobarbital | (fee noe bar′ bi tal) |

| Drug Name | Pronunciation |
|---|---|
| pentoxifylline | (pen toks i′ fi leen) |
| tamoxifen | (ta moks′ i fen) |
| Pentrax® | (pen′ traks) |
| Permax® | (per′ max) |
| Perative® | (per ah′ tive) |
| Periactin® | (pear ee ak′ tine) |
| Perceptin™ | (per cep′ tin) |
| Herceptin® | (her cep′ tin) |
| Percocet® | (per′ koe set) |
| Percodan® | (per′ koe dan) |
| Percodan® | (per′ koe dan) |
| Decadron® | (dek′ ah dron) |
| Percodan® | (per′ koe dan) |
| Percocet® | (per′ koe set) |
| Percodan® | (per′ koe dan) |
| Percogesic® | (per coe gese′ ik) |
| Percodan® | (per′ koe dan) |
| Periactin® | (pear ee ak′ tine) |
| Percogesic® | (per coe gese′ ik) |
| Paregoric® | (pare eh gor′ ik) |
| Percogesic® | (per coe gese′ ik) |
| Percodan® | (per′ koe dan) |
| Perdiem® | (per dee′ em) |
| Pyridium® | (pye rid′ dee um) |
| Periactin® | (pear ee ak′ tine) |
| Perative® | (per ah′ tive) |
| Periactin® | (pear ee ak′ tine) |
| Percodan® | (per′ koe dan) |
| Periactin® | (pear ee ak′ tine) |
| Persantine® | (per san′ teen) |
| Permax® | (per′ max) |
| Bumex® | (byoo′ mex) |
| Permax® | (per′ max) |
| Pentrax® | (pen′ traks) |
| Permitil® | (per′ mi till) |
| Persantine® | (per san′ teen) |
| Peroxyl® | (per ox′ ill) |
| Benoxyl® | (ben ox′ ill) |
| Persantine® | (per san′ teen) |
| Periactin® | (pear ee ak′ tine) |
| Persantine® | (per san′ teen) |
| Permitil® | (per′ mi till) |
| Persantine® | (per san′ teen) |
| Pertofrane® | (per′ toe frane) |
| Pertofrane® | (per′ toe frane) |
| Persantine® | (per san′ teen) |
| Phazyme® | (fay′ zeem) |
| Pherazine® | (fer′ ah zeen) |

| Drug Name | Pronunciation |
|---|---|
| Phenaphen® | (fen′ ah fen) |
| Phenergan® | (fen′ er gan) |
| phenelzine | (fen′ el zeen) |
| phenytoin | (fen′ i toyn) |
| Phenergan® | (fen′ er gan) |
| Phenaphen® | (fen′ ah fen) |
| Phenergan® | (fen′ er gan) |
| Phrenilin® | (fren′ ni lin) |
| Phenergan® | (fen′ er gan) |
| Theragran® | (ther′ ah gran) |
| phenobarbital | (fee noe bar′ bi tal) |
| pentobarbital | (pen toe bar′ bi tal) |
| phentermine | (fen′ ter meen) |
| phentolamine | (fen tole′ ah meen) |
| Phentermine® | (fen′ ter meen) |
| phenytoin | (fen′ i toyn) |
| phentolamine | (fen tole′ ah meen) |
| phentermine | (fen′ ter meen) |
| phentolamine | (fen tole′ ah meen) |
| Ventolin® | (ven′ to lin) |
| phenytoin | (fen′ i toyn) |
| mephenytoin | (me fen′ i toyn) |
| phenytoin | (fen′ i toyn) |
| phenelzine | (fen′ el zeen) |
| phenytoin | (fen′ i toyn) |
| Phentermine® | (fen′ ter meen) |
| Pherazine® | (fer′ ah zeen) |
| Phazyme® | (fay′ zeem) |
| pHisoHex® | (fye′ so heks) |
| Fostex® | (fos′ teks) |
| PhosChol® | (fos′ kol) |
| PhosLo® | (fos′ lo) |
| PhosChol® | (fos′ kol) |
| Phosphocol® | (fos′ fo kol) |
| Phos-Flur® | (fos′ flur) |
| PhosLo® | (fos′ lo) |
| PhosLo® | (fos′ lo) |
| PhosChol® | (fos′ kol) |
| PhosLo® | (fos′ lo) |
| Phos-Flur® | (fos′ flur) |
| PhosLo® | (fos′ lo) |
| ProSom™ | (pro′ som) |
| Phosphocol® | (fos′ fo kol) |
| PhosChol® | (fos′ kol) |
| Phrenilin® | (fren′ ni lin) |
| Phenergan® | (fen′ er gan) |
| Phrenilin® | (fren′ ni lin) |
| Trinalin® | (tri′ na lin) |

| Drug Name | Pronunciation |
|---|---|
| physostigmine | (fye zoe stig′ meen) |
| Prostigmin® | (pro stig′ min) |
| physostigmine | (fye zoe stig′ meen) |
| pyridostigmine | (peer id oh stig′ meen) |
| pindolol | (pin′ doe lole) |
| Panadol® | (pa′ nah dol) |
| pindolol | (pin′ doe lole) |
| Parlodel® | (par′ loe dell) |
| pindolol | (pin′ doe lole) |
| Plendil® | (plen′ dill) |
| pipercuronium | (pi pe kur oh′ nee um) |
| pancuronium | (pan kyoo roe′ nee um) |
| Pitocin® | (pi toe′ sin) |
| Pitressin® | (pi tres′ sin) |
| Pitressin® | (pi tres′ sin) |
| Pitocin® | (pi toe′ sin) |
| Plaquenil® | (pla′ kwe nil) |
| Platinol® | (pla′ ti nol) |
| Platinol® | (pla′ ti nol) |
| Paraplatin® | (pare ah pla′ tin) |
| Platinol® | (pla′ ti nol) |
| Patanol® | (pa′ ta nol) |
| Platinol® | (pla′ ti nol) |
| Plaquenil® | (pla′ kwe nil) |
| Plavix® | (plah′ viks) |
| Elavil® | (el′ ah vil) |
| Plavix® | (plah′ viks) |
| Paxil® | (paks′ ol) |
| Plendil® | (plen′ dill) |
| Isordil® | (eye′ sor dil) |
| Plendil® | (plen′ dill) |
| pindolol | (pin′ doe lole) |
| Plendil® | (plen′ dil) |
| Pletal® | (ple′ tal) |
| Plendil® | (plen′ dil) |
| Prilosec™ | (pry′ lo sek) |
| Plendil® | (plen′ dill) |
| Prinivil® | (pri′ ni vill) |
| Pletal® | (ple′ tal) |
| Plendil® | (plen′ dil) |
| Ponstel® | (pon′ stel) |
| Pronestyl® | (pro nes′ til) |
| pralidoxime | (pra li dox′ eem) |
| pramoxine | (pra moks′ een) |
| pralidoxime | (pra li dox′ eem) |
| pyridoxine | (peer i dox′ een) |
| Pramosone® | (pra′ mo sone) |
| prednisone | (pred′ ni sone) |

| Drug Name | Pronunciation |
|---|---|
| pramoxine | (pra moks′ een) |
| pralidoxime | (pra li dox′ eem) |
| Prandin™ | (pran′ din) |
| Avandia® | (ah van′ de a) |
| Pravachol® | (prav′ ah kol) |
| Prevacid® | (prev′ ah sid) |
| Pravachol® | (prav′ ah kol) |
| propranolol | (proe pran′ oh lole) |
| prazepam | (pra′ ze pam) |
| prazosin | (pra′ zoe sin) |
| prazosin | (pra′ zoe sin) |
| prazepam | (pra′ ze pam) |
| prazosin | (pra′ zoe sin) |
| prednisone | (pred′ ni sone) |
| Precare® | (pre′ kare) |
| Precose® | (pre′ kose) |
| Precose® | (pre′ kose) |
| Precare® | (pre′ kare) |
| prednisolone | (pred nis′ oh lone) |
| prednisone | (pred′ ni sone) |
| prednisone | (pred′ ni sone) |
| methylprednisolone | (meth il pred nis′ oh lone) |
| prednisone | (pred′ ni sone) |
| Pramosone® | (pra′ mo sone) |
| prednisone | (pred′ ni sone) |
| prazosin | (pra′ zoe sin) |
| prednisone | (pred′ ni sone) |
| prednisolone | (pred nis′ oh lone) |
| prednisone | (pred′ ni sone) |
| Prilosec™ | (pry′ lo sek) |
| prednisone | (pred′ ni sone) |
| primidone | (pri′ mi done) |
| prednisone | (pred′ ni sone) |
| promethazine | (proe meth′ ah zeen) |
| Prelone® | (pree′ lone) |
| Pedia Profen® | (pe′ de ah pro′ fen) |
| Premarin® | (prem′ ah rin) |
| Primaxin® | (pri maks′ in) |
| Premarin® | (prem′ ah rin) |
| Provera® | (pro ver′ ah) |
| Premphase® | (prem′ fase) |
| Prempro™ | (prem′ pro) |
| Prempro™ | (prem′ pro) |
| Premphase® | (prem′ fase) |
| Prepidil® | (pre′ pi dil) |
| Bepridil® | (be′ pri dil) |
| Prevacid® | (prev′ ah sid) |
| Pravachol® | (prav′ ah kol) |

| Drug Name | Pronunciation |
|---|---|
| Prevacid® | (prev′ ah sid) |
| Prinivil® | (pri′ ni vill) |
| PREVEN™ | (pre′ ven) |
| Preveon™ | (pre′ vee on) |
| Preveon™ | (pre′ vee on) |
| PREVEN™ | (pre′ ven) |
| prilocaine | (pril′ oh kane) |
| Prilosec™ | (pry′ lo sek) |
| Prilosec™ | (pry′ lo sek) |
| Plendil® | (plen′ dill) |
| Prilosec™ | (pry′ lo sek) |
| prednisone | (pred′ ni sone) |
| Prilosec™ | (pry′ lo sek) |
| prilocaine | (pril′ oh kane) |
| Prilosec™ | (pry′ lo sek) |
| Prinivil® | (pri′ ni vill) |
| Prilosec™ | (pry′ lo sek) |
| Prozac® | (proe′ zak) |
| Primaxin® | (pri maks′ in) |
| Premarin® | (prem′ ah rin) |
| primidone | (pri′ mi done) |
| prednisone | (pred′ ni sone) |
| Prinivil® | (pri′ ni vill) |
| Plendil® | (plen′ dill) |
| Prinivil® | (pri′ ni vill) |
| Prevacid® | (prev′ ah sid) |
| Prinivil® | (pri′ ni vill) |
| Prilosec™ | (pry′ lo sek) |
| Prinivil® | (pri′ ni vill) |
| Proventil® | (pro ven′ till) |
| Priscoline® | (pris′ coe leen) |
| Apresoline® | (aye press′ sow leen) |
| probenecid | (proe ben′ e sid) |
| Procanbid® | (proe can′ bid) |
| Procanbid® | (proe can′ bid) |
| probenecid | (proe ben′ e sid) |
| procarbazine | (proe kar′ ba zeen) |
| dacarbazine | (da kar′ ba zeen) |
| prochlorperazine | (proe klor per′ ah zeen) |
| chlorpromazine | (klor proe′ ma zeen) |
| Proctocort® | (prok′ toe kort) |
| ProctoCream HC® | (prok′ toe cream aych see) |
| ProctoCream HC® | (prok′ toe cream aych see) |
| Proctocort® | (prok′ toe kort) |
| Prograf® | (pro′ graf) |
| Gengraf™ | (gen′ graf) |
| Proleukin® | (pro lu′ kin) |
| oprelvekin | (op rel′ ve kin) |
| Proloprim® | (pro′ low prim) |
| Prolixin® | (pro liks′ in) |
| Proloprim® | (pro′ low prim) |
| Protropin® | (proe tro′ pin) |
| Prolixin® | (pro liks′ in) |
| Proloprim® | (pro′ low prim) |
| promazine | (proe′ ma zeen) |
| promethazine | (proe meth′ ah zeen) |
| promethazine | (proe meth′ ah zeen) |
| chlorpromazine | (klor proe′ ma zeen) |
| promethazine | (proe meth′ ah zeen) |
| prednisone | (pred′ ni sone) |
| promethazine | (proe meth′ ah zeen) |
| promazine | (proe′ ma zeen) |
| Pronestyl® | (pro nes′ til) |
| Ponstel® | (pon′ stel) |
| proparacaine | (proe par′ ah kane) |
| propoxyphene | (proe poks′ i feen) |
| propoxyphene | (proe poks′ i feen) |
| proparacaine | (proe par′ ah kane) |
| propranolol | (proe pran′ oh lole) |
| Pravachol® | (prav′ ah kol) |
| propranolol | (proe pran′ oh lole) |
| Propulsid® | (pro pul′ sid) |
| Propulsid® | (pro pul′ sid) |
| propranolol | (proe pran′ oh lole) |
| Proscar® | (pros′ car) |
| ProSom® | (pro′ som) |
| Proscar® | (pros′ car) |
| Prozac® | (proe′ zak) |
| Pro-Sof® Plus | (proe′ sof plus) |
| ProSom® | (pro′ som) |
| ProSom® | (pro′ som) |
| PhosLo® | (fos′ lo) |
| ProSom® | (pro′ som) |
| Proscar® | (pros′ car) |
| ProSom® | (pro′ som) |
| Pro-Sof® Plus | (proe′ sof plus) |
| ProSom® | (pro′ som) |
| Prozac® | (proe′ zak) |
| ProStep® | (proe′ step) |
| Prozac® | (proe′ zak) |
| Prostigmin® | (pro stig′ min) |
| physostigmine | (fye zoe stig′ meen) |
| protamine | (proe′ ta meen) |
| Protopam® | (proe′ toe pam) |

| Drug Name | Pronunciation |
|---|---|
| protamine | (proe′ ta meen) |
| Protropin® | (proe tro′ pin) |
| Protopam® | (proe′ toe pam) |
| Proloprim® | (pro′ low prim) |
| Protopam® | (proe′ toe pam) |
| protamine | (proe′ ta meen) |
| Protopam® | (proe′ toe pam) |
| Protropin® | (proe tro′ pin) |
| Protropin® | (proe tro′ pin) |
| Proloprim® | (pro′ low prim) |
| Protropin® | (proe tro′ pin) |
| protamine | (proe′ ta meen) |
| Protropin® | (proe tro′ pin) |
| Protopam® | (proe′ toe pam) |
| Proventil® | (pro ven′ till) |
| Bentyl® | (ben′ til) |
| Proventil® | (pro ven′ till) |
| Prinivil® | (pri′ ni vill) |
| Provera® | (pro ver′ ah) |
| Covera® | (co ver′ ah) |
| Provera® | (pro ver′ ah) |
| Parlodel® | (par′ loe dell) |
| Provera® | (pro ver′ ah) |
| Premarin® | (prem′ ah rin) |
| Provera® | (pro ver′ ah) |
| Provir® | (pro′ vir) |
| Provir® | (pro′ vir) |
| Provera® | (pro ver′ ah) |
| Prozac® | (proe′ zak) |
| Prilosec™ | (pry′ lo sek) |
| Prozac® | (proe′ zak) |
| Proscar® | (pros′ car) |
| Prozac® | (proe′ zak) |
| ProSom® | (pro′ som) |
| Prozac® | (proe′ zak) |
| ProStep® | (proe′ step) |
| Psorcon® | (sore′ kon) |
| Psorion® | (sore′ ee on) |
| Psorion® | (sore′ ee on) |
| Psorcon® | (sore′ kon) |
| Pyridium® | (pye rid′ dee um) |
| Dyrenium® | (dye ren′ e um) |
| Pyridium® | (pye rid′ dee um) |
| Perdiem® | (per dee′ em) |
| Pyridium® | (pye rid′ dee um) |
| pyridoxine | (peer i dox′ een) |
| Pyridium® | (pye rid′ dee um) |
| pyrithione | (peer i thye′ one) |
| pyridostigmine | (peer id oh stig′ meen) |
| physostigmine | (fye zoe stig′ meen) |
| pyridoxine | (peer i dox′ een) |
| paroxetine | (pa roks′ e teen) |
| pyridoxine | (peer i dox′ een) |
| Pyridium® | (pye rid′ dee um) |
| pyridoxine | (peer i dox′ een) |
| pralidoxime | (pra li dox′ eem) |
| pyrithione | (peer i thye′ one) |
| Pyridium® | (pye rid′ dee um) |
| Quarzan® | (kwar′ zan) |
| quazepam | (kway′ ze pam) |
| Quarzan® | (kwar′ zan) |
| Questran® | (kwes′ tran) |
| quazepam | (kway′ ze pam) |
| oxazepam | (oks a′ ze pam) |
| quazepam | (kway′ ze pam) |
| Quarzan® | (kwar′ zan) |
| Questran® | (kwes′ tran) |
| Quarzan® | (kwar′ zan) |
| quinidine | (kwin′ i deen) |
| clonidine | (kloe′ ni deen) |
| quinidine | (kwin′ i deen) |
| quinine | (kwye′ nine) |
| quinine | (kwye′ nine) |
| quinidine | (kwin′ i deen) |
| ramipril | (ra mi′ pril) |
| enalapril | (e nal′ ah pril) |
| ramipril | (ra mi′ pril) |
| Monopril® | (mon′ oh pril) |
| ranitidine | (ra ni′ ti deen) |
| amantadine | (ah man′ ta deen) |
| ranitidine | (ra ni′ ti deen) |
| rimantadine | (ri man′ ta deen) |
| ranitidine | (ra ni′ ti deen) |
| ritodrine | (ri′ toe dreen) |
| ratgam | (rat′ gam) |
| Atgam® | (at′ gam) |
| Reglan® | (reg′ lan) |
| Megace® | (me′ gase) |
| Reglan® | (reg′ lan) |
| Regonol® | (reg′ oh nol) |
| Regonol® | (reg′ oh nol) |
| Reglan® | (reg′ lan) |
| Regonol® | (reg′ oh nol) |
| Regroton® | (re gro′ ton) |
| Regroton® | (re gro′ ton) |
| Regonol® | (reg′ oh nol) |

| Drug Name | Pronunciation |
|---|---|
| Regranex® | (re gra′ neks) |
| Granulex® | (gran′ u lecks) |
| Remegel® | (reh′ me gel) |
| Renagel® | (reh′ na gel) |
| Remeron® | (reh′ me ron) |
| Zemuron™ | (zeh′ mu ron) |
| remifentanil | (rem i fen′ ta nil) |
| alfentanil | (al fen′ ta nil) |
| Renagel® | (reh′ na gel) |
| Remegel | (reh′ me gel) |
| Repan® | (ree′ pan) |
| Riopan® | (rye′ oh pan) |
| reserpine | (re ser′ peen) |
| Risperdal® | (ris per′ dal) |
| reserpine | (re ser′ peen) |
| risperidone | (ris per′ i done) |
| Restore® | (res tore′) |
| Restoril® | (res′ tor ril) |
| Restoril® | (res′ tor ril) |
| Restore® | (res tore′) |
| Restoril® | (res′ tor ril) |
| Vistaril® | (vis′ tar ril) |
| Retrovir® | (re′ tro vir) |
| ritonavir | (ri ton′ oh vir) |
| Revex® | (rev′ ex) |
| Nimbex® | (nim′ beks) |
| Revex® | (rev′ ex) |
| ReVia® | (rev′ ve ah) |
| ReVia® | (rev′ ve ah) |
| Revex® | (rev′ ex) |
| Rhythmin® | (rith′ min) |
| Rythmol® | (rith′ mol) |
| ribavirin | (rye ba vye′ rin) |
| riboflavin | (rye′ boe flay vin) |
| riboflavin | (rye′ boe flay vin) |
| ribavirin | (rye ba vye′ rin) |
| Ridaura® | (ri dur′ ah) |
| Cardura® | (kar dur′ ah) |
| rifabutin | (rif ah byoo′ tin) |
| rifampin | (rif′ am pin) |
| Rifadin® | (rif′ ah din) |
| Ritalin® | (ri′ ta lin) |
| rifampin | (rif′ am pin) |
| rifabutin | (rif ah byoo′ tin) |
| Rimactane® | (ri mak′ tane) |
| rimantadine | (ri man′ ta deen) |
| rimantadine | (ri man′ ta deen) |
| amantadine | (ah man′ ta deen) |
| rimantadine | (ri man′ ta deen) |
| ranitidine | (ra ni′ ti deen) |
| rimantadine | (ri man′ ta deen) |
| Rimactane® | (ri mak′ tane) |
| Riopan® | (rye′ oh pan) |
| Repan | (ree′ pan) |
| Risperdal® | (ris per′ dal) |
| lisinopril | (lyse in′ oh pril) |
| Risperdal® | (ris per′ dal) |
| reserpine | (re ser′ peen) |
| Risperdal® | (ris per′ dal) |
| risperidone | (ris per′ i done) |
| risperidone | (ris per′ i done) |
| reserpine | (re ser′ peen) |
| risperidone | (ris per′ i done) |
| Risperdal® | (ris per′ dal) |
| Ritalin® | (ri′ ta lin) |
| Ismelin® | (is′ meh lin) |
| Ritalin® | (ri′ ta lin) |
| Rifadin® | (rif′ ah din) |
| Ritalin® | (ri′ ta lin) |
| ritodrine | (ri′ toe dreen) |
| ritodrine | (ri′ toe dreen) |
| ranitidine | (ra ni′ ti deen) |
| ritodrine | (ri′ toe dreen) |
| Ritalin® | (ri′ ta lin) |
| ritonavir | (ri ton′ oh vir) |
| Retrovir® | (re′ tro vir) |
| Robaxin® | (roe baks′ in) |
| Rubex® | (rue′ beks) |
| Rocephin® | (roe sef′ fen) |
| Roferon® | (roe fer′ on) |
| Roferon® | (roe fer′ on) |
| Rocephin® | (roe sef′ fen) |
| Roferon-A® | (roe fer′ on ay) |
| Imferon® | (im′ fer on) |
| ropivacaine | (roe piv′ a kane) |
| bupivacaine | (byoo piv′ ah kane) |
| Roxanol® | (roks′ ah noll) |
| Roxicet® | (roks′ ih set) |
| Roxicet® | (roks′ ih set) |
| Roxanol® | (roks′ ah noll) |
| Rubex® | (rue′ beks) |
| Robaxin® | (roe baks′ in) |
| Rynatan® | (rye′ na tan) |
| Rynatuss® | (rye′ na tuss) |
| Rynatuss® | (rye′ na tuss) |
| Rynatan® | (rye′ na tan) |

| Drug Name | Pronunciation |
|---|---|
| Rythmol® | (rith' mol) |
| Rhythmin® | (rith' min) |
| Salacid® | (sal as' sid) |
| Salagen® | (sal' ah gen) |
| Salagen® | (sal' ah gen) |
| Salacid® | (sal as' sid) |
| salbutamol | (sal byu' tu mol) |
| salmeterol | (sal me' te role) |
| salmeterol | (sal me' te role) |
| salbutamol | (sal byu' tu mol) |
| salsalate | (sal' sa late) |
| sucralfate | (soo kral' fate) |
| salsalate | (sal' sa late) |
| sulfasalazine | (sul fa sal' ah zeen) |
| Sandimmune® | (san' di mune) |
| Sandoglobulin® | (san doe glo' byu line) |
| Sandimmune® | (san' di mune) |
| Sandostatin® | (san doe sta' tin) |
| Sandoglobulin® | (san doe glo' byu line) |
| Sandimmune® | (san' di mune) |
| Sandoglobulin® | (san doe glo' byu line) |
| Sandostatin® | (san doe sta' tin) |
| Sandostatin® | (san doe sta' tin) |
| Sandimmune® | (san' di mune) |
| Sandostatin® | (san doe sta' tin) |
| Sandoglobulin® | (san doe glo' byu line) |
| saquinavir | (sa kwin' ah veer) |
| Sinequan® | (si' ne kwan) |
| Sarafem™ | (sar' ah fem) |
| Serophene® | (ser' oh feen) |
| Sebex® | (see' beks) |
| Sebutone® | (se' byu tone) |
| Sebex® | (see' beks) |
| Surbex® | (sir' beks) |
| Sebutone® | (se' byu tone) |
| Sebex® | (see' beks) |
| Seconal™ | (sek' oh nal) |
| Sectral® | (sek' tral) |
| Sectral® | (sek' tral) |
| Factrel® | (fak' trel) |
| Sectral® | (sek' tral) |
| Seconal™ | (sek' oh nal) |
| Sectral® | (sek' tral) |
| Septra® | (sep' trah) |
| selegiline | (seh ledge' ah leen) |
| Serentil® | (se ren' till) |
| selegiline | (seh ledge' ah leen) |
| sertraline | (ser' tra leen) |
| selegiline | (seh ledge' ah leen) |
| Serzone® | (ser zone') |
| selegiline | (seh ledge' ah leen) |
| Stelazine® | (stel' ah zene) |
| Senexon® | (sen' e son) |
| Cenestin® | (se nes' tin) |
| Senokot® | (sen' oh kot) |
| Depakote® | (dep' ah kote) |
| Septa® | (sep' tah) |
| Septra® | (sep' trah) |
| Septra® | (sep' trah) |
| Ceptaz® | (sep' taz) |
| Septra® | (sep' trah) |
| Sectral® | (sek' tral) |
| Septra® | (sep' trah) |
| Septa® | (sep' tah) |
| Seracult® | (ser' a cult) |
| Hemoccult® | (he' mo cult) |
| Serax® | (sear' aks) |
| Eurax® | (yoor' aks) |
| Serax® | (sear' aks) |
| Urex® | (yur' eks) |
| Serax® | (sear' aks) |
| Xerac® | (zear' ak) |
| Serax® | (sear' aks) |
| Zyrtec® | (zir' tec) |
| Serentil® | (se ren' till) |
| selegiline | (seh ledge' ah leen) |
| Serentil® | (se ren' till) |
| sertraline | (ser' tra leen) |
| Serentil® | (se ren' till) |
| Seroquel® | (seer' oh kwel) |
| Serentil® | (se ren' till) |
| Serzone® | (ser zone') |
| Serentil® | (se ren' till) |
| Sinequan® | (si' ne kwan) |
| Serentil® | (se ren' till) |
| Surgicel® | (sir' gee cell) |
| Serophene® | (ser' oh feen) |
| Sarafem™ | (sar' ah fem) |
| Seroquel® | (seer' oh kwel) |
| Serentil® | (se ren' till) |
| Seroquel® | (seer' oh kwel) |
| Serzone® | (ser zone') |
| Seroquel® | (seer' oh kwel) |
| Sinequan® | (si' ne kwan) |
| Serzone® | (ser zone') |
| selegiline | (seh ledge' ah leen) |

| Drug Name | Pronunciation |
|---|---|
| Serzone® | (ser zone′) |
| Serentil® | (se ren′ till) |
| Serzone® | (ser zone′) |
| Seroquel® | (seer′ oh kwel) |
| Serzone® | (ser zone′) |
| sertraline | (ser′ tra leen) |
| simethicone | (sye meth′ i kone) |
| cimetidine | (sye met′ i deen) |
| Sinarest® | (sy′ na rest) |
| Allerest® | (al′ e rest) |
| Sinequan® | (si′ ne kwan) |
| saquinavir | (sa kwin′ ah veer) |
| Sinequan® | (si′ ne kwan) |
| Serentil® | (se ren′ till) |
| Sinequan® | (si′ ne kwan) |
| Seroquel® | (seer′ oh kwel) |
| Sinequan® | (si′ ne kwan) |
| Singulair® | (sin′ gu lare) |
| Singulair® | (sin′ gu lare) |
| Sinequan® | (si′ ne kwan) |
| Slo-bid™ | (slo′ bid) |
| Dolobid® | (dol′ ah bid) |
| Slo-bid™ | (slo′ bid) |
| Lopid® | (lo′ pid) |
| Slo-bid™ | (slo′ bid) |
| Lorabid® | (lor′ ah bid) |
| Solu-Medrol® | (sol′ yu med′ role) |
| Depo-Medrol® | (dep′ oh med′ role) |
| Somatrem® | (sow′ mah trem) |
| somatropin | (sow mah troh′ pin) |
| somatropin | (sow mah troh′ pin) |
| Somatrem® | (sow′ mah trem) |
| Soriatane® | (sor′ e ah tane) |
| Loxitane® | (loks′ e tane) |
| Stadol® | (stay′ dol) |
| Haldol® | (hal′ dol) |
| Stelazine® | (stel′ ah zene) |
| selegiline | (seh ledge′ ah leen) |
| Stilphostrol® | (stil phos′ trol) |
| Disophrol® | (dye′ so frol) |
| streptomycin | (strep toe mye′ sin) |
| streptozocin | (strep toe zoe′ sin) |
| streptozocin | (strep toe zoe′ sin) |
| streptomycin | (strep toe mye′ sin) |
| sucralfate | (soo kral′ fate) |
| salsalate | (sal′ sa late) |
| Sudafed® | (sue′ da fed) |
| Sufenta® | (sue fen′ tah) |

| Drug Name | Pronunciation |
|---|---|
| Sufenta® | (sue fen′ tah) |
| Alfenta® | (al fen′ tah) |
| Sufenta® | (sue fen′ tah) |
| Sudafed® | (sue′ da fed) |
| sufentanil | (sue fen′ ta nil) |
| alfentanil | (al fen′ ta nil) |
| sufentanil citrate | (sue fen′ ta nil sit′ rate) |
| fentanyl citrate | (fen′ ta nil sit′ rate) |
| sulfadiazine | (sul fa dye′ ah zeen) |
| sulfasalazine | (sul fa sal′ ah zeen) |
| sulfamethizole | (sul fa meth′ i zole) |
| sulfamethoxazole | (sul fa meth oks′ ah zole) |
| sulfamethoxazole | (sul fa meth oks′ ah zole) |
| sulfamethizole | (sul fa meth′ i zole) |
| sulfamethoxazole | (sul fa meth oks′ ah zole) |
| sulfisoxazole | (sul fi soks′ ah zole) |
| sulfasalazine | (sul fa sal′ ah zeen) |
| salsalate | (sal′ sa late) |
| sulfasalazine | (sul fa sal′ ah zeen) |
| sulfadiazine | (sul fa dye′ ah zeen) |
| sulfasalazine | (sul fa sal′ ah zeen) |
| sulfisoxazole | (sul fi sox′ ah zole) |
| sulfisoxazole | (sul fi soks′ ah zole) |
| sulfamethoxazole | (sul fa meth oks′ ah zole) |
| sulfisoxazole | (sul fi sox′ ah zole) |
| sulfasalazine | (sul fa sal′ ah zeen) |
| sumatriptan | (soo ma trip′ tan) |
| zolmitriptan | (zohl mi trip′ tan) |
| Suprax® | (su′ prax) |
| Surbex® | (sir′ beks) |
| Surbex® | (sir′ beks) |
| Sebex® | (see′ beks) |
| Surbex® | (sir′ beks) |
| Suprax® | (su′ prax) |
| Surbex® | (sir′ beks) |
| Surfak® | (sur′ fak) |
| Surfak® | (sur′ fak) |
| Surbex® | (sir′ beks) |
| Surgicel® | (sir′ gee cell) |
| Serentil® | (se ren′ till) |
| Surgilube® | (sur′ gi lube) |
| Lacrilube® | (lac′ ri lube) |
| Symmetrel® | (sim′ et trell) |
| Synthroid® | (sin′ throid) |
| Synagis® | (si na′ gis) |
| Synvisc® | (sin′ visc) |
| Synthroid® | (sin′ throid) |
| Symmetrel® | (sim′ et trell) |

| Drug Name | Pronunciation |
|---|---|
| Synvisc® | (sin′ visc) |
| Synagis® | (si na′ gis) |
| Sytobex® | (sye′ toe beks) |
| Cytotec® | (sye′ toe tek) |
| Talacen® | (tal′ ah sen) |
| Tegison® | (teg′ i son) |
| Talacen® | (tal′ ah sen) |
| Timoptic® | (tim op′ tik) |
| Talacen® | (tal′ ah sen) |
| Tinactin® | (tin ak′ tin) |
| Tambocor® | (tam′ bo kor) |
| tamoxifen | (ta moks′ i fen) |
| Tamiflu™ | (tam′ eh flu) |
| Theraflu® | (ther′ ah flu) |
| tamoxifen | (ta moks′ i fen) |
| Tambocor® | (tam′ bo kor) |
| tamoxifen | (ta moks′ i fen) |
| pentoxifylline | (pen toks i′ fi leen) |
| Taxol® | (tacks′ ol) |
| Paxil® | (paks′ ol) |
| Taxol® | (tacks′ ol) |
| Taxotere® | (taks′ oh tere) |
| Taxotere® | (taks′ oh tere) |
| Taxol® | (tacks′ ol) |
| Tegison® | (teg′ i son) |
| Talacen® | (tal′ ah sen) |
| Tegretol® | (teg′ ree tol) |
| Mebaral® | (meb′ ah ral) |
| Tegretol® | (teg′ ree tol) |
| Tegrin® | (teg′ rin) |
| Tegretol® | (teg′ ree tol) |
| Toradol® | (tor′ ah doll) |
| Tegrin® | (teg′ rin) |
| Tegretol® | (teg′ ree tol) |
| temazepam | (te maz′ e pam) |
| flurazepam | (flure az′ e pam) |
| temazepam | (te maz′ e pam) |
| lorazepam | (lor a′ ze pam) |
| Tenex® | (ten′ eks) |
| Entex® | (en′ teks) |
| Tenex® | (ten′ eks) |
| Ten-K® | (ten′ kay) |
| Tenex® | (ten′ eks) |
| Xanax® | (zan′ aks) |
| Ten-K® | (ten′ kay) |
| Tenex® | (ten′ eks) |
| Tenormin® | (ten or′ min) |
| Imuran® | (im′ yu ran) |
| Tenormin® | (ten or′ min) |
| Norpramin® | (nor′ pra min) |
| Tenormin® | (ten or′ min) |
| thiamine | (thye′ ah min) |
| Tenormin® | (ten or′ min) |
| Trovan® | (tro′ van) |
| terbinafine | (ter′ bin ah feen) |
| terfenadine | (ter fen′ na deen) |
| terbinafine | (ter′ bin ah feen) |
| terbutaline | (ter byoo′ ta leen) |
| terbutaline | (ter byoo′ ta leen) |
| terbinafine | (ter′ bin ah feen) |
| terbutaline | (ter byoo′ ta leen) |
| tolbutamide | (tole byoo′ ta mide) |
| terconazole | (ter kone′ ah zole) |
| tioconazole | (tye oh kone′ ah zole) |
| terfenadine | (ter fen′ na deen) |
| terbinafine | (ter′ bin ah feen) |
| Terramycin® | (tehr ah mye′ sin) |
| Garamycin® | (gar ah mye′ sin) |
| Testoderm® | (tes′ toh derm) |
| Estraderm® | (es′ tra derm) |
| testolactone | (tess toe lak′ tone) |
| testosterone | (tess toss′ ter one) |
| testosterone | (tess toss′ ter one) |
| testolactone | (tess toe lak′ tone) |
| tetracycline | (tet ra sye′ kleen) |
| tetradecyl sulfate | (tetra dek′ il sul′ fate) |
| tetradecyl sulfate | (tetra dek′ il sul′ fate) |
| tetracycline | (tet ra sye′ kleen) |
| Theolair™ | (thee′ oh lare) |
| Thiola™ | (thye oh′ la) |
| Theolair® | (thee′ oh lare) |
| Thyrolar® | (thye′ roe lar) |
| Theraflu® | (ther′ ah flu) |
| Tamiflu™ | (tam′ eh flu) |
| Theragran® | (ther′ ah gran) |
| Phenergan® | (fen′ er gan) |
| thiamine | (thye′ ah min) |
| Thorazine® | (thor′ ah zene) |
| thiamine | (thye′ ah min) |
| Tenormin® | (ten or′ min) |
| Thiazide® | (thye′ ah zide) |
| Dyazide® | (dye′ ah zide) |
| Thiola™ | (thye oh′ la) |
| Theolair™ | (thee′ oh lare) |
| thioridazine | (thye oh rid′ ah zeen) |
| Thorazine® | (thor′ ah zene) |

| Drug Name | Pronunciation |
|---|---|
| thioridazine | (thye oh rid′ ah zeen) |
| thiothixene | (thye oh thix′ een) |
| thiothixene | (thye oh thix′ een) |
| thioridazine | (thye oh rid′ ah zeen) |
| Thorazine® | (thor′ ah zene) |
| thiamine | (thye′ ah min) |
| Thorazine® | (thor′ ah zene) |
| thioridazine | (thye oh rid′ ah zeen) |
| Thyrolar® | (thye′ roe lar) |
| Theolair™ | (thee′ oh lare) |
| Thyrolar® | (thye′ roe lar) |
| Thytropar® | (thye′ troe par) |
| Thytropar® | (thye′ troe par) |
| Thyrolar® | (thye′ roe lar) |
| tiagabine | (tye ag′ a bene) |
| tizanidine | (tye zan′ i deen) |
| Tiazac® | (tye′ ah zak) |
| Tigan® | (tye′ gan) |
| Tiazac® | (tye′ ah zak) |
| Ziac™ | (zye′ ak) |
| Ticar® | (tye′ kar) |
| Tigan® | (tye′ gan) |
| Tigan® | (tye′ gan) |
| Tiazac® | (tye′ ah zak) |
| Tigan® | (tye′ gan) |
| Ticar® | (tye′ kar) |
| timolol | (tye′ moe lole) |
| atenolol | (ah ten′ oh lole) |
| timolol | (tye′ moe lole) |
| Tylenol® | (tye′ le nole) |
| Timoptic® | (tim op′ tik) |
| Talacen® | (tal′ ah sen) |
| Timoptic® | (tim op′ tik) |
| Viroptic® | (vir op′ tik) |
| Tinactin® | (tin ak′ tin) |
| Talacen® | (tal′ ah sen) |
| tioconazole | (tye oh kone′ ah zole) |
| terconazole | (ter kone′ ah zole) |
| tizanidine | (tye zan′ i deen) |
| tiagabine | (tye ag′ a bene) |
| TNKase™ | (tee en case′) |
| t-PA | (tee′ pee ay) |
| TobraDex® | (toe′ bra deks) |
| Tobrex® | (toe′ breks) |
| tobramycin | (toe bra mye′ sin) |
| Trobicin® | (troe′ bi sin) |
| Tobrex® | (toe′ breks) |
| TobraDex® | (toe′ bra deks) |

| Drug Name | Pronunciation |
|---|---|
| tolazamide | (tole az′ ah mide) |
| tolazoline | (tole az′ oh leen) |
| tolazamide | (tole az′ ah mide) |
| tolbutamide | (tole byoo′ ta mide) |
| tolazoline | (tole az′ oh leen) |
| tolazamide | (tole az′ ah mide) |
| tolbutamide | (tole byoo′ ta mide) |
| terbutaline | (ter byoo′ ta leen) |
| tolbutamide | (tole byoo′ ta mide) |
| tolazamide | (tole az′ ah mide) |
| Tolinase® | (tole′ i nase) |
| Orinase® | (or′ in ase) |
| tolnaftate | (tole naf′ tate) |
| Tornalate® | (tor′ na late) |
| Tonocard® | (ton′ oh kard) |
| Torecan® | (tor′ e kan) |
| Topic® | (top′ ik) |
| Topicort® | (top′ ih kort) |
| Topicort® | (top′ ih kort) |
| Topic® | (top′ ik) |
| Toradol® | (tor′ ah doll) |
| Inderal® | (in′ der al) |
| Toradol® | (tor′ ah doll) |
| Tegretol® | (teg′ ree tol) |
| Toradol® | (tor′ ah doll) |
| Torecan® | (tor′ eh kan) |
| Toradol® | (tor′ ah doll) |
| tramadol | (tra′ ma dole) |
| Torecan® | (tor′ e kan) |
| Tonocard® | (ton′ oh kard) |
| Torecan® | (tor′ eh kan) |
| Toradol® | (tor′ ah doll) |
| Tornalate® | (tor′ na late) |
| tolnaftate | (tole naf′ tate) |
| torsemide | (tor′ se mide) |
| furosemide | (fyoor oh′ se mide) |
| t-PA | (tee′ pee ay) |
| TNKase™ | (tee en case′) |
| tramadol | (tra′ ma dole) |
| Toradol® | (tor′ ah doll) |
| tramadol | (tra′ ma dole) |
| Voltaren® | (vol tare′ en) |
| Trandate® | (tran′ date) |
| Trendar® | (tren′ dar) |
| Trandate® | (tran′ date) |
| Trental® | (tren′ tal) |
| Trandate® | (tran′ date) |
| Tridrate® | (trye′ date) |

| Drug Name | Pronunciation |
|---|---|
| Trendar® | (tren′ dar) |
| Trandate® | (tran′ date) |
| Trental® | (tren′ tal) |
| Bentyl® | (ben′ til) |
| Trental® | (tren′ tal) |
| Trandate® | (tran′ date) |
| tretinoin | (tret′ i noyn) |
| trientine | (trye′ en teen) |
| Tri-Levlen® | (trye′ lev len) |
| Trilafon® | (tri′ la fon) |
| triacetin | (trye ah see′ tin) |
| Triacin® | (trye′ ah sin) |
| Triacin® | (trye′ ah sin) |
| triacetin | (trye ah see′ tin) |
| triamcinolone | (trye am sin′ oh lone) |
| Triaminicin® | (trye ah min′ ih sin) |
| triamcinolone | (trye am sin′ oh lone) |
| Triamoline® | (trye am′ oh lene) |
| Triaminic® | (trye ah min′ ik) |
| Triaminicin® | (trye ah min′ ih sin) |
| Triaminic® | (trye ah min′ ik) |
| TriHemic® | (trye hee′ mik) |
| Triaminicin® | (trye ah min′ ih sin) |
| Triaminic® | (trye ah min′ ik) |
| Triaminicin® | (trye ah min′ ih sin) |
| triamcinolone | (trye am sin′ oh lone) |
| Triamoline® | (trye am′ oh lene) |
| triamcinolone | (trye am sin′ oh lone) |
| triamterene | (trye am′ ter een) |
| trimipramine | (trye mi′ pra meen) |
| Triapin® | (trye ah pin) |
| Triban® | (trye′ ban) |
| triazolam | (trye ay′ zoe lam) |
| alprazolam | (al pray′ zoe lam) |
| Triban® | (trye′ ban) |
| Triapin® | (trye ah pin) |
| Tridrate® | (trye′ date) |
| Trandate® | (tran′ date) |
| trientine | (trye′ en teen) |
| Trental® | (tren′ tal) |
| trientine | (trye′ en teen) |
| tretinoin | (tret′ i noyn) |
| trifluoperazine | (trye floo oh per′ ah zeen) |
| trihexyphenidyl | (trye heks ee fen′ i dil) |
| TriHemic® | (trye hee′ mik) |
| Triaminic® | (trye ah min′ ik) |

| Drug Name | Pronunciation |
|---|---|
| trihexyphenidyl | (trye heks ee fen′ i dil) |
| trifluoperazine | (trye floo oh per′ ah zeen) |
| Trilafon® | (tri′ la fon) |
| Tri-Levlen® | (trye′ lev len) |
| trimeprazine | (trye mep′ ra zeen) |
| trimipramine | (trye mi′ pra meen) |
| trimethaphan | (trye meth′ ah fan) |
| trimethoprim | (trye meth′ oh prim) |
| trimethoprim | (trye meth′ oh prim) |
| trimethaphan | (trye meth′ ah fan) |
| trimipramine | (trye mi′ pra meen) |
| triamterene | (trye am′ ter een) |
| trimipramine | (trye mi′ pra meen) |
| trimeprazine | (trye mep′ ra zeen) |
| Trimox® | (trye′ moks) |
| Diamox® | (dye′ ah moks) |
| Trimox® | (trye′ moks) |
| Tylox® | (tye′ loks) |
| Trinalin® | (tri′ na lin) |
| Phrenilin® | (fren′ ni lin) |
| Tri-Norinyl® | (tri nor′ ih nil) |
| Triphasil® | (tri fay′ sil) |
| Triphasil® | (tri fay′ sil) |
| Tri-Norinyl® | (tri nor′ ih nil) |
| Trobicin® | (troe′ bi sin) |
| tobramycin | (toe bra mye′ sin) |
| Tronolane® | (tron′ oh lane) |
| Tronothane® | (tron′ oh thane) |
| Tronothane® | (tron′ oh thane) |
| Tronolane® | (tron′ oh lane) |
| Trovan® | (tro′ van) |
| Tenormin® | (ten or′ min) |
| Tuinal® | (tu′ i nal) |
| Luminal® | (lu′ mi nal) |
| Tuinal® | (tu′ i nal) |
| Tylenol® | (tye′ le nole) |
| Tussafed® | (tus′ ah fed) |
| Tussafin® | (tus′ ah fin) |
| Tussafin® | (tus′ ah fin) |
| Tussafed® | (tus′ ah fed) |
| Tylenol® | (tye′ le nole) |
| atenolol | (ah ten′ oh lole) |
| Tylenol® | (tye′ le nole) |
| timolol | (tye′ moe lole) |
| Tylenol® | (tye′ le nole) |
| Tuinal® | (tu′ i nal) |
| Tylenol® | (tye′ le nole) |
| Tylox® | (tye′ loks) |

| Drug Name | Pronunciation |
|---|---|
| Tylox® | (tye′ loks) |
| Trimox® | (trye′ moks) |
| Tylox® | (tye′ loks) |
| Tylenol® | (tye′ le nole) |
| Tylox® | (tye′ loks) |
| Wymox® | (wye′ moks) |
| Tylox® | (tye′ loks) |
| Xanax® | (zan′ aks) |
| Ultane® | (uhl′ tane) |
| Ultram® | (uhl′ tram) |
| Ultram® | (uhl′ tram) |
| Ultane® | (uhl′ tane) |
| Ultram® | (uhl′ tram) |
| Voltaren® | (vol tare′ en) |
| Ultravate® | (ul′ trah vate) |
| Cutivate™ | (kyu′ te vate) |
| Urex® | (yur′ eks) |
| Erex® | (err′ eks) |
| Urex® | (yur′ eks) |
| Eurax® | (yoor′ aks) |
| Urex® | (yur′ eks) |
| Serax® | (sear′ aks) |
| Uricit-K® | (yur′ ah sit kay′) |
| Urised® | (yur′ ih sed) |
| Uridon® | (yur′ ih don) |
| Vicodin® | (vye′ co din) |
| Urised® | (yur′ ih sed) |
| Uricit-K® | (yur′ ah sit kay′) |
| Urised® | (yur′ ih sed) |
| Urispas® | (yur′ ih spas) |
| Urispas® | (yur′ ih spas) |
| Urised® | (yur′ ih sed) |
| valsartan | (val sar′ tan) |
| losartan | (loe sar′ tan) |
| Vancenase® | (van′ sen ase) |
| Vanceril® | (van′ ser il) |
| Vanceril® | (van′ ser il) |
| Vancenase® | (van′ sen ase) |
| vancomycin | (van koe mye′ sin) |
| vecuronium | (ve kyoo′ roe nee um) |
| Vantin® | (van′ tin) |
| Ventolin® | (ven′ tow lin) |
| Vasocidin® | (vay so sye′ din) |
| Vasodilan® | (vay so di′ lan) |
| Vasodilan® | (vay so di′ lan) |
| Vasocidin® | (vay so sye′ din) |
| Vasosulf® | (vay′ so sulf) |
| Velosef® | (vel′ oh sef) |
| vecuronium | (ve kyoo′ roe nee um) |
| vancomycin | (van koe mye′ sin) |
| Velosef® | (vel′ oh sef) |
| Vasosulf® | (vay′ so sulf) |
| Ventolin® | (ven′ tow lin) |
| Benylin® | (ben′ eh lin) |
| Ventolin® | (ven′ to lin) |
| phentolamine | (fen tole′ ah meen) |
| Ventolin® | (ven′ tow lin) |
| Vantin® | (van′ tin) |
| VePesid® | (veh′ pe sid) |
| Versed® | (ver′ sed) |
| verapamil | (ver ap′ a mil) |
| Verelan® | (ver′ e lan) |
| Verelan® | (ver′ e lan) |
| verapamil | (ver ap′ a mil) |
| Verelan® | (ver′ e lan) |
| Virilon® | (vir′ ih lon) |
| Verelan® | (ver′ e lan) |
| Vivarin® | (vye′ va rin) |
| Verelan® | (ver′ e lan) |
| Voltaren® | (vol tare′ en) |
| Versed® | (ver′ sed) |
| VePesid® | (veh′ pe sid) |
| Versed® | (ver′ sed) |
| Vistaril® | (vis′ tar ril) |
| Vexol® | (veks′ ole) |
| VoSol® | (voe′ sol) |
| Viagra® | (vye ag′ ra) |
| Allegra® | (al leg′ ra) |
| Vicodin® | (vye′ co din) |
| Hycodan® | (hye′ co dan) |
| Vicodin® | (vye′ co din) |
| Hycomine® | (hye′ co meen) |
| Vicodin® | (vye′ co din) |
| Uridon® | (yur′ ih don) |
| vidarabine | (vye dare′ ah been) |
| cytarabine | (sye tare′ ah been) |
| Videx® | (vye′ deks) |
| Lidex® | (lye′ deks) |
| vinblastine | (vin blas′ teen) |
| vincristine | (vin kris′ teen) |
| vincristine | (vin kris′ teen) |
| vinblastine | (vin blas′ teen) |
| Vioxx® | (vye′ oks) |
| Zyvox™ | (zye′ voks) |
| Viracept® | (vir′ uh sept) |
| Viramune® | (vir′ ah myune) |

| Drug Name | Pronunciation |
|---|---|
| Viramune® | (vir′ ah myune) |
| Viracept® | (vir′ uh sept) |
| Virilon® | (vir′ ih lon) |
| Verelan® | (ver′ e lan) |
| Viroptic® | (vir op′ tik) |
| Timoptic® | (tim op′ tik) |
| Visine® | (vye′ seen) |
| Visken® | (vis′ ken) |
| Visken® | (vis′ ken) |
| Visine® | (vye′ seen) |
| Vistaril® | (vis′ tar ril) |
| Restoril® | (res′ tor ril) |
| Vistaril® | (vis′ tar ril) |
| Versed® | (ver′ sed) |
| Vistaril® | (vis′ tar ril) |
| Zestril® | (zes′ tril) |
| Vivarin® | (vye′ va rin) |
| Verelan® | (ver′ e lan) |
| Volmax® | (vol′ maks) |
| Flomax® | (flo′ maks) |
| Voltaren® | (vol tare′ en) |
| tramadol | (tra′ ma dole) |
| Voltaren® | (vol tare′ en) |
| Ultram® | (uhl′ tram) |
| Voltaren® | (vol tare′ en) |
| Verelan® | (ver′ e lan) |
| VoSol® | (voe′ sol) |
| Vexol® | (veks′ ole) |
| Vytone® | (vye′ tone) |
| Hytone® | (hye′ tone) |
| Vytone® | (vye′ tone) |
| Zydone® | (zye′ doan) |
| Wellbutrin® | (well byu′ trin) |
| Wellcovorin® | (well coe vor′ in) |
| Wellbutrin® | (well byu′ trin) |
| Wellferon® | (well′ fer on) |
| Wellcovorin® | (well coe vor′ in) |
| Wellbutrin® | (well byu′ trin) |
| Wellcovorin® | (well coe vor′ in) |
| Wellferon® | (well′ fer on) |
| Wellferon® | (well′ fer on) |
| Wellbutrin® | (well byu′ trin) |
| Wellferon® | (well′ fer on) |
| Wellcovorin® | (well coe vor′ in) |
| Wyamine® | (wye′ ah meen) |
| Wydase® | (wye′ dase) |
| Wycillin® | (wye sil′ lin) |
| Bicillin® | (bye sil′ lin) |

| Drug Name | Pronunciation |
|---|---|
| Wydase® | (wye′ dase) |
| Lidex® | (lye′ deks) |
| Wydase® | (wye′ dase) |
| Wyamine® | (wye′ ah meen) |
| Wymox® | (wye′ moks) |
| Tylox® | (tye′ loks) |
| Xalatan® | (za la′ tan) |
| Zarontin® | (za ron′ tin) |
| Xanax® | (zan′ aks) |
| Lanoxin® | (lan oks′ in) |
| Xanax® | (zan′ aks) |
| Tenex® | (ten′ eks) |
| Xanax® | (zan′ aks) |
| Tylox® | (tye′ loks) |
| Xanax® | (zan′ aks) |
| Zantac® | (zan′ tak) |
| Xanax® | (zan′ aks) |
| Zyrtec® | (zir′ tec) |
| Xerac® | (zear′ ak) |
| Serax® | (sear′ aks) |
| Xylo-Pfan® | (zye′ lo fan) |
| Zyloprim® | (zye′ lo prim) |
| Yocon® | (yo′ con) |
| Zocor® | (zoe′ cor) |
| Zagam® | (za′ gam) |
| Zyban™ | (zye′ ban) |
| Zantac® | (zan′ tak) |
| Xanax® | (zan′ aks) |
| Zantac® | (zan′ tak) |
| Zarontin® | (za ron′ tin) |
| Zantac® | (zan′ tak) |
| Zofran® | (zoe′ fran) |
| Zantac® | (zan′ tak) |
| Zyrtec® | (zir′ tec) |
| Zarontin® | (za ron′ tin) |
| Xalatan® | (za la′ tan) |
| Zarontin® | (za ron′ tin) |
| Zantac® | (zan′ tak) |
| Zarontin® | (za ron′ tin) |
| Zaroxolyn® | (za roks′ oh lin) |
| Zaroxolyn® | (za roks′ oh lin) |
| Zarontin® | (za ron′ tin) |
| Zebeta® | (ze′ bay tah) |
| Diaβeta® | (dye ah bay′ tah) |
| Zemuron™ | (zeh′ mu ron) |
| Remeron® | (reh′ me ron) |
| Zerit® | (zer′ it) |
| Ziac™ | (zye′ ak) |

| Drug Name | Pronunciation |
|---|---|
| Zestril® | (zes' trill) |
| Desyrel® | (des' e rell) |
| Zestril® | (zes' trill) |
| Vistaril® | (vis' tar ril) |
| Ziac™ | (zye' ak) |
| Tiazac® | (tye' ah zak) |
| Ziac™ | (zye' ak) |
| Zerit® | (zer' it) |
| Zinacef® | (zin' ah sef) |
| Zithromax® | (zith' roe maks) |
| Zithromax® | (zith' roe maks) |
| Zinacef® | (zin' ah sef) |
| Zocor® | (zoe' cor) |
| Cozaar® | (koe' zar) |
| Zocor® | (zoe' cor) |
| Yocon® | (yo' con) |
| Zocor® | (zoe' cor) |
| Zoloft® | (zoe' loft) |
| Zofran® | (zoe' fran) |
| Zantac® | (zan' tak) |
| Zofran® | (zoe' fran) |
| Zosyn® | (zoe' sin) |
| Zoloft® | (zoe' loft) |
| Zocor® | (zoe' cor) |
| zolmitriptan | (zohl mi trip' tan) |
| sumatriptan | (soo ma trip' tan) |

| Drug Name | Pronunciation |
|---|---|
| Zonalon® | (zon' ah lon) |
| Zone-A Forte® | (zone' ah for' tay) |
| Zone-A Forte® | (zone' ah for' tay) |
| Zonalon® | (zon' ah lon) |
| Zosyn® | (zoe' sin) |
| Zofran® | (zoe' fran) |
| Zyban™ | (zye' ban) |
| Zagam® | (za' gam) |
| Zydone® | (zye' doan) |
| Vytone® | (vye' tone) |
| Zyloprim® | (zye' lo prim) |
| Xylo-Pfan® | (zye' lo fan) |
| Zyprexa® | (zye preks' a) |
| Celexa® | (se lex' a) |
| Zyprexa® | (zye preks' ah) |
| Zyrtec® | (zir' tec) |
| Zyrtec® | (zir' tec) |
| Serax® | (sear' aks) |
| Zyrtec® | (zir' tec) |
| Xanax® | (zan' aks) |
| Zyrtec® | (zir' tec) |
| Zantac® | (zan' tak) |
| Zyrtec® | (zir' tec) |
| Zyprexa® | (zye preks' ah) |
| Zyvox™ | (zye' voks) |
| Vioxx® | (vye' oks) |

# NEW DRUGS INTRODUCED OR APPROVED BY THE FDA IN 2001

| Brand Name | Generic Name | Use |
|---|---|---|
| ---- | argatroban | Prophylaxis or treatment of thrombocytopenia |
| Abreva™ | docosanol | Herpes simplex |
| Angiomax™ | bivalirudin | Anticoagulant |
| Axert™ | almotriptan | Migraine |
| BenzaClin™ | clindamycin and benzoyl peroxide | Acne vulgaris |
| Campath® | alemtuzumab | B-cell chronic lymphocytic leukemia |
| Cancidas® | caspofungin | *Aspergillus* infection |
| Gleevec™ | imatinib | Chronic myeloid leukemia (CML) |
| Lumigan™ | bimatoprost | Glaucoma |
| Lunelle™ | estradiol and medroxyprogesterone acetate | Prevention of pregnancy |
| Micardis® HCT | telmisartan and hydrochlorothiazide | Hypertension |
| Myobloc® | botulinum toxin type B | Cervical dystoni |
| Nexium™ | esomeprazole | Erosive esophagitis |
| PEG-Intron™ | peginterferon alfa-2b | Treatment of chronic hepatitis C |
| Pepcid® Complete | famotidine, calcium carbonate, and magnesium hydroxide | Heartburn |
| Protonix® | pantoprazole | Proton pump inhibitor |
| Reminyl® | galantamine | Alzheimer's disease |
| Starlix® | nateglinide | Management of type 2 diabetes mellitus |
| TriHIBit® | diphtheria, tetanus toxoids, and acellular pertussis vaccine and haemophilus B conjugate vaccine | Prevention of diphtheria, tetanus, pertussis, and invasive disease caused by *H. influenzae* type b |
| Trizivir® | abacavir, lamivudine, and zidovudine | Treatment of HIV infection |
| Twinrix® | hepatitis A inactivated and hepatitis B (recombinant) vaccine | Active immunization against disease caused by hepatitis A virus and hepatitis B virus |
| Venofer® | iron sucrose | Iron-deficiency anemia |
| Yasmin® | ethinyl estradiol and drospirenone | Prevention of pregnancy |
| Zyrtec-D 12 Hour™ | cetirizine and pseudoephedrine | Treatment of symptoms of seasonal or perennial allergic rhinitis |

# PENDING DRUGS OR DRUGS IN CLINICAL TRIALS

| Proposed Brand Name | Generic Name | Use |
|---|---|---|
| Alredase® | tolrestat | Aldose reductase inhibitor |
| Amdray® | valspodar | P-glycoprotein inhibitor |
| Amsidyl® | amsacrine | Acute leukemia |
| Aptosyn® | exisulind | Antineoplastic |
| Aranesp® | darbepoetin | Hematopoietic agent |
| Arixtra® | fondaparinex | Anticoagulant |
| Arkin-Z® | vesnarinone | Congestive heart failure agent |
| Berotec® | fenoterol | $Beta_2$ agonist |
| Catatrol® | viloxazine | Bicyclic antidepressant |
| Cipralan® | cifenline succinate | Antiarrhythmic agent |
| Cytolex® | pexiganan | Diabetic foot ulcers |
| Decabid® | indecainide hydrochloride | Antiarrhythmic agent |
| Delaprem® | hexoprenaline sulfate | Tocolytic agent |
| Dirame® | propiram | Opioid analgesic |
| Eldisine® | vindesine | Antineoplastic |
| Eloxatin® | oxaliplatin | Treatment of colorectal cancer |
| Enable® | tenidap sodium | Arthritis |
| Freedox® | tirilazad | Antioxidant |
| Frisium® | clobazam | Benzodiazepine |
| Gastrozepine® | pirenzepine | Antiulcer drug |
| Isoprinosine® | inosiplex | Immunomodulating drug |
| Lacipil® | lacidipine | Hypertension |
| Maxicam® | isoxicam | NSAID |
| Mentane® | velnacrine | Alzheimer's disease agent |
| Micturin® | terodiline hydrochloride | Agent for urinary incontinence |
| Mogadon® | nitrazepam | Benzodiazepine |
| Motilium® | domperidone | Antiemetic |
| Napa® | acecainide | Antiarrhythmic agent |
| Natrecor® | nesiritide | Congestive heart failure |
| Orzel® | tegafur and uracil | Treatment of metastatic colorectal cancer |
| Pindac® | pinacidil | Antihypertensive |
| Prothiaden® | dothiepin hydrochloride | Tricyclic antidepressant |
| Rimadyl® | carprofen | NSAID |
| Roxiam® | remoxipride | Antipsychotic agent |
| Roxin® | roxatidine | Peptic ulcers |
| Selecor® | celiprolol | Hypertension and angina |
| Serlect® | sertindole | Antipsychotic agent |
| Simdax® | levosimendan | Treatment of heart failure |
| SNX-111 | ziconotide | Non-narcotic analgesic |
| Spexil® | trospectomycin | Antibiotic |
| Stemgen® | ancestim | Growth factor |
| Symlin® | pramlintide | Diabetes |
| Targocoid® | teicoplanin | Antibiotic, similar to vancomycin |
| Therafectin® | amiprilose hydrochloride | Synthetic carbohydrate |
| Unicard® | dilevalol | Hypertension |
| Vestra® | reboxetine | Antidepressant |
| Xigris® | drotrecogin | Recombinant human activated protein C |
| Xolair® | omalizumab | Monoclonal antibody |
| Xyvion® | tibolone | Synthetic steroid |
| Zeldox® | ziprasidone | Treatment of schizophrenia |
| Zelmac® | tegaserod | Treatment of irritable bowel syndrome |

# DRUG PRODUCTS NO LONGER AVAILABLE (U.S.)

| Brand Name | Generic Name |
|---|---|
| Absorbine® Antifungal | tolnaftate |
| Absorbine® Jock Itch | tolnaftate |
| Absorbine Jr® Antifungal | tolnaftate |
| Achromycin® Parenteral | tetracycline |
| Achromycin® V Capsule | tetracycline |
| Achromycin® V Oral Suspension | tetracycline |
| Actagen-C® | triprolidine, pseudoephedrine, and codeine |
| Actagen® Syrup | triprolidine and pseudoephedrine |
| Actagen® Tablet | triprolidine and pseudoephedrine |
| ACTH-40® | corticotropin |
| Actidil® | triprolidine |
| Actifed® Syrup | triprolidine and pseudoephedrine |
| Actifed® With Codeine | triprolidine, pseudoephedrine, and codeine |
| Actinex® | masoprocol |
| Acutrim® 16 Hours | phenylpropanolamine |
| Acutrim® Late Day | phenylpropanolamine |
| Acutrim® II, Maximum Strength | phenylpropanolamine |
| Adalat® | nifedipine |
| Adipost® | phendimetrazine tartrate |
| Adphen® | phendimetrazine tartrate |
| Adrin® | nylidrin hydrochloride |
| Adsorbocarpine® Ophthalmic | pilocarpine |
| Aeroaid® | thimerosal |
| Aerodine® | povidone-iodine |
| Aerolate® Oral Solution | theophylline |
| Aerosporin® Injection | polymyxin B |
| Agoral® Plain | mineral oil |
| Ak-Chlor® Ophthalmic | chloramphenicol |
| Ak-Homatropine® Ophthalmic | homatropine |
| Akoline® C.B. Tablet | vitamin |
| AK-Zol® | acetazolamide |
| Ala-Tet® | tetracycline |
| Alazide® | hydrochlorothiazide and spironolactone |
| Aldoclor® | chlorothiazide and methyldopa |
| Allercon® Tablet | triprolidine and pseudoephedrine |
| Allerest® 12 Hour Capsule | chlorpheniramine and phenylpropanolamine |
| Allerfrin® Syrup | triprolidine and pseudoephedrine |
| Allerfrin® Tablet | triprolidine and pseudoephedrine |
| Allerfrin® w/Codeine | triprolidine, pseudoephedrine, and codeine |
| Alor® 5/500 | hydrocodone and aspirin |
| Amen® | medroxyprogesterone acetate |
| Amin-Aid® | amino acid |
| Ami-Tex LA® | guaifenesin and phenylpropanolamine |
| Amonidrin® Tablet | guaifenesin |
| AMO Vitrax® | sodium hyaluronate |
| Amvisc® | sodium hyaluronate |
| Amvisc® Plus | sodium hyaluronate |
| Anabolin® | nandrolone |
| Anacin-3® (all products) | acetaminophen |
| Anaids® Tablet | alginic acid and sodium bicarbonate |
| Anatuss® | guaifenesin, phenylpropanolamine, and dextromethorphan |
| Androlone® | nandrolone |
| Androlone®-D | nandrolone |
| Anergan® 25 Injection | promethazine hydrochloride |
| Antagon™ | ganirelix |

*(continued)*

| Brand Name | Generic Name |
|---|---|
| Antiben® | antipyrine and benzocaine |
| Antihist-1® | clemastine |
| Antihist-D® | clemastine and phenylpropanolamine |
| Antilirium® | physostigmine |
| Antiminth® | pyrantel pamoate |
| Antinea® Cream | benzoic acid and salicylic acid |
| Antivert® Chewable Tablet | meclizine hydrochloride |
| Antrocol® Capsule & Tablet | atropine and belladonna |
| Anxanil® Oral | hydroxyzine |
| ---- | apomorphine (now available as an orphan drug only) |
| Apresazide® | hydralazine and hydrochlorothiazide |
| Aquaphyllin® | theophylline |
| Aralen® Phosphate With Primaquine Phosphate | chloroquine phosphate and primaquine phosphate |
| Arcotinic® Tablet | iron and liver combination |
| Argyrol® S.S. | silver protein, mild |
| Arlidin® | nylidrin (all products) |
| A.R.M® Caplet | chlorpheniramine and phenylpropanolamine |
| Arm-a-Med® Isoetharine | isoetharine |
| Arm-a-Med® Isoproterenol | isoproterenol |
| Arm-a-Med® Metaproterenol | metaproterenol sulfate |
| Arrestin® | trimethobenzamide |
| Artha-G® | salsalate |
| Arthritis Foundation® Ibuprofen | ibuprofen |
| Arthritis Foundation® Nighttime | acetaminophen and diphenhydramine |
| Arthritis Foundation® Pain Reliever, Aspirin Free | acetaminophen |
| Arthritis Strength Bufferin® | aspirin (buffered) |
| Articulose-50® Injection | prednisolone |
| Asbron-G® Elixir | theophylline and guaifenesin |
| Asbron-G® Tablet | theophylline and guaifenesin |
| Asmalix® | theophylline |
| Asproject® | sodium thiosalicylate |
| Atabrine® Tablet | quinacrine hydrochloride |
| Atozine® Oral | hydroxyzine |
| Atrohist® Plus | chlorpheniramine, phenylephrine, phenylpropanolamine, and belladonna alkaloids |
| ---- | atropine soluble tablet |
| Aureomycin® | chlortetracycline |
| Avlosulfon® | dapsone |
| Axotal® | butalbital compound and aspirin |
| Azdone® | hydrocodone and aspirin |
| Azlin® Injection | azlocillin |
| Azo Gantanol® | sulfamethoxazole and phenazopyridine |
| Azo Gantrisin® | sulfisoxazole and phenazopyridine |
| Azulfidine® Suspension | sulfasalazine |
| B-A-C® | butalbital compound with aspirin |
| Bactocill® | oxacillin |
| Bancap® | butalbital compound with acetaminophen |
| Banesin® | acetaminophen |
| Banthine® | methantheline |
| Bantron® | lobeline (all products) |
| Barbita® | phenobarbital |
| Baycol® | cerivastatin |
| Baypress® | nitrendipine |
| Becomject-100® | vitamin B complex |
| Beepen-VK® | penicillin V potassium |
| Beesix® | pyridoxine hydrochloride |

*(continued)*

| Brand Name | Generic Name |
|---|---|
| Bellafoline® | levorotatory alkaloids of belladonna (all products) |
| Bemote® | dicyclomine |
| Bena-D® | diphenhydramine |
| Benadryl® 50 mg Capsule | diphenhydramine hydrochloride |
| Benadryl® Cold/Flu | acetaminophen, diphenhydramine, and pseudoephedrine |
| Benahist® Injection | diphenhydramine hydrochloride |
| Benoject® | diphenhydramine hydrochloride |
| Beta-2® | isoetharine |
| Betachron® | propranolol |
| Betalin® S | thiamine |
| Betapen-VK® | penicillin V potassium |
| Beta-Val® Ointment | betamethasone |
| Betoptic® | betaxolol |
| Bexophene® | propoxyphene and aspirin |
| Biamine® Injection | thiamine hydrochloride |
| Bilezyme® Tablet | pancrelipase |
| Biodine® | povidone-iodine |
| Biomox® | amoxicillin |
| Biozyme-C® | collagenase |
| Biphetamine® | amphetamine and dextroamphetamine |
| Blanex® Capsule | chlorzoxazone and acetaminophen |
| Brethaire® | terbutaline |
| Bretylol® | bretylium |
| Bricanyl® | terbutaline |
| Bromaline® Elixir | brompheniramine and phenylpropanolamine |
| Bromanate® DC | brompheniramine, phenylpropanolamine, and codeine |
| Bromanate® Elixir | brompheniramine and phenylpropanolamine |
| Bromatapp® | brompheniramine and phenylpropanolamine |
| Bromphen® DC With Codeine | brompheniramine, phenylpropanolamine, and codeine |
| Bromphen® Tablet | brompheniramine and phenylpropanolamine |
| Bronchial® | theophylline and guaifenesin |
| Bronkephrine® | ethylnorepinephrine hydrochloride |
| Bronkometer® | isoetharine |
| Bronkosol® | isoetharine |
| Bucladin®-S Softab® | buclizine |
| Buffered®, Tri-buffered | aspirin |
| Bufferin® Arthritis Strength | aspirin |
| Bufferin® Extra Strength | aspirin |
| Buf-Puf® Acne Cleansing Bar | salicylic acid |
| Butace® | butalbital compound |
| Caladryl® Spray | diphenhydramine and calamine |
| Calcimar® | calcitonin |
| Calciparine® Injection | heparin calcium |
| Camalox® Suspension & Tablet | aluminum hydroxide, calcium carbonate, and magnesium hydroxide |
| Cantharone® | cantharidin |
| Cantharone Plus® | cantharidin |
| Cardem® | celiprolol |
| Cardilate® | erythrityl tetranitrate |
| Cardio-Green® | indocyanine green |
| Caroid® | cascara sagrada and phenolphthalein |
| Catarase® 1:5000 | chymotrypsin (all products) |
| Cedilanid-D® Injection | deslanoside |
| Celectol® | celiprolol |
| Cenocort® A-40 | triamcinolone |
| Cenocort® Forte | triamcinolone |
| Centrax® Capsule & Tablet | prazepam |
| Cerespan® | papaverine hydrochloride |

*(continued)*

| Brand Name | Generic Name |
|---|---|
| Cesamet® | nabilone |
| Cetane® | ascorbic acid |
| Chenix® Tablet | chenodiol |
| Chlorgest-HD® Elixir | chlorpheniramine, phenylephrine, and hydrocodone |
| Chlorofon-A® Tablet | chlorzoxazone |
| Chloromycetin® Cream | chloramphenicol |
| Chloromycetin® Kapseals® | chloramphenicol |
| Chloromycetin® Ophthalmic | chloramphenicol |
| Chloromycetin® Otic | chloramphenicol |
| Chloromycetin® Palmitate Oral Suspension | chloramphenicol |
| Chloroserpine® | reserpine and hydrochlorothiazide |
| Chlor-Rest® Tablet | chlorpheniramine and phenylpropanolamine |
| Chlortab® | chlorpheniramine maleate |
| Choledyl® | oxtriphylline |
| Choloxin® | dextrothyroxine |
| Chymex® | bentiromide (all products) |
| Cibacalcin® | calcitonin |
| Cithalith-S® Syrup | lithium citrate |
| Citro-Nesia™ Solution | magnesium citrate |
| Clindex® | clidinium and chlordiazepoxide |
| Clistin® Tablet | carbinoxamine maleate |
| Clopra® | metoclopramine |
| Clorpactin® XCB Powder | oxychlorosene sodium |
| Cloxapen® | cloxacillin |
| Cobalasine® Injection | adenosine phosphate |
| Codamine® | hydrocodone and phenylpropanolamine |
| Codamine® Pediatric | hydrocodone and phenylpropanolamine |
| Codimal-A® Injection | brompheniramine maleate |
| Codimal® Expectorant | guaifenesin and phenylpropanolamine |
| Coldlac-LA® | guaifenesin and phenylpropanolamine |
| Coldloc® | guaifenesin, phenylpropanolamine, and phenylephrine |
| Cold & Allergy® Elixir | brompheniramine and phenylpropanolamine |
| Coly-Mycin® S Oral | colistin sulfate |
| Conex® | guaifenesin and phenylpropanolamine |
| Congestant D® | chlorpheniramine, phenylpropanolamine, and acetaminophen |
| Constant-T® Tablet | theophylline |
| Control® | phenylpropanolamine |
| Control-L® | pyrethrins |
| Contuss® | guaifenesin, phenylpropanolamine, and phenylephrine |
| Contuss® XT | guaifenesin and phenylpropanolamine |
| Corgonject® | chorionic gonadotropin |
| Corliprol® | celiprolol |
| Cortaid® Ointment | hydrocortisone |
| Cortone® Acetate | cortisone acetate |
| Cotrim® | co-trimoxazole |
| Cotrim® DS | co-trimoxazole |
| Cortrophin-Zinc® | corticotropin |
| Crysticillin® 300 A.S. | penicillin G procaine |
| Crysticillin® 600 A.S. | penicillin G procaine |
| Crystodigin® | digitoxin |
| Cyclospasmol® | cyclandelate (all products) |
| Cycrin® 10 mg Tablet | medroxyprogesterone acetate |
| Dalgan® | dezocine |
| D-Amp® | ampicillin |
| Danex® Shampoo | pyrithione zinc |
| Dapacin® Cold Capsule | chlorpheniramine, phenylpropanolamine, and acetaminophen |

*(continued)*

| Brand Name | Generic Name |
|---|---|
| Darbid® Tablet | isopropamide iodide (all products) |
| Daricon® | oxyphencyclimine (all products) |
| Darvon® 32 mg Capsule | propoxyphene hydrochloride |
| Darvon-N® Oral Suspension | propoxyphene napsylate |
| Datril® Extra Strength | acetaminophen |
| Dayto Himbin® | yohimbine |
| Decadron® Phosphate Ophthalmic Ointment | dexamethasone |
| Decadron® 0.25 mg & 6 mg Tablets | dexamethasone |
| Decaspray® | dexamethasone |
| Decholin® | dehydrocholic acid |
| Dehist® | brompheniramine maleate |
| Deltalin® Capsule | ergocalciferol |
| Demazin® Syrup | chlorpheniramine and phenylpropanolamine |
| Depo-Provera® 100 mg/mL | medroxyprogesterone |
| Deprol® | meprobamate and benactyzine hydrochloride |
| Dermoxyl® Gel | benzoyl peroxide |
| Despec® Liquid | guaifenesin, phenylpropanolamine, and phenylephrine |
| Dexacen-4® | dexamethasone |
| Dexacen® LA-8 | dexamethasone |
| Dexatrim® Pre-Meal | phenylpropanolamine |
| Dexchlor® | dexchlorpheniramine |
| Dexedrine® Elixir | dextroamphetamine sulfate |
| Dey-Dose® Isoproterenol | isoproterenol |
| Dey-Dose® Metaproterenol | metaproterenol sulfate |
| Dey-Lute® Isoetharine | isoetharine |
| Dialose® Capsule | docusate sodium |
| Diaparene® Cradol® | methylbenzethonium |
| Diapid® Nasal Spray | lypressin |
| Diar-aid® | loperamide |
| Dilantin-30® Pediatric Suspension | phenytoin |
| Dilantin® With Phenobarbital | phenytoin with phenobarbital |
| Dilaudid® 1 mg & 3 mg Tablet | hydromorphone hydrochloride |
| Dimaphen® Elixir | brompheniramine and phenylpropanolamine |
| Dimaphen® Tablets | brompheniramine and phenylpropanolamine |
| Dimetane® | brompheniramine maleate |
| Dimetane®-DC | brompheniramine, phenylpropanolamine, and codeine |
| Dimetapp® 4-Hour Liqui-Gel Capsule | brompheniramine and phenylpropanolamine |
| Dimetapp® Elixir | brompheniramine and phenylpropanolamine |
| Dimetapp® Extentabs® | brompheniramine and phenylpropanolamine |
| Dimetapp® Tablet | brompheniramine and phenylpropanolamine |
| Diphenylan Sodium® | phenytoin |
| Dispos-a-Med® Isoproterenol | isoproterenol |
| Dital® | phendimetrazine |
| Diupress® | chlorothiazide and reserpine |
| Diurigen® | chlorothiazide |
| Dizymes® Tablet | pancreatin |
| Dolene® | propoxyphene |
| Dolorac™ | capsaicin |
| Dommanate® Injection | dimenhydrinate |
| Donphen® Tablet | hyoscyamine, atropine, scopolamine, and phenobarbital |
| Dopar® | levodopa |
| Dopastat® Injection | dopamine hydrochloride |
| Doriden® Tablet | glutethimide |
| Doxinate® Capsule | docusate sodium |

*(continued)*

| Brand Name | Generic Name |
|---|---|
| Dramamine® Injection | dimenhydrinate |
| Dramocen® | dimenhydrinate |
| Dramoject® | dimenhydramine |
| D-S-S Plus® | docusate and casanthranol |
| Duadacin® Capsule | chlorpheniramine, phenylpropanolamine, and acetaminophen |
| Duo-Medihaler® | isoproterenol and phenylephrine |
| Duotrate® | pentaerythritol tetranitrate |
| Duracid® | aluminum hydroxide, magnesium carbonate, and calcium carbonate |
| Duract® | bromfenac (all products) |
| Dura-Gest® | guaifenesin, phenylpropanolamine, and phenylephrine |
| Dura-Vent® | guaifenesin and phenylpropanolamine |
| Durrax® Oral | hydroxyzine |
| Duvoid® | bethanechol |
| Dycill® | dicloxacillin |
| Dyflex-400® Tablet | dyphylline |
| Efodine® | povidone-iodine |
| Elase®-Chloromycetin® Ointment | fibrinolysin and desoxyribonuclease |
| Eldepryl® Tablet (only) | selegiline |
| Eldoquin® Lotion | hydroquinone |
| Elixomin® | theophylline |
| Elixophyllin SR® | theophylline |
| E-Lor® Tablet | propoxyphene and acetaminophen |
| Emete-Con® Injection | benzquinamide |
| ---- | emetine hydrochloride |
| Emitrip® | amitriptyline |
| Endep® 25 mg, 50 mg, 100 mg | amitriptyline hydrochloride |
| Enduron® 2.5 mg Tablet | methyclothiazide |
| Enkaid® | encainide |
| Enomine® | guaifenesin, phenylpropanolamine, and phenylephrine |
| Enovid® | mestranol and norethynodrel |
| Enovil® | amitriptyline |
| E.N.T.® | brompheniramine and phenylpropanolamine |
| Entex® | guaifenesin, phenylpropanolamine, and phenylephrine |
| Entex® LA | guaifenesin and phenylpropanolamine |
| Entozyme® | pancreatin |
| E.P. Mycin® Capsule | oxytetracycline |
| Ercaf® | ergotamine |
| Ergostat® | ergotamine |
| Eridium® | phenazopyridine hydrochloride |
| Ery-Sol® Topical Solution | erythromycin, topical |
| Esidrix® 100 mg Tablet | hydrochlorothiazide |
| Estradurin® Injection | polyestradiol phosphate |
| Estroject-2® Injection | estradiol |
| Estroject-L.A.® Injection | estradiol |
| Estronol® Injection | estrone |
| Estrovis® | quinestrol |
| Ethaquin® | ethaverine hydrochloride |
| Ethatab® | ethaverine hydrochloride |
| Euthroid® Tablet | liotrix |
| Eutron® | methyclothiazide and pargyline |
| Evac-Q-Mag® | magnesium citrate |
| Exna® | benzthiazide |
| Fastin® | phentermine |
| FemCare® | clotrimazole |
| Femguard® | sulfabenzamide, sulfacetamide, and sulfathiazole |
| Femstat® | butoconazole nitrate |

*(continued)*

| Brand Name | Generic Name |
|---|---|
| Fergon Plus® | iron with vitamin B |
| Fer-In-Sol® Capsule | ferrous sulfate |
| Fermalox® | ferrous sulfate, magnesium hydroxide, and docusate |
| Ferndex | dextroamphetamine sulfate |
| Fiorital® | butalbital compound and aspirin |
| Flaxedil® | gallamine triethiodide |
| Flexaphen® | chlorzoxazone |
| Flonase® 9 g | fluticasone |
| Floropryl® Ophthalmic | isoflurophate |
| Fluonid® Topical | fluocinolone |
| Fluothane® | halothane |
| Flurosyn® Topical | fluocinolone |
| Folex® Injection | methotrexate |
| Folex® PFS™ | methotrexate |
| Follutein® | chorionic gonadotropin |
| Formula Q® | quinine |
| FS Shampoo® Topical | fluocinolone |
| Furalan® | nitrofurantoin |
| Furamide® | diloxanide furoate |
| Furan® | nitrofurantoin |
| Furanite® | nitrofurantoin |
| Gamastan® | immune globulin, intramuscular |
| Gammagard® Injection | immune globulin, intravenous |
| Gammar® | immune globulin, intramuscular |
| Gamulin® Rh | $Rh_o$(D) immune globulin (intramuscular) |
| Gantanol® | sulfamethoxazole |
| Gantrisin® Ophthalmic | sulfisoxazole |
| Gantrisin® Tablet | sulfisoxazole |
| Gelusil® Liquid | aluminum hydroxide, magnesium hydroxide, and simethicone |
| Genabid® | papaverine hydrochloride |
| Genagesic® | guaifenesin and phenylpropanolamine |
| Genamin® Cold Syrup | chlorpheniramine and phenylpropanolamine |
| Genamin® Expectorant | guaifenesin and phenylpropanolamine |
| Genatap® Elixir | brompheniramine and phenylpropanolamine |
| Gen-D-phen® | diphenhydramine hydrochloride |
| Geridium® | phenazopyridine |
| GG-Cen® | guaifenesin |
| Glukor® | chorionic gonadotropin |
| Glycerol-T® | theophylline and guaifenesin |
| G-myticin® | gentamicin |
| Gonic® | chorionic gonadotropin |
| Grisactin® Ultra | griseofulvin |
| Guaifenex® | guaifenesin, phenylpropanolamine, and phenylephrine |
| Guaifenex® PPA 75 | guaifenesin and phenylpropanolamine |
| Guaipax® | guaifenesin and phenylpropanolamine |
| Guiatex® | guaifenesin, phenylpropanolamine, and phenylephrine |
| Guiatuss CF® | guaifenesin, phenylpropanolamine, and dextromethorphan |
| G-well® | lindane |
| Gyne-Sulf® | sulfabenzamide, sulfacetamide, and sulfathiazole |
| Gynogen® Injection | estradiol |
| ---- | halazone tablet |
| Haldrone® | paramethasone acetate |
| Halenol® Tablet | acetaminophen |
| Halotex® | haloprogin |
| Harmonyl® | deserpidine |
| H-BIG® | hepatitis B immune globulin |
| Healon® | sodium hyaluronate |

*(continued)*

| Brand Name | Generic Name |
|---|---|
| Healon® GV | sodium hyaluronate |
| HemFe® | iron with vitamins |
| Hep-B-Gammagee® | hepatitis B immune globulin |
| Herplex® | idoxuridine |
| Hetrazan® | diethylcarbamazine citrate |
| Hismanal® | astemizole |
| Histaject® | brompheniramine maleate |
| Histalet Forte® Tablet | chlorpheniramine, pyrilamine, phenylephrine, and phenylpropanolamine |
| Hista-Vadrin® Tablet | chlorpheniramine, phenylephrine, and phenylpropanolamine |
| Hycomine® | hydrocodone and phenylpropanolamine |
| Hycomine® Pediatric | hydrocodone and phenylpropanolamine |
| Hydeltra-T.B.A.® | prednisolone |
| Hydramine® | diphenhydramine hydrochloride |
| Hydrobexan® Injection | hydroxocobalamin |
| Hydro Cobex® | hydroxocobalamin |
| Hydrocodone PA® Syrup | hydrocodone and phenylpropanolamine |
| Hydro-Crysti-12® | hydroxocobalamin |
| Hydromox® | quinethazone |
| Hydro-Par® | hydrochlorothiazide |
| Hydrophed® | theophylline, ephedrine, and hydroxyzine |
| Hydropres® 25 mg Tablet | hydrochlorothiazide and reserpine |
| Hydroxacen® | hydroxyzine |
| Hygroton® | chlorthalidone |
| Hy-Pam® Oral | hydroxyzine |
| Hyperab® | rabies immune globulin (human) |
| Hyper-Tet® | tetanus immune globulin (human) |
| HypRho®-D | $Rh_o$(D) immune globulin (intramuscular) |
| HypRho®-D Mini-Dose | $Rh_o$(D) immune globulin (intramuscular) |
| Hyprogest® 250 | hydroxyprogesterone caproate |
| Ilopan-Choline® Oral | dexpanthenol |
| Ilopan® Injection | dexpanthenol |
| Inocor® | inamrinone (amrinone) |
| Intal® Inhalation Capsule | cromolyn sodium |
| Intercept™ | nonoxynol 9 |
| Intropin® | dopamine |
| Iodo-Niacin® Tablet | potassium iodide and niacinamide hydroiodide |
| Iophen® | iodinated glycerol |
| Iophen-C® | iodinated glycerol and codeine |
| Iophen-DM® | iodinated glycerol and dextromethorphan (all products) |
| Iophylline® | iodinated glycerol and theophylline |
| Iotuss® | iodinated glycerol and codeine |
| Iotuss-DM® | iodinated glycerol and dextromethorphan (all products) |
| I-Picamide® | tropicamide |
| Ismotic® | isosorbide |
| Iso-Bid® | isosorbide dinitrate |
| Isopto® Eserine | physostigmine |
| Isopto® P-ES | pilocarpine and physostigmine |
| Isovex® | ethaverine hydrochloride |
| Isuprel® Glossets® | isoproterenol |
| Janimine® | imipramine |
| Jenamicin® | gentamicin |
| Kalcinate® | calcium gluconate |
| Kaochlor-Eff® | potassium bicarbonate, potassium chloride, and potassium citrate |
| Kaopectate® Children's Tablet | attapulgite |
| Kaopectate® II | loperamide |
| Kato® Powder | potassium chloride |
| Keflin® | cephalothin sodium |

*(continued)*

| Brand Name | Generic Name |
|---|---|
| Kestrin® Injection | estrone |
| Koate®-HS Injection | antihemophilic factor (human) |
| Koate®-HT Injection | antihemophilic factor (human) |
| Kolyum® Powder | potassium chloride and potassium gluconate |
| Konakion® Injection | phytonadione |
| Kondon's Nasal® | ephedrine |
| Konyne-HT® Injection | factor IX complex (human) |
| Kwell® | lindane |
| LA-12® | hydroxocobalamin |
| Lamprene® 100 mg | clofazimine |
| Laniazid® Tablet | isoniazid |
| Lanorinal® | butalbital compound and aspirin |
| Largon® | propiomazine |
| Lasan™ HP-1 Topical | anthralin |
| Lasan™ Topical | anthralin |
| Ledercillin VK® | penicillin V potassium |
| Libritabs® (all products) | chlordiazepoxide |
| Liquaemin® | heparin |
| Liquid Pred® | prednisone |
| Listerex® Scrub | salicylic acid |
| Lithane® | lithium |
| Lithonate® | lithium |
| Lithotabs® | lithium |
| Logen® | diphenoxylate and atropine |
| Lomanate® | diphenoxylate and atropine |
| Lorcet® | hydrocodone and acetaminophen |
| Lorelco® | probucol |
| Lotronex® | alosetron |
| Malatal® | hyoscyamine, atropine, scopolamine, and phenobarbital |
| Mallisol® | povidone-iodine |
| Malotuss® Syrup | guaifenesin |
| Mantadil® Cream | chlorcyclizine |
| Maolate® | chlorphenesin |
| Marax® | theophylline, ephedrine, and hydroxyzine |
| Marezine® Injection | cyclizine hydrochloride |
| Marthritic® | salsalate |
| Max-Caro® | beta-carotene |
| Maximum Strength Dex-A-Diet® | phenylpropanolamine |
| Maximum Strength Dexatrim® | phenylpropanolamine |
| Maxolon® | metoclopramide |
| Mazanor® | mazindol |
| Meclan® Topical | meclocycline |
| Meclomen® | meclofenamate sodium |
| Medihaler-Epi® | epinephrine |
| Medihaler Ergotamine® | ergotamine |
| Medihaler-Iso® | isoproterenol |
| Medrapred® | prednisolone and atropine |
| Medrol® Acetate Topical | methylprednisolone |
| Melfiat® Tablet | phendimetrazine tartrate |
| Mellaril-S® | thioridazine |
| Meprospan® | meprobamate |
| Mesantoin® | mephenytoin |
| Metahydrin® | trichlormethiazide |
| Metaprel® Aerosol | metaproterenol sulfate |
| Metaprel® Inhalation Solution | metaproterenol sulfate |
| Metaprel® Syrup | metaproterenol sulfate |

*(continued)*

| Brand Name | Generic Name |
|---|---|
| Metaprel® Tablet | metaproterenol sulfate |
| Metizol® Tablet | metronidazole |
| Metra® | phendimetrazine tartrate |
| Metubine® Iodide | metocurine iodide |
| Miflex® Tablet | chlorzoxazone and acetaminophen |
| Milkinol® | mineral oil |
| Milontin® | phensuximide |
| Milophene® | clomiphene |
| Milprem® | meprobamate and conjugated estrogens |
| Mini-Gamulin® Rh | $Rh_0$(D) immune globulin (intramuscular) |
| Minocin® Tablet | minocycline |
| Miochol® | acetylcholine |
| Mitran® Oral | chlordiazepoxide |
| Moisturel® Lotion | dimethicone |
| Monocete® Topical Liquid | monochloroacetic acid |
| Moxam® Injection | moxalactam |
| Mus-Lax® | chlorzoxazone |
| Myconel® Topical | nystatin and triamcinolone |
| Mylaxen® Injection | hexafluorenium bromide |
| Myminic® Expectorant | guaifenesin and phenylpropanolamine |
| Myochrysine® | gold sodium thiomalate |
| Myotonachol™ | bethanechol |
| Myphetane DC® | brompheniramine, phenylpropanolamine, and codeine |
| Nafcil™ | nafcillin |
| Naldecon® | chlorpheniramine, phenyltoloxamine, phenylpropanolamine, and phenylephrine |
| Naldecon® DX Adult Liquid | guaifenesin, phenylpropanolamine, and dextromethorphan |
| Naldecon-EX® Children's Syrup | guaifenesin and phenylpropanolamine |
| Naldelate® | chlorpheniramine, phenyltoloxamine, phenylpropanolamine, and phenylephrine |
| Nalgest® | chlorpheniramine, phenyltoloxamine, phenylpropanolamine, and phenylephrine |
| Nalspan® | chlorpheniramine, phenyltoloxamine, phenylpropanolamine, and phenylephrine |
| Nandrobolic® Injection | nandrolone phenpropionate |
| Navane® Concentrate & Injection | thiothixene |
| N-B-P® Ointment | bacitracin, neomycin, and polymyxin B |
| Neo-Castaderm® | resorcinol, boric acid, acetone |
| Neo-Cortef® Ophthalmic | neomycin and hydrocortisone |
| Neo-Cortef® Topical | neomycin and hydrocortisone |
| NeoDecadron® Topical | neomycin and dexamethasone |
| Neo-Durabolic® | nandrolone |
| Neo-Medrol® Acetate Topical | methylprednisolone and neomycin |
| Neoquess® Injection | dicyclomine hydrochloride |
| Neoquess® Tablet | hyoscyamine sulfate |
| Neo-Synalar® Topical | neomycin and fluocinolone |
| Nestrex® | pyridoxine |
| Netromycin® | netilmicin |
| Neucalm-50® Injection | hydroxyzine |
| Neuramate® | meprobamate |
| Neutra-Phos® Capsule | potassium phosphate and sodium phosphate |
| New Decongestant® | chlorpheniramine, phenyltoloxamine, phenylpropanolamine, and phenylephrine |
| Niac® | niacin |
| Niacels™ | niacin |
| Niclocide® | niclosamide |
| Nidryl® | diphenhydramine hydrochloride |

(continued)

| Brand Name | Generic Name |
|---|---|
| Niferex Forte® | iron with vitamins |
| Niloric® | ergoloid mesylates |
| Nipride® Injection | nitroprusside sodium |
| Nisaval® | pyrilamine maleate |
| Nitro-Bid® Oral | nitroglycerin |
| Nitrocine® Oral | nitroglycerin |
| Nitrodisc® Patch | nitroglycerin |
| Nitrostat® 0.15 mg Tablet | nitroglycerin |
| Noctec® | chloral hydrate |
| Nolamine® | chlorpheniramine, phenindamine, and phenylpropanolamine |
| Nolex® LA | guaifenesin and phenylpropanolamine |
| Noludar® | methyprylon |
| No Pain-HP® | capsaicin |
| Norlutate® | norethindrone |
| Norlutin® | norethindrone |
| Normiflo® | ardeparin |
| Norzine® | thiethylperazine |
| Novafed® | pseudoephedrine |
| Novahistine DMX® Liquid | guaifenesin, pseudoephedrine, and dextromethorphan |
| Novahistine® Elixir | chlorpheniramine and phenylephrine |
| Novahistine® Expectorant | guaifenesin, pseudoephedrine, and codeine |
| Nursoy® | enteral nutritional therapy |
| Octamide® | metoclopramide |
| Octocaine® | lidocaine and epinephrine |
| OmniHIB™ | *Haemophilus* B conjugate vaccine |
| Omnipen® | ampicillin |
| Omnipen®-N | ampicillin |
| Oncet® | hydrocodone and homatropine |
| Ophthaine® | proparacaine |
| Ophthochlor® Ophthalmic | chloramphenicol |
| Ophthocort® | chloramphenicol, polymyxin B, and hydrocortisone |
| Oradex-C® | dyclonine |
| Orasone® | prednisone |
| Oratect® | benzocaine |
| Ordrine AT® Extended Release Capsule | caramiphen and phenylpropanolamine |
| Oreticyl® | deserpidine and hydrochlorothiazide |
| Oreton® Methyl | methyltestosterone |
| Organidin® | iodinated glycerol |
| Orinase® Oral | tolbutamide |
| Ormazine® | chlorpromazine |
| Ornade® Spansule® | chlorpheniramine and phenylpropanolamine |
| Osteocalcin® | calcitonin |
| Otic Tridesilon® | desonide and acetic acid |
| O-V Staticin® | nystatin |
| Oxsoralen® Oral | methoxsalen |
| ---- | oxyphenbutazone |
| Panasal® 5/500 | hydrocodone and aspirin |
| Pantopon® | opium alkaloids |
| Panwarfarin® | warfarin sodium |
| Paplex® | salicylic acid |
| Paradione® | paramethadione |
| Paraflex® | chlorzoxazone |
| Para-Hist AT® | promethazine, phenylephrine, and codeine |
| Par Decon® | chlorpheniramine, phenyltoloxamine, phenylpropanolamine, and phenylephrine |
| Paredrine® | hydroxyamphetamine |
| Parepectolin® | kaolin and pectin with opium |

*(continued)*

| Brand Name | Generic Name |
|---|---|
| Pargen Fortified® | chlorzoxazone |
| Par Glycerol® | iodinated glycerol |
| Parsidol® | ethopropazine (all products) |
| Partuss® LA | guaifenesin and phenylpropanolamine |
| Pathilon® | tridihexethyl |
| Pathocil® | dicloxacillin |
| Pavabid® (all products) | papaverine hydrochloride |
| Pavasule® | papaverine hydrochloride |
| Pavatine® | papaverine hydrochloride |
| Pavatym® | papaverine hydrochloride |
| Pavesed® | papaverine hydrochloride |
| Pavulon® | pancuronium |
| Paxene® | paclitaxel |
| PBZ® (all products) | tripelennamine |
| Pediatric Triban® | trimethobanzamide |
| Pentids® | penicillin G potassium, oral (all products) |
| Pen.Vee® K | penicillin V potassium |
| Peptavlon® | pentagastrin |
| Pepto® Diarrhea Control | loperamide |
| Peritrate® | pentaerythritol tetranitrate |
| Peritrate® SA | pentaerythritol tetranitrate |
| Pfizerpen-AS® | penicillin G procaine |
| Phenahist-TR® | chlorpheniramine, phenylephrine, phenylpropanolamine, and belladonna alkaloids |
| Phenaphen® | acetaminophen |
| Phenaphen®/Codeine #4 | acetaminophen and codeine |
| Phenaseptic® | phenol |
| Phencen-50® | promethazine |
| Phenchlor® S.H.A. | chlorpheniramine, phenylephrine, phenylpropanolamine, and belladonna alkaloids |
| Phenerbel-S® | belladonna, phenobarbital, and ergotamine tartrate |
| Phenetron® | chlorpheniramine |
| ---- | phenolsulfonphthalein |
| Phenoxine® | phenylpropanolamine |
| Phenurone® | phenacemide |
| Phenyldrine® | phenylpropanolamine |
| Phenylfenesin® L.A. | guaifenesin and phenylpropanolamine |
| Phos-Ex® 62.5 | calcium acetate |
| Phos-Ex® 125 | calcium acetate |
| Phos-Ex® 167 | calcium acetate |
| Phos-Ex® 250 | calcium acetate |
| pHos-pHaid® | ammonium biphosphate, sodium biphosphate, and sodium acid pyrophosphate |
| Phosphaljel® | aluminum phosphate |
| Pilagan® Ophthalmic | pilocarpine |
| Pilostat® Ophthalmic | pilocarpine |
| Pin-Rid® | pyrantel pamoate |
| Plasmatein® | plasma protein fraction |
| Poladex® | dexchlorpheniramine |
| Polargen® | dexchlorpheniramine maleate |
| Poliovax® Injection | poliovirus vaccine, inactivated |
| Polycillin-N® Injection | ampicillin |
| Polycillin® Oral | ampicillin |
| Polycillin-PRB® | ampicillin and probenecid (all products) |
| Polyflex® Tablet | chlorzoxazone |
| Polygam® Injection | immune globulin, intravenous |
| Poly-Histine CS® | brompheniramine, phenylpropanolamine, and codeine |
| Poly-Histine-D® Capsule | phenyltoloxamine, phenylpropanolamine, pyrilamine, and pheniramine |

*(continued)*

| Brand Name | Generic Name |
|---|---|
| Polymox® | amoxicillin |
| Pondimin® | fenfluramine |
| Posicor® | mibefradil (all products) |
| Predair® | prednisolone |
| Predaject-50® | prednisolone |
| Predalone® | prednisolone |
| Predcor® | prednisolone |
| Predcor-TBA® | prednisolone |
| Predicort-50® | prednisolone |
| Prednicen-M® | prednisone |
| Preludin® | phenmetrazine hydrochloride |
| Proampacin® | ampicillin and probenecid (all products) |
| Pro-Banthine® | propantheline |
| Procan SR® | procainamide |
| Profenal® | suprofen |
| Profen II® | guaifenesin and phenylpropanolamine |
| Profen II DM® | guaifenesin, phenylpropanolamine, and dextromethorphan |
| Profen LA® | guaifenesin and phenylpropanolamine |
| Profilate-HP® | antihemophilic factor (human) |
| Progestaject® Injection | progesterone |
| ProHIBiT® | *Haemophilus* B conjugate vaccine |
| Prokine™ Injection | sargramostim |
| Prolamine® | phenylpropanolamine |
| Proloid® | thyroglobulin |
| Prometa® | metaproterenol sulfate |
| Prometh® | promethazine |
| Propacet® | propoxyphene and acetaminophen |
| Propagest® | phenylpropanolamine |
| Proplex® SX-T Injection | factor IX complex (human) |
| Pro-Sof® | docusate sodium |
| Prostaphlin® | oxacillin |
| Protenate® | plasma protein fraction |
| Protopam® Tablet | pralidoxime chloride |
| Provatene® | beta-carotene |
| Pyridium Plus® | phenazopyridine, hyoscyamine, and butabarbital |
| Questran® Tablet | cholestyramine resin |
| Quiess® Injection | hydroxyzine |
| Quinamm® | quinine sulfate |
| Quiphile® | quinine sulfate |
| Q-vel® | quinine sulfate |
| Raudixin® | *Rauwolfia serpentina* |
| Rauverid® | *Rauwolfia serpentina* |
| Raxar® | grepafloxacin |
| Rectacort® Suppository | hydrocortisone |
| Redux® | dexfenfluramine |
| Regitine® | phentolamine |
| Regutol® | docusate |
| Relefact® TRH | protirelin |
| Renoquid® | sulfacytine |
| Reposans-10® Oral | chlordiazepoxide |
| Rep-Pred® | methylprednisolone |
| Resa® | reserpine |
| Resaid® | chlorpheniramine and phenylpropanolamine |
| Rescaps-D® S.R. Capsule | caramiphen and phenylpropanolamine |
| Rescon Liquid | chlorpheniramine and phenylpropanolamine |
| Rexigen Forte® | phendimetrazine |
| Rezulin® | troglitazone |

*(continued)*

| Brand Name | Generic Name |
|---|---|
| R-Gel® | capsaicin |
| R-Gen® | iodinated glycerol |
| Rhesonativ® Injection | $Rh_o$(D) immune globulin |
| Rhindecon® | phenylpropanolamine |
| Rhinolar® | chlorpheniramine, phenylpropanolamine, and methscopolamine |
| Rhuli® Cream | benzocaine, calamine, and camphor |
| Riobin® | riboflavin |
| Robafen® CF | guaifenesin, phenylpropanolamine, and dextromethorphan |
| Robicillin® Tablet | penicillin V potassium |
| Robitet® | tetracycline |
| Robitussin-CF® | guaifenesin, phenylpropanolamine, and dextromethorphan |
| Romycin® Solution | erythromycin, topical |
| Rondomycin® Capsule | methacycline hydrochloride (all products) |
| RotaShield® | rotavirus vaccine |
| Roxiprin® | oxycodone and aspirin |
| Rufen® | ibuprofen |
| Ru-Tuss® | chlorpheniramine, phenylephrine, phenylpropanolamine, and belladonna alkaloids |
| Rymed-TR® | guaifenesin and phenylpropanolamine |
| Salgesic® | salsalate |
| Salmonine® | calcitonin |
| Salsitab® | salsalate |
| Salutensin® | hydroflumethiazide and reserpine |
| Salutensin-Demi® | hydroflumethiazide and reserpine |
| SangCya™ | cyclosporine |
| Sanorex® | mazindol |
| Scabene® | lindane |
| Sclavo - PPD® Solution | tuberculin purified protein derivative |
| Sclavo Test - PPD® | tuberculin purified protein derivative |
| Seldane® | terfenadine |
| Seldane-D® | terfenadine and pseudoephedrine |
| Selectol® | celiprolol |
| Selestoject® | betamethasone |
| Senolax® | senna |
| Septisol® | hexachlorophene |
| Ser-Ap-Es® | hydralazine, hydrochlorothiazide, and reserpine |
| Serpalan® | reserpine |
| Serpasil® | reserpine |
| Serpatabs® | reserpine |
| Siblin® | psyllium |
| Silain® | simethicone |
| Silaminic® Cold Syrup | chlorpheniramine and phenylpropanolamine |
| Silaminic® Expectorant | guaifenesin and phenylpropanolamine |
| Sildicon-E® | guaifenesin and phenylpropanolamine |
| Siltussin-CF® | guaifenesin, phenylpropanolamine, and dextromethorphan |
| Sinubid® | phenyltoloxamine, phenylpropanolamine, and acetaminophen |
| Skelex® | chlorzoxazone |
| Slo-Salt® | salt substitute |
| Snaplets-EX® | guaifenesin and phenylpropanolamine |
| Sodium P.A.S.® | aminosalicylate sodium |
| Sofarin® | warfarin sodium |
| Solatene® | beta-carotene |
| Solfoton® | phenobarbital |
| Sparine® | promazine |
| Spasmoject® | dicyclomine |
| Spectrobid® Tablet | bacampicillin |
| Spironazide® | hydrochlorothiazide and spironolactone |

*(continued)*

| Brand Name | Generic Name |
|---|---|
| Spirozide® | hydrochlorothiazide and spironolactone |
| Stahist® | chlorpheniramine, phenylephrine, phenylpropanolamine, and belladonna alkaloids |
| Staphcillin® | methicillin (all products) |
| Statobex® | phendimetrazine tartrate |
| Stemex® | paramethasone acetate |
| Sucostrin® | succinylcholine chloride |
| Sudafed® Children | pseudoephedrine |
| Sudafed® Cough | guaifenesin, pseudoephedrine, and dextromethorphan |
| Sudafed Plus® Liquid | chlorpheniramine and pseudoephedrine |
| Sulfa-Gyn® | sulfabenzamide, sulfacetamide, and sulfathiazole |
| Sulfamethoprim® | co-trimoxazole |
| Sulfa-Trip® | sulfabenzamide, sulfacetamide, and sulfathiazole |
| Sultrin™ | sulfabenzamide, sulfacetamide, and sulfathiazole |
| Superchar® | charcoal |
| Superchar® With Sorbitol | charcoal |
| Surital® | thiamylal sodium |
| Sustaire® | theophylline |
| Symadine® | amantadine hydrochloride |
| Symmetrel® Capsule | amantadine hydrochloride |
| Synalar-HP® Topical | fluocinolone |
| Synkayvite® | menadiol sodium |
| Syntocinon® Nasal | oxytocin |
| Tabron® | vitamins, multiple |
| Tacaryl® | methdilazine hydrochloride (all products) |
| TACE® | chlorotrianisene |
| Tamine® | brompheniramine and phenylpropanolamine |
| Taractan® | chlorprothixene |
| Tavist-D® | clemastine and phenylpropanolamine |
| T-Caine® Lozenge | benzocaine |
| Tebamide® | trimethobenzamide |
| Tedral® | theophylline, ephedrine, and phenobarbital |
| Tegopen® | cloxacillin |
| Teline® | tetracycline |
| Temaril® | trimeprazine tartrate |
| Temazin® Cold Syrup | chlorpheniramine and phenylpropanolamine |
| Tepanil® | diethylpropion hydrochloride |
| Tepanil® TenTabs® | diethylpropion hydrochloride |
| ---- | terpin hydrate |
| ---- | terpin hydrate and codeine |
| Terra-Cortril® Ophthalmic Suspension | oxytetracycline and hydrocortisone |
| Terramycin® Oral | oxytetracycline |
| Tes-Tape® | diagnostic aids (*in vitro*), urine |
| Tetralan® | tetracycline |
| Tetram® | tetracycline |
| T-Gen® | trimethobenzamide |
| Theelin® Aqueous Injection | estrone |
| Theobid® | theophylline |
| Theobid® Jr Duracaps® | theophylline |
| Theoclear-80® | theophylline |
| Theoclear®-L.A. | theophylline |
| Theo-Dur® Sprinkle® | theophylline |
| Theo-Organidin® | iodinated glycerol and theophylline |
| Theo-Sav® | theophylline |
| Theospan®-SR | theophylline |
| Theostat-80® | theophylline |
| Theovent® | theophylline |

*(continued)*

| Brand Name | Generic Name |
|---|---|
| Theo-X® | theophylline |
| Thera-Hist® Syrup | chlorpheniramine and phenylpropanolamine |
| Theramine® Expectorant | guaifenesin and phenylpropanolamine |
| Thiacide® | methenamine and potassium acid phosphate |
| Thrombinar® | thrombin (topical) |
| Thrombostat® | thrombin (topical) |
| Thypinone® | protirelin |
| Thyrar® | thyroid |
| Thyroid Strong® | thyroid |
| Ticon® | trimethobenzamide |
| Tiject-20® | trimethobenzamide |
| Tindal® | acetophenazine maleate |
| Tinver® | sodium thiosulfate |
| Torecan® Suppository | thiethylperazine |
| Totacillin® | ampicillin |
| Totacillin-N® | ampicillin |
| Tral® | hexocyclium methylsulfate |
| Travase® | sutilains |
| Triaminic® Allergy Tablet | chlorpheniramine and phenylpropanolamine |
| Triaminic® Cold Tablet | chlorpheniramine and phenylpropanolamine |
| Triaminic® Expectorant | guaifenesin and phenylpropanolamine |
| Triaminic® Oral Infant, Drops | pheniramine, phenylpropanolamine, and pyrilamine |
| Triaminic® Syrup | chlorpheniramine and phenylpropanolamine |
| Triaminicol® Multi-Symptom Cold Syrup | chlorpheniramine, phenylpropanolamine, and dextromethorphan |
| Triavil® 4-50 | amitriptyline and perphenazine |
| Tri-Clear® Expectorant | guaifenesin phenylpropanolamine |
| Tridione® | trimethadione |
| Tridione® Suppository | trimethadione |
| Trifed-C® | triprolidine, pseudoephedrine, and codeine |
| TRIKOF-D® | guaifenesin, phenylpropanolamine, and dextromethorphan |
| Trimazide® | trimethobenzamide |
| Trimox® 500 mg | amoxicillin |
| Tri-Nefrin® Extra Strength Tablet | chlorpheniramine and phenylpropanolamine |
| Triofed® Syrup | triprolidine and pseudoephedrine |
| Tri-P® Oral Infant Drops | pheniramine, phenylpropanolamine, and pyrilamine |
| Tri-Phen-Chlor® | chlorpheniramine, phenyltoloxamine, phenylpropanolamine, and phenylephrine |
| Triphenyl® Expectorant | guaifenesin and phenylpropanolamine |
| Triphenyl® Syrup | chlorpheniramine and phenylpropanolamine |
| Tri-Statin® II Topical | nystatin and triamcinolone |
| Trofan® | L-tryptophan |
| Trofan DS® | L-tryptophan |
| Tryptacin® | L-tryptophan |
| Trysul® | sulfabenzamide, sulfacetamide, and sulfathiazole |
| Tucks® Cream | witch hazel |
| Tusal® | sodium thiosalicylate |
| Tuss-Allergine® Modified T.D. Capsule | caramiphen and phenylpropanolamine |
| Tussi-Organidin® | iodinated glycerol and codeine |
| Tussi-Organidin® DM | iodinated glycerol and dextromethorphan (all products) |
| Tusso-DM® | iodinated glycerol and dextromethorphan (all products) |
| Tussogest® Extended Release Capsule | caramiphen and phenylpropanolamine |
| Tuss-Ornade® | caramiphen and phenylpropanolamine |
| Tylenol® Cold Effervescent Medication Tablet | chlorpheniramine, phenylpropanolamine, and acetaminophen |

*(continued)*

| Brand Name | Generic Name |
|---|---|
| ULR-LA® | guaifenesin and phenylpropanolamine |
| Ultralente® U | insulin zinc suspension, extended |
| Ultrase® MT24 | pancrelipase |
| Uni-Decon® | chlorpheniramine, phenyltoloxamine, phenylpropanolamine, and phenylephrine |
| Unipen® | nafcillin |
| Unipres® | hydralazine, hydrochlorothiazide, and reserpine |
| Unitrol® | phenylpropanolamine |
| Urabeth® | bethanechol |
| Uracel® | sodium salicylate |
| Ureacin®-40 Topical | urea |
| Uri-Tet® | oxytetracycline |
| Urobak® | sulfamethoxazole |
| Urobiotic-25® | oxytetracycline and sulfamethizole |
| Urodine® | phenazopyridine |
| Uroplus® DS | co-trimoxazole |
| Uroplus® SS | co-trimoxazole |
| Uticort® | betamethasone (all products) |
| Vagitrol® | sulfanilamide |
| Valadol® | acetaminophen |
| Valergen® Injection | estradiol |
| Valmid® Capsule | ethinamate |
| Valpin® 50 | anisotropine methylbromide |
| Valrelease® | diazepam |
| Vamate® Oral | hydroxyzine |
| Vanex-LA® | guaifenesin and phenylpropanolamine |
| Vanseb-T® Shampoo | coal tar, sulfur, and salicylic acid |
| Vansil™ | oxamniquine |
| Vasoxyl® | methoxamine |
| V-Cillin K® | penicillin V potassium |
| Velsar® Injection | vinblastine sulfate |
| Vercyte® | pipobroman |
| Vermizine® | piperazine |
| Verr-Canth™ | cantharidin |
| Verrex-C&M® | podophyllin and salicylic acid |
| Verrusol® | salicylic acid, podophyllin, and cantharidin |
| V-Gan® Injection | promethazine hydrochloride |
| Vibazine® | buclizine |
| Vicks® DayQuil® Allergy Relief 4 Hour Tablet | brompheniramine and phenylpropanolamine |
| Vicks® DayQuil® Sinus Pressure & Congestion Relief | guaifenesin and phenylpropanolamine |
| Vicks® Vatronol® | ephedrine |
| Vioform® | clioquinol |
| Vioform®-Hydrocortisone Topical | clioquinol and hydrocortisone |
| Vistacon-50® Injection | hydroxyzine |
| Vistaject-25® | hydroxyzine |
| Vistaject-50® | hydroxyzine |
| Vistaquel® Injection | hydroxyzine |
| Vistaril® Injection | hydroxyzine |
| Vistazine® Injection | hydroxyzine |
| Vontrol® | diphenidol |
| Wehamine® Injection | dimenhydrinate |
| Wehdryl® | diphenhydramine |
| Wesprin® Buffered | aspirin |
| Wolfina® | *Rauwolfia serpentina* |

*(continued)*

| Brand Name | Generic Name |
|---|---|
| Wyamycin S® | erythromycin |
| Zantryl® | phentermine |
| Zartan® | cephalexin |
| Zeasorb-AF® | tolnaftate |
| Zebrax® | clidinium and chlordiazepoxide |
| Zefazone® | cefmetazole |
| Zetran® | diazepam |
| Zolyse® | chymotrypsin alpha (all products) |
| Zyban™ 100 mg | bupropion |

# PHARMACEUTICAL MANUFACTURERS AND DISTRIBUTORS

**Abana Pharmaceuticals, Inc**
(see Jones Pharma, Inc)

**Abbott Laboratories**
**(Pharmaceutical Product Division)**
100 Abbott Park Road
Abbott Park, IL 60064-3500
(800) 441-4987
www.abbott.com

**Able Laboratories, Inc**
6 Hollywood Court
South Plainfield, NJ 07080
(908) 754-2253

**Academic Pharmaceuticals, Inc**
25720 Saunders Road North
Lake Forest, IL 60045
(847) 735-1170

**Acme United Corp**
1931 Black Rock Turnpike
Fairfield, CT 06432
(800) 835-2263
www.acmeunited.com

**Adams Laboratories, Inc**
14801 Sovereign Road
Ft Worth, TX 76155-2645
(800) 770-5270
www.adamslaboratories.com

**Adria Laboratories** (see Pharmacia Corp)

**Advance Biofactures Corp**
(See Biospecifics Technologies Corp)

**Advanced Nutritional Technology**
6988 Sierra Court
Dublin, CA 94568
(800) 624-6543

**Advanced Polymer Systems**
123 Saginaw Drive
Redwood City, CA 94063
(650) 366-2626
www.advancedpolymer.com

**Advanced Tissue Sciences, Inc**
10933 North Torrey Pines Road
La Jolla, CA 92037-1005
(858) 713-7300
www.advancedtissue.com

**Advanced Vision Research**
7 Alfred Street
Suite 330
Woburn, MA 01801
(800) 579-8327
www.theratears.com

**Agouron Pharmaceuticals**
10350 North Torrey Pines Road
La Jolla, CA 92037-1020
(858) 223-0432
www.agouron.com

**A. H. Robins Consumer Products**
(See Whitehall-Robins Healthcare)

**A. H. Robins, Inc**
(See Whitehall-Robins Healthcare)

**Akorn, Inc**
2500 Millbrook Drive
Buffalo Grove, IL 60089
(800) 535-7155
www.akorn.com

**AkPharma, Inc**
6840 Old Egg Harbor Road
Pleasantville, NJ 08232
(800) 994-4711
www.akpharma.com

**Alcon Laboratories, Inc**
6201 South Freeway
Ft Worth, TX 76134-2099
www.alconlabs.com

**Alimenterics, Inc**
301 American Road
Morris Plains, NJ 07950
(973) 285-3100

**ALK**
27 Village Lane
Wallingford, CT 06492
(800) 252-9778
www.alk-abello.net

**A. L. Labs** (See Alpharma USPD, Inc)

**Allen & Hanburys** (See GlaxoWellcome, Inc)

**Allercreme** (See Carme, Inc)

**Allerderm Laboratories**
PO Box 2070
Petaluma, CA 94953-2070

**Allergan Herbert** (see Allergan)

**Allergan, Inc**
2525 DuPont Drive
Irvine, CA 92612
(800) 433-8871
www.allergan.com

**Alliance Pharmaceutical Corp**
3040 Science Park Road
San Diego, CA 92121
(858) 410-5275
www.allp.com

**Allied Pharmacy**
801 Stadium Drive
Suite 111
Arlington, TX 76111
(817) 226-5050

**Allscripts, Inc**
2401 Commerce Drive
Libertyville, IL 60048-4464
(800) 654-0889
www.allscripts.com

**Almay, Inc**
1501 Williamsboro Street
Oxford, NC 27565
(800) 473-8566

**Alpha 1 Biomedicals, Inc**
6707 Democracy Boulevard
Suite 111
Bethesda, MD 20817
(301) 564-4400

**Alpharma**
**(US Pharmaceuticals)**
7205 Windsor Boulevard
Baltimore, MD 21244

**Alpharma USPD, Inc**
333 Cassell Drive
Suite 3500
Baltimore, MD 21224
(800) 638-9096
www.alpharmaUSPD.com

**Alpha Therapeutic Corp**
5555 Valley Boulevard
Los Angeles, CA 90032
(800) 421-0008
www.alphather.com

**Alra Laboratories, Inc**
3850 Clearview Court
Gurnee, IL 60031
(800) 248-2572

**Altana, Inc**
60 Baylis Road
Melville, NY 11747
(800) 432-6673

**AltaRex Corp**
610 Lincoln Street
Waltham, MA 02451
(888) 801-6665

**Alto Pharmaceuticals, Inc**
PO Box 1910
Land O'Lakes, FL 34639-1910
(800) 330-2891

**Alza Corp**
1900 Charleston Road
PO Box 7210
Mt View, CA 94039
(800) 634-8977
www.alza.com

**Amarin Pharmaceuticals**
25 Independence Boulevard
Warren, NJ 07059
(908) 580-5535

**Ambix Laboratories**
210 Orchard Street
East Rutherford, NJ 07073
(201) 939-2200

**Amcon Laboratories**
40 North Rock Hill Road
St Louis, MO 63119
(800) 255-6161

**Americal Pharmaceutical, Inc**
(see Akorn, Inc)

**American Dermal Corp** (see Aventis)

**American Drug Industries, Inc**
5810 South Perry Avenue
Chicago, IL 60621

**American Home Products**
(see Whitehall-Robins Healthcare)

**American Lecithin Company**
115 Hurley Road
Unit 2B
Oxford, CT 06478
(800) 364-4416

**American Medical Industries**
330 1/2 East Third Street
Dell Rapids, SD 57022
(605) 428-5501

**American Pharmaceutical, Company**
12 Dwight Place
Fairfield, NJ 07004-3434
(973) 276-1310

**American Pharmaceutical Partners, Inc**
10866 Wilshire Boulevard
Suite 1270
Los Angeles, CA 90024
(800) 551-7176

**American Red Cross**
1616 North Fort Myers Drive
Arlington, VA 22209
(800) 446-8883
www.redcross.org/plasma

**American Regent Labs, Inc**
One Luitpold Drive
Shirley, NY 11967
(800) 645-1706
www.luitpold.com

**Ames** (see Miles Biological Products)

**Amgen Inc**
One Amgen Center Drive
Thousand Oaks, CA 91320-1799
(800) 282-6436
www.amgen.com

**Amide Pharmaceuticals, Inc**
101 East Main Street
Little Falls, NJ 07424
(973) 890-1440
amide@ix.netcom.com

**AMSCO Scientific** (see Steris Labs)

**Anaquest** (see Baxter)

**Andrew Jergens Company**
2535 Spring Grove Avenue
Cincinnati, OH 45214
(800) 222-3553
www.jergens.com

**Andrulis Pharmaceutical Corp**
PO Box 2135
Bethesda, MD 20817
(301) 419-2400

**Andrx Pharmaceuticals, Inc**
4001 Southwest 47th Avenue
Fort Lauderdale, FL 33314
(800) 621-7143
www.andrx.com

**Angelini Pharmaceuticals, Inc**
70 Grand Avenue
River Edge, NJ 07661
(201) 646-1697

**Anthra Pharmaceuticals, Inc**
103 Carnegie Center
Suite 102
Princeton, NJ 08540
(609) 514-1060
www.anthra.com

**Antibodies, Inc**
PO Box 1560
Davis, CA 95617
(800) 824-8540
www.antibodiesinc.com

**Aplicare, Inc**
50 East Industrial Road
Branford, CT 06405
(800) 760-3236
www.aplicare.com

**Apollon, Inc**
One Great Valley Parkway
Malvern, PA 19355
(610) 647-9452

**Apotex Corp**
50 Lakeview Parkway
Suite 127
Vernon Hills, IL 60061

**Apotex USA**
1776 Broadway
Suite 1900
New York, NY 10019
(800) 700-3092

**Apothecary Products, Inc**
11750 12th Avenue South
Burnsville, MN 55337
(800) 328-2742

**Apothecon, Inc**
**(Bristol-Myers Squibb Company)**
PO Box 4500
Princeton, NJ 08543-4500
(800) 321-1335
www.apothecon.com

**Apothecus, Inc**
20 Audrey Avenue
Oyster Bay, NY 11771
(800) 227-2393

**Applied Analytical Industries**
1200 North 23rd Street
Wilmington, NC 28405
(800) 575-4224

**Applied Biotech, Inc**
10237 Flanders Court
San Diego, CA 92121
(858) 587-6771

**Applied Genetics**
205 Buffalo Avenue
Freeport, NY 11520
(516) 868-9026
www.agiderm.com

**Applied Medical Research**
308 15th Avenue North
Nashville, TN 37203
(615) 327-0676

**Approved Drug**
(see Health for Life Brands, Inc)

**Arcola Laboratories**
500 Arcola Road
Collegeville, PA 19426
(800) 472-4467

**Arco Pharmaceuticals, Inc**
90 Orville Drive
Bohemia, NY 11716
(800) 645-5412

**Armour Pharmaceutical**
(see Aventis Behring)

**Aronex Pharmaceuticals, Inc**
8707 Technology Forest Place
The Woodlands, TX 77381
(281) 367-1666
aronex-pharm.com

**Arrow International Corp Headquarters**
2400 Bernville Road
Reading, PA 19605
(800) 523-8446

**Ascent Pediatrics, Inc**
187 Ballardvale Street
Suite B125
Wilmington, MA 01887
(978) 658-2500
www.ascentpediatrics.com

**AstraZeneca Pharmaceuticals, LP**
1800 Concord Pike
PO Box 15437
Wilmington, DE 19850-5437
(800) 456-3669
www.astrazeneca-us.com

**Athena Neurosciences, Inc**
700 Gateway Boulevard
South San Francisco, CA 94080
(888) 638-7605
www.athenaneuro.com

**Atley Pharmaceuticals, Inc**
14433 North Washington Highway
Ashland, VA 23005
(804) 752-8400
www.atley.com

**AutoImmune, Inc**
128 Spring Street
Lexington, MA 02173
(781) 860-0710

**Aventis Behring LLC**
1020 First Avenue
King of Prussia, PA 19406
(800) 504-5434
www.aventisbehring.com

**Aventis Pasteur, Inc**
Discovery Drive
Swiftwater, PA 18370-0187
(800) 822-2463
www.aventispasteur.com

**Aventis Pharmaceuticals, Inc**
10236 Marion Park Drive
Kansas City, MO 64137
(800) 207-8049

**Axcan Scandipharm, Inc**
22 Inverness Center Parkway
Suite 310
Birmingham, AL 35242
(800) 950-8085
www.scandipharm.com

**Bajamar Chemical Company, Inc**
9609 Dielman Rock Island
St Louis, MO 63132
(888) 242-3414
www.vesselvite.com

**Baker Cummins Dermatologicals**
(see Baker Norton)

**Baker Norton Pharmaceuticals**
4400 Biscayne Boulevard
Miami, FL 33137
(800) 735-2315
www.ivax.com

**Ballard Medical Products**
12050 South Lone Peak Parkway
Draper, UT 84020
(800) 528-5591
www.bmed.com

**Banner Pharmacaps**
4125 Premier Drive
High Point, NC 27265
(800) 447-1140
www.banpharm.com

**Barr Laboratories, Inc**
2 Quaker Road
Pomona, NY 01970
(800) 222-0190
www.barrlabs.com

**Bartor Pharmacal Company**
70 High Street
Rye, NY 10580
(914) 967-4219

**Basel Pharmaceuticals**
(see Novartis Pharmaceuticals)

**Bausch & Lomb Pharmaceuticals**
8500 Hidden River Parkway
Tampa, FL 33637
(800) 323-0000
www.bausch.com

**Baxa Corp**
13760 East Arapahoe Road
Englewood, CO 80112
(800) 567-2292
www.baxa.com

**Baxter Healthcare Corp**
**Corp Headquarters**
One Baxter Parkway DF4-1W
Deerfield, IL 60015
(800) 422-9837
www.baxter.com

**Baxter Hyland Immuno**
550 North Brand Boulevard
Glendale, CA 91203
(800) 423-2862
www.baxter.com

**Baxter Pharmaceutical Products, Inc**
**(Baxter PPI)**
110 Allen Road
Liberty Corner, NJ 07938-0804
(800) 782-9375

**Bayer Corp**
**(Biological & Pharmaceutical Division)**
400 Morgan Lane
West Haven, CT 06516-4175
(800) 288-8371
www.bayer.com

**Bayer, Inc**
77 Belfield Road
Toronto, Ontario, Canada M9W 1G6
(800) 268-1331
www.bayerdiag.com

**B. Braun**
PO Box 19791
Irvine, CA 92713-9791
(800) 227-2862
www.bbraunusa.com

**B. Braun Medical, Inc**
PO Box 19791
Irvine, CA 92613-9791
(800) 854-6851
www.bbraunusa.com

**BD (Becton Dickinson & Company)**
One Becton Drive
Franklin Lakes, NJ 07417
(888) 237-2762
www.bd.com

**BD Biosciences**
2350 Qume Drive
San Jose, CA 95131
(800) 223-8226
www.bdbiosciences.com

**BDI Pharmaceuticals, Inc**
9700 North Michigan Road
Carmel, IN 46220
(800) 428-1717
www.bdip.com

**Beach Pharmaceuticals**
5220 South Manhattan Avenue
Tampa, FL 33611
(800) 322-8210

**Beckman Coulter, Inc**
4300 North Harbor Boulevard
PO Box 3100
Fullerton, CA 92834
(714) 871-4848
www.beckman.com

**Becton Dickinson Microbiology Systems**
7 Loveton Circle
Sparks, MD 21152
(800) 638-8663

**Bedford Laboratories**
300 Northfield Road
Bedford, OH 44146
(800) 562-4797
www.benvenue.com

**Beecham** (see SmithKline Beecham)

**Beiersdorf, Inc**
Wilton Corporate Center
187 Danbury Road
Wilton, CT 06897
(203) 563-5800
www.beiersdorf.com

**Bergen Brunswig Drug Company**
4000 Metropolitan Drive
Orange, CA 92868
(714) 385-4000

**Berlex Laboratories, Inc**
300 Fairfield Road
Wayne, NJ 07470
(888) 237-5394
www.berlex.com

**Berna Products**
4216 Ponce de Leon Boulevard
Coral Gables, FL 33146
(800) 533-5899
www.bernaproducts.com

**Bertek**
**Pharmaceuticals, Inc**
PO Box 4310
Morgantown, WV 26504
(800) 986-9526
www.bertek.com

**Best Generics** (see Goldline Consumer, Inc)

**Beta Dermaceuticals, Inc**
PO Box 691106
San Antonio, TX 78216-1106

**Beutlich Pharmaceuticals**
1541 Shields Drive
Waukegan, IL 60085
(800) 238-8542
www.beutlich.com

**B. F. Ascher & Company**
PO Box 717
Shawnee Mission, KS 66201
(800) 324-1880

**Biocare International, Inc**
2643 Grand Avenue
Bellmore, NY 11710
(516) 781-5800

**Biocraft Laboratories, Inc**
(see Teva Pharmaceuticals)

**BioCryst Pharmaceuticals, Inc**
2190 Parkway Lake Drive
Birmingham, AL 35244
(205) 444-4600
www.biocryst.com

**Biofilm, Inc**
3121 Scott Street
Vista, CA 92083-8323
(800) 848-5900
www.astroglide.com

**Biogen**
14 Cambridge Center
Cambridge, MA 02142
(800) 456-2255
www.biogen.com

**BioGenex Laboratories**
4600 Norris Canyon Road
Suite 400
San Ramon, CA 94583
(800) 421-4149
www.biogenex.com

**Bioglan Pharma**
7 Great Valley Parkway
Suite 301
Malvern, PA 19355
(888) 246-4526

**Bioline Labs, Inc** (see Ivax Pharmaceuticals)

**Biomedical Frontiers, Inc**
1095 10th Avenue, Southeast
Minneapolis, MN 55414
(612) 378-0228

**Biomerica, Inc**
1533 Monrovia Avenue
Newport Beach, CA 92663
(800) 854-3002
www.biomerica.com

**Biomira USA, Inc**
1002 East Park Boulevard
Cranbury, NJ 08512
(609) 655-5300
www.biomira.com

**Biopharmaceutics, Inc** (see Feminique Corp)

**Biopure Corp**
11 Hurley Street
Cambridge, MA 02141
(617) 234-6500
www.biopure.com

**Biospecifics Technologies Corp**
35 Wilbur Street
Lynbrook, NY 11563
(516) 593-7000
www.biospecifics.com

**BioStar, Inc**
6655 Lookout Road
Boulder, CO 80301
(800) 637-3717
www.biostar.com

**Bio-Technology General Corp**
70 Wood Avenue South
Iselin, NJ 08830
(800) 284-2480
www.btgc.com

**BIO-TECH Pharmacal, Inc**
PO Box 1992
Fayetteville, AR 72702
(800) 345-1199
www.bio-tech-pharm.com

**BIRA Corp**
2525 Quicksilver
McDonald, PA 15057
(724) 796-1820

**Birchwood Laboratories, Inc**
7900 Fuller Road
Eden Prairie, MN 53344
(800) 328-6156

**Bird Products Corp**
1100 Bird Center Drive
Palm Springs, CA 92262
(800) 328-4139
www.thermoresp.com

**Blaine Pharmaceuticals**
1515 Production Drive
Burlington, KY 41005
(800) 633-9353
www.blainepharma.com

**Blairex Labs, Inc**
PO Box 2127
Columbus, IN 47202-2127
(800) 252-4739
www.blairex.com

**Blair Laboratories** (see Purdue Frederick)

**Blansett Pharmacal Company, Inc**
PO Box 638
North Little Rock, AR 72115
(501) 758-8635

**Blistex, Inc**
1800 Swift Drive
Oak Brook, IL 60523
(800) 837-1800
www.blistex.com

**Block Drug Company, Inc**
257 Cornelison Avenue
Jersey City, NJ 07302
(800) 365-6500
www.blockdrug.com

**Bluco, Inc**
28350 Schoolcraft
Livonia, MI 48150
(800) 832-4464

**Bock Pharmacal Company**
(see Sanofi-Synthelabo, Inc)

**Boehringer Ingelheim Pharmaceuticals, Inc**
900 Ridgebury Road
Ridgefield, CT 06877-0368
(800) 542-6257
www.boehringer-ingelheim.com

**Boehringer Mannheim** (see Roche)

**Bone Care International**
**Bone Care Center**
1600 Aspen Commons
Middleton, WI 53562
(888) 389-3300
www.bonecare.com

**Boots Pharmaceuticals, Inc**
(see Knoll Laboratories)

**Bracco Diagnostics, Inc**
PO Box 5225
Princeton, NJ 08543
(800) 631-5244
www.bracco.com

**Bradley Pharmaceutical**
(see Kenwood Laboratories)

**Braintree Laboratories, Inc**
60 Columbian Street West
Braintree, MA 02185-0929
(800) 874-6756
www.braintreeLabs.com

**Breath Asure**
31280 Oak Crest Drive
Suite 1
Westlake Village, CA 91361
(800) 827-3284
www.breathasure.com

**Breckenridge Pharmaceutical, Inc**
1141 South Rogers Circle
Suite 3
Boca Raton, FL 33487
(800) 466-2700

**Brightstone Pharma, Inc**
109 MacKenan Drive
Cary, NC 27511
(888) 460-7300

**Brimms, Inc**
425 Fillmore Avenue
Tonawanda, NY 14150
(800) 828-7669

**Bristol-Myers Squibb Company (Pharmaceutical Division)**
PO Box 4500
Princeton, NJ 08540
(800) 321-1335
www.bms.com

**Bryan Corp**
4 Plympton Street
Woburn, MA 01801
(800) 343-7711
www.bryancorporation.com

**BTG** (see Bio-Technology General Corp)

**Burroughs Wellcome Company**
(see GlaxoWellcome)

**Calmoseptine, Inc**
5901 Warner Avenue
Suite 100
Huntington Beach, CA 92649
(800) 800-3405
www.calmoseptineointment.com

**Cal-White Mineral Company**
PO Box 7890
Klamath Falls, OR 97602
(800) 944-8096

**Camall Company, Inc**
PO Box 307
Romeo, MI 48065-0307
(800) 521-6720
www.camall.com

**Cambridge NeuroScience**
One Kendall Square
Building 700
Cambridge, MA 02139
(617) 225-0600

**Cambridge Nutraceuticals**
294 Washington Street
Suite 601
Boston, MA 02108
(800) 265-2202
www.cambridgenutra.com

**Can-Am Care Corp**
Cimetra Industrial Park
PO Box 98
Chazy, NY 12921
(800) 461-7448

**Capellon Pharmaceuticals, Inc**
7462 Dogwood Drive
Fort Worth, TX 76118
(817) 595-5820
www.capellon.com

**Caraco Pharmaceutical Laboratories**
1150 Elijah McCoy Drive
Detroit, MI 48202
(800) 818-4555
www.caraco.com

**Cardinal Health, Inc**
5555 Glendon Court
Dublin, OH 43016
(800) 234-8701

**Care Technologies, Inc**
PO Box 82
10 Corbin Drive
Darien, CT 06820
(800) 783-1919
www.clearcare.com

**Carma Labs, Inc**
5801 West Airways Avenue
Franklin, WI 53132
(414) 421-7707

**Carme, Inc**
84 Galli
Novato, CA 94949
(800) 447-6758

**Carnation**
800 North Brand Boulevard
Glendale, CA 91203
(800) 628-2229
www.carnationbaby.com

**Carnrick Laboratories**
45 Horse Hill Road
Cedar Knolls, NJ 07927
(973) 267-2670
www.elan.ie

**Carolina Medical Products**
PO Box 147
Farmville, NC 27828
(800) 227-6637
www.carolinamedical.com

**Carrington Labs**
2001 Walnut Hill Lane
(800) 527-5216
www.carringtonlabs.com

**C. B. Fleet Company, Inc**
4615 Murray Place
Lynchburg, VA 24506
(800) 999-9711
www.cbfleet.com

**CCA Industries, Inc**
200 Murray Hill Parkway
East Rutherford, NJ 07073
(800) 524-2720

**Celgene Corp**
7 Powder Horn Drive
Warren, NJ 07059
(800) 890-4619
www.celgene.com

**Cellcor, Inc**
200 Wells Avenue
Newton, MA 02159
(617) 332-2500

**Cellegy Pharmaceuticals, Inc**
349 Oyster Point Boulevard
Suite 200
San Francisco, CA 94080
(650) 616-2200

**Celltech**
755 Jefferson Road
Rochester, NY 14623-0000
(800) 234-5535

**Cell Therapeutics**
201 Elliott Avenue West
Seattle, WA 98119
(800) 215-2355

**Centeon** (see Aventis Behring)

**Center Pharmaceuticals, Inc**
3620 Park Central Boulevard North
Pompano Beach FL, 33064
(800) 223-6837
www.centerpharm.com

**Centers for Disease Control and Prevention**
1600 Clifton Road Northeast
Atlanta, GA 30333
(800) 311-3435
www.cdc.gov

**Centocor, Inc**
200 Great Valley Parkway
Malvern, PA 19355
(888) 457-6399
www.centocor.com

**Central Pharmaceuticals, Inc**
(see Schwarz Pharma)

**Century Pharmaceuticals, Inc**
10377 Hague Road
Indianapolis, IN 46256-3399
(317) 849-4210

**Cephalon, Inc**
145 Brandywine Parkway
West Chester, PA 19380
(800) 782-3656
www.cephalon.com

**Cerenex Pharmaceuticals**
(see GlaxoWellcome)

**Cetylite Industries, Inc**
9051 River Road
PO Box 90006
Pennsauken, NJ 08110
(800) 257-7740
www.cetylite.com

**Chase Laboratories**
(see Banner Pharmacaps)

**Chattem Consumer Products**
1715 West 38th Street
Chattanooga, TN 37409
(800) 366-6833
www.chattem.com

**Cheesebrough-Ponds USA, Inc**
(see Unilever Home and Personal Care)

**Chemrich Laboratories**
5211 Telegraph Road
Los Angeles, CA 90022

**ChemTrak, Inc**
929 East Arques Avenue
Sunnyvale, CA 94086-4520
(800) 927-7776

**Chesapeake Biological Labs, Inc**
111 South Paca Street
Baltimore, MD 21230
(410) 843-5000

**Cheshire Pharmaceutical Systems**
6225 Shiloh Road
Alpharetta, GA 30005
(800) 582-3194
www.cpsrx.com

**Chew-Rite Company**
265 South Pioneer Boulevard
Springboro, OH 45066
(513) 746-5509

**Chiesi Pharmaceuticals, Inc**
150 Danbury Road
Ridgefield, CT 06877
(203) 438-3390

**Children's Hospital of Columbus**
700 Children's Drive
Columbus, OH 43205
(614) 722-2000
www.childrenshospital.columbus.oh.us

**Chilton Labs, Inc**
23 Fairfield Place
West Caldwell, NJ 07006
(973) 575-1990

**Chiron Corp**
4560 Horton Street
Emeryville, CA 94608-2916
(800) 244-7668
www.chiron.com

**Chronimed, Inc**
10900 Red Circle Drive
Minnetonka, MN 55343
(800) 444-5951
www.chronimed.com

**Ciba-Geigy Pharmaceuticals**
(see Novartis Pharmaceuticals)

**Ciba Vision Corp**
11460 Johns Creek Parkway
Duluth, GA 30097
(800) 845-6585
www.cibavision.com

**Circa Pharmaceuticals, Inc** (see Watson)

**Cirrus Healthcare Products, LLC**
PO Box 469
Locust Valley, NY 11560
(800) 327-6151
www.earplanes.com

**CIS-US, Inc**
10 DeAngelo Drive
Bedford, MA 01730
(800) 221-7554

**Claragen, Inc**
387 Technology Drive
College Park, MD 20742
(301) 405-8593
www.claragen.com

**Clay-Park Labs, Inc**
1700 Bathgate Avenue
Bronx, NY 10457
(800) 933-5550
www.claypark.com

**Clear Technologies**
10 Corbin Drive
Darien, CT 06820
(203) 655-9680
www.clearcare.com

**Clintec Nutrition**
3 Parkway North
Suite 500
(800) 422-2751
www.baxter.com

**Clint Pharmaceutical**
629 Shute Lane
Old Hickory, TN 63718
(800) 677-5022

**C & M Pharmacal, Inc**
1721 Maple Lane Avenue
Hazel Park, MI 48030-1215
(800) 423-5173

**CNS, Inc**
PO Box 1985
South Hackensack, NJ 07606
(877) 553-4237
www.cns.com

**Coast Labs, Inc**
521 West 17th Street
Long Beach, CA 90813-1513

**Colgate Oral Pharmaceuticals**
One Colgate Way
Canton, MA 02021
(800) 962-2345
www.colgate.com/pro/index.html

**Colgate-Palmolive Company**
300 Park Avenue
New York, NY 10022
(800) 221-4607
www.colgate.com

**CollaGenex Pharmaceuticals, Inc**
41 University Drive
Suite 200
Newtown, PA 18940
(888) 339-5678
www.collegenex.com

**Columbia Laboratories, Inc**
2875 Northeast 191st Street
Suite 400
Aventura, FL 33180
(800) 749-1919
www.columbialabs.com

**Combe, Inc**
1101 Westchester Avenue
White Plains, NY 10604
(800) 873-7400
www.combe.com

**Complimed Medical Research Group**
1441 West Smith Road
Ferndale, WA 98248
(888) 977-8008
www.complimed.com

**Conair Interplak Division**
One Cummings Point Road
Stamford, CT 06904
(800) 726-6247
www.conair.com

**Concord Laboratories**
140 New Dutch Lane
Fairfield, NJ 07704
(973) 227-6757

**Connaught Labs** (see Aventis Pasteur)

**Connetics Corp**
3294 West Bayshore Road
Palo Alto, CA 94303
(800) 280-2879
www.connetics.com

**Consep, Inc**
213 Southwest Columbia Street
Bend, OR 97702
(800) 367-8727
www.consep.com

**Consolidated Midland Corp**
20 Main Street
Brewster, NY 10509
(845) 279-6108

**Consumers Choice Systems, Inc**
2891 152nd Avenue Northeast
Redmond, WA 98052
(800) 479-5232
www.womenswellness-uti.com

**Continental Consumer Products**
770 Forest
Suite B
Birmingham, MI 48009
(800) 542-5903

**Continental Quest Research**
220 West Carmel Drive
Carmel, IN 46032
(800) 451-5773
contlquest@aol.com

**Contract Pharmacal Corp**
160 Commerce Drive
Hauppauge, NY 11788
(516) 231-4610

**ConvaTec**
**(Bristol-Myers Squibb Company)**
PO Box 5254
Princeton, NJ 08543-5254
(800) 422-8811
www.convatec.com

**Cooke Pharma, Inc**
1404 Old Country Road
Belmont, CA 94002
(888) 808-6838
www.cookepharma.com

**CooperVision**
200 Willowbrook Office Park
Fairport, NY 14450
(800) 538-7850
www.coopervision.com

**Copley Pharmaceutical**
**(Teva)**
25 John Road
Canton, MA 02021
(800) 325-6111
www.copleypharm.com

**Cord Labs** (see Geneva Pharmaceuticals)

**COR Therapeutics**
256 East Grand Avenue
South San Francisco, CA 94080
(888) 267-4633
www.corr.com

**Corixa**
1124 Columbia Street
Suite 200
Seattle, WA 98104
(206) 754-5711
www.corixa.com

**C. O. Truxton, Inc**
PO Box 1594
Camden, NJ 08101
(609) 365-4118

**Coulter Corp**
**(Beckman Coulter, Inc)**
11800 Southwest 147th Avenue
PO Box 169015
Miami, FL 33116
(800) 327-6531
www.coulter.com

**C. R. Bard, Inc**
**(Urological Division)**
8195 Industrial Boulevard
Covington, GA 30014
(800) 526-4455
www.bardmedical.com

**C. S. Dent & Company**
1820 Airport Exchange Boulevard
Erlanger, KY 41018
(800) 684-1468

**CTEX Pharmaceuticals, Inc**
PO Box 1549
Madison, MS 39130
(888) 898-0751
www.ctex.com

**Curatek Pharmaceuticals**
(see 3M Pharmaceuticals)

**Cutter Biologicals**
(see Bayer Corp, Biological and Pharmaceutical Division)

**CVS Procare Direct**
3651 Ridge Mill Drive
Columbia, OH 43026
(800) 252-6245

**Cyanotech Corp**
73-4460 Queen Kaahamanu Highway
Suite 102
Kailua-Kona, HI 96740
(800) 395-1353
www.cyanotech.com

**Cyclin Pharmaceuticals, Inc**
429 Gammon Place
Madison, WI 53715
(800) 982-1186
www.womenshealth.com

**Cygnus, Inc**
400 Penobscot Drive
Redwood City, CA 94063
(650) 369-4300
www.cygn.com

**Cynacon/OCuSOFT**
5311 Avenue North
Rosenburg, TX 77471
(800) 233-5469
www.ocusoft.com

**Cypress Pharmaceutical, Inc**
135 Industrial Boulevard
Madison, MS 39110
(800) 856-4393
www.cypressrx.com

**Cypros Pharmaceutical Corp**
(see Questcor Pharmaceuticals, Inc)

**Cytogen Corp**
600 College Road East
Princeton, NJ 08540
(800) 833-3533
www.cytogen.com

**Cytosol Laboratories**
55 Messina Drive
Braintree, MA 02184
(800) 288-3858

**CytRx Corp**
154 Technology Parkway
Suite 200
Norcross, GA 30092
(770) 368-9500
www.cytrx.com

**Daiichi Pharmaceutical Corp**
11 Philips Parkway
Montvale, NJ 07648
(877) 324-4244
www.daiichipharm.co.jp

**Dakryon Pharmaceuticals**
(see Medco Pharmaceuticals)

**Danbury Pharmacal, Inc**
**(Schein Pharmaceutical, Inc)**
131 West Street
Danbury, CT 06810
(203) 744-7200
www.schein-rx.com

**Danco Labs, LLC**
PO Box 4816
New York, NY 10185
(877) 432-7596

**Daniels Pharmaceuticals, Inc**
(see Jones Pharma)

**Dartmouth Pharmaceuticals, Inc**
**(Elan)**
38 Church Avenue
Wareham, MA 02571
(800) 414-3566
www.ilovemynails.com

**Davis and Geck** (see Kendall Healthcare)

**Davol, Inc**
100 Sockanossett Crossroad
Cranston, RI 02920
(401) 463-7000
www.davol.com

**Dayton Laboratories**
3337 Northwest 74th Avenue
Miami, FL 33122
(800) 446-0255
www.daytonlab.com

**Deacrin Corp Development**
Building 96 13th Street
Charlestown, MA 02129
(617) 242-9100

**Debio Pharm**
1747 Pennsylvania Ave Northwest
Suite 300
Washington, DC 20006
(703) 751-7777

**Degussa Corp**
379 Enterpace Parkway
Parsippany, NJ 07054-0677
(877) 273-2668
www.degussa.com

**Del Laboratories, Inc**
178 EAB Plaza
Uniondale, NY 11556
(800) 952-5080
www.dellabs.com

**Delmont Laboratories, Inc**
715 Harvard Avenue
PO Box 269
Swarthmore, PA 19081
(800) 562-5541
www.delmont.com

**Del-Ray Laboratories, Inc**
22-20th Avenue Northwest
Birmingham, AL 35215
(205) 853-8247

**Denison Labs, Inc**
60 Dunnell Lane
Pawtucket, RI 02862
(401) 723-5500

**Den-Mat Corp**
2727 Skyway Drive
Santa Maria, CA 93455
(800) 445-0345
www.den-mat.com

**Dental Herb Company**
Tower Suite 6900
405 Lexington Avenue
New York, NY 10174
(800) 747-4372

**DepoTech Corp**
**(SkyePharma)**
10450 Science Center Drive
Suite 100
San Diego, CA 92121
(619) 625-2424
www.skyepharma.com

**Derma Science**
214 Carnegie Center
Suite 100
Princeton, NJ 08540
(800) 825-4325
www.dermasciences.com

**Dermik Laboratories**
500 Arcola Road
Collegeville, PA 19426-0107
(800) 523-6674
www.dermik.com

**DeRoyal Industries, Inc**
200 DeBusk Lane
Powell, TN 37849
(800) 337-6925

**DexGen Pharmaceuticals**
PO Box 675
Manasquan, NJ 08736
(877) DEXGEN1

**Déy Laboratories**
2751 Napa Valley Corporate Drive
Napa, CA 94558
(800) 755-5560
www.deyinc.com

**Diacrin**
Building 96 13th Street
Charlestown, MA 02129
(617) 242-9100

**DiaPharma Group, Inc**
8948 Beckett Road
West Chester, OH 45069-2939
(800) 526-5224
www.diapharma.com

**Diatide, Inc**
9 Delta Drive
Londonderry, NH 03053
(603) 437-8970
www.diatide.com

**Dickinson Brands, Inc**
31 East High Street
East Hampton, CT 06424
(888) 860-2279

**Digestive Care, Inc**
1120 Win Drive
Bethlehem, PA 18017
(610) 882-5950

**Discovery Laboratories, Inc**
350 South Main Street
Suite 307
Doylestown, PA 18901
(215) 340-4699
www.discoverylabs.com

**Discus Dental, Inc**
8550 Higuera Street
Culver City, CA 90232
(800) 273-2847
www.discusdental.com

**Dista Products Company**
(see Eli Lilly)

**DJ Pharma, Inc**
12730 High Bluff Drive
Suite 160
San Diego, CA 92130
(877) 357-4276

**Doak Dermatologics**
383 Route 46 West
Fairfield, NJ 07004-2402
(800) 405-3625
www.bradpharm.com

**Donell DerMedex**
342 Madison Avenue
Suite 1422
New York, NY 10173
(212) 697-3800
www.CxProducts.com

**Dow Hickam, Inc**
(see Bertek Pharmaceuticals, Inc)

**Dreir Pharmaceuticals, Inc**
9602 North 122nd Place
Scottsdale, AZ 85259
(800) 541-4044
www.dreirpharmaceuticals.com

**DuPont Pharmaceuticals Company**
974 Centre Road
Room 158
Wilmington, DE 19805
(800) 474-2762
www.dupontpharma.com

**Duramed Pharmaceuticals**
5040 Duramed Drive
Cincinnati, OH 45213
(800) 543-8338
www.duramed.com

**Dura Pharmaceuticals**
7475 Lusk Boulevard
San Diego, CA 92121-4202
(800) 859-8585
www.durapharm.com

**Durex Consumer Products**
3585 Engineering Drive
Suite 200
Norcross, GA 30092
(888) 566-3468
www.durex.com

**Durham Pharmacal Corp**
Route 145
Oak Hill, NY 12460
(888) 438-7426

**DUSA Pharmaceuticals, Inc**
25 Upton Drive
Wilmington, MA 01887
(978) 657-7500
www.dusapharma.com

**DynaGen, Inc** (see Able Labs)

**Eagle Vison, Inc**
6263 Poplar Avenue
Suite 650
Memphis, TN 38119
(800) 222-7584
www.eaglevis.com

**(Eastman) Kodak Company**
10 Indigo Creek Drive
Rochester, NY 14650-0862
(800) 242-2424
www.kodak.com

**Eaton Medical Corp**
1401 Heistan Place
Memphis, TN 38104
(800) 253-4740

**Eckerd Drug Corp**
PO Box 4689
Clearwater, FL 33758
(800) 325-3737
www.eckerd.com

**Ecological Formulas, Inc**
1061-B Shary
Concord, CA 94518
(800) 888-4585

**Econolab**
PO Box 85543
Westland, MI 48185-0543
(561) 391-5245

**EconoMed Pharmaceuticals**
4305 Sartin Road
Burlington, NC 27217-7522
(800) 327-6007

**ECR Pharmaceuticals**
3981 Deep Rock Road
Richmond, VA 23233
(800) 527-1955

**Edwards Pharmaceuticals, Inc**
111 Mulberry Street
Ripley, MS 38663
(800) 543-9560

**Effcon Laboratories**
1800 Sandy Plains Parkway
Marietta, GA 30066-7499
(800) 722-2428
www.effcon.com

**E. Fougera & Company**
60 Baylis Road
Melville, NY 11747
(800) 645-9833
www.fougera.com

**Eisai, Inc**
500 Frank W. Burr Boulevard
Teaneck, NJ 07666
(888) 793-4724

**Elan Pharmaceuticals**
800 Gateway Boulevard
South San Francisco, CA 94080
(888) 638-7605
www.elanpharma.com

**Eli Lilly & Company**
Lilly Corporate Center
Indianapolis, IN 46285
(800) 545-5979
www.elililly.com

**Elkins-Sinn, Inc** (see Wyeth-Ayerst)

**Emerson Laboratories**
7400 Alumax Drive
Texarkana, TX 75501
(800) 662-3435

**EM Industries, Inc**
7 Skyline Drive
Hawthorne, NY 10532
(800) 831-3662
www.emindustries.com

**Enamelon, Inc**
7 Cedar Brook Drive
Cranbury, NJ 08512
(888) 432-3535

**Endo Pharmaceuticals, Inc**
223 Wilmington Westchester Pike
Chadds Ford, PA 19317
(800) 462-3636
www.endo.com

**EnviroDerm Pharmaceuticals, Inc**
PO Box 32370
Louisville, KY 40232-2370
(800) 991-3376

**Enzon, Inc**
20 Kingsbridge Road
Piscataway, NJ 08854-3998
(732) 980-4500
www.enzon.com

**Eon Labs Manufacturing, Inc**
227-15 North Conduit Avenue
Laurelton, NY 11413
(800) 526-0225
www.eonlabs.com

**Epitope, Inc**
8505 Southwest Creekside Place
Beaverton, OR 97008
(800) 234-3786
www.epitope.com

**E. R. Squibb & Sons, Inc**
(see Bristol-Myers Squibb)

**ESI Lederle Generics**
PO Box 8299
Philadelphia, PA 19101-8299
(610) 688-4400
www.ahp.com

**Ethex Corp**
10888 Metro Court
St Louis, MO 63043-2413
(800) 321-1705
www.ethex.com

**Ethicon, Inc**
**(Johnson & Johnson)**
US Route 22 West
PO Box 151
Somerville, NJ 08876-0151
(800) 255-2500
www.ethiconinc.com

**Eurand America, Inc**
845 Center Drive
Vandalia, OH 45377
(937) 898-9669

**Everett Laboratories, Inc**
29 Spring Street
West Orange, NJ 07052
(973) 324-0200
www.everettlabs.com

**E-Z-EM**
717 Main Street
Westbury, NY 11590
(800) 544-4624

**Falcon Ophthalmics, Inc**
6201 South Freeway
Fort Worth, TX 76134
(800) 343-2133
www.alconlabs.com

**Farmacon, Inc**
90 Grove Street
Suite 109
Ridgefield, CT 06877-4118
(203) 431-9989

**Faro Pharmaceuticals, Inc**
4287 A Beltline Road LB351
Addison, TX 75244
(800) 480-1985

**Faulding USA**
200 Elmora Avenue
Elizabeth, NJ 07207
(800) 432-8534
www.faulding.com/au

**Female Health Company**
875 North Michigan Avenue
Suite 3660
Chicago, IL 60611-9267
(800) 635-0844
www.femalehealth.com

**Feminique Corp**
990 Station Road
Bellport, NY 11713
(516) 286-5900
www.feminique.com

**Ferndale Laboratories, Inc**
780 West Eight Mile Road
Ferndale, MI 48220-1218
(800) 621-6003

**Ferring Pharmaceuticals, Inc**
120 White Plains Road
Suite 400
Tarrytown, NY 10591
(888) 337-7464
www.ferringusa.com

**Fibertone** (see Naturally Vitamins Company)

**Fidia Pharmaceutical Corp**
2000 K Street Northwest
Suite 700
Washington, DC 20006
(202) 371-9898
www.fidiapharma.com

**Fielding Pharmaceutical Company**
11551 Adie Road
Maryland Heights, MO 63043
(800) 776-3435
www.fieldingcompany.com

**First Horizon Pharmaceutical Corp**
660 Hembree Parkway
Suite 106
Roswell, GA 30076
(800) 849-9707
www.horizonpharm.com

**First Scientific, Inc**
Lake Forest Plaza
2222 Francisco Drive 510-174
El Dorado Hills, CA 95762
(800) 767-2208

**Fischer Pharmaceuticals, Inc**
3707 Williams Road
San Jose, CA 95117
(800) 782-0222
www.dr-fischer.com

**Fiske Industries**
527 Route 303
Orangeburg, NY 10962
(800) 248-8033
www.irenegari.com

**Fisons Corp** (see Celltech)

**Flanders, Inc**
PO Box 39143
Charleston, SC 29407-9143
(843) 571-3363

**Fleming & Company**
1733 Gilsinn Lane
Fenton, MO 63026-2918
(636) 343-8200
www.flemingco.com

**Fluoritab Corp**
8151 Brentwood Lane
Temperance, MI 48182-0507
(734) 847-3985

**Forest/Inwood Laboratories Inc**
500 Commack Road
Commack, NY 11725-5000

**Forest Pharmaceutical, Inc**
13600 Shoreline Drive
St Louis, MO 63045
(800) 678-1605
www.forestpharm.com

**Forte Pharma**
220 Lake Drive
Newark, DE 19702
(877) 993-6783

**Fournier Research**
9 Law Drive
Fairfield, NY 07004
(973) 575-1010

**Freeda Vitamins, Inc**
36 East 41st Street
New York, NY 10017-6203
(800) 777-3737
www.imall.com/stores/freeda

**Free Radical Sciences, Inc**
245 First Street
Cambridge, MA 02142
(617) 374-1200

**Fuisz Technologies, Ltd**
3701 Concorde
Suite 800
Chantilly, VA 20151
(703) 803-3260

**Fujisawa Healthcare, Inc**
3 Parkway North Center
Deerfield, IL 60015-2548
(800) 888-7704
www.fujisawa.com

**Galagen Nutrition Medical, Inc**
4001 Lexington Avenue North
PO Box 64314
St Paul, MN 55164-0314
(800) 569-7828
www.galagen.com

**Galderma Laboratories, Inc**
14501 North Freeway
Fort Worth, TX 76177
(800) 582-8225
www.galderma.com

**Gallipot, Inc**
2020 Silver Bell Road
St Paul, MN 55122
(800) 423-6967

**Gambro, Inc**
810 Collins Avenue
Lakewood, CO 80215
(800) 525-2623
www.gambro.com

**Gate Pharmaceuticals**
650 Chethill
Sellerville, PA 18960
(800) 292-4283
www.tevapharmusa.com

**Gebauer Company**
9410 St Catherine Avenue
Cleveland, OH 44104
(800) 321-9348
www.gebauerco.com

**Geigy Pharmaceuticals**
(see Novartis Pharmaceuticals)

**Gel-Tech**
6430 Varil Avenue
Suite 102B
Woodland Hills, CA 91367
(877) 942-2626

**GenDerm Corp** (see Medicis)

**Gen-King** (see Kinray)

**Genentech, Inc**
One DNA Way
South San Francisco, CA 94080
(800) 551-2231
www.gene.com

**General Injectables & Vaccines**
US Highway 52 South
PO Box 9
Bastian, VA 24314-0009
(540) 688-4121
www.giv.com

**General Medical Corp**
8741 Landmark Road
Richmond, VA 23261
(800) 753-4633
www.mckgenmed.com

**General Nutrition, Inc**
300 6th Avenue
Pittsburgh, PA 15222
(888) 462-2548
www.gnc.com

**Genesis Nutrition**
1816 Wall Street
Florence, SC 29501
(800) 451-7933
www.genesisnutrition.com

**Genetco, Inc**
711 Union Parkway
Ronkonkama, NY 11779

**Genetics Institute**
87 Cambridge Park Drive
Cambridge, MA 02140
(888) 446-3344

**Genetic Therapy, Inc**
938 Clopper Road
Gaithersburg, MD 20878
(301) 590-2626

**Geneva Pharmaceuticals, Inc**
2655 West Midway Boulevard
PO Box 446
Broomfield, CO 80038-0446
(800) 525-8747
www.genevarx.com

**Geneva Pharmaceutical Technology Corp**
2400 Route 130N
Dayton, NJ 08810
(732) 274-2400

**GenPharm International, Inc (Medarex)**
2350 Qume Drive
San Jose, CA 95131-1807
(408) 526-1290
www.genpharm.com

**Gensia Automedics, Inc**
9360 Town Center Drive
San Diego, CA 92121
www.gensia.com

**Gensia Sicor Pharmaceuticals, Inc**
19 Hughes
Irvine, CA 92618
(800) 729-9991
www.gensiasicor.com

**GenVec, Inc**
65 West Watkins Mill Road
Gaithersburg. MD 20878
(240) 632-0740

**Genzyme Pharmaceuticals**
One Kendall Square
Cambridge, MA 02139
(617) 252-7500

**Geodesic MediTech, Inc**
2921 Sandy Pointe No. 3
Del Mar, CA 92014
(888) 357-9399

**Gerber Products Company**
445 State Street
Fremont, MI 49413-0001
(800) 443-7237

**Geriatric Pharmaceutical Corp**
(see Roberts Pharmaceuticals)

**Gilead Sciences**
333 Lakeside Drive
Foster City, CA 94404
(800) 445-3235
www.gilead.com

**Glades Pharmaceuticals**
500 Satellite Boulevard
Suwanee, GA 30174
(888) 4-GLADES
www.glades.com

**GlaxoSmithKline**
5 Moore Drive
PO Box 13398
Research Triangle Park, NC 27709
(888) 825-5249
www.gsk.com

**GlaxoWellcome, Inc** (see GlaxoSmithKline)

**Glenwood, LLC**
19 Empire Boulevard
South Hackensack, NJ 07606
(201) 221-0050
www.glenwood-llc.com

**Glenwood-Palisades**
One New England Avenue
Piscataway, NJ 08855

**Global Pharmaceuticals, Inc**
3735 Castor Avenue
Philadelphia, PA 19124
(215) 289-2220
www.globalphar.com

**Global Source**
3001 North 29th Street
Hollywood, FL 33020
(800) 662-7556
www.globalvitamin.com

**GML Industries, LLC**
Denison, TX 75020
(877) 828-4633
www.gml-industries.com

**GM Pharmaceutical**
PO Box 150312
Arlington, TX 76015
(817) 461-8230

**Goldenstate Medical Supply**
27644 North Newhall Ranch Road
Suite 40
Valencia, CA 91355
(800) 284-8633

**Goldline Consumer**
1900 West Commercial Boulevard
Fort Lauderdale, FL 33309
(800) 327-4114

**Goldline Laboratories, Inc**
(see Zenith Goldline)

**Goody's Manufacturing Corp**
(see Block Drug Company, Inc)

**Gordon Laboratories**
6801 Ludlow Street
Upper Darby, PA 19082-2408
(800) 356-7870
www.gordonlabs.com

**Graham Field**
81 Spence Street
Bay Shore, NY 11706
(800) 645-1023
www.grahamfield.com

**Grandpa Brands Company**
1820 Airport Exchange Boulevard
Erlanger, KY 41018
(800) 684-1468
www.grandpabrands.com

**Gray Pharmaceutical Company** (see Purdue Frederick)

**Great American Nutrition**
2002 South 5070 West
Salt Lake City, UT 84104
(800) 223-5326

**Great Southern Laboratories**
10863 Rockley Road
Houston, TX 77099
(281) 530-3077

**Greenstone Limited**
**(Pharmacia)**
8225 Moors Bridge Road
Portage, MI 49002
(800) 447-3360
www.pnu.com

**Green Turtle Bay Vitamin Company**
56 High Street
Summit, NJ 07901
(800) 887-8535
www.energywave.com

**Greer Laboratories, Inc**
639 Nuway Circle
PO Box 800
Lenoir, NC 28645-0800
(800) 438-0088
www.greerlabs.com

**Guardian Drug Company**
72 Prince Street
Trenton, NJ 08638

**Guardian Laboratories**
230 Marcus Boulevard
Hauppauge, NY 11788
(800) 645-5566
www.u-g.com

**Guilford Pharmaceuticals, Inc**
6611 Tributary Street
Baltimore, MD 21224
(800) 453-3746
www.guilford.com

**Gum-Tech Industries, Inc**
246 East Watkins
Phoenix, AZ 85004
(800) 676-4769

**G & W Laboratories**
111 Coolidge Street
South Plainfield, NJ 07080
(800) 922-1038
www.gwlabs.com

**Gynetics**
PO Box 8509
Somerville, NJ 08876
(800) 311-7378
www.gynetics.com

**Gynex** (see BTG)

**Halocarbon Products Corp**
887 Kinderkamack Road
River Edge, NJ 07661
(201) 262-8899
http://halocarbon.com/

**Halsey Drug Company** (see Watson)

**Hannan Ophthalmic Marketing Services, Inc**
163 Meetinghouse Road
Duxbury, MA 02332
(781) 834-8111

**Harmony Laboratories**
1109 South Main
Landis, NC 28088
(800) 245-6284
www.harmonylabs.com

**Hart Health & Safety**
4310 South 131st Place
Seattle, WA 98168
(800) 234-4278

**Harvard Drug Group**
Oxford, MS 38655
(601) 234-0130

**Hauser Pharmaceutical, Inc**
4401 East US Highway 30
Valparaiso, IN 46383-9573
(800) 441-2309
www.hauserpharmaceutical.com

**Hawthorn Pharmaceuticals, Inc**
(see Cypress Pharmaceuticals)

**HDC Corp**
2109 O'Toole Avenue
San Jose, CA 95131
(800) 227-8162
www.hdccorp.com

**Health Care Products**
369 Bayview Avenue
Amityville, NY 11701
(800) 899-3116

**Healthfirst Corp**
22316 70th Avenue West
Unit A
Mountlake Terrace, WA 98043-2184
(800) 331-1984

**Health for Life Brands, Inc**
1643 East Genesee Street
Syracuse, NY 13210
(800) 448-5255

**Healthline Laboratories, Inc**
2805 Danbar Drive
Green Bay, WI 54313
(715) 434-9710

**Health-Mark Diagnostics**
3333 Southwest 15th Street
Pompano Beach, FL 33069
(954) 979-0400
www.health-mark.com

**Health & Medical Techniques**
(see Graham Field)

**Healthpoint Medical**
2600 Airport Freeway
Fort Worth, TX 76111
(800) 441-8227
www.healthpoint.com

**Health Products Corp**
1060 NepperHan
Yonkers, NY 10703
(914) 423-2900

**Heartland Healthcare Services**
4755 South Avenue
Toledo, OH 43615

**Helena Laboratories**
1530 Lindbergh Drive
Beaumont, TX 77707
(800) 231-5663
www.helena.com

**Hemacare Corp**
4954 Van Nuys Boulevard
Sherman Oaks, CA 91403
(888) 481-1538
www.hemacare.com

**Hemagen Diagnostics, Inc**
9033 Red Branch Road
Columbia, MD 21045
(800) 495-2180
www.hemagen.com

**Hemispherx**
One Penn Center
1617 John F. Kennedy Boulevard
Suite 660
Philadelphia, PA 19103
(215) 988-8800
www.hemispherx.com

**Hemotec Medical Products, Inc**
PO Box 19255
Johnston, RI 02919
(401) 934-2571

**Henry Schein, Inc**
135 Duryea Road
Melville, NY 11747
(800) 472-4346
www.henryschein.com

**Herald Pharmacal, Inc** (see Allergan, Inc)

**Herbert Laboratories** (see Allergan, Inc)

**Hercon Laboratories, Inc**
460 Park Avenue
New York, NY 10022
(212) 751-5600

**Heritage Consumer Products, LLC**
Brookfield Commons
Suite CL-41
246 Federal Road
Brookfield, CT 06804
(800) 797-7969
www.cnewsusa.com

**H & H Laboratories**
4701 25 Mile Road
Shelby Township, MI 48316

**Hill Dermaceuticals, Inc**
2650 South Mellonville Avenue
Sanford, FL 32773
(800) 344-5707

**Himmel Pharmaceuticals, Inc**
1926 10th Avenue North
Suite 303
Lake Worth, FL 33461
(800) 535-3823

**Hind Health Care, Inc**
3707 Williams Road
Suite 101
Campbell, CA 96117
(408) 615-4140

**Hi-Tech Pharmaceutical, Inc**
369 Bayview Avenue
Amityville, NY 11701
(800) 262-9010
www.diabeticproducts.com

**H. L. Moore Drug Exchange, Inc**
(see Moore Medical Corp)

**Hoechst-Marion Roussel, Inc** (see Aventis)

**Hoechst-Roussel**
(see Hoechst Marion Roussel)

**Hoffmann-LaRoche**
(see Roche Laboratories)

**Hogil Pharmaceutical Corp**
2 Manhattanville Road
Purchase, NY 10577
(914) 696-7600
www.hogil.com

**Holles Laboratories, Inc**
30 Forest Notch
Cohasset, MA 02025-1198
(800) 356-4015

**Hollister-Stier Laboratories LLC**
3525 North Regal Street
Spokane, WA 99207-5788
(800) 992-1120
www.hollister-stier.com

**Home Access Health Corp**
2401 West Hassell Road
Suite 1510
Hoffman Estates, IL 60195-5200
(847) 781-2500
www.homeaccess.com

**Hope Pharmaceuticals**
8260 East Gelding Drive
Suite 104
Scottsdale, AZ 85260
(800) 755-9595
www.hopepharm.com

**Horizon Pharmaceutical Corp**
(see First Horizon Pharmaceutical)

**Huckaby Pharmacal, Inc**
6316 Old La Grange Road
Crestwood, KY 40014
(888) 206-5525
www.huckabypharmacal.com

**Humco Holding Group, Inc**
7400 Alumax
Texarkana, TX 75501
(800) 662-3435

**Hybritech**
PO Box 269006
San Diego, CA 92196-9006
(800) 854-1957
www.beckmancoulter.com

**Hyland Immuno**
**(Baxter)**
550 North Brand Boulevard
Glendale, CA 91203
(800) 423-2090
http://baxdb1.baxter.com

**Hyland Laboratories, Inc**
**(Standard Homeopathic Company)**
210 West 131st Street
Los Angeles, CA 90061
(800) 624-9659
www.hylands.com

**Hyland Therapeutics**
(see Baxter Hyland Immuno)

**Hynson, Westcott & Dunning**
(see Becton Dickinson Microbiology Systems)

**Hyrex Pharmaceuticals**
3494 Democrat Road
Memphis, TN 38118
(800) 238-5282

**ICI Pharmaceuticals**
(see Zeneca Pharmaceuticals)

**ICN Canada Ltd**
Montreal, Quebec Canada

**ICN Pharmaceuticals, Inc**
3300 Hyland Avenue
Costa Mesa, CA 92626
(800) 556-1937
www.icnpharm.com

**IDEC Pharmaceuticals**
11011 Torreyana Road
San Diego, CA 92121
(858) 431-8500

**Ilex Oncology, Inc**
14960 Omicron Drive
San Antonio, TX 78245
(210) 667-8000
www.ilexonc.com

**Immcel Pharmaceuticals, Inc**
79-55 Albion Avenue
Elmhurst, NY 11373

**Immucell Corp**
56 Evergreen Drive
Portland, ME 04103
(207) 878-2770
www.immucell.com

**Immunex Corp**
51 University Street
Seattle, WA 98101-2936
(800) 466-8639
www.immunex.com

**Immunobiology Research Institute**
Route 22 East
PO Box 999
Annandale, NJ 08801-0999
(908) 730-1700

**ImmunoGen**
148 Sidney Street
Cambridge, MA 02139
(617) 497-1113
www.immunogen.com

**Immunomedics, Inc**
300 American Road
Morris Plains, NJ 07950
(973) 605-8200
www.immunomedics.com

**Immuno-US, Inc**
(see Baxter Healthcare Corp)

**Impax Laboratories, Inc**
30831 Huntwood Avenue
Hayward, CA 95444
(510) 471-3600

**I.M.S., Ltd** (see Medeva)

**IMX Pharmaceuticals, Inc**
2295 Corporate Boulevard
Boca Raton, FL 33431
(561) 998-5660
www.imxn.com

**Infusaid, Inc** (see Aero International)

**InKine Pharmaceutical Company, Inc**
1787 Sentry Parkway
West Building 18
Suite 440
Blue Bell, PA 19422
(215) 283-6850

**Inner Health Group**
6203 Woodlake Center
San Antonio, TX 78244
(800) 381-4697

**INO Therapeutics, Inc**
54 Old Highway 22
Clinton, NJ 08809
(908) 238-6600

**Inspire Pharmaceuticals, Inc**
4222 Emperor Boulevard
Suite 470
Durham, NC 27703
(919) 941-9777
www.inspirepharm.com

**Interchem Corp**
120 Route 17 North
Suite 115
PO Box 1579
Paramus, NJ 07653
(800) 261-7332
www.interchem.com

**Interfalk US, Inc**
25 Margaret
Plattsburgh, NY 12901

**Interferon Sciences**
783 Jersey Avenue
New Brunswick, NJ 08901
(888) 728-4372
www.interferonsciences.com

**Intermax Pharmaceuticals, Inc**
228 Sherwood Avenue
Farmingdale, NY 11735
(631) 777-3318

**InterMune Pharmaceuticals, Inc**
1710 Gilbreth Road
Suite 301
Burlingame, CA 94010
(888) 696-8036

**International Laboratory Technology Corp**
3389 Sheridan Street
Suite 149
Hollywood, FL 33021
(954) 893-1118

**International Medication Systems, Ltd (IMS) (Amphastar Pharmaceuticals, Inc)**
1886 Santa Anita Avenue
South El Monte, CA 91733
(800) 423-4136
www.ims-limited.com

**Interneuron Pharmaceuticals, Inc**
One Ledgemont Center
99 Hayden Avenue
Lexington, MA 02421
(781) 861-8444
www.interneuron.com

**Interpharm, Inc**
3 Fairchild Avenue
Plainview, NY 11803

**Interstate Drug Exchange**
(see Henry Schein, Inc)

**Intramed**
102 Tremont Way
Augusta, GA 30907

**Invamed, Inc** (see Geneva Pharmaceuticals)

**Inveresk**
4470 Redwood Highway
San Rafael, CA 94903
(415) 491-6460
www.inveresk-research.com

**Inverness Medical**
200 Prospect Street
Waltham, MA 02154
(781) 647-3900

**Inwood Laboratories (Forest)**
321 Prospect Street
Inwood, NY 11096
(800) 284-6966

**Iolab Pharmaceuticals** (see Ciba Vision)

**Iomed**
7425 Pebble Drive
Fort Worth, TX 76118
(817) 589-7257
www.iomed.com

**ION Laboratories, Inc**
7431 Pebble Drive
Fort Worth, TX 76118
(817) 284-8044
www.ionlaboratories.com

**Iopharm**
7549 Pebble Drive
Fort Worth, TX 76118
(817) 284-8044

**IOP, Inc**
3151 Airway Avenue
Suite I-1
Costa Mesa, CA 92626
(800) 535-3545
www.iopinc.com

**Isis Pharmaceuticals**
2292 Faraday Avenue
Carlsbad, CA 92008
(760) 931-9200
www.isip.com

**Iso-Tex Diagnostics, Inc**
1511 County Road 129
Friendswood, TX 77546
(800) 447-4839

**Ivax Pharmaceuticals, Inc**
4400 Biscayne Boulevard
Miami, FL 33178
(800) 327-4114

**Ivy Corp**
23 Fairfield Place
West Caldwell, NJ 07006
(800) 443-8856

**Jacobus Pharmaceutical Company**
37 Cleveland Lane
Princeton, NJ 08540
(609) 921-7447

**Janssen Pharmaceutical**
1125 Trenton-Harbourton Road
Titusville, NJ 08560-0200
(800) 526-7736
www.janssen.com

**J. B. Williams Company, Inc**
65 Harristown Road
3rd Floor
Glen Rock, NJ 07452-3317
(800) 254-8656

**Jerome Stevens Pharmaceuticals, Inc**
60 Da Vinci Drive
Bohemia, NY 11716
(631) 567-1113

**J. J. Balan, Inc**
5725 Foster Avenue
Brooklyn, NY 11234
(800) 552-2526
www.jjbalan.com

**J & J Merck Consumer Pharmaceutical Company**
Camp Hill Road
Fort Washington, PA 19034
(800) 523-3484
www.jnj-merck.com

**JMI-Canton Pharmaceuticals**
(see Jones Pharma)

**Johnson & Johnson**
One Johnson & Johnson Plaza
New Brunswick, NJ 08933
(732) 524-0400
www.jnj.com

**Jones Pharma, Inc**
1945 Craig Road
St Louis, MO 63146-6903
(800) 525-8466
www.jmedpharma.com

**J. R. Carlson Laboratories**
15 College Drive
Arlington Heights, IL 60004-1985
(888) 234-5656
www.carlsonlabs.com

**J. T. Baker, Inc** (see Mallinckrodt-Baker)

**KabiVitrum, Inc** (see Pharmacia)

**Kanetta Pharmacal**
90 Park Avenue
New York, NY 10016
(800) 372-6634

**Keene Pharmaceuticals, Inc**
303 South Mockingbird
Keene, TX 76059-0007
(800) 541-0530

**Kendall Health Care Products**
15 Hampshire Street
Mansfield, MA 02048
(508) 261-8000
www.kendallhq.com

**Kendall-McGaw Labs, Inc** (see B. Braun)

**Kenwood Laboratories**
(see Doak Dermatologics)

**Key Pharmaceuticals** (see Schering Plough)

**Kiel Laboratories, Inc**
Gainesville, GA 30504
(770) 534-0079

**King Pharmaceuticals, Inc**
501 Fifth Street
Bristol, TN 37620
(800) 776-3637
www.kingpharm.com

**Kingswood Laboratories, Inc**
10375 Hague Road
Indianapolis, IN 46256
(800) 968-7772

**Kinray**
152-35 10th Avenue
Whitestone, NY 11357
(800) 854-6729

**Kirkman Laboratories, Inc**
PO Box 1009
Wilsonville, OR 97070-1009
(800) 245-8282

**Kiwi Brands, Inc**
447 Old Swede Road
Douglassville, PA 19518-1239
(610) 385-3041

**KLI Corp**
1119 Third Avenue Southwest
Carmel, IN 46032
(800) 308-7452
www.entertainers-secret.com

**Knoll Pharmaceuticals**
3000 Continental Drive North
Mt Olive, NJ 07828-1234
(800) 526-0221
www.basf.com

**Konsyl Pharmaceuticals, Inc**
4200 South Hulen
Suite 513
Fort Worth, TX 76109
(800) 356-6795
www.konsyl.com

**Kos Pharmaceutics, Inc**
1001 Brickell Bay Drive
25th Floor
Miami, FL 33131
(305) 577-3464
www.kospharm.com

**Kramer Laboratories, Inc**
8778 Southwest 8th Street
Miami, FL 33174-9990
(800) 824-4894
www.kramerlabs.com

**Kremers Urban**
PO Box 427
Mequon, WI 53092
(800) 625-5710

**K-Tech USA, Inc**
80 Southwest 8th Street
Miami, FL 33130
(305) 372-3363
ww.ktechusa.com

**K. V. Pharmaceutical Company**
2503 South Hanley Road
St Louis, MO 63144
(314) 645-6600

**Lacrimedics, Inc**
PO Box 1209
Eastsound, WA 98245
(800) 367-8327
www.lacrimedics.com

**Lactaid, Inc**
7050 Camp Hill Road
Fort Washington, PA 19034
(800) 522-8243
www.lactaid.com

**Lafayette Pharmaceuticals, Inc**
526 North Earl Avenue
Lafayette, IN 47904-2819
(800) 428-7843
www.lafayettepharm.com

**La Haye Laboratories, Inc**
2205 152nd Avenue Northeast
Redmond, WA 98052
(800) 344-2020
www.lahaye.com

**Lake Consumer Products**
625 Forest Edge Drive
Vernon Hills, IL 60061
(800) 635-3696

**Lannett Company, Inc**
9000 State Road
Philadelphia, PA 19136
(800) 325-9994
www.lannett.com

**Laser, Inc**
2200 West 97th Place
Crown Point, IN 46307
(800) 325-0925

**Lavoptik Company, Inc**
661 Western Avenue
St Paul, MN 55103
(612) 489-1351

**LecTec Corp**
10701 Red Circle Drive
Minnetonka, MN 55343
(877) 587-2824
www.lectec.com

**Lederle Consumer Health & Pharmaceutical Division**
North Middletown Road
Pearl River, NY 10965-1299
(800) 322-3129

**Lederle-Praxis Biologicals**
555 East Lancaster Avenue
St Davids, PA 19087
(800) 999-9384

**Leeming**
(see Pfizer US Pharmaceutical Group)

**Lee Pharmaceuticals**
1434 Santa Anita Boulevard
South Elmonte, CA 91733
(800) 950-5337
www.leepharma.com

**Legere Pharmaceuticals, Inc**
7326 East Evans Road
Scottsdale, AZ 85260
(800) 528-3144

**Lehn & Fink** (see Reckitt & Colman)

**Leiner Health Products**
901 East 233rd Street
Carson, CA 90745
(310) 835-8400
www.leiner.com

**Leiras Pharmaceuticals, Inc**
2345 Waukegan Road
Suite N-135
Bonnockburn, IL 60015

**Lemmon Company** (see Teva Pharmaceuticals)

**Life Cycle Ventures, Inc**
220 Lake Drive
Newark, DE 19702
(866) 645-4528

**LifeScan, Inc**
**(Johnson & Johnson Company)**
1000 Gibraltar Drive
Milpitas, CA 95035-6312
(800) 227-8862
www.lifescan.com

**LifeSign LLC**
71 Veronica Avenue
PO Box 218
Somerset, NJ 08875-0218
(800) 526-2125
www.lifesignmed.com

**Ligand Pharmaceuticals, Inc**
10275 Science Center Drive
San Diego, CA 92121
(800) 964-5836
www.ligand.com

**Lilly & Company** (see Eli Lilly)

**Lincoln Diagnostics**
PO Box 1128
Decatur, IL 62525
(217) 877-2531

**Lipha Pharmaceuticals, Inc**
1114 Avenue of the Americas
New York, NY 10036-7703
(800) 547-4299

**Liposome Company**
One Research Way
Princeton, NJ 08540
(800) 335-5476
www.liposome.com

**LNK International, Inc**
60 Arkay Drive
Hauppauge, NY 11788
(631) 435-3500

**Lobana Laboratories**
**(Ulmer Pharmacal)**
2440 Fernbrook Lane
Plymouth, MN 55447
(800) 848-5637

**Loch Pharmaceuticals**
(see Bedford Laboratories)

**L'Oreal Suncare Research**
575 Fifth Avenue
26th Floor
New York, NY 10017
(212) 984-4109

**Lorvic Corp** (see Young Dental Mfg)

**Lotus Biochemical Corp**
7335 Lee Highway
Radford, VA 24141
(423) 989-9192

**L. Perrigo Company**
515 Eastern Avenue
Allegan, MI 49010
www.perrigo.com

**LSI America Corp**
4732 Twin Valley Drive
Austin, TX 78731-3537
(800) 720-5936
www.ondrox.com

**Luitpold Pharmaceuticals, Inc**
One Luitpold Drive
Shirley, NY 11967
(516) 924-4000

**Lyne Laboratories**
10 Burke Drive
Brockton, MA 02401
(800) 525-0450

**Lyphomed** (see Fujisawa)

**3M Pharmaceuticals**
3M Center
Building 275-3W-01
St Paul, MN 55133
(800) 328-0255
3m.com/pharma

**Magno-Humphries Laboratories, Inc**
8800 Southwest Commercial Street
Tigard, OR 97223
(503) 684-5464

**Major Pharmaceuticals, Inc**
31778 Enterprise Drive
Livonia, MI 48150
(800) 688-9696

**Mallinckrodt Baker, Inc**
222 Red School Lane
Phillipsburg, NJ 08865
(908) 859-2151
www.mallinckrodt.com

**Mallinckrodt Chemical**
16305 Swingley Ridge Drive
Chesterfield, MO 63017
(800) 325-8888
www.mallinckrodt.com

**Mallinckrodt, Inc**
**(Corp Headquarters)**
675 McDonnell Boulevard
Hazelwood, MO 63042
(888) 744-1414
www.mallinckrodt.com

**Manloe Labs, Inc**
6320 South Sandhill Road
Suite 10
Las Vegas, NV 89120
(800) 777-4876

**Manne**
PO Box 825
Johns Island, SC 29457
(800) 517-0228

**Marathon Biopharmaceuticals**
97 South Street
Hopkinton, MA 01748
(508) 497-0700
www.marathonbio.com

**Marion Merrell Dow**
(see Hoechst Marion Roussel)

**Marlex Pharmaceuticals, Inc**
50 McCullough Drive
Southgate Center
New Castle, DE 10135
(302) 328-3355

**Marlin Industries**
PO Box 560
Grover City, CA 93483-0560
(800) 423-5926

**Marlop Pharmaceuticals, Inc**
230 Marshall Street
Elizabeth, NJ 07206
(908) 355-8854

**Marlyn Nutraceuticals, Inc**
14851 North Scottsdale Road
Scottsdale, AZ 85254
(800) 462-7596

**Marnel Pharmaceuticals, Inc**
206 Luke Drive
Lafayette, LA 70506
(337) 232-1396

**Marsam Pharmaceuticals, Inc**
24 Olney Avenue
Building 31
Cherry Hill, NJ 08034
(800) 883-2600
www.schein-rx.com

**Martec Pharmaceutical, Inc**
**(Ratiopharm, GmbH)**
1800 North Topping Avenue
Kansas City, MO 64120-3510
(800) 822-6782
www.martec-kc.com

**Mason Pharmaceuticals, Inc**
4425 Jamboree Road
Suite 250
Newport Beach, CA 92660
(800) 366-2454

**Mason Vitamins, Inc**
5105 Northwest 159th Street
Miami Lakes, FL 33014-6370
(800) 327-6005

**Massachusetts Public Health Biological Laboratories**
305 South Street
Jamaica Plains, MA 02130-3597
(617) 983-6400

**Matrix Pharmaceutical, Inc**
34700 Campus Drive
Fremont, CA 94555
(510) 742-9900
www.matx.com

**Mayo Foundation**
200 1st Street Southwest
Rochester, MN 55905
www.mayo.edu

**Mayrand, Inc** (see Merz Pharmaceuticals)

**McDonnell Douglas Corp**
PO Box 516, 107/2 MS10
St Louis, MO 63166

**McGaw, Inc** (see B. Braun)

**McGregor Pharmaceuticals, Inc**
8420 Ulmenton Road
Suite 305
Largo, FL 33771
(727) 530-4361

**McGuff Company, Inc**
3524 West Lake Center Drive
Santa Ana, CA 92704
(800) 854-7220

**McNeil Consumer Healthcare**
Camp Hill Road
Mail Stop 278
Fort Washington, PA 19034-2292
(800) 962-5357
www.ortho-mcneil.com

**McNeil Pharmaceutical**
1000 US Highway Route 202
Raritan, NJ 08869-0602
(800) 631-5273

**MCR American Pharmaceuticals**
15355 Flight Path Drive
Brooksville, FL 34604
(352) 754-8587

**Mead Johnson Laboratories** (see Bristol-Myers Squibb)

**Mead Johnson Nutritionals (Bristol-Myers Squibb Company)**
2400 West Lloyd Expressway
Evansville, IN 47721-7189
(812) 429-5000
www.meadjohnson.com

**Medco Pharmaceuticals, Inc**
2015 Highway 190 Bypass
PO Box 2088
Covington, LA 70433
(800) 793-8740
www.dry-eye-institute.org

**Med-Derm Pharmaceuticals**
PO Box 5193
Kingsport, TN 37663
(800) 334-4286

**Med-Pro, Inc**
210 East 4th Street
Lexington, NE 68850
(800) 447-6060

**Medac GmbH c/o Princeton Regulatory Association**
65 South Main Street
Pennington, NJ 08534
(609) 951-9596

**Medarex**
1545 Route 22 East
PO Box 992
Annandale, NJ 08801-0992
(908) 713-6000
www.medarex.com

**Medco Lab, Inc**
716 West 7th Street
Sioux City, IA 51103-5333
(712) 255-8770
www.medcolab.com

**Medco Pharmaceuticals**
Covington, LA 70433
(800) 793-8740

**Medco Research, Inc**
PO Box 13886
Research Triangle Park, NC 27709
(919) 549-8117

**Medea Research Laboratories**
200 Wilson Street
Port Jefferson, NY 11776
(516) 474-8014

**Medeva Pharmaceuticals**
(see Celltech Pharmaceutical)

**Medi Aid Corp**
8250 South Akron Street
Suite 205
Englewood, CO 80155
(800) 525-9567

**Medical Action Industries**
150 Motor Parkway
Suite 205
Hauppauge, NY 11788
(800) 645-7042

**Medical Products Panamericana**
647 West Flagler Street
Miami, FL 33130
(305) 545-6524

**Medicis Dermatologics, Inc**
8125 North Hayden Drive
Scottsdale, AZ 85258
(800) 550-5115

**Medicis Pharmaceutical Corp**
4343 East Camelback Road
Suite 150
Phoenix, AZ 85018
(800) 845-1313

**MedImmune, Inc**
35 West Watkins Mill Road
Gaithersburg, MD 20878
(800) 934-7426
(877) 633-4411
www.medimmune.com

**Medi-Plex Pharm, Inc**
(see ECR Pharmaceuticals)

**Medirex, Inc**
20 Chapin Road
Pine Brook, NJ 07058
(800) 343-3848

**Medisan**
400 Lanidex Plaza
Parsippany, NJ 07054
(800) 763-3472

**Medisca, Inc**
661 Route 3, Unit C
Plattsburgh, NY 12901
(800) 932-1039

**MediSense, Inc**
**(Abbott Laboratories)**
4A Crosby Drive
Bedford, MA 01730
(800) 323-9100

**Medix Pharmaceuticals Americas, Inc (MPA)**
12505 Starkey Road
Suite M
Largo, FL 33773
www.biafine.com

**MedPointe, Inc**
Half Acre Road
Cranbury, NJ 08512
(609) 655-6000
www.medpointeinc.com

**Medtech Laboratories, Inc**
3510 North Lake Creek
Jackson, WY 83001-1108
(800) 443-4908

**Medtronic, Inc**
800 53rd Avenue Northeast
Minneapolis, MN 55421
(800) 328-0810

**Melville Biologics**
155 Duryea Road
Melville, NY 11747
(516) 752-7314

**Menicon USA**
333 West Pontiac Way
Clovis, CA 93612
(800) 636-4266
www.menicon.com

**Mennen Company** (see Colgate-Palmolive)

**Mentholatum Company, Inc**
**(Rohto Pharmaceutical Company)**
1360 Niagra Street
Buffalo, NY 14213
(800) 688-7660
www.mentholatum.com

**ME Pharmaceuticals, Inc**
2800 Southeast Parkway
Richmond, IN 47374
(800) 637-4276

**Merck & Company**
PO Box 4
West Point, PA 19486
(866) 448-7590
www.merck.com

**Mericon Industries, Inc**
8819 North Pioneer Road
Peoria, IL 61615
(800) 242-6464

**Meridian Chemical & Equipment**
4015 River Road
Amarillo, TX 79108
(800) 687-7850

**Meridian Medical Technologies, Inc**
10240 Old Columbia Road
Columbia, MD 21046
(800) 638-8093
www.meridianmeds.com

**Merieux Institute, Inc** (see Aventis)

**Merit Pharmaceuticals**
2611 San Fernando Road
Los Angeles, CA 90065
(800) 421-9657

**Merrell Dow** (see Hoechst Marion Roussel)

**Merz Pharmaceuticals**
4215 Tudor Lane
Greensboro, NC 27410
(800) 334-0514
www.merzusa.com

**Methapharm, Inc**
2825 University Drive
Suite 240
Coral Springs, FL 33065
(800) 287-7686

**MGI Pharma, Inc**
9900 Bren Road East
Suite 300E
Minnetonka, MN 55343-9667
(800) 562-0679
www.mgipharma.com

**Michigan Department of Health**
PO Box 30035
Lansing, MI 48909
(517) 335-8000

**MicroGeneSys, Inc**
(see Protein Sciences Corp)

**Mikart, Inc**
1750 Chattahoochee Avenue
Atlanta, GA 30318
(404) 351-4510
www.mikart.com

**Miles Allergy** (see Bayer Corp)

**Miles, Inc** (see Bayer Corp)

**Milex Products, Inc**
4311 North Normandy
Chicago, IL 60634-1403
(800) 621-1278

**Miller Pharmacal Group, Inc**
350 Randy Road
Unit #2
Carol Stream, IL 60188
(800) 323-2935

**Misemer Pharmaceuticals, Inc**
(see Edwards Pharmaceuticals)

**Mission Pharmacal Company**
10999 IH-10 West
Suite 1000
San Antonio, TX 78230
(800) 531-3333
www.missionpharmacal.com

**Miza Pharmaceuticals, Inc**
**(Corp Office)**
4950 Yonge Street
Suite 2001
PO Box 118
Toronto, Ontario
Canada M2N 6K1 (416) 927-0600
www.miza.com

**Miza Pharmaceuticals USA, Inc**
40 Main Street
Fairton, NJ 08320-0210
(856) 451-9350
www.miza.com

**Monaghan Medical Corp**
Plattsburgh, NY 12901

**Monarch** (see King Pharm)

**Monarch Pharmaceuticals**
**(King Pharmaceuticals, Inc)**
355 Beecham Street
Bristol, TN 37620
(800) 776-3637
www.monarchpharm.com

**Montgomery Medical Ventures**
600 Montgomery Street
San Francisco, CA 94111

**Monticello Drug Company**
1604 Stockton Co
Jacksonville, FL 32204
(800) 735-0666
www.monticellocompanies.com

**Moore Medical Corp**
389 John Downey Drive
PO Box 1500
New Britain, CT 06050-1500
(800) 234-1464
www.mooremedical.com

**Morton Grove Pharmaceuticals, Inc**
6451 West Main Street
Morton Grove, IL 60053
(800) 346-6854
www.mgp-online.com

**Morton International**
**(Rohm & Haas Company)**
1275 Lake Avenue
Woodstock, IL 60098-7499
(815) 338-1800
www.rohmhaas.com

**Morton Salt**
100 North Riverside Plaza
Chicago, IL 60606-1597
(312) 807-2000
www.mortonsalt.com

**Mount Sinai Medical Center**
5th Avenue and 100th Street
New York, NY 10029-6574
(212) 241-6944

**Mova Pharmaceutical**
214 Carnegie Center
Princeton, NJ 08540
(609) 514-9600

**MSD** (see Merck & Company)

**Mt Vernon Foods, Inc**
13246 Wooster Road
Mt Vernon, OH 43050
(800) 932-5525

**Murdock, Madaus, Schwabe**
**(Nature's Way)**
10 Mountain Springs Parkway
Springville, UT 84663
(801) 489-1500
www.naturesway.com

**Muro Pharmaceuticals, Inc**
**(ASTA Medica)**
890 East Street
Tewksbury, MA 01876-9987
(800) 225-0974
www.muropharm.com

**Murray Drug Corp**
415 South 4th Street
Murray, KY 42071
(502) 753-6654

**Mutual Pharmaceutical Company,**
**Inc/United Research Laboratories**
1100 Orthodox Street
Philadelphia, PA 19124
(800) 523-3684
www.urlmutual.com

**Mylan Pharmaceuticals, Inc**
781 Chestnut Ridge Road
P0 Box 4310
Morgantown, WV 26505
(800) 826-9526
www.mylan.com

**Nabi**
**(Corp Headquarters)**
5800 Park of Commerce Boulevard Northwest
Boca Raton, FL 33487
(561) 989-5800
www.nabi.com

**Nastech Pharmaceutical Company, Inc**
45 Adams Avenue
Hauppauge, NY 11788
(631) 273-0252
www.nastech.com

**NATREN, Inc**
3105 Willow Lane
Westlake Village, CA 91361
(800) 992-3323
www.natren.com

**Natrol, Inc**
21411 Prairie Street
Chatsworth, CA 91311
(800) 326-1520
www.natrol.com

**Natural Nutritionals Company**
200 Webro Road
Parsippany, NJ 07054
(973) 276-1310

**Natures Bounty, Inc**
**(NBTY, Inc)**
90 Orville Drive
Bohemia, NY 11716
(631) 244-2055
www.naturesbounty.com

**Nature Smart**
1500 East 128th Avenue
Thornton, CO 80241
(303) 474-2300

**Nature's Sunshine Products, Inc**
75 East 1700 South
Provo, UT 84606
(800) 223-8225
www.nsponline.com

**Natures' Way**
2400 Kirkwood Highway
Wilmington, DE 19805
(800) 888-2176
www.natway.com

**NBTY, Inc**
90 Orville Drive
Bohemia, NY 11716
(800) 645-5412
www.nbty.com

**NCI Medical Foods**
5801 Ayala Avenue
Irwindale, CA 91706
(800) 869-1515

**NeoPharm, Inc**
225 East Deerpath
Suite 250
Lake Forest, IL 60045
(708) 295-8678

**NeoRx Corp**
410 West Harrison Street
Seattle, WA 98119
(206) 281-7001
www.neorx.com

**Nephron Pharmaceuticals Corp**
4121 34th Street
Orlando, FL 32811-6458
(800) 443-4313
www.nephronpharm.com

**Nephro-Tech, Inc**
PO Box 16106
Shawnee, KS 66203
(800) 879-4755

**Neurex Pharmaceuticals**
**(Elan Pharmaceuticals, Inc)**
3760 Haven Avenue
Menlo Park, CA 94025
(888) 638-7605
www.elanpharma.com

**NeuroGenesis/Matrix Tech, Inc**
100 Louisiana
Suite 600
Houston, TX 77002
(800) 345-8912
www.neurogenesis.com

**Neuromuscular Adjuncts**
University Hospital
Orthopedic Center
HSCT-18020
Stony Brook, NY 11790
(516) 444-7830

**Neutrogena Corp**
5760 West 96th Street
Los Angeles, CA 90045-5595
(800) 582-4048
www.neutrogena.com

**Neutron Technology Corp**
1205 North 11th
Biose, ID 83702
(208) 863-4847

**New Halsey Drug Company, Inc**
(see Halsey Drug Company)

**New Mark Laboratories**
PO Box 6321
Edison, NJ 08818
(800) 338-8079

**New World Trading Corp**
PO Box 952
DeBary, FL 32713
(407) 668-7520

**NeXstar Pharmaceuticals, Inc**
**(Gilead Sciences)**
2860 Wilderness Place
Boulder, CO 80301
(303) 444-5893
www.gilead.com

**Niche Pharmaceuticals, Inc**
200 North Oak Street
PO Box 449
Roanoke, TX 76262
(800) 677-0355
www.niche-inc.com

**Nnodum Corp**
**(Ziks)**
886 Clinton Springs Avenue
Cincinnati, OH 45229
(513) 861-2329
www.zikspain.com

**Nomax, Inc**
40 North Rock Hill Road
St Louis, MO 63119
(314) 961-2500
www.nomax.com

**Noramco, Inc**
**(Johnson & Johnson)**
1440 Olympic Drive
Athens, GA 30608
www.noramco.com

**Norcliff Thayer**
(see SmithKline Beecham Consumer Healthcare)

**Norstar Consumer Products Company, Inc**
5517 95th Avenue
Kenosha, WI 53144
(262) 652-8505

**North American Biologicals, Inc** (see Nabi)

**North American Vaccine, Inc**
12103 Indian Creek Court
Beltsville, MD 21046
(888) 628-2829

**Northern Research Laboratories, Inc**
8400 Normandale Lake Boulevard
Suite 920
Minneapolis, MN 55437
(888) 884-4675

**Norwich Eaton** (see Procter & Gamble)

**Novartis Pharmaceuticals Corp**
One Health Plaza
Building 161
East Hanover, NJ 07936-1080
(888) 669-6682
www.pharma.us.novartis.com

**Novel Pharmaceutical, Inc**
6 E.V. Hogan Drive
Hamlet, NC 28345
(910) 582-8800

**Noven Pharmaceuticals**
11960 Southwest 144th Street
Miami, FL 33186
(888) 253-5099
www.noven.com

**Novocol**
**(Septodont, Inc)**
PO Box 11926
Wilmington, DE 19850
(800) 872-8305
www.septodontinc.com

**Novo Nordisk Pharmaceuticals, Inc**
100 College Road West
Princeton, NJ 08540-7810
(800) 727-6500
www.novonordisk-us.com

**Novopharm USA, Inc**
165 East Commerce Drive
Suite 100
Schaumburg, IL 60173-5326
(800) 635-5067

**Numark Laboratories, Inc**
164 North Field Avenue
Edison, NJ 08818
(800) 338-8079
www.numarklabs.com

**NutraMax Laboratories, Inc**
2208 Lakeside Boulevard
Edgewood, MD 21040
(800) 925-5187
www.nutramaxlabs.com

**NutraMax Products**
51 Blackburn Drive
Gloucester, MA 01930-2237
(978) 282-1800

**Nutricept, Inc**
11220 Grader
Dallas, TX 75238
(214) 221-3400

**Nutricia, Inc** (see Mt Vernon Foods, Inc)

**NutriSoy International, Inc**
424 South Kentucky Avenue
Evansville, IN 47714
(888) 769-0769
www.nutrisoy.com

**Nutrition Medical, Inc** (see Galagen, Inc)

**Nutri Vention**
6991 Alamos Downs Parkway
San Antonio, TX 78238
(210) 661-8589

**Nutro Laboratories**
South Plainfield, NJ 07080

**Nycomed Amersham**
101 Carnegie Center
Princeton, NJ 08540-6231
(800) 654-0118
www.nycomed-amersham.com

**Oakhurst Company**
3000 Hempstead Turnpike
Levittown, NY 11756
(800) 831-1135

**7 Oaks Pharmaceutical Corp**
161 Harry Stanley Drive
Easley, SC 29640
(864) 850-1700

**Oclassen Pharmaceuticals, Inc**
220 South Orange Avenue
2nd Floor
Livingston, NJ 07039
(800) 808-5208

**O'Connor, Inc**
(see Columbia Laboratories, Inc)

**Ocumed, Inc**
119 Harrison Avenue
Roseland, NJ 07068
(973) 226-2330

**Odyssey Pharmaceuticals, Inc**
72 DeForest Avenue
East Hanover, NJ 07936
(877) 427-9068

**Ohmeda Pharmaceuticals** (see Baxter)

**OHM Laboratories, Inc**
600 College Road
Suite 2100
Princeton, NJ 08540
(800) 527-6481

**OMJ Pharmaceuticals, Inc**
PO Box 367
San German, Puerto Rico 00683

**Omnii Products**
1500 North Florida Mango Road
Suite 1
West Palm Beach, FL 33409
(800) 445-3386
www.omniiproducts.com

**ONY, Inc**
1576 Sweet Home Road
Amherst, NY 14228
(877) 274-4669

**Optics Laboratory, Inc**
9480 Telstar Avenue #3
El Monte, CA 91731
(626) 350-1926

**Optikem International, Inc**
2172 South Jason Street
Denver, CO 80223
(303) 936-1137

**Optimox Corp**
PO Box 3378
Torrance, CA 90510-3378
(800) 223-1601
www.optimox.com

**Optopics Laboratories Corp**
40 Main Street
PO Box 210
Fairton, NJ 08320-0210
(856) 451-9350

**Oread, Inc**
Palo Alto, CA 94304

**Organogenesis, Inc**
Canton, MA 02021

**Organon, Inc**
375 Mt Pleasant Avenue
West Orange, NJ 07052
(800) 241-8812
www.organoninc.com

**Organon Teknika Corp**
100 Akzo Avenue
Durham, NC 27712
(800) 682-2666

**Orion Diagnostica**
71 Veronica Avenue
PO Box 218
Somerset, NJ 08875-0218
(800) 526-2125

**Orphan Medical, Inc**
13911 Ridgedale Drive
Minnetonka, MN 55305
(888) 867-7426
www.orphan.com

**Orphan Pharmaceuticals USA**
1101 Kermit Drive
Suite 608
Nashville, TN 37217
(615) 399-0700
www.orphanusa.com

**Ortho Biotech, Inc**
**(Johnson & Johnson)**
700 US Highway 202
P0 Box 670
Raritan, NJ 08869-0670
(800) 325-7504
www.jnj.com

**Ortho-Clinical Diagnostics**
100 Indigo Creek Drive
Rochester, NY 14626
(800) 828-6316

**Ortho-McNeil Pharmaceutical**
**(Johnson & Johnson)**
Route 202
Raritan, NJ 08869
(800) 631-5273
www.ortho-mcneil.com

**Ortho Pharmaceutical Corp - Dermatological**
199 Grandview Road
Shillman, NJ 08555
(800) 426-7762

**Otsuka America Pharmaceutical, Inc**
2440 Research Boulevard
Suite 250
Rockville, MD 20850
(800) 562-3974
www.otsuka.com

**Owen/Galderma**
(see Galderma Laboratories, Inc)

**Oxford Pharmaceutical Services, Inc**
One US Highway 46 West
Totowa, NJ 07512
(877) 284-9120
www.oxfordpharm.com

**OXIS International, Inc**
6040 North Cutter Circle
Suite 317
Portland, OR 97212
(503) 283-3911
www.oxis.com

**Oxypure, Inc**
3550 Morris Street North
St Petersburg, FL 33713
(888) 216-8930

**Paddock Laboratories, Inc**
3940 Quebec Avenue North
Minneapolis, MN 55427
(800) 328-5113
www.paddocklabs.com

**Palisades Pharmaceuticals, Inc**
(see Glenwood)

**Pan American Laboratories, Inc**
PO Box 8950
Mandeville, LA 70470-8950
www.panamericanlabs.com

**Parkedale Pharmaceuticals**
870 Parkedale Road
Rochester, MI 84307
(800) 336-7783

**Parke-Davis**
**Pfizer Pharmaceuticals**
201 Tabor Road
Morris Plains, NJ 07950
(800) 223-0432

**Parmed Pharmaceuticals, Inc (Alpharma)**
4220 Hyde Park Boulevard
Niagra Falls, NY 14305-6714

**Parnell Pharmaceuticals, Inc**
PO Box 5130
Larkspur, CA 94977
(800) 457-4276
www.parnellpharm.com

**Par Pharmaceutical, Inc**
One Ram Ridge Road
Spring Valley, NY 10977
(800) 727-0923
www.parpharm.com

**Parthenon Company, Inc**
3311 West 2400 South
Salt Lake City, UT 84119
(800) 453-8898

**Pasadena Research Labs**
(see Taylor Pharmaceuticals)

**Pasteur Merieux Connaught** (see Aventis)

**PathoGenesis Corp** (see Chiron Corp)

**PBH Wesley Jessen**
810 Kifer Road
Sunnyvale, CA 94086
(800) 538-1680

**PDRx Pharmaceuticals, Inc**
72 North Ann Arbor
Oklahoma City, OK 73127
(800) 299-7379
www.pdrx.com

**Pecos Pharmaceutical**
25301 Cabot Road
Suites 212-213
Laguna Hills, CA 92653

**Pediatric Pharmaceuticals, Inc**
120 Wood Avenue South
Suite 300
Iselin, NJ 08830
(732) 603-7708
www.pediatricpharm.com

**Pedinol Pharmacal, Inc**
30 Banfi Plaza North
Farmingdale, NY 11735
(800) 733-4665
www.pedinol.com

**Pegasus Laboratories, Inc**
Pensacola, FL 32514

**Pegasus Medical, Inc**
PO Box 6101
Irvine, CA 92618
(949) 823-9636

**Pennex Pharmaceutical, Inc**
(see Morton Grove Pharmaceuticals)

**Pentech Pharmaceuticals, Inc**
417 Harvester Court
Wheeling, IL 60090
(847) 459-9122

**Permeable Technologies, Inc**
712 Ginesi Drive
Morganville, NJ 07751
(800) 622-7376
www.lifestylecompany.com

**Perrigo Company**
515 Eastern Avenue
Allegan, MI 49010
(616) 673-9399

**Person & Covey, Inc**
616 Allen Avenue
PO Box 25018
Glendale, CA 91221-5018
(800) 423-2341

**Personal Care**
One Paragon Drive
Montvale, NJ 07645
(800) 816-5742

**Personal Products Company (Johnson & Johnson)**
Route 202
PO Box 610
Raritan, NJ 08869
(800) 582-6097
www.jnj.com

**Pfeiffer Company**
71 University Avenue
Atlanta, GA 30315
(800) 342-6450

**Pfipharmecs**
(see Pfizer US Pharmaceutical Group)

**Pfizer Pharmaceuticals Group (PPG)**
235 East 42nd Street
New York, NY 10017-5755
(800) 438-1985
www.pfizer.com

**Pharma 21**
4850 Scholls Ferry Road
Portland, OR 97225-1686
(503) 297-3349

**Pharmacel Laboratory, Inc**
203 South Coolidge Avenue
Tampa, FL 33609
(813) 289-2750

**Pharmaceutical Associates, Inc**
201 Delaware Street
Greenville, SC 29605
(800) 845-8210

**Pharmaceutical Basics, Inc**
(see Rosemont Pharmaceutical)

**Pharmaceutical Corp of America**
12348 Hancock Street
Carmel, IN 46032
(800) 722-0772

**Pharmaceutical Formulations, Inc**
460 Plainfield Avenue
Edison, NJ 08818

**Pharmaceutical Labs, Inc**
6704 Ranger Avenue
Corpus Christi, TX 78415
(800) 856-7040

**Pharmaceutical Specialties, Inc**
PO Box 6298
Rochester, MN 55903-6298
(800) 325-8232
www.psico.com

**Pharmacia & Upjohn Company (Ophthalmics Division)**
701 East Milham Road
Kalamazoo, MI 49001
(800) 423-4866

**Pharmacia Corp**
100 Route 206 North
Peapack, NJ 07977
(888) 768-5501
www.pharmacia.com

**Pharmadigm, Inc**
2401 Foothill Drive
Salt Lake City, UT 84109
(801) 464-6100
www.pharmadigm.com

**Pharmafair**
(see Bausch & Lomb Pharmaceuticals)

**Pharmakon Labs, Inc**
6050 Jet Port Industrial Boulevard
Tampa, FL 33634
(800) 888-4045

**Pharmanex**
75 West Center
Provo, UT 84601
(800) 487-1000
www.pharmanex.com

**Pharmanex, Inc**
625 Cochran Street
Simi Valley, CA 93065-1939
(805) 582-9300
www.pharmanex.com

**Pharmascience Laboratories, Inc**
175 Ranco Street
Suite 200
Buffalo, NJ 14207
(800) 340-9735

**Pharma-Tek, Inc**
PO Box 1148
Elmira, NY 14902
(800) 645-6655
www.pharma-tek.com

**Pharmavite Corp (Otsuka Pharmaceutical Company)**
15451 San Fernando Mission Boulevard
Mission Hills, CA 91345
(800) 423-2405
www.pharmavite.com

**Pharmics, Inc**
2350 South Redwood Road
Salt Lake City, UT 84119
(800) 456-4138
www.pharmics.com

**Phillips Gulf Corp**
PO Box 270692
Tampa, FL 33688
(800) 729-8446
www.phillipsgulf.com

**Phoenix Laboratories**
140 Lauman Lane
Hicksville, NY 11801

**Physician's Total Care**
5415 South 125th East Avenue
Suite 205
Tulsa, OK 74146

**PhytoPharmica, Inc**
825 Challenger Drive
Green Bay, WI 54311-8328
(800) 553-2370
www.phytopharmica.com

**Plantex USA, Inc**
482 Hudson Terrace
Englewood Cliffs, NJ 07632

**Playtex Company**
74 Commerce Drive
Allendale, NJ 07401-1600
(800) 816-5742
www.playtex.com

**Plough, Inc**
(see Schering-Plough Healthcare Products)

**PolyMedica Corp**
11 State Street
Woburn, MA 01801
(781) 933-2020
www.polymedica.com

**Polymer Technology Corp**
100 Research Drive
Wilmington, MA 01887
(800) 885-1241

**Poly Pharmaceuticals, Inc**
PO Box 93
Quitman, MS 39355
(800) 882-1041

**Porton Product Limited**
(see Speywood Pharmaceuticals, Inc)

**Pratt Pharmaceuticals**
235 East 42nd Street
New York, NY 10017-5755
(800) 438-1985

**Premier** (see Advanced Polymer Systems)

**Press Chemical & Pharmaceutical Laboratories**
Columbus, OH
(614) 258-7620

**Primedics Laboratories**
14131 South Avalon
Los Angeles, CA 90061
(800) 599-0173

**Princeton Pharmaceutical Products**
(see Bristol-Myers Squibb)

**Procter & Gamble Pharmaceuticals**
P0 Box 231
Norwich, NY 13815-0191
(800) 448-4878
www.pg.com

**ProCyte Corp**
PO Box 808
Redmond, WA 98073-0808
(425) 869-1239
www.procyte.com

**ProMetic Pharma USA, Inc**
5436 West 78th Street
Indianapolis, IN 46268
(888) 313-2520

**Propst Pharmaceuticals**
1236 Jordan Road
Huntsville, AL 35811
(256) 704-6394

**Protein Design Labs, Inc**
34801 Campus Drive
Fremont, CA 94555
(510) 574-1400
www.pdl.com

**Protein Sciences Corp**
1000 Research Parkway
Meriden, CT 06450
(800) 488-7099
www.proteinsciences.com

**Protherics, Inc**
1207 17th Avenue South
Suite 103
Nashville, TN 37212
(615) 327-1027
www.protherics.com

**P & S Laboratories, Inc**
210 West 131st Street
Los Angeles, CA 90061
(800) 624-9659
www.hylands.com

**Psychemedics Corp (Laboratory Operations)**
5832 Uplander Way
Culver City, CA 90230
(800) 522-7424
www.psychemedics.com

**Purdue Pharm LP (Corporate Headquarters)**
One Stamford Forum
201 Tresser Boulevard
Stamford, CT 06901-3431
(203) 588-8000
www.pharma.com

**Purepac Pharmaceutical Company (F. H. Faulding & Company Ltd)**
200 Elmora Avenue
Elizabeth, NJ 07207
(800) 432-8534
www.purepac.com

**Puritan's Pride**
1233 Montauk Highway
PO Box 9001
Oakdale, NY 11769-9001
(800) 645-9584
www.puritanspride.com

**QLT Phototherapeutics, Inc**
887 Great Northern Way
Vancouver, BC
Canada V5T 4T5
(800) 663-5486
www.qlt-pdt.com

**Qualitest Pharmaceuticals, Inc**
1236 Jordan Road
Huntsville, AL 35811
(800) 444-4011

**Quality Research Pharmaceuticals, Inc**
1117 Third Avenue South West
Carmel, IN 46032

**Questcor Pharmaceuticals, Inc**
3260 Whipple Road
Union City, CA 94587
(510) 400-0700
www.questcor.com

**Quidel Corp**
10165 McKellar Court
San Diego, CA 92121
(800) 874-1517
www.quidel.com

**Ranbaxy Pharmaceuticals, Inc USA**
600 College Road East
Princeton, NJ 08540
(609) 720-9200
www.ranbaxy.com

**Randob Laboratories, Limited**
6 Walnut Street
Cornwall, NY 12518
(845) 534-2197

**R & D Laboratories, Inc**
4640 Admiralty Way
Suite 710
Marina Del Ray, CA 90292
(800) 338-9066
www.rndlabs.com

**Reckitt Benckiser, Inc**
1655 Valley Road
PO Box 943
Wayne, NJ 07470-0943
(973) 633-3600
www.reckitt.com

**Recsei Laboratories**
330 South Kellogg
Building M
Goleta, CA 93117-3875
(805) 964-2912

**Reed & Carnrick** (see Schwarz Pharma)

**Reese Pharmaceutical Company, Inc**
10617 Frank Avenue
Cleveland, OH 44106-0157
(800) 321-7178
www.reesechemical.com

**Redi-Products Labs, Inc** (see Aplicare, Inc)

**Regeneron Pharmaceuticals, Inc**
777 Old Saw Mill River Road
Tarrytown, NY 10591-6707
(800) 637-8322
www.regeneron.com

**Regent Laboratories**
700 West Hillsboro Boulevard
#2-206
Deerfield Beach, FL 33441
(800) 872-1526

**Reid Rowell** (see Solvay)

**Remel, Inc**
12076 Santa Fe Drive
PO Box 14428
Lenexa, KS 66215
(800) 255-6730
www.remelinc.com

**Republic Drug Company**
175 Great Arrow Avenue
Suite 4
Buffalo, NY 14207
(800) 828-7444

**Requa, Inc**
One Seneca Place
Greenwich, CT 06830
(800) 321-1085
www.requa.com

**Research Industries Corp**
6864 South 300 West
Midvale, UT 84047
(800) 453-8432

**Research Triangle Institute**
PO Box 12194
Research Triangle Park, NC 27709
(800) 263-5428
www.rti.org

**Respa Pharmaceuticals, Inc**
PO Box 88222
Carol Stream, IL 60188
(630) 462-9986

**Rexall Group**
4031 Northeast 12th Terrace
Fort Lauderdale, FL 33334
(800) 255-7399

**Rexall Sundown, Inc**
**(Royal Numico, N.V.)**
6111 Broken Sound Parkway Northwest
Boca Raton, FL 33487
(800) 327-0908
www.rexallsundown.com

**Rgene Therapeutics, Inc**
2170 Buckthorne Place
Suite 230
The Woodlands, TX 77380
(713) 367-5443

**Rhone-Poulenc Rorer Pharmaceuticals, Inc**
500 Arcola Road
PO Box 1200
Collegeville, PA 19426-0998
(800) 340-7502

**RH Pharmaceuticals, Inc**
104 Chancellor Matheson Road
Winnipeg R3T 2N2
Canada
(204) 989-6850

**Ribi Immunochem Research, Inc**
553 Old Corvallis Road
Hamilton, MT 59840-3131
(406) 363-6214

**Richardson-Vicks, Inc**
(see Procter & Gamble Company)

**Richie Pharmacal, Inc**
119 State Avenue
PO Box 460
Glasgow, KY 42141
(800) 627-0250

**Richwood** (see Shire Richwood)

**Ricola, Inc**
51 Gibraltar Drive
Morris Plains, NJ 07950
(973) 984-6811
www.ricolausa.com

**R.I.D., Inc**
609 North Mednik Avenue
Los Angeles, CA 90022-1320
(323) 268-0635

**Ridgebury Pharmaceuticals, Inc**
Danbury, CT 06810

**Rite Aid Corp**
30 Hunter Lane
Camp Hill, PA 17011
(717) 761-2633

**Robins** (see Wyeth-Ayerst)

**Roberts Pharmaceuticals Corp**
4 Industrial Way West
Eatontown, NJ 07724
(800) 828-2088

**Roche Laboratories**
340 Kingsland Street
Nutley, NJ 07110-1199
(800) 526-0625
www.rocheusa.com

**Roerig**
235 East 42nd Street
New York, NY 10017
(800) 438-1985

**Rorer** (see Rhone-Poulenc Rorer)

**Rosemont Pharmaceutical Corp**
301 South Cherokee Street
Denver, CO 80223
(800) 445-8091

**Ross Laboratories**
6480 Busch Boulevard
Columbus, OH 43229
(800) 624-7677

**Ross Products Division, Abbott Labs**
625 Cleveland Avenue
Columbus, OH 43215
(614) 624-7677
www.abbott.com

**Roxane Laboratories, Inc**
PO Box 16532
Columbus, OH 43216
(800) 520-1631
www.roxane.com

**Royce Laboratories, Inc**
16600 Northwest 54th Avenue
Miami, FL 33014
(800) 677-6923

**R. P. Scherer, Inc**
645 Martinsville Road
Suite 200
Basking Ridge, NJ 07920
(888) 636-1919
www.rpscherer.com

**R & R Registrations**
PO Box 262069
San Diego, CA 92196
(858) 586-0751

**Rugby Labs, Inc**
2170 Satellite Boulevard
Suite 300
Duluth, GA 30097
(800) 645-2158

**Russ Pharmaceuticals**
(see UCB Pharmaceuticals)

**Rydelle Laboratories**
1525 Howe Street
Racine, WI 53403-5011
(800) 558-5252

**Rystan, Inc**
PO Box 214
Little Falls, NJ 07424-0214
(973) 256-3737

**Salix Pharmaceuticals, Inc**
3600 West Bayshore Road
Palo Alto, CA 94303
(650) 849-5900

**Sandoz Pharmaceuticals** (see Novartis Pharmaceuticals)

**SangStat Medical Corp**
6300 Dunbarton Circle
Fremont, CA 94555
(510) 789-4300
www.sangstat.com

**Sanitube Company**
19 Concord Street
South Norwalk, CT 06854
(203) 853-7856

**Sankyo Parke-Davis**
2 Hilton Court
Parsippany, NJ 07054-1296
(800) 726-5961

**Sanofi-Synthelabo, Inc**
90 Park Avenue
New York, NY 10016
(212) 551-4000
www.sanofi-synthelabous.com

**Santen, Inc**
555 Gateway Road
Napa, CA 94558
(707) 254-1750

**Savage Laboratories**
**(Altana Inc)**
60 Baylis Road
Melville, NY 11747-2006
(800) 231-0206
www.savagelabs.com

**Scandinavian Natural Health & Beauty Products**
13 North 7th Street
Perkasie, PA 18944
(800) 288-2844
scandinaviannaturals.com

**Scandipharm, Inc**
(see Axcan Scandipharm, Inc)

**Schaffer Laboratories**
1058 North Allen Avenue
Pasadena, CA 91104
(800) 231-6725

**Schein Pharmaceutical, Inc**
**(Watson Pharmaceuticals, Inc)**
100 Campus Drive
Florham Park, NJ 07932
(800) 356-5790
www.schein-rx.com

**Scherer Laboratories, Inc**
2301 Ohio Drive
Suite 234
Plano, TX 75093
(800) 449-8290

**Schering-Plough Corp**
**(World Headquarters)**
2000 Galloping Hill Road
Kenilworth, NJ 07033-0530
(908) 298-4000
www.sch-plough.com

**Schering-Plough Healthcare Products**
3 Oak Way
Berkeley Heights, NJ 07922-0603
(800) 842-4090
www.schering-plough.com

**Schmid Products Company**
(see Durex Consumer Products)

**Scholl, Inc**
(see Schering-Plough Healthcare Products)

**Schwarzkopf & Dep, Inc**
2101 East Via Arado
Rancho Dominguez, CA 90220
(800) 326-2855

**Schwarz Pharma, Inc**
PO Box 2038
Milwaukee, WI 53201
(800) 558-5114
www.schwarzusa.com

**SciClone Pharmaceuticals**
901 Mariner's Island Boulevard
Suite 205
San Mateo, CA 94404
(650) 358-3456
www.sciclone.com

**Scios Nova**
**(Corp Headquarters)**
820 West Maude Avenue
Sunnyvale, CA 94085
(408) 616-8200
www.sciosinc.com

**Scot-Tussin Pharmacal Company, Inc**
50 Clemence Street
PO Box 8217
Cranston, RI 02920-0217
(800) 638-7268
www.scottussin.com

**Searle** (see Pharmacia Corp)

**Seatrace Pharmaceuticals**
PO Box 363
Gadsden, AL 35902-0363
(256) 442-5023

**Seneca Pharmaceutical, Inc**
PO Box 25021
8621 Barefoot Industrial Road
Raleigh, NC 27613

**Sepracor**
**(Corp Headquarters)**
111 Locke Drive
Marlborough, MA 01752
(877) SEPRACOR
www.sepracor.com

**Septodont, Inc**
PO Box 11926
Wilmington, DE 19850
(800) 872-8305
www.septodontinc.com

**Sequus Pharmaceuticals, Inc**
980 Hamilton Court
Menlo Park, CA 94025
(800) 323-9051

**Seres Laboratories, Inc**
3331-B Industrial Drive
PO Box 470
Santa Rosa, CA 95403
(707) 526-4526
www.sereslabs.com

**Serono Laboratories, Inc**
100 Longwater Circle
Norwell, MA 02061
(800) 283-8088

**SG Labs, Inc**
500 North Broadway
Jericho, NY 11753
(516) 822-2900

**Shaklee Corporation (Corp Headquarters)**
4747 Willow Road
Pleasanton, CA 94588
(925) 924-2000
www.shaklee.com

**Sheffield Laboratories (Faria Ltd LLC)**
170 Broad Street
New London, CT 06320
(800) 222-1087
www.sheffield-labs.com

**Sherwood Davis & Geck**
(see Kendall Healthcare)

**Sherwood Medical** (see Kendall Healthcare)

**Shionogi USA**
3848 Carson Street
Suite 206
Torrance, CA 90503
(310) 540-1161

**Shire US, Inc**
7900 Tanners Gate Drive
Florence, KY 41042
(859) 282-2100
www.shiregroup.com

**SHS North America**
9600 Medical Center Drive
Suite 102
Rockville, MD 20850
(800) 636-2283
www.SHSNA.com

**Sidmak Laboratories, Inc**
17 West Street
East Hanover, NJ 07936
(800) 922-0547
www.sidmaklab.com

**Sigma-Tau Pharmaceuticals, Inc**
800 South Frederick Avenue
Suite 300
Gaithersburg, MD 20877-4150
(800) 447-0169

**Silarx Pharmaceuticals, Inc**
19 West Street
Spring Valley, NY 10977
(914) 352-4020

**SkyePharma, Inc**
10450 Science Center Drive
San Diego, CA 92121
(858) 625-2424
www.skyepharma.com

**Slim Fast Foods Company**
PO Box 3625
West Palm Beach, FL 33402
(877) 375-4632

**Smith & Nephew, Inc**
160 Dascomb Road
Andover, MA 01810
www.smithnephew.com

**SmithKline Beecham Pharmaceuticals**
P0 Box 7929
One Franklin Plaza
Philadelphia, PA 19101-7920
(800) 366-8900
www.sb.com

**SmithKline Diagnostics**
225 Baypoint Parkway
San Jose, CA 95134-1622
(800) 877-6242

**Sola/Barnes** (see Pilkington Barnes Hind)

**SoloPak Pharmaceuticals Inc**
6001 Broken Sound Parkway
Suite 600
Boca Raton, FL 33487

**Solvay Pharmaceuticals**
901 Sawyer Road
Marietta, GA 30062-2224
(770) 578-9000
www.solvaypharmaceuticals.com

**Somerset Pharmaceuticals**
2202 Northwest Shore Boulevard
Suite 450
Tampa, FL 33602
(800) 892-8889

**Southward Pharmaceuticals, Inc**
33 Hammond Street
Suite 201
Irvine, CA 92718

**Sovereign Pharmaceuticals**
7590 Sand Street
Fort Worth, TX 76118
(817) 284-0429

**Sparta Pharmaceuticals**
111 Rock Road
Horsham, PA 19044-2310
(215) 442-1700

**Spectrum Chemical Manufacturing Corp**
14422 South San Pedro Street
Gardena, CA 90248-9985
(800) 772-8786
www.spectrumchemical.com

**Speywood Pharmaceuticals, Inc**
27 Maple Street
Milford, MA 01757-3650
(508) 478-8900

**S.S.S. Company**
65-71 University Avenue Southwest
Atlanta, GA 30315
(800) 237-3843

**St Jude Medical, Inc**
One Lillehei Plaza
St Paul, MN 55117-1761
(612) 483-2000

**Stanback Company (Block Drug)**
PO Box 1669
Salisbury, NC 28145-1669
(800) 338-5428

**Standard Drug Company**
1279 North 7th Street
Riverton, IL 62561
(217) 629-9884

**Standard Homeopathic Company**
210 West 131st Street
PO Box 61067
Los Angeles, CA 90061
(800) 624-9659

**Star Pharmaceuticals, Inc**
1990 Northwest 44th Street
Pompano Beach, FL 33064-8712
(800) 845-7827
www.starpharm.com

**Stellar Pharmacal Corp** (see Star Pharmaceuticals, Inc)

**Stephan Company**
1850 West McNab Road
Fort Lauderdale, FL 33300
(800) 327-4963

**Squibb** (see Bristol-Myers Squibb)

**Steris Laboratories, Inc**
(Schein)
620 North 51st Avenue
Phoenix, AZ 85043
(800) 692-9995

**Sterling Health**
(see Bayer Consumer Care Division)

**Sterling Winthrop** (see Sanofi-Synthelabo)

**Stewart-Jackson Pharmacal**
4200 Lamar
Suite 103
Memphis, TN 38118
(800) 367-1395

**Stiefel Laboratories, Inc**
255 Alhambra Circle
Coral Gables, FL 33134
(888) 784-3335
www.stiefel.com

**Storz** (see Bausch & Lomb Surgical)

**Stratus Pharmaceuticals, Inc**
14377 Southwest 142nd Street
Miami, FL 33186-6727
(800) 442-7882

**Stuart Pharmaceuticals**
(see AstraZeneca Pharmaceuticals)

**Summa Rx Laboratories**
Mineral Wells, TX 76067

**Summers Laboratories, Inc**
103 G.P. Clement Drive
Collegeville, PA 19426-2044
(800) 533-7546
www.sumlab.com

**Summit Pharmaceuticals**
(see Novartis Pharmaceuticals)

**SuperGen, Inc**
4140 Dublin Boulevard
Suite 200
Dublin, CA 94568
(800) 905-5474
www.supergen.com

**Superior Pharmaceutical Company**
1385 Kemper Meadow Drive
Cincinnati, OH 45240-1635
(800) 826-5035
www.superiorpharm.com

**Survival Technical, Inc**
(see Meridian Medical Technologies)

**Swiss-American Products, Inc**
4315 Alpha Road
Dallas, TX 75244
(800) 633-8872

**Syncom Pharmaceuticals, Inc**
155 Passaic Avenue
Fairfield, NJ 07004
(201) 822-9222

**Syncor Pharmaceuticals, Inc**
1313 Washington Avenue
Golden, CO 80401
(800) 539-1503

**Synergen, Inc** (see Amgen)

**Syntex Laboratories** (see Roche)

**Syntex-Synergen Neuroscience**
1885 33rd Street
Boulder, CO 80301
(303) 442-1926

**Syva Company**
929 Queensbridge
St Louis, MO 63021
(800) 227-9948

**Takeda Pharmaceuticals America, Inc**
475 Half Day Road
Suite 500
Lincolnshire, IL 60069
(847) 383-3000

**Tambrands, Inc**
777 Westchester Avenue
White Plains, NY 10604
(914) 696-6000

**Tanox, Inc**
10301 Stella Link
Houston, TX 77025-5497
(713) 664-2288

**Tap Pharmaceuticals**
2355 Waukegan Road
Deerfield, IL 60015
(800) 622-2011
www.tapholdings.com

**Targeted Genetics Corp**
1100 Olive Way
Suite 100
Seattle, WA 98101
(206) 623-7612
www.targen.com

**Taro Pharmaceuticals USA, Inc**
5 Skyline Drive
Hawthorne, NY 10532-9998
(800) 544-1449
www.taropharma.com

**Taylor Pharmacal**
1222 West Grand
Decatur, IL 62525

**Taylor Pharmaceuticals**
942 Calle Negocio
Suite 150
San Clemente, CA 92673-5136
(800) 223-9851

**Tec Laboratories, Inc**
615 Water Avenue Northeast
PO Box 1958
Albany, OR 97321-0512
(800) 482-4464
www.teclabsinc.com

**Telluride Pharmaceuticals Corp**
146 Flanders Drive
Hillsborough, NJ 08876-4059
(908) 359-1375

**Tel-Test, Inc**
Friendswood, TX
(800) 631-0600

**Teva Marion Partners**
10236 Marion Park Drive
Kansas City, MO 64137-1405
(800) 221-4026

**Teva Pharmaceuticals USA**
1090 Horsham Road
PO Box 1090
North Wales, PA 19454-1090
(215) 591-3000
www.tevapharmusa.com

**Textilease Medique Products Company**
900 Lively Boulevard
Wood Dale, IL 60191
(800) 634-7680

**Thames Pharmacal, Inc**
2100 5th Avenue
Ronkonkama, NY 11779-6906
(800) 225-1003

**The Medicines Company**
One Cambridge Center
Cambridge, MA 02142
(800) 264-4662

**Therakos, Inc**
437 Creameway
Exton, PA 19341
(610) 280-1000

**Therapeutic Antibodies, Inc**
1207 17th Avenue South
Suite 103
Nashville, TN 37212
(615) 327-1027

**Therasense**
1370 South Loop Road
Alameda, CA 95402
(510) 748-5400

**Ther-Rx Corp**
13622 Lakefront Drive
Earth City, MO 63045
(877) 859-9361

**Thompson Medical Company, Inc**
777 South Flagler
Suite 1500, West Tower
West Palm Beach, FL 33401
(561) 820-9900

**T/I Pharmaceuticals, Inc**
(see Fischer Pharmaceuticals)

**Time-Cap Labs, Inc**
7 Michael Avenue
Farmingdale, NY 11735
(631) 753-9090

**Tishcon Corp**
30 New York Avenue
Westbury, NY 11590
(516) 338-0829

**Tompix Pharmaceuticals**
5200 New Horizons Boulevard
North Amityville, NY 11701-1144
(800) 445-2595

**Tom's of Maine, Inc**
302 LaFayette Center
PO Box 710
Kennebunk, ME 04043
(800) 367-8667
www.tomsofmaine.com

**Trask Industries, Inc**
163 Farrell Street
Somerset, NJ 08873
(800) 579-3131

**Triage Pharmaceuticals**
(see Health for Life Brands, Inc)

**Tri Tec Laboratories**
1000 Robins Road
Lynchburg, VA 24504-3558
(804) 845-7073

**Triton Consumer Products, Inc**
561 West Golf Road
Arlington Heights, IL 60005-3904
(800) 942-2009

**Tweezerman**
55 Sea Cliff Avenue
Glen Cove, NY 11542-3695
(800) 645-3340

**TwinLab Corp**
2120 Smithtown Avenue
Ronkonkama, NY 11779
(631) 467-3140
www.twinlab.com

**Tyson Nutraceuticals**
12832 South Chadron Avenue
Hawthorne, CA 90250-5525
(800) 367-7744

**UAD Laboratories, Inc**
(see Forest Pharmaceuticals, Inc)

**UCB Pharmaceuticals, Inc**
1950 Lake Park Drive
Smyrna, GA 30080
(800) 477-7877

**UDL Laboratories, Inc**
1718 Northrock Court
Rockford, IL 61103
(800) 435-5272

**Ulmer Pharmacal Company**
1614 Industry Avenue
Park Rapid, MN 56470
(800) 848-5637

**Unico Holdings, Inc**
1830 2nd Avenue North
Lake Worth, FL 33461
(800) 367-4477

**Unilever Home and Personal Care USA** (see Unilever HPC USA)

**Unilever HPC USA**
33 Benedict Place
Greenwich, CT 06830
(800) 243-5320
www.unilever.com

**Unimed Pharmaceuticals**
4 Park Way North
Deerfield, IL 60015
(800) 864-6330
www.unimed.com

**Unipath Diagnostics Company**
47 Hulfish Street
Suite 400
Princeton, NJ 08542
(800) 321-3279
www.unipath.com

**United Guardian Laboratories**
230 Marcus Boulevard
Hauppauge, NY 11788
(800) 645-5566

**United Research Laboratories**
1100 Orthodox Street
Philadelphia, PA 19124
(800) 523-3684
www.urlmutual.com

**Univax Biologics**
(see North American Biologicals, Inc)

**Upjohn** (see Pharmacia Corp)

**Upsher-Smith Labs, Inc**
14905 23rd Avenue North
Minneapolis, MN 55447-4709
(800) 654-2299
www.upsher-smith.com

**UroCor, Inc**
840 Research Parkway
Oklahoma City, OK 73104
(800) 634-9330

**Urologix**
14405 21st Avenue North
Minneapolis, MN 55447
(888) 229-0772
www.urologix.com

**USA Nutritionals**
513 Adams Boulevard
Conway, NY 11729
(800) 722-7570
www.USANutritionals.com

**US Bioscience**
100 Front Street
Suite 400
West Conshohocken, PA 19428
(800) 447-3969
www.usbio.com

**US DenTek**
1460 Cedar Lane
Suite A
Petaluma, CA 94954
(800) 433-6835

**US Dermatologics**
133 Franklin Corner Drive
Lawrenceville, NJ 08648
(877) 873-3762

**US Pharmaceutical Corp**
2401-C Mellon Court
Decatur, GA 30035
(800) 330-3040

**US Surgical Corp**
150 Glover Avenue
Norwalk, CT 06856
(800) 722-8772
www.ussurg.com

**ValMed, Inc**
100 Otis Street
Suite 4A
Northboro, MA 01532
(800) 477-0487

**Value in Pharmaceuticals**
3000 Alt Boulevard
Grand Island, NY 14702
(800) 724-3784
www.vippharm.com

**Van Den Bergh Foods Company**
75 Merritt Boulevard
Trumbull, CT 06611
(203) 381-3500

**Vertex Pharmaceuticals, Inc**
130 Waverly Street
Cambridge, MA 02139-4211
(617) 576-3111
www.vpharm.com

**VHA, Inc**
220 East Las Colinas Boulevard
Irving, TX 75039
(800) 842-7587

**Vicks Health Care Products**
(see Procter & Gamble)

**Vicks Pharmacy Products**
(see Procter & Gamble)

**Viratek** (see AstraZeneca)

**Virco Pharmaceuticals, Inc**
1121 Virginia Avenue
Bluefield, VA 24605
(888) 968-4726

**Vision Pharmaceuticals, Inc**
PO Box 400
Mitchell, SD 57301-0400
(800) 325-6789
www.visionpharm.com

**VistaPharm**
1200 Corporate Drive
Suite 174
Birmingham, AL 35242
(205) 981-1387
www.vistapharm.com

**Vitaline Corp**
385 Williamson Way
Ashland, OR 97520
(800) 648-4755
www.vitaline.com

**Vitamin Research Product, Inc**
3579 Highway 50 East
Carson City, NV 89701
(800) 877-2447
www.vrp.com

**Vivus, Inc**
545 Middlefield Road
Suite 200
Menlo Park, CA 94025
(888) 345-6873
www,vivus.com

**Wakefield Pharmaceuticals, Inc**
310 Maxwell Road
Suite 100
Alpharetta, GA 30004
(770) 664-1661

**Walgreen Company**
200 Wilmont Road
Dearfield, IL 60015
(847) 940-2500
www.walgreens.com

**Wallace Laboratories**
**(Carter Wallace)**
Half Acre Road
Cranbury, NJ 08512-0181
(800) 526-3840
www.wallacelabs.com

**Wal-Mart Stores, Inc**
702 Southwest 8th Street
Bentonville, AR 72716
(501) 273-4000
www.wal-mart.com

**Wampole Laboratories**
Half Acre Road
PO Box 1001
Cranbury, NJ 08512-0181
(800) 257-9525
www.wampolelabs.com

**Warner Chilcott Laboratories**
100 Enterprise Drive
Suite 280
Rockaway, NJ 07866
(800) 521-8813
www.wclabs.com

**Warner Lambert Consumer Healthcare**
201 Tabor Road
Morris Plains, NJ 07950
(800) 223-0182
www.warner-lambert.com

**Warrick Pharmaceuticals**
**(Schering Plough Corp)**
1095 Morris Avenue
Union, NJ 07083-7137
(800) 547-3869

**Watson Laboratories, Inc**
311 Bonnie Circle Drive
Corona, CA 91720
(800) 272-5525
www.watsonpharm.com

**WE Pharmaceuticals, Inc**
PO Box 1142
Ramona, CA 92065
(800) 262-9555

**Weider Nutrition International, Inc**
2002 South 5070 West
Salt Lake City, UT 84104
(801) 975-5000
www.weider.com

**Wellspring Pharmaceutical**
1430 Route 40
Colts Neck, NJ 07722
(732) 938-5885

**Wendt Laboratories**
PO Box 128
Belle Plaine, MN 56011
(800) 328-5890

**Wesley Pharmacal, Inc**
114 Railroad Drive
Ivyland, PA 18974
(800) 634-4922

**West Point Pharma**
(see Endo Pharmaceuticals)

**West-Ward Pharmaceutical Corp**
465 Industrial Way West
Eatontown, NJ 07724
(800) 631-2174

**Westwood-Squibb Pharmaceuticals (Bristol-Myers Squibb)**
100 Forest Avenue
Buffalo, NY 14213
(800) 333-0950
www.westwood-squibb.com

**W. F. Young, Inc**
111 Lyman Street
Springfield, MA 01102
(800) 628-9653
www.absorbine.com

**Whitby Pharmaceuticals, Inc**
(see UCB Pharmaceuticals, Inc)

**Whitehall-Robins Healthcare (American Home Products)**
5 Giralda Farms
Madison, NJ 07940-0871
(800) 322-3129
www.whitehallrobins.com

**Willen Pharmaceuticals**
(see Baker Norton Pharmaceuticals)

**Winthrop Pharmaceuticals**
(see Sanofi-Synthelabo)

**Wisconsin Pharmacal Company (WPC Brands)**
One Repel Road
Jackson, WI 53037
(800) 558-6614

**Wm. Wrigley Jr Company**
410 North Michigan Avenue
Chicago, IL 60611
(866) 787-7277

**Women First Healthcare, Inc**
12220 El Camino Real
Suite 400
San Diego, CA 92130
(858) 509-1171
www.womenfirst.com

**Women's Capital Corp**
11808 Northup Way
Suite W290
Bellevue, WA 98005
(800) 330-1271
www.go2planb.com

**Wonderful Dream Salve Corp**
46219 Baldwin Drive
Macomb, MI 48044-5220
(810) 226-9975

**Woodside Biomedical, Inc**
1915 Aston Avenue
Suite 102
Carlsbad, CA 92008
(888) 297-9728
www.woodsidebiomedical.com

**Woodward Laboratories, Inc**
11132 Winners Circle #100
Los Alamitos, CA 90720
(562) 598-0800
www.woodwardlabs.com

**Wyeth-Ayerst**
555 Lancaster Avenue
St David's, PA 19087
(800) 666-7248
www.ahp.com/wyeth

**Xactdose, Inc** (see Alpharma USPD)

**Xoma**
2910 7th Street
Berkely, CA 94710
(800) 544-9662
www.xoma.com

**Xttrium Laboratories, Inc**
415 West Pershing Road
Chicago, IL 60609
(800) 587-3721
www.xttrium.com

**Young Again Products**
3608-B Oleander Drive #310
Wilmington, NC 28403
(910) 392-6775

**Young Dental Manufacturing**
13705 Shoreline Court East
Earth City, MO 63045
(800) 325-1881
www.youngdental.com

**Zanfel Laboratories, Inc**
Morton, IL 61550
(800) 401-4002
www.zanfel.com

**Zeneca Pharmaceuticals**
(see AstraZeneca Pharmaceuticals LP)

**Zenith Goldline Pharmaceuticals**
(see Ivax Pharmaceutical)

**Zila Pharmaceuticals, Inc**
5227 North 7th Street
Phoenix, AZ 85014-2800
(800) 922-7887
www.zila.com

**Zonagen, Inc**
2408 Timberloch Place, B-4
Phoenix, AZ 77380
(281) 367-5892
www.zonagen.com

**ZymeTx, Inc**
800 Research Parkway
Suite 100
Oklahoma City, OK 73104
(888) 817-1314
www.zymetx.com

**Zymogenetics, Inc**
1201 Eastlake Avenue East
Seattle, WA 98102
(206) 547-8080
www.bio.com

# INDICATION/THERAPEUTIC CATEGORY INDEX

## ACQUIRED IMMUNODEFICIENCY SYNDROME (AIDS)

### Antiretroviral Agent, Non-nucleoside Reverse Transcriptase Inhibitor (NNRTI)



### Antiretroviral Agent, Nucleoside Reverse Transcriptase Inhibitor (NRTI)



### Antiviral Agent



### Non-nucleoside Reverse Transcriptase Inhibitor (NNRTI)



### Protease Inhibitor



## ACROMEGALY

### Ergot Alkaloid and Derivative



### Somatostatin Analog



## ACUTE CORONARY SYNDROME

### Antiplatelet Agent



## ADAMS-STOKES SYNDROME

### Adrenergic Agonist Agent



## ADDISON'S DISEASE *see also* ADRENOCORTICAL FUNCTION ABNORMALITIES

### Adrenal Corticosteroid



### Adrenal Corticosteroid (Mineralocorticoid)



### Diagnostic Agent



## ADENOSINE DEAMINASE DEFICIENCY

### Enzyme



## ADRENOCORTICAL FUNCTION ABNORMALITIES

### Adrenal Corticosteroid

### Adrenal Corticosteroid (Mineralocorticoid)



## ALCOHOLISM

### Aldehyde Dehydrogenase Inhibitor Agent



### Phenothiazine Derivative



## ALCOHOL WITHDRAWAL

### Alpha-Adrenergic Agonist



### Antihistamine



### Benzodiazepine



### Beta-Adrenergic Blocker



### Phenothiazine Derivative



(Continued)

(Continued)

### General Anesthetic *(Continued)*



## ANESTHESIA (LOCAL)

### Local Anesthetic

(Continued)

(Continued)

## Nonsteroidal Anti-inflammatory Drug (NSAID) *(Continued)*

(Continued)

(Continued)

(Continued)

### Corticosteroid, Topical *(Continued)*



### Local Anesthetic



## BITES (SNAKE)

### Antivenin



## BITES (SPIDER)

### Antivenin



### Electrolyte Supplement, Oral



### Skeletal Muscle Relaxant



## BLADDER IRRIGATION

### Antibacterial, Topical



## BLASTOMYCOSIS

### Antifungal Agent

(Continued)

(Continued)

(Continued)

## Antineoplastic Agent *(Continued)*



## Antineoplastic Agent, Anthracycline



## Antiviral Agent

(Continued)

## COLONIC EVACUATION

### Laxative



## CONDYLOMA ACUMINATUM

### Antiviral Agent



### Biological Response Modulator



### Keratolytic Agent



## CONGENITAL SUCRASE-ISOMALTASE DEFICIENCY

### Enzyme



## CONGESTION (NASAL)

### Adrenergic Agonist Agent



(Continued)

## Adrenergic Agonist Agent *(Continued)*



## Antihistamine



## Antihistamine/Antitussive



## Antihistamine/Decongestant/Anticholinergic

(Continued)

## Antihistamine/Decongestant Combination *(Continued)*



## Antitussive/Decongestant



## Antitussive/Decongestant/Expectorant



## Cold Preparation

### Decongestant/Analgesic



### Phenothiazine Derivative



## CONJUNCTIVITIS (ALLERGIC)

### Adrenal Corticosteroid



### Antihistamine


(Continued)

**Laxative/Stool Softner**



**Stool Softener**



## COPROPORPHYRIA

**Beta-Adrenergic Blocker**



## CORNEAL EDEMA

**Lubricant, Ocular**



## COUGH

**Antihistamine**



**Antihistamine/Antitussive**



(Continued)

### Antitussive/Decongestant



### Antitussive/Decongestant/ Expectorant



### Antitussive/Expectorant



### Cold Preparation



(Continued)

(Continued)

## Dietary Supplement *(Continued)*



### Topical Skin Product



## DERMATOLOGIC DISORDERS

### Adrenal Corticosteroid



## DERMATOMYCOSIS

### Antifungal Agent

(Continued)

## DIGITALIS GLYCOSIDE POISONING

### Antidote



### Chelating Agent



## DIPHTHERIA

### Antitoxin



## DISCOID LUPUS ERYTHEMATOSUS (DLE)

### Aminoquinoline (Antimalarial)



### Corticosteroid, Topical

(Continued)

(Continued)

## EDEMA

### Antihypertensive Agent, Combination



(Continued)

## EMPHYSEMA

### Adrenergic Agonist Agent



### Anticholinergic Agent



### Expectorant



### Mucolytic Agent



### Theophylline Derivative



## ENCEPHALITIS (HERPESVIRUS)

### Antiviral Agent



## ENDOCARDITIS TREATMENT

### Aminoglycoside (Antibiotic)



### Antibiotic, Miscellaneous



### Antibiotic, Penicillin



### Antifungal Agent



### Cephalosporin (First Generation)

## EPILEPSY

### Anticonvulsant



### Anticonvulsant, Miscellaneous



### Anticonvulsant, Sulfonamide



### Antidepressant



### Barbiturate



### Benzodiazepine



(Continued)

## FAMILIAL ADENOMATOUS POLYPOSIS

### Nonsteroidal Anti-inflammatory Drug (NSAID), COX-2 Selective



## FATTY ACID DEFICIENCY

### Intravenous Nutritional Therapy



### Nutritional Supplement



## FEBRILE NEUTROPENIA

### Quinolone



## FEVER

### Antipyretic

(Continued)

(Continued)

(Continued)

### Nonsteroidal Anti-inflammatory Drug (NSAID) *(Continued)*



### Uricosuric Agent



### Xanthine Oxidase Inhibitor



## GRAFT VS HOST DISEASE

### Immunosuppressant Agent



## GRAM-NEGATIVE INFECTION

### Aminoglycoside (Antibiotic)



### Antibiotic, Miscellaneous



### Antibiotic, Penicillin



### Antibiotic, Quinolone



### Carbapenem (Antibiotic)



### Cephalosporin (First Generation)

### Cephalosporin (Second Generation)



### Cephalosporin (Third Generation)



### Cephalosporin (Fourth Generation)



### Genitourinary Irrigant



### Macrolide (Antibiotic)



### Penicillin



(Continued)

## HEADACHE (SINUS)

### Analgesic, Non-narcotic


(Continued)

(Continued)

## HEMOLYTIC DISEASE OF THE NEWBORN

### Immune Globulin



## HEMOPHILIA

### Antihemophilic Agent



### Coagulation Factor



### Vasopressin Analog, Synthetic



## HEMOPHILIA A

### Antihemophilic Agent



### Blood Product Derivative



## HEMOPHILIA B

### Antihemophilic Agent



### Blood Product Derivative



## HEMORRHAGE

### Adrenergic Agonist Agent



### Antihemophilic Agent



(Continued)

(Continued)

### Electrolyte Supplement, Oral



## HYPERACTIVITY *see* ATTENTION-DEFICIT/HYPERACTIVITY DISORDER (ADHD)

## HYPERAMMONEMIA

### Ammonium Detoxicant



## HYPERCALCEMIA

### Antidote



### Bisphosphonate Derivative



### Chelating Agent

(Continued)

(Continued)

## Antihypertensive Agent, Combination *(Continued)*



## Beta-Adrenergic Blocker



## Calcium Channel Blocker

(Continued)

(Continued)

## LUNG SURFACTANT

### Lung Surfactant



## LYME DISEASE

### Antibiotic, Penicillin



### Cephalosporin (Third Generation)



### Macrolide (Antibiotic)



### Penicillin



### Tetracycline Derivative



### Vaccine



## LYMPHOMA

### Antineoplastic Agent

(Continued)

(Continued)

### Antidepressant, Tricyclic (Tertiary Amine)



### Antimigraine Agent



### Beta-Adrenergic Blocker



### Calcium-entry Blocker (Selective)



### Decongestant/Analgesic



### Ergot Alkaloid and Derivative



### Serotonin 5-HT$_{1D}$ Receptor Agonist



### Serotonin Agonist



## MIGRAINE (PROPHYLAXIS)

### Antimigraine Agent



## MIOSIS

### Alpha-Adrenergic Blocking Agent



### Cholinergic Agent



(Continued)

(Continued)

(Continued)

## Antiemetic *(Continued)*



### Antihistamine



### Gastrointestinal Agent, Prokinetic



### Phenothiazine Derivative



### Selective 5-HT$_3$ Receptor Antagonist



## NEOPLASTIC DISEASE (TREATMENT ADJUNCT)

### Adrenal Corticosteroid

(Continued)

(Continued)

(Continued)

(Continued)

(Continued)

## Local Anesthetic



## Otic Agent, Analgesic

(Continued)

## Analgesic, Narcotic *(Continued)*

## Analgesic, Non-narcotic


(Continued)

## Analgesic, Non-narcotic *(Continued)*

### Decongestant/Analgesic



### Local Anesthetic



### Neuroleptic Agent



### Nonsteroidal Anti-inflammatory Drug (NSAID)



### Nonsteroidal Anti-inflammatory Drug (NSAID), COX-2 Selective



### Nonsteroidal Anti-inflammatory Drug (NSAID), Oral



## PAIN (ANOGENITAL)

### Anesthetic/Corticosteroid

(Continued)

(Continued)

(Continued)

(Continued)

## PSEUDOGOUT

### Antigout Agent



### Nonsteroidal Anti-inflammatory Drug (NSAID)



## PSEUDOHYPOPARATHYROIDISM

### Vitamin D Analog



## PSORIASIS

### Antibiotic/Corticosteroid, Topical



### Antineoplastic Agent



### Antipsoriatic Agent



### Corticosteroid, Topical

### Keratolytic Agent



### Psoralen



### Retinoid-like Compound



## PSYCHOSES

### Antipsychotic Agent



### Antipsychotic Agent, Benzisoxazole



### Antipsychotic Agent, Butyrophenone



(Continued)

(Continued)

(Continued)

(Continued)

(Continued)

### Corticosteroid, Topical *(Continued)*



## SARCOMA

### Antineoplastic Agent



## SCABIES

### Scabicides/Pediculicides



## SCHISTOSOMIASIS

### Anthelmintic



## SCHIZOPHRENIA

### Antipsychotic Agent



### Antipsychotic Agent, Benzisoxazole



### Antipsychotic Agent, Dibenzodiazepine



### Neuroleptic Agent



### Thioxanthene Derivative



## SCLERODERMA

### Aminoquinoline (Antimalarial)

(Continued)

(Continued)

## SMOKING CESSATION

### Antidepressant, Monoamine Oxidase Inhibitor



### Smoking Deterrent



## SOFT TISSUE INFECTION

### Aminoglycoside (Antibiotic)



### Antibiotic, Carbacephem



### Antibiotic, Miscellaneous



### Antibiotic, Penicillin



### Antibiotic, Quinolone



### Antifungal Agent



### Cephalosporin (First Generation)



### Cephalosporin (Second Generation)



### Cephalosporin (Third Generation)



### Cephalosporin (Fourth Generation)

(Continued)

(Continued)

(Continued)

(Continued)

(Continued)

(Continued)